ISBN 978-0-260-11361-0
PIBN 10928753

THE PRINCIPLES AND PRACTICE OF MEDICINE

DESIGNED FOR THE USE OF PRACTITIONERS AND STUDENTS OF MEDICINE

BY

THE LATE SIR WILLIAM OSLER, BT., M.D., F.R.S.

FELLOW OF THE ROYAL COLLEGE OF PHYSICIANS, LONDON; REGIUS PROFESSOR OF MEDICINE, OXFORD UNIVERSITY; HONORARY PROFESSOR OF MEDICINE, JOHNS HOPKINS UNIVERSITY, BALTIMORE; FORMERLY PROFESSOR OF THE INSTITUTES OF MEDICINE, McGILL UNIVERSITY, MONTREAL, AND PROFESSOR OF CLINICAL MEDICINE IN THE UNIVERSITY OF PENNSYLVANIA, PHILADELPHIA

AND

THOMAS McCRAE, M.D.

FELLOW OF THE ROYAL COLLEGE OF PHYSICIANS, LONDON; PROFESSOR OF MEDICINE, JEFFERSON MEDICAL COLLEGE, PHILADELPHIA; PHYSICIAN TO THE JEFFERSON AND PENNSYLVANIA HOSPITALS, PHILADELPHIA; FORMERLY ASSOCIATE PROFESSOR OF MEDICINE, JOHNS HOPKINS UNIVERSITY

NINTH THOROUGHLY REVISED EDITION

Walter W Palmer.

NEW YORK AND LONDON
D. APPLETON AND COMPANY
1920

PRINTED IN THE UNITED STATES OF AMERICA

TO THE

Memory of Three Teachers of William Osler:

WILLIAM ARTHUR JOHNSON

PRIEST OF THE PARISH OF WESTON, ONTARIO

JAMES BOVELL

OF THE TORONTO SCHOOL OF MEDICINE, AND OF THE UNIVERSITY OF TRINITY COLLEGE, TORONTO

ROBERT PALMER HOWARD

DEAN OF THE MEDICAL FACULTY AND PROFESSOR OF MEDICINE, McGILL UNIVERSITY, MONTREAL

PREFACE

The death of Sir William Osler takes from medicine—and from medical literature—one of its greatest masters. A prolific writer, he never wrote for the mere sake of writing but because he had something worthy of being written. With the art of extracting and condensing the essentials of a subject went the ability to present them clearly. His use of the telling phrase often drove home a point more strongly than a long description could do. To promote sound knowledge was one of his ambitions and that he succeeded there is no question. It is doubtful if any man of his generation exercised a greater influence. From all who knew him has come the tribute to the man even more than to his learning.

This *Text Book of Medicine* was one of the great interests in his life; as he said, it brought him "mind to mind" with members of the profession in many parts of the world. It was interesting to find the number of letters concerning it which he had kept. He regretted greatly the interruption in the usual triennial appearance of a new edition caused by the war. At its ending he turned actively to work on his part of the revision for this edition and had practically completed it at the onset of his last illness. It is a grim coincidence that at the time of my association as assistant author in 1912 he planned to give up active participation in the revision when he reached seventy years of age.

My association with the book began as a student in 1892 when the first edition was used as my text-book of medicine. In my copy of this edition are many additions picked up in the wards of the Johns Hopkins Hospital from the author himself. A study of successive editions represents a record of the advance of medicine during a period of nearly thirty years.

In this edition many changes have been made throughout the whole book, which has been recast. Many parts have been re-written. New sections have been added on Paratyphoid Fever, Focal Infection, Trench Fever, Gas Poisoning, Brass Poisoning, Acidosis, Diverticulitis, Infectious Jaundice, Torsion of the Omentum, Foreign Bodies in the Bronchi, Hæmothorax, Mediastinitis, and Diseases of the Diaphragm. Additions have been made to the discussion of Diseases of the Circulation, with a new section on Aortitis. In the section on the Nervous System, certain familial and hereditary diseases have been grouped together. Epidemic Encephalitis represents new material and the section on Cerebral Arterio-sclerosis is entirely rewritten. The description of the Sympathetic Nervous System and the discussion of Cervical Rib, the Pineal and Sex Glands, Lipodystrophia, Osteomalacia and Chondrodysplasia represent added material.

One problem is ever present in a text-book—the matter of arrangement. Should poliomyelitis, for example, be placed with the acute infectious diseases or in the section on Diseases of the Nervous System? Should syphilis in all its aspects be discussed together or some parts, for example, the nervous system features, be separated and taken up with the other diseases of that system? There are points for and against any rigid plan and it is difficult to be consistent. The effort has been made to consider the student and make such arrangement as seems to be most helpful for him.

Thanks are due to many friends for suggestions and aid in various ways. Dr. H. M. Thomas of Baltimore has given valuable assistance in the section dealing with diseases of the nervous system in every edition and not least with this one. To my associates, Dr. Ross V. Patterson, Dr. E. H. Funk and Dr. M. H. Rehfuss, I am under many obligations, and Dr. A. Malloch helped in many ways. To practitioners and students in many lands thanks are due for criticism and suggestions.

THOMAS McCRAE.

CONTENTS

SECTION I

Specific Infectious Diseases

SECTION VII

Diseases of the Respiratory System

SECTION VIII

Diseases of the Kidneys

SECTION IX

Diseases of the Blood-forming Organs

SECTION X

Diseases of the Circulatory System

SECTION XI

Diseases of the Ductless Glands

SECTION XII

Diseases of the Nervous System

SECTION XIII

Diseases of the Locomotor System

CHARTS AND ILLUSTRATIONS

THE PRINCIPLES AND PRACTICE OF MEDICINE

SECTION I

SPECIFIC INFECTIOUS DISEASES

A. BACTERIAL DISEASES

I. TYPHOID FEVER

Definition.—A general infection caused by the *Bacillus typhosus*, characterized anatomically by hyperplasia and ulceration of the intestinal lymph-follicles, swelling of the mesenteric glands and spleen, and parenchymatous changes in the other organs. There are cases in which the local changes are slight or absent, and there are others with intense localization in the lungs, spleen, kidneys, or cerebro-spinal system. Clinically the disease is marked by fever, rose-colored eruption, abdominal tenderness, tympanites, and enlargement of the spleen; but these symptoms are extremely inconstant, and even the fever varies in its character.

Historical Note.—Huxham, in his remarkable Essay on Fevers, had "taken notice of the very great difference there is between the *putrid malignant* and the *slow nervous fever*." In 1813 Pierre Bretonneau, of Tours, distinguished "dothiénentérite" as a separate disease; and Petit and Serres described entero-mesenteric fever. In 1829 Louis' great work appeared, in which the name "typhoid" was given to the fever. At this period typhoid fever alone prevailed in Paris and many European cities, and it was universally believed to be identical with the continued fever of Great Britain, where in reality typhoid and typhus coëxisted. The intestinal lesion was regarded as an accidental occurrence in the course of ordinary typhus. Louis' students, returning to their homes in different countries, had opportunities for studying the prevalent fevers in the thorough and systematic manner of their master. Among these were certain young American physicians, to one of whom, Gerhard, of Philadelphia, is due the great honor of having first clearly laid down the differences between the two diseases. His papers in the American Journal of the Medical Sciences, 1837, are the first which give a full and satisfactory account of their clinical and anatomical distinctions. The studies of James Jackson, Sr. and Jr., of Enoch Hale and of George C. Shattuck, of

Boston, and of Alfred Stillé and Austin Flint made the subject very familiar in American medicine. In 1842 Elisha Bartlett's work appeared, in which, for the first time in a systematic treatise, typhoid and typhus fever were separately considered with admirable clearness. In Great Britain the recognition of the difference between the two diseases was slow, and due largely to A. P. Stewart, and to the studies of Jenner between 1849 and 1850.

Etiology.—GENERAL PREVALENCE.—Typhoid fever prevails especially in temperate climates, in which it constitutes the most common continued fever. Widely distributed throughout all parts of the world, it probably presents everywhere the same essential characteristics, and is everywhere an index of the sanitary intelligence of a community. *Imperfect sewerage* and *contaminated water-supply* are two special conditions favoring the distribution of the bacilli; *filth, overcrowding,* and *bad ventilation* are accessories in lowering the resistance of the individuals exposed. While from an infected person the disease may be spread by *fingers, food* and *flies.*

In *England and Wales* in 1916 the disease was fatal to 1,122 persons, a mortality of 30 per million of living persons. It destroys more lives in proportion to population in towns than in the country. The rate was lower in 1916 than in any year since 1869. In *India* the disease is very prevalent; no race or creed is exempt, and 80 per cent. of the cases of continued fever lasting three weeks prove to be typhoid fever (L. Rogers).

In the *United States* there has been a marked decrease in the last twenty years. The death rate per 100,000 population in the registration areas has fallen from 35.9 in 1900 to 13.4 in 1917. In 1919 the death rate in the sixty largest cities was 4.2 per 100,000. It is more prevalent in country districts than in cities, and, as Fulton showed, the propagation is largely from the country to the town. What is needed both in Canada and the United States is a realization by the public that certain primary laws of health must be obeyed.

Typhoid fever has been one of the great scourges of armies, and killed and maimed more than powder and shot. The recent war shows the results of preventive inoculation in a striking way. In the Spanish-American War the report of the Commission (Reed, Vaughan, and Shakespeare) showed that in the national encampments among 107,973 men there were 20,738 cases of typhoid fever with 1,580 deaths. In 90 per cent. of the volunteer regiments the disease broke out within eight weeks after going into camp. In the opinion of the Commission the most important factors were camp pollution, flies as carriers of contagion, and the contamination through the air in the form of dust. In the South African War the British army, 557,653 officers and men, had 57,684 cases of typhoid fever, with 8,225 deaths (Simpson), while only 7,582 men died of wounds received in battle. The disease was essentially one of the standing camps; troops constantly on the move were rarely much affected. While contaminated water was no doubt an important factor, as it always is in camp pollution, yet certain of the conditions in Africa were peculiar. Fæcal and urinary contamination must have been very common, as in the cooking, performed in the open air, sand "entered largely into every article of food." As there was a perfect plague of flies, they were without doubt a very important factor in the infection of both food and drink.

On the other hand, the Japanese and Russian War demonstrated the remarkable efficiency of modern hygiene, if carried out in an intelligent manner. In the great European war typhoid fever did not prevail to any extent in the Western armies. The efficacy of inoculation has been demonstrated. The large proportion of paratyphoid cases is remarkable.

Season.—Almost without exception the disease is everywhere more prevalent in the autumn, hence the old popular name autumnal fever. The exhaustive study of this question by Sedgwick and Winslow shows everywhere a striking parallelism between the monthly variations in temperature and the prevalence of the disease. In a few cities the curves are irregular, showing, in addition to the usual summer rise, two secondary maxima in the winter and spring, and these authors suggest that epidemics at these seasons are characteristic of cities whose water-supply is most subject to pollution. In their opinion "the most reasonable explanation of the seasonal variations of typhoid fever is a direct effect of the temperature upon the persistence in nature of the germs which proceed from previous victims of the disease."

Of 1,500 cases at the Johns Hopkins Hospital (upon the study of which this section is based), 840 were in August, September, and October.

Sex.—Males and females are equally liable to the disease, but males are much more frequently admitted into hospitals, 2.4 to 1 in our series.

Age.—Typhoid fever is a disease of youth and early adult life. The greatest susceptibility is between the ages of fifteen and twenty-five. Of 1,500 cases treated in the Johns Hopkins Hospital there were under fifteen years of age, 231; between fifteen and twenty, 253; between twenty and thirty, 680; between thirty and forty, 227; between forty and fifty, 88; between fifty and sixty, 8; above sixty, 11; age not given, 1. Cases in advanced life are not uncommon, but as the course is often atypical the diagnosis may be uncertain and the disease not recognized until autopsy. It is not very infrequent in childhood, but infants are rarely attacked. Murchison saw a case at the sixth month.

Immunity.—Not all exposed to the infection take the disease. Some families seem more susceptible than others. One attack usually protects. Two attacks have been described within a year. In 500 of our cases in which special inquiry was made as to a previous attack, it was found to have occurred in 11 (2.2 per cent.) but some of those were probably paratyphoid fever. The interval varied from nine months to thirty years. It is well known that usually within a short time after recovery the immune substances disappear from the blood, yet in most cases the immunity lasts a long time, frequently for life. An experimental explanation for this fact has been given in the demonstration that animals which have once reacted to the typhoid infection, react in throwing out immune substances more quickly and in larger amounts when danger again threatens (Cole).

BACILLUS TYPHOSUS.—(*a*) *General Characters.*—It is a rather short, thick, flagellated, motile bacillus, with rounded ends, in one of which, sometimes in both (particularly in cultures), there can be seen a glistening round body, at one time believed to be a spore; but these polar structures are probably only areas of degenerated protoplasm. There are various strains which show antigenic differences. This organism fulfills all the requirements of Koch's law—it is constantly present, and grows outside the body in a specific manner; the third requirement, the production of the disease experimentally, has been successfully met by its conveyance to chimpanzees. The bacilli or their toxins inoculated in large quantities into the blood of rabbits are pathogenic, and in some instances ulcerative and necrotic lesions in the intestine may be produced. But similar intestinal lesions may be caused by other bacteria, including *Bacillus coli.*

Cultures are killed within ten minutes by a temperature of 60° C. They may live for eighteen weeks at —5° C., although most die within two weeks, and all within twenty-two weeks (Park). The typhoid bacillus resists ordinary drying for months, unless in very thin layers, when it is killed in five to fifteen days. The direct rays of the sun completely destroy them in from four to ten hours' exposure. Bouillon cultures are destroyed by carbolic acid, 1 to 200, and by corrosive sublimate, 1 to 2,500.

(*b*) *Distribution in the Body.*—Our ideas in regard to this have been much modified, owing to the demonstration that in practically all cases the bacilli enter the circulating blood and are carried throughout the body. During life they may be demonstrated in the circulating blood in a large proportion of cases, in 75 per cent. of 604 collected cases (Coleman and Buxton). They occur in the urine in from 25 to 30 per cent. of the cases. They may be isolated from the stools in practically all cases at some stage. They are probably always present in the rose spots. They are reported to have been cultivated from the sweat, and occur with considerable frequency in the sputum (Richardson, Rau, and others). They have been found in the milk of nursing women. At autopsy they are found widely distributed, most numerous and constant usually in the mesenteric glands, spleen, and gall-bladder, but are found in almost all organs, even the muscles, uterus, and lungs (von Drigalski). Cultures made from the intestines at autopsy (according to von Jürgens, and von Drigalski) show that they are very numerous in the duodenum and jejunum, and practically constant in cultures made from the mucous membrane of the stomach. They are present in the œsophagus and frequently on the tongue and tonsils. From endocardial vegetations, from meningeal and pleural exudates and from foci of suppuration in various parts of the body, the bacilli have been isolated. A most important fact is that at times they may be present in the stools of persons who show no symptoms of typhoid fever, but who have lived in very close association with typhoid-fever patients. This is especially true of children.

(*c*) *The Bacilli outside the Body.*—In sterile water the bacilli retain their vitality for weeks, but under ordinary conditions, in competition with saprophytes, disappear within a few days. The question of the longevity of the typhoid bacillus in water is of great importance, and was much discussed in connection with the supposed pollution of the water of the Mississippi by the Chicago drainage canal. The experiments of E. O. Jordan would indicate that the vitality was retained as a rule not longer than three days after infection. Whether an increase can occur in water is not finally settled. Their detection in water is difficult, and although they undoubtedly have been found, many such discoveries are not certain on account of the inaccurate differentiation of the typhoid bacillus and varieties of intestinal bacilli closely resembling it. Both Prudden and Ernst found it in water filters.

There are cities deriving their ice supply from polluted streams with low death rates from typhoid fever. Sedgwick and Winslow conclude from their careful study that very few typhoid germs survive in ice. The Ogdensburg epidemic in 1902-'03 was apparently due to infection from ice. Typhoid bacilli were grown from frozen material in it (Hutchins and Wheeler).

In *milk* the bacilli undergo rapid development without changing its appearance. They may persist for three months in sour milk, and may live for several days in butter made from infected cream.

Robertson has shown that under entirely natural conditions typhoid bacilli may live in the upper layers of the soil for eleven months. Von Drigalski says if stools which contain typhoid bacilli are kept at room temperature the *B. typhosus* disappears in a few days.

The direct infection of exposed food-stuffs by dust is very probable. The bacilli retain their vitality for many weeks; in garden earth 21 days, in filter-sand 82 days, in street dust 30 days, on linen 60 to 70 days, on wood 32 days, on thread kept under suitable conditions for a year.

Modes of Conveyance.—(*a*) *Contagion.*—Direct aerial transmission does not seem probable. Each case should be regarded as a possible source of infection, and in houses, hospitals, schools, and barracks a widespread epidemic may arise from it. Fingers, food, and flies are the chief means of local propagation. It is impossible for a nurse to avoid finger contamination, and without scrupulous care the germs may be widely distributed in a ward or throughout a house. Cotton or rubber gloves are used in some institutions. Even with special precautions and an unusually large proportion of nurses to patients, it was not possible to avoid "house" infection at the Johns Hopkins Hospital. T. B. Futcher analyzed the 31 cases contracted in the hospital among the first 1,500 cases; physicians, 5* among a total of 288; nurses, 15 of a total of 407; patients, 8 out of a total of 47,956 admissions; 4 of these occurred in a small ward epidemic. Two orderlies were infected while caring for typhoid patients, and one woman in charge of a supply room, where she handled clean linen only. Newman concluded from his study of typhoid fever in London that direct personal infection and infection through food are the two common channels for its propagation.

(*b*) *Infection of water* is the most common source of widespread epidemics, many of which have originated in the contamination of a well or a spring. A striking one occurred at Plymouth, Pa., in 1885. The town, with a population of 8,000, was in part supplied with drinking-water from a reservoir fed by a mountain stream. During January, February, and March, in a cottage by the side of and at a distance of from 60 to 80 feet from this stream, a man was ill with typhoid fever. The attendants were in the habit at night of throwing out the evacuations on the ground toward the stream. During these months the ground was frozen and covered with snow. In the latter part of March and early in April there was considerable rainfall and a thaw, in which a large part of the three months' accumulation of discharges was washed into a brook, not 60 feet distant. At the time of this thaw the patient had numerous and copious discharges. About the 10th of April cases of typhoid fever broke out in the town, appearing for a time at the rate of 50 a day. In all about 1,200 people were attacked. An immense majority of all the cases

* Only three of these were in attendance on typhoid cases. Two of the five died.—Oppenheimer and Ochsner.

were in the part of the town which received water from the infected reservoir.

The experience of Maidstone in 1897 illustrates the widespread and serious character of an epidemic when the water-supply becomes badly contaminated. The outbreak began about the middle of September, and within the first two weeks 509 cases were reported. By October 27th there were 1,748 cases, and by November 17th 1,848 cases. In all, in a population of 35,000, about 1,900 persons were attacked.

(*c*) *Typhoid Carriers.*—The bacilli may persist for years in the bile passages and intestines of persons in good health. They have been found in the urinary bladder and in the gall-bladder, ten and twenty years after the fever, and there have been cases of typhoid bone lesion from which the bacilli were isolated many years after the primary attack. The work of Strassburg observers called attention to a group of chronic typhoid carriers of the first importance in the spread of the disease. The majority of carriers are females. One woman, a baker, had typhoid fever ten years previously. The bacilli were found in large numbers in her stools. Every new employee in the bakery sooner or later became ill with typhoid-like symptoms, and in two persons the disease proved fatal. Many localized epidemics have been traced to carriers. Soper reported an instance in which a cook, apparently in perfect health, but in whose stools bacilli were present in large numbers, had been responsible for the occurrence of typhoid in seven households in five years. Apparently there is no limit to the length of time in which the bacilli may persist. One carrier had the attack of typhoid fever forty-seven years before. The paratyphoid bacillus may be carried in the same way. An epidemic of 19 cases in a French barrack was traced to a cook.

(*d*) *Infection of Food.*—Milk may be the source of infection. One of the most thoroughly studied epidemics due to this cause was that investigated by Ballard in Islington. The milk may be contaminated by the infected water used in cleaning the cans. The milk epidemics have been collected by Ernest Hart and by Kober. The germs may be conveyed in ice, salads of various sorts, spaghetti, etc. The danger of eating celery and other uncooked vegetables, which have grown in soil on which infected material has been used as a fertilizer, must not be forgotten.

Much attention has been paid to the *oyster* as a source of infection. In several epidemics, such as that in Middletown, reported by Conn, that in Naples, by Lavis, and the outbreak which occurred at Winchester, the chain of circumstantial evidence seems complete. Most suggestive sporadic cases have been recorded by Broadbent and others. Foote showed that oysters taken from the feeding-grounds in rivers contain a larger number of micro-organisms of all sorts than those from the sea. Chantemesse found typhoid bacilli in oysters which had lain in infected sea-water, even after they had been transferred to and kept in fresh water for a time. Mosny, in his report to the French Government (1900), admits the possibility of oyster infection, but thinks that the oyster plays a very small *rôle* in relation to the total morbidity of the disease. Mussels have been found contaminated with typhoid bacilli, and it is stated that dried fish have carried the infection.

(*e*) *Flies.*—The importance of flies in the transmission of the disease was brought out very strongly in the Spanish-American War in 1898. The Report of the Commission states that "flies were undoubtedly the most active agents in the spread of typhoid fever. Flies alternately visited and fed on the infected fæcal matter and the food in the mess-tent. . . . Typhoid fever was much less frequent among members of the messes who had their mess-tents screened than it was among those who took no such precautions." In the South African War there was a perfect plague of flies, particularly in the typhoid fever tents, and among the army surgeons the opinion was universal that they had a great deal to do with the dissemination of the disease. Firth and Horrocks demonstrated the readiness with which flies, after feeding on typhoid stools or fresh cultures of typhoid bacilli, could infect sterile media. One of the most interesting studies on the question was made in the Chicago epidemic of 1902 by Alice Hamilton. Flies caught in two undrained privies, on the fences of two yards, on the walls of two houses, and in the room of a typhoid fever patient, were used to inoculate eighteen tubes, and from five of these tubes typhoid bacilli were isolated.

(*f*) *Contamination of the Soil.*—Filth, bad sewers, or cesspools can not in themselves cause typhoid fever, but they furnish the conditions suitable for the preservation of the bacillus, and possibly for its propagation.

Dust may be an important factor, though it has been shown that the bacilli die very quickly when desiccated. Possibly, as Barringer suggested, the dust on the railway tracks may become contaminated. Men working on the tracks are very liable to infection.

Types of Infection.—We may recognize the following groups: (*a*) *Ordinary typhoid fever with marked enteric lesions.* An immense majority of all cases are of this character; and while the spleen and mesenteric glands are involved the lymphatic apparatus of the intestinal walls bears the brunt of the attack. (*b*) *Cases in which the intestinal lesions are very slight,* and may be found only after a very careful search. In reviewing the cases of "typhoid fever without intestinal lesions," Opie and Bassett call attention to the fact that in many negative cases slight lesions really did exist, while in others death occurred so late that the lesions might have healed. In some cases the disease is a general septicæmia with symptoms of severe intoxication and high fever and delirium. In others the main lesions may be in organs—liver, gall-bladder, pleura, meninges, or even the endocardium. (*c*) *Cases in which the typhoid bacillus enters the body without causing any lesion of the intestine.* In a number of the earlier cases reported as such the demonstration of the typhoid bacillus was inconclusive. In others the intestine showed tuberculous ulcers, through which the organisms may have entered. But after excluding all these, a few cases remain in which the demonstration of the typhoid bacillus was conclusive, cases in which death occurred early, and yet after a very careful search no intestinal lesions could be found. There were 4 cases in this series. Undoubtedly the intestinal lesions may be so slight as not to be recognizable at autopsy. (*d*) *Mixed infections.* It is well to distinguish, as Dreschfeld pointed out, between double infections, as with bacillus tuberculosis, the diphtheria bacillus, and the plasmodia of Laveran, in which two different diseases are present and can be distinguished, and the true mixed or secondary infections, in which the conditions induced by one organism favor the growth of other pathogenic forms; thus in ordinary typhoid fever secondary infection with the colon bacillus, the streptococcus, staphylococcus, or the pneumococcus, may occur. (*e*) *Paratyphoid infections.* (Page 43.)

(*f*) *Local infections.* The typhoid bacillus may cause a local abscess, cystitis, or cholecystitis without evidence of a general infection. (*g*) *Terminal typhoid infections.* In rare instances the bacillus causes a fatal infection towards the end of other diseases. The subjects may, of course, be typhoid carriers. In two cases of malignant disease at the Johns Hopkins Hospital the bacilli were isolated from the blood, and there were no intestinal lesions.

Products of the Growth of the Bacilli.—According to Pfeiffer, the chief poison belongs to the intracellular group of toxins. Sidney Martin isolated a poison which is in the nature of a secretion, but does not differ from that contained within the bacterial cell. Injected into animals it causes lowering of temperature, diarrhœa, loss of weight, and degeneration of the myocardium. Its chemical nature is not known. Similar, but weaker, poisons may be isolated from cultures of *Bacillus coli* and other members of this group. No toxins have been isolated which cause changes in animals at all comparable to typhoid fever in human beings.

Morbid Anatomy.—INTESTINES.—A catarrhal condition exists throughout the small and large bowel. Specific changes occur in the lymphoid elements, chiefly at the lower end of the ileum. The alterations which occur are most conveniently described in four stages:

(*a*) *Hyperplasia,* which involves the glands of Peyer in the jejunum and ileum, and to a variable extent those in the large intestine. The follicles are swollen, grayish-white, and the patches may project 3 to 5 mm., or may be still more prominent. The solitary glands, which range in size from a pin's head to a pea, are usually deeply imbedded in the submucosa, but project to a variable extent. Occasionally they are very prominent, and may be almost pedunculated. Microscopic examination shows at the outset a condition of hyperæmia of the follicles. Later there is a great increase and accumulation of cells of the lymph-tissue which may even infiltrate the adjacent mucosa and the muscularis; and the blood-vessels are more or less compressed, which gives the whitish, anæmic appearance to the follicles. The cells have all the characters of ordinary lymph-corpuscles, but some are larger, epithelioid, and contain several nuclei. Occasionally cells containing red blood-corpuscles are seen. This so-called medullary infiltration, always more intense toward the lower end of the ileum, reaches its height from the eighth to the tenth day and then undergoes one of two changes, *resolution* or *necrosis.* Death very rarely takes place at this stage. Resolution is accomplished by a fatty and granular change in the cells, which are destroyed and absorbed. A curious condition of the patches is produced at this stage, in which they have a reticulated appearance. The swollen follicles in the patch undergo resolution and shrink more rapidly than the surrounding framework, or what is more probable the follicles alone, owing to the intense hyperplasia, become necrotic and disintegrate, leaving the little pits. In this process superficial hæmorrhages may result, and small ulcers may originate by the fusion of these superficial losses of substance.

Except histologically there is nothing distinctive in the hyperplasia of the lymph-follicles; but apart from typhoid fever we rarely see in adults a marked affection of these glands with fever. In children, however, it is not uncommon when death has occurred from intestinal affections, and it is also met with in measles, diphtheria, and scarlet fever.

(*b*) *Necrosis and Sloughing.*—When the hyperplasia of the lymph-follicles reaches a certain grade, resolution is no longer possible. The blood-vessels become choked, there is a condition of anæmic necrosis, and sloughs form which must be separated and thrown off. The necrosis is probably due in great part to the direct action of the bacilli. According to Mallory, there occurs a proliferation of endothelial cells due to the action of a toxin. These cells are phagocytic in character, and the swelling of the intestinal lymphoid tissue is due almost entirely to their formation. The necrosis, he thinks, is due to the occlusion of the veins and capillaries by fibrinous thrombi, which owe their origin to degeneration of phagocytic cells beneath the lining endothelium of the vessels. The process may be superficial, affecting only the upper part of the mucous coat, or it may extend to and involve the submucosa. The "slough" may sometimes lie upon the Peyer's patch, scarcely involving more than the epithelium (Marchand). It is always more intense toward the ileo-cæcal valve, and in very severe cases the greater part of the mucosa of the last foot of the ileum may be converted into a brownish-black eschar. The necrotic area in the solitary glands forms a yellowish cap which often involves only the most prominent point of a follicle. The extent of the necrosis is very variable. It may pass deep into the muscular coat, reaching to or even perforating the peritoneum.

(*c*) *Ulceration.*—The separation of the necrotic tissue—the sloughing—is gradually effected from the edges inward, and results in the formation of an ulcer, the size and extent of which are directly proportionate to the amount of necrosis. If this be superficial, the entire thickness of the mucosa may not be involved and the loss of substance may be small and shallow. More commonly the slough in separating exposes the submucosa and muscularis, particularly the latter, which forms the floor of a majority of all typhoid ulcers. It is not common for an entire Peyer's patch to slough away, and a perfectly ovoid ulcer opposite to the mesentery is rarely seen. Irregularly oval and rounded forms are most common. A large patch may present three or four ulcers divided by septa of mucous membrane. The terminal 6 or 8 inches of the mucous membrane of the ileum may form a large ulcer, in which are here and there islands of mucosa. The edges of the ulcer are usually swollen, soft, sometimes congested, and often undermined. The base of a typhoid ulcer is smooth and clean, being usually formed of the submucosa or of the muscularis.

(*d*) *Healing.*—This begins with the development of a thin granulation tissue which covers the base. Occasionally an appearance is seen as if an ulcer had healed in one place and was extending in another. The mucosa gradually extends from the edge, and a new growth of epithelium is formed. The glandular elements are reformed; the healed ulcer is somewhat depressed and is usually pigmented. In death during relapse healing ulcers may be seen in some patches with fresh ulcers in others.

We may say, indeed, that healing begins with the separation of the sloughs, as, when resolution is impossible, the removal of the necrosed part is the first step in the process of repair. In fatal cases, we seldom meet with evidences of cicatrization, as the majority of deaths occur before this stage is reached. It is remarkable that no matter how extensive the ulceration has been, healing is never associated with stricture, and typhoid fever does not appear as one of the causes of intestinal obstruction. Within a very short time all traces of the old ulcers disappear.

LARGE INTESTINE.—The cæcum and colon are affected in about one-third of the cases. Sometimes the solitary glands are greatly enlarged. The ulcers are usually larger in the cæcum than in the colon.

PERFORATION OF THE BOWEL.—*Incidence at Autopsy.*—J. A. Scott's figures, embracing 9,713 cases, give 351 deaths from perforation among 1,037 deaths from all causes, a percentage of 33.8 of the deaths and 3.6 of the cases. The German statistics give a much lower proportion of deaths from perforation; Munich in 2,000 autopsies, 5.7 per cent. from perforation; Basle in 2,000 autopsies, 1.3 per cent. from perforation; Hamburg in 3,686 autopsies, 1.2 per cent. from perforation (Hector Mackenzie, Lancet, 1903). At the Johns Hopkins Hospital among 1,500 cases of typhoid fever there were 43 with perforation. Twenty of these were operated upon, with 7 recoveries. One died of toxæmia on the eighth day after operation. At the Pennsylvania Hospital there were 139 cases of perforation among 5,891 cases. Chomel remarks that "the accident is sometimes the result of ulceration, sometimes of a true eschar, and sometimes it is produced by the distention of the intestine, causing the rupture of tissues weakened by disease." As a rule, sloughs are adherent about the site of perforation. The site is usually in the ileum, 232 times in Hector Mackenzie's collection of 264 cases; the jejunum twice, the large intestine 22 times, and the appendix 9 times in his series. As a rule, the perforation occurs within twelve inches of the ileo-cæcal valve. There may be two or three separate perforations. J. A. Scott described two distinct varieties: first, the more common single, circular, pin-point in size, due to the extension of a necrotic process through the base of a small ulcer. The second variety, produced by a large area of tissue becoming necrotic, ranges in size from the finger-tip to 3 cm. in diameter.

Death from hæmorrhage occurred in 99 of the Munich cases, and in 12 of 137 deaths in our 1,500 cases. The bleeding seems to result directly from the separation of the sloughs. It is unusual to find the bleeding vessel. In one case only a single patch had sloughed, and a firm clot was adherent to it. The bleeding may come from the soft swollen edges of the patch.

The *mesenteric glands* show hyperæmia and subsequently become greatly swollen. Spots of necrosis are common. In several of our cases suppuration had occurred, and in one a large abscess of the mesentery was present. The rupture of a softened or suppurating mesenteric gland, of which there are only a few cases in the literature, may cause either fatal hæmorrhage or peritonitis. Le Conte has successfully operated upon the latter condition. The bunch of glands in the mesentery, at the lower end of the ileum, is especially involved. The retroperitoneal glands are also swollen.

The *spleen* is invariably enlarged in the early stages of the disease. In 11 of our series it exceeded 20 ounces (600 grams) in weight, in one 900 grams. The tissue is soft, even diffluent. Infarction is not infrequent. Rupture may occur spontaneously or as a result of injury. In the Munich autopsies there were 5 instances of rupture of the spleen, one of which resulted from a gangrenous abscess.

The *bone-marrow* shows changes very similar to those in the lymphoid tissues, and there may be foci of necrosis (Longcope).

The *liver* shows signs of parenchymatous degeneration. Early in the disease it is hyperæmic, and in a majority of instances it is swollen, somewhat pale, on section turbid, and microscopically the cells are very granular and loaded with fat. Nodular areas (microscopic) occur in many cases. Some of the nodules are lymphoid, others are necrotic. In 12 of the Munich autopsies liver abscess was found, and in 3, acute yellow atrophy. In 3 of this series liver abscess occurred. Pylephlebitis may follow abscess of the mesentery or perforation of the appendix. Affections of the gall-bladder are not uncommon, and are described under the clinical features.

Kidneys.—Cloudy swelling, with granular degeneration of the cells of the convoluted tubules, less commonly an acute nephritis, may be present. Rayer, Wagner, and others described the occurrence of numerous small areas infiltrated with round cells, which may have the appearance of lymphomata, or may pass on to softening and suppuration, producing the so-called *miliary abscesses*, of which there were 7 cases in this series. The typhoid bacilli have been found in these areas. The kidneys in cases of typhoid bacilluria may show no changes other than cloudy swelling. Diphtheritic inflammation of the pelvis of the kidney may occur. It was present in 3 of our cases, in one of which the tips of the papillæ were also affected. Catarrh of the bladder is not uncommon. Diphtheritic inflammation of this viscus may also occur. Orchitis is occasionally met with.

Respiratory Organs.—Ulceration of the larynx occurs in a certain number of cases; in the Munich series it was noted 107 times. It may come on at the same time as the ulceration in the ileum. It occurs in the posterior wall, at the insertion of the cords, at the base of the epiglottis, and on the ary-epiglottidean folds. The cartilages are very apt to become involved. In the later periods ulcers may be present.

Œdema of the glottis was present in 20 of the Munich cases, in 8 of which tracheotomy was performed. Diphtheritis of the pharynx and larynx is not very uncommon. It occurred in a most extensive form in 2 of our cases. Lobar pneumonia may be found early (see Pneumo-typhus), or it may be a late event. Hypostatic congestion and the condition of the lung spoken of as splenization occur. Gangrene of the lung occurred in 40 cases in the Munich series; abscess of the lung in 14; hæmorrhagic infarction in 129. Pleurisy is not a common event. Fibrinous pleurisy occurred in about 6 per cent. of the Munich cases, and empyema in nearly 2 per cent.

Changes in the Circulatory System.—*Heart Lesions.—Endocarditis*, while not common, is probably more frequent than is generally supposed. It was present without being suspected in 3 out of 105 autopsies in this series, while in 3 other cases the clinical symptoms suggested its presence. Typhoid bacilli have been found in the vegetations. *Pericarditis* was present in 14 cases of the Munich autopsies. *Myocarditis* is not very infrequent. In protracted cases the muscle-fibre is usually soft, flabby, and of a pale yellowish-brown color. The softening may be extreme, though rarely of the grade described by Stokes in typhus fever, in which, when held apex up by the vessels, the organ collapsed over the hand, forming a mushroom-like cap. Microscopically, the fibres may show little or no change, even when the impulse of the heart has been extremely feeble. A granular parenchymatous degeneration is common. Fatty degeneration may be present, particularly in long-standing cases with anæmia. The hyaline change is not common.

Lesions of the Blood-vessels.—Changes in the arteries are not infrequent. In 21 of 52 cases in our series, in which there were notes on the state of the aorta, fresh endarteritis was present, and in 13 of 62 cases in which the condition of the coronary arteries was noted similar changes were found (Thayer). *Arteritis* of a peripheral vessel with thrombus formation is not uncommon. Bacilli have been found in the thrombi. The artery may be blocked by a thrombus of cardiac origin—an embolus—but in the great majority of instances they are autochthonous and due to arteritis, obliterating or partial. *Thrombosis* in the veins is very much more frequent than in the arteries, but is not such a serious event. It is most frequent in the femoral, and in the left more often than the right.

Nervous System.—There are very few obvious changes met with. *Meningitis* is rare and occurred in only 11 of the 2,000 Munich cases. The exudation may be either serous, sero-fibrinous, or purulent, and typhoid bacilli have been isolated. Five cases of serous and one of purulent meningitis occurred in our series (Cole). Optic neuritis, which occurs sometimes in typhoid fever, has not been described in connection with the meningitis. The anatomical lesion of the *aphasia*—seen not infrequently in children—is not known, possibly it is an encephalitis. Parenchymatous changes have been met with in the periphereal nerves, and appear to be not very uncommon, even when there have been no symptoms of neuritis.

The *voluntary muscles* show, in certain instances, the changes described by Zenker, which occur in all long-standing febrile affections, and are not peculiar to typhoid fever. The muscle substance undergoes either a granular degeneration or a hyaline transformation. The abdominal muscles, the adductors of the thighs, and the pectorals are most commonly involved. Rupture of a rectus abdominis has been found post mortem. Hæmorrhage may occur. Abscesses may develop in the muscles during convalescence.

Symptoms.—In a disease so complex as typhoid fever it will be well first to give a general description, and then to study more fully the symptoms, complications, and sequelæ according to the individual organs.

General Description.—The period of incubation lasts from "eight to fourteen days, sometimes twenty-three" (Clinical Society), during which there are feelings of lassitude and inaptitude for work. The average is about ten days. The onset is rarely abrupt. In the 1,500 cases chills occurred at onset in 334, headache in 1,117, anorexia in 825, diarrhœa (without purgation) in 516, epistaxis in 323, abdominal pain in 443, constipation in 249, pain in right iliac fossa in 10. The patient at last takes to his bed, from which event, in a majority of cases, the definite onset may be dated. During the *first week* there is, in some cases (but by no means in all, as has long been taught), a steady rise in the fever, the evening record rising a degree or a degree and a half higher each day, reaching 103° or 104°. The pulse is not rapid when compared with the temperature, full in volume, but of low tension and often dicrotic; the tongue is coated and white; the abdomen is slightly distended and tender. Unless the fever is high there is no delirium, but the patient complains of headache, and there may be mental confusion at night. The bowels may be constipated or there may be loose movements.

Toward the end of the week the spleen becomes enlarged and the rash appears in the form of rose-colored spots, seen first on the skin of the abdomen. Cough and bronchitic symptoms are not uncommon at the outset.

In the *second week,* in cases of moderate severity, the symptoms become aggravated; the fever remains high and the morning remission is slight. The pulse is rapid and loses its dicrotic character. There is no longer headache, but there are mental torpor and dullness. The face looks heavy; the lips are dry; the tongue, in severe cases, becomes dry also. The abdominal symptoms, if present—diarrhœa, tympanites, and tenderness—become aggravated. Death may occur during this week, with pronounced nervous symptoms, or, toward the end of it, from hæmorrhage or perforation. In mild cases the temperature declines, and by the fourteenth day may be normal.

In the *third week,* in cases of moderate severity, the pulse ranges from 110 to 130; the temperature shows marked morning remissions, and there is a gradual decline in the fever. The loss of flesh is more noticeable, and the weakness pronounced. Diarrhœa and meteorism may occur for the first time. Unfavorable symptoms at this stage are the pulmonary complications, increasing feebleness of the heart, and pronounced delirium with muscular tremor. Special dangers are perforation and hæmorrhage.

With the *fourth week,* in a majority of instances, convalescence begins. The temperature gradually reaches the normal point, the diarrhœa stops, the tongue cleans, and the desire for food returns. In severe cases the fourth and even the fifth week may present an aggravated picture of the third; the patient grows weaker, the pulse is more rapid and feeble, the tongue dry, and the abdomen distended. He lies in a condition of profound stupor, with low muttering delirium and subsultus tendinum, and passes the fæces and urine involuntarily. Failure of the circulation and secondary complications are the chief dangers of this period.

In the *fifth and sixth weeks* protracted cases may still show irregular fever, and convalescence may not set in until after the fortieth day. In this period we meet with relapses in the milder forms or slight recrudescence of the fever. At this time, too, occur many of the complications and sequelæ.

Special Features and Symptoms.—*Mode of Onset.*—As a rule, the symptoms come on insidiously, and the patient is unable to fix definitely the time at which he began to feel ill. The following are the most important deviations from this common course:

(*a*) *Onset with Pronounced, Sometimes Sudden, Nervous Manifestations.*—Headache, of a severe and intractable nature, is by no means an infrequent initial symptom. Again, a severe facial neuralgia may for a few days put the practitioner off his guard. In cases in which the patients have kept about and, as they say, fought the disease, the very first manifestation may be pronounced delirium. Such patients may even leave home and wander about for days. In rare cases the disease sets in with the most intense cerebro-spinal symptoms, simulating meningitis—severe headache, photophobia, retraction of the head, twitching of the muscles, and even convulsions. Occasionally drowsiness, stupor, and signs of basilar meningitis may exist for ten days or more before the characteristic symptoms develop; the onset may be with mania and marked mental symptoms.

(*b*) *With Pronounced Pulmonary Symptoms.*—The initial bronchial catarrh may be of great severity and obscure the other features of the disease. More striking still are those cases in which the disease sets in with a single chill, with pain in the side and all the characteristic features of lobar pneumonia or of acute pleurisy; or tuberculosis is suspected.

(*c*) *With Intense Gastro-intestinal Symptoms.*—The incessant vomiting and pain may lead to a suspicion of poisoning, or the patient may be sent to the surgical wards for appendicitis.

(*d*) *With symptoms of an acute nephritis,* smoky or bloody urine, with much albumin and tube-casts.

(*e*) *Ambulatory Form.*—Deserving of especial mention are those cases in which the patient keeps about and attempts to work, or perhaps takes a long journey to his home. He may come under observation for the first time with a temperature of 104° or 105°, and the rash well out. Many of these cases run a severe course, and in general hospitals contribute largely to the mortality. Finally, there are rare instances in which typhoid is unsuspected until perforation or a profuse hæmorrhage from the bowels occurs.

Facial Aspect.—Early in the disease the cheeks are flushed and the eyes bright. Toward the end of the first week the expression becomes more listless, and when the disease is well established the patient has a dull and heavy look. There is never the rapid anæmia of malarial fever, and the color of the lips and cheeks may be retained even to the third week.

Fever.—(*a*) *Regular Course.* (Chart I.)—In the stage of invasion the fever rises steadily during the first five or six days. The evening temperature is about a degree or a degree and a half higher than the morning remission, so that a temperature of 104° or 105° is not uncommon by the end of the first week. Having reached the fastigium or height, the fever then persists with very slight daily remissions. The fever may be singularly persistent and but little influenced by bathing or other measures. At the end of the second and throughout the third week the temperature becomes more distinctly remittent. The difference between the morning or evening record may be 3° or 4°, and the morning temperature may even be normal. It falls by lysis, and the temperature is not considered normal until the evening record is at 98.4°.

(*b*) *Variations from the typical temperature curve* are common. We do not always see the gradual step-like ascent in the early stage; the patients do not often come under observation at this time. When the disease sets in with a chill, or in children with a convulsion, the temperature may rise at once to 103° or 104°. In many cases defervescence occurs at the end of the second week and the temperature may fall rapidly, reaching the normal within twelve or twenty hours. An inverse type of temperature, high in the morning and low in the evening, is occasionally seen, but has no especial significance.

Sudden falls in the temperature may occur, thus, as shown in Chart II, a drop of 6.4° may follow an intestinal hæmorrhage, and the fall may be apparent before the blood has appeared in the stools. Sometimes during the anæmia which follows a severe hæmorrhage from the bowels there are remarkable oscillations in the temperature. Hyperpyrexia is rare. In only 58 of 1,500 cases did the fever rise above 106°. Before death the fever may rise; the highest we have known was 109.5°.

(*c*) *Post-typhoid Variations.*—(1) *Recrudescences.*—After a normal tem-

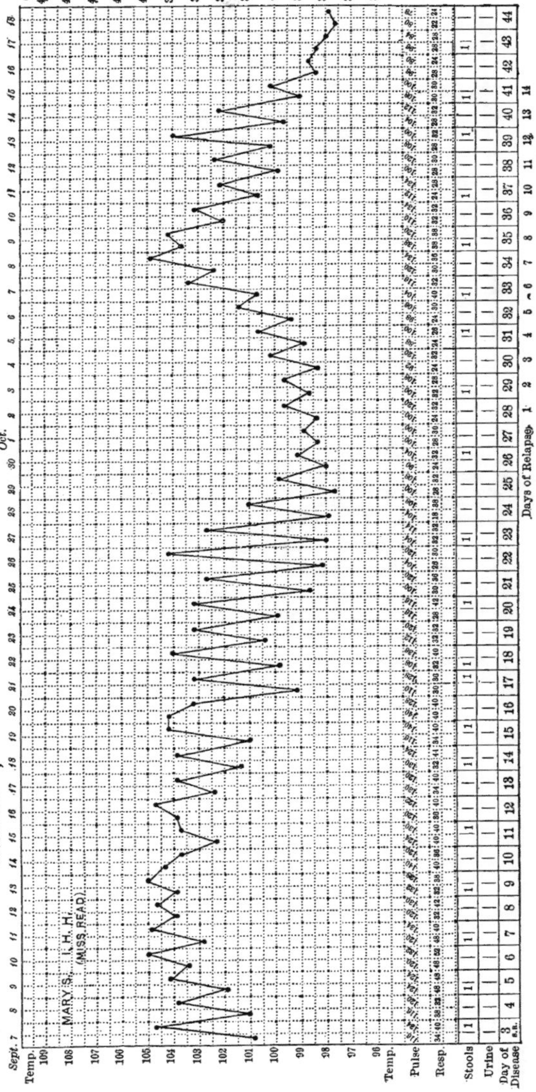

CHART I.—TYPHOID FEVER WITH RELAPSE.

perature of perhaps five or six days, the fever may rise suddenly to 102° or 103°, without constitutional disturbance, furring of the tongue, or abdominal symptoms. After persisting for from two to four days the temperature falls. Of 1,500 cases, 92 presented these elevations, notes of which are given in the Studies on Typhoid Fever (Johns Hopkins Hospital Reports). Constipation, errors in diet, or excitement may cause them. These attacks are a frequent source of anxiety; they are common, and it is not always possible to say upon what they depend. In some cases typhoid or colon bacilli are found in the blood. As a rule, if the rise in temperature is the result of a complication, such as thrombosis, there is an increase in the leucocytes. Naturally one suspects a relapse, but there is an absence of the step-like ascent, and, as a rule, the fever falls after a few days.

(2) *The Sub-febrile Stage of Convalescence.*—In children, in very nervous patients, and in cases of anæmia, the evening temperature may keep up for weeks after the tongue has cleaned and the appetite has returned. This may usually be disregarded, and is often best treated by allowing the patient to get up, and by stopping the use of the thermometer. Of course, it is important not to overlook any latent complications.

(3) *Hypothermia.*—Low temperatures in typhoid fever are common, following baths, or spontaneously in the third and fourth week in the periods of marked remissions, and following hæmorrhage. An interesting form is the persistent hypothermia of convalescence. For ten days or more, particularly in the protracted cases with great emaciation, the temperature may be 96.5° or 97°. It is of no special significance.

(*d*) *The Fever of the Relapse.*—This is a repetition in many instances of the original fever, a gradual ascent and maintenance for a few days at a certain height and then a decline. It is usually shorter than the original pyrexia, and rarely continues more than two or three weeks. (Chart I.)

(*e*) *Afebrile Typhoid.*—The occurrence of this is doubtful and the cases so termed are probably mild attacks with slight fever for a few days.

(*f*) *Chills* occur (1) sometimes with the fever of onset; (2) occasionally at intervals throughout the course, and followed by sweats (so-called sudoral form); (3) with the advent of complications, pleurisy, pneumonia, otitis media, phlebitis, etc.; (4) with active antipyretic treatment by the coal-tar remedies; (5) occasionally during the period of defervescence without relation to any complication, sometimes due to a septic infection; (6) after the injection of vaccines or serum; (7) according to Herringham, chills may result from constipation. There are cases in which throughout the latter half of the disease chills recur with great severity. (See Chills in Typhoid Fever, Studies II.)

SKIN.—The characteristic rash consists of hyperæmic spots, which appear from the seventh to the tenth day, usually at first upon the abdomen. They are slightly raised, flattened papules, which can be felt distinctly, of a rose-red color, disappearing on pressure, and ranging in diameter from 2 to 4 mm. They were present in 93.2 per cent. of the white patients and 20.6 per cent. of the colored. They come out in successive crops, and after persisting for two or three days they disappear, occasionally leaving a brownish stain. The spots may be present upon the back, and not upon the abdomen. The eruption may be very abundant over the whole skin of the trunk, and on the extremities. There were 81 in which they occurred on the arms, 17 on the forearms, 43 on the thighs, legs 15, face 5, hands 3. The cases with very abundant eruption are not necessarily more severe. Typhoid bacilli have been found in the spots. Of variations in the rash, frequently the spots are capped by small vesicles. A profuse miliary or sudaminal rash is not uncommon. In 38 cases in our series there were purpuric spots. Three of the cases were true hæmorrhagic typhoid fever. The rash may not appear until the relapse. In 21 cases in our series the rose spots came out after the patient was afebrile.

A branny desquamation is not rare in children, and common in adults after hydrotherapy. Occasionally the skin peels off in large flakes. A yellow color of the palms of the hands and soles of the feet is not uncommon.

Among other skin lesions the following may be mentioned:

Erythema.—It is not very uncommon in the first week of the disease to find a diffuse erythematous blush—E. typhosum. Sometimes the skin may have a peculiar mottled pink and white appearance. E. exudativum, E. nodosum, and urticaria may be present.

Herpes.—Herpes is rare in typhoid fever in comparison with its great frequency in malarial fever and in pneumonia. It was noted in 20 of our 1,500 cases, usually on the lips.

The Tâches bleuâtres—Peliomata—Maculæ ceruleæ.—These are pale-blue or steel-gray spots, subcuticular, from 4 to 10 mm. in diameter, and of irregular outline. They are due to lice (see PEDICULOSIS).

Skin Gangrene.—Areas of superficial gangrene may follow the prolonged use of an ice-bag. In children noma may occur; as reported by McFarland in the Philadelphia epidemic of 1898, there were many cases with multiple areas of gangrene of the skin. The nose, ears, and genitals may be attacked.

Sweats.—At the height of the fever the skin is usually dry. Profuse sweating is rare, but it is not very uncommon to see the abdomen or chest moist with perspiration, particularly in the reaction which follows the bath. Sweats in some instances constitute a striking feature and may be associated with chilly sensations or actual chills. In this *sudoral* form of typhoid fever there may be recurring paroxysms of chill, fever, and sweats (even several in twenty-four hours), and the case may be mistaken for one of malarial fever. Profuse sweats may occur with hæmorrhage or perforation.

Œdema of the skin occurs: (1) As the result of vascular obstruction, most commonly of a vein, as in femoral thrombosis. (2) In connection with nephritis, very rarely. (3) In association with the anæmia and cachexia. *The hair* falls out after the attack, but complete baldness is rare. The nutrition of the nails suffers, and during and after convalescence transverse ridges may occur. A peculiar *odor* is exhaled from the skin in some cases. Whether due to a cutaneous exhalation or not, there is a very distinctive smell connected with many patients. Nathan Smith described it as of a "semi-cadaverous, musty character."

Lineæ atrophicæ.—Lines of atrophy may appear on the skin of the abdomen, lateral aspects of the thighs and about the knees, similar to those seen after pregnancy. They have been attributed to neuritis, and Duckworth has reported a case in which the skin adjacent to them was hyperæsthetic.

Bed-sores are not uncommon in protracted cases, with great emaciation.

In some cases the necrosis begins in the deeper structures but, as a rule, they result from pressure and are seen upon the sacrum, more rarely the ilia, the shoulders, and the heels. These are less common since the introduction of hydrotherapy and scrupulous care does much for their prevention, but in cases with profound involvement of the nerve centres acute bed-sores of the back and heels may occur with very slight pressure, and with astonishing rapidity.

Boils and superficial abscesses constitute a common and troublesome sequel.

CIRCULATORY SYSTEM.—The *blood* presents important changes. The following statements are based on studies made by W. S. Thayer (Studies I and III): During the first two weeks there may be little or no change in the blood. Profuse sweats or copious diarrhœa may cause the corpuscles—as in the collapse stage of cholera—to rise above normal. In the third week a fall usually takes place in corpuscles and hæmoglobin, and the number may sink rapidly even to 1,300,000 per c. mm., gradually rising to normal during convalescence. When the patient first gets up, there may be a slight fall in the corpuscles. The average maximum loss is about 1,000,000 to the c. mm.

The amount of hæmoglobin is always reduced, and usually in a greater relative proportion than the red corpuscles, and during recovery the normal color standard is reached at a later period. Leucopenia is present throughout the course. Cold baths increase temporarily the number of leucocytes in the peripheral circulation. The absence of leucocytosis is of value in distinguishing typhoid fever from various septic fevers and acute inflammatory processes. The large mononuclears are relatively increased. When an acute inflammatory process occurs in typhoid fever the leucocytes show an increase in the polynuclear forms, and this may be of great diagnostic moment.

The post-typhoid anæmia may reach an extreme grade. In one of our patients the blood-corpuscles sank to 1,300,000 per c. mm. and the hæmoglobin to about 20 per cent. but these severe grades of anæmia are not common. In the Munich statistics there were 54 cases with general and extreme anæmia. Of changes in the blood plasma very little is known.

The *pulse* presents no special characters. It is increased in rapidity, but not always in proportion to the fever, and this may be a special feature in the early stages. There is no acute disease with which, in the early stage, a dicrotic pulse is so frequently associated. Even with high fever the pulse may not be greatly accelerated. As the disease progresses the pulse becomes more rapid, feebler, and small. In 15 per cent. of our cases the pulse rate rose above 140. In the extreme prostration of severe cases it may reach 150 or more, and is a mere undulation—the so-called running pulse. The lowered arterial pressure is manifest in the dusky lividity of the skin and coldness of the hands and feet.

During convalescence the pulse gradually returns to normal, and occasionally becomes very slow. After no other acute fever do we so frequently meet with bradycardia. The pulse may be as low as 30, and instances are on record of still fewer beats to the minute. Some of these are probably due to temporary heart-block. Tachycardia, while less common, may be a very troublesome and persistent feature of convalescence.

Blood Pressure.—There is a gradual fall during the course to about 100-110 mm. Hg at the beginning of apyrexia. In two or three weeks later the pressure has usually returned to normal. Hæmorrhage usually produces a marked fall both in the systolic and diastolic pressure. In some cases of perforation there may be a sharp rise in systolic pressure. Tubs and ice sponges usually cause a rise of 10-20 mm. Hg.

The *heart-sounds* may be normal throughout. In severe cases, the first sound becomes feeble and there is often heard, at the apex and along the left sternal margin, a soft systolic murmur, which was present in 22 per cent. of our cases. Absence of the first sound is rare. Gallop rhythm is not uncommon. In the extreme feebleness of the graver forms, the first and second sounds become similar, and the long pause is shortened (embryocardia).

Pericarditis is rare and has been met with chiefly in children and in association with pneumonia. It was present in 3 of our series and occurred in only 14 of the 2,000 Munich post mortems. *Endocarditis* was found post mortem in 3 cases, and the physical signs suggested its presence in 3 other cases in the series. *Myocarditis* is more common, and is indicated by a progressive weakening of the heart-sounds and enfeeblement of the action of the organ.

Complications in the Arteries.—Arteritis with thrombus formation occurred in four cases in the series, one in the branches of the middle cerebral, two in the femoral, and one in the brachial. In one case gangrene of the leg followed. In a similar case seen with Roddick, in Montreal, obliteration of the left femoral artery occurred on the sixteenth day, and of the vessel on the right side on the twentieth day, with gangrene of both feet. Pain, tenderness and swelling occur over the artery, with diminution or disappearance of the pulsations and coldness and blueness of the extremity. In two of the cases these symptoms gradually disappeared, and the pulsation returned not only in the peripheral, but in the affected vessels (Thayer). Keen refers to 46 cases of arterial gangrene, of which 8 were bilateral, 19 on the right side, and 19 on the left.

Thrombi in the Veins.—In our series there were 43 instances, distributed in the following veins: femoral 23, popliteal 5, iliac 5, veins of the calf 5, internal saphenous 3, pulmonary artery and common iliac 1, axillary vein 1 (Thayer). In one case it occurred in the right circumflex iliac vein. Femoral thrombosis is the most common, and almost invariably in the left vessel, due probably to the fact that the left iliac vein is crossed by the right iliac artery, and the blood flow is not so free. The symptoms are very definite—the fever may increase or recur. Chills occurred in 11 of the cases. Pain and swelling at the site are constantly present, and the thrombotic mass can be felt, not always at first, nor is it well to feel for it. Swelling of the leg follows as a rule, but it is rarely so extreme, and not so painful as in the puerperal cases. In iliac thrombosis the pain may be severe and lead to the suspicion of perforation, as in one of our cases. Leucocytosis is usually present; in 12 cases it rose above 10,000. Five of the 43 patients died, 2 only as a result of the thrombus; in the case of axillary thrombosis from pulmonary embolism, in one from embolism of the inferior cava and right auricle from the dislocation of a piece of thrombus from the left iliac vein. Thayer examined 16 of the patients at varying periods after convalescence, and found in every case more or less disability from the varices and persistent swelling. In some cases, however, the recovery is complete.

Conner has emphasized the frequency of thrombosis in the small veins of the legs and feet and suggests that pulmonary embolism of slight extent is a common result.

Digestive System.—Loss of appetite is early, and, as a rule, the relish for food is not regained until convalescence. The *tongue* presents the changes inevitable in a prolonged fever. Early in the disease it is moist, swollen, and coated with a thin white fur, which, as the fever progresses, becomes denser. It may remain moist throughout. In severe cases, particularly those with delirium, the tongue becomes very dry, partly owing to the fact that such patients breathe with the mouth open. It may be covered with a brown or brownish-black fur, or with crusts between which are cracks and fissures. In these cases the teeth and lips may be covered with a dark brownish matter called *sordes*—a mixture of food, epithelial *débris,* and micro-organisms. By keeping the mouth and tongue clean from the outset, the fissures may be prevented. Acute *glossitis* occurred in one case at the onset of the relapse. During convalescence the tongue gradually becomes clean, and the fur is thrown off, almost imperceptibly or occasionally in flakes.

The secretion of saliva is often diminished; salivation is rare.

Parotitis was present in 45 of the 2,000 Munich cases. It occurred in 14 cases in our series; of these, 5 died. It is most frequent in the third week in very severe cases. Extensive sloughing may follow in the tissues of the neck. Usually unilateral, and in a majority of cases going on to suppuration, it is regarded as a very fatal complication, but recovery followed in nine of our cases. It may arise from extension of inflammation along Steno's duct. This is probably not so serious a form as when it arises from metastatic inflammation. In four cases the submaxillary glands were involved alone, in one a cellulitis of the neck extended from the gland and proved fatal. Parotitis may occur after the fever has subsided. A remarkable localized sweating in the parotid region is an occasional sequel.

The *pharynx* may be the seat of catarrh or ulceration. Sometimes the fauces are deeply congested. Membranous pharyngitis, a serious and fatal complication, may come on in the third week. Difficulty in swallowing may result from ulcers of the œsophagus, and in one of our cases stricture followed. The *thyroid* gland is often enlarged in the acute stages. Thyroiditis may occur with abscess formation years after the attack of typhoid fever. Typhoid bacilli have been found in the pus.

The *gastric symptoms* are extremely variable. Nausea and vomiting are not common. There are instances, however, in which vomiting, resisting all measures, is a marked feature from the outset, and may directly cause death from exhaustion. Vomiting does not often occur in the second and third weeks, unless associated with some serious complication. Ulcers have been found in the stomach. Hæmatemesis occurred in 4 of our cases.

Intestinal Symptoms.—Diarrhœa is a very variable symptom, occurring in from 20 to 30 per cent. of the cases. Of 1,500 cases, 516 had diarrhœa before entering, 260 during their stay in hospital. It frequently follows the giving of purgatives and the small percentage in the hospital may be due to the fact that we used no purges or intestinal antiseptics. Its absence must not be taken as an indication that the intestinal lesions are of slight extent. The most extensive infiltration and ulceration of the small intestine may be seen with the colon filled with solid fæces. The diarrhœa is caused less by the ulcers than by the associated catarrh, and, as in tuberculosis, it is probable that when this is in the large intestine the discharges are more frequent. It is most common toward the end of the first and throughout the second week, but it may not occur until the third or even the fourth week. The number of

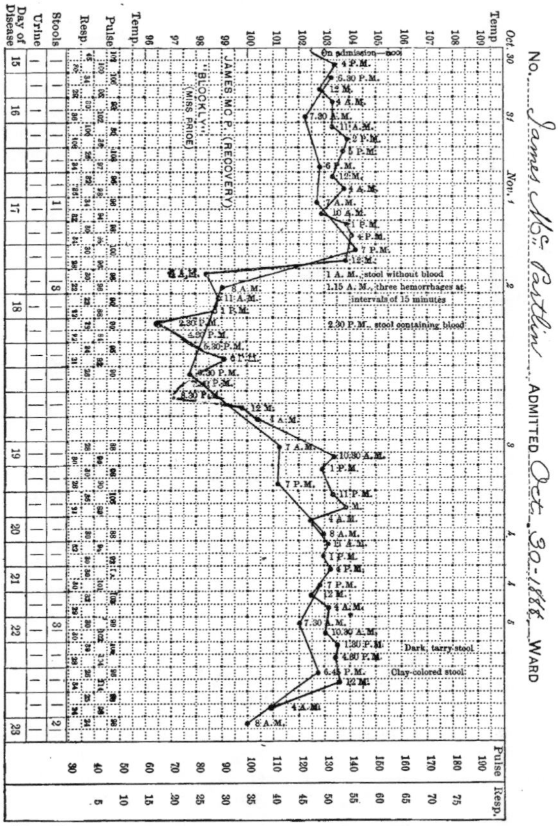

CHART II.—HÆMORRHAGE FROM THE BOWELS. RAPID FALL OF TEMPERATURE.

discharges ranges from 3 to 8 or 10 in the twenty-four hours. They are usually abundant, thin, grayish-yellow, granular, of the consistency and appearance of pea-soup, and resemble, as Addison remarked, the normal contents of the small bowel. Blood may be in small amount and only recognized by the microscope. Sloughs of the Peyer's glands occur as grayish-yellow fragments or occasionally as ovoid masses, an inch or more in length, in which portions of bowel tissue may be found. The bacilli are not found in the stools until the end of the first or the middle of the second week. Constipation was present in 51 per cent. of this series.

Hæmorrhage from the bowels is a serious complication, occurring in about 7 per cent. of all cases. It had occurred in 99 of the 2,000 fatal Munich cases. In 1,500 cases of our series hæmorrhage occurred in 118, and in 12 death followed the hæmorrhage. It occurred in 1,641 (7 per cent.) of 23,721 collected cases. There may be only a slight trace of blood in the stools, but often it is a profuse, free hæmorrhage. It occurs most commonly between the end of the second and the beginning of the fourth week, the time of the separation of the sloughs. Occasionally, early in the course, it results simply from the intense hyperæmia. It usually comes on without warning. A sensation of sinking or collapse is experienced by the patient, the temperature falls, and may, as in the annexed chart, drop 6° or 7° in a few hours. Fatal collapse may supervene before the blood appears in the stool. Hæmorrhage usually occurs in cases of considerable severity, but Graves and Trousseau held that it was not a very dangerous symptom.

It must not be forgotten that melæna may also be part of a general hæmorrhagic tendency (to be referred to later), in which cases it is associated with petechiæ and hæmaturia. There may be a special family predisposition to intestinal hæmorrhages in typhoid fever.

Meteorism, a frequent symptom, is not serious if of moderate grade, but when excessive is usually of ill omen. Owing to defective tone in the walls, in severe cases to their infiltration with serum, gas accumulates in the stomach, small and large bowel, particularly in the last. Pushing up the diaphragm, it interferes very much with the action of the heart and lungs, and may also favor perforation. Gurgling in the right iliac fossa exists in a large proportion of the cases, and indicates simply the presence of gas and fluid fæces in the colon and cæcum.

Abdominal pain and tenderness were present in three-fifths of a series of 500 cases studied with special reference to the point (McCrae). In some it was only present at the onset. Pain occurred during the course in about one-third of the cases. This is due in some instances to conditions apart from the bowel lesions, such as pleurisy, distention of the bladder, and phlebitis. It may be associated with diarrhœa, severe constipation, perisplenitis, or acute abdominal complications. Pain occurs with some cases of hæmorrhage, but is most constantly present with perforation. In a large group no cause could be found for the pain, and if other symptoms be associated the condition may lead to error in diagnosis. Operation for appendicitis has been performed in the early stage of typhoid fever, owing to the combination of pain in the right iliac fossa, fever and constipation.

PERFORATION.—From one-fourth to one-third of the deaths are due to perforation. Among 34,916 collected cases perforation occurred in 3.1 per cent. While it may occur as early as the first week, in the great majority it is at the height of the disease in the third week, and much more frequently in the severe cases, particularly those associated with tympanites, diarrhœa, and hæmorrhage. It may occur, however, in very mild attacks and with great suddenness, when the patient is apparently progressing favorably.

Symptoms of Perforation.—By far the most important single indication is a sudden, sharp pain of increasing severity, often paroxysmal in character. It is rarely absent, except in the small group of cases with profound toxæmia. The situation is most frequent in the hypogastric region and to the right of the middle line. Tenderness on pressure is present in the great majority of cases, usually in the hypogastric and right iliac regions, sometimes diffuse; it may only be brought out on deep pressure. As LeConte points out, when the perforation happens to be in contact with the parietal peritoneum the local features on palpation are much more marked than when the perforated ulcer is next to a coil or to the mesentery. There may be early irritability of the bladder, with frequent micturition, and pain extending toward the penis. A third important sign is muscle rigidity, increased tension, and spasm on any attempt to palpate. The temperature may rise for a few hours to fall later or may drop at once. The pulse and respiration rate are usually increased. Following these features in a few hours there is usually a reaction, and then the features of general peritonitis become manifest to a more or less marked degree. Among the general features, the facies of the patient shows changes; there is increased pallor, a pinched expression, and as the symptoms progress and toward the end a marked Hippocratic facies, a dusky suffusion, and the forehead bathed in a clammy perspiration. The temperature rises with the increase of the peritonitis. The pulse quickens, is running and thready, the heart's action becomes more feeble, and there is an increase in the respiration rate. Vomiting is a variable feature; it is present in a majority of the cases. Hiccough is common and may occur early, but more frequently late.

The local abdominal features are often more important than the general, as it is surprising to notice how excellent the condition of a patient may be with perforative peritonitis. Limitation of the respiratory movements is usually present, perhaps confined to the hypogastric area. Increasing distention is the rule, but perforation and peritonitis may occur, it is to be remembered, with an abdomen flat or even scaphoid. Increasing pain on pressure, increasing muscle spasm and tension of the wall are important signs. Percussion may reveal a flat note in the flanks, due to exudate. A friction may be present within a few hours of the onset of the perforation. Obliteration of the liver flatness in the nipple line may be caused by excessive tympany, but rapid obliteration of liver flatness in a flat, or a not much distended abdomen, is a valuable sign. Examination of the rectum may show fullness or tenderness in the pelvis. Advance in the abdominal signs is an important point.

In some cases there is a rise in the leucocytes, and when present may be a valuable help, but it is not constant. Increase in the blood pressure is not constant.

General peritonitis, without perforation of the bowel, may occur by extension from an ulcer, or by rupture of a softened mesenteric gland, or, as in one case in our series, from inflammation of the Fallopian tubes. It was present in 2.2 per cent. of the Munich autopsies.

Perforation is almost invariably fatal without operation. In a few cases healing takes place spontaneously or the orifice may be closed by a tag of omentum. There is a group of cases in which hæmorrhage complicates the perforation and adds to the difficulty in diagnosis. In 7 of our 43 cases hæmorrhage accompanied the perforation; in 3 others the hæmorrhage had occurred some days before.

The *diagnosis* of perforation, easy enough at times, is not without serious difficulties. The conditions for which it was mistaken in our series were: appendicitis, occurring during the course of the typhoid fever, phlebitis of the iliac vein with great pain, hæmorrhage, and in one case a local peritonitis without perforation, for which no cause was found. Recovery followed the exploratory operation in all but one (hæmorrhage case) of the cases. Exploration is justifiable and better than delay in suspicious cases.

ASCITES occurs in rare instances (McPhedran).

The SPLEEN is usually enlarged, and the edge was felt below the costal margin in 71.6 per cent. of our cases. Percussion is uncertain, as, owing to distention of the stomach and colon, even the normal area of dulness may not be obtainable. Enlargement is often not marked in elderly patients. Rupture of the spleen occurs occasionally.

LIVER.—Symptoms on the part of this organ are rare.

(*a*) *Jaundice* of marked grade was present in only 8 cases of our series, but slight icterus is not uncommon. Catarrh of the ducts, toxæmia, abscess, and occasionally gall-stones are the usual causes.

(*b*) *Abscess.*—Solitary abscess is exceedingly rare and occurred in but 3 cases in our series. It may occur early in the disease, but most frequently is a sequel. Eberts collected 30 cases, in 9 of which the typhoid bacillus was isolated from the pus. In about half the cases the right lobe was affected. Eighteen of the patients recovered. Abscess may follow the intestinal lesion or a complication as parotitis. Suppurative pylephlebitis may follow perforation of the appendix. Suppurative cholangitis has been described.

(*c*) *Cholecystitis* occurred in 19 cases of the series. Pain in the region of the gall-bladder is the most constant symptom. Tenderness, muscle spasm with rigidity, and a gall-bladder tumor are present in a majority of the cases. Jaundice is inconstant. Leucocytosis usually occurs. With perforation there may be a marked drop in the fever and the onset of signs of peritonitis. In simple cholecystitis the urgency of the symptoms may abate, and recovery follow. Suppuration may occur with infection of the bile passages. Months or years later the bacilli may cause cholecystitis or gall-stones. Typhoid bacilli have been found in the gall-bladder in patients who never had typhoid fever.

(*d*) *Gall-stones.*—Bernheim called attention to the frequency of cholelithiasis after typhoid fever. It is probably associated with the presence of typhoid bacilli in the gall-bladder (see under Gall-Stones).

PANCREAS.—Hæmorrhagic pancreatitis has occurred rarely.

RESPIRATORY SYSTEM.—*Epistaxis,* an early symptom, precedes typhoid fever more commonly than any other febrile affection. It is occasionally profuse and serious and may occur during the course.

Laryngitis is not very common and œdema, apart from ulceration, is rare. In the United States the laryngeal complications of typhoid fever seem much less frequent than on the Continent. We have twice seen severe perichondritis; both of the patients recovered, one after the expectoration of large portions of the thyroid cartilage. Keen and Lüning collected 221 cases of serious surgical complications of the larynx. General emphysema may follow the perforation of an ulcer. Stenosis is a very serious sequence. It would appear that paralysis of the laryngeal muscles is more common than we have supposed. Przedborski (Volkmann's Sammlung, No. 182) examined the larynx in 100 consecutive cases and found 25 with paralysis. This is nearly always due to neuritis, sometimes in connection with affections of other nerves.

Bronchitis is one of the most frequent initial symptoms. It is indicated by the presence of sibilant râles. The sputum is usually scanty. The smaller tubes may be involved, producing urgent cough and even slight cyanosis. Collapse and lobular pneumonia may also occur.

Lobar pneumonia is met with under two conditions:

(*a*) At the outset, the *pneumo-typhus* of the Germans. This occurred in three of our cases. After an indisposition of a day or so, the patient is seized with a chill, has high fever, pain in the side, and within forty-eight hours there are signs of consolidation and the evidences of an ordinary lobar pneumonia. The intestinal symptoms may not occur until toward the end of the first week or later; the pulmonary symptoms persist, crisis does not occur; the aspect of the patient changes, and by the end of the second week the clinical picture is that of typhoid fever. Spots may then be present and doubts as to the nature of the case are solved. In other instances, in the absence of a characteristic eruption, the case remains doubtful, and it is impossible to say whether the disease has been pneumonia, in which the so-called typhoid symptoms have developed, or whether it was typhoid fever with early implication of the lungs. This condition may depend upon an early localization of the typhoid bacillus in the lung.

(*b*) Lobar pneumonia forms a serious and not infrequent complication of the second or third week—in 19 of our cases. It was present in over 8 per cent. of the Munich cases. The symptoms are usually not marked. There may be no rusty sputum, and, unless sought for, the condition is frequently overlooked. The etiological agent is still in dispute. Typhoid bacilli have been isolated from the sputum and also from the consolidated lungs at autopsy, but in such cases the pneumococci may have been originally present, and the typhoid bacilli secondary invaders. In all cases of pneumonia during typhoid fever in the Johns Hopkins Hospital and coming to autopsy, the pneumococcus could be demonstrated in the consolidated lung. Infarction, abscess, and gangrene are occasionally pulmonary complications.

Hypostatic congestion of the lungs and œdema, due to enfeebled circulation, occur in the later periods. The physical signs are defective resonance at the bases, feeble breath sounds, and moist râles on deep inspiration. Dulness at the right base is not uncommon.

Hæmoptysis may occur. Creagh reports a case in which it caused death.

Pleurisy was present in about 8 per cent. of the Munich autopsies. It occurred in 2 per cent. of our series. It may occur at the outset—pleuro-typhoid —or slowly during convalescence, in which case it is almost always purulent and due to the typhoid bacillus.

Pneumothorax is rare. Hale White has reported two cases, in both of which pleurisy existed. After death, no lesions of the lungs or bronchi were discovered. The condition may be due to straining, or to the rupture of a small pyæmic abscess. It may occur also during convalescence.

NERVOUS SYSTEM.—*Cerebro-spinal Form.*—The disease may set in with intense and persistent headache, or an aggravated form of neuralgia. Kernig's sign is often present without any evidence of meningeal reaction. There are cases in which the effect of the poison is manifested on the nervous system early and with the greatest intensity. There are headache, photophobia, retraction of the neck, marked twitchings of the muscles, rigidity, and even convulsions. In such cases the diagnosis of meningitis is invariably made. The cases showing marked *meningeal features* during the course may be divided into three groups. First, those with symptoms suggestive of meningitis, but without localizing features and without the anatomical lesions of meningitis at post mortem (meningism). In every series of cases numerous such examples occur. Secondly, the cases of so-called *serous* meningitis. There is a localization of typhoid bacilli in the cerebro-spinal fluid and a mild inflammatory reaction, but without suppurative meningitis. Cole in 1904 collected 13 such cases, 5 of them occurring in our series, and Bayne-Jones has collected 17 cases from the literature since 1904. Probably more frequent lumbar punctures will show that this occurs not infrequently. Thirdly, true typhoid *suppurative* meningitis due to *B. typhosus*. Only one such case occurred in our series, and Cole collected 13 from the literature. Bayne-Jones has collected 18 additional cases. Meningitis in typhoid fever is occasionally due to other organisms, as the tubercle bacillus, or the meningococcus. Marked convulsive movements, local or general, with coma and delirium, are seen also in thrombosis of the cerebral veins and sinuses.

Delirium, usually present in very severe cases, is much less frequent under a rigid plan of hydrotherapy. It may exist from the outset, but usually does not occur until the second and sometimes not until the third week. It may be slight and only nocturnal. It is, as a rule, a quiet delirium, though there are cases in which the patient is very noisy and constantly tries to get out of bed, and, unless carefully watched, may escape. The patient does not often become maniacal. In heavy drinkers the delirium may have the character of delirium tremens. Even in patients who have no positive delirium, the mental processes are usually dulled and the aspect is listless and apathetic. In severe cases the patient passes into a condition of unconsciousness. The eyes may be open, but he is oblivious to all surrounding circumstances and neither knows nor can indicate his wants. The urine and fæces are passed involuntarily. In this pseudo-wakeful state, or coma vigil, as it is called, the eyes are open and the patient is constantly muttering. The lips and tongue are tremulous; there are twitchings of the fingers and wrists—subsultus tendinum and carphologia. He picks at the bedclothes or grasps at invisible objects. These are among the most serious symptoms of the disease and always indicate danger.

Convulsions are rare. There were 7 instances in our series, with 3 deaths. They occur: first, at the onset, particularly in children; secondly, as a manifestation of the toxæmia; and thirdly, as a result of severe cerebral complications—thrombosis, meningitis, or acute encephalitis. Occasionally in convalescence convulsions may occur from unknown causes.

Neuritis, which is not uncommon—11 cases in the series—may be multiple or local. *Multiple neuritis* comes on usually during convalescence. The legs may be affected, or the four extremities. The cases are often difficult to differentiate from those with subacute poliomyelitis. Recovery is the rule.

Local Neuritis.—This may occur during the height of the fever or after convalescence is established. It may set in with agonizing pain, and with sensitiveness of the affected nerve trunks. The local neuritis may affect the nerves of an arm or of a leg, and involve chiefly the extensors, so that there is wrist-drop or foot-drop. The arm or leg may be much swollen and the skin over it erythematous. A curious condition, probably a local neuritis in some but in others due to phlebitis, is that described by Handford as *tender toes.* The tips and pads of the toes, rarely the pads at their bases, become exquisitely sensitive, so that the patient can not bear the weight of the bed-clothes. There is no discoloration or swelling, and the pain disappears usually within a week or ten days.

Poliomyelitis may occur with the symptoms of acute ascending paralysis and prove fatal in a few days. More frequently it is less acute, and causes either a paraplegia or a limited atrophic paralysis of one arm or leg.

Hemiplegia is a rare complication. Smithies (1907) collected 40 cases in 26 of which aphasia occurred and in 10 the hemiplegia was preceded by convulsions. In 21 cases the paralysis was on the right side. The lesion is usually thrombosis of the arteries, less often a meningo-encephalitis. The aphasia usually disappears. *Aphasia,* apart from hemiplegia, occurs rarely and usually in children. The prognosis is good.

The superficial abdominal reflexes may disappear early in the course and not return until convalescence, but this is not constant and can not be regarded as important in diagnosis.

True *tetany* occurs sometimes, and has been reported in connection with certain epidemics. It may set in during the height of the disease.

Typhoid Psychoses.—There are three groups of cases: first, an initial delirium, which may be serious, and cause the patient to wander away from his home, or he may even become maniacal; secondly, the psychosis associated directly with the pyrexia and the toxæmia; in a few cases this outlasts the disappearance of the fever for months or even years; and, lastly, the asthenic psychosis of convalescence, more common after typhoid than after any other fever. The prognosis is usually good. Edsall studied the condition in children, finding 69 cases, of which 43 recovered.

There is a distressing post-typhoid neurasthenia, in which for months or even for years the patient is unable to get into harmony with his surroundings.

Special Senses.—*Eye.*—Conjunctivitis, simple or phlyctenular, sometimes with keratitis and iritis, may develop. Panophthalmitis has been reported in one case in association with hæmorrhage (Finlay). Loss of accommodation may occur, usually in the asthenia of convalescence. Oculo-motor paralysis has been seen, due probably to neuritis. Retinal hæmorrhages may occur alone or in association with other hæmorrhagic features. Double optic neuritis has been described and may be independent of meningitis. Atrophy may follow, but these complications are excessively rare. Cataract may follow inflammation of the uveal tract. Other rare complications are thrombosis of the orbital veins and orbital hæmorrhage. (See de Schweinitz in Keen's monograph for full consideration of the subject.)

Ear.—Deafness is common during the course but usually is not permanent. Otitis media is not infrequent, 2.5 per cent. in Hengst's collected cases. We never found the typhoid bacillus in the discharge. Serious results are rare; only one case of mastoid disease occurred in our series. The otitis may set in with a chill and an aggravation of the fever.

Renal System.—*Retention of urine* is an early symptom and may be the cause of abdominal pain. It may recur throughout the attack. *Suppression of urine* is rare. The urine is usually diminished at first, has the ordinary febrile characters, and the pigments are increased. *Polyuria* is not very uncommon. While most common during convalescence, the increase may be sudden in the second week at the height of the fever. The amount of urine depends very much on the fluid taken. Patients treated by what is known as the washing-out method, in which large quantities of water are taken, may pass enormous amounts, 18 or 19 litres. One of our patients passed 33 litres in one day!

Bacilluria caused by the typhoid bacilli occurs in about one-third of the cases. The urine may be turbid from their presence and in the test-tube give a peculiar shimmer. There may be millions of bacilli to the cubic millimetre without pyuria or any symptoms of renal or bladder trouble. The routine administration of hexamine diminishes the occurrence of typhoid bacilluria. The bacilli may be present in the urine for years after the attack (see Gwyn, Studies III).

The renal complications in typhoid fever may be thus grouped:

(*a*) Febrile *albuminuria* is common and of no special significance. It was present in 999 of 1,500 cases, 66 per cent. Tube casts were present in 568 cases, 37.8 per cent. *Hæmoglobinuria* occurred in one case.

(*b*) *Acute nephritis* at the onset or during the height of the disease—the *nephro-typhus* of the Germans, the *fièvre typhoïd à forme rénale* of the French—may set in, masking in many instances the true nature of the malady. After an indisposition of a few days there may be fever, pain in the back, and the passage of a small amount of bloody urine.

(*c*) Nephritis during convalescence is rare, and is usually associated with anæmia and œdema. Chronic nephritis is a most exceptional sequel.

(*d*) The lymphomatous nephritis, described by E. Wagner, and referred to in the section on morbid anatomy, produces, as a rule, no symptoms.

(*e*) *Pyuria*, a not uncommon complication, may be associated with the typhoid or the colon bacillus, less often with staphylococci. It disappears during convalescence. It is usually due to a simple catarrh of the bladder, rarely to an intense cystitis, sometimes to pyelitis.

(*f*) *Post-typhoid Pyelitis.*—One or both kidneys may be involved, either at the height of the disease or during convalescence. There may be blood and pus at first, later pus alone, varying in amount. A severe pyelonephritis may follow. The colon bacillus is often the organism present. *Perinephric abscess* is a rare sequel.

Generative System.—*Orchitis* is occasionally met with. Kinnicutt collected 53 cases in the literature. It may be associated with a catarrhal urethritis. Induration or atrophy may occur, and more rarely suppuration. It was present in 4 cases of our series. In 1 case double hydrocele developed suddenly on the nineteenth day (Dunlap). *Prostatitis* occurs rarely.

Acute mastitis, which may go on to suppuration, is rare. It was present in 3 cases of our series during the fever and in one late in convalescence.

Osseous System.—Among the most troublesome of the sequelæ are the *bone lesions* which in a few cases occur at the height of the disease or even earlier. Of 237 cases collected by Keen there was periostitis in 110, necrosis in 85, and caries in 13. They are much more frequent than the figures indicate. Six cases came under personal notice in the course of a year, and formed the basis of Parsons' paper (Studies II). The legs are chiefly involved. In Keen's series the tibia was affected in 91 cases, the ribs in 40. The typhoid bone lesion is apt to form what the old writers called a cold abscess. Only a few of the cases are acute. Chronicity, indolence, and a remarkable tendency to recurrence are perhaps the three most striking features. A bony node may be left by the typhoid periostitis.

Arthritis was present in 8 cases of our series. Keen collected 84 cases from the literature. It may be monarticular or polyarticular. One of the most important points relating to it is the frequency with which spontaneous dislocations occur, particularly of the hip.

Typhoid Spine (Gibney).—During the disease but more often during convalescence, the patient complains of pain in the lumbar and sacral regions, perhaps after a slight jar or shock. Stiffness of the back, pain on movement, sometimes radiating, and tenderness on pressure are the chief features, but there are in addition marked nervous manifestations. There is rigidity and fixation of the spine, usually in the lower part. Kyphosis occurs in some cases. The X-ray plates may show definite bony change. There is usually spondylitis or perispondylitis. The duration is weeks or months, but the outlook is good.

The *muscles* may be the seat of degeneration but it rarely causes any symptoms. Hæmorrhage occasionally occurs into the muscles, and late in protracted cases abscesses may follow. Rupture of a muscle, usually the rectus abdominis, may occur, possibly associated with acute hæmorrhagic myositis. *Painful muscles* are not uncommon, particularly in the calves (Studies III). Painful cramps may also occur. In some of the cases of painful legs the condition is a myositis; in others the swelling and pain may be due to thrombosis in the deeper veins.

Post-typhoid Septicæmia and Pyæmia.—In very protracted cases after defervescence a slight fever (100°-101° F.) may recur with sweats, which is possibly septic. In other cases for two or three weeks there are recurring chills, often of great severity. They are usually of no moment in the absence of signs of complication. (See Studies II and III.)

Typhoid pyæmia is not common. (*a*) Extensive furunculosis may be associated with irregular fever and leucocytosis. (*b*) Following the fever there may be multiple subcutaneous "cold" abscesses, often with a dark, thin bloody pus. A score or more of these may appear in different parts. Pratt isolated the bacillus in pure culture from the subcutaneous abscesses. (*c*) A crural thrombus may suppurate and cause a widespread pyæmia. (*d*) In rare instances suppuration of the mesenteric glands, of a splenic infarct, a sloughing parotid bubo, a perinephric or perirectal abscess, acute necrosis of the bones, or a multiple suppurative arthritis may cause pyæmia. In other cases following bed-sores or a furunculosis a general infection with pyogenic organisms occurs with fatal result. In three such cases in our series staphylococci were cultivated from the blood. In one case with many chills late in the disease, and the general condition excellent, typhoid bacilli were cultivated from the blood. The colon bacillus may also be found in blood cultures.

Association of Other Diseases.—Erysipelas is a rare complication, most commonly met with during convalescence. Measles or scarlet fever may develop during the fever or in convalescence. Chicken-pox and noma have been reported in children. Pseudo-membranous inflammations may occur in the pharynx, larynx, or genitals.

Malarial and typhoid fevers may be associated, but a majority of the cases of so-called typho-malarial fever are either remittent malarial fever or true typhoid. It is interesting to note that among 1,500 cases of typhoid fever plasmodia were found in the blood in only 3 cases. (See Lyon, Studies III.) Many of the typhoid fever patients came from malarious regions.

The symptoms of influenza may precede the typhoid fever, or the two diseases may run concurrently. There are cases of chronic influenza which simulate typhoid fever very closely.

Typhoid Fever and Tuberculosis.—(*a*) The diseases may coexist. A person with chronic tuberculosis may contract the fever. Of 105 autopsies in typhoid fever, 7 presented marked tuberculous lesions. Miliary tuberculosis and typhoid fever may occur together. (*b*) Cases of typhoid fever with pulmonary and pleuritic symptoms may suggest tuberculosis at the onset. (*c*) There are types of tuberculosis infection which may simulate typhoid fever: the acute miliary form; the acute septicæmic form; tuberculous meningitis; tuberculous peritonitis; the acute toxæmia of certain local lesions; and forms of ordinary pulmonary tuberculosis. And, lastly, pulmonary tuberculosis may follow typhoid. In a large majority of such cases from the onset the disease has been tuberculosis, which has begun with a low fever and features suggestive of typhoid fever.

In epilepsy and in chronic chorea the fits and movements usually cease during an attack, and in typhoid fever in a diabetic subject the sugar may be absent during the height of the disease.

Varieties.—Typhoid fever presents an extremely complex symptomatology. Many forms have been described, some of which present exaggeration of common symptoms, others modification in the course, others again greater intensity of action of the poison on certain organs. When the nervous system is specially involved, it has been called the cerebro-spinal form; when the kidneys are early and severely affected, nephro-typhoid; when the disease begins with pulmonary symptoms, pneumo-typhoid; with pleurisy, pleuro-typhoid; when characterized throughout by profuse sweats, the sudoral form of the disease. It is enough to remember that typhoid has no fixed and constant course, that it may set in occasionally with symptoms localized in certain organs, and that many of its symptoms are extremely variable—in one epidemic uniform and text-book-like, in another slight or not met with. This diversified symptomatology has led to many clinical errors, and in the absence of the salutary lessons of morbid anatomy it is not surprising that practitioners have so often been led astray. We may recognize the following varieties:

(*a*) The *mild* and *abortive* forms. Much attention has been paid to the milder varieties—the typhus levissimus of Griesinger. Woodruff called special attention to the great danger of neglecting these mild forms, which are often spoken of as mountain fever and malarial fever, "acclimation," "ground," and "miasmatic" fevers. During an epidemic there may be cases so mild that the patient does not go to bed. The onset may be sudden, particularly in children. The general symptoms are slight, the pulse rate not high, the fever rarely above 102°. Rose spots are usually present, with splenic enlargement. Diarrhœa is rare. The Widal reaction is present in a majority of the patients. There may be a marked tendency to relapse. While infrequent, characteristic complications and sequelæ may give the first positive clue to the nature of the trouble. Briggs studied 44 of these mild cases from our series in which the fever lasted 14 days or less. Rose spots were present in 24, and the Widal reaction in 26. There were three relapses. It can not be too forcibly impressed upon the profession that it is just by these mild cases, to which so little attention is paid, that the disease may be kept up in a community.

(*b*) The *grave* form is usually characterized by high fever and pronounced nervous symptoms. In this category come the very severe cases, setting in with pneumonia and nephritis, and with the very intense gastro-intestinal or cerebro-spinal symptoms.

(*c*) The *latent* or *ambulatory* form is particularly common in hospital practice. The symptoms are usually slight, and the patient scarcely feels ill enough to go to bed. He has languor, perhaps slight diarrhœa, but keeps about and may even attend to his work throughout the entire attack. In other instances delirium sets in. The worst cases of this form are seen in sailors, who keep up and about, though feeling ill and feverish. When brought to the hospital they often have symptoms of a most severe type. Hæmorrhage or perforation may be the first marked symptom of this ambulatory type. Sir W. Jenner called attention to the dangers of this form, and particularly to the grave prognosis in the case of persons who have travelled far with the disease in progress.

(*d*) *Hæmorrhagic Typhoid Fever.*—This is excessively rare. Among Ouskow's 6,513 cases there were 4 fatal cases with general hæmorrhagic features. Only three instances were present in our series. Hæmorrhages may be marked from the outset, but more commonly they come on during the course. The condition is not necessarily fatal. (See Hamburger, Studies III.)

(*e*) An *afebrile* typhoid fever is recognized by some authors, but there is usually slight fever. The patients presented lassitude, depression, headache, furred tongue, loss of appetite, slow pulse, and even the spots and enlarged spleen.

Typhoid Fever in Children.—Griffith collected a series of 325 cases in children under two and a half years; 111 of these were in the first year. Out of a total of 278 cases in which the result was recorded, 142 died. The cases are not very uncommon. The high mortality in Griffith's series was probably due to the fact that only the more serious cases are reported. The abdominal symptoms are usually mild; fatal hæmorrhage and perforation are rare. Among sequelæ, aphasia, noma, and bone lesions are stated to be more common in children than in adults. Two of our cases were under one year of age.

Typhoid Fever in the Aged.—After the sixtieth year the disease runs a less favorable course, and the mortality is high. The fever is less, but complications are more common, particularly pneumonia and heart-failure.

Typhoid Fever in Pregnancy.—Pregnancy affords no immunity against typhoid. In 1,500 of our cases, 438 of which were females, there were 6 cases. Goltdammer noted 26 pregnancies in 600 cases of typhoid fever in the female. It is more commonly seen in the first half of pregnancy. The pregnancy is interrupted in about 65 per cent. of the cases, usually in the second week of the disease. In the obstetrical department of the Johns Hopkins Hospital (J. W. Williams) there were (to January, 1905) three cases of puerperal infection with bacillus typhosus. One showed a localized lesion of the chorion, from which bacilli were obtained (Little).

TYPHOID FEVER IN THE FETUS.—The typhoid bacillus may pass through the placenta to the child, causing a typhoid septicæmia, without intestinal lesions. Lynch collected 16 such cases. Infection of the fetus does not necessarily follow, but when infected the child dies, either *in utero* or shortly after birth. The Widal reaction has been obtained with fetal blood. Its presence does not indicate that the child has survived infection, as the agglutinating substances may filter through the placenta. They may also be transmitted to the nursling through the milk, and cause a transient reaction. The reaction could not be obtained with fetal blood from which typhoid bacilli were cultivated (Lynch).

RELAPSE.—Relapses vary in frequency in different epidemics, and, it would appear, in different places. The percentages of different authors range from 3 to 15 or 18 per cent. In 1,500 cases there were 172 relapses, 11.4 per cent. Among 28,057 collected cases 8.8 per cent. had a relapse. We may recognize the ordinary, the intercurrent, and the spurious relapse.

The *ordinary relapse* sets in after complete defervescence. The average duration of the interval of normal temperature is five or six days. In one of our cases there was complete apyrexia for twenty-three days, followed by a relapse of forty-one days' duration; then apyrexia for forty-two days, followed by a second relapse of two weeks' duration. As a rule, two of the three important symptoms—step-like temperature at onset, roseola, an enlarged spleen—should be present to justify the diagnosis of a relapse. The intestinal symptoms are variable. The onset may be abruptly with a chill, or the temperature may have a typical ascent. The number of relapses ranges from 1 to 5. In a case at the Pennsylvania Hospital in 1904 the disease lasted eleven months and four days, during which there were six relapses. The relapse is usually less severe, of shorter duration and the mortality is low.

The *intercurrent relapse* is common, often most severe, and is responsible for a great many of the most protracted cases. The temperature drops and the patient improves; but after remaining between 100° and 102° for a few days, the fever again rises and the patient enters upon another attack, which may be more protracted, and of much greater intensity than the original one.

Spurious relapses are very common. They have already been mentioned as post-typhoid elevations of temperature. They are recrudescences of the fever due to a number of causes. It is not always easy to determine whether a relapse is present, particularly in cases in which the fever persists for only five or seven days without rose-spots and without enlargement of the spleen.

Undoubtedly a reinfection from within, yet of the conditions favoring the occurrence of relapse we know little. Durham advanced an interesting theory: Every typhoid infection is a complex phenomenon caused by groups of bacilli alike in species but not identical, as shown by their serum reactions. The antibodies formed in the blood during the primary attack neutralize only one (or several) groups, the remaining groups still preserving their pathogenic power. From some cause these latter groups may multiply sufficiently to cause a reinfection. Multiple relapses may be similarly explained.

Diagnosis.—There are several points to note. In the first place, typhoid fever is the most common of all continued fevers. Secondly, it is extraordinarily variable in its manifestations. Thirdly, there is no such hybrid malady as typho-malarial fever. Fourthly, errors in diagnosis are inevitable, even under the most favorable conditions.

Data for Diagnosis.—(*a*) *General.*—No single symptom or feature is characteristic. The onset is often suggestive, particularly the occurrence of epistaxis, and (if seen from the start) the ascending fever. The steadiness of the fever for a week or longer after reaching the fastigium is an important point. The irregular remittent character in the third week, and the intermittent features with chills, are common sources of errors. While there is nothing characteristic in the pulse, dicrotism is so much more common early in typhoid fever that its presence is always suggestive. The rash is the most valuable single sign, and with the fever usually clinches the diagnosis. The enlarged spleen is of less importance, since it occurs in all febrile conditions, but with the fever and the rash it completes a diagnostic triad. The absence of leucocytosis is a valuable accessory sign. Typhoid should be suspected in every doubtful fever.

(*b*) *Specific.*—(1) *Isolation of Typhoid Bacilli from the Blood.*—This is especially useful early in the disease, in doubtful cases and in the acute septic forms.

(2) *Isolation of Typhoid Bacilli from the Stools.*—Cultures from the stools are of diagnostic value at all stages.

(3) *Isolation of Typhoid Bacilli from the Urine.*—In some cases positive cultures may be obtained before the Widal test is positive. Routine cultures are frequently of diagnostic value.

(4) *Isolation of Typhoid Bacilli from the Rose-spots.*—This may be done but as the procedure causes considerable discomfort it can not be used as a routine method.

(5) *The Agglutination Test.*—In 1894 Pfeiffer showed that cholera spirilla, when introduced into the peritoneum of an immunized animal, or when mixed with the serum of immunized animals, lose their motion and break up. This "Pfeiffer's phenomenon" was thoroughly studied by Durham and the specificity of the reaction demonstrated. A. S. Grünbaum and Widal made the method available in clinical work.

Macroscopic Method.—This may be done with living or dead organisms and has the advantage of use away from a laboratory. The diluted serum and organisms are mixed in a tube of small calibre (dilution 1 to 50 or 1 to 100). With a positive reaction there should be complete precipitation leaving a clear fluid above in twenty-four hours.

Microscopic Method.—If the reaction is positive the bacilli lose their motility and collect in clumps. With Dreyer's method of standard cultures of constant and known sensitiveness it is possible to follow the patient's serum changes in typhoid or paratyphoid infection. Whatever be the infection the agglutination for that bacillus will show (*a*) a marked rise in an early stage and (*b*) a marked fall later in the infection. If the patient's serum already contains agglutinins for one or more of the bacilli (owing to inoculation), the following phenomena will be noted (*a*) there is no change in the inoculation agglutinins or (*b*) a slight rise occurs, followed by a slight fall—an alteration which may be caused by a number of non-specific stimuli. A well marked rise or fall of the titre is the only positive evidence of active infection that can be obtained with the agglutination test and is probably the best evidence afforded by any test except a successful blood culture.

On the whole the serum reaction is of great value, in spite of certain difficulties and objections, and with the newer methods the reactions of equal importance in inoculated and uninoculated persons and in the paratyphoids.

(6) *Ophthalmo-Reaction.*—A solution of one-third to one-half of a milligram of "typho-protein" derived from many different strains of typhoid bacilli is instilled into the conjunctival sac. A typical reaction is marked by deep congestion of the conjunctiva of the lower lid and the caruncle. It reaches its maximum in six hours. A positive reaction is obtained most often during the febrile period, frequently before the agglutination reaction is given. The simplicity of the method and the absence of discomfort are valuable features. A cutaneous method has also been employed.

(*c*) *Atropine Test* (*Marris*).—The patient should remain as quiet as possible during the test, which should not be done until at least an hour after the last feeding. The pulse rate is counted until it is found to be steady. Atropine gr. 1/33 (0.002 gm.) is given hypodermically, and 25 minutes later the pulse is counted each minute until any rise which follows the injection has begun to pass off. The difference between the average pulse rate before the injection and the maximum after it gives the acceleration due to the atropine. The highest average count is usually about thirty minutes after the injection. If the "escape" is 14 or less, the diagnosis is probably typhoid or para-typhoid fever; if 15 or more the reaction is negative. Three negative reactions within the first fortnight of a febrile illness exclude the typhoid group. A negative reaction after the end of the second week or when the fever has fallen may be unreliable. This test is most useful from the fifth to the fourteenth day, but a series of negative reactions later than the fourteenth day may be generally taken as evidence against typhoid infection. A positive reaction may be obtained in those over fifty years of age, especially if arteriosclerotic. In patients with a pulse rate of 100 or over, a positive reaction has to be taken with caution and the test repeated; a negative reaction in patients who are very toxic is not necessarily conclusive.

Common Sources of Error in Diagnosis.—An early and intense localization of the infection in certain organs may give rise to doubt at first.

Cases coming on with severe headache, photophobia, delirium, twitching of the muscles and retraction of the head are almost invariably regarded as *cerebro-spinal meningitis*. Under such circumstances it may for a few days be impossible to make a satisfactory diagnosis. The senior author has performed autopsies on cases of this kind in which no suspicion of typhoid fever had been present, the intense cerebro-spinal manifestations having dominated the scene. Until the appearance of abdominal symptoms, or the rash, it may be quite impossible to determine the nature of the case. Cerebro-spinal meningitis is, however, a rare disease; typhoid fever a very common one, and the onset with severe nervous symptoms is by no means infrequent. The lumbar puncture is a great help.

The misleading pulmonary symptoms, which occasionally occur at the very outset of the disease, have been mentioned. The bronchitis rarely causes error, though it may be intense and attract the chief attention. More difficult are the cases setting in with chill and followed rapidly by *pneumonia.* Such a case may be shown to a class one week as typical pneumonia, and a fortnight later as typhoid fever. There is less danger of mistaking the pneumonia which occurs at the height of the disease, and yet this is possible, as in the case of a man aged seventy, insensible, with a dry tongue, tremor, ecchymoses upon the wrists and ankles, no rose-spots, enlargement of the spleen, and consolidation of the right lower lobe. It was very natural, particularly since there was no history, to regard such a case as senile pneumonia with profound constitutional disturbance, but the autopsy showed the characteristic lesions of typhoid fever. Early involvement of the pleura or the kidneys may for a time obscure the diagnosis.

Of diseases with which typhoid fever may be confounded, malaria, certain forms of pyæmia, acute tuberculosis, and tuberculous peritonitis are the most important.

From *malarial fever,* typhoid is, as a rule, readily recognized. There is no such disease as typho-malarial fever—that is, a separate and distinct malady. Typhoid fever and malarial fever may coexist in the same patient but this is rare. The term typho-malarial fever should be abandoned. The autumnal type of malarial fever may present a striking similarity to typhoid fever and differentiation may be made only by the blood examination. There may be no chills, the remissions may be extremely slight, there is a history perhaps of *malaise,* weakness, diarrhœa, and sometimes vomiting. The tongue is furred and white, the cheeks flushed, the spleen slightly enlarged, and the temperature continuous, or with very slight remissions. The æstivo-autumnal variety of the malarial parasite may not be present in the circulating blood for several days. Every year in Baltimore we had one or two cases in which the diagnosis was in doubt for a few days.

Pyæmia.—The long-continued fever of obscure, deep-seated suppuration, without chills or sweats, may simulate typhoid. The more chronic cases of ulcerative endocarditis are usually diagnosed typhoid fever. The presence or absence of leucocytosis is an important aid. The Widal reaction and the blood cultures offer valuable help.

Acute miliary tuberculosis is not infrequently mistaken for typhoid fever. The points in differential diagnosis will be discussed under that disease. *Tuberculous peritonitis* in certain of its forms may closely simulate typhoid fever, and will be referred to in another section.

The early abdominal pain, etc., may lead to the diagnosis of appendicitis.

The mild endemic form of typhus fever described by Brill may be regarded as typhoid fever, but the character of the rash, the absence of the agglutination reaction, negative results of blood cultures and the course are against this. The majority of cases are probably diagnosed as typhoid fever.

Prognosis.—(*a*) DEATH-RATE.—The mortality is very variable, ranging in private practice from 5 to 12 and in hospital practice from 7 to 20 per cent. In some large epidemics the death-rate has been very low. In the Maidstone epidemic it was between 7 and 8 per cent. In recent years the mortality from typhoid fever has diminished, and hydrotherapy has reduced the death-rate in a remarkable manner, even as low as 5 or 6 per cent. Of the 1,500 cases in our series, 9.1 per cent. died.

(*b*) Special Features.—Unfavorable symptoms are high fever, toxic symptoms with delirium, meteorism, and hæmorrhage. Perforation renders the outlook hopeless unless operation is done early. Fat subjects stand typhoid fever badly. The mortality in women is greater than in men. The complications and dangers are more serious in the ambulatory form in which the patient has kept about for a week or ten days. Early involvement of the nervous system is a bad indication; and the low, muttering delirium with tremor means a close fight for life. Prognostic signs from the fever alone are deceptive. A temperature above 104° may be well borne if the nervous system is not involved. The degree of bacteræmia is of value; the greater this is the worse the prognosis.

(*c*) Sudden Death.—It is difficult in many cases to explain this most lamentable of accidents. There are cases in which neither cerebral, renal, nor cardiac changes have been found; there are instances too in which it does not seem likely that there could have been a special localization of the toxins in the pneumogastric centres. Fibrillation of the ventricle may be the cause in some cases. Under conditions of abnormal nutrition a state of *delirium cordis* is sometimes induced, which may occur spontaneously, or, in the case of animals, on slight irritation of the heart, with the result of extreme irregularity and finally failure of action. Sudden death occurs more frequently in men than in women, according to Dewèvre's statistics, in a proportion of 114 to 26. It may occur at the height of the fever, and, as pointed out by Graves, also during convalescence. There were four cases in our series.

Prophylaxis.—In cities the prevalence of typhoid fever is directly proportionate to the inefficiency of the drainage and the water-supply. With their improvement the incidence has been reduced materially. Fulton has shown that in the United States, at least, the disease exists to a proportionately greater extent in the country than it does in the city, and that the propagation is in general from the country to the town. In the water-supply of the latter the chances for dilution of the contaminating fluids are much greater than in the country, where the privy vault is often in close proximity to the well.

But it is not only through water that the disease is transmitted. Other methods play an important though not so frequent rôle. The bacilli may be carried by milk, oysters, uncooked vegetables, etc. Flies play an important part in the spread of the disease. Many cases undoubtedly arise by direct infection. But through whatever channel the infection occurs, for new cases to arise the bacilli must be obtained from another patient. Under ordinary circumstances the bacilli do not live and thrive long outside the body. To stamp out typhoid fever requires (1) *the recognition of all cases, including the typhoid carriers* and (2) *the destruction of all typhoid bacilli as they leave the patient.* It is as much a part of the physician's duty to look after these points as to take care of the patient. Mild cases of fever are to be regarded with suspicion.

From the standpoint of prophylaxis, the question practically narrows down to disinfection of the urine, stools, sputum (in the few cases where bacilli are present), and of objects which may be contaminated accidentally by these excretions. The nurse or attendant should be taught to regard every specimen of urine as a pure culture of typhoid bacilli, and to exercise the greatest care in preventing the scattering of drops of urine over the patient, bedding or floor, or over the hands of the attendant.

To disinfect the *urine* the best solutions are carbolic acid, 1-20, in an amount equal to that of the urine, or bichloride of mercury, 1-1,000, in an amount one-fifth that of the fluid to be sterilized. These mixtures with the urine should stand at least two hours. Hexamine causes disappearance of the bacilli from the urine when bacilluria is present, but under no circumstances should its administration permit the disinfection of the urine to be neglected. For the *stools,* heat is the most efficient and can be employed in hospitals by special hoppers in which steam is used. Of solutions, carbolic acid or freshly prepared milk of lime is most useful. The stool should be mixed with at least thrice its volume of these solutions and allowed to stand for several hours. For the disinfection of the bath water chloride of lime is the best and even when the water contains coarse fæcal matter, 250 gm. (one-half pound) of chloride of lime will render the ordinary bath of 200 litres sterile in one-half hour.

If there be any expectoration, the *sputum* should receive the same care as in tuberculosis. It is best to collect it in small cloths, which may be burned.

All the *linen* from the patient's bed or person should be soaked for two hours in 1-20 carbolic acid solution or 1-2000 bichloride solution, and then sent to the laundry, where it should be boiled. All dishes should be boiled before leaving the patient's room.

The nurse should wear a rubber apron when giving tubs or working over a typhoid patient, and this should be washed frequently with a carbolic acid or bichloride of mercury solution. The nurse should wear rubber gloves when giving tubs, or else soak her hands thoroughly in 1-1,000 bichloride solution after she has finished.

It is impossible here to deal with all the possible modes of spread of the infection. Keeping in mind that everything leaving the patient should be sterilized, a nurse of ordinary intelligence, even one of the family, can carry out very satisfactory prophylaxis. Those nursing the patient should not handle food for others.

Should the typhoid fever patient be isolated? To prevent direct infection of others a moderate degree of isolation should be carried out, though this need not be absolute as in the exanthemata. The windows should have fly screens in summer. After recovery the room should be disinfected.

An important question is as to the necessity for the isolation of typhoid patients in special wards in hospitals. At present this is not generally done in the United States. When, however, in a hospital with as good sanitary arrangements as the Johns Hopkins possesses, and in which all possible precautions are taken to prevent the infection spreading from patient to patient, 1.8 per cent. of all the cases have been of hospital origin, the advisability of isolation of typhoid fever patients is certainly worth considering. On the other hand, in the general hospital, with students in the wards, the cases are more thoroughly studied, and in the graver complications, as perforation, it is of the greatest advantage to have the early co-operation of the house surgeon.

When the disease is prevalent the drinking-water and the milk should be boiled. Travellers should drink mineral water rather than ordinary water or milk. Care should be taken to thoroughly cook oysters which have been fattened or freshened in streams contaminated with sewage. While in camps it is easy to boil and filter the water, with troops on the march it is a very different matter. Various chemical methods have been recommended of which chlorination has proved the most satisfactory.

During an epidemic the early recognition of all cases followed by isolation and thorough disinfection is most important. Preventive inoculation should be given as generally as possible. Every effort should be made to find the source of infection with a thorough search for carriers, especially in local outbreaks. In the search for carriers the agglutination test is not sufficient and cultural studies of the contents of the duodenum, of the fæces and urine should be made.

PROTECTIVE INOCULATION.—Introduced by Wright this has proved of inestimable value in reducing the occurrence of typhoid fever. The experience of the European War gives ample proof of this. The material used is a bouillon or agar culture of bacilli heated to a temperature of 53° to 55° C. in order to kill them. Lysol or tricresol may be added. Three inoculations are given at intervals of ten days. The use of a sensitized vaccine has some advantages.

A triple vaccine against typhoid and paratyphoid A and B should be used. Untoward results are rare. Of 31,000 inoculated at the Valcartier camp, Quebec, only one had a local abscess and there were no serious sequels. The inoculation fever begins in from four to six hours and may reach 101° or even 103° to 104°. Headache, chilliness, pains in the back and limbs, and vomiting may occur. In many there is only a transient indisposition. More severe symptoms may occur, such as arthritis, fugitive erythema, diarrhœa, abdominal pains, septicæmia, with pneumonia, pleurisy and pericarditis. In a few cases a fever resembling typhoid has followed. No case of a fatality due directly to the inoculation was found. A light diet, avoidance of stimulants and rest lessen the possibility of serious sequels. The evidence so far points to a persistence of the protective effect for at least two years after inoculation. The typhoidin skin reaction is a guide to the duration of immunity. If infection results after proper inoculation it is probably due to a very large dose of typhoid bacilli.

Treatment.—(*a*) GENERAL MANAGEMENT.—The profession was long in learning that typhoid fever is not a disease to be treated mainly with drugs. Careful nursing, a proper diet, and hydrotherapy are the essentials in a majority of cases. The patient should be in a well-ventilated room (or in summer out of doors during the day), strictly confined to bed from the outset, and there remain until convalescence is well established. The bed should be single, not too high, and the mattress should not be too hard. The woven wire bed, with soft hair mattress, upon which are two folds of blanket, combines the two great qualities of a sick-bed, smoothness and elasticity. A rubber cloth should be placed under the sheet. An intelligent nurse should be in charge. When this is impossible, the physician should write out specific instructions regarding diet and treatment of the discharges and bed-linen.

(*b*) DIET.—More liberality is now generally practised, as was advised years ago by Austin Flint and strongly supported by Shattuck, Kinnicutt and others. The patient should be nourished as well as possible and food given with a value of 2,500 to 3,000 calories and containing about 70 grams of protein if conditions permit. The bulk of the food should be liquid and milk or its modifications form the largest part. Milk in any form, cream, ice cream, cocoa, tea or coffee with cream, strained soups, eggs, either the white or the whole egg, raw or soft boiled, gruels and jellies may be given. The milk may be boiled or diluted, or some modification given—peptonised milk, fermented milk, malted milk, buttermilk or whey. Soft food is often permissible, such as milk toast, custard, junket, crackers and milk, bread and butter, and mashed potatoes. It is important to give carbohydrate freely to spare the body proteins, and this is aided by the addition of milk sugar to the diet; it can be given with each feeding of milk. Cane sugar can also be given freely. The food should be chosen for each patient and a routine diet not allowed. In case of digestive disturbance—undigested food in the stools, diarrhœa, meteorism—the diet should be made very simple, buttermilk, whey, peptonised milk or albumin water usually being suitable. The beef extracts, meat juices, and artificially prepared foods are unnecessary, and sometimes harmful. *Water* should be given freely at fixed intervals. A good plan is to have a jug of water beside the patient and tubing with a glass mouthpiece, so that he can drink as much as he wishes. It is desirable to have the patient take at least four litres of water daily and larger amounts are an advantage. This causes polyuria, and is a sort of internal hydrotherapy by which the toxins are washed out. Barley water, lemonade, soda water, or iced-tea may be used. It is doubtful if alcohol is of any value except when the addition of small amounts enables the patient to take nourishment more freely.

Special care must be given to the mouth, which should be cleaned after each feeding. A mouth wash should be used freely (such as phenol ʒ i, 4 c. c., glycerine ℥ i, 30 c. c., and boric acid, saturated solution, to ℥ x, 300 c. c.).

(*c*) Hydrotherapy.—The use of water, inside and outside, was no new treatment in fevers at the end of the eighteenth century, when James Currie (a friend of Burns and the editor of his poems) wrote his Medical Reports on the Effects of Water, Cold and Warm, as a Remedy in Fevers and other Diseases. In the United States it was used with great effect and recommended strongly by Nathan Smith, of Yale. Since 1861 the value of bathing in fevers has been specially emphasized by the late Dr. Brand, of Stettin.

Hydrotherapy may be carried out in several ways, of which, the most satisfactory are sponging, the wet pack, the ice rub, and the full bath.

(1) *Cold Sponging.*—The water may be tepid or cold, according to the height of the fever. A thorough sponge-bath should take from fifteen to twenty minutes. The cold sponging and the ice-rub are not quite as formidable as the full bath, for which, when there is an insuperable objection in private practice, they are excellent alternatives. But frequently it is difficult to get the friends to appreciate the advantages of the sponging. When such is the case, and in children and delicate persons, it can be made a little less formidable by sponging limb by limb and then the back and abdomen.

(2) The *cold pack* is not so generally useful in typhoid fever, but in cases with very pronounced nervous symptoms, if the tub is not available, the patient may be wrapped in a sheet wrung out of water at 60° or 65°, and then cold water sprinkled over him with an ordinary watering-pot.

(3) *The Bath.*—The tub should be long enough so that the patient can be completely covered except his head. Our rule has been to give a bath every

third hour when the temperature was above 102.5°. The patient remains in the tub for fifteen or twenty minutes, is taken out, wrapped in a dry sheet, and covered with a blanket. While in the tub the limbs and trunk are rubbed thoroughly, either with the hand or with a suitable rubber. It is well to give the first one or two baths at a temperature of 80° to 85°. There is no routine temperature and that between 70° and 85° which suits best is chosen. It is important to see that the canvas supports are properly arranged, and that the rubber pillow is comfortable for the patient's head. The amount of complaint made by the patient is largely dependent upon the skill and care with which the baths are given. The blueness and shivering, which may follow the bath, are not serious features. The rectal temperature is taken immediately after the bath, and again three-quarters of an hour later. Contra-indications are peritonitis, hæmorrhage, phlebitis, abdominal pain, and great prostration.

The good effects of the baths are: (i) The influence on the nervous system; delirium lessens, tremor diminishes and toxic features are less marked. (ii) Increased excretion of toxins by the kidney. (iii) The tonic effect on the circulation; the heart rate falls, the pulse becomes smaller and harder, and the blood pressure rises. Vaso-motor paresis is lessened. (iv) With hydrotherapy the initial bronchitis is benefited, and there is less chance of passive congestion of the bases of the lungs. (v) The liability to bed-sores is diminished and the frequent cleansing of the skin is beneficial. The addition of half a pound of alum to the water is an advantage. Should boils occur, one bath-tub should be used for that patient alone. (vi) Reduction of the temperature may occur but is not an important effect. (vii) The mortality is reduced. In general hospitals from six to eight patients in every hundred are saved by this plan of treatment. At the Brisbane Hospital, where F. E. Hare used it so thoroughly, the mortality was reduced from 14.8 to 7.5 per cent. There is a remarkable uniformity in the death-rate of institutions using the method—usually from 6 to 8 per cent.

(*d*) Medicinal Treatment.—There is no specific drug treatment, but it is usually advisable to give hexamine after the second week, twenty to thirty grains (1.3 to 2 gm.) daily. In private practice it may be safer, for the young practitioner especially, to order an acid or a mild fever mixture. The question of medicinal antipyretics is important: they are used far too often and too rashly in typhoid fever. An occasional dose may do no harm but the daily use of these drugs is most injurious. Quinine in moderate doses is sometimes given but its value is doubtful. In the various antiseptic drugs which have been advised we have no faith. Most of them do no harm, except that in private practice their use has too often diverted the practitioner from more rational and safer courses.

(*e*) Vaccine and Serum Therapy.—Treatment by vaccines during the height of the disease is still in an experimental stage. Various forms of vaccines are used and given subcutaneously or intravenously. Doses varying from 50 to 500 million bacilli are given, usually three or four days apart. A moderate reaction should be produced. As patients react very differently, the smaller doses are safer at first, especially if given intravenously. Gay reports good results from the intravenous injection of sensitized vaccine sediment. His initial dose is 1/50 mg., corresponding to 150 million bacteria. In long-continued attacks when progress is slow, for complications due to the presence of typhoid bacilli in organs or tissues, and for carriers, vaccine therapy is helpful. No serum of proved value has been obtained.

(*f*) Treatment of Special Symptoms.—For severe *toxæmia* water should be given freely by mouth if possible, otherwise by the bowel or subcutaneously. Hydrotherapy should be used actively, best by tub baths. For headache and delirium an ice-bag or cold compresses should be kept to the head. If the patient is delirious and restless a dose of morphia hypodermically is the best treatment. Lumbar puncture is also useful, the fluid being allowed to run as long as it flows under pressure. Every delirious patient should be constantly watched. It is important to secure sleep for these patients, for which morphia is most reliable. Hydrotherapy, internal and external, is our greatest aid in the treatment of the nervous conditions. The abdominal *pain* and *tympanites* are best treated with fomentations or turpentine stupes. The latter, if well applied, give great relief. Sir William Jenner used to lay great stress on the advantages of a well-applied turpentine stupe. He directed it to be applied as follows: A flannel roller was placed beneath the patient, and then a double layer of thin flannel, wrung out of very hot water, with a dram of turpentine mixed with the water, was applied to the abdomen and covered with the ends of the roller. When the stomach is greatly distended the passage of a stomach tube gives relief. When the gas is in the large bowel, a rectal tube may be passed or a turpentine enema given. For tympanites, with a dry tongue, turpentine may be given, ♏ xv (1 c. c.) every three hours. If whey and albumen-water are substituted for milk, the distention lessens, Pituitary extract or eserine $^1/_{50}$ gr. (0.0013 gm.) hypodermically, may be tried. Opium should not be given.

For the *diarrhœa,* if severe—that is, if there are more than three or four stools daily—a starch and opium enema may be given; or, by the mouth, a combination of bismuth, in large doses, with Dover's powder; or the acid diarrhœa mixture, acetate of lead (gr. ii, 0.13 gm.), dilute acetic acid (♏ xv, 1 c. c.), and acetate of morphia (gr. $^1/_6$, 0.01 gm.). Repeated saline irrigations are sometimes helpful. The amount of food should be reduced, and whey and albumen-water in small amounts substituted for the milk. An ice-bag or cold compresses relieve the soreness which sometimes accompanies diarrhœa.

Constipation is present in many cases and it is well to give an ordinary enema every second day. The addition of turpentine (℥ ss, 15 c. c.) is advisable if there is meteorism.

Hæmorrhage.—As absolute rest is essential, the greatest care should be taken in the use of the bed-pan. It is perhaps better to allow the patient to pass the motions into a large pad. Ice may be given and a light ice-bag placed on the abdomen. The amount of food should be restricted for eight or ten hours. If there is a tendency to collapse, stimulants should be given, and, if necessary, hypodermic injections of camphor (gr. iii, 0.2 gm. in oil). Injection of salt solution beneath the skin or into a vein may revive a failing heart, but should only be done in case of emergency. Turpentine is warmly recommended by certain authors. Should opium be given? One-fifth of the cases of perforation occur with hæmorrhage, and the opium may obscure the features upon which alone the diagnosis of perforation may be made. Opium increases any tendency to tympanites. We have abandoned the use of opium. The injection of human or horse serum (10 to 20 c. c.) is sometimes of value. Transfusion should be done in serious cases.

Perforation and Peritonitis.—Early diagnosis and early operation mean the saving of one-third of the cases of this otherwise fatal complication. The aim should be to operate for the perforation, and not to wait until a general peritonitis diminishes the chances of recovery. An incessant, intelligent watchfulness on the part of the medical attendant and the early co-operation of the surgeon are essentials. Every case of more than ordinary severity should be watched with special reference to this complication. Thorough preparation by early observation, careful notes, and knowledge of the conditions will help to prevent needless exploration. No case is too desperate; we had a recovery after three operations. Twenty cases of perforation in our series were operated upon with seven recoveries; in an eighth case the patient died of toxæmia on the eighth day after the laparotomy. In doubtful cases it is best to operate, as experience shows that patients stand an exploration very well.

Cholecystitis.—A majority of the cases recover, but if the symptoms are very severe and progressive, operation should be advised. For chronic cholecystitis hexamine should be given in large doses and the vaccine treatment employed.

With signs of failure of the *circulation*, hydrotherapy should be carried on actively and strychnine given hypodermically (gr. $^1/_{50}$ to $^1/_{20}$, 0.001 to 0.003 gm.) every three hours. Saline infusions (500 c. c.) are useful especially if the patient is not taking much water by mouth. Digitalis may be given as the tincture (♏ xv, 1 c. c.) but if collapse or severe symptoms occur, strophanthin gr. $^1/_{100}$ (0.00065 gm.) intramuscularly or intravenously is better. For collapse, camphor (gr. ii, 0.13 gm.) or epinephrine (♏ xv, 1 c. c.) should be given intramuscularly. The bath treatment is the best preventive of circulatory failure. For *phlebitis* the limb should be kept absolutely at rest and wrapped in raw cotton. The application of a sedative lotion may relieve pain.

Bacilluria.—When bacilli are present, hexamine may be given in ten-grain (0.65 gm.) doses and kept up, if necessary, for several weeks. If the urine is alkaline sodium benzoate gr. x (0.6 gm.) should be added. A patient should not be discharged with bacilli in his urine. *Pyelitis* should be treated in the same way, large amounts of water being given. For *cystitis*, irrigations of bichloride of mercury (1/100,000 solution and gradually increased in strength) may be given.

For *orchitis, mastitis, parotitis*, etc., an ice-bag should be applied. Incision and drainage are advisable on the first signs of suppuration. Vaccine treatment may be helpful.

In protracted cases special care should be taken to guard against *bed-sores*. Absolute cleanliness and careful drying of the parts after an evacuation should be enjoined. Pressure should be avoided by the use of rubber rings. The patient should be turned from side to side and propped with pillows, and the back sponged with alcohol.

Bone Lesions.—The use of a typhoid vaccine is well worthy of trial. Typhoid periostitis does not always go on to suppuration, though, as a rule, it requires operation. This should be done very thoroughly and the diseased parts completely removed, as otherwise recurrence is inevitable. For *typhoid spine* fixation by a plaster jacket or some form of apparatus is advisable. Trauma should be guarded against. In the milder cases active counter-irritation is useful. If pain is severe, large doses of sedatives are necessary.

(*g*) Convalescence.—The diet can be gradually increased, but it is usually best to wait at least a week after the temperature is normal before giving ordinary meats or coarse vegetables. Solid food sometimes disagrees if it is given too early. Whether an error in diet may cause relapse is doubtful. The patient may be allowed to sit up for a short time about the end of the first week of convalescence, and the period may be prolonged with a gradual return of strength. He should move about slowly, and when the weather is favorable should be in th open air as much as possible. He should be guarded at this period against all unnecessary excitement. Emotional disturbance not infrequently is the cause of recrudescence of the fever. Constipation is not uncommon in convalescence and is best treated by enemata. A protracted diarrhœa, which is usually due to ulceration in the colon, may retard recovery. In such cases the diet should be restricted to milk and the patient confined to bed; large doses of bismuth and astringent injections will prove useful. The recrudescence of the fever does not require special measures. The treatment of the relapse is essentially that of the original attack.

Post-typhoid insanity requires the judicious care of an expert. The cases usually recover. The swollen leg after phlebitis is a source of great worry. A bandage or a well-fitting elastic stocking should be worn during the day. The outlook depends on the completeness with which the collateral circulation is established. In a good many cases there is permanent disability.

The *post-typhoid neuritis,* a cause of much alarm and distress, usually gets well, though it may take months, or even a couple of years, before the paralysis disappears. After the subsidence of the acute symptoms systematic massage of the paralyzed and atrophic muscles is the best treatment.

Typhoid Carriers.—Treatment of these is difficult. Hexamine should be given persistently and in large doses. Drainage or removal of the gall bladder and X-ray exposures over it have been successful in some cases. The employment of an autogenous vaccine offers the best chance of success. Doses increasing from 25 to 1,000 or 1,500 million bacilli are given at intervals of 10 days. Carriers should not be allowed to handle or prepare food.

Lastly, no patient should be discharged from observation until we are certain that he can not infect others.

II. PARATYPHOID FEVER

Definition.—An acute infection caused by the *Bacillus paratyphosus A* and *B,* which are closely related to the typhoid bacillus and cause a clinical picture much like typhoid fever.

Historical.—In 1896 Achard and Bensaude reported a case of "typhoid fever" in which they found an organism which was not *B. typhosus* and to which they gave the name of paratyphoid. In 1898 Gwyn isolated an organism to which he gave the name of paracolon bacillus. In 1902 Buxton described the two varieties A and B. Since then many reports on this disease have been made and the experience of the great war added much to our knowledge of these infections.

Occurrence.—Before the recent war paratyphoid A was more common in the United States and paratyphoid B in Europe. During the recent war the relative proportions have varied in different places, but as a rule the B form has been the more common. As regards the relative incidence of typhoid and paratyphoid fever in soldiers, one army series of 4,218 cases showed 1,684 of typhoid and 2,534 of paratyphoid fever, and in another series of 5,700 cases, 93 per cent. were paratyphoid. The inoculation in the majority had been against typhoid fever only.

Etiology.—The paratyphoid organisms differ from *B. typhosus* in cultural and agglutination properties. The A form is nearer to the typhoid bacillus and the B form closer to *B. suipestifer and enteritidis.* The general problems of infection are the same as those of typhoid fever with particular importance on the part played by carriers, especially in paratyphoid B. The B form at times occurs with outbreaks of meat poisoning.

Pathology.—The toxins of the paratyphoid organisms do not show the same tendency to attack lymphoid tissues as the toxin of the typhoid bacillus and appear to cause a greater variety of lesions elsewhere. As there is a bacteræmia there is a possibility of any part of the body being attacked. In general the intestinal lesions are much like those of typhoid fever but show a tendency to superficial necrosis rather than to deep ulceration. In some cases the intestines are acutely inflamed without involvement of the lymphoid tissue. Some statistics suggest that the colon frequently shows ulceration. Hæmorrhage and perforation are not so common as in typhoid fever. There are several forms: (1) A septicæmia with little or no change in the bowels; (2) cases not distinguishable from ordinary typhoid; (3) a dysenteric form, in which the lesions are chiefly in the large bowel, and (4) cases in which the lesions are particularly in one part of the body. In Dawson and Whittingdon's study of 17 fatal cases, in 10 the large bowel was involved.

Symptoms.—The average incubation period is about ten days and an acute onset is common. Headache and abdominal pain may occur at the onset, to be followed by the usual signs of an infection, malaise, chilly sensations, and general pains. Bronchitis is common early in the attack. The clinical features are variable, as in typhoid fever, and various forms have been described depending on the predominant symptoms, such as typhoid, septicæmic, dysenteric, biliary, urinary, respiratory, arthritic, etc. Apathy is often marked, especially early, and severe headache is common. The striking point about the fever curve is the irregularity. It may be of the classical typhoid type with remissions beginning about the end of the second week, the duration of fever may be short, there may be constant remissions or the fever may be irregular throughout. The pulse rate is usually slow and with a rising temperature may be a suggestive point. The blood pressure is usually low. The *rash* is generally like the roseola of typhoid fever, but sometimes consists of large irregular spots, raised and not fading completely on pressure, leaving areas of pigmentation. It is sometimes general. Sweating is common especially in patients with a remittent type of fever. The *spleen* is usually enlarged. Intestinal disturbance may be marked, more particularly at the onset, especially in the B form. Hæmorrhage is rarely profuse and perforation is rare. Relapse rarely occurs. The *course* as a rule is shorter than in typhoid fever. Some writers comment on the slow improvement after the acute features are over and emphasize mental depression in convalescence.

Complications.—These are much like those of typhoid fever with more tendency to involvement of the respiratory tract, jaundice with infection of the bile passages, nephritis, abscess formation and arthritis. The sequelæ are the same as typhoid fever, even to the bone lesions.

Diagnosis.—For practical purposes typhoid and paratyphoid fever may be considered as one disease; clinically the diagnosis is based on the same findings and only a bacteriological diagnosis can be regarded as absolutely beyond doubt. The agglutination tests are fairly reliable if markedly positive.

Prognosis.—In civil life the death rate is very low, about one per cent., but in the armies it has been higher.

Prophylaxis.—This is the same as for typhoid fever and the use of preventive inoculation has had the same success. The triple vaccine (typhoid and both paratyphoids) should be used. The importance of carriers should be kept in mind.

Treatment.—This is the same as in typhoid fever.

III. COLON BACILLUS INFECTIONS

The colon bacillus, or more properly speaking the group of colon bacilli, in their biological and pathological peculiarities are closely related to the organisms of the typhoid group. Normal inhabitants of the intestines, where in all probability they serve a useful function, the *Bacillus coli communis* may be taken as the typical member of the group. There are great difficulties in determining the extent of the lesions caused by this organism, which varies extraordinarily in virulence. To it has been attributed a host of maladies from appendicitis to old age, but more conservative pathologists limit very much its pathogenic scope. It is not easy to separate the effects of the *B. coli* from those of other organisms with which it is so often associated. The needful bacteriological distinction must be considered in connection with agglutination tests.

Recognized infections may be classed as follows:

A. General Hæmic Infections.—There are several groups of cases:

(*a*) *Terminal Infections.*—After death the colon bacillus swarms in the body, invading the blood and contaminating all parts. In protracted illnesses, in acute intestinal and peritoneal affections it may be present in the blood some time before death and may be responsible for the terminal fever.

(*b*) Cases running a course resembling typhoid fever.

(*c*) Cases of general infection with secondary abscesses.

(*d*) Secondary infection in other diseases, as for example typhoid fever.

B. Sub-infections.—Adami suggested that a number of chronic diseases have their origin in a mild, continuous infection with *B. coli* and he brought forward evidence to show that such affections as anæmia and cirrhosis of the liver may be due to it. Metchnikoff induced the lesions of early cirrhosis and of arterio-sclerosis by administering the products of the growth of the *B. coli*. The question is far from settled.

C. Local Infections.—Here we are on safer ground and have definite lesions produced by the organism.

(*a*) *Peritonitis.*—In perforation of the bowel, in strangulated hernia, in obstruction, in various types of ulcer, the associated peritonitis may be due to *B. coli.*

(*b*) *Cholecystitis* and *cholangitis,* either of the simple catarrhal type or suppurative, may be caused by it.

(*c*) *Infection of the Urinary Tract.*—The bladder and the pelvis of the kidneys are chiefly affected. There are three possible channels of infection—by the ureter, the blood stream, and the lymphatics. Hæmatogenous infection is the most common but lymphatic infection from the bowel plays an important rôle in many cases. Bowel troubles have been present, constipation or diarrhœa, and with very slight abrasion of the mucosa of the colon the bacilli may enter the lymphatics. An interesting point is the relative frequency of involvement of the right kidney; Franke states that the cæcum and ascending colon are connected by a train of lymphatics with the right kidney, an anatomical communication not present with the left. There are several groups of cases. (1) In children, in whom it seems by no means uncommon. In Jeffrey's study of 60 cases at the Hospital for Sick Children a large proportion occurred in females (53). Death followed in 9 cases. (2) In connection with pregnancy. The cases are common and important and may occur at any time during pregnancy or follow delivery. The pelvis of the right kidney is most often attacked. (3) As a secondary infection in other diseases, especially typhoid fever. (4) The group of cases in adults, men and women, in whom, without any obvious cause, and in the majority of cases without any previous intestinal trouble, acute pyelitis or pyelocystitis comes on. The infection is obstinate and very difficult to treat. A distressing sequel is a chronic arthritis. In one instance the condition was very similar to that of a gonorrhœal synovitis and peri-arthritis. The clinical picture presents nothing peculiar. (5) *Cystitis* and *urethritis* in newly married women are sometimes due to colon infection. Care should be taken not to regard them as gonorrhœal.

(*d*) *Intestines.*—To the *bacillus coli* almost all the diseases of the bowels from ulcers of the duodenum to appendicitis have been attributed. Ulcers of the stomach and of the duodenum have been produced by feeding cultures of *B. coli* to dogs, and from the peptic ulcers of very young infants Helmholz isolated the organism in pure culture. There is great difficulty in determining the precise etiological relationship of *B. coli* to the various lesions of the gastro-intestinal tract.

(*e*) Other local infections with which the *colon bacillus* has been associated are acute meningitis, abscess of the brain, endocarditis, and suppuration in various parts. Only in a small proportion of these cases has the association been demonstrated by cultural and biological tests.

Treatment.—In the cases of general infection, rest, careful diet, and large amounts of water are indicated. In the local infections the treatment is that of the condition present, as peritonitis and cholecystitis. For infection of the urinary tract the diet should be simple and large amounts of water should be given with urinary antiseptics, especially hexamine (gr. xl to lx a day, 2.6

to 4 gm.). Local treatment by irrigations is helpful in cystitis and in some cases of pyelitis. The use of an autogenous vaccine is an aid in some cases but is often disappointing.

IV. TYPHUS FEVER

Definition.—An acute infectious disease characterized by sudden onset, maculated and hæmorrhagic rash, marked nervous symptoms, and a cyclical course terminating by crisis, usually about the end of the second week.

The disease is known by the names of hospital fever, spotted fever, jail fever, camp fever, and ship fever, and in Germany is called *exanthematic* typhus, in contradistinction to *abdominal* typhus. The word signifies "smoke" or "mist" in Greek and was used by Hippocrates to describe any condition with a tendency to stupor. In the eighteenth century the name was given by de Sauvages to the common putrid or pestilential fever, and the general use came in through its adoption by Cullen.

Etiology.—Typhus has been one of the great *epidemics* of the world, whose history, as Hirsch remarks, is written in those dark pages which tell of the grievous visitations of mankind by war, famine, and misery. It now exists in a few endemic areas, where from time to time sporadic cases occur. Ireland was terribly scourged by the disease between the years 1817 and 1819, and again in 1846. It prevailed extensively in all the large cities of Great Britain and the Continent. In 1875 in England and Wales there were 1,499 deaths from the disease. Of late years the name typhus has rarely appeared in the Registrar-General's report. In the United States and Canada it prevailed extensively in the early years of the nineteenth century, and there were severe epidemics in the wake of the Irish immigrations in '46 and '47. It is endemic in parts of Russia and in the Slav countries, and there have been extensive epidemics in the recent war.

Sporadic typhus fever offers peculiarities which are apt to make its recognition difficult. There may be outbreaks of a few cases, the origin of which may be very difficult to trace. Two such limited outbreaks came under observation, one at the House of Refuge, Montreal, in 1877, in which eleven persons were affected, and the second in 1901 at the Johns Hopkins Hospital, where three cases occurred.

A question of interest has arisen as to the relation of typhus fever to the cases of fever studied by Brill in New York. This is a sporadic type of typhus, confirmed by the studies of Anderson and Goldberger. Beginning with the usual prodromes, the fever increases rapidly and reaches a maximum about the third or fourth day, where it remains fairly constant between 103° and 104°. On the 5th or 6th day an eruption appears, maculo-papular in type, dull red in color, rarely hæmorrhagic, not appearing in crops, not disappearing on pressure, and neither profuse as in measles nor diffuse as in typical typhus; there may be only a few hundred spots. The rash persists until the crisis and then fades rapidly. The patients are much prostrated, with severe headache, but no abdominal symptoms. Constipation is usually a marked feature. After persisting for 12 to 15 days, the fever declines rapidly, usually with a critical fall, and there is a speedy convalescence. It is rarely fatal.

The typhus fever prevailing in Mexico City, where it is known as Tabardillo, is more severe, and in its study Ricketts of Chicago fell a victim. Neither the Rocky Mountain spotted fever, nor the Flood or River fever of Japan is identical with typhus.

The disease is transmitted by the body louse and possibly by the head louse and so is associated with filth and overcrowding. In epidemics it is one of the most dangerous of all diseases, and those in attendance upon patients are almost invariably attacked unless special precautions are taken to guard against lice. In a period of twenty-five years in Ireland, among 1,230 physicians attached to institutions, 550 died of this disease. The disease has been transmitted to animals.

Plotz and his co-workers have isolated a small slender bacillus, *Bacillus typhi-exanthematici*. It was found in the blood throughout the course of the disease and the percentage of successful cultures was highest in the severe forms. The organism has been isolated from monkeys and guinea-pigs to which the disease had been conveyed. The same organism has been found in infected lice. Specific antibodies are formed and the agglutination and complement fixation tests are important aids in diagnosis.

Morbid Anatomy.—The anatomical changes are those which result from intense fever. The blood is dark and fluid; the muscles are of a deep red color, and often show a granular degeneration, particularly in the heart; the liver is enlarged and soft and may have a dull clay-like lustre; the kidneys are swollen; there is moderate enlargement of the spleen, and a general hyperplasia of the lymph-follicles. Peyer's glands are not ulcerated. Bronchial catarrh is usually, and hypostatic congestion of the lungs often, present. The skin shows the petechial rash.

Symptoms.—Incubation.—This is placed at about twelve days, but it may be less. There may be ill-defined feelings of discomfort. As a rule, however, the *invasion* is abrupt and marked by chills or a single rigor, followed by fever. The chills may recur during the first few days, and there is headache with pains in the back and legs. There is early prostration, and the patient is glad to take to his bed at once. The temperature is high at first, and may attain its maximum on the second or third day. The pulse is full, rapid, and not so frequently dicrotic as in typhoid. The tongue is furred and white, and there is an early tendency to dryness. The face is flushed, the eyes congested, and the expression dull and stupid. Vomiting may be a distressing symptom. In severe cases mental symptoms are present from the outset, either a mild febrile delirium or an excited, active, almost maniacal condition. Bronchial catarrh is common.

Stage of Eruption.—From the third to the fifth day the eruption appears—first upon the abdomen and upper part of the chest, and then upon the extremities and face; occurring so rapidly that in two or three days it is all out. There are two elements in the eruption: a subcuticular mottling, "a fine, irregular, dusky red mottling, as if below the surface of the skin some little distance, and seen through a semi-opaque medium" (Buchanan); and distinct papular rose-spots which change to petechiæ. In some instances the petechial rash comes out with the rose-spots. Collie describes the rash as consisting of three parts: rose-colored spots which disappear on pressure, dark-red spots which are modified by pressure, and petechiæ upon which pressure produces no effect. In children the rash at first may present a striking resemblance to that of measles and give as a whole a curiously mottled appearance to the skin. The term mulberry rash is sometimes applied to it. In mild cases the eruption is slight, but even then is largely petechial in character. As the rash is hæmorrhagic, it does not disappear after death. Usually the skin is dry, so that sudaminal vesicles are not common. It is stated by some authors that a distinctive odor is present. During the second week the general symptoms are much aggravated. The prostration becomes more marked, the delirium more intense, and the fever rises. The patient lies on his back

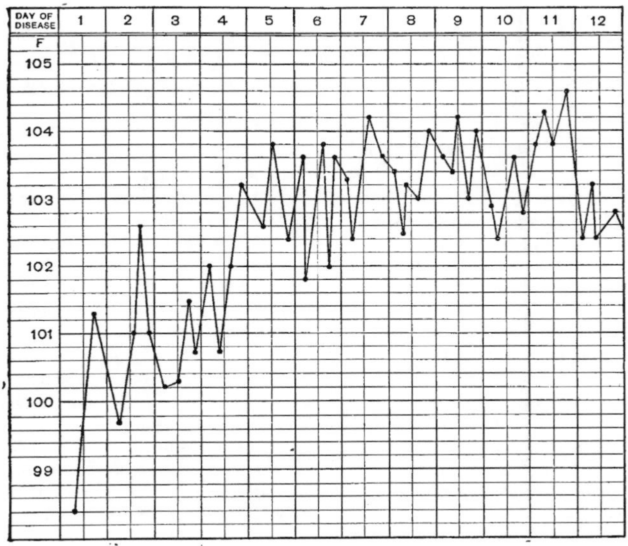

CHART III.—TYPHUS FEVER (Murchison).

with a dull, expressionless face, flushed cheeks, injected conjunctivæ, and contracted pupils. The pulse increases in frequency and is feebler; the face is dusky, and the condition becomes more serious. Retention of urine is common. Coma-vigil is frequent, a condition in which the patient lies with open eyes, but quite unconscious; with it there may be subsultus tendinum and picking at the bedclothes. The tongue is dry, brown, and cracked, and there are sordes on the teeth. Respiration is accelerated, the heart's action becomes more and more enfeebled, and death takes place from exhaustion. In favorable cases about the end of the second week occurs the crisis, in which, often after a deep sleep, the patient awakes feeling much better and with a clear mind. The temperature falls, and although the prostration may be extreme convalescence is rapid and relapse very rare. This abrupt termination by crisis is in striking contrast to the mode of termination in typhoid fever.

FEVER.—The temperature rises steadily during the first four or five days, and the morning remissions are not marked. The maximum is usually attained by the fifth day, when the temperature may be 105°, 106°, or 107° F. In mild cases it seldom rises above 103° F. After reaching its maximum the fever generally continues with slight morning remissions until the twelfth or fourteenth day, when the crisis occurs, during which the temperature may fall below normal within twelve or twenty-four hours. Preceding a fatal termination, there is usually a rapid rise in the fever to 108° or even 109° F.

The heart may early show signs of weakness. The first sound becomes feeble and almost inaudible, and a systolic murmur at the apex is not infrequent. Hypostatic congestion of the lungs occurs in all severe cases. The brain symptoms are usually more pronounced than in typhoid, and the delirium is more constant. A slight leucocytosis is common.

The urine shows the usual febrile characteristics. The chlorides diminish or disappear. Albumin is present in a large proportion of the cases, but nephritis seldom occurs.

Variations in the course of the disease are naturally common. There are malignant cases which rapidly prove fatal within two or three days; the so-called *typhus siderans*. On the other hand, during epidemics there are extremely mild cases in which the fever is slight, the delirium absent, and convalescence is established by the tenth day.

Complications and Sequelæ.—Broncho-pneumonia is perhaps the most common complication. It may pass on to gangrene. In certain epidemics gangrene of the toes, the hands, or the nose, and in children noma or cancrum oris, have occurred. Meningitis is rare. Paralyses, which are probably due to a post-febrile neuritis, are not very uncommon. Septic processes, such as parotitis and abscesses in the subcutaneous tissues and in the joints, are occasionally met with. Nephritis is rare. Hæmatemesis may occur.

Prognosis.—The mortality ranges in different epidemics from 12 to 20 per cent. It is very slight in the young. Children, who are quite as frequently attacked as adults, rarely die. After middle age the mortality is high, in some epidemics 50 per cent. Death usually occurs toward the close of the second week and is due to the toxæmia. In the third week it more commonly results from pneumonia.

Diagnosis.—During an epidemic there is rarely any doubt, for the disease presents distinctive general characters. Isolated cases and the form described by Brill may be very difficult to distinguish from typhoid fever. While in typical instances the eruption in the two affections is very different, yet taken alone it may be deceptive, since in typhoid fever a roseolous rash may be abundant and there may be occasionally a subcuticular mottling and even petechiæ. The difference in the onset, particularly in the temperature, is marked; but cases in which it is important to make an accurate diagnosis are not usually seen until the fourth or fifth day. The suddenness of the onset, the greater frequency of the chill, and the early prostration are the distinctive features in typhus. The brain symptoms, too, are earlier. It is easy to put down on paper elaborate differential distinctions, which are practically useless at the bedside. The Widal reaction and blood cultures are important aids, but in sporadic cases the diagnosis is sometimes extremely difficult. Severe cerebro-spinal fever may closely simulate typhus at the outset, but the diagnosis is usually clear within a few days. Malignant variola also has certain features in common with severe typhus, but the greater extent of the hæmorrhages and the bleeding from the mucous membranes make the diagnosis clear within a short time. The rash at first resembles that of measles, but in the latter the eruption is brighter red in color, often crescentic or irregular in arrangement, and appears first on the face.

The agglutination test with the organism is positive. What is termed the Weil-Felix reaction is positive in many cases. This consists in the agglutination of a proteus-like organism obtained from the urine of patients with the disease. It is not given till the sixth or seventh day.

Prophylaxis.—This involves measures against lice. The patient's clothing should be sterilized by heat. Removal of the patient to an isolation hospital is important. During epidemics when this can not be done, those attending the patients should take special precautions to prevent infection by lice and wear louse-proof clothing.

Treatment.—The general management is like that of typhoid fever. Hydrotherapy should be thoroughly and systematically employed; water should be given freely. Judging from the good results which we have obtained by this method in typhoid cases with nervous symptoms, much may be expected from it. Medicinal antipyretics are even less suitable than in typhoid, as the tendency to heart-weakness is often more pronounced. As a rule, the patients require from the outset a supporting treatment.

The bowels may be kept open by mild aperients. The so-called specific medication, by sulphocarbolates, the sulphides, carbolic acid, etc., is not commended by those who have had the largest experience. The special nervous symptoms and the pulmonary symptoms should be dealt with as in typhoid fever. In epidemics, when the conditions of the climate are suitable, the patients are best treated in tents in the open air.

V. THE PYOGENIC INFECTIONS

(*Sapræmia, Septicæmia, Pyæmia, Focal Infection, Terminal Infections*)

Definition.—A group of non-specific diseases, induced by a number of micro-organisms, of which the pyogenic cocci are the most important, characterized by fever, chills, leucocytosis, often a profound intoxication and sometimes by foci of suppuration. A hard-and-fast line can not be drawn between an infection and an intoxication, but agents of infection alone are capable of reproduction, whereas those of intoxication are chemical poisons, some of which are produced by the agency of bacteria, or by vegetable and animal cells. There are five chief clinical types of pyogenic infection:

1. LOCAL INFECTIONS WITH THE DEVELOPMENT OF TOXINS

This is the common mode of invasion of many of the infectious diseases. Tetanus, diphtheria and erysipelas are diseases which have sites of local infection in which the pathogenic organisms develop; but the constitutional effects are caused by the absorption of the poisonous products. The diphtheria toxin produces all the general symptoms, the tetanus toxin every feature of the disease without the presence of their respective bacilli. Certain of the symptoms following the absorption of the toxins are general to all; others are special and peculiar, according to the organism which produces them. A chill, fever, general malaise, prostration, rapid pulse, restlessness, and headache are the most frequent. With but few exceptions the febrile disturbance is the most common feature. The most serious effects are upon the nervous system and the circulation, and the gravity of the symptoms on the part of these organs is to some extent a measure of the intensity of the intoxication. The organisms of certain local infections produce poisons which have special actions; thus, the diphtheria toxin is especially prone to attack the nervous system and to cause peripheral neuritis. The tetanus toxin has a specific action on the motor neurones.

2. SEPTICÆMIA

Formerly, and in a surgical sense, the term "septicæmia" was used to designate the invasion of the blood and tissues of the body by the organisms of suppuration, but in the medical sense the term may be applied to any condition in which, with or without a local site of infection, there is microbic invasion of the blood and tissues, but without metastatic foci of suppuration. Owing to the development of bacteria in the blood, and to separate it sharply from local infectious processes with toxic invasion of the body, this condition is termed bacteræmia; toxæmia denotes the latter state.

(a) Progressive Septicæmia from Local Infection.—The common streptococcus and staphylococcus infection is, as a rule, first local, and the toxins alone pass into the blood. In other instances the cocci appear in the blood and throughout the tissues, causing a septicæmia which intensifies greatly the severity of the case. The clinical features of this form are well seen in the cases of puerperal septicæmia or in dissection wounds, in which the course of the infection may be traced along the lymphatics. The symptoms usually set in within twenty-four hours, and rarely later than the third or fourth day. There is a chill or chilliness, with moderate fever at first, which gradually rises and is marked by daily remissions and even intermissions. The pulse is small and compressible, and may reach 120 or higher. Gastro-intestinal disturbances are common, the tongue is red at the margin, and the dorsum is dry and dark. There may be early delirium or marked mental prostration and apathy. As the disease progresses there may be pallor of the face or a yellowish tint. Capillary hæmorrhages are not uncommon.

In streptococcus cases we now recognize that these infections are not always so serious as we thought. Death may occur within twenty-four hours or be delayed for several days, even for weeks, and recovery may occur. One patient showed streptococci in the blood for six weeks, but recovered (Cole). On post-mortem examination there may be no gross focal lesions in the viscera, and the seat of infection may present only slight changes. The spleen is enlarged and soft, the blood may be extremely dark in color, and hæmorrhages are common, particularly on the serous surfaces. Neither thrombi nor emboli are found. Certain clinical features separate the streptococcus from the staphylococcus infection, chiefly the absence of delirium, a rather abnormal mental acuteness, and the presence of a greater degree of anæmia.

Many instances of septicæmia are combined infections; thus in diphtheria streptococcus septicæmia is a common, and the most serious, event. The local disease and the symptoms produced by absorption of the toxins dominate the clinical picture; but the features are usually much aggravated by the systemic invasion. A similar infection may occur in typhoid fever and tuberculosis, and obscure the typical picture. These secondary septicæmias are caused most frequently by the streptococcus, but may be due to other bacteria.

(b) General Septicæmia without Recognizable Local Infection.—*Cryptogenetic Septicæmias.*—This is a group of very great interest to the physician, the full importance of which we have only recently recognized.

The subjects when attacked may be in perfect health; more commonly they are already weakened by acute or chronic illness. The pathogenic organisms are varied. *Streptococcus pyogenes* is the most common; the forms of staphylococcus more rare. Other occasional causal agents are the pneumococcus, *Bacillus proteus, Bacillus pyocyaneus* and *Bacillus influenzæ.* Between May 1, 1892, and June 1, 1895, from the medical wards of the Hopkins Hospital, 21 cases of general infection came to autopsy, of which 13 were due to *Streptococcus pyogenes,* 2 to *Staphylococcus pyogenes,* and 6 to the pneumococcus. In 19 of these cases the patients were already the subjects of some other malady, which was aggravated, or in most instances terminated, by the septicæmia. The symptoms vary somewhat with the character of the micro-organisms. In the streptococcus cases there may be chills with high, irregular fever, and a more characteristic *septic* state than in the pneumococcus infection.

These cases come correctly under the term "cryptogenetic septicæmia" as employed by Leube, inasmuch as the local focus of infection is not evident during life and may not be found after death. Although most of these cases are terminal infections, yet there are instances of this type of affection coming on in apparently healthy persons. The fever may be extremely irregular, characteristically septic, and persist for many weeks. Foci of suppuration may not develop, and may not be found even at autopsy. There are cases of an intermittent pyrexia persisting for weeks, in which it is impossible to give any explanation of the phenomena, which ultimately recover, and in which tuberculosis and malaria can be excluded. These cases require to be carefully studied bacteriologically. Local symptoms may be absent, though there may be enlargement of the liver, in some due to a diffuse suppurative hepatitis. The pyocyanic disease, or cyano-pyæmia, is an extremely interesting form of infection with *Bacillus pyocyaneus,* of which a number of cases have been reported.

3. SEPTICO-PYÆMIA

The pathogenic micro-organisms which invade the blood and tissues may settle in certain foci and there cause suppuration. When multiple abscesses are thus produced in connection with a general infection, the condition is known as pyæmia or, perhaps better, septico-pyæmia. There are no specific organisms of suppuration, and the condition of pyæmia may be produced by organisms other than the streptococci and staphylococci, though these are the most common. Other forms which may invade the system and cause foci of suppuration are the pneumococcus, the gonococcus, *Bacillus coli, Bacillus typhosus, Bacillus proteus, Bacillus pyocyaneus, Bacillus influenzæ.* In a large proportion of all cases of pyæmia there is a focus of infection, either a suppurating external wound, an osteomyelitis, a gonorrhœa, an otitis media, an empyema, or an area of suppuration in a lymph-gland or about the appendix. In a large majority of all these cases the common pus cocci are present.

In a suppurating wound, for example, the pus organisms induce hyaline necrosis in the smaller vessels with the production of thrombi and purulent phlebitis. The entrance of pus organisms in small numbers into the blood does not necessarily produce pyæmia. Commonly the transmission to various parts from the local focus takes place by the fragments of thrombi which pass as emboli to different parts, where, if the conditions are favorable, the pus organisms excite suppuration. A thrombus which is not septic or contaminated, when dislodged and impacted in a distant vessel, produces at most only a simple infarction; but, coming from an infected source and containing pus microbes, an independent centre of infection is established wherever the embolus may lodge. These independent suppurative centres in pyæmia, known as *embolic or metastatic abscesses,* have the following distribution:

(*a*) In external wounds, in osteomyelitis, and in acute phlegmon of the skin, the embolic particles very frequently excite suppuration in the lungs, producing wedge-shaped pyæmic infarcts; from these, or rarely by paradoxical embolism, or direct passage of bacteria or minute emboli through the pulmonary capillaries, metastatic foci of inflammation may occur in other parts.

(*b*) Suppurative foci in the territory of the portal system, particularly in the intestines, produce metastatic abscesses in the liver with or without suppurative pylephlebitis.

Endocarditis is an event which is very liable to occur in all forms of septicæmia, and modifies materially the character of the clinical features. Streptococci and staphylococci are the most common organisms in the vegetations, but pneumococci, gonococci, tubercle bacilli, typhoid bacilli, and other forms have been isolated. The vegetations which grow at the site of the valve lesion become covered with thrombi, particles of which may be dislodged and carried as emboli to different parts of the body, causing multiple abscesses or infarcts.

Symptoms of Septico-pyæmia.—In a case of wound infection, prior to the onset of the characteristic symptoms, there may be signs of local trouble, and in the case of a discharging wound the pus may change in character. The onset of the disease is marked by a severe rigor, during which the temperature rises to 103° or 104° and is followed by a profuse sweat. These chills are repeated at intervals, either daily or every other day. In the intervals there may be slight pyrexia. The constitutional disturbance is marked and there are loss of appetite, nausea, and vomiting, and, as the disease progresses, rapid emaciation. Local symptoms usually occur. If the lungs become involved there are dyspnœa and cough. The physical signs may be slight. Involvement of the pleura and pericardium is common. The anæmia, often profound, causes great pallor of the skin, which later may be bile-tinged. The spleen is enlarged, and there may be intense pain in the side, pointing to perisplenitis from embolism. Usually in the rapid cases a typhoid state supervenes, and the patient dies comatose.

Skin Lesions.—These are very numerous. *Erythema,* the so-called "surgical scarlet fever," may extend from the infected wound or appear on the face or chest and spread widely. *Purpura* occurs as a widespread lesion in all hyper-intense types of septicæmia and is met with in the later stages as a remarkable discrete rash in various parts of the body. In the acute purpura of septicæmia the skin may be completely covered within 36 hours, usually preceded by a dusky erythema. Pustules, vesicles, ecthyma, urticaria and papular rashes are occasional complications. Ordinary herpes is rare.

In the chronic cases the disease may be prolonged for months; the chills recur at long intervals, the temperature is irregular, and the condition of the patient varies from month to month. The course is usually slow and progressively downward.

Diagnosis.—Septicæmia and pyæmia are frequently overlooked and often mistaken for other affections. Cases following a wound, an operation, or parturition are readily recognized. On the other hand, the following conditions may be overlooked:

Osteo-myelitis.—Here the lesion may be limited; the constitutional symptoms severe, and the course of the disease very rapid. The cause of the trouble may be discovered only post mortem

So, too, acute septico-pyæmia may follow *gonorrhœa* or a *prostatic abscess.*

Cases are sometimes confounded with *typhoid fever,* paticularly the more chronic instances, in which there are diarrhœa, great prostration, delirium, and irregular fever. The spleen, too, is often enlarged. The marked leucocytosis is an important differential point.

In some of the instances of *ulcerative endocarditis* the diagnosis is very difficult, particularly in what is known as the typhoid, in contradistinction to the septic, type. In *acute miliary tuberculosis* the symptoms may resemble those of septicæmia, more commonly those of typhoid fever.

The *post-febrile arthritides,* such as occur after scarlet fever and gonorrhœa, are really instances of mild septic infection. The joints may sometimes suppurate and pyæmia develop. So, also, in *tuberculosis of the kidneys* and *calculous pyelitis* recurring rigors and sweats due to septic infection are common. In some latitudes septic and pyæmic processes are too often confounded with *malaria.* In early tuberculosis, or even when signs of excavation are present in the lungs, and in cases of suppuration in various parts, particularly empyema and abscess of the liver, the diagnosis of malaria is made. The practitioner may take it as a safe rule, to which he will find very few exceptions, that *an intermittent fever which resists quinine is not malaria.*

Other conditions associated with chills which may be mistaken for pyæmia are profound anæmia, infective sinus thrombosis, certain cases of Hodgkin's disease, cholecystitis, the hepatic intermittent fever associated with the lodgment of gall-stones at the orifice of the common duct, rare cases of essential fever in nervous women, and the intermittent fever sometimes seen in rapidly growing cancer.

Treatment.—(*a*) GENERAL.—Nourishment should be given liberally in the form of liquids and soft foods up to 3,000 calories with 80 grams of protein a day. Water should be forced and it is well to give it by the drop method into the bowel and by infusion if there is any difficulty in taking it by mouth.

Free purgation is advisable especially by calomel and salines. Hydrotherapy by tub baths is useful. Sedatives should be given for sleep.

(*b*) Surgical.—In pyæmia, when the pus is accessible, free evacuation and drainage is often the only treatment required. In a case of empyema with weeks of high and irregular fever the day after operation the temperature may be normal, and remain so. Unfortunately, in only too many cases the focus of infection is not accessible; it then is a septicæmia, and for such cases we have the treatment with serums and vaccines.

(*c*) Vaccine and Serum Treatment.—By blood cultures or by cultures from the focus of infection the organism is isolated, and an autogenous vaccine prepared. "Stock" vaccines may be used, but are not as useful as an autogenous vaccine. In many cases in which the germ cannot be isolated and the condition is one of septic fever the ordinary antistreptococcus serum or one of the polyvalent serums is used. Good results are not infrequently obtained.

(*d*) Drugs.—There are none which control septic fever. The coal-tar products are of doubtful service. Quinine may be used. The intravenous injection of antiseptic drugs has not been proved to be of value.

4. FOCAL INFECTION

A local focus of infection may be the source of acute septicæmia, but in addition a variety of chronic infections may arise with distant and important manifestations. The resulting infection may be either local or general. The importance and frequency of focal sepsis have been emphasized in recent years and it gives the clue to the etiology of many obscure conditions. Foci of infection may be primary and secondary. The latter are usually the result of infection through the blood or lymph.

Etiology.—The organism most often concerned is some variety of streptococcus, such as *S. hæmolyticus, mucosus, viridans.* These organisms vary in virulence and especially in their hæmolytic properties. The colon bacillus is sometimes responsible. The foci may be situated in many parts of the body and may be open to the surface or closed. An example of the former is seen in pyorrhœa alveolaris and of the latter in the closed abscess at the root of a tooth. The local infection may be situated in many parts of the body but in a majority the situation is in the mouth or tonsils. Investigation has shown the frequency of deep tonsillar infection, which may show no indication on the surface, and of suppuration about the roots of teeth. Infection of the nose or sinuses, bronchi, gall-bladder, appendix, intestine, pelvic organs in the male and female and the urinary tract may be the source.

Pathology.—The lesions may be varied and situated in almost any part of the body. Perhaps the most frequent sites are in the joints and fibrous tissues. Arthritis is common and many of the obscure pains, termed myalgia, neuritis, "chronic and muscular rheumatism," are really due to fibrositis secondary to a focal infection. Among other resulting lesions are endocarditis, myocarditis, gastric ulcer, cholecystitis, appendicitis and nephritis. The resulting disturbance is due to absorbed toxins or to bacteria which reach the blood stream or lymph and are carried to other parts. Systemic intoxication from absorption is not rare. In some cases the individual becomes sensitized to the protein of the organism concerned. The lesions produced do not show any particular characteristic. In general they are those of a chronic inflammatory process with occasional acute exacerbations, but on the whole tending to chronicity. The organisms are usually of low virulence. The disparity between the frequency of foci of infection and resulting disease is apparently largely due to natural resistance and immunity.

Symptoms.—These cannot be stated in detail as so many different structures may be involved. In general, however, there are some statements that can be made. (1) The condition is usually chronic and may vary much from time to time. Thus secondary arthritis is generally sub-acute or chronic, although there are occasional cases with an acute course and more with acute exacerbations. (2) The onset of symptoms may be determined by some intercurrent disease or debilitating condition. (3) The general health is apt to be affected. (4) Active reaction as shown by marked fever is unusual, as the process is too chronic. (5) There is a tendency to anæmia and disturbance of nutrition.

Diagnosis.—This cannot be stated in any exact terms. The first essential is the recognition of the important part that focal infection plays. Chronic arthritis and fibrositis are not primary maladies; they are secondary to infection somewhere. We know that if a patient has gonorrhœal arthritis there is a primary local process. The primary focus has often to be searched for; it may give no symptoms. This may involve the examination of many organs. If there is no localizing indication, the teeth and tonsils may be examined first. The nose and sinuses, bronchi, gall bladder, etc., have all to be considered. Duodenal cultures are important in the recognition of biliary tract infection. Nor is it safe to conclude that a focus when found is the responsible one. There may be multiple foci.

Prognosis.—Many factors enter into this, especially the resistance of the individual and the virulence of the organism. The degree of anatomical change must be considered, thus if extensive joint changes have occurred the removal of a focus of infection cannot alter these although it may prevent further damage. Naturally the earlier proper treatment is instituted the better the outlook.

Treatment.—(1) Removal of the cause, the focus of infection. This demands proper diagnosis and should not be done until this is as definite as possible. A man with mouth infection may have the real focus in his prostate. Caution should be exercised in the treatment of foci if the general symptoms are acute. (2) Vaccine therapy. In some cases this is of value and, if possible, an autogenous vaccine should be used. (3) Injection of non-specific protein, for example fifty millions of killed typhoid bacilli intravenously. This has proved useful, particularly in cases of chronic arthritis, but is to be employed with caution. (4) Helping the patient's powers of resistance by attention to the general health. Fresh air and sunlight, sufficient food, and proper treatment for anæmia, are indicated.

5. TERMINAL INFECTIONS

There is truth in the paradoxical statement that persons rarely die of the disease with which they suffer. Secondary *terminal* infections carry off many incurable cases. Flexner analyzed 255 cases of chronic renal and cardiac disease in which complete bacteriological examinations were made at autopsy. Excluding tuberculous infection, 213 gave positive and 42 negative results. The infections may be local or general. The former are extremely common, and are found in a large proportion of all cases of nephritis, arterio-sclerosis, heart disease, cirrhosis of the liver, and other chronic disorders. Affections of the serous membranes (acute pleurisy, pericarditis, or peritonitis), meningitis, and endocarditis are the most frequent lesions. It is perhaps safe to say that the majority of cases of advanced arterio-sclerosis and of nephritis succumb to these intercurrent infections. The infective agents are very varied. The streptococcus is the most common, but the pneumococcus, staphylococcus and gonococcus, and the proteus, pyocyaneus, and gas bacillus are also found. It is surprising in how many instances of arterio-sclerosis, of chronic heart disease, of nephritis, and particularly of cirrhosis of the liver in Flexner's series the fatal event was determined by an acute tuberculosis of the peritoneum or pleura.

The general terminal infections are somewhat less common. Of 85 cases of chronic renal disease in which Flexner found micro-organisms at autopsy, 38 exhibited general infections; of 48 cases of chronic cardiac disease, in 14 the distribution of bacteria was general. The blood-serum of persons suffering from advanced chronic disease was found by him to be less destructive to the staphylococcus aureus than normal human serum. Other diseases in which general terminal infection may occur are Hodgkin's disease, leukæmia, and chronic tuberculosis. And, lastly, probably of the same nature is the terminal entero-colitis so frequently met with in chronic disorders.

VI. ERYSIPELAS

Definition.—A special pyogenic infection caused by the *Streptococcus erysipelatis*, characterized by inflammation of the skin with fever and toxæmia.

Etiology.—Erysipelas is a widespread affection, endemic in most communities, and at certain seasons epidemic. We are as yet ignorant of the atmospheric or telluric influences which favor the diffusion of the poison.

It is particularly prevalent in the spring of the year. Of 2,012 cases collected by Anders, 1,214 occurred during the first five months of the year. April had the largest number of cases. The affection prevails extensively in old, ill-ventilated hospitals and institutions in which the sanitary conditions are defective. With improved sanitation the number of cases has materially diminished. It has been observed, however, to break out in new institutions under the most favorable hygienic circumstances. Erysipelas is both infectious and inoculable; but, except under special conditions, the poison is not very virulent and does not seem to act at any great distance. It can be conveyed by a third person. The virus attaches itself to the furniture, bedding, and walls of rooms in which patients have been confined.

The disposition to the disease is widespread, but the susceptibility is specially marked in the case of individuals with wounds or abrasions of any sort. Recently delivered women and persons who have been the subjects of surgical operations are particularly prone to it. A wound, however, is not necessary, and in the so-called idiopathic form, although it may be difficult to say that there was not a slight abrasion about the nose or lips, in very many cases there certainly is no observable external lesion. In some cases the infection apparently spreads through the tissues from the nasal cavity to the skin.

Chronic alcoholism, debility, and nephritis are predisposing agents. Certain persons show a special susceptibility to erysipelas, and it may recur in them repeatedly. There are instances, too, of a family predisposition.

The specific agent of the disease is a streptococcus growing in long chains, which is included under the group name *Streptococcus pyogenes,* with which *Streptococcus erysipelatis* appears to be identical. The fever and constitutional symptoms are due in great part to the toxins; the more serious visceral complications are the result of secondary metastatic infection.

Morbid Anatomy.—Erysipelas is a simple inflammation. In its uncomplicated forms there is seen, post mortem, little else than inflammatory œdema. Investigations have shown that the cocci are found chiefly in the lymph-spaces and most abundantly in the zone of spreading inflammation. In the uninvolved tissue beyond the inflamed margin they are to be found in the lymph-vessels, and it is here, according to Metschnikoff and others, that an active warfare goes on between the leucocytes and the cocci (phagocytosis). In more extensive and virulent forms there is usually suppuration.

Infarcts occur in the lungs, spleen, and kidneys, and there may be the general evidences of pyæmic infection. Some of the worst cases of malignant endocarditis are secondary to erysipelas; thus, of 23 cases, 3 occurred in connection with this disease. Septic pericarditis and pleuritis also occur. The disease may in rare cases extend to and involve the meninges. Pneumonia is not a very common complication. Acute nephritis is also met with; it is often ingrafted upon an old chronic trouble.

Symptoms.—The following description applies specially to erysipelas of the face and head; the form of the disease which is most common.

The *incubation* is variable, probably from three to seven days.

The stage of *invasion* is often marked by a rigor, and followed by a rapid rise in the temperature and other characteristics of an acute fever. When there is a local abrasion, the spot is slightly reddened; but if the disease is idiopathic, there is seen within a few hours slight redness over the bridge of the nose and on the cheeks. The swelling and tension of the skin increase and within twenty-four hours the external symptoms are well marked. The skin is smooth, tense, and œdematous. It looks red, feels hot, and the superficial layers of the epidermis may be lifted as small blebs. The patient complains of an unpleasant feeling of tension in the skin; the swelling rapidly increases; and during the second day the eyes are usually closed. The first-affected parts gradually become pale and less swollen as the disease extends at the periphery. When it reaches the forehead it progresss as an advancing ridge perfectly well defined and raised; and often, on palpation, hardened extensions can be felt beneath the skin which is not yet reddened. Even in a case of moderate severity, the face is enormously swollen, the eyes are closed, the lips greatly œdematous, the ears thickened, the scalp is swollen, and the patient's features are quite unrecognizable. The formation of blebs is common on the eyelids, ears, and forehead. The cervical lymph-glands are swollen, but are usually masked in the œdema of the neck. The temperature keeps high without marked remissions for four or five days and then defervescence takes place by crisis. Leucocytosis is present. The general condition of the patient varies much with his previous state of health. In old and debilitated persons, particularly in those addicted to alcohol, the constitutional depression from the outset may be very great. Delirium is present, the tongue becomes dry, the pulse feeble, and there is marked tendency to death from toxæmia. In the majority of cases, however, even with extensive lesions, the constitutional disturbance, considering the height of the fever, is slight. The mucous membrane of the mouth and throat may be swollen and reddened. The process may extend to the larynx, but the severe œdema of this part occasionally met with is commonly due to the extension of the inflammation from without inward.

There are cases in which the inflammation extends from the face to the neck, and over the chest, and may gradually migrate or wander over the greater part of the body (*E. migrans*).

The close relation between the erysipelas coccus and the pus organisms is shown by the frequency with which suppuration occurs in facial erysipelas. Small cutaneous abscesses are common about the cheeks and forehead and neck, and beneath the scalp large collections of pus may accumulate. Suppuration seems to occur more frequently in some epidemics than in others, and at the Philadelphia Hospital during one year nearly all the cases in the erysipelas wards presented local abscesses.

Complications.—Meningitis is rare. The cases in which death occurs with marked brain symptoms do not usually show, post mortem, meningeal affection. Pneumonia is an occasional complication. Ulcerative endocarditis and septicæmia are more common. Albuminuria is almost constant, particularly in persons over fifty. True nephritis is occasionally seen. Da Costa called attention to curious irregular returns of the fever which occur during convalescence without any aggravation of the local condition.

Diagnosis.—This rarely presents any difficulty. The mode of onset, the rapid rise in fever, and the characters of the local disease are distinctive.

Prognosis.—Healthy adults rarely die. The general mortality in hospitals is about 7 per cent.; in private practice about 4 per cent. (Anders.) In the new-born, when the disease attacks the navel, it is almost always fatal. In drunkards and in the aged erysipelas is a serious affection, and death may result either from the intensity of the fever or, more commonly, from toxæmia. The wandering or ambulatory erysipelas, which has a more protracted course, may cause death from exhaustion.

Treatment.—Isolation should be strictly carried out, particularly in hospitals. A practitioner in attendance upon a case of erysipelas should not attend cases of confinement.

The disease is self-limited and a large majority of the cases get well without any internal medication. The diet should be nutritious and light. Large amounts of water should be given. For the restlessness, delirium, and insomnia, chloral or the bromides may be given; or, if these fail, opium. When the fever is high the patient may be bathed or sponged, or, in private practice, if there is an objection to this, antipyrin or antifebrin may be given. Of internal remedies believed to influence the disease, the tincture of the perchloride of iron has been highly recommended but it is doubtful if any medicine, given internally, has a definite control over the course of the disease.

Antistreptococcic serum may be tried or, better still, an autogenous vaccine, with the use of which good results have been obtained.

Of local treatment, the injection of antiseptic solutions at the margin of the spreading areas has been much practised. Two-per-cent. solutions of phenol, corrosive sublimate (1 to 4,000), and the biniodide of mercury have been much used. The injection should be made not into but just a little beyond the border of the inflamed patch.

Of local applications, ichthyol (as a salve, 1 to 4 of lanolin), bichloride of mercury solution (1 to 5,000), salicylic acid (1 to 500), phenol in oil (5 per cent.), a saturated solution of magnesium sulphate, powdered stearate of zinc, collodion, or ichthyol in collodion (1 to 4), may be used. Painting the skin ahead of the advancing area with tincture of iodine is sometimes effectual. Perhaps as good an application as any is cold water, which was highly recommended by Hippocrates. If the disease involves the eyelids boric acid compresses should be applied and one or two drops of argyrol solution (10 per cent.) instilled several times a day.

VII. DIPHTHERIA

Definition.—A specific infectious disease, characterized by a local fibrinous exudate, usually upon the mucous membrane of the throat, and by constitutional symptoms due to toxins produced at the site of the lesion. The presence of the Klebs-Loeffler bacillus is the etiological criterion by which true diphtheria is distinguished from other forms of membranous inflammation.

Cases of angina, diagnosed as diphtheria, may be due to other organisms and to these the term diphtheroid is applied. Though usually milder, severe constitutional disturbance, and even paralysis, may follow these forms.

History.—Known in the East for centuries, and referred to in the Babylonian Talmud, it is not until the first century A. D. that an accurate clinical account appears in the writings of Aretæus. The paralysis of the palate was recognized by Ætius (sixth century A. D.). Throat pestilences are mentioned in the Middle Ages. Severe epidemics occurred in Europe in the sixteenth and seventeenth centuries, particularly in Spain. In England in the latter part of the eighteenth century it was described by Fothergill and Huxham, and in America by Bard. Washington died of the disease. Ballonius recognized the affection of the larynx and trachea in 1762, Home in Scotland described it as croup. The modern description dates from Bretonneau, of Tours (1826), who gave to it the name *diphthérite*. Throughout the nineteenth century it prevailed extensively in all known countries, and it is at present everywhere epidemic. After innumerable attempts, in which Klebs took a leading part, the organism was isolated by Loeffler. The toxin was determined by the work of Roux, Yersin, and others, and finally the antitoxin was discovered by Behring.

Etiology.—Everywhere endemic in large centres of population, the disease becomes at times epidemic. It is more prevalent on the continent of Europe than in Great Britain, and Ireland has less than other countries. In England and Wales in 1916, 5,358 persons died of the disease. In the registration area in the United States the death rate per 100,000 has fallen from 43 in 1900 to 16.5 in 1917. In the tropics it is not a very serious disease. Pandemics occur cyclically, at irregular intervals, under conditions as yet imperfectly known. Dry seasons seem to favor the disease, which shows an autumnal prevalence.

Modes of Infection.—The disease is highly infectious. The bacilli may be transmitted (*a*) from one person to another; few diseases have proved more fatal to physicians and nurses. (*b*) Infected articles may convey the bacilli, which may remain alive for many months; scores of well-attested instances have been recorded of this mode of transmission. (*c*) Persons suffering from atypical forms of diphtheria may convey the disease; nasal catarrh, membranous rhinitis, mild tonsillitis, otorrhœa may be caused by the diphtheria bacilli, and from each of these sources cases have been traced. (*d*) From the throats of healthy contacts—diphtheria carriers, persons who present no signs of the disease—the bacilli have been obtained by culture. (*e*) Even healthy children without any naso-pharyngeal catarrh, who have not been in contact with the disease, may harbor the bacilli. In 1,000 children from the New York tenements Shelley found 18 with virulent and 38 with non-virulent bacilli, and the percentage has been sometimes much higher. Long after recovery virulent bacilli have been isolated from the throat. It is important to bear in mind under *d* and *e* that it is only persons who harbor the virulent forms who are capable of transmitting the disease. In schools the interchange of articles, such as sweets, pencils, etc., and the habit which children have of putting everything into their mouths afford endless opportunities for the transmission of the disease. As Wesbrook remarked, diphtheria is transmitted usually by almost direct exchange of the flora of the nose and mouth. (*f*) Numerous epidemics have been traced to milk, since Power in 1878 determined this method of spread. Virulent bacilli have been found in milk, and Dean and Todd and Ashby found virulent organisms in the acquired lesions on the teats of cows. (*g*) A few instances of accidental infection from cultures and through animals are on record.

Predisposing Causes.—*Age* is the most important. Sucklings are not often attacked, but Jacobi saw three cases in the new-born. Early in the second year the disposition increases rapidly, and continues at its height until the fifth year. At Baginsky's clinic, Berlin, among 2,711 cases, 1,235 occurred from the second to the fifth years inclusive. In New York between 1891-1900 among the deaths 80.8 per cent. occurred under five, 17 per cent. between five and ten—figures which show the extraordinary preponderance of the disease among children. Girls are attacked in slightly larger numbers than boys. November, December, and January are the months of greatest prevalence in the United States; in London October and November. *Soil* and *altitude* have little or no influence; nor does race play an important rôle.

Individual susceptibility is a very special factor; not only do many of those exposed escape, but even those, too, in whose throats virulent bacilli lodge and grow. Probably about 70 per cent. of all persons have antitoxin in the blood and so are protected. The Schick reaction (intradermic injection of diphtheria toxin) is of great value in determining the presence of immunity. A negative reaction indicates the presence of antitoxin as when it is not present the toxin causes a reaction on the skin.

The Klebs-Loeffler Bacillus occurs in a large number of all suspected cases. It is found chiefly in the false membrane, and does not extend into the subjacent mucosa. The organisms are localized, and only a few penetrate into the interior. Post mortem the bacilli may be found in the blood and in the internal organs. Occasionally they are found in the blood during life. It may be the predominating or sole organism in the broncho-pneumonia so common in the disease. Outside the throat, the Klebs-Loeffler bacillus has been found in diphtheritic conjunctivitis, in otitis media, sometimes in wound diphtheria, upon the genitals, in fibrinous rhinitis, and in ulcerative endocarditis.

Morphological Characters.—The bacillus is non-motile, varies from 2 to 6 μ in length and from 0.3 to 0.8 μ in thickness. In appearance it is multiform, varying from short, rather sharply pointed rods to irregular bizarre forms, with one or both ends swollen, and staining more or less unevenly and intensely. Wesbrook recognized three main types—granular, barred, and solid staining. Branching forms are occasionally met with. The bacillus stains in sections or on the cover-glass by the Gram method.

The bacillus is very resistant, and cultures have been made from a bit of membrane preserved for five months in a dry cloth. Incorporated with dust and kept moist, the bacilli were still cultivable at the end of eight weeks; kept in a dried state they no longer grew at the end of this period (Ritter).

The Klebs-Loeffler bacillus has very varying grades of virulence down even to complete absence of pathogenic effects. The name pseudo-bacillus of diphtheria should not be given to this avirulent organism.

The Presence of the Klebs-Loeffler Bacillus in Non-membranous Angina and in Healthy Throats.—The bacillus has been isolated from cases which show nothing more than a simple catarrhal angina, of a mild type without any membrane, with diffuse redness, and perhaps huskiness and signs of catarrhal laryngitis. In other cases the anatomical picture may be that of a lacunar tonsillitis. The organisms may be met with in perfectly healthy throats (diphtheria carriers), particularly in persons in the same house, or the ward attendants and nurses in fever hospitals. Following an attack of diphtheria the bacilli may persist in the throat or nose after all the membrane has disappeared for weeks or months—even 15 months. In explanation of this persistence Councilman has called attention to the frequency with which the antrum is affected.

Toxins of the Klebs-Loeffler Bacillus.—Roux and Yersin showed that a fatal result following the inoculation with the bacillus was not caused by any extension of the micro-organisms within the body; and they were enabled in bouillon cultures to separate the poison from the bacilli. The toxin so separated killed with very much the same effects as those caused by the inoculation of the bacilli; the pseudo-membrane, however, is not formed.

Susceptible animals may be rendered immune from diphtheritic infection by injecting weakened cultures of the bacillus or, what is better, suitable doses of the diphtheria toxin. The result is a febrile reaction which soon passes away and leaves the animal less susceptible to the poison or the living bacilli. By repeating and gradually increasing the quantity of poison injected a high degree of immunity can be produced in large animals.

The Bacteria Associated with the Diphtheria Bacillus.—The most common is the streptococcus pyogenes. Others, in addition to the organisms constantly found in the mouth, are the pneumococcus, the bacillus coli, and the staphylococcus aureus and albus. Of these, probably the streptococcus pyogenes is the most important, as cases of general infection with this organism have been found in diphtheria. The suppuration in the lymph-glands and the broncho-pneumonia are usually caused by this organism.

Pseudo-Diphtheria Bacillus.—The Klebs-Loeffler bacillus varies very much in its virulence, and may exist in a form entirely devoid of pathogenic properties. This organism should not, however, be designated pseudo-diphtheria bacillus. The name should be confined to bacilli, which, though resembling the diphtheria bacillus morphologically and in their cultural reactions, do not produce diphtheria toxin. They may be found both in healthy and diseased throats. Another bacillus, showing certain cultural differences from the pseudo-diphtheria bacillus, has been repeatedly found in the conjunctival sac in health and disease (*B. xerosis*). *Hoffmann's Bacillus,* which is also spoken of as pseudo-diphtheria bacillus, is a common organism in the throats of healthy persons and is found also in cases of diphtheria; but how far it is responsible for pathological conditions is not settled. *Vincent's Bacillus* is a fusiform organism associated with a diphtheroid angina (Vincent's angina), which occurs in two forms: a membranous and an ulcerative and destructive. The fusiform bacilli have been found in healthy throats and also in association with true diphtheria.

Diphtheroid Inflammations.—Under the term *diphtheroid* may be grouped those membranous inflammations which are not associated with the Klebs-Loeffler bacillus. It is perhaps a more suitable designation than pseudo-diphtheria or secondary diphtheria. Streptococci and pneumococci are the organisms most often found. The name "diphtheritis" is best used in an anatomical sense to designate an inflammation of a mucous membrane or integumentary surface characterized by necrosis and a fibrinous exudate, whereas the term "diphtheria" should be limited to the disease caused by the Klebs-Loeffler bacillus. The proportion of cases of diphtheroid inflammation varies greatly in the different statistics. Of the observations made by Park and Beebe (5,611) in New York, 40 per cent. were diphtheroid. Figures from other sources do not show so high a percentage.

Conditions under Which the Diphtheroid Affection Occurs.—Of 450 cases (Park and Beebe), 300 occurred in the autumn months and 150 in the spring; 198 occurred in children from the first to the seventh year. In a large proportion of all the cases the disease develops in children, and can be differentiated from diphtheria proper only by the bacteriological examination. It may be simply an acute catarrhal angina with lacunar tonsillitis. Some of the cases are due to Hoffmann's bacillus, a few to Vincent's fusiform bacillus. The diphtheroid inflammations are particularly prone to develop in connection with the acute fevers.

(*a*) *Scarlet Fever.*—In a large proportion of the cases of angina in scarlet fever the Klebs-Loeffler bacillus is not present. Streptococci are usually found, but the angina is not always due to the streptococcus. Where diphtheria is prevalent and opportunities are favorable for exposure, a large proportion of the cases of membranous throats in scarlet fever may be genuine diphtheria.

(*b*) *Measles.*—Membranous angina is much less common in this disease. It occurred in 6 of the 450 diphtheroid cases in New York. Of 4 cases with severe membranous angina at the Boston City Hospital, only 1 presented the Klebs-Loeffler bacillus.

(*c*) *Whooping-cough* may be complicated with membranous angina. Escherich records 4 cases, the Klebs-Loeffler bacillus being found in all.

(*d*) *Typhoid Fever.*—Membranous inflammations in this disease are not very infrequent; they may occur in the throat, the pelvis of the kidney, the bladder, or the intestines. The complication may be caused by the Klebs-Loeffler bacillus, but it is frequently a streptococcus infection. Ernst Wagner has remarked upon the greater frequency of these membranous inflammations in typhoid fever when diphtheria is prevailing.

Clinical Features of the Diphtheroid Affection.—The cases, as a rule, are milder, and the mortality is low, only 2.5 per cent. in the 450 cases of Park and Beebe. The diphtheroid inflammations complicating the specific fevers are often very fatal, and a general streptococcus infection is not infrequent. As in the Klebs-Loeffler angina, there may be only a simple catarrhal process. In other instances the tonsils are covered with a creamy, pultaceous exudate, without any actual membrane. An important group may begin as a simple lacunar tonsillitis, while in others the entire fauces and tonsils are covered by a continuous membrane, and there is a foul sloughing angina with intense constitutional disturbance.

Are the diphtheroid cases contagious? General clinical experience warrants the statement that the membranous angina associated with the fevers is rarely communicated to other patients. The health department of New York does not keep the diphtheroid cases under supervision. Their investigation of the 450 diphtheroid cases seems to justify this conclusion. Park and Beebe say that "it did not seem that the secondary cases were any less liable to occur when the primary case was isolated than when it was not."

Sequelæ of the Diphtheroid Angina.—The usual mildness of the disease is in part, no doubt, due to the less frequent systemic invasion. Some of the worst forms of general streptococcus infection are, however, seen in this disease. There are no peculiarities, local or general, which are distinctive; and even the most extensive paralysis may follow an angina caused by it.

Morbid Anatomy.—Distribution of Membrane.—A definite membrane was found in 127 of the 220 fatal Boston cases, distributed as follows: tonsils, 65 cases; epiglottis, 60; larynx, 75; trachea, 66; pharynx, 51; mucous membrane of nares, 43; bronchi, 42; soft palate, including uvula, 13; œsophagus, 12; tongue, 9; stomach, 5; duodenum, 1; vagina, 2; vulva, 1; skin of ear, 1; conjunctiva, 1. An interesting point in the Boston investigation was the great frequency with which the accessory sinuses of the nose were found to be infected. In the fatal cases, the exudation is very extensive, involving the uvula, the soft palate, the posterior nares, and the lateral and posterior walls of the pharynx. These parts are covered with a dense pseudo-membrane, in places firmly adherent, in others beginning to separate. In extreme cases the necrosis is advanced and there is a gangrenous condition of the parts. The membrane is of a dirty greenish or gray color, and the tonsils and palate may be in a state of necrotic sloughing. The erosion may be deep enough in the tonsils to open the carotid artery, or a false aneurism may be produced in the deep tissues of the neck. The nose may be completely blocked by the membrane, which may extend into the conjunctivæ and through the Eustachian tubes into the middle ear. In laryngeal diphtheria the exudate in the pharynx may be extensive. In many cases it is slight upon the tonsils and fauces and abundant upon the epiglottis and the larynx, which may be completely occluded by false membrane. In severe cases the exudate extends into the trachea and to the bronchi of the third or fourth dimension.

In all these situations the membrane varies very much in consistence, depending greatly upon the stage at which death has taken place. If death has occurred early, it is firm and closely adherent; if late, it is soft, shreddy, and readily detached. When firmly adherent it is torn off with difficulty and leaves an abraded mucosa. In the most extreme cases, in which there is extensive necrosis, the parts look gangrenous. In fatal cases the lymphatic glands of the neck are enlarged, and there is a general infiltration of the tissues with serum; the salivary glands, too, may be swollen. In rare instances the membrane extends to the gullet and stomach.

On inspection of the larynx of a child dead of laryngeal diphtheria the *rima* is seen filled with mucus or with a shreddy material which, when washed off, leaves the mucosa covered by a thin grayish-yellow membrane, which may be uniform or in patches. It covers the ary-epiglottic folds and the true cords, and may be continued into the ventricles or even into the trachea. Above, it may involve the epiglottis. It varies much in consistency. In some fatal cases the exudation is not actually membranous, but rather friable and granular. The exudation may extend down the trachea and into the bronchi, and may pass beyond the epiglottis to the fauces. Usually it is readily stripped off from the mucous membrane of the larynx and leaves the swollen and injected mucosa exposed. The fibrinous material involves chiefly the epithelial lining and does not greatly infiltrate the subjacent tissues.

We owe largely to Wagner, Weigert, and more particularly to Oertel, our knowledge of the *histological changes*. The beginning of the lesion is due to the toxic action of the bacilli growing in the throat. The primary lesion is a necrosis and degeneration of the epithelial tissues. The organisms grow, not in the living, but in the necrotic tissues. The first step is necrosis of the epithelium, often preceded by active proliferation of the nuclei of the cells, which become changed into refractive hyaline masses. From the structures below an inflammatory exudate rich in fibrin factors is poured out, and fibrin is formed when this comes in contact with the necrotic epithelium.

The following are the important changes in the other organs:

HEART.—Fatty degeneration is found in a majority of the cases. It may precede the more advanced degeneration, in which the sarcous elements become swollen and converted into hyaline masses. There is a primary, acute, interstitial myositis, and also a form secondary to degeneration of the heart muscle, to which some of the cases of fibrous myocarditis may be due. Pericarditis and endocarditis are rare; endocarditis was present in 7 of 220 cases at the Boston City Hospital. The diphtheria bacilli have been found in the vegetations.

The PULMONARY COMPLICATIONS are the most important, and death is due to them as often as to the throat lesion. Broncho-pneumonia, or, as Councilman terms it, acinous pneumonia, is the most common, and was present in 131 of the 220 Boston cases. Acute lobar pneumonia is rare. The pneumococcus is the principal agent in producing the lung infection. The streptococci and the diphtheria bacilli are frequently met with.

Kidneys.—The lesions, which are due to the action of the toxins, not to the presence of bacteria, vary from simple degeneration to an intense nephritis. There is no specific type of lesion. Interstitial and glomerular nephritis are most common in the older subjects. Degenerative changes are present in a large proportion of all the fatal cases. The liver and spleen show the degenerative lesions of acute infections.

General infection is common, and is about equal with the streptococcus and the diphtheria bacillus. It occurs generally in the grave septic cases, in which type of cases the former organism is more frequently met with.

Symptoms.—The period of incubation is "from two to seven days, oftenest two." The initial symptoms are those of an ordinary febrile attack—slight chilliness, fever, and aching pains in the back and limbs. In mild cases these symptoms are trifling, and the child may not feel ill enough to go to bed. Usually the temperature rises within the first twenty-four hours to 102.5° or 103° F.; in severe cases to 104° F. In young children there may be convulsions at the outset.

Pharyngeal Diphtheria.—In a typical case there is at first redness of the fauces, and the child complains of slight difficulty in swallowing. The membrane first appears upon the tonsils, and it may be a little difficult to distinguish a patchy diphtheritic pellicle from the exudate of the tonsillar crypts. The pharyngeal mucous membrane is reddened, and the tonsils themselves are swollen. By the third day the membrane has covered the tonsils, the pillars of the fauces, and perhaps the uvula, which is thickened and œdematous, and may fill completely the space between the swollen tonsils. The membrane may extend to the posterior wall of the pharynx. At first grayish-white in color, it changes to a dirty gray, often to a yellow-white. It is firmly adherent, and when removed leaves a bleeding, slightly eroded surface, which is soon covered by fresh exudate. The glands in the neck are swollen, and may be tender. The general condition of a patient in a case of moderate severity is usually good; the temperature not very high, in the absence of complications ranging from 102° to 103° F. The pulse range is from 100 to 120. The local condition of the throat is not of great severity, and the constitutional depression is slight. The symptoms gradually abate, the swelling of the neck diminishes, the membranes separate, and from the seventh to the tenth day the throat becomes clear and convalescence sets in.

Clinically atypical forms are common, and we follow Koplik's division:

(*a*) There may be no local manifestation of membrane, but a simple catarrhal angina associated sometimes with a croupy cough. The detection in these cases of the Klebs-Loeffler bacillus can alone determine the diagnosis. Such cases are of great moment, inasmuch as they may communicate the severer disease to other children.

(*b*) There are cases in which the tonsils are covered by a pultaceous exudate, not a consistent membrane.

(*c*) Cases presenting a punctate form of membrane, isolated, and usually on the surface of the tonsils.

(*d*) Cases which begin and often run their entire course with the local picture of a typical lacunar amygdalitis. They may be mild, and the local exudate may not extend, but in other cases there is rapid development of membrane, and extension of the disease to the pharynx and the nose, with severe septic and constitutional symptoms.

(*e*) Under the term "latent diphtheria" Heubner has described cases, usually secondary, occurring chiefly in hospital practice, in young persons the subject of wasting affections, such as rickets and tuberculosis. There are fever, naso-pharyngeal catarrh, and gastro-intestinal disturbances. Diphtheria may not be suspected until severe laryngeal complications develop, or the condition may not be determined until autopsy.

Systemic Infection.—The constitutional disturbance in mild diphtheria is very slight. There are instances, too, of extensive local disease without grave systemic symptoms. As a rule, the general features bear a definite relation to the severity of the local disease. There are rare instances in which from the outset the constitutional prostration is extreme, the pulse frequent and small, the fever high, and the nervous phenomena are pronounced; the patient may sink in two or three days overwhelmed by the intensity of the toxæmia. There are cases of this sort in which the exudate in the throat may be slight, but usually the nasal symptoms are pronounced. The temperature may be very slightly raised or even subnormal. More commonly the severe systemic symptoms appear at a later date when the pharyngeal lesion is at its height. They are constantly present in extensive disease, and when there is a sloughing, fetid condition. The lymphatic glands become greatly enlarged; the pallor is extreme; the face has an ashen-gray hue; the pulse is rapid and feeble, and the temperature sinks below normal. In the most aggravated forms there are gangrenous processes in the throat, and in rare instances, extensive sloughing of the tissues of the neck.

Escherich accounts for the discrepancy sometimes observed between the severity of the constitutional disturbance and the intensity of the local process, by assuming varying degrees of susceptibility to the diphtheria bacillus on the one hand, and to its toxin on the other hand. With high local susceptibility to the action of the bacillus, with little general susceptibility to the toxin, there is extensive local exudate with mild constitutional symptoms, or *vice versa,* severe systematic disturbance with limited local inflammation.

A leucocytosis is present in diphtheria. Morse does not think it of any prognostic value, since it is present and may be pronounced in mild cases.

Nasal Diphtheria.—In cases of pharyngeal diphtheria the Klebs-Loeffler bacillus is found on the mucous membrane of the nose and in the secretions, even when no membrane is present, but it may apparently produce two affections similar enough locally but widely differing in their general features.

In *membranous or fibrinous rhinitis,* a very remarkable affection seen usually in children, the nares are occupied by thick membranes, but there is an entire absence of any constitutional disturbance. Ravenel collected 77 cases, in 41 of which a bacteriological examination was made, in 33 the Klebs-Loeffler bacillus being present. All the cases ran a benign course, and in all but a few the membrane was limited to the nose, and the constitutional symptoms were either absent or very slight. Remarkable and puzzling features are that the disease runs a benign course, and that infection of other children in the family is extremely rare.

On the other hand, *nasal diphtheria* is apt to present a most malignant type of the disease. The infection may be primary in the nose, and in one case there was otitis media, and the Klebs-Loeffler bacillus was separated from the discharge before the condition of nasal diphtheria was suspected. While some cases are of mild character, others are very malignant, and the constitutional symptoms most profound. The glandular inflammation is usually very intense, owing, as Jacobi points out, to the great richness of the nasal mucosa in lymphatics. From the nose the inflammation may extend through the tear-ducts to the conjunctivæ and into the antra.

Laryngeal Diphtheria (*Membranous Croup*).—With a very large proportion of all the cases of membranous laryngitis the Klebs-Loeffler bacillus is associated; in a smaller number other organisms, particularly the streptococcus, are found. Of 286 cases in which the disease was confined to the larynx or bronchi, in 229 the Klebs-Loeffler bacilli were found. In 57 they were not present, but 17 of these cultures were unsatisfactory (Park and Beebe). The streptococcus cases are more likely to be secondary to other acute diseases.

Symptoms.—Naturally, the clinical symptoms are almost identical in the non-specific and specific forms of membranous laryngitis.

The affection begins like an acute laryngitis with slight hoarseness and rough cough, to which the term croupy has been applied. After these symptoms have lasted for a day or two with varying intensity, the child suddenly becomes worse, usually at night, and there are signs of impeded respiration. At first the difficulty in breathing is paroxysmal, due probably to more or less spasm of the muscles of the glottis. Soon the dyspnœa becomes continuous, inspiration and expiration become difficult, particularly the latter, and with the inspiratory movement the epigastrium and lower intercostal spaces are retracted. The voice is husky and may be reduced to a whisper. The color gradually changes and the imperfect äeration of the blood is shown in the lividity of the lips and finger-tips. Restlessness comes on and the child tosses from side to side, vainly trying to get breath. Occasionally, in a severer paroxysm, portions of membrane are coughed out. The fever in membranous laryngitis is rarely very high and the condition of the child is usually good at the time of the onset. The pulse is always increased in frequency and is small if cyanosis be present. In favorable cases the dyspnœa is not very urgent, the color of the face remains good, and after one or two paroxysms the child goes to sleep and wakes in the morning, perhaps without fever and feeling comfortable. The attack may recur the following night with greater severity. In unfavorable cases the dyspnœa becomes more and more urgent, the cyanosis deepens, the child, after a period of intense restlessness, sinks into a semi-comatose state, and death finally occurs from poisoning of the nerve centres. In other cases the onset is less sudden and is preceded by a longer period of indisposition. As a rule, there are pharyngeal symptoms. The constitutional disturbance may be more severe, the fever higher, and there may be swelling of the glands of the neck. Inspection of the fauces may show the presence of false membranes on the pillars or on the tonsils. Bacteriological examination can alone determine whether these are due to the Klebs-Loeffler bacillus or to the streptococcus. Fagge held that non-contagious membranous croup may spread upward from the larynx just as diphtheritic inflammation is in the habit of spreading downward from the fauces. Ware, of Boston, whose essay on croup is one of the most solid contributions to the subject, reported the presence of exudate in the fauces in 74 out of 75 cases of croup. These observations were made prior to 1840, during periods in which diphtheria was not epidemic to any extent in Boston. In protracted cases pulmonary symptoms may occur, which are sometimes due to the difficulty in expelling the muco-pus from the tubes; in others, the false membrane extends into the trachea and even into the bronchial tubes. During the paroxysm the vesicular murmur is scarcely audible, but the laryngeal stridor may be loudly communicated along the bronchial tubes.

Diphtheria of Other Parts.—Primary diphtheria occurs occasionally in the *conjunctiva*. It follows in some instances the affection of the nasal mucous membrane. Some of the cases are severe and serious, but it has been shown that the diphtheria bacilli may be present in a conjunctivitis catarrhal in character, or associated with only slight croupous deposits.

Diphtheria of the *external auditory meatus* is seen when a diphtheritic otitis media has extended through the tympanic membrane.

Diphtheria of the *skin* is most frequently seen in the severer forms of pharyngeal diphtheria, in which the membrane extends to the mouth and lips, and invades the adjacent portions of the skin of the face. The skin about the anus and genitals may also be attacked. Pseudo-membranous inflammation is not uncommon on ulcerated surfaces and wounds. In very many of these cases it is a streptococcus infection, but in a majority, perhaps, in which the patient is suffering with diphtheria, the Klebs-Loeffler bacillus will be found in the fibrinous exudate. As proposed by Welch, the term "wound diphtheria" should be limited to infection of a wound by the Klebs-Loeffler bacillus. Paralysis may follow wound diphtheria. Pseudo-membranous inflammations of wounds are caused more frequently by other micro-organisms, particularly the streptococcus pyogenes, than by the Klebs-Loeffler bacillus. The fibrinous membrane so common in the neighborhood of the tracheotomy wound in diphtheria is rarely associated with the Klebs-Loeffler bacillus. Diphtheria of the genitals is occasionally seen.

Complications and Sequelæ.—Of local complications, hæmorrhage from the nose or throat may occur in the severe ulcerative cases. Skin rashes are not infrequent, particularly the diffuse erythema. Occasionally there is urticaria and in the severe cases purpura. Fatal cases almost invariably show capillary bronchitis with broncho-pneumonia and large patches of collapse, or the septic particles may reach the bronchi and excite gangrenous processes which may lead to severe and fatal hæmorrhage. Jaundice, usually a feature of the toxæmia, is rarely of serious import. Local gangrene may occur.

Albuminuria, present in all severe cases, is alarming only when the albumin is in considerable quantity and associated with epithelial or blood casts. *Nephritis* may appear quite early, setting in occasionally with complete suppression of urine. In comparison with scarlet fever the renal changes lead less frequently to general dropsy. In rare instances there may be coma, and even convulsions, without albumin in the urine, and without dropsy.

Of the sequelæ, *paralysis* is by far the most important. It can be experimentally produced in animals by the inoculation of the toxins. The process is a toxic neuritis, due to the absorption of the toxin which probably travels in the perineural channels of the cranial nerves to the centres in the medulla. The generalized neuritis, usually a later manifestation, appears to be part of a systemic toxæmia through the blood stream. The proportion of the cases in which it occurs ranges from 10 to 15 and even to 20 per cent. It usually comes on in the second or third week of convalescence. It may follow very mild cases; indeed, the local lesion may be so trifling that the onset of the paralysis alone calls attention to the true nature of the trouble. It is proportionately less frequent in children than in adults. J. D. Rolleston's study of the subject indicates that the early use of antitoxin diminishes the liability to paralysis. In 494 cases collected by Woodhead, the palate was involved in 155, the ocular muscles in 197, in 10 other muscles. Ninety-one of the patients died.

Of the local paralyses the most common is that which affects the *palate.* This gives a nasal character to the voice, and, owing to a return of liquids through the nose, causes a difficulty in swallowing. The palate is seen to be relaxed and motionless, and the sensation in it is also much impaired. The affection may extend to the constrictors of the pharynx, and deglutition become embarrassed. Within two or three weeks or even a shorter time the paralysis disappears. In many cases the affection of the palate is only part of a general neuritis. Of other local forms perhaps the most common are paralyses of the *eye-muscles,* intrinsic and extrinsic. There may be strabismus, ptosis, and loss of power of accommodation. Facial paralysis is rare. The neuritis may be confined to the nerves of one limb, though more commonly the legs or the arms are affected together. Very often with the palatal paralysis is associated a weakness of the legs without definite palsy but with loss of the knee-jerk.

The *multiple* form of diphtheritic neuritis may begin with the palatal affection, or with loss of power of accommodation and loss of the tendon reflexes. This last is an important sign, which may occur early, but is not necessarily followed by other symptoms of neuritis. There is paraplegia, which may be complete or involve only the extensors of the feet. The paralysis may extend and involve the arms and face and render the patient entirely helpless. The muscles of respiration may be spared. Sensory is less common than motor disturbance.

Heart.—Irregularity is common and was present in 60 per cent. of the Boston cases of White and Smith. A murmur at the apex or base of the heart is present in 94 per cent. of all cases. This means, of course, that a majority of young children with fever have a heart murmur. Only a few cases of diphtheria have serious heart symptoms, 36 out of the 946 cases specially studied. Rapid action of the heart with gallop rhythm and epigastric pain and tenderness are serious symptoms. The cases in which the pulse drops from 110 to 40 or 30 are usually very serious. Some are due to heart block. The heart symptoms are more common in the second or third week of the disease, and fatal dilatation may come on as late as the sixth or seventh week. It seems probable that the heart weakness is due to degeneration of the muscle. Possibly in some of the cases there is degeneration of the vagus, a view which is supported by the frequency of paralysis of the palate with vomiting and epigastric pain and tenderness. Experimental evidence is against the vasomotor centre being impaired.

Diagnosis.—The presence of the Klebs-Loeffler bacillus is regarded by bacteriologists as the sole criterion of true diphtheria, and as this organism may be associated with all grades of throat affections, from a simple catarrh to a sloughing, gangrenous process, it is evident that in many instances there will be a striking discrepancy between the clinical and the bacteriological diagnosis.

The bacteriological diagnosis is simple. The plan adopted by the New York Health Department is a model which may be followed with advantage in other cities. Outfits for making cultures, consisting of a box containing a tube of blood-serum and a sterilized swab in a test-tube, are distributed at convenient points. The directions are as follows: "The patient should be placed in a good light, and, if a child, properly held. In cases where it is possible to get a good view of the throat, depress the tongue and rub the cotton swab gently but freely against any visible exudate. In other cases, including those in which the exudate is confined to the larynx, avoiding the tongue, pass the swab far back and rub it freely against the mucous membrane of the pharynx and tonsils. Without laying the swab down, withdraw the cotton plug from the culture-tube, insert the swab, and rub that portion of it which has touched the exudate gently but thoroughly all over the surface of the blood-serum. Do not push the swab into the blood-serum, nor break the surface in any way. Then replace the swab in its own tube, plug both tubes, put them in the box, and return the culture outfit at once to the station from which it was obtained." The culture-tubes which have been inoculated are kept in an incubator at 37° C. for twelve hours and are then ready for examination. Some prefer a method by which the material from the throat collected on a sterile swab, or on small pieces of sterilized sponge, is sent to the laboratory.

An immediate diagnosis may be possible by making a smear preparation of the exudate. The Klebs-Loeffler bacilli may be present in sufficient numbers, and may be quite characteristic. In this connection may be given the following statement by Park, who has had an exceptional experience: "The examination by a competent bacteriologist of the bacterial growth in a blood-serum tube which has been properly inoculated and kept for fourteen hours at the body temperature can be thoroughly relied upon in cases where there is visible membrane in the throat, if the culture is made during the period in which the membrane is forming, and no antiseptic, especially no mercurial solution, has lately been applied. In cases in which the disease is confined to the larynx or bronchi, surprisingly accurate results can be obtained from cultures, but in a certain proportion of cases no diphtheria bacilli will be found in the first culture, and yet will be abundantly present in later cultures. We believe, therefore, that absolute reliance for a diagnosis can not be placed upon a single culture from the pharynx in purely laryngeal cases."

Where a bacteriological examination can not be made, the practitioner must regard as suspicious all forms of throat affections in children, and carry out measures of isolation and disinfection. In this way alone can serious errors be avoided. It is not, of course, in the severer forms of membranous angina that mistake is likely to occur, but in the various lighter forms, many of which are in reality due to the Klebs-Loeffler bacillus.

A large proportion of the cases of diphtheroid inflammation of the throat are due to the streptococcus pyogenes. They are usually milder, and the liability to general infection is less intense; still, in scarlet fever and other specific fevers some of the most virulent cases of throat disease which we see, with intense systemic infection, are caused by this micro-organism. These streptococcus cases are probably much less numerous than the figures given would indicate. The more careful examinations in the diphtheria pavilions of hospitals, particularly in Europe, have shown that in the large majority of cases admitted the Klebs-Loeffler bacillus is present. The question of the diagnosis between scarlet fever with severe angina and diphtheria is discussed in the section on scarlet fever.

Prognosis.—The outlook in any case depends on the promptness and thoroughness with which antitoxin treatment is carried out. In hospital practice the mortality was formerly from 30 to 50 per cent. In the Boston City Hospital the death-rate between 1888 and 1894 was only once below 40 per cent., and in 1892 and 1893 rose to nearly 50 per cent. Following the introduction of antitoxin from 1895 to 1912 the death-rate has not once been above 15 per cent., and in 6,080 recent cases has been 7.8 per cent. (McCollom). In country places the disease may display an appalling virulence. In cases of ordinary severity the outlook is usually good. Death results from involvement of the larynx, septic infection, sudden heart-failure, diphtheritic paralysis, occasionally from uræmia, and sometimes from broncho-pneumonia occurring during convalescence. Of late years the mortality has been steadily falling.

Prophylaxis.—Isolation of the sick, disinfection of the clothing and of everything that has come in contact with the patient, careful scrutiny of the milder cases of throat disorder, and more stringent surveillance in the period of convalescence are the essential measures to prevent the spread of the disease. Suspected cases in families or schools should be at once isolated or removed to a hospital for infectious disorders. When a death has occurred from diphtheria, the body should be wrapped in a sheet which has been soaked in a corrosive-sublimate solution (1 to 2,000), and placed in a closely sealed coffin. The funeral should always be private.

In cases of well-marked diphtheria these precautions are usually carried out, but the chief danger is from the milder cases, particularly the ambulatory form, in which the disease has perhaps not been suspected. But from such patients mingling with susceptible children the disease is often conveyed. The healthy children in a family in which diphtheria exists may carry the disease. The question of the influence of isolation hospitals on the spread of the disease has been solved in Boston, a city which has suffered terribly from diphtheria. The ratio of mortality per 10,000 living in 1893 was 11+, and in 1894 it was 18+. In 1895 the infectious pavilion was opened. Prior to that year only about 10 per cent. of the reported cases were treated in hospital; in succeeding years 50 per cent. were treated in hospital. In 1898 the mortality per 10,000 had fallen to 3, and in 1912 it was 1.5.

A very important matter relates to the period of convalescence as after all the membrane has cleared away, virulent bacilli may persist in the throat from periods ranging from six weeks to six months, or even longer. The disease may be communicated by these *carriers* and they should be isolated and the throat carefully treated, but there are cases very resistant to all forms of throat antiseptics. Antitoxin may be applied locally to the throat and spraying the throat and nose with a culture of lactic acid bacilli is sometimes efficient. Among other measures is the use of kaolin, which is blown over the nasal surfaces every two hours. The application of iodized phenol (phenol 60, iodine crystals 20, glycerine 20) every second day is sometimes effectual. In some patients the organisms are deep in the tonsils and their removal may be advisable.

It cannot be too strongly emphasized that the important elements in the prophylaxis of diphtheria are the rigid scrutiny of the milder types of throat affection, and the thorough isolation and disinfection of the individual patients. During an epidemic there should be repeated examinations made of all those exposed to infection to detect carriers.

Careful attention should be given to the throats and mouths of children, particularly to the teeth and tonsils. Swollen and enlarged tonsils should be removed. Cats and dogs may carry infection and should be excluded from contact with patients. In persons exposed, the antiseptic mouth washes, such as corrosive sublimate (1 to 10,000), hydrogen peroxide, or swabbing the throat with a diluted Loeffler's solution, should be employed. Physicians and nurses should wear gowns and caps, and cover the nose and mouth with gauze.

IMMUNIZATION.—The giving of antitoxin as a preventive measure has an important place. Its value is well shown in the children's hospitals in which it is given as a routine prophylactic measure. The usual dose for adults is 1,000 units, for older children 750 units, and for children under two years of age 500 units. The immunity lasts about three weeks. The same precautions should be taken as in giving antitoxin to those with the disease.

Toxin-antitoxin inoculations have been used in those found susceptible by the Schick test. Three injections are given at weekly intervals. Park and Zingher suggest that it would be well to immunize susceptible children at the beginning of the second year of age to protect them during the years of greatest prevalence. The immunity may last for two years.

Treatment.—The important points are hygienic measures to prevent the spread of the malady, local treatment of the throat to destroy the bacilli, medication, general or specific, to counteract the effects of the toxins, and, lastly, to meet the complications and sequelæ.

(*a*) HYGIENIC MEASURES.—The patient should be in a room from which the carpets, curtains, and superfluous furniture have been removed. The temperature should be about 68°, and thorough ventilation should be secured. The air may be kept moist by a kettle or a steam-atomizer. If possible, only the nurse, the child's mother, and the doctor should come in contact with the patient. During the visit the physician should wear a gown and cap, and on leaving the room he should thoroughly wash his hands and face in corrosive sublimate solution. The strictest quarantine should be employed against other members in the house.

(*b*) LOCAL TREATMENT.—In mild cases the throat symptoms are alone prominent. Local treatment should be carried out, taking especial care to avoid mechanical injury to the tissues. Since the introduction of antitoxin, this is much less important than formerly and many patients do perfectly well with little or no local treatment. There are a large number of solutions recommended which may be employed locally by a swab, by spraying, or by irrigation. In the use of the last, the temperature of the solution should be as hot as is comfortable. In all cases the frequency of local treatment should be determined by the local lesion. Of the solutions to be applied by swabbing, the following are examples: Loeffler's solution: Menthol, 10 grams dissolved in toluol to 36 c. c.; Liq. ferri sesquichlorati, 4 c. c.; alcohol absol., 60 c. c. Another solution is: The tincture of the perchloride of iron, ʒ iss (6 c. c.), glycerine, ℥i (30 c. c.), water, ℥i (30 c. c.) with ♏ xv (1 c. c.) of phenol. Boric acid and peroxide of hydrogen may be used.

Boracic acid solutions, peroxide of hydrogen, Dobell's solution, and bichloride of mercury (1-2000) may be employed in the form of sprays, but in many cases the use of irrigations is the most satisfactory. This should always be done very gently with the patient lying on the side. Either a saline solution or a 2 per cent. boric acid solution is satisfactory.

Nasal diphtheria requires prompt and thorough disinfection of the passages. Jacobi recommends chloride of sodium, saturated boric acid, or 1 part of bichloride of mercury, 35 of chloride of sodium, and 1,000 of water, or the 1-per-cent. solution of phenol. Loeffler's solution may be diluted and applied with a syringe or spray. To be effectual the injection must be properly given. The nozzle of the syringe should be passed horizontally, not vertically; otherwise the fluid will return through the same nostril.

When the larynx becomes involved, a steam tent may be arranged, so that the child may breathe an atmosphere saturated with moisture. When the signs of obstruction are marked there should be no delay in the performance of intubation or tracheotomy. The choice between these must depend on the circumstances in each case. Intubation may be regarded as the operation of choice in the majority of cases. Tracheotomy is preferable in adults and may be the operation of necessity. The patient requires more skilful care after intubation than after tracheotomy.

Hot applications to the neck are usually very grateful, particularly to young children, though in the case of older children and adults the ice poultices are to be preferred.

(*c*) General Measures.—Every effort should be made to nourish the patient. The food should be liquid—milk, beef juices, barley water, ice cream, albumen water, and soups. If there is difficulty in swallowing, these should be given by a tube. The patient should be encouraged to drink water freely. If there is difficulty in taking it by mouth, it should be given by the bowel or subcutaneously. The bowels should be freely opened, for which a calomel and saline purge is usually best. When the pharyngeal involvement is very great and swallowing painful, a 5 per cent. glucose solution can be given by the bowel.

Medicines given internally are of little avail, but there is a widespread belief that forms of mercury are beneficial. The tincture of the perchloride of iron is also warmly recommended. We must rely on general measures of feeding and stimulation to support the strength. For the circulation the early giving of antitoxin is the best preventive of trouble. When symptoms arise, circulatory stimulants, such as digitalis, camphor, and epinephrine are indicated. Saline solution by rectum or subcutaneously is useful.

(*d*) ANTITOXIN TREATMENT.—As the years go on experience has shown that, thoroughly carried out, this method of treatment is both safe and efficacious. There are no reasonable grounds for skepticism on the part of intelligent practitioners, and still less on the part of those in charge of the hospitals for infectious diseases.

The principle of action depends on the circumstance that the blood-serum of an animal rendered immune, when introduced into another animal, protects it from infection with the diphtheria bacilli, and has also an important curative influence upon diphtheria, whether artificially given to animals, or spontaneously acquired by man. In the preparation of the serum a uniform standard strength is procured. The antitoxin unit is the amount of antitoxin which, injected into a guinea-pig of 250 grams in weight, neutralizes 100 times the minimum fatal dose of toxin of standard strength.

Dosage.—This is one of the most important questions relating to the use of the antitoxin. J. H. McCollom, of the Boston City Hospital, who probably had a richer experience with the disease than any man in the United States, insisted that the guiding practice in the use of the antitoxin is to give it until the characteristic effects are produced, whether 4,000 or 70,000 units be required for this result. He very rightly said that in the case of a patient ill with diphtheria there is no way of estimating the quantity of toxin generated by the membrane, and therefore one must administer the agent until the characteristic effect is produced—viz., the shriveling of the membrane, the diminution of the nasal discharge, the correction of the fetid odor, and a general improvement in the condition of the patient. No case, he says, in the acute stage should be considered hopeless. "When one sees a patient in whom the intubation tube has been repeatedly clogged, when the hopeless condition of the patient changes for the better after the administration of 50,000 units, one can not help but be convinced of the importance of giving large doses of antitoxin in the very severe and apparently hopeless cases. In the majority of instances these large doses are not required, particularly if the patients are seen early in the attack, 4,000 to 6,000 units being enough to produce the characteristic effect on the membrane." The initial dose in ordinary cases should be from 3,000 to 10,000 units and the result must determine the frequency of repetition. In severe cases and in laryngeal diphtheria the first dose should be from 10,000 to 15,000 units, repeated in six hours. The danger is in giving too small and not too large a dose.

Administration.—Antitoxin may be injected subcutaneously, intramuscularly or intravenously. The last is advisable in severe cases. Intramuscular is better than subcutaneous injection. The skin and needle should be thoroughly clean.

Favorable effects are seen in the improvement in both the local and general condition. The swelling of the fauces subsides, the membrane begins to disappear, the temperature falls, and the pulse becomes slower.

Untoward Effects.—"Serum Disease."—This may appear in any normal individual and is due to the serum and not to the antitoxin. Following the injection after a varying interval, which varies from one to eighteen days, but is usually between seven and ten days, a local reaction appears which may be accompanied by general symptoms. The site of injection shows œdema, urticaria or erythema, which may become more or less general. Malaise, vomiting, fever, adenitis, albuminuria, and arthralgia may accompany this. The symptoms are usually not severe and disappear in three or four days. Calcium lactate (gr. xv, 1 gm. three times a day) may be given as a prophylactic or when the symptoms have appeared. There is another reaction which is much more serious. In individuals who have been given antitoxin previously, even at a long interval—who have been sensitized—in some who have had asthma and in some of those who are affected by the smell or proximity of horses, an acute dangerous condition may be caused by the injection of serum—*anaphylaxis*. This comes on very suddenly and with acute symptoms, among which are extreme distress, dyspnœa, cyanosis, œdema, collapse, respiratory failure and convulsions; death may follow rapidly. Fortunately this occurs rarely, but its possibility should be kept in mind, and before giving antitoxin the patient should be asked as to a history of asthma, an idiosyncrasy to horses and previous administration of antitoxin. This must be kept in mind in the case of patients who have a relapse, as if seven days have elapsed since the first dose the patient may be sensitized. If there is any reason to suspect the possibility of a reaction, the patient should be tested by the administration of two or three drops of antitoxin, which will not give a dangerous reaction. If he is susceptible a reaction usually occurs in an hour, but it is safer to wait three hours. The skin reaction may also be tried (Moss), but this demands twenty-four hours, too long to wait if the diphtheria is severe. If the patients are sensitive and the need of antitoxin is great, small doses (2 to 4 c. c.) should be given at hourly intervals. In the absence of reaction it is safe to give the usual dose, for a sensitized individual, after receiving a small dose, is refractory to larger doses some hours later. Children seem to be much less liable to sensitization than adults. If anaphylaxis should occur, morphia (gr. 1/4, 0.016 gm.) and atropine (gr. 1-100, 0.0006 gm.) hypodermically should be given at once. Artificial respiration should be done if there is respiratory failure.

Results.—Of 183,256 cases treated in 150 cities previous to the serum period, the mortality was 38.4 per cent. Since the introduction of serum among 132,548 cases, there was a mortality of 14.6 per cent. Leaving out those not treated with the serum, the mortality was 9.8 per cent. (Edwin Rosenthal).

Convalescence.—This demands special care, particularly if there are signs of cardiac disturbance. In this event the patient should be kept absolutely at rest and this may be necessary for a long period. Nourishment should be given freely, strychnine administered in full doses, and iron with arsenic if there is anæmia. If swallowing becomes difficult it is wise to use the stomach tube for feeding. With the post-diphtheritic paralysis the patients should be kept in bed, fed liberally and given strychnine hypodermically. Antitoxin is valuable in doses of 1,000 to 3,000 units daily. In the chronic forms with muscular wasting, electricity and massage should be used. The patient should not be discharged from quarantine until two successive cultures from the throat and nose, two days apart, have been negative.

VIII. THE PNEUMONIAS AND PNEUMOCOCCIC INFECTIONS

A variety of diseases are caused by the pneumococcus, among which lobar and lobular pneumonia are the most important. Various inflammatory affections of the lungs may be caused by other organisms, but the pneumococcus plays the important rôle in the common lobar pneumonia and in the ordinary broncho-pneumonia. It may set up also many local affections and is the cause of many terminal infections in chronic diseases.

A. LOBAR PNEUMONIA

(*Croupous or Fibrinous Pneumonia, Lung Fever*)

Definition.—An infection caused by the pneumococcus, characterized by inflammation of the lungs, a toxæmia of varying intensity and a fever which usually terminates by crisis. Secondary infective processes are common.

History.—The disease was known to Hippocrates and the old Greek physicians, by whom it was confounded with pleurisy. Among the ancients, Aretæus gave a remarkable description. "Ruddy in countenance, but especially the cheeks; the white of the eyes very bright and fatty; the point of the nose flat; the veins in the temples and neck distended; loss of appetite; pulse, at first, large, empty, very frequent, as if forcibly accelerated; heat indeed, externally, feeble, and more humid than natural, but, internally, dry and very hot, by means of which the breath is hot; there is thirst, dryness of the tongue, desire of cold air, aberration of mind; cough mostly dry, but if anything be brought up it is a frothy phlegm, or slightly tinged with bile, or with a very florid tinge of blood. The blood-stained is of all others the worst." At the end of the seventeenth and the beginning of the eighteenth century Morgagni and Valsalva made many accurate clinical and anatomical observations on the disease. Our modern knowledge dates from Laënnec (1819), whose masterly description of the physical signs and morbid anatomy left very little for subsequent observers to add or modify.

Incidence.—One of the most widespread and fatal of all acute diseases, pneumonia has become the "Captain of the Men of Death," to use the phrase applied by John Bunyan to consumption. In England and Wales in 1916 there were 37,916 deaths from this cause. In the United States in the registration area in 1917 there were 112,821 deaths, a rate of 149.8 per 100,000; of these 65,438 were due to lobar pneumonia, 37,947 to broncho-pneumonia, and 9,436 were unclassified. It is a disease of cities, in the overcrowded districts of which there has been an increase of late, particularly in America.

Careful studies of tropical pneumonia have been made at Panama. At the Ancon Hospital among 574 cases the mortality was 37 per cent.; among the mixed races, natives of the Isthmus, from 50 to 60 per cent. The same high death rate prevails at the Colon Hospital. Among the natives employed in the Transvaal mines the disease was very fatal, killing a larger number than any other disease, tuberculosis coming second. It is more particularly among the natives during the first month of work in the mines, 443 per thousand of all deaths during this period. There is a marked decline in succeeding periods of six months—from 16 per thousand in the first six months to 9.24 per thousand in the second six months, and 5.5 per thousand in the third six months. Of a total of 6,333 deaths in 1909-1910 in the labor area, 2,264, more than one-third, were due to pneumonia (G. D. Maynard). The case mortality is not extraordinarily high. In Johannesburg the deaths among the colored people fell from 1,196 in 1912-13 (a rate of 10.79 per 1,000 population) to 325 in 1913-14 (a rate of 3.09 per 1,000) coincident with improvement in the sanitary condition of the dwellings.

Etiology.—Age.—To the sixth year the predisposition to pneumonia is marked; it diminishes to the fifteenth year, but then for each subsequent decade it increases. For children Holt's statistics of 500 cases give: First year, 15 per cent.; from the second to the sixth year, 62 per cent.; from the seventh to the eleventh year, 21 per cent.; from the twelfth to the fourteenth year, 2 per cent. Lobar pneumonia has been met with in the newborn. The relation to age is well shown in the U. S. Census Report for 1900. The death-rate in persons from fifteen to forty-five years was 100.05 per 100,000 of population; from forty-five to sixty-five years it was 263.12; and in persons sixty-five years of age and over it was 733.77. Pneumonia may well be called the friend of the aged. Taken off by it in an acute, short, not often painful illness, the old escape those "cold gradations of decay" that make the last stage of all so distressing.

Sex.—Males are more frequently affected than females—533 to 125 in the Johns Hopkins Hospital series.

Race.—In the United States pneumonia is more fatal in negroes than among the whites. This was not so marked in our figures at the Johns Hopkins Hospital, but at the Charité Hospital, New Orleans, and at the Ancon and Colon hospitals of the Canal Zone the death rate among the negroes is much higher. It is rare among the Chinese.

Social Condition.—The disease is more common in the cities. Overcrowding probably is a factor. Individuals who are much exposed to hardship and cold are particularly liable to the disease. Newcomers and immigrants are stated to be less susceptible than native inhabitants.

Personal Condition.—Debilitating causes of all sorts render individuals more susceptible. Alcoholism is perhaps the most potent predisposing factor. Robust, healthy men are, however, often attacked.

Previous Attack.—No other acute disease recurs in the same individual with such frequency. Instances are on record of individuals who have had ten or more attacks. The percentage of recurrences has been placed as high as 50. Netter gives it as 31, and he has collected the statistics of eleven observers who place the percentage at 26.8. Among the highest figures for recurrences are those of Benjamin Rush, 28, and Andral, 16.

Trauma—Contusion-pneumonia.—Pneumonia may follow directly upon injury, particularly of the chest, without necessarily any lesion of the lung. Litten gives 4.4 per cent., Stern 2.8 per cent. Stern describes three clinical varieties: first, the ordinary lobar pneumonia following a contusion of the chest wall; secondly, atypical cases, with slight fever and not very characteristic physical signs; thirdly, cases with the physical signs and features of bronchopneumonia. The last two varieties have a favorable prognosis. According to

Ballard, workers in certain phosphate factories, where they breathe a very dusty atmosphere, are particularly prone to pneumonia.

COLD has been for years regarded as an important etiological factor. The frequent occurrence of an initial chill has been one reason for this widespread belief. As to the close association of pneumonia with exposure there can be no question. We see the disease occur promptly after a wetting or a chilling due to some unusual exposure, or come on after an ordinary catarrh of one or two days' duration. Cold is now regarded simply as a factor in lowering the resistance of the bronchial and pulmonary tissues.

CLIMATE AND SEASON.—Climate does not appear to have very much influence, as pneumonia prevails equally in hot and cold countries. It is stated to be more prevalent in the Southern than in the Northern States, but the Census Reports show that there is little difference in the various State groups. The disease is less prevalent in England than in the United States, where the dry, overheated air of the houses favors catarrhal processes in the air passages.

Much more important is the influence of *season*. Statistics are almost unanimous in placing the highest incidence of the disease in the winter and spring months. In Montreal, January, the coldest month of the year, but with steady temperature, has usually a comparatively low death-rate from pneumonia. The large statistics of Seitz from Munich and of Seibert of New York give the highest percentage in February and March.

Bacteriology.—(*a*) MICROCOCCUS LANCEOLATUS, PNEUMOCOCCUS OR DIPLOCOCCUS PNEUMONIÆ OF FRAENKEL AND WEICHSELBAUM.—In September, 1880, Sternberg inoculated rabbits with his own saliva and isolated a micrococcus. The publication was not made until April, 1881. Pasteur discovered the same organism in the saliva of a child dead of hydrophobia in December, 1880, and the priority of the discovery belongs to him, as his publication is dated January, 1881. There was, however, no suspicion that this organism was concerned in the etiology of lobar pneumonia, and it was not really until April, 1884, that Fraenkel determined that the organism found by Sternberg and Pasteur in the saliva, and known as the coccus of sputum septicæmia, was the most frequent germ in pneumonia.

The organism is a somewhat elliptical, lance-shaped coccus, usually occurring in pairs; hence the term diplococcus. About the organism in the sputum a capsule can always be demonstrated. Its kinship to *Streptococcus pyogenes* is regarded by many as very close. R. Cole and his co-workers recognize four groups based upon well defined immunological differences. Types I and II each comprise about one third of the cases with a mortality of 25-30 per cent. Type III comprises 10-15 per cent. with a mortality about 50 per cent. and Type IV, the remainder with a mortality about 12 per cent. Organisms of Type IV are the commonest forms in the mouths of healthy individuals. A fifth well-marked strain has been determined in South Africa by Lister.

Distribution in the Body.—In the bronchial secretions and in the affected lung the pneumococcus is readily demonstrated in smears, and in the latter in sections. It is possible to isolate the pneumococcus from the blood in a large proportion of all cases.

PNEUMOCOCCUS UNDER NORMAL CONDITIONS.—(1) *In the Mouth.*—

The pneumococcus is present in the mouths of a large proportion of healthy individuals, various observers giving 80 to 90 per cent. of positive results. The virulence is not always uniform, and Longcope and Fox showed that the saliva of the same individual increased in virulence during the winter months. Some persons always harbor a virulent variety. Buerger studied the communicability of the organism from one person to another and it was found repeatedly that normal individuals—*i. e.,* persons in whose mouths the pneumococcus was proved by repeated examinations to be absent—acquired the organisms by association with cases of pneumonia, or with healthy persons in whose saliva pneumococci were present.

(2) *Outside the Body.*—The viability of the pneumococcus is not great. It has been found occasionally in the dust and sweepings of rooms, but Wood has shown (New York Commission Report) that the germs exposed to sunlight die in a very short time—an hour and a half being the limit. In moist sputum kept in a dark room the germs lived ten days, and in a badly ventilated room in which a person with pneumonia coughed, the germs suspended in the air retained their vitality for several hours.

(*b*) Bacillus pneumoniæ of Friedländer.—This is a larger organism than the pneumococcus, and appears in the form of plump, short rods. It also shows a capsule, but presents marked differences from Fraenkel's pneumococcus. It may cause broncho-pneumonia and other affections, and is not a cause of genuine lobar pneumonia. The exudate caused by this bacillus is usually more viscid and poorer in fibrin than that in diplococcus pneumonia.

(*c*) Other Organisms.—Various bacteria may be associated with the pneumococcus in lobar pneumonia, the most common of these being *Streptococcus pyogenes,* the pyogenic staphylococci, and Friedländer's pneumobacillus; but while these latter may cause broncho-pneumonia, they have not been satisfactorily demonstrated to be other than secondary invaders in lobar pneumonia. Likewise the pneumonias caused by *Bacillus typhosus, Bacillus diphtheriæ,* and the influenza bacillus are not to be identified with true lobar pneumonia.

Clinically, the *infectious nature* of pneumonia was recognized long before we knew anything of the pneumococcus. It may occur in endemic form, localized in certain houses, in barracks, jails, and schools. As many as ten occupants of one house have been attacked. We have seen several members of a family consecutively attacked with a most malignant type of pneumonia. Among the more remarkable endemic outbreaks is that reported by W. B. Rodman, of Frankfort, Ky. In a prison with a population of 735 there occurred in one year 118 cases of pneumonia with 25 deaths. The disease may assume epidemic proportions. In the Middlesborough epidemic, studied by Ballard, 682 persons were attacked, with a mortality of 21 per cent. During some years pneumonia is so prevalent that it is practically pandemic. Direct contagion is suggested by the fact that a patient in the next bed to a pneumonia case may take the disease, or 2 or 3 cases may follow in rapid succession in a ward. It is very exceptional, however, for nurses or doctors to be attacked.

Infection, the Symptoms and Immunity.—A majority of persons harbor the germ in mouth, nose, or throat, but the virulence of the ordinary mouth form is low and varies with the season. A virulent germ may be constant and such persons are true carriers and play an important rôle in the spread of the disease. Some individuals are less resistant, and in no other acute disease may so many successive attacks occur in the same person. The negro race in the United States, in the Canal Zone, and in South Africa shows an extreme susceptibility; on the other hand the Chinese workmen, when in South Africa, showed an extraordinary resistance to the disease.

There are three phases in the infection—a period of incubation and onset, the clinical manifestations, and the immunization characterized by the crisis. The attack is usually attributed to lowered general resistance, but experimentally there is basis for the view that local conditions in the lung, such as the catarrhal processes, favor the development of pneumococci. Changes leading to lobar consolidation may be regarded as local defensive reactions. The explosive onset bears a certain resemblance to the anaphylactic reaction.

The clinical features are a toxæmia, plus disturbances of respiratory and circulatory functions. The intoxication bears no proportion to the local lesion. There are profound general infections with little or no pulmonary involvement. Some of the most toxic cases, particularly in the aged, have very slight lesions, while a lung may be solid and the patient show no signs of poisoning. The nature of the toxæmia is unknown, nor whether due to absorption of the products of digestion of the local exudate, which does not seem likely, as the symptoms abate after crisis when this absorption is most active. To regard the symptoms as due to absorption of a toxin is natural but no special substance has been discovered in the culture fluids of pneumococci; the problem is under discussion. Studies on the oxygen and carbon dioxide contents of the blood by Peabody show no change in the reaction of the body tissues beyond the mild grade of acidosis present in all fevers. Probably, as Pfeifer suggests, it is an endotoxin produced from the bodies of the pneumococci.

The explanation of the crisis is obscure. Immune bodies are not constantly increased after it, or they may not appear for several days. Upon what the neutralization of the toxins depends is doubtful.

The serum of a horse actively immunized will protect a mouse against a million lethal doses when injected together; but if injected only a few hours after the lethal dose it is not possible to save the animal (Cole). Insufficient dosage may account for the common failure and in each case the special strain must be determined. A univalent serum was efficient to protect animals against about 40 per cent. of cultures obtained from the blood of patients. Up to the present the serum has been found useful in the treatment of infections with Type I. No effective serum has been obtained for Type III (*Pneumococcus Mucosus*).

Morbid Anatomy.—Since the time of Laënnec, pathologists have recognized three stages in the inflamed lung: engorgement, red hepatization, and gray hepatization.

In the stage of *engorgement* the lung tissue is deep red in color, firmer to the touch, and more solid, and on section the surface is bathed with blood and serum. It still crepitates, though not so distinctly as healthy lung, and excised portions float. The air-cells can be dilated by insufflation from the bronchus. The capillary vessels are greatly distended, the alveolar epithelium swollen, and the air-cells occupied by a variable number of blood corpuscles and detached alveolar cells. In the stage of *red hepatization* the lung tissue is solid, firm, and airless. If the entire lobe is involved it looks voluminous, and shows indentations of the ribs. On section, the surface is dry, reddish-brown in color, and has lost the deeply congested appearance of the first stage. One of the most remarkable features is the friability; in striking contrast to the healthy lung, which is torn with difficulty. The surface has a granular appearance due to the fibrinous plugs filling the air-cells. The distinctness of this appearance varies greatly with the size of the alveoli, which are about 0.10 mm. in diameter in the infant, 0.15 or 0.16 in the adult, and from 0.20 to 0.25 in old age. On scraping the surface with a knife a reddish viscid serum is removed, containing small granular masses. The smaller bronchi often contain fibrinous plugs. If the lung has been removed before the heart, it is not uncommon to find solid moulds of clot filling the blood-vessels. Microscopically, the air-cells are seen to be occupied by coagulated fibrin in the meshes of which are red blood-corpuscles, leucocytes, and alveolar epithelium. The alveolar walls are infiltrated and leucocytes are seen in the interlobular tissues. Cover-glass preparations from the exudate, and thin sections show, as a rule, the diplococci, many of which are contained within cells. Staphylococci and streptococci may also be seen in some cases. In the stage of *gray hepatization* the tissue has changed from a reddish-brown to a grayish-white color. The surface is moister, the exudate obtained on scraping is more turbid, the granules in the acini are less distinct, and the lung tissue is still more friable. The air-cells are densely filled with leucocytes, the fibrin network and the red blood-corpuscles have largely disappeared. A more advanced condition of gray hepatization is that known as *purulent infiltration,* in which the lung tissue is softer and bathed with a purulent fluid. Small abscess cavities may form, and by their fusion larger ones, though this is a rare event in ordinary pneumonia.

Resolution.—The changes in the exudate which lead to its resolution are due to an autolytic digestion by proteolytic enzymes which are present much more abundantly in gray hepatization than in the preceding stage. The dissolved exudate is for the most part excreted by the kidneys. By following the nitrogen excess in the urine the progress of resolution may be followed and even an estimate formed of the amount of the exudate thus eliminated. H. W. Cook found in cases of delayed resolution that the nitrogen excess in the urine (which persisted until the lung was clear) was very large, and he suggests that delayed resolution may really be a matter of continued exudation.

General Details of the Morbid Anatomy.—In 100 autopsies at the General Hospital, Montreal, in 51 cases the right lung was affected, at 32 the left, in 17 both organs. In 27 cases the entire lung, with the exception, perhaps, of a narrow margin at the apex and anterior border, was consolidated. In 34 cases, the lower lobe alone was involved; in 13 cases, the upper lobe alone. When double, the lower lobes were usually affected together, but in three instances the lower lobe of one and the upper lobe of the other were attacked. In 3 cases, also, both upper lobes were affected. Occasionally the disease involves the greater part of both lungs. In a third of the cases, red and gray hepatization existed together. In 22 instances there was gray hepatization. As a rule the unaffected portion of the lung is congested or œdematous. When the greater portion of a lobe is attacked, the uninvolved part may be in a state of almost gelatinous œdema. The unaffected lung is usually congested, particularly at the posterior part. This may be largely due to post mortem subsidence. The uninflamed portions are not always congested and œdematous. The upper lobe may be dry and bloodless when the lower lobe is uniformly consolidated. The average weight of a normal lung is about 600 grams, while that of an inflamed organ may be 1,500, 2,000, or even 2,500 grams.

The bronchi contain, as a rule, at the time of death a frothy serous fluid, rarely the tenacious mucus so characteristic of pneumonic sputum. The mucous membrane is usually reddened, rarely swollen. In the affected areas the smaller bronchi often contain fibrinous plugs, which may extend into the larger tubes, forming perfect casts. The bronchial glands are swollen and may even be soft and pulpy. The pleural surface of the inflamed lung is invariably involved when the process becomes superficial. Commonly, there is only a thin sheeting of exudate, producing slight turbidity of the membrane. The pleura was not involved in only two of the hundred instances. In some cases the fibrinous exudate may form a creamy layer an inch in thickness. A serous exudation of variable amount is not uncommon.

Lesions in Other Organs.—The heart, particularly its right chamber, is distended with firm, tenacious coagula, which can be withdrawn from the vessels as dendritic moulds. In no other acute disease do we meet with coagula of such solidity. The spleen is often enlarged, though in only 35 of the 100 cases was the weight above 200 grams. The kidneys show parenchymatous swelling, turbidity of the cortex, and, in a very considerable proportion of the cases—25 per cent.—chronic interstitial changes.

Pericarditis was present in 35 of 658 cases in our series (Chatard). *Endocarditis* occurred in 16 of the 100 post mortems. In 5 of these the endocarditis was of the simple character; in 11 the lesions were ulcerative. Of 209 cases of malignant endocarditis collected from the literature, 54 occurred in pneumonia. Kanthack found an antecedent pneumonia in 14.2 per cent. of cases of infective endocarditis. In the figures collected by E. F. Wells, of 517 fatal cases of acute endocarditis, 22.3 per cent. were in pneumonia. It is more common on the left than on the right side of the heart. Among 658 cases of pneumonia in the Johns Hopkins Hospital endocarditis occurred in 15 (Marshall). *Myocarditis* and fatty degeneration of the heart may be present in protracted cases.

Meningitis, which is not infrequent, may be associated with malignant endocarditis. It was present in 8 of the 100 autopsies. Of 20 cases of meningitis in ulcerative endocarditis 15 occurred in pneumonia.

Croupous or diphtheritic inflammation may occur in other parts. A *croupous colitis,* as pointed out by Bristowe, is not very uncommon. It occurred in 5 of the 100 post mortems. It is usually a thin, flaky exudation, most marked on the tops of the folds of the mucous membrane. In one case there was a patch of *croupous gastritis,* covering an area 2 by 8 cm., situated to the left of the cardiac orifice. The liver shows parenchymatous changes, and often extreme engorgement of the hepatic veins.

Symptoms.—Course of the Disease in Typical Cases.—We know but little of the incubation period, but it is probably very short. There are sometimes slight catarrhal symptoms for a day or two. As a rule, the disease sets in abruptly with a severe *chill*, which lasts from fifteen to thirty minutes or longer. In no acute disease is an initial chill so constant or so severe. The patient may be taken abruptly in the midst of his work, or may awaken out of a sound sleep in a rigor. The temperature taken during the chill shows that the fever has already begun. If seen shortly after the onset, the patient usually has features of an acute fever, and complains of headache and general pains. Within a few hours there is pain in the side, often of an agonizing character; a short, dry, painful cough begins, and the respirations are increased in frequency. When seen on the second or third day, the picture in typical pneumonia is more distinctive than that presented by any other acute disease. The patient lies often on the affected side; the face is flushed, particularly one or both cheeks; the breathing is hurried, accompanied often with a short expiratory grunt; the alæ nasi dilate with each inspiration; herpes is usually present on the lips or nose; the eyes are bright, the pupils are often unequal, the expression is anxious, and there is a frequent short cough which makes the patient wince and hold his side. The expectoration is blood-tinged and extremely tenacious. The temperature may be 104° or 105°. The pulse is full and bounding and the pulse-respiration ratio much disturbed. Examination of the lungs shows the physical signs of consolidation with blowing breathing and fine râles. After persisting for from seven to ten days the crisis occurs, and with a fall in the temperature the patient passes from the condition of extreme distress and anxiety to one of comparative comfort.

Special Features.—The fever rises rapidly, and the height may be 104° F. or 105° F. within twelve hours. Having reached the fastigium, it is remarkably constant. Often the two-hour temperature chart will not show more than a degree of variation for several days. In children and in cases without chill the rise is more gradual. In old persons and in drunkards the temperature range is lower than in children and in healthy individuals; one occasionally meets with an afebrile pneumonia.

The Crisis.—After the fever has persisted for from five to nine or ten days there is an abrupt drop, known as the crisis, which is one of the most characteristic features of the disease. The day of the crisis is variable. It is very uncommon before the third day, and rare after the twelfth. We have seen it as early as the third day. From the time of Hippocrates it has been thought to be more frequent on the uneven days, particularly the fifth and seventh; the latter has the largest number of cases (Musser and Norris). A *precritical rise* of a degree or two may occur. In one case the temperature rose from 105° to nearly 107°, and then in a few hours fell to normal. Not even after the chill in malarial fever do we see such a prompt and rapid drop in the temperature. The usual time is from five to twelve hours, but often in an hour there may occur a fall of six or eight degrees (S. West). The temperature may be subnormal after the crisis, as low as 96° or 97°. Usually there is an abundant sweat, and the patient sinks into a comfortable sleep. The day after the crisis there may be a slight post-critical rise. A *pseudo-crisis* is not very uncommon, in which on the fifth or sixth day the temperature drops from 104° or 105° to 102°, and then rises again. When the fall takes place gradually within twenty-four hours it is called a protracted crisis. If the fever persists beyond the twelfth day, the fall is likely to be by lysis. In children this mode of termination is common, and occurred in one-third of a series of 183 cases reported by Morrill. Occasionally in debilitated individuals the temperature drops rapidly just before death; more frequently there is an ante-mortem elevation. In delayed resolution the fever may persist for six or eight weeks. The crisis, the most remarkable phenomenon of pneumonia, appears to represent the stage of active immunity to the toxin of the pneumococcus. The fever, dyspnœa and general symptoms disappear when the immunity reaches a certain stage. With the fall in the fever the respirations become reduced almost to normal, the pulse slows, and the patient passes from perhaps a state of extreme hazard and distress to one of safety and comfort, and yet, so far as the physical examination indicates, there is with the crisis no special change in the condition in the lung. For a study of the problem see Emerson, Johns Hopkins Hospital Reports, Vol. XV.

Pain.—There is early a sharp, agonizing pain, generally referred to the region of the nipple or lower axilla of the affected side, and much aggravated on deep inspiration and on coughing. It is associated, as Aretæus remarks, with involvement of the pleura. It is absent in central pneumonia, and much less frequent in apex pneumonia. The pain may be severe enough to require a hypodermic injection of morphia. As has been recognized for many years, the pain may be altogether abdominal, either central or in the right iliac fossa, suggesting appendicitis. The operation for appendicitis has been performed.

Dyspnœa is almost constant and even early in the disease the respirations may be 30 in the minute, and on the second or third day between 40 and 50. The movements are shallow, evidently restrained, and if the patient is asked to draw a deep breath he cries out with the pain. Expiration is frequently interrupted by an audible grunt. At first with the increased respiration there may be no sensation of distress. Later this may be present in a marked degree. In children the respirations may be 80 or even 100. Many factors combine to produce the shortness of breath—the pain in the side, the toxæmia, the fever, acidosis possibly, and the loss of function in a considerable area of the lung tissue. Sometimes there appear to be nervous factors at work. That it does not depend upon the consolidation is shown by the fact that after the crisis, without any change in the condition of the lung, the number of respirations may drop to normal. The ratio between the respirations and the pulse may be 1 to 2 or even 1 to 1.5, a disturbance rarely so marked in any other disease.

Cough.—This usually comes on with the pain in the side, and at first is dry, hard, and without any expectoration. Later it becomes very characteristic—frequent, short, restrained, and associated with great pain in the side. In old persons, in drunkards, in the terminal pneumonias, and sometimes in young children, there may be no cough. After the crisis the cough usually becomes much easier and the expectoration more easily expelled. The cough is sometimes persistent, continuous, and by far the most aggravated and distressing symptom of the disease. Paroxysms of coughing of great intensity after the crises suggest a pleural exudate.

Sputum.—A brisk hæmoptysis may be the initial symptom. At first the sputum may be mucoid, but usually after twenty-four hours it becomes blood-tinged, viscid, and very tenacious. At first quite red from the unchanged blood, it gradually becomes rusty or of an orange yellow. The tenacious viscidity of the sputum is remarkable; it often has to be wiped from the lips of the patient. When jaundice is present it may be green or yellow. In low types of the disease the sputum may be fluid and of a dark brown color, resembling prune juice. The amount is very variable, ranging from 100 to 300 c. c. in the twenty-four hours. In 100 cases studied by Emerson, in 16 there was little or no sputum; in 32 it was typically rusty; in 33 blood-streaked; in 3 cases the sputum was very bloody. In children and very old people there may be no sputum whatever. After the crisis the quantity is variable, abundant in some cases, absent in others.

Microscopically, the sputum consists of leucocytes, mucus corpuscles, red blood-corpuscles in all stages of degeneration, and bronchial and alveolar epithelium. Hæmatoidin crystals are occasionally met with. Of micro-organisms the pneumococcus is usually present, and sometimes Friedländer's bacillus, the influenza bacillus, streptococci and the colon bacillus. Very interesting constituents are small cell moulds of the alveoli and the fibrinous casts of the bronchioles; the latter may be plainly visible to the naked eye; and sometimes may form good-sized dendritic casts. Chemically, the expectoration is particularly rich in calcium chloride.

Physical Signs.—*Inspection.*—The position of the patient is not constant. He usually rests more comfortably on the affected side, or he is propped up with the spine curved toward it. Orthopnœa is rare.

In a small lesion no differences may be noted between the sides; as a rule, movement is much less on the affected side, which may look larger. With involvement of a lower lobe, the apex on the same side may show greater movement. The compensatory increased movement on the sound side is sometimes very noticeable even before the patient's chest is bared. The intercostal spaces are not usually obliterated. When the cardiac lappet of the left upper lobe is involved there may be a marked increase in the area of visible cardiac pulsation. Pulsation of the affected lung may cause a marked movement of the chest wall (Graves). Other points to be noticed in the inspection are the frequency of the respiration, the action of the accessory muscles, such as the sterno-cleido-mastoids and scaleni, and the dilatation of the nostrils with each inspiration. Asynchronous contractions of the respiratory muscles occur in many cases. When fully developed the diaphragm and thoracic respiratory muscles contract alternately (Coleman). It is of grave significance.

Mensuration may show a definite increase in the volume of the side affected, rarely more, however, than 1 or 1½ cm.

Palpation.—The lack of expansion on the affected side is sometimes more readily perceived by touch than by sight. The pleural friction may be felt. The voice fremitus is greatly increased in comparison with the corresponding point on the healthy side. It is to be noted that if the bronchi are filled with thick secretion, or if, in what is known as massive pneumonia, they are filled with fibrinous exudate, the tactile fremitus may be diminished. It is always well to ask the patient to cough before testing the fremitus.

Percussion.—In the stage of engorgement the note is higher pitched and may have a somewhat tympanitic quality. This can often be obtained over the lung tissue just above a consolidated area. L. A. Conner calls attention to a point which all observers must have noticed, that, when the patient is lying on his side, the percussion at the dependent base is "deeper and more resonant than that of the upper side," which by contrast may seem abnormal, and there may even be a faint tubular element added to the vesicular breathing on the compressed side. When the lung is hepatized, the percussion note is dull, the quality varying a good deal from a note which has in it a certain tympanitic quality to one of absolute flatness. There is not the wooden flatness of effusion and the sense of resistance is not so great. During resolution the tympanitic quality of the percussion note usually returns. For weeks or months after convalescence there may be a higher-pitched note on the affected side. Wintrich's change in the percussion note when the mouth is open may be very well marked in pneumonia of the upper lobe. Occasionally there is an almost metallic quality over the consolidated area, and when this exists with a very pronounced amphoric quality in the breathing the presence of a cavity may be suggested. In deep-seated pneumonias there may be no change in the percussion note for several days.

Auscultation.—Quiet, suppressed breathing in the affected part is often a marked feature in the early stage, and is always suggestive. Only in a few cases is the breathing harsh or puerile. Very early there is heard at the end of inspiration the fine crepitant râle, a series of minute cracklings heard close to the ear, and perhaps not audible until a full breath is drawn. This is possibly a fine pleural crepitus, as J. B. Leaming maintained; it is usually believed to be produced in the air-cells and finer bronchi by the separation of the sticky exudate. In the stage of red hepatization and when dulness is well defined, the respiration is tubular. It is heard first with expiration (a point noted by James Jackson, Jr.), and is soft and of low pitch. Gradually it becomes more intense, and finally presents an intensity unknown in any other pulmonary affection—of high pitch, perfectly dry, and of equal length with inspiration and expiration. It is simply the propagation of the laryngeal and tracheal sounds through the bronchi and the consolidated lung tissue. The permeability of the bronchi is essential to its production. Tubular breathing is absent in the excessively rare cases of massive pneumonia in which the larger bronchi are completely filled with exudation. When resolution begins mucous râles of all sizes can be heard. At first they are small and have been called the *redux-crepitus.* The voice-sounds and the expiratory grunt are transmitted through the consolidated lung with great intensity. This bronchophony may have a curious nasal quality, to which the term ægophony has been given. There are cases in which the consolidation is deeply seated—so-called central pneumonia, in which the physical signs are slight or even absent, yet the cough, the rusty expectoration, and general features make the diagnosis certain.

Circulatory Symptoms.—During the chill the *pulse* is small, but in the succeeding fever it becomes full and bounding. In cases of moderate severity it ranges from 100 to 120. It is not often dicrotic. In strong, healthy individuals and in children there may be no sign of failing pulse throughout the attack. With extensive consolidation the left ventricle may receive a very much diminished amount of blood and the pulse in consequence may be small. In the old and feeble it may be small and rapid from the outset.

The pulse may be full, soft, very deceptive, and of no value whatever in prognosis.

Blood Pressure.—During the first few days there is no change. The extent of involvement seems to have no effect upon the peripheral blood pressure. In the toxic cases the pressure may begin to fall early; a drop of 15-20 mm. Hg is perfectly safe, but a progressive fall indicates the need of stimulation. A sudden drop is rarely seen except just before death. A slow, gradual fall of more than 20 mm. Hg means cardio-vascular asthenia, and calls for an increase in the stimulation. The crisis has no effect on the blood pressure. The opinion commonly held, that when the blood pressure as expressed in millimeters of Hg does not fall below the pulse rate expressed in beats per minute, the outlook is good, and *vice versa,* is by no means always correct. The *heart sounds* are usually loud and clear. During the intensity of the fever, particularly in children, murmurs are not uncommon both in the mitral and in the pulmonic areas. The second sound over the pulmonary artery is accentuated. Attention to this sign gives a valuable indication as to the condition of the lesser circulation. With distention of the right chambers and failure of the right ventricle to empty itself completely, the pulmonary second sound becomes much less distinct. When the right heart is engorged there may be an increase in the dulness to the right of the sternum. With gradual heart weakness and signs of dilatation the long pause is greatly shortened, the sounds approach each other in tone and have a fetal character (embryocardia).

There may be a sudden early collapse of the heart with very feeble, rapid pulse and increasing cyanosis. This may happen on the third day. Even when these symptoms are very serious recovery may take place. In other instances without any special warning death may occur even in robust, previously healthy men. The heart weakness may be due to paralysis of the vaso-motor centre and consequent lowering of the general arterial pressure. The soft, easily compressed pulse, with the gray, ashy facies, cold hands and feet, the clammy perspiration, and the progressive prostration tell of a toxic action on the circulation. Endocarditis and pericarditis will be considered under complications.

Blood.—Pneumococci are present in the blood in a large proportion of all cases. Anæmia is rare. A decrease in the red cells may occur at the time of the crisis. There is in most cases a leucocytosis, which appears early, persists, and disappears with the crisis. The leucocytes may number from 12,000 to 40,000 or even 100,000 per cubic millimetre. The fall in the leucocytes is often slower than the drop in the fever, particularly when resolution is delayed or complications are present. The annexed chart gives a study by Chatard of the leucocytes in 582 cases at the Johns Hopkins Hospital. More than half of the patients, about 350, had a leucocytosis of between 15,000 and 35,000, and nearly one-third (198) between 20,000 and 30,000. The broken line represents the mortality which is high when the leucocytes are below 10,000, but steadily decreases and is lowest when they are between 20,000 and 30,000. With the leucocytes between 30,000 and 60,000 the mortality is again higher. The two patients with the highest leucocytosis of the series, 95,000 and 105,000 respectively, recovered. A striking feature in the blood-slide is the richness and density of the fibrin network. This corresponds to the great increase in the fibrin elements, the proportion rising from 4 to 10 parts per thousand. The blood-plates are greatly increased.

Digestive Organs.—The tongue is white and furred, and in severe toxic cases rapidly becomes dry. Vomiting is not uncommon at the onset in children. The appetite is lost. Constipation is more common than diarrhœa.

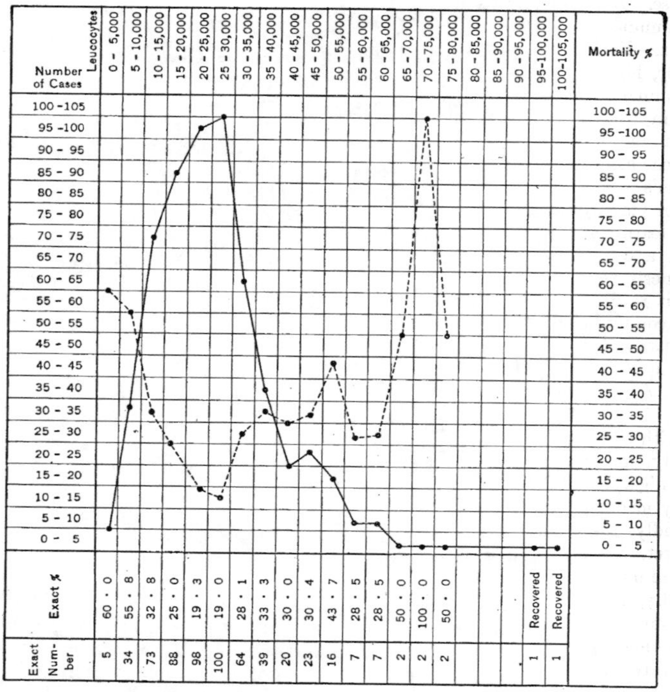

Chart IV.—Blood Count in Pneumonia and Comparative Mortality. Continuous Line Represents Number of Cases of Pneumonia. Broken Line Represents Mortality Percentage of Same.

A distressing and sometimes dangerous symptom is meteorism. Fibrinous, pneumococcic exudates may occur in the conjunctivæ, nose, mouth, prepuce, and anus (Cary). The liver may be depressed by the large right lung, or enlarged from the engorged right heart or as a result of the infection. The spleen is usually enlarged, and the edge can be felt during a deep inspiration.

Skin.—Among *cutaneous* symptoms one of the most interesting is the association of *herpes* with pneumonia. Not excepting malaria, we see labial herpes more frequently in this than in any other disease, occurring, as it does, in from 12 to 40 per cent. of the cases. It is supposed to be of favorable prognosis, and figures have been quoted in proof of this assertion. It may also occur on the nose, genitals, and anus. Its significance and relation to the disease are unknown. At the height of the disease sweats are not common, but at the crisis they may be profuse. Redness of one cheek is a phenomenon long recognized in pneumonia, and is usually on the same side as the disease. A diffuse erythema is occasionally seen, and in rare cases purpura. Jaundice is referred to among the complications.

Urine.—Early in the disease it presents the usual febrile characters of high color, high specific gravity, and increased acidity. A trace of albumin is very common. There may be tube-casts, and in a few instances the existence of albumin, tube-casts, and blood indicates the presence of an acute nephritis. The urea and uric acid are usually increased at first, but may be much diminished before the crisis, to increase greatly with its onset. Robert Hutchison's researches show that a true retention of chlorides within the body takes place, the average amount being about 2 grams daily. It is a more constant feature of pneumonia than of any other febrile disease, and this being the case, a diminution of the chlorides in the urine may be of value in the diagnosis from pleurisy with effusion or empyema. It is to be remembered that in dilatation of the stomach chlorides may be absent. Hæmaturia is a rare complication.

Cerebral Symptoms.—Headache is common. In children vomiting or convulsions may occur at the outset. Apart from meningitis, considered separately, one may group the cases with marked cerebral features into:

First, the so-called cerebral pneumonias of children, in which the disease sets in with a convulsion, and there are high fever, headache, delirium, great irritability, muscular tremor, and perhaps retraction of the head and neck with Kernig's sign and an extensor plantar reflex. The diagnosis of meningitis is usually made, and the local affection may be overlooked.

Secondly, the cases with maniacal symptoms. These may occur at the very outset, and there may be no suspicion whatever that the disease is other than acute mania.

Thirdly, alcoholic cases with the features of delirium tremens. It should be an invariable rule, even if fever be not present, to examine the lungs in a case of *mania a potu*.

Fourthly, cases with toxic features, rather resembling those of uræmia. Without a chill and without cough or pain in the side, a patient may have fever, a little shortness of breath, and then gradually grow dull mentally, and within three days be in profound toxæmia with low, muttering delirium.

It is stated that apex pneumonia is more often accompanied with severe delirium. Occasionally the cerebral symptoms occur immediately after the crisis. Mental disturbance may persist during and after convalescence, and in a few instances delusional insanity follows, the outlook in which is favorable.

Hemiplegia may be due to thrombosis, embolism, abscess or œdema. Withington called attention to a form associated with encephalitis. It may be transient and recovery complete. Transient *aphasia,* with or without hemiplegia, may occur and there are cases in which no gross lesions have been found, so that it has been suggested that it is due to œdema or to a relative ischæmia. Inequality of the pupils is not uncommon but has no special significance.

Complications.—Compared with typhoid fever, pneumonia has but few complications and still fewer sequelæ. The most important are the following:

Pleurisy is an inevitable event when the inflammation reaches the surface of the lung, and thus can scarcely be termed a complication. But there are cases in which the pleuritic features take the first place. The exudation may be sero-fibrinous with copious effusion, differing from that of an ordinary acute pleurisy in the greater richness of the fibrin, which may form thick, tenacious, curdy layers. Pneumonia on one side with extensive pleurisy on the other is sometimes a puzzling complication to diagnose, and an aspirating needle may be required to settle the question. *Empyema* is a most common complication occurring in 2.2 per cent. of clinical cases collected by Musser and Norris and in 3.6 per cent. of the Johns Hopkins Hospital series. During the eight years, 1883-'90, there were at Guy's Hospital 7 cases of empyema among 445 cases of pneumonia, while in the eight years, 1891-'98, there were 38 cases among 896 cases of pneumonia (Hale White). Influenza may be responsible for the increase. The pneumococcus is usually present; in a few the streptococcus, in which case the prognosis is not so good. Some cases may be due to extension from or rupture of a small lung abscess. Recurrence of the fever after the crisis or persistence of it after the tenth day, with sweats, leucocytosis, and an aggravation of the cough, are suspicious symptoms. The dulness persists at the base, or may extend. The breathing is feeble and there are no râles. Such a condition may be closely simulated, of course, by a thickened pleura. Exploratory aspiration may settle the question at once. There are obscure cases in which the pus has been found only after operation, as the collection may be very small. The X-rays often give aid.

Pericarditis, one of the most serious of complications, was present in 35 of 658 patients in the Johns Hopkins Hospital (Chatard). It is often a terminal affair and overlooked. The mortality is very high; 31 of the 35 patients died. It was most frequently associated with pneumonia of the right lung. In only three instances was the amount of fluid above 500 c. c. Pleurisy is an almost constant accompaniment, being present in 28 of the 29 autopsies in my series.

Endocarditis.—The valves on the left side are more commonly attacked, and particularly if the seat of arterio-sclerosis. It is especially liable to attack persons with old valvular disease. There may be no symptoms indicative of this complication even in very severe cases. It may, however, be suspected in cases (1) in which the fever is protracted and irregular; (2) when signs of septic mischief arise, such as chills and sweats; (3) when embolic phenomena appear. The frequent complication of meningitis with the endocarditis of pneumonia gives prominence to the cerebral symptoms in these cases. The physical signs may be deceptive. There are instances in which no cardiac murmurs have been heard. In others the occurrence under observation of a loud, rough murmur, particularly if diastolic, is extremely suggestive.

Ante-mortem clotting in the heart, upon which the old writers laid great stress, is very rare. *Thrombosis* in the peripheral veins is also uncommon. Three cases occurred in the Hopkins clinic, which have been reported by Steiner, who was able to collect only 54 cases from the literature. In 35 out of 44 cases which were fully reported, the thrombosis occurred during convalescence. It is almost always in the femoral veins. A rare complication is *embolism* of one of the larger arteries. The senior author saw an instance of embolism of the femoral artery at the height of pneumonia, which necessitated amputation at the thigh. The patient recovered.

Meningitis is perhaps the most serious complication and varies very much at different times and in different regions. The Montreal series is rather exceptional, as 8 per cent. of the fatal cases had this complication. In twenty years at the Johns Hopkins Hospital there were 25 cases of pneumococcus meningitis, in 18 of which pneumonia was present. In 16 of the cases the organism was demonstrated in the cerebro-spinal fluid. Endocarditis was present in 7 of the 18 cases. The percentage of meningitis in the pneumonia cases was 2.4, which is lower than the figures of Musser and Norris of 3.5 per cent. in 4,883 autopsies. It usually comes on at the height of the fever, and in the majority of the cases is not recognized unless the base is involved, which is not common. Occurring later in the disease, it is more easily diagnosed. The prognosis is bad; all of our patients died. A few instances of recovery are on record.

Peripheral neuritis is a rare complication, of which several cases have been described.

Gastric complications are rare. Fussell has drawn attention to the occurrence of acute *dilatation of the stomach*. Persistent vomiting, sudden abdominal distention and collapse are the most common features. A croupous gastritis has been mentioned. The *croupous colitis* may induce severe diarrhœa. It is by no means uncommon to have early *pain*, either in the region of the umbilicus or in the right iliac fossa, and a suspicion of appendicitis is aroused; indeed, a catarrhal form of this disease may occur coincidently with the pneumonia. In other instances so localized may the pain be in the region of the pancreas, associated with meteorism and high fever, that the diagnosis of acute hæmorrhagic pancreatitis is made. Such a case occurred in the wards of our colleague Dr. Halsted. The patient was admitted in a desperate condition, all the symptoms were abdominal, and the apex pneumonia was not discovered. *Peritonitis* is a rare complication, of which we have had only two or three instances. It is sometimes in the upper peritoneum, and a direct extension through the diaphragm. It is usually in the severer cases and not easy to recognize. In one case, indeed, in which there was a friction along the costal border, which we thought indicated a peritonitis, it was communicated from the diaphragmatic pleura. *Meteorism* is not infrequent, and is sometimes serious. In some cases it may be due to a defect in the mechanical action of the diaphragm, in others to an acute septic catarrh of the bowels, or to a toxic paresis of the walls, occasionally to peritonitis. *Jaundice* occurs with curious irregularity in different outbreaks of the disease. In Baltimore it was more common among the negro patients. It sets in early, is rarely very intense, and has not the characters of obstructive jaundice. There are cases in which it assumes a very serious form. The mode of production is not well ascertained. It does not appear to bear any definite relation to the degree of hepatic engorgement, and it is not always due to catarrh of the ducts. Possibly it may be, in great part, hæmatogenous.

Parotitis occasionally occurs, commonly in association with endocarditis. In children, middle-ear disease is not an infrequent complication.

Nephritis does not often follow pneumonia.

Arthritis occurred in 5 of 658 cases at the Johns Hopkins Hospital (Howard). It may precede the onset, and the pneumonia, possibly with endocarditis and pleurisy, may occur as a complication. In other instances at the height of the pneumonia one or two joints may become red and sore or after the crisis has occurred pain and swelling may come on in the joints. It is a serious complication as recovery is often slow and a stiff joint may follow.

Relapse.—There are cases in which from the ninth to the eleventh day the fever subsides, and after the temperature has been normal for a day or two a rise occurs and fever may persist for another ten days or even two weeks. Though this might be termed a relapse, it is more correct to regard it as an instance of an anomalous course or delayed resolution. Wagner, who has studied the subject carefully, says that in his experience of 1,100 cases he met with only 3 doubtful cases. When it does occur, the attack is usually abortive and mild. In one case, with pneumonia of the right lower lobe, crisis occurred on the seventh day, and after a normal temperature for thirteen days he was discharged. That night he had a shaking chill, followed by fever, and he had recurring chills with reappearance of the pneumonia. In a second case the crisis occurred on the third day, and there was recurrence of pneumonia on the thirteenth day.

Recurrence is more common in pneumonia than in any other acute disease. Rush gives an instance in which there were 28 attacks. Other authorities narrate cases of 8, 10, and even more attacks.

Convalescence in pneumonia is usually rapid, and sequelæ are rare. After the crisis, sudden death has occurred when the patient has got up too soon. With the onset of fever and persistence of the leucocytosis the affected side should be very carefully examined for pleurisy. With a persistence of the dulness the physical signs may be obscure, but the use of a small exploratory needle or the X-rays will help to clear the diagnosis.

Clinical Varieties.—Local variations are responsible for some of the most marked deviations from the usual type. *Apex pneumonia* is said to be more often associated with adynamic features and with marked cerebral symptoms. The expectoration and cough may be slight. *Migratory* or *creeping pneumonia* is a form which successively involves one lobe after the other. *Double pneumonia* has no peculiarities other than the greater danger connected with it. *Massive pneumonia* is a rare form, in which not alone the air-cells but the bronchi of an entire lobe or even of a lung are filled with the fibrinous exudate. The auscultatory signs are absent; there is neither fremitus nor tubular breathing, and on percussion the lung is absolutely flat. It closely resembles pleurisy with effusion. The moulds of the bronchi may be expectorated in violent fits of coughing.

Central Pneumonia.—The inflammation may be deep-seated at the root of the lung or centrally placed in a lobe, and for several days the diagnosis may be in doubt. It may not be until the third or fourth day that a pleural friction is detected, or that dulness or blowing breathing and râles are recognized. The senior author saw with Drs. H. Adler and Chew a young, thin-chested girl in whom at the end of the fourth day all the usual symptoms of pneumonia were present without any physical signs other than a few clicking râles at the left apex behind. The thinness of the patient greatly facilitated the examination. The general features of pneumonia continued, and the crisis occurred on the seventh day.

Pneumonia in Infants.—It is sometimes seen in the new-born. In infants it very often sets in with a convulsion. The apex of the lung seems more frequently involved than in adults, and the cerebral symptoms are more marked. The torpor and coma, particularly if they follow convulsions, and the preliminary stage of excitement, may lead to the diagnosis of meningitis. Pneumonic sputum is rarely seen in children.

Pneumonia in the Aged.—The disease may be latent and set in without a chill; the cough and expectoration are slight, the physical signs ill-defined and changeable, and the constitutional symptoms out of all proportion to the extent of the local lesion.

Pneumonia in Alcoholic Subjects.—The onset is insidious, the symptoms masked, the fever slight, and the clinical picture usually that of delirium tremens. The thermometer alone may indicate the presence of an acute disease. Often the local condition is overlooked, as the patient makes no complaint, and there may be very little dyspnœa, no cough, and no sputum.

Terminal Pneumonia.—The wards and the post mortem room show a very striking contrast in their pneumonia statistics, owing to the occurrence of what may be called terminal pneumonia. During the winter months patients with chronic pulmonary tuberculosis, arterio-sclerosis, heart disease, nephritis, and diabetes are not infrequently carried off by a pneumonia which may give few or no signs. In the Johns Hopkins Hospital series of 658 cases, there were 35 cases of this variety, 20 of which were associated with cardiovascular and 14 with renal disease. It is nearly always of the lobar form. There may be slight fever, with increase in the respirations, but the patient is near the end and perhaps not in a condition in which a thorough physical examination can be made. In our series the right lung was involved in 19 cases and 9 had a low leucocyte count. In diabetic patients the disease often runs a rapid and severe course, and may end in abscess or gangrene.

Secondary Pneumonia.—This is met with chiefly in the specific fevers, particularly diphtheria, typhoid fever, typhus, influenza, and the plague. Anatomically, it rarely presents the typical form of red or gray hepatization. The surface is smoother, not so dry, and it is often a pseudo-lobar condition, a consolidation caused by closely set areas of lobular involvement. Histologically, it is characterized in many instances by a more cellular, less fibrinous exudate, which may also infiltrate the alveolar walls. Bacteriologically, the pneumococcus may be the dominant organism; but Friedländer's bacillus, streptococci, staphylococci, the influenza and colon bacillus have been found.

The symptoms of the secondary pneumonias often lack the striking definiteness of the primary lobar pneumonia. The pulmonary features may be latent or masked altogether. There may be no cough and only a slight increase in the number of respirations. The lower lobe of one lung is most commonly involved, and the physical signs are obscure and rarely amount to more than impaired resonance, feeble breathing, and a few crackling râles.

Epidemic Pneumonia is, as a rule, more fatal, and often displays minor complications which vary in different outbreaks. In some the cerebral manifestations are marked; in others, the cardiac; in others again, the gastro-intestinal.

Larval Pneumonia.—Mild, abortive types are seen, particularly in institutions when pneumonia is prevailing extensively. A patient may have the initial symptoms of the disease, a slight chill, moderate fever, a few indefinite local signs, and herpes. The whole process may only last for two or three days; some authors recognize even a one-day pneumonia.

Asthenic, Toxic, or Typhoid Pneumonia.—The toxæmic features dominate the scene throughout. The local lesions may be slight in extent and the subjective phenomena of the disease absent. The nervous symptoms usually predominate. There are delirium, prostration, and early weakness. Very frequently there is jaundice. Gastro-intestinal symptoms may be present, particularly diarrhœa and meteorism. In such a case, seen about the end of the first week, it may be difficult to say whether the condition is one of asthenic pneumonia or one of typhoid fever which has set in with early localization in the lung. Here the Widal reaction and blood cultures are important aids. Possibly, too, there is a mixed infection, and the streptococcus pyogenes may be in large part responsible for the toxic features.

Association of Pneumonia with Other Diseases.—(*a*) *With Malaria.*—A malarial pneumonia is described and thought to be particularly prevalent in some parts of the United States. One hears of it, indeed, even where true malaria is rarely seen. Pneumonia is a common disease in the tropics and often attacks the subjects of malaria. The prognosis is bad in the æstivo-autumnal infections. A special form of pneumonia due to the malarial parasite is unknown. Yet there are cases reported by Craig and others in which in an acute malarial infection the features suggest pneumonia at the onset, but the parasites are found in the blood, and under the use of quinine the fever drops rapidly and the pneumonia symptoms clear up. In some instances we have found a chill in the course of an ordinary pneumonia to be associated with a malarial infection.

(*b*) *Pneumonia and Acute Arthritis.*—We have already spoken under complications of this association, which is more frequently seen in children.

(*c*) *Pneumonia and Tuberculosis.*—Subjects of chronic pulmonary tuberculosis may die of an acute lobar pneumonia. A point to be specially borne in mind is the fact that acute tuberculous pneumonia may set in with all the features and physical signs of lobar pneumonia.

For the consideration of the association of pneumonia with typhoid fever and influenza, the reader is referred to the sections on those diseases.

Post-operation Pneumonia.—Before the days of anæsthesia, lobar pneumonia was a well-recognized cause of death after surgical injuries and operations. Norman Cheevers, in an early number of the Guy's Hospital Reports, called attention to it as one of the most frequent causes of death after surgical procedures, and Erichsen states that of 41 deaths after surgical injuries 23 cases showed signs of pneumonia. In the statistics collected by Homans the mortality due to lung complications after laparotomies ranged from 0.56 to 12.5. Operations on the stomach seem to be peculiarly liable to be followed by pneumonia. The low figure, 0.56, in Krönlein's clinic may be attributed to the use of ether by the open method, to the absence of all preparation on the table and to shortening as much as possible the period of anæsthesia. The cases may be divided into three groups: (1) Inhalation or anæsthesia pneumonia which may be lobar or broncho-pneumonia. (2) Hypostatic pneumonia due to enfeebled circulation. (3) Embolic cases with sudden onset. The route may be lymphatic or by the veins.

Anæsthesia Pneumonia.—The cases appear to be quite as frequent after chloroform as after ether. The vapor of the anæsthetic may itself have a damaging influence on the bronchial and alveolar epithelium, but a more important influence is the aspiration of mucus and saliva into the air passages during the anæsthesia. Thorough disinfection of the mouth and throat before operation is a useful preventive measure. W. Pasteur called attention to a condition of massive collapse of the lungs due to deflation of the lower lobes, owing to imperfect action or paralysis of the diaphragm. He published the statistics of lung complications at the Middlesex Hospital; following 3,559 abdominal operations there were 201 pulmonary complications, with 45 deaths. Among these pneumonia heads the list with 88 cases and 31 deaths. The complications are much more numerous in operations above the umbilicus. The pneumonia is usually patchy, involving both lungs; sometimes it is lobar, and as a rule the signs are well marked within the first two days after operation. The collapse, to which Pasteur calls attention, may involve both lower lobes or only one lung, and it may simulate pneumonia very closely, or may initiate it. When unilateral, the mediastinum and heart are drawn towards the affected side. It may come on with great suddenness, and when widespread it may prove fatal.

Delayed Resolution.—The lung is restored to its normal state by the liquefaction and absorption of the exudate. There are cases in which resolution takes place rapidly without any increase in (or, indeed, without any) expectoration; on the other hand, during resolution it is not uncommon to find in the sputum the little plugs of fibrin and leucocytes which have been loosened from the air-cells and expelled by coughing. A variable time is taken in the restoration of the lung.. Sometimes within a week or ten days the dulness is greatly diminished, the breath-sounds become clear, and, so far as physical signs are any guide, the lung seems perfectly restored. Delayed resolution occurs in from 3 to 4 per cent. of cases. Of 40 cases at the Johns Hopkins Hospital, 33 were males and 7 females; 23 of the patients were negroes, a very high incidence. The lower lobe is most frequently involved, 37 cases in this series, usually the right one and as a rule only one lobe. The duration was to the fourth week 5 cases, fifth week 10 cases, sixth week 4 cases, ninth week 3 cases, tenth, eleventh and twelfth weeks each one case. In one patient the left lung, except a small portion of the upper lobe, remained solid for eleven weeks and then cleared perfectly.

Clinically, there are several groups of cases: First, those in which the crisis occurs naturally, the temperature falls and remains normal; but the local features persist—well-marked flatness with tubular breathing and râles. Resolution may occur very slowly and gradually, taking from two to three weeks. In a second group of cases the temperature falls by lysis, and with the persistence of the local signs there is slight fever, sometimes sweats and rapid pulse. The condition may persist for three or four weeks and during all this time there may be little or no sputum. The practitioner is naturally much exercised, and he dreads lest tuberculosis should supervene. In a third group the crisis occurs or the fever falls by lysis; but the consolidation persists, and there may be intense bronchial breathing, with few or no râles, or the fever may recur and the patient may die exhausted.

TERMINATION IN CHRONIC PNEUMONIA.—The exudate may organize and the alveolar walls thicken with the gradual production of a chronic interstitial or fibroid pneumonia. In one pneumonia autopsy on a patient aged 58, dead on the thirty-second day from the initial chill, the right lung was solid and the cut surface grayish in color with a smooth, translucent appearance. This is most frequently seen as a sequence of delayed resolution in debilitated subjects. Milne found 10 instances of organization of the exudate among 150 fatal cases. The shortest duration in the series was twenty-three days.

Ordinary lobar pneumonia never terminates in tuberculosis. The instances of caseous pneumonia and softening which have followed an acute pneumonic process have been tuberculous from the outset.

TERMINATION IN ABSCESS.—This occurred in 4 of the 100 autopsies. Usually the lung breaks down in limited areas and the abscesses are not large, but they may fuse and involve a considerable proportion of a lobe. The condition is recognized by the sputum, which is usually abundant and contains pus and elastic tissue, sometimes cholesterin crystals and hæmatoidin crystals. The cough is often paroxysmal and of great severity; usually the fever is remittent, or in protracted cases intermittent in character, and there may be pronounced hectic symptoms. When a case is seen for the first time it may be difficult to determine whether it is one of abscess of the lung or a local empyema which has perforated the lung.

GANGRENE.—This is most commonly seen in old debilitated persons. It was present in 3 of the 100 autopsies. It very often occurs with abscess. The gangrene is associated with the growth of the saprophytic bacteria on a soil made favorable by the presence of the pneumococcus or the streptococcus. Clinically, the gangrene is rendered very evident by the horribly fetid odor of the expectoration and its characteristic features. In some instances the gangrene may be found post mortem when clinically there has not been any evidence of its existence.

Prognosis.—Pneumonia is one of the most fatal of all acute diseases, outranking even tuberculosis as a cause of death in some years. In America the mortality appears to be increasing.

The statistics of the clinic at the Johns Hopkins Hospital from 1889 to 1905 have been analyzed by Chatard. There were 658 cases with 200 deaths, a mortality of 30.4 per cent. Excluding 35 cases of terminal pneumonia, the percentage is 26.4. The death rate among 245 negroes was very little above that of the whites. Greenwood and Candy in a study of the pneumonia statistics at the London Hospital from 1854-1903, a total of 5,097 cases, conclude that the fatality of the disease has not appreciably changed in this period. In comparing the collected figures of these authors with those from other institutions, there is an extraordinary uniformity in the mortality rate. Between the ages of 21-30 the mortality is everywhere about 20 per cent.; between the ages of 31-40, 30 per cent.; and then after each decade it rises, until above the age of 60 more than one-half of the persons attacked die.

The mortality in private practice varies greatly. R. P. Howard treated

170 cases with only 6 per cent. of deaths. Fussell reported 134 cases with a mortality of 17.9 per cent. The mortality in children is sometimes very low. Morrill reported 6 deaths in 123 cases of frank pneumonia. On the other hand, Goodhart had 25 deaths in 120 cases.

The following are among the factors which influence prognosis:

Age.—As Sturges remarks, the old are likely to die, the young to recover. Under one year it is more fatal than between two and five. Of 50 cases under 10 years of age, 4 died; of 119 cases under 20, 16 died (Chatard). Above sixty the death rate is very high, amounting to 60 or 80 per cent.; 33 of 44 cases in our series. From the reports of its fatality in some places, one may say that to die of pneumonia is almost the natural end of old people.

Previous habits of life and the condition of bodily health at the time of the attack are most important factors. In analyzing a series of fatal cases one is very much impressed with the number of cases in which the organs show signs of degeneration. In 25 of the 100 autopsies at the Montreal General Hospital the kidneys showed extensive interstitial changes. Individuals debilitated from sickness or poor food, hard drinkers, and that large class of hospital patients, composed of robust-looking laborers between the ages of forty-five and sixty, whose organs show signs of wear and tear, and who have by excesses in alcohol weakened the reserve power, fall an easy prey to the disease. Very few fatal cases occur in robust, healthy adults. Some of the statistics given by army surgeons show the low mortality from pneumonia in healthy picked men. The death rate in the German army in over 40,000 cases was only 3.6 per cent.

Certain *complications* and terminations are particularly serious. The meningitis of pneumonia is almost always fatal. Endocarditis is extremely grave, more so than pericarditis. Much stress has been laid upon the factor of *leucocytosis* as an element in the prognosis. A very slight or complete absence of a leucocytosis is rightly regarded as very unfavorable.

Toxæmia is the important prognostic feature, to which in a majority of the cases the degree of pyrexia and the extent of consolidation are entirely subsidiary. It is not at all proportionate to the degree of lung involved. A severe and fatal toxæmia may occur with the consolidation of only a small part of one lobe. On the other hand, a patient with complete solidification of one lung may have no signs of a general infection. The question of individual resistance seems to be the most important one, and one sees robust-looking individuals fatally stricken within a few days.

The determination of the *type* of organism is of assistance. The death rate in Types I and II is from 25 to 30 per cent; in Type III about 50 per cent., and in Type IV 12 per cent. A high degree of blood infection as shown by cultures is a bad omen.

Death is rarely due to direct interference with the function of respiration, even in double pneumonia. Sometimes it seems to be caused by the extensive involvement with œdema of the other parts of the lungs, an engorgement with progressive weakness of the right heart. But death is most frequently due to the action of the toxin on the circulation, with progressive lowering of the blood pressure.

Diagnosis.—No disease is more readily recognized in a large majority of the cases. The external characters, the sputum, and the physical signs combine to make one of the clearest of clinical pictures. The ordinary lobar pneumonia of adults is rarely overlooked. Errors are particularly liable to occur in the intercurrent pneumonias, in those complicating chronic affections, and in the disease as met with in children, the aged, and drunkards. Acute pneumonic tuberculosis is frequently confounded with pneumonia. Pleurisy with effusion is not often mistaken except in children. The diagnostic points will be referred to under pleurisy.

In diabetes, nephritis, chronic heart-disease, pulmonary tuberculosis, and cancer, an acute pneumonia often ends the scene, and is frequently overlooked. In these cases the temperature is perhaps the best index, and should, more particularly if cough occurs, lead to a careful examination of the lungs. The absence of expectoration and of pulmonary symptoms may make the diagnosis very difficult.

In children there are two special sources of error: the disease may be entirely masked by the cerebral symptoms and the case mistaken for one of *meningitis*. It is remarkable in these cases how few indications there are of pulmonary trouble. Lumbar puncture is of great aid in these cases. The other condition is *pleurisy with effusion*, which in children often has deceptive physical signs. The breathing may be intensely tubular and tactile fremitus may be present. The exploratory needle is sometimes required to decide the question. In the old and debilitated a knowledge that the onset of pneumonia is insidious, and that the symptoms are ill-defined and latent, should put the practitioner on his guard and make him very careful in the examination of the lungs in doubtful cases. In chronic alcoholism the cerebral symptoms may completely mask the local process. As mentioned, the disease may assume the form of violent mania, but more commonly the symptoms are those of delirium tremens. In any case, rapid pulse, rapid respiration, and fever are symptoms which should invariably excite suspicion of pneumonia. The acute signs due to a foreign body in a bronchus are often mistaken for those of pneumonia.

Pneumonia is rarely confounded with pulmonary tuberculosis, but to differentiate acute pneumonic tuberculosis is often difficult. The attack may set in with a chill. It may be impossible to determine which condition is present until softening occurs and elastic tissue and tubercle bacilli appear in the sputum. A similar mistake is sometimes made in children. With typhoid fever, pneumonia is not infrequently confounded. There are instances of pneumonia with the local signs well marked in which the patient rapidly sinks into what is known as the typhoid state, with dry tongue, rapid pulse, and diarrhœa. Unless the case is seen from the outset it may be very difficult to determine the true nature of the malady. On the other hand, there are cases of typhoid fever which set in with symptoms of lobar pneumonia—the so-called pneumo-typhus. It may be impossible to make a differential diagnosis in such a case unless the characteristic eruption occurs, a blood culture is positive, or the Widal reaction is given.

Prophylaxis.—We do not know the percentage of individuals who harbor the pneumococcus normally in the secretions of the mouth and throat. In a great majority of cases it is an auto-infection, and the lowered resistance due to exposure or to alcohol, or a trauma or anæsthetization, simply furnishes conditions which favor the spread and growth of an organism already present.

Individuals who have already had pneumonia should be careful to keep the teeth in good condition, and the mouth and throat in as healthy a state as possible. Antiseptic mouth washes may be used.

The experimental evidence suggests that there may be value in vaccines as a preventive. When done it should be regarded as an experiment and careful records kept. The question requires much further study.

We know practically nothing of the conditions under which the pneumococcus lives outside the body, or how it gains entrance in healthy individuals. The sputum of each case should be very carefully disinfected. In institutions the patients should be isolated.

Treatment.—Pneumonia is a self-limited disease and even under the most unfavorable circumstances it may terminate abruptly and naturally. So also, under the favoring circumstances of good nursing and careful diet, the experience of many physicians in different lands has shown that pneumonia runs its course in a definite time, terminating sometimes spontaneously on the third or the fifth day, or continuing until the tenth or twelfth.

Morgenroth and Levy claim for optochin, a quinine derivative, a specific action on the pneumococcus. It has a well-marked protective action against experimental infection in mice; encouraging, but scarcely good enough results to use the term specific have been reported clinically. It is given in amounts of 1.5 gm. per day in doses of 0.2 to 0.25 gm. Over-dosage is usually manifested by disturbances of vision.

(*a*) General Management of a Case.—The same careful hygiene of the bed and of the sick-room should be carried out as in typhoid fever. Everything should be done to make the patient comfortable and to save him exertion. Whenever possible the patient should be in the open air. In cold weather he should have sufficient covering to keep him warm, but should not be overburdened by a heavy weight of clothes. A blanket and rubber sheet, under the mattress, which can be folded up over the bed prevent chilling from below. A hot-water bag should be kept at the feet. The patient is brought indoors when necessary for hydrotherapy. For the heavy undershirts should be substituted a thin, light flannel jacket, open in front, which enables the physician to make his examinations without unnecessarily disturbing the patient. If the patient is indoors the room should be bright and light, letting in the sunshine if possible, and thoroughly well ventilated. Only one or two persons should be allowed in the room at a time. Even when not called for on account of the high fever, the patient should be carefully sponged each day with tepid water. This should be done with as little disturbance as possible. Special care should be taken to keep the mouth and nose clean. The giving of an alkali, such as potassium citrate (gr. xv, 1 gm. four times a day) is advisable.

(*b*) Diet.—Plain water, a pleasant table water, or lemonade should be given freely. When the patient is delirious the water should be given at fixed intervals and by the bowel or subcutaneously if it is not taken by mouth. The food should be liquid, consisting chiefly of milk, either alone or, better, mixed with food prepared from some one of the cereals, and eggs, either soft boiled or raw. Carbohydrate, as milk sugar, can be added to each feeding of milk, and as cane sugar to lemonade.

(*c*) Bowels.—At the onset it is well to give a calomel and saline purge.

The bowels can be kept open by salines or enemata. Drastic purgation is not advisable. It is important to prevent *meteorism,* if possible, by care in the diet, giving water freely and preventing constipation. If present, measures for relief should be begun at once. Turpentine stupes, turpentine (℥ ss, 15 c. c.) added to an enema, and the use of the rectal tube, are helpful. Strychnine and pituitary extract hypodermically are also useful. If the stomach is distended a stomach tube should be passed.

(*d*) Bleeding.—The reproach of Van Helmont, that "a bloody Moloch presides in the chairs of medicine," can not be brought against this generation of physicians. Before Louis' iconoclastic paper on bleeding in pneumonia it would have been regarded as almost criminal to treat a case without venesection. We employ it much more than we did a few years ago, but more often late in the disease than early. To bleed at the very onset in robust, healthy individuals in whom the disease sets in with great intensity and high fever is good practice. Late in the course marked dilatation of the right heart is the common indication. The quantity of blood removed must be decided by the effect; small amounts are often sufficient.

(*e*) Antipneumococcic Serum.—The value of this method of treatment is established for Type I. The type of infection must be determined. In Type I, the serum should be given as soon as possible in doses of 50-100 c. c. diluted one half with freshly prepared salt solution. This is repeated twice daily, four or five doses usually being necessary. A rise in temperature indicates further dosage. Immune bodies are found in the blood after the first injection and remain if the treatment is continued. There is no proof that the use of vaccines is of value in treatment.

(*f*) Hydrotherapy.—This—internal and external—is our principal means of combating toxæmia and circulatory failure. Cold sponging is usually the best measure, done every three hours and with the least possible disturbance of the patient. With marked toxæmia or hyperpyrexia a bath at 80° with constant friction may be given for five minutes if it does not increase distress or dyspnœa. The application of linen compresses covered by flannel is an excellent measure. They should be cut to the size of the body, in the shape of a jacket, with the opening at one side instead of in the front, which can be applied from the side of the body with the patient turned, and fastened over the other shoulder and in the axilla. They should be wrung out of water at 50° to 60° and be changed every hour. The compress should cover the thorax and upper abdomen. A large flat ice bag may be kept to the side or back constantly, unless it causes distress. Probably the best effect of hydrotherapy is on the vaso-motor system.

(*g*) Symptomatic Treatment.—(1) *To Relieve the Pain.*—The stitch in the side at onset, which is sometimes so agonizing, is best relieved by a hypodermic injection of morphia (gr. ¼, 0.016 gm.). When the pain is less intense and diffuse over one side, the Paquelin cautery applied lightly is very helpful, but the ice bag is usually efficacious. When the disease is fairly established the pain is not, as a rule, distressing, except when the patient coughs, and for this codein (gr. ½, 0.03 gm.) may be used, heroin (gr. 1/12, 0.005 gm.), or morphia given hypodermically (gr. 1/6, 0.01 gm.), according to the patient's needs. Hot poultices relieve the pain, though not more than the cold applications. For children they are often preferable.

(2) *To Combat the Toxæmia.*—Abundance of water should be given to promote the flow of urine, and saline subcutaneously seems to act helpfully in this way, but care must be taken not to give too large an amount if the circulation is failing; 500 c. c. is usually sufficient. External hydrotherapy should be kept up actively. The bowels should be kept freely open by saline laxatives.

(3) An all-important indication is *to support the circulation.* Hydrotherapy and keeping the patient out of doors are of great value for this. Mechanical disturbance, as from meteorism, should be prevented if possible. Drugs should not be given in any routine way and not until they are required. Strychnine is useful (also for its effects on the respiratory centre). It should be given hypodermically and in full doses (gr. 1/20, 0.003 gm., and even gr. 1/10, 0.006 gm., for short periods) every two or three hours. Atropine is useful, especially when there is stasis, and should be given in full doses hypodermically. In severe cases it is well to begin the use of digitalis early in the form of the tincture (♏ xv, 1 c. c.) three or four times a day. With signs of weakness of the circulation, intramuscular injections of one of the digitalis preparations are advisable. In severe conditions the use of strophanthus is often more efficient, given as the tincture (♏ xv, 1 c. c.) or strophanthin (gr. 1/100, 0.0006 gm.) intramuscularly or intravenously. This may be repeated once in twelve or twenty-four hours. For severe circulatory failure, camphor gr. iii, 0.2 gm. in olive oil, caffeine (sodiobenzoate) gr. v. (0.3 gm.), or epinephrine (♏ xv, 1 c. c.) may be given hypodermically. Pituitary extract (posterior lobe) has been warmly recommended. An injection of hot saline solution given high in the bowel or a saline infusion is helpful.

(4) *Respiratory Tract.*—The most comfortable position, avoidance of exertion, and abundance of fresh air are important aids in preventing dyspnœa. Pain should be relieved as much as possible. The value of the administration of oxygen is doubtful. If used, it should be given slowly and through a funnel held over the mouth and nose. The effect is the best guide as to its continuance. Expectorant drugs are not indicated and often upset the stomach. When the cough is severe it is well to give sedatives, of which codein or heroin are the best. Morphia in small doses may be required, but these drugs should be given only when necessary. For *œdema* of the lungs digitalis or strophanthus should be given intramuscularly and atropine (gr. 1/100, 0.0006 gm.) and caffeine hypodermically. Venesection is advisable if the right heart be dilated.

(5) *Nervous System.*—The patient with delirium should be constantly watched. An ice bag to the head and frequent ice packs or cold sponges are useful. *Sleep* is important for every patient and the need for this is often forgotten. While such drugs as the bromides and chloral hydrate may be effectual, it is wiser, as a rule, to give morphia hypodermically in a sufficient dose (gr. ¼, 0.016 gm.) to secure rest and sleep.

(6) *Crisis.*—As this approaches constant watch should be kept for signs of collapse. If sweating is profuse and the patient feeble, atropine (gr. 1/100, 0.0006 gm.) should be given hypodermically as often as necessary, with camphor and epinephrine.

(*h*) Treatment of Complications.—If the fever persists it is important to look out for pleurisy, particularly for the empyema. The exploratory needle should be used if necessary. A sero-fibrinous effusion should be aspirated, a purulent opened and drained. In a complicating pericarditis with a large effusion aspiration may be necessary. Delayed resolution is a difficult condition to treat. The use of the X-rays is perhaps the most effective treatment, but tuberculosis should be excluded.

(*i*) CONVALESCENCE.—The diet should be increased as rapidly as possible, the patient kept out of doors and after an ordinary attack allowed up in about a week. If the heart has suffered rest should be more prolonged.

B. BRONCHO-PNEUMONIA

(*Lobular Pneumonia, Capillary Bronchitis*)

Definition.—A bacterial infection of the finer bronchi and their related lobules. The process begins with inflammation of the bronchioles and smaller bronchi, a capillary bronchitis, which extends to the alveoli and the whole lobule or a group of lobules becomes filled with exudate, cellular and hæmorrhagic but distinctly less fibrinous than in lobar pneumonia.

Etiology.—Broncho-pneumonia occurs either as a primary or as a secondary affection. The relative frequency in 443 cases is thus given by Holt: Primary, without previous bronchitis, 154; secondary to bronchitis of the larger tubes, 41; to measles, 89; to whooping-cough, 66; to diphtheria, 47; to scarlet fever, 7; to influenza, 6; to varicella, 2; to erysipelas, 2; and to acute ileo-colitis, 19. The proportion of primary to secondary forms as shown in this list is probably too low.

PRIMARY ACUTE BRONCHO-PNEUMONIA, like the lobar form, attacks those of any age. The etiological factors are very much those of lobar pneumonia, and probably the pneumococcus is often associated with it.

SECONDARY BRONCHO-PNEUMONIA occurs in two great groups: (a) As a sequence of the infectious fevers—measles, diphtheria, influenza, whooping-cough, scarlet fever, and, less frequently smallpox, erysipelas, and typhoid fever. In children it forms the most serious complication of these diseases, and in reality causes more deaths than are due directly to the fevers. In large cities it ranks next in fatality to infantile diarrhœa. Following, as it does, the contagious diseases which principally affect children, we find that a large majority of cases occur during early life. According to Morrill's Boston statistics, it is most fatal during the first two years of life. The number of cases increases or decreases with the prevalence of measles, scarlet fever, and diphtheria. It is most prevalent in the winter and spring months. In the febrile affections of adults broncho-pneumonia is not very common. Thus in typhoid fever it is not so frequent as lobar pneumonia, though isolated areas of consolidation at the bases are by no means rare in protracted cases of this disease. In old people it may follow debilitating causes of any sort, and is met with in chronic nephritis and various acute and chronic maladies.

(*b*) In the second division of this affection are embraced the cases of so-called aspiration or deglutition pneumonia. Whenever the sensitiveness of the larynx is benumbed, as in the coma of apoplexy or uræmia, minute particles of food or drink are allowed to pass the *rima,* and, reaching finally the smaller tubes, excite an intense inflammation similar to the vagus pneumonia which follows the section of the pneumogastrics in the dog. Cases are common after operations about the mouth and nose, after tracheotomy, and in cancer of the larynx and œsophagus. The aspirated particles in some instances induce such an intense broncho-pneumonia that suppuration or gangrene supervenes. The ether pneumonia may be lobular in type.

An aspiration broncho-pneumonia may follow hæmoptysis, the aspiration of material from a bronchiectatic cavity, and occasionally the material from an empyema which has ruptured into the lung. A common and fatal form of broncho-pneumonia is that excited by the tubercle bacillus.

Among general predisposing causes may be mentioned *age*. It is prone to attack infants, and a majority of cases of pneumonia in children under five years of age are of this form. Of 370 cases in children under five years of age, 75 per cent. were broncho-pneumonia (Holt). At the opposite extreme of life it is also common, in association with influenza and with various debilitating circumstances and chronic diseases. In children, rickets and diarrhœa are marked predisposing causes, and broncho-pneumonia is one of the most frequent post mortem lesions in infants' homes and foundling asylums. The disease prevails most extensively among the poorer classes.

Morbid Anatomy.—On the pleural surfaces, particularly toward the base, are seen depressed bluish or blue-brown areas of collapse, between which the lung tissue is of a lighter color. Here and there are projecting portions over which the pleura may be slightly turbid or granular. The lung is fuller and firmer than normal, and, though in great part crepitant, solid, nodular bodies can be felt in places throughout the substance. The dark depressed areas may be isolated or a large section of one lobe may be in the condition of collapse. Gradual inflation by a blow-pipe inserted in the bronchus will distend a great majority of these collapsed areas. On section, the general surface has a dark reddish color and usually drips blood. Projecting above the level of the section are lighter red or reddish-gray areas representing the patches of broncho-pneumonia. These may be isolated and separated from each other by tracts of uninflamed tissue or they may be in groups; or the greater part of a lobe may be involved. Study of a favorable section of an isolated patch shows: (*a*) A dilated central bronchiole full of tenacious purulent mucus. A fortunate section parallel to the long axis may show a racemose arrangement—the alveolar passages full of muco-pus. (*b*) Surrounding the bronchus for from 3 to 5 mm. or even more, an area of grayish-red consolidation, usually elevated above the surface and firm to the touch. It may present a perfectly smooth surface, though in some instances it is distinctly granular. In a late stage small grayish-white points may be seen, which on pressure may be squeezed out as purulent droplets. A section in the axis of the lobule may present a somewhat grape-like arrangement, the stalks and stems representing the bronchioles and alveolar passages filled with a yellowish or grayish-white pus, while surrounding them is a reddish-brown hepatized tissue. (*c*) In the immediate neighborhood of this peribronchial inflammation the tissue is dark in color, smooth, airless, at a somewhat lower level than the hepatized portion, and differs distinctly in color and appearance from the other portions of the lung. This is the condition to which the term *splenization* has been given. It really represents a tissue in the early stage of inflammation, and it would be well to give up the use of this term and also that of *carnification,* which is only a more advanced stage.

There are three groups of cases: (1) Those in which the bronchitis and bronchiolitis are most marked, and in which there may be no definite consolidation, and yet on microscopic examination many of the alveolar passages and adjacent air-cells appear filled with inflammatory products. (2) The disseminated broncho-pneumonia, in which there are scattered areas of peribronchial hepatization with patches of collapse, while a considerable proportion of the lobe is still crepitant. This is by far the most common condition. (3) The pseudo-lobar form, in which the greater portion of the lobe is consolidated, but not uniformly, for intervening strands of dark congested lung tissue separate the groups of hepatized lobules.

Microscopically, the centre of the bronchus is seen filled with a plug of exudation, consisting of leucocytes and swollen epithelium. Section in the long axis may show irregular dilatations of the tube. The bronchial wall is swollen and infiltrated with cells. The air-cells next the bronchus are mostly densely filled, while toward the periphery the alveolar exudation becomes less. The contents of the air-cells are made up of leucocytes and swollen epithelial cells in varying proportions. Red corpuscles are not often present and a fibrin network is rarely seen, though it may be present in some alveoli. In the swollen walls are seen distended capillaries and numerous leucocytes. As Delafield pointed out, the interstitial inflammation of the bronchi and alveolar walls is the special feature of broncho-pneumonia.

The histological changes in the aspiration or deglutition broncho-pneumonia differ from the ordinary post-febrile form in a more intense infiltration of the air-cells with leucocytes, producing suppuration and foci of softening; even gangrene may be present.

Bacteriology.—The organisms most commonly found in broncho-pneumonia are the pneumococcus, *Streptococcus pyogenes* (either alone or with the pneumococcus), *Staphylococcus aureus et albus,* Friedländer's *Bacillus pneumoniæ,* and the influenza bacillus. The Klebs-Loeffler bacillus is not infrequently found in the secondary lesions of diphtheria. Except the pneumococcus these microbes are rarely found in pure cultures. In the lobular type the streptococcus is the most constant organism, in the pseudo-lobar the pneumococcus. Mixed infections are almost the rule in broncho-pneumonia.

Terminations of Broncho-pneumonia.—(*a*) In *resolution,* which when it once begins goes on more rapidly than in fibrinous pneumonia. Broncho-pneumonia of the apices, in a child, persisting for three or more weeks, particularly if it follow measles or diphtheria, is often tuberculous. In these instances, when resolution is supposed to be delayed, caseation has in reality taken place. (*b*) In *suppuration,* which is rarely seen apart from the aspiration and deglutition forms, in which it is extremely common. (*c*) In *gangrene,* which occurs under the same conditions. (*d*) In *fibroid changes*—*chronic broncho-pneumonia*—a rare termination in the simple, a common sequence of the tuberculous, disease. Formerly it was thought that one of the most common changes in broncho-pneumonia, particularly in children, was caseation, but this is really a tuberculous process, the natural termination of an originally specific broncho-pneumonia.

Symptoms.—The *primary* form sets in abruptly with a chill or a convulsion. The patient has not had a previous illness, but there may have been slight exposure. The temperature rises rapidly and is more constant; the physical signs are more local and there is not the widespread diffuse catarrh of the smaller tubes. Many cases are mistaken for lobar pneumonia. In others the pulmonary features are in the background or are overlooked in the intensity of the general or cerebral symptoms. The termination is often by crisis, and the recovery is prompt. The mortality of this form is slight. S. West has called attention to the importance of recognizing these primary cases and to their resemblance in clinical features to acute lobar pneumonia. The *secondary* form begins usually as a bronchitis of the smaller tubes. Much confusion has arisen from the description of capillary bronchitis as a separate affection, whereas it is only a part, though a primary and important one, of broncho-pneumonia. At the outset it may be said that if in convalescence from measles or whooping-cough a child has an accession of fever with cough, rapid pulse, and rapid breathing, and if, on auscultation, fine râles are heard at the bases, or widely spread throughout the lungs, even though neither consolidation nor blowing breathing can be detected, the diagnosis of broncho-pneumonia may safely be made. We have never seen in a fatal case after diphtheria or measles a capillary bronchitis as the sole lesion. The onset is rarely sudden, or with a distinct chill; but after a day or so of indisposition the child becomes feverish and begins to cough and be short of breath. The fever is extremely variable; a range of from 102° to 104° F. is common. The skin is very dry and hot. The cough is hard, distressing, and may be painful. Dyspnœa gradually becomes a prominent feature. Expiration may be jerky and grunting. The respirations may rise as high as 60 or even 80 per minute. Within the first forty-eight hours the percussion resonance is not impaired; the note, indeed, may be very full at the anterior borders of the lungs. On auscultation, many râles are heard, chiefly the fine subcrepitant variety, with sibilant rhonchi. There may really be no signs indicating that the parenchyma of the lung is involved, and yet even at this early stage, within forty-eight hours of the onset of the pulmonary symptoms, scattered nodules of lobular hepatization may be found. Northrup, in a case in which death occurred within the first twenty-four hours, in addition to the extensive involvement of the smaller bronchi, found the intralobular tissue also involved in places. The dyspnœa is constant and progressive and soon signs of deficient aëration of the blood are noted. The face becomes a little suffused and the finger-tips bluish. The patient has an anxious expression and gradually enters upon the most distressing stage of asphyxia. At first the urgency of the symptoms is marked, but soon the influence of the toxins is seen and there are no longer strenuous efforts to breathe. The cough subsides, and, with a gradual increase in lividity and a drowsy restlessness, the right ventricle becomes more and more distended, the bronchial râles become more liquid as the tubes fill with mucus, and death follows. These are symptoms of a severe case of broncho-pneumonia, or what the older writers called *suffocative catarrh*.

The PHYSICAL SIGNS may at first be those of capillary bronchitis, as indicated by the absence of dulness and the presence of fine subcrepitant and whistling râles. In many cases death takes place before any definite pneumonic signs are detected. When these exist they are much more frequent at the bases, where there may be areas of impaired resonance or even of positive dulness. When numerous foci involve the greater part of a lobe the breathing may become tubular, but in the scattered patches of ordinary broncho-pneumonia, following the fevers, the breathing is more commonly harsh than blowing. In grave cases there is retraction of the base of the sternum and of the lower costal cartilages during inspiration, pointing to deficient lung expansion. There is a group in which an area of consolidation at the base may persist for some time, weeks or months.

Diagnosis.—With lobar pneumonia it may readily be confounded if the areas of consolidation are large and merged together. It is to be remembered, as Holt's figures well show, that in children broncho-pneumonia occurs chiefly under one year, whereas lobar pneumonia is more common after the third year. No writer has so clearly brought out the difference between pneumonia at these periods as Gerhard,* of Philadelphia, whose papers on this subject have the freshness and accuracy which characterized all the writings of that eminent physician. Between lobar pneumonia and the secondary form of broncho-pneumonia the diagnosis is easy. The mode of onset is essentially different in the two infections, the one developing insidiously in the course or at the conclusion of another disease, the other setting in abruptly in a person in good health. In lobar pneumonia the disease is usually unilateral, in broncho-pneumonia bilateral. The chief trouble arises in cases of primary broncho-pneumonia, which by aggregation of the foci involves the greater part of one lobe. Here the difficulty is very great, and the physical signs may be practically identical, but in broncho-pneumonia it is much more likely that a lesion, however slight, will be found on the other side. In children the signs caused by a foreign body in a bronchus, especially a peanut, may be mistaken for those of broncho-pneumonia.

A still more difficult question to decide is whether an existing broncho-pneumonia is simple or tuberculous. In many instances the decision cannot be made, as the circumstances under which the disease occurs, the mode of onset, and the physical signs may be identical. A case may be sent down from the children's ward to the dead house with the diagnosis of broncho-pneumonia in which there was no suspicion of the existence of tuberculosis; but the section shows tuberculous bronchial glands and scattered areas of broncho-pneumonia, some of which are distinctly caseous, while others show signs of softening. It is well to emphasize the fact that there are many cases of broncho-pneumonia which time alone enables us to distinguish from tuberculosis. The existence of extensive disease at the apices or central regions is a suggestive indication, and signs of softening may be detected. In the vomited matter, which is brought up after severe spells of coughing, sputum may be picked out and elastic tissue and tubercle bacilli detected.

It must not be forgotten that, as in lobar pneumonia, cerebral symptoms may mask the true nature of the disease, and may even lead to the diagnosis of meningitis. Without an autopsy it may not be possible to determine whether the infant had tuberculous meningitis or a cerebral complication of an acute pulmonary affection.

Prognosis.—In the primary form the outlook is good. In children enfeebled by constitutional disease and prolonged fevers broncho-pneumonia is

* American Journal of Medical Sciences, vols. xiv and xv.

terribly fatal, but in cases coming on in connection with whooping-cough or after measles recovery may take place in the most desperate cases. It is in this disease that the truth of the old maxim is shown—"Never despair of a sick child." The death rate in children under five has been variously estimated at from 30 to 50 per cent. After diphtheria and measles thin, wiry children seem to stand broncho-pneumonia much better than fat, flabby ones. In adults the aspiration or deglutition pneumonia is a very fatal disease.

Prophylaxis.—Much can be done to reduce the probability of attack after febrile affections. Thus, in the convalescence from measles and whooping-cough, it is very important that the child should not be exposed to cold, particularly at night, when the temperature of the room naturally falls. The use of light flannel "combinations" obviates this nocturnal chill, which is an important factor in the colds and pulmonary affections of young children. The catarrhal troubles of the nose and throat should be carefully attended to, and during fevers the mouth should be washed two or three times a day with an antiseptic solution.

Treatment.—The frequency and the seriousness of broncho-pneumonia render it a disease which taxes to the utmost the resources of the practitioner. There is no acute pulmonary affection over which he at times so greatly despairs. On the other hand, there is not one in which he will be more gratified in saving patients who have seemed past all succor. The general measures are much as in lobar pneumonia. The patient should be in the open air if a trial shows that he is more comfortable than inside; if indoors, the windows should be wide open with the patient protected from drafts.

(*a*) Diet.—As much food as possible should be given. Milk and its modifications, ice cream, eggs, broths, cocoa, and gruels are suitable. Water should be given freely by mouth and if this is not possible by the bowel or subcutaneously. The *bowels* should be opened by castor oil or calomel and care taken to secure a daily movement.

(*b*) Hydrotherapy.—This may be given by various methods to be chosen for each patient, depending on the condition and results. Sponges may be given to any patient. Packs are useful, hot if there is much restlessness or cold if the temperature is high, or baths may be given to children for short periods, using water at 95° F. and gradually reducing to 75° or 80° F. Compresses, made out of linen covered by flannel or of flannel alone, wrung out of water 60° to 70°, are often useful. They should not be covered by oiled silk. A mustard bath is of value for children, especially early in the attack. Hydrotherapy is especially indicated for patients with high fever, delirium or stupor, severe toxæmia, or circulatory failure.

(*c*) Local Applications.—Poultices have gone out of fashion but are sometimes of value. They should be light and are best kept in place by being slipped in pockets in a flannel jacket which is constantly worn so that the poultice can be replaced without disturbing the patient. The use of dry cups is often advised; they should be applied frequently. The ice bag should be used if it gives comfort.

(*d*) Medicinal.—The indications must be carefully studied and drugs which may disturb the stomach given with care. If cough is distressing the use of the compound tincture of benzoin in an inhalation should be tried. The expectorant drugs may aid and of these ammonium chloride (gr. ii to v,

0.13 to 0.3 gm.) and the wine of ipecacuanha (♏ x to xx, 0.6 to 1.3 c. c.) are the most useful. To these a sedative, such as paregoric (ʒ i, 4 c. c.), codein (gr. $\frac{1}{4}$, 0.016 gm.) or heroin (gr. 1-20, 0.0032 gm.) should be added if the cough is very distressing. Strychnine hypodermically (gr. 1-40 to 1-20, 0.0016 to 0.0032 gm.) is an aid to the respiratory centre and to the circulation. For circulatory failure the treatment is the same as described under lobar pneumonia. With increasing difficulty in getting up the secretions an emetic may be given, but only to robust patients. Ipecacuanha or apomorphine hypodermically should be employed. Inhalations of oxygen are advisable if they give relief to the dyspnœa and lessen cyanosis.

In old persons early stimulation is usually advisable and every effort should be made to persuade them to take nourishment. Cold applications must be used with caution and the use of heat is generally better. At all ages frequent change in position is advisable and in young children this may be done by taking them out of bed and holding them in the arms.

C. OTHER PNEUMOCOCCIC INFECTIONS

The organism is widely distributed and causes a number of affections other than pulmonary, of which the following are the most important:

1. **Acute Septicæmia.**—Without any recognized local lesion there may be a general infection with the pneumococcus. In Townsend's case, a girl, aged six, had pain in the abdomen, vomiting and a temperature of 104.2° F. without any throat affection. Death occurred in thirty hours, and a general infection with the organism was found in the blood, spleen, lungs and kidneys.

2. **Local Affections.**—The local affections caused by the pneumococcus are very numerous and will be described under their appropriate sections. In the *mouth*, erosions, gingivitis and glossitis; in the *pharynx*, inflammation and tonsillitis; in the *ear*, acute and chronic suppuration; in the accessory sinuses, of which it is a common habitant, inflammation and suppuration; in the *membrane of the brain* it is a common cause of primary and secondary meningitis; in the *bronchi* it has been found associated with acute and chronic bronchitis, and bronchiectasis; in the *lungs*, in addition to the two important diseases already considered, it may cause acute œdema and is associated with tuberculosis and many chronic affections. It has been found in acute pleurisy and it is one of the common causes of empyema; acute arthritis, primary and secondary forms; acute peritonitis, particularly in children; appendicitis; endocarditis; pyelitis and local abscesses in various parts may be caused by it.

IX. CEREBRO-SPINAL FEVER

Definition.—An infectious disease, occurring sporadically and in epidemics, caused by the *Meningococcus,* characterized by inflammation of the cerebro-spinal meninges and a clinical course of great irregularity.

The affection is also known by the names of malignant purpuric fever, petechial fever, spotted fever and epidemic cerebro-spinal meningitis.

History.—Vieusseux first described a small outbreak in Geneva in 1805. In 1806 L. Danielson and E. Mann (Medical and Agricultural Register, Boston) gave an account of "a singular and very mortal disease which lately made its appearance in Medfield, Mass." The Massachusetts Medical Society, in 1809, appointed James Jackson, Thomas Welch, and J. C. Warren to investigate it. Elisha North's little book (1811) gives a full account of the early epidemics. Stillé's monograph (1867) and the elaborate section in vol. i of Joseph Jones' works contain details of the later American outbreaks. In his Geographical Pathology, Hirsch divides the outbreaks into four periods: From 1805 to 1830, in which the disease was most prevalent throughout the United States; a second period, from 1837 to 1850, when the disease prevailed extensively in France, and there were a few outbreaks in the United States; a third period, from 1854 to 1874, when there were outbreaks in Europe and several extensive epidemics in America. During the Civil War there were comparatively few cases. It prevailed extensively in the Ottawa Valley early in the seventies. In the fourth period, from 1875 to the present time, the disease has broken out in a great many regions. In the United States, during 1898-1899, it prevailed in mild form in 27 states. Since 1899 there have been extensive outbreaks in the cities of the United States on the Atlantic coast. In New York in 1904-5 there were 6,755 cases and 3,455 deaths. In Glasgow in 1907 there were nearly 1,000 cases with 595 deaths (Chalmers). In Belfast in the eighteen months ending June, 1908, there were 725 cases with 548 deaths (Robb). There were 1,974 deaths in England and Wales in 1915, the average for the five years before being 153. In the winter of 1914-15 the disease appeared among the Canadian troops and was carried by them to England. It broke out in many home camps and, spreading to the civil population, for the first time in its history the disease prevailed widely in England.

Etiology.—Cerebro-spinal fever occurs in epidemic and in sporadic forms. The *epidemics* are localized and are rarely very widespread. Only in the tropics have there been extensive killing pandemics. As a rule, country districts have been more afflicted than cities. Mining districts and seaports have suffered most severely. The outbreaks have occurred most frequently in the winter and spring. The concentration of individuals, as of troops in barracks, is a special factor; recruits and young soldiers are specially liable. In civil life children and young adults are most susceptible. Over-exertion, long marches in the heat, depressing mental and bodily surroundings, and the misery and squalor of the large tenement houses in cities are predisposing causes. The disease is not highly infectious. It is very rare to have more than one or two cases in a house, and in a city epidemic the distribution of the cases is very irregular. The organism enters and leaves the body by the naso-pharnygeal mucous membrane, and hence infection may be by contact or by coughing and sneezing. Meningitis *carriers* play an important rôle in transmitting the disease. They are found also when the disease is not epidemic.

Sporadic cerebro-spinal fever.—The disease lingers indefinitely after an outbreak, and in all large cities cases occur. There are two types, one the posterior basic meningitis of Gee and Barlow and the other the meningococcus meningitis of young adults met with in periods during which the disease is not specially prevalent; two, three, and even five cases may occur in succession in one family. The meningitis in children, known as the *simple* or *posterior basic,* is the sporadic form. Still determined the identity of the organism with the meningococcus, and the view has been confirmed by Koplik and many others.

Bacteriology.—In 1877 Weichselbaum described the *meningococcus* or *Diplococcus intracellularis meningitidis.* In the tissues the organism is almost constantly within the polynuclear leucocytes. Investigations have shown that there are two fixed types, and others which are less fixed, distinguishable from one another by immune reactions. They are comparable to the different types of pneumococci causing pneumonia (Ellis). The type of organism in the cerebro-spinal fluid is the same as in the naso-pharynx and apparently if one variety infects the mucous membrane it is not likely that another will be superimposed on it. The use of agglutination tests has been of great value in identifying the organism. The occurrence of the organism in the blood before the signs of meningitis appear has been specially emphasized by Herrick. Three important facts have been brought out—the presence of the germ in many cases in the naso-pharynx, the existence of it in healthy contacts, and the preparation of a curative serum.

Morbid Anatomy.—In malignant cases there may be no characteristic changes, the brain and spinal cord showing only extreme congestion, which was the lesion described by Vieusseux. In a majority of the acutely fatal cases death occurs within the first week. There is intense injection of the pia-arachnoid. The exudate is usually fibrino-purulent, most marked at the base of the brain, where the meninges may be greatly thickened and plastered over with it. On the cortex there may be much lymph along the larger fissures and in the sulci; sometimes the entire cortex is covered with a thick, purulent exudate. It deserves to be recorded that Danielson and Mann made five autopsies and were the first to describe "a fluid resembling pus between the dura and pia mater." The cord is always involved with the brain. The exudate is more abundant on the posterior surface, and involves, as a rule, the dorsal and lumbar regions more than the cervical portion.

In the more chronic cases there is general thickening of the meninges and scattered yellow patches mark where the exudate has been. The ventricles in the acute cases are dilated and contain a turbid fluid, or in the posterior cornua pure pus. In the chronic cases the dilatation may be very great. The brain substance is usually a little softer than normal and has a pinkish tinge; foci of hæmorrhage and of encephalitis may be found. The cranial nerves are usually involved, particularly the second, fifth, seventh, and eighth. The spinal nerve roots are also found imbedded in the exudate.

Microscopically, the exudate consists largely of polynuclear leucocytes closely packed in a fibrinous material. In some instances there are foci of purulent infiltration and hæmorrhage. The neuroglia cells are swollen, with large, clear, and vesicular nuclei. The ganglion cells show less marked changes. Diplococci are found in variable numbers in the exudate, being more numerous in the brain than in the cord.

The nasal secretion during life may show diplococci. The sphenoidal sinuses may be full of pus and the surrounding bone inflamed. The frequency of catarrhal and other changes in the naso-pharynx and sinuses suggests that the infection reaches the meninges through this route.

Pneumonia and pleurisy have been described in the disease. Councilman reports that in 13 cases there was congestion with œdema, in 7 broncho-pneumonia, in 2 characteristic croupous pneumonia with pneumococci; in 8 pneumonia due to the meningococcus was present.

The *spleen* varies a good deal in size. In only three of the Boston fatal cases was it much enlarged. The *liver* is rarely abnormal. Acute *nephritis* may be present. The intestines sometimes show swelling of the follicles.

Symptoms.—Cases differ remarkably in their characters. Many different forms have been described. These are perhaps best grouped into three classes:

(*a*) Malignant Form.—This fulminant or apoplectic type is found with variable frequency in epidemics. It may occur sporadically. The onset is sudden, usually with violent chills, headache, somnolence, spasms in the muscles, great depression, moderate elevation of temperature, and feeble pulse, which may fall to fifty or sixty in the minute. Usually a purpuric rash develops. In a Philadelphia case, in 1888, a young girl, apparently quite well, died within twenty hours of this form. There are cases on record in which death has occurred within a shorter time. Stillé tells of a child of five years, in whom death occurred after an illness of ten hours; and refers to a case reported by Gordon, in which the entire duration of the illness was only five hours. Two of Vieusseux's cases died within twenty-four hours.

(*b*) Ordinary Form.—The stage of incubation is not known. The disease usually sets in suddenly. There may be premonitory symptoms: headache, pains in the back, and loss of appetite. More commonly, the onset is with headache, severe chill, and vomiting. The temperature rises to 101° or 102°. The pulse is full and strong. An early and important symptom is a painful stiffness of the muscles of the neck. The headache increases, and there are photophobia and great sensitiveness to noises. Children become very irritable and restless. In severe cases the contraction of the muscles of the neck sets in early, the head is drawn back, and when the muscles of the back are also involved, there is orthotonos, which is more common than opisthotonos. The pains in the back and in the limbs may be very severe. The motor symptoms are most characteristic. Tremor of the muscles may be present, with tonic or clonic spasms in the arms or legs. Rigidity of the muscles of the back or neck is very common, and the patient lies with the body stiff and the head drawn so far back that the occiput may be between the shoulder-blades. Except in early childhood convulsions are not common. Strabismus is a frequent and important symptom. Spasm of the muscles of the face may also occur. Cases have been described in which the general rigidity and stiffness was such that the body could be moved like a statue. Paralysis of the trunk muscles is rare, but paralysis of the muscles of the eye and the face is not uncommon.

Of *sensory* symptoms, headache is the most dominant and persists from the outset. It is chiefly in the back of the head, and the pain extends into the neck and back. There may be great sensitiveness along the spine, and in many cases there is general hyperæsthesia.

The *psychical* symptoms are pronounced. Delirium occurs at the onset, occasionally of a furious and maniacal kind. The patient may display marked erotic symptoms at the onset. The delirium gives place in a few days to stupor, which, as the effusion increases, deepens to coma.

The temperature is irregular and variable. Remissions occur frequently, and there is no uniform or typical curve during the disease. In some instances there has been little or no fever. In others the temperature may reach 105° or 106° F., or, before death, 108° F. The pulse may be very rapid in children; in adults it is at first usually full and strong. In some cases it is remarkably slow, and may not be more than fifty or sixty in the minute. Sighing respirations and Cheyne-Stokes breathing are met with in some instances. Unless there is pneumonia the respirations are not often increased in frequency.

The *cutaneous* features are important. Herpes occurs with a frequency almost equal to that in pneumonia or intermittent fever. The petechial rash, which has given the name spotted fever to the disease, is very variable. Stillé states that of 98 cases in the Philadelphia Hospital, no eruption was observed in 37. In the Montreal cases petechiæ and purple spots were common. They appear to have been more frequent in the epidemics in America than in Europe. The petechiæ may be numerous and cover the entire skin. An erythema or dusky mottling may be present. In some instances there have been rose-colored hyperæmic spots like the typhoid rash. Urticara or erythema nodosum, ecthyma, pemphigus, and in rare instances gangrene of the skin have been noted.

Leucocytosis is an early and constant feature, and ranges from 25,000 to 40,000 per cubic millimetre. It persists even in the most protracted cases. The meningococcus is present in the blood during life and has been demonstrated in the leucocytes.

Vomiting may be a special feature at the onset; but, as a rule, it gradually subsides. In some instances, however, it persists and becomes the most serious and distressing of the symptoms. Diarrhœa is not common, the bowels being usually constipated. The abdomen is not tender. In the acute form the spleen is usually enlarged. The urine is sometimes albuminous and the quantity may be increased. Glycosuria has been noted in some instances, and hæmaturia in the malignant types.

The duration of the disease is extremely variable. Hirsch rightly states that it may range between a few hours and several months. More than half of the deaths occur within the first five days. In favorable cases, after the symptoms have persisted for five or six days, improvement is indicated by a lessening of the spasm, reduction of the fever, and a return of the intelligence. A sudden fall in the temperature is of bad omen. Convalescence is extremely tedious, and may be interrupted by complications and sequelæ.

(*c*) Anomalous Forms.—(1) *Abortive Type.*—The attack sets in with great severity, but in a day or two the symptoms subside and convalescence is rapid. Strümpell would distinguish between this abortive variety, which begins with such intensity, and the mild ambulant cases described by certain writers. He reports a case in which the meningeal symptoms set in with the greatest intensity and persisted for four days, the temperature rising to 105.6° F. On the fifth day the patient entered upon a rapid convalescence. In the mild cases, as distinguished from the abortive, the patients complain of headache, nausea, sensations of discomfort in the back and limbs, and stiffness in the neck. There is little or no fever, and only moderate vomiting. These cases could be recognized only during the prevalence of an epidemic.

(2) *An intermittent* type has been observed in many epidemics, and was recognized by von Ziemssen and Stillé. It is characterized by exacerbations of fever, which may recur daily or every second day, or follow a curve of an intermittent or remittent character. The pyrexia resembles that of pyæmia rather than malaria.

(3) *Chronic Form.*—Heubner states that this is a relatively frequent form, though it does not seem to be recognized by many writers on the subject. An attack may be protracted for from two to five or even six months, and may cause the most intense marasmus. It is characterized by a series of recurrences of the fever, and may present the most complex symptomatology. It is not improbable that in these protracted cases chronic hydrocephalus or abscess of the brain is present. This form differs distinctly from the intermittent type. Three cases in our series were of this chronic form; in one the disease persisted for ninety days.

Complications.—Pleurisy, picarditis, and parotitis are not uncommon.

Pneumonia is described as frequent in certain outbreaks. Immermann found many instances of the combination of pneumonia with meningitis, but it does not seem possible to determine whether, in such cases, pneumonia is the primary disease and the meningitis secondary, or *vice versa.* The frequency with which inflammation of the meninges of the brain complicates pneumonia is well known. Councilman suggests that the pneumonia of the disease is not the true lobar form, but due to the meningococcus. This was found in eight of the Boston cases, and in one it was so extensive that it could have been mistaken for the ordinary lobar pneumonia. Cerebro-spinal fever sometimes prevails extensively with ordinary pneumonia, as in New York in the winter of 1903-'04. *Arthritis* has been the most frequent complication in certain epidemics. Many joints are affected simultaneously, and there are swelling, pain, and exudation, sometimes serous, sometimes purulent. This was first observed by James Jackson, Sr., in the epidemic which he described. Enteritis is rarer. Epididymitis is common in some epidemics.

Headache may persist for months or years after an attack. Chronic *hydrocephalus* occurs in certain instances in children. The symptoms of this are "paroxysms of severe headache, pains in the neck and extremities, vomiting, loss of consciousness, convulsions, and involuntary discharges of fæces and urine" (von Ziemssen). On percussion of the skull behind the junction of the frontal, parietal and temporal bones there is a tympanitic quality to the note (Macewen). Mental feebleness and aphasia have occasionally been noted. Paralysis of individual cranial nerves or of the lower extremities may persist for some time. In some of these cases there may be peripheral neuritis, as Mills suggested.

Special Senses.—*Eye.*—Optic neuritis may follow involvement of the nerve in the exudation at the base. Acute papillitis was found in 6 out of 40 cases examined by Randolph. The inflammation may extend directly into the eye along the pia-arachnoid of the optic nerve, causing purulent choroido-iritis or even keratitis. A neuritis of the fifth nerve may be followed by keratitis and purulent conjunctivitis.

Ear.—Deafness very often follows inflammation of the labyrinth. Otitis media, with mastoiditis, may occur from direct extension. In 64 cases of meningitis which recovered, Moos found that 55 per cent. were deaf. He suggests that the abortive form of the disease may be responsible for many cases of early acquired deafness. In children this not infrequently leads to deafmutism. Von Ziemssen states that in the deaf and dumb institutions of Bamberg and Nuremberg, in 1874, a majority of the pupils had become deaf from epidemic cerebro-spinal meningitis.

Nose.—Coryza is not infrequent early in the disease, probably associated with the presence of the organism on the nasal mucous membrane. In carriers the organism may persist for several weeks, in a small number over three months.

Diagnosis.—(*a*) General Features.—The fever, headache, delirium, retraction of the neck, tremor, and rigidity of the muscles are most important signs. In the meningitis of cerebro-spinal fever the spinal symptoms are very much more marked than in the other forms. One has constantly to bear in mind that certain cases of typhoid fever and of pneumonia closely simulate cerebro-spinal meningitis.

(*b*) Among the special diagnostic features may be mentioned:

Kernig's Sign.—When the thigh is flexed at right angles to the abdomen, the leg can be extended upon the thigh nearly in a straight line. If meningitis be present, strong contractures of the flexors prevent the full extension of the leg on the thigh.

Brudzinski's Sign.—Flexing the head on the chest causes flexion of the legs at the hip and knee joints, and flexing one leg on the trunk produces the same movement in the other leg.

Lumbar Puncture.—The procedure in a majority of cases can be done without general anæsthesia. The fluid runs, as a rule, with increased pressure which may reach 250-300 mm., the normal being about 120 mm., and when meningitis is present it is usually turbid, sometimes purulent, occasionally bloody. Meningitis may be present with a clear fluid. The cytology of the fluid is important. The polymorphonuclear leucocytes are in great excess while in the tuberculous form the lymphocytes are the more abundant. In the late stages and throughout the course of the posterior basic form the formula may be reversed. There is rarely any difficulty in determining between the pneumococcus and the meningococcus. If there is any doubt as to the organism the agglutination test should be done or the meningococcus searched for in the naso-pharynx. For the serological tests necessary to determine the type, monovalent serums are required, best prepared from rabbits. Careful search will usually show tubercle bacilli in cases of tuberculous meningitis or a guinea-pig may be inoculated.

Prognosis.—The mortality before the use of serum was about 75 per cent. In children the death rate is higher than in adults. The earlier the serum is given the better the outlook.

Prophylaxis.—The patient should be isolated, seen only by the doctor, nurses, and one or two special members of the family. Cultures from the naso-pharynx of those in immediate contact should be taken and *carriers* should be isolated until proved to be free of infection. The use of chloramin (1 per cent.) and zinc sulphate (1.2 per cent.) solution has been helpful in some cases. These may be applied directly to the mucous membrane or the chloramin used in an oil spray after thorough cleansing with saline solution. Another method is to use a watery solution of chloramin (2 per cent.) and zinc sulphate (1.2 per cent.). A litre of this solution is sprayed by steam into a small room and inhaled. A 1 per cent. solution of peroxide or a solution of iodine and glycerine may be used as a spray. Some carriers prove very resistant; in others the germs disappear after a few days. Hexamine, 30 to 50 grains daily, may be given. Protective vaccination was tried extensively in the last English epidemic.

Treatment.—The patient should be kept as quiet as possible, handled gently, and all causes of irritation removed. Special attention should be given to the care of the skin owing to the danger of bedsores. The hair should be clipped close and an ice-bag applied to the head. The diet should be liquid, as concentrated as possible, and given at short intervals. If swallowing is difficult the patient can be fed through a tube. Water should be given freely. The bowels are to be opened by a calomel and saline purge, and laxatives or enemata used later if necessary. For severe headache, general pains or vomiting, morphia hypodermically is usually best. The administration of hexamine, sixty grains (4 gm.) a day, is worthy of a trial.

Serum Therapy.—To Flexner we owe the specific serum which has reversed the mortality and recovery rates—one of the most striking advances in modern therapy. The serum should be given as early as possible and also in doubtful cases. It should be given intravenously in doses of 100 c. c. every eight hours, first desensitizing by giving 5 c. c. subcutaneously. Whenever the fluid obtained by lumbar puncture is purulent the serum should be given, but repeated only if the meningococcus is found. Before giving the serum as much cerebro-spinal fluid as possible should be withdrawn. If this has been large in amount (over 40 c. c.) and in severe cases, 45 c. c. of the serum should be introduced through the needle. In ordinary cases 30 c. c. of the serum should be given. In all cases with abnormal resistance to the injection of serum after an amount equal to the fluid removed has been injected, it is well to stop. If the symptoms are very severe or increasing, the injection should be repeated in twelve hours. Otherwise the usual dose (30 c. c.) should be given daily for four days. If diplococci are found after this, daily injections should be continued. Continuance or exacerbation of the symptoms demands further injections. If the condition remains stationary after four days' interval, the four daily injections should be given again and this repeated until the diplococci disappear and the symptoms abate. An average dosage of serum is 400-600 c. c. intravenously and 100 c. c. intraspinally. The failure of the serum in many hands during the recent epidemic may have been due to its preparation from different strains and the need of a polyvalent serum is evident. In the chronic forms the serum should be given if diplococci are present and in the posterior basic form in the hope of benefit.

Hydrotherapy.—This may give relief to the symptoms. Hot baths or hot packs may be given for fifteen minutes every three hours.

Lumbar Puncture.—Done for injection of the serum it is often of value in itself. Severe headache and marked cerebral features are indications. As much fluid as possible should be removed and if it escapes under high pressure early repetition is advisable. It should be done early and frequently with signs of accumulation of fluid in the ventricles.

Complications.—Conditions due to extension to the cranial nerves are not influenced by treatment. *Otitis* requires early incision and *arthritis* rest, local applications and incision if suppuration occurs. With signs of dilatation of the ventricles, drainage with injection of serum may be tried, or the serum may be introduced by ventricular puncture. This is readily done if the fontanelle is still open, the ventricle being reached at a depth of about 3 cm. In the chronic cases every effort should be made to nourish the patient well and especial precautions taken against bed-sores. For the pain and stiffness sometimes occurring in convalescence, hot baths and massage are useful.

X. INFLUENZA

(*La Grippe*)

Definition.—A pandemic disease, appearing at irregular intervals, characterized by extraordinary rapidity of extension and the large number of people attacked. Following the pandemic there are, as a rule, for several years endemic, epidemic, or sporadic outbreaks in different regions. Clinically, the disease has protean aspects, but a special tendency to attack the respiratory mucous membranes. A special organism, *Bacillus influenzæ,* is found.

History.—Great pandemics have been recognized since the sixteenth century. There were four with their succeeding epidemics during the last century—1830-'33, 1836-'37, 1847-'48, and 1889-'90. The last seems to have begun, as many others had before, in the far East. The pandemic of 1918 far exceeded any of its predecessors in its intensity. It is unusual to have the culmination in the summer months as was the case in some countries. A special feature was the high mortality in young adults, the very young and the old being comparatively immune. The accompanying pneumonia was very virulent. Pregnant women seemed particularly susceptible. The epidemic was severe in the American camps and on the transports. The *Olympic* arrived in port with 5,951 troops. On the day of arrival 571 cases of acute respiratory disease developed and within three weeks there were 1,668 cases. Of these, 534 (32 per cent.) had pneumonia, of whom 317 died, 59 per cent.

The duration of an epidemic in any one locality is from six to eight weeks. With the exceptions, perhaps, of dengue, there is no disease which attacks indiscriminately so large a portion of the inhabitants, about 40 per cent., as a rule. Fortunately, as in dengue, the rate of mortality is low if all cases are included. Leichtenstern's article in Nothnagel's Handbuch is a masterly and systematic consideration of the disease.

Etiology.—What relation has the epidemic influenza to the ordinary influenza cold or catarrhal fever (commonly also called the *grippe*), which is constantly present in the community? Leichtenstern answers this question by making the following divisions: (*a*) Epidemic *influenza vera;* (*b*) endemic-epidemic *influenza vera,* which often occurs for several years in succession after a pandemic; (*c*) endemic *influenza nostras,* pseudo-influenza or catarrhal fever, commonly called the *grippe,* is caused by various organisms, alone or in combination, and bears the same relation to the true influenza as cholera nostras does to Asiatic cholera.

Since the pandemic of 1889-'90 we have not been free from local outbreaks in some part of the world. In some places the disease seems to have been continually present. The reports are sufficiently numerous to show that the influenza bacillus is constantly with us. Many observations show that it is a frequent invader of the respiratory tract in the inter-epidemic periods and is probably responsible for many of the cases of influenza nostras. It seems to bear a similar relation to the acute infections of the respiratory tract as other common organisms.

The disease is highly infectious; it spreads with remarkable rapidity, which, however, is not greater than modern methods of conveyance. In the great pandemics some of the large prisons escaped entirely. The outbreak of epidemics is independent of all seasonal and meteorological conditions. One attack does not necessarily protect from a subsequent one. A few persons appear not to be liable to the disease.

Bacteriology.—In 1892 Pfeiffer isolated a bacillus from the nasal and bronchial secretions, which by some is recognized as the cause of the disease. It is a small, non-motile organism, which stains well in Loeffler's methylene blue, or in a dilute, pale-red solution of carbol-fuchsin in water. It has been found in the blood in a number of cases. The bacilli are present in enormous numbers in the nasal and bronchial secretions of patients, in the latter almost in pure cultures. They persist often after the severe symptoms have subsided. The experience of the pandemic of 1918 has raised the question as to the relation of the influenza bacillus to the disease. Is it the responsible organism or a secondary invader? The evidence is conflicting but does not seem to justify the conclusion that this organism is not causal. There are many secondary invading organisms, which vary in prevalence in different localities.

Symptoms.—The incubation period is from one to four days and has an average of two days. The onset is usually abrupt, with fever and its associated phenomena, headache, general pains, prostration and sometimes sore throat and an irritating cough.

Types of the Disease.—The manifestations are so extraordinarily complex that it is best to describe them under types of the disease.

(*a*) Respiratory.—The mucous membrane of the respiratory tract from the nose to the air-cells of the lungs may be regarded as the seat of election of the infection. In the simple forms the disease sets in with coryza, and presents the features of an acute catarrhal fever, with perhaps rather more prostration and debility than is usual. In other cases after catarrhal symptoms bronchitis occurs, the fever increases, there is delirium and much prostration, and the picture is that of severe toxæmia. The graver respiratory conditions are bronchitis, pleurisy, and pneumonia. The bronchitis has really no special peculiarities but the sputum is supposed by many to be distinctive. Sometimes it is in extraordinary amounts, very thin, and containing purulent masses. Pfeiffer regards sputum of a greenish-yellow color and in coin-like lumps as almost characteristic of influenza. In other cases there may be a dark red, bloody sputum. It occasionally happens that the bronchitis is of great intensity and reaches the finer tubes, so that the patient becomes cyanosed or even asphyxiated.

Influenza *pneumonia* is one of the most serious manifestations, and may depend upon Pfeiffer's bacillus itself, or be the result of a mixed infection. The true influenza pneumonia is lobular and probably never lobar. It was a special feature of the 1918 pandemic and responsible for many of the deaths. It may be present from the onset of the attack or develop after some days of general infection. The clinical course is often atypical and the signs obscure. The signs were often atypical for several days and suppression of breath sounds with fine crackling râles were the common early signs. Severe cough with bloody sputum or hæmoptysis is common. Cyanosis is usually marked. There is a special tendency to the secretion of fluid so that the lungs are "water-logged." Abscess or gangrene follows not infrequently. The toxæmia is often extreme but the circulation shows remarkably little change in many cases. The blood pressure is usually low. *Subcutaneous emphysema* was common in the 1918 epidemic, usually over the neck and upper thorax but sometimes very widespread. In many of these cases there was extreme emphysema of the lungs. Probably the air escaped, after rupture of a surface bleb, into the mediastinum and then reached the tissues of the neck.

Influenza *pleurisy* is more rare, but cases of primary involvement of the pleura are reported. It is very apt to lead to empyema. Pulmonary tuberculosis is usually much aggravated by an attack of influenza.

(*b*) Nervous Form.—Without any catarrhal symptoms there are severe headache, pain in the back and joints, with profound prostration. Among the more serious complications may be mentioned meningitis and encephalitis, the latter leading to hemiplegia or monoplegia. Abscess of the brain has followed in acute cases. Myelitis, with symptoms like an acute Landry's paralysis, has occurred, and spastic paraplegia or a pseudo-tabes may follow an attack. In the recent epidemic there were cases of widespread hæmorrhage into the spinal thecæ.

The influenza bacillus has been demonstrated by lumbar puncture during life and in the meninges after death. All forms of neuritis are not uncommon, and in some cases are characterized by marked disturbance of motion and sensation. Judging from the accounts in the literature, almost every form of disease of the nervous system may follow influenza. Among the most important of the nervous sequelæ are depression, melancholia, and in some cases dementia.

(*c*) Gastro-intestinal Form.—With the onset of the fever there may be nausea and vomiting, or the attack may set in with abdominal pain, profuse diarrhœa, and collapse. In some epidemics jaundice has been a common symptom. In a considerable number of the cases there is enlargement of the spleen, depending chiefly upon the intensity of the fever.

(*d*) Febrile Form.—The fever in influenza is very variable, but it is important to recognize that it may be the only manifestation of the disease. It is sometimes markedly remittent, with chills; or in rare cases there is a protracted, continued fever of several weeks' duration, which simulates typhoid closely. The blood shows a leucopenia which is often marked. Sometimes the fever resembles that of a tertian malaria.

Complications.—The *pericarditis* is apt to be latent. Of *endocarditis,* a number of cases have been reported in which micro-organisms morphologically like influenza bacilli have been isolated from the vegetations. The malignant form may occur. Myocarditis may follow, and has been a cause of sudden death. Functional disturbances are common, palpitation, bradycardia, tachycardia, and angina-like attacks. Phlebitis and thrombosis of various vessels have been described. *Meningitis* occurs occasionally.

Peritonitis is rare. *Cholelithiasis* may follow an attack. The increased prevalence of *appendicitis* has been attributed to influenza.

Various renal affections have been noted, but nephritis was rare in the 1918 pandemic. Orchitis has been seen. Herpes is common. A diffuse erythema sometimes occurs, occasionally purpura. Catarrhal conjunctivitis is a frequent event. Iritis, and in rare instances optic neuritis, have been met with. Acute otitis media is a common complication and infection of the sinuses is not rare. Severe and persistent vertigo may follow influenza, probably from involvement of the labyrinth. Bronchiectasis may follow. We have seen several cases; in a fatal one of three years' duration the influenza bacilli were present in the sputum.

Since the late severe epidemics it has been the fashion to date various ailments or chronic ill health from influenza. In many cases this is correct. It is astonishing the number of people who have been crippled in health for years after an attack, particularly with nervous or circulatory disturbances. Alopecia is a common sequel but is rarely permanent.

Diagnosis.—During a pandemic the cases offer but slight difficulty. The profoundness of the prostration, out of all proportion to the intensity of the disease, is one of the most characteristic features. In the respiratory form the diagnosis may be made by the bacteriological examination of the sputum, a procedure which should be resorted to early in a suspected epidemic. The more chronic pulmonary infections are sometimes mistaken for tuberculosis. The differentiation of the various forms has been sufficiently considered.

Treatment.—Isolation should be practised when possible, and old people should be guarded against all possible sources of infection. There is no conclusive proof that vaccines have any preventive effect or that they are useful in treatment. The secretions, nasal and bronchial, should be thoroughly disinfected. In every case the disease should be regarded as serious, and the patient should be confined to bed until the fever has completely disappeared. In this way alone can serious complications be avoided. From the outset the treatment should be supporting, and the patient carefully fed and well nursed. The bowels should be opened by a dose of calomel or a saline draught. At night 10 grains (0.65 gm.) of Dover's powder may be given. At the onset a warm bath is sometimes grateful in relieving the pain in the back and limbs, but great care should be taken to have the bed well warmed, and the patient should be given a hot drink after it. If the fever is high and there is delirium, acetyl-salicylic acid (gr. x, 0.6 gm.) may be given and an ice-cap applied to the head. The medicinal antipyretics should be used with caution, as profound prostration sometimes occurs after their employment. An alkali, such as potassium citrate (gr. xv, 1 gm.) four times a day should be given. Too much stress should not be laid upon the mental features. Delirium may be marked even with slight fever. In the cases with great cardiac weakness stimulants should be given freely, and during convalescence strychnia in full doses.

The intense bronchitis, pneumonia, and other complications should receive their appropriate treatment. The convalescence requires careful management, and it may be weeks or months before the patient is restored to full health. A good nutritious diet, change of air, and pleasant surroundings are essential. The depression following this disease is one of its most unpleasant and obstinate features.

XI. WHOOPING COUGH

Definition.—A specific affection due to the *Bacillus pertussis,* characterized by catarrh of the respiratory passages and a series of convulsive coughs which end in a long-drawn inspiration or "whoop."

History.—Ballonius, in his *Ephemerides,* describes the disease as it appeared in 1578. Glisson and Sydenham in the following century gave brief accounts. Willis (Pharmaceutice Rationalis, second part, 1674) gave a much better description and called it an "epidemical disorder."

Etiology.—The disease occurs in epidemic form, but sporadic cases appear in a community from time to time. It is directly contagious from person to person; but dwelling-rooms, houses, school-rooms, and other localities may be infected by a sick child. It is, however, in this way less contagious than other diseases, and is probably most often taken by direct contact. Epidemics prevail for two or three months, usually during the winter and spring, and have a curious relation to other diseases, often preceding or following epidemics of measles, less frequently of scarlet fever.

Children between the first and second dentitions are most liable to be attacked. Sucklings are not exempt, and there may be very severe attacks in infants under six weeks. Congenital cases are described. It is stated that girls are more subject to the disease than boys. Adults and old people are sometimes attacked, and in the aged it may be a very serious affection. It appears to be most contagious in the catarrhal period. A natural immunity has been mentioned, but it must be remembered that a child may have the disease in a very mild form. As a rule, one attack protects; second attacks are rare. The disease is more than twice as fatal in the negro race as in others. There were 6,075 deaths from it in 1916 in England.

The *Bacillus pertussis* resembles in certain features the influenza bacillus. It is found in early stages of the disease and not later than two weeks after the appearance of the "whoop." In convalescents the deviation of complement reaction is present and the serum is stated to agglutinate the organism. The complement fixation test is not given early and so is not of great value in diagnosis. Apes have been inoculated with the production of a characteristic pertussis.

Morbid Anatomy.—Whooping cough itself has no special pathological changes. In fatal cases pulmonary complications, particularly broncho-pneumonia, are usually present. Collapse and compensatory emphysema, vesicular and interstitial, are found, and the tracheal and bronchial glands are enlarged.

There is a constant lesion of the trachea with the presence of bacilli between the columnar cells.

Symptoms.—There is a variable period of incubation of from seven to ten days. Catarrhal and paroxysmal stages can be recognized. In the *catarrhal stage* the child has the symptoms of an ordinary cold, which may begin with slight fever, running at the nose, injection of the eyes, and a bronchial cough, usually dry, and sometimes giving indications of a spasmodic character. Trousseau calls attention to the *incessant* character of the early cough. The fever is usually not high, and slight attention is paid to the symptoms, which are thought to be those of a simple catarrh. After a week or ten days, instead of subsiding, the cough becomes worse and more convulsive in character.

The *paroxysmal stage,* marked by the characteristic cough, dates from the first appearance of the "whoop." The fit begins with a series of from fifteen to twenty forcible short coughs of increasing intensity, between which no inspiratory effort is made. The child gets blue in the face, and then with a deep inspiration the air is drawn into the lungs, making the "whoop," which may be heard at a distance, and from which the disease takes its name. A deep inspiration may precede the series of spasmodic expiratory efforts. Several coughing fits may succeed each other until a tenacious mucus is ejected, usually small in amount, but after a series of coughing spells a considerable quantity may be expectorated. Vomiting often takes place at the end of a paroxysm, and may recur so frequently that the child does not get enough food and becomes emaciated. There may be only four or five attacks in the day; an average is twenty attacks daily. In severe and fatal cases the paroxysms may exceed one hundred daily. During the paroxysm the thorax is very strongly compressed by the powerful expiratory efforts, and, as very little air passes in through the glottis, there are signs of defective aëration of the blood; the face becomes swollen and congested, the veins are prominent, the eyeballs protrude, and the conjunctivæ become deeply engorged. Suffocation indeed seems imminent, when with a deep, crowing inspiration air enters the lungs and the color is quickly restored. The child knows for a few moments when the attack is coming on, and tries in every way to check it, but failing to do so, runs terrified to the nurse or mother to be supported, or clutches anything near by. Few diseases are more painful to witness. In severe paroxysms the sphincters may be opened. An ulcer may form under the tongue from rubbing on the teeth (Riga's disease). Among circumstances which precipitate a paroxysm are emotion, such as crying, and any irritation about the throat. Even the act of swallowing sometimes seems sufficient. In a close dusty atmosphere the coughing fits are more frequent. After lasting for three or four weeks the attacks become lighter and finally cease. In cases of ordinary severity the course of the disease is rarely under six weeks.

During the attack, if the chest be examined, the resonance is defective in the expiratory stage, full and clear during the deep, crowing inspiration; but on auscultation during the latter there may be no vesicular murmur heard, owing to the slowness with which the air passes the narrowed glottis. Bronchial râles are occasionally heard.

Complications and Sequelæ.—During the extensive venous congestion hæmorrhages are very apt to occur in the form of petechiæ, particularly about the forehead, ecchymosis of the conjunctivæ, and even bleeding tears of blood (Trousseau) from the rupture of the vessels, epistaxis, bleeding from the ears, and occasionally hæmoptysis. Hæmorrhage from the bowels is rare. Glycosuria occurs occasionally. Convulsions are not very uncommon, due perhaps to the extreme engorgement of the cerebral cortex. Death has occurred from spasm of the glottis. Sudden death has been caused by extensive subdural hæmorrhage. Choked disk, relieved by decompression, has occurred. Paralysis is a rare event. It was associated with 3 in a series of 120 cases, but in none of them did the hemiplegia come on during the paroxysm, as in a case reported by S. West. Valentine (1901) collected 79 cases, chiefly hemiplegias. A spastic paraplegia may follow. Acute polyneuritis is a rare sequel.

The persistent vomiting may induce marked anæmia and wasting. The pulmonary complications are extremely serious. During the severe coughing spells interstitial emphysema may be induced, more rarely pneumothorax. In one instance rupture occurred, evidently near the root of the lung, and the air passed along the trachea and reached the subcutaneous tissues of the neck, a condition which has been known to become general. Capillary bronchitis, lobular and pseudo-lobar pneumonia are the dangerous complications, responsible for nine out of ten deaths in the disease. In some cases the process is tuberculous. Pleurisy is sometimes met with and occasionally lobar pneumonia. Enlargement of the bronchial glands is very common in whooping cough, and has been thought to cause the disease. It may sometimes be sufficient to produce dulness over the manubrium. During the spasm the radial pulse is small, the right heart engorged, and during and after the attack the cardiac action is very much disturbed. Serious damage may result, and possibly some of the cases of severe valvular disease in children who have had neither rheumatic nor scarlet fever may be attributed to the terrible heart strain during a prolonged attack. Koplik regards the swelling about the face and eyes as an important sign of the heart strain. Serious renal complications are very uncommon, but albumin sometimes and sugar frequently are found in the urine. A distressing sequel in adults is asthma, which may recur at intervals for a year or more. A leucocytosis sometimes appears early, chiefly of the lymphocytes (Meunier).

Diagnosis.—So distinctive is the "whoop" that the diagnosis is easy; but occasionally there are doubtful cases, particularly during epidemics, in which a series of expiratory coughs occurs without any inspiratory crow. The spasmodic cough due to enlarged bronchial glands may cause difficulty.

Prognosis.—If we include its complications, whooping cough is a very fatal affection, ranking one of the first among the acute infections as a cause of death in children under five years of age.

Prophylaxis.—The disease should be placed on the list of reportable infections. When possible the sputum should be collected and disinfected. As the organism usually disappears within two weeks from the appearance of the characteristic cough there seems little danger of contagion in the later stages. A prophylactic vaccine has been used with success, three injections of 500 million, 2 and 3 billion, being given every third day.

Treatment.—The gravity of the disease is scarcely appreciated by the public. Children with the disease should not be sent to school or exposed in public in any way. There is more reprehensible neglect in connection with this than with any other disease. The patient should be isolated, and if the paroxysms are at all severe, at rest in bed. Fresh air, night and day, is important, but in cities in the winter this is not easy to manage. Stock vaccine has been used for treatment with benefit; some patients are promptly cured. The average initial dose is 500 million for children over one year. With two day intervals doses of 1 and 2 billion are given. Antiseptic measures have been extensively tried. Quinine holds its own with many practitioners; a sixth of a grain (0.01 gm.) may be given three times a day for each month of age, and a grain and a half (0.1 gm.) for each year in children under five. The use of benzoin and eucalyptus inhalations is often helpful. Sedatives are by far the most trustworthy drugs in severe cases, and paregoric may be given freely, particularly to give rest at night. Codein and heroin in doses proper for the age often give much relief. Jacobi advised belladonna in full doses until a flush appears on the cheeks. Children can often be taught to inhibit an attack. The wearing of a tight abdominal binder is sometimes of value.

Other remedies, such an antipyrin and chloral hydrate, may be tried. In older children and in adults it would be worth while to try the intratracheal injections of olive-oil and iodoform, which are sometimes so useful in allaying severe paroxysmal cough.

After the severity of the attack has passed and convalescence has begun, the child should be watched with the greatest care. It is just at this period that the fatal broncho-pneumonias are apt to develop. The cough sometimes persists for months and the child remains weak and delicate. Change of air should be tried. Such a patient should be fed with care and given tonics and cod-liver oil.

XII. GONOCOCCUS INFECTION

Definition.—An acute infection with a primary lesion, usually urethritis, and numerous secondary and systemic manifestations, of which prostatitis and epididymitis, salpingitis, arthritis, synovitis and endocarditis are the most important. The *Micrococcus gonorrhϾ* (gonococcus) was described by Neisser, in 1879.

Gonorrhœa, one of the most widespread and serious of infectious diseases, presents many features for consideration. It is not a killing disease; only 61 fatal cases are recorded in the Registrar General's Report, 1915, for England and Wales, but as a cause of ill-health and disability the gonococcus occupies a position of the very first rank among its fellows. While the local lesion is too often thought to be trifling, in its singular obstinacy, in the possibilities of permanent sexual damage to the individual himself and still more in the "grisly troop" which may follow in its train, gonorrhœa does not fall very far short of syphilis in importance.

Etiology.—The organism is a biscuit-shaped micrococcus, occurring in pairs, usually within the leucocytes, and is always found in the primary and systemic lesions. Two types of gonococci are described, corresponding to the adult and infant forms of infection. The disease has been reproduced by inoculation of the pure culture.

The disease is seen in men and women as a result of impure sexual intercourse, in the new-born from vaginal contamination, and in older children by accidental infection. Ophthalmia neonatorum is one of the great causes of blindness, but an active campaign of education is rapidly reducing the number of cases. The gonococcus vaginitis and the ophthalmia are very serious diseases in children's hospitals and in infants' homes. The story of the gonococcus infection in the Babies' Hospital, New York, for eleven years, as told by Holt (N. Y. Med. Jour., March, 1905), illustrates the singular obstinacy of the infection. In spite of the greatest care and precaution, there were, in 1903, 65 cases of vaginitis, with 2 of ophthalmia and 12 of arthritis. In 1904 there were 52 cases of vaginitis, only 16 of which would have been recognized without the bacteriological examination. In all, in the eleven years, there were 273 cases of vaginitis, only 6 with ophthalmia and 26 with arthritis. Other institutions have had equally sad experiences. Isolation and prolonged quarantine are the only measures to combat the disease successfully.

The immediate and remote effects of the gonococcus may be considered under—

I. The primary infection.
II. The spread in the genito-urinary organs by direct continuity.
III. Systemic gonococcus infection.

The primary lesion we need not here consider, but we may call attention to the frequency of the complications, such as periurethral abscess, gonorrhœal prostatitis and seminal vesiculitis in the male, and vaginitis, endocervicitis, and inflammation of the glands of Bartholin in the female.

Perhaps the most serious of all the sequels are those which result from the **spread** by direct continuity of tissue. Gonococcus salpingitis is not infrequent. Metritis and ovaritis are also met with, and peritonitis. The gonococcus has been found in pure culture in cases of acute general peritonitis. Equally important is the cystitis, which is probably much more frequently the result of a mixed infection than due to the gonococcus itself. There is some danger of extension upward through the ureters to the kidneys. The pyelitis, like the cystitis, is usually a mixed infection.

Systemic Gonococcus Infection.—(1) GONOCOCCUS SEPTICÆMIA AND PYÆMIA.—Thayer and Blumer first cultivated the gonococci from the blood in a case in the senior author's wards, and the septicæmia has been studied by them and by Cole, who divided the cases into four groups: (1) Those with *endocarditis,* 11 of the 29 cases collected by him. The clinical features are those of malignant endocarditis; two recovered. (2) Cases with *local suppuration* and the general features of a *pyæmia*—of the six cases three died. The septicæmia associated with a small focus of suppuration may be very intense. A man ten days after the onset of urethritis had chills and high fever; he became profoundly toxæmic and died on the morning of the fourth day from the chill. There was a small prostatic abscess. (3) Cases *with no metastatic local affections* or perhaps only slight arthritis. In a remarkable case at the Johns Hopkins Hospital, three months after an acute gonorrhœa the patient had a fever resembling typhoid, which lasted seven weeks. Gonococci were cultivated from the blood. He recovered and, as Cole suggests, such cases are probably more common than we suspect. (4) Cases of *gonorrhœal puerperal septicæmia,* of which several instances have been reported. Of the 29 cases in which the septicæmia was demonstrated by the cultivation of the organism from the blood, 12 died. The endocarditis will be considered later.

(2) Gonococcus Arthritis.—In many respects this is the most damaging, disabling, and serious of all the complications of gonorrhœa, occurring in from 2 to 5 per cent. of the cases. It occurs more frequently in males than in females; 43 to 7 in one series at the Johns Hopkins Hospital (Cole). In a series of 252 cases collected by Northrup, 230 were in males; 130 cases were between twenty and thirty years of age. It occurs, as a rule, during an acute attack of gonorrhœa. In 208 of Northrup's series there was a urethral discharge while in hospital. It may occur as the attack subsides, or even when it has become chronic. A gonorrhœal-arthritis of great intensity may occur in a newly married woman infected by an old gleet in her husband. In women it is not always easy to find evidence of local infection. As a rule, many joints are affected. In an analysis by Cole and McCrae of the involvement of the joints in gonococcus arthritis and in rheumatic fever, the average number in the former was double that in the latter. In Northrup's series three or more joints were affected in 175 cases, one joint in 56 cases.

The *anatomical changes* are variable. The inflammation is often peri-articular, and extends along the sheaths of the tendons. When effusion occurs in the joints it rarely becomes purulent. It has more commonly the characters of a synovitis. About the wrist and hand suppuration sometimes occurs in the sheaths. The gonococcus itself is present in the inflamed joint or in the peri-arthritic exudate, and may often be obtained in pure culture. Sometimes the cultures are negative. Mixed infection with staphylococci or streptococci is very rare.

Clinical Course.—Variability and obstinacy are the two most distinguishing features. The following are the most important clinical forms:

(*a*) *Arthralgic,* in which there are wandering pains about the joints, without redness or swelling. These persist for a long time.

(*b*) *Polyarthritic,* in which several joints become affected. The fever is slight; the local inflammation may fix itself in one joint, but more commonly several become swollen and tender. In this form cerebral and cardiac complications may occur. In other cases one joint is especially involved, the others subsiding rapidly. The pain is severe, the swelling extensive, and due chiefly to peri-articular œdema. The general fever is not at all proportionate to the intensity of the local signs. The exudate usually resolves, though suppuration occasionally supervenes.

(*d*) *Chronic Hydrarthrosis.*—This is usually mono-articular, and is particularly apt to involve the knee. It comes on often without pain, redness, or swelling. Formation of pus is rare. It occurred only twice in 96 cases tabulated by Nolen.

(*e*) *Bursal and Synovial Form.*—This attacks chiefly the tendons and their sheaths and the bursæ and the periosteum. The articulations may not be affected. The bursæ of the patella, the olecranon, and the tendo Achillis are most apt to be involved.

(*f*) *Septicæmic.*—In this the gonococci invade the blood, and the picture is that of an intense septico-pyæmia, usually with endocarditis.

(*g*) The *Painful Heel of Gonorrhœa.*—This is due to local periosteal thickening and exostosis on the os calcis, causing pain and great disability. Baer has demonstrated the gonococcus in the periosteal lesion.

Complications.—Iritis is not infrequent and may recur with successive attacks. The visceral complications are serious. Endocarditis, pericarditis, and pleurisy may occur. Renal infections are rare. There may be a mixed infection with the colon bacillus.

Treatment.—The primary infection—usually urethritis—should be actively treated. Of special measures, the use of antigonococcus serum and vaccine treatment are worthy of trial; either will help some cases, both fail in many. Good food, fresh air, and open bowels are important. Drugs are of little value, especially sodium salicylate and potassium iodide. Phenacetine or acetyl-salicylic acid may be given for the pain.

The local treatment is very important. In acute cases, fixation of the joints for a short period is beneficial, and in the chronic forms, massage and passive motion. Counter-irritation by the cautery or blisters, active hyperæmia by baking or passive by the Bier method are all useful. A distended joint may be tapped and then tightly bandaged. The surgical treatment is more satisfactory in severe cases and good results usually follow incision and irrigation.

XIII. BACILLARY DYSENTERY

Definition.—A form of intestinal flux, usually of an acute type, occurring sporadically and in severe epidemics, attacking children as well as adults, characterized by pain, frequent passages of blood and mucus, and due to the action of a specific bacillus, of which there are various strains.

Etiology.—Owing to improved sanitation, dysentery has become less frequent. In temperate climates sporadic cases occur from time to time, and at intervals epidemics prevail, particularly in overcrowded institutions. Records of widespread epidemics have been collected by Woodward. The most serious was that which prevailed from 1847 to 1856. In Great Britain and Ireland epidemics of the disease have become less frequent. In institutions, particularly in overcrowded asylums, dysentery is very common, and this form has been made the subject of a valuable report by Mott and Durham. In the tropics "dysentery is a destructive giant compared to which strong drink is a mere phantom" (Macgregor). Dysentery is one of the great camp diseases, and it has been more destructive to armies than powder and shot. In the Federal service during the civil war, according to Woodward,* there were 259,071 cases of acute and 28,451 cases of chronic dysentery. The disease prevails in Porto Rico, the Philippines, and to a less extent in Cuba. In the South African campaign dysentery prevailed widely. For many years a very fatal form of dysentery has prevailed in Japan, particularly in the summer and autumn months, having a mortality of from 26 to 27 per cent.; in 1899 there were 125,989 cases, with 26,709 deaths (Eldridge). It is now generally conceded that the severe epidemics of acute dysentery occurring

* Medical and Surgical History of the War of the Rebellion, Medical, vol. ii. The most exhaustive treatise extant on intestinal fluxes—an enduring monument to the industry and ability of the author.

in the tropics are of the bacillary type, and the same form prevails in temperate climates.

Bacillus Dysenteriæ.—In 1898, Shiga, a Japanese observer, found in the dysentery prevailing in his country a bacillus with special characters, which he considered to be the specific cause of the disease.

Flexner and Barker, of the Johns Hopkins Commission for the Study of Tropical Diseases, found in the dysentery in the Philippine Islands an identical organism, and it has been made the subject of very careful study by Flexner, and also by R. P. Strong, Musgrave, and Craig, of the United States army. The organism appears to be constantly present in the acute dysentery of the tropics. In Manila, according to Strong and Musgrave, of 1,328 cases, 712 were of the acute specific variety, 55 suspected specific cases, and 561 of amœbic dysentery. Kruse, in an outbreak at Laar, in Germany, in which 300 persons were attacked, isolated an identical bacillus. Vedder and Duval demonstrated that sporadic cases in adults in Philadelphia, as well as epidemics of dysentery in the Lancaster County Asylum, Pennsylvania, and in the almshouse at New Haven, were due to this organism. Duval and Bassett demonstrated that certain forms of summer diarrhœas of infants were due to infection with *B. dysenteriæ*. The Rockefeller Institute conducted a collective investigation into the cause of infantile diarrhœas; several observers, under Flexner's direction, studied 412 cases and found the dysentery bacillus present in 279 or 63.2 per cent.

The strain of the bacillus most frequently found in the United States is the "Flexner-Harris" type. It is now conceded that a number of strains of the bacillus occur. This fact has been determined by the relative agglutinative power of immune serum upon the bacilli isolated, as well as by the action of the latter upon various sugars. The lesions produced by the different strains are identical. The organism agglutinates with the blood serum of cases with acute dysentery as well as with the serum of immunized animals.

Infection takes place by the mouth. The organisms are widely distributed by the fæces of persons suffering with the disease and also by dysentery "carriers." In institutions food and drink readily become contaminated. Possibly, too, the germs are distributed by flies and dust.

Morbid Anatomy.—In the acute cases, when death has occurred on the fourth to the seventh day, the mucous membrane of the large intestine is swollen, of a deep-red color, and presents elevated, coarse corrugations and folds. In addition to the intense hyperæmia there are hæmorrhagic areas. Over the surface there is usually a superficial necrotic layer, which can be brushed off lightly with the finger. This may be in patches, or uniform over large areas. There is no ulceration, only the superficial, general necrosis of the mucosa. The solitary follicles are swollen and red, but the prominence is obscured in the involvement of the entire mucosa. In cases of great intensity the entire coats of the colon may be stiff and thick, and the mucous membrane enormously increased in thickness, grayish black, extensively necrotic, and, in places, gangrenous. The serous surface is often deeply injected. The ileum may be involved, having a deeply hæmorrhagic mucosa, with a superficial necrosis. In the subacute cases there is not the same great thickening of the intestinal wall, the solitary follicles are more swollen, there is less necrosis, and, while there are no ulcers, there are superficial erosions.

Symptoms.—According to Strong and Musgrave, the period of incubation is not more than forty-eight hours. The onset, which is usually sudden, is characterized by slight fever, pain in the abdomen, and frequent stools. At first mucus is passed, but within twenty-four hours blood appears with it, or there is pure blood. There is a constant desire to go to stool, with great straining and tenesmus; every hour or half hour there may be a small amount of blood and mucus passed. The temperature rises and may reach 103° or 104°. The pulse increases in frequency, and in the severer cases becomes very small. The tongue is coated with a white fur, and there is excessive thirst. In the very acute cases the patient becomes seriously ill within forty-eight hours, the movements increase in frequency, the pain is of great intensity, the patient becomes delirious, and death may occur on the third or fourth day. In cases of moderate severity the urgency of the symptoms abates, the stools lessen, the temperature falls, and within two or three weeks the patient is convalescent. The mortality in the severe forms is very high. There is a subacute form which lasts for many weeks or months. The patients become greatly emaciated, having from three to five stools in the twenty-four hours. The *Bacillus dysenteriæ* is found in the stools, and it agglutinates readily with the blood serum.

Other Clinical Types.—The foregoing account describes the essential features of bacillary dysentery as seen in Japan, the Philippines, and the tropics. The clinical features of bacillary dysentery in adults in temperate climates differ in no essential manner from those already described. Although the evidence hardly warrants us at present in making the sweeping statement that all non-amœbic cases of dysentery are bacillary in origin, yet experience will probably demonstrate eventually that this is the case. What is known as the acute catarrhal dysentery is probably a sporadic form due to the *Bacillus dysenteriæ*. Diphtheritic dysentery is a type of the bacillary form with great necrosis and infiltration of the mucosa. There may be rapid gangrene and a fatal termination within twenty-four hours. A secondary diphtheritic dysentery is a common terminal event in many acute and chronic diseases, and a bacillus of the Shiga type has been isolated from these cases.

Complications and Sequelæ.—*Peritonitis* is rare, due either to extension through the wall of the bowel or to perforation. When this occurs about the cæcal region, perityphlitis results; when low down in the rectum, periproctitis. In 108 autopsies collected by Woodward perforation occurred in 11. Abscess of the liver, so common in the amœbic form, is very rare. It is interesting to note, as illustrating the probable type of the disease, how comparatively rare abscess of the liver was during the American civil war. Very few cases occurred in the South African War (Rolleston).

In the tropics malaria and acute dysentery very often coexist. With reference to typhoid fever, as a complication, Woodward mentions that the combination was exceedingly frequent during the civil war, and characteristic lesions of both diseases coexisted. In civil practice it is extremely rare.

Sydenham noted that dysentery was sometimes associated with rheumatic pains, and in certain epidemics a secondary arthritis has been especially prevalent. In severe cases there may be pleurisy, thrombosis, pericarditis, endocarditis, and occasionally pyæmic manifestations, among which may be mentioned pylephlebitis. Chronic nephritis is also an occasional sequel. In protracted cases there may be an anæmic œdema. An interesting sequel of dysentery is paralysis. Woodward reports 8 cases. Weir Mitchell mentioned it as not uncommon, occurring chiefly in the form of paraplegia. As in other acute fevers, this is due probably to a neuritis. Remlinger, in two cases of non-amœbic dysentery in Tunis, observed an epididymitis during convalescence; gonorrhœa was excluded. In a third case the dysentery was complicated by an abscess of the spleen, which ruptured, causing death. Intestinal stricture is a rare sequence—so rare that no case was reported at the Surgeon-General's office during the civil war. It appears to be not uncommon in the East. Among the sequelæ of chronic dysentery, in persons who have recovered a certain measure of health, may be mentioned persistent dyspepsia and irritability of the bowels.

Diagnosis.—In the acute specific form the blood serum agglutinates the dysentery bacillus. The "Flexner-Harris" type of the organism agglutinates in dilutions of from 1 to 1,000 up to 1 to 1,500. The "Shiga" type agglutinates less readily. The blood serum of a dysenteric patient will agglutinate both types, but the former more readily than the latter. In all non-amœbic dysenteries efforts should be made to isolate the dysentery bacillus from the stools.

Treatment.—Flint showed that sporadic dysentery is, in its slighter grades at least, a self-limited disease, which runs its course in eight or nine days. Reading the report of his cases, one is struck, however, with their comparative mildness.

Prophylactic.—The same precautions should be followed as are adopted in typhoid fever. Flexner and Gay have shown that animals can be protected from infection by a previous treatment with immune serum. Protective and curative serums have been prepared.

I. Acute Dysentery.—The patient should be absolutely at rest in bed. He should be kept warm and have a flannel abdominal binder applied. The diet should be very simple—whey, egg albumen, barley or rice water, and strained gruels. Milk and lactose may be added later. Enough water should be given to relieve thirst. If vomiting occurs, nothing should be given by mouth for some hours, and if the patient requires fluid this can be given subcutaneously. Hot applications to the abdomen are useful. If the patient is seen early in the attack, free purgation is advisable, for which sodium sulphate and Rochelle salts are best. Either may be given in doses of two drams (8 gm.) for two doses an hour apart and later half the amount every three hours until the bowels have moved freely. By this treatment the course is sometimes cut short. If the attack is well established, the use of purgatives must be determined by the conditions present. If solid fæcal matter is being passed, a purgative is indicated, castor oil being the best (ʒ vi, 25 c. c.). Until the bowels have been thoroughly cleared, purgation is indicated.

Medicinal.—Bismuth in large doses often has a beneficial effect. Thirty to sixty grains (2 to 4 gm.) should be given every hour. Minute doses of bichloride of mercury, gr. 1/100 (0.0006 gm.) every two hours, were recommended by Ringer. For the relief of pain and to quiet the bowel, morphia is the most useful drug and is to be preferred to opium by mouth. It should be given hypodermically in large doses (gr. 1-4 to 1-3, 0.016 to 0.022 gm.), and repeated according to the needs of the patient. If tenesmus is not marked, opium can be given as the starch and laudanum enema, in which thirty minims (2 c. c.) of laudanum are given.

Local Treatment.—During the acute stages this may be out of the question, but should be employed whenever possible. Normal saline or sodium bicarbonate (1 per cent.) solution at the body temperature can be used as an irrigation. This should be given very gently and with the hips elevated. If there is rectal irritation, a cocaine or morphia suppository should be given beforehand. As the symptoms lessen, the quantity of fluid can be increased and other solutions used, such as boric acid (5 per cent.), salicylic acid (1 per cent.) or alum (1 to 200).

With convalescence the diet should be increased very gradually and only simple foods allowed. The patient should be kept quiet until all danger of a relapse is over. This is most important in the prevention of a chronic dysentery.

Serum Therapy.—Shiga produced a polyvalent serum by immunizing horses, by which he claims to have reduced the mortality in "endemic" dysentery in Japan from about 35 per cent. to 9 per cent. Good results have been reported from the use of the Pasteur Institute and Lister Institute serums, which should be given in doses of 20 c. c. two or three times a day.

II. Chronic Dysentery.—The patient should be at rest in bed and on simple diet, milk, boiled, peptonized or fermented, whey, beef juice, and eggs. In some cases milk may have to be given well diluted or in small amounts, but it usually agrees well. It is well to give an occasional purge (castor oil, ℥ ss, 15 c. c.) to empty the bowels. Drugs by mouth are not of great value. Bismuth, if used, should be in large doses (ʒ i, 4 gm.) every three hours while the patient is awake. Opium should not be given as a routine measure, as there is great danger of forming a habit. If employed, it is best given in the starch and laudanum enema.

Local Treatment.—This is most rational and should be carried out thoroughly. If the rectum is irritable, a cocaine or morphine suppository should be given half an hour previously. The irrigation, at the body temperature, should be given very gently, the patient encouraged to retain it as long as possible, and the amount gradually increased up to two litres if possible. One irrigation a day is usually enough. Silver nitrate solution is probably the best (1 to 5,000 at first and increased to 1 to 500). Boric acid (5 per cent.), salicylic acid (2 per cent.), alum, or tannic acid (3 per cent.) may also be used. With any of these an occasional irrigation of saline solution is useful. With improvement the frequency of the irrigations should be reduced. To any ulcers in the bowel which can be reached silver nitrate solution (25 per cent.) should be applied. In the obstinate cases an appendicostomy may be done and the bowel irrigated through the opening.

XIV. MALTA FEVER

(*Undulant Fever, Mediterranean Fever, Goat Fever*)

Definition.—A specific fever, caused by the *Micrococcus melitensis* (and *M. paramelitensis*) characterized by undulatory pyrexial relapses, profuse sweats, arthritis, and an enlarged spleen. It is spread, as a rule, through the agency of goat's milk.

Distribution.—The disease prevails in the Mediterranean littoral, and endemic foci exist in India, Africa, China, and Manila. In the goat raising sections of Texas the disease is endemic (Gentry and Ferenbaugh). In the Malta garrison in the seven years 1898-1904, there were 2,229 cases, with an average case duration of one hundred and twenty days and with 77 deaths. About the same number of cases occurred in the fleet. Since the introduction of prophylactic measures the disease has practically disappeared from the Army and Navy, and has diminished greatly in the civil population.

Etiology.—The greater part of our knowledge of this remarkable disease we owe to the work of British army surgeons, particularly to Marston, Bruce, and Hughes. In 1886 Bruce isolated an organism, *Micrococcus melitensis,* from the spleen and blood. Hughes, Wright, Semple, and others confirmed this. In 1904-1905 a Government Commission began a study of the problems of the disease. It was shown to be a septicæmia, due to the above-named organism, which had an unusually prolonged saprophytic existence. Zamit showed that the goats, the most important animals in the domestic life of Malta, were largely infected, from 10 to 15 per cent. having the micrococcus in their milk. Monkeys were successfully infected with milk which contained the organisms. Steps were at once taken to stop the use of goat's milk for the troops, with the result that the disease has disappeared in the garrison and in the fleet.

The micrococcus enters the system through the gastro-intestinal tract. It may spread by the infection of food by flies or by the fingers. Ambulant carriers may pass organisms by the urine.

Symptoms.—There is no specific fever which presents the same remarkable group of phenomena. The period of incubation is from six to ten days. "Clinically the fever has a peculiar irregular temperature curve, consisting of intermittent waves or undulations of pyrexia, of a distinctly remittent character. These pyrexial waves or undulations last, as a rule, from one to three weeks, with an apyrexial interval lasting for two or more days. In rare cases the remissions may become so marked as to give an almost intermittent character to the febrile curve, clearly distinguishable, however, from the paroxysms of paludic infection. This pyrexial condition is usually much prolonged, having an uncertain duration, lasting for even six months or more. Unlike paludism, its course is not markedly affected by the administration of quinine. Its course is often irregular and even erratic in nature. This pyrexia is usually accompanied by obstinate constipation, progressive anæmia, and debility. It is often complicated with and followed by neuralgic symptoms referred to the peripheral or central nervous system, arthritic effusions, painful inflammatory conditions of certain fibrous structures, of a localized nature, or swelling of the testicles" (Hughes). There is a malignant type, in which the disease may prove fatal within a week or ten days; an undulatory type—the common variety—in which the fever is marked by intermittent waves or undulations of variable length, separated by periods of apyrexia and freedom from symptoms. In this really lie the peculiar features of the disease, and the victim may suffer a series of relapses which may extend from three months, the average time, to two years. Lastly, there is an intermittent type, in which the patient may simply have daily pyrexia toward evening, without any special complications, and may do well and be able to work, and yet at any time the other serious features of the disease may develop. The mortality is slight, only about 2 per cent.

Diagnosis.—In early cases the organism can usually be cultivated from the blood. The agglutination reaction and urine cultures are of value. Clinically the disease may be diagnosed as typhoid fever, infective arthritis or gastro-intestinal catarrh.

The *prophylaxis* is self-evident, and the brilliant work of the commission has reduced the incidence of the disease to a minimum. The disease has disappeared from Gibraltar since the importation of goats from Malta has been stopped.

Treatment.—General measures suitable to typhoid fever are indicated. Fluid food should be given during the febrile period. Vaccines may be used and good results have been reported. Hydrotherapy, either the bath or the cold pack, should be used every third hour when the temperature is above 103° F. Otherwise the treatment is symptomatic. No drugs appear to have any special influence on the fever. A change of climate seems to promote convalescence.

XV. CHOLERA ASIATICA

Definition.—A specific, infectious disease, caused by the comma bacillus of Koch, and characterized clinically by violent purging and rapid collapse.

Historical Summary.—Cholera has been endemic in India from a remote period, but only within the last century did it make inroads into Europe and America. An extensive epidemic occurred in 1832, in which year it was brought in immigrant ships from Great Britain to Quebec. It travelled along the lines of traffic up the Great Lakes, and finally reached as far west as the military posts of the upper Mississippi. In the same year it entered the United States by way of New York. There were recurrences of the disease in 1835-'36. In 1848 it entered the country through New Orleans, and spread widely up the Mississippi Valley and across the continent to California. In 1849 it again appeared. In 1854 it was introduced by immigrant ships into New York and prevailed widely throughout the country. In 1866 and in 1867 there were less serious epidemics. In 1873 it again appeared in the United States, but did not prevail widely. In 1884 there was an outbreak in Europe, and again in 1892 and 1893. Although occasional cases have been brought by ship to the quarantine stations of Great Britain and the United States, the disease has not gained a foothold in either country since 1873. It has prevailed extensively in the Philippines. For the past fifteen years it has prevailed widely in the near and far East. In 1911 cholera prevailed in Italy, North Africa and Madeira. There were outbreaks in Asia Minor, Arabia and Turkey, and the usual prevalence in India. To the United States, during 1911, cholera was frequently conveyed by ships from Italy, but there was no difficulty in controlling it. A number of cholera "carriers" were found.

Etiology.—In 1884 Koch announced the discovery of the specific organism. Subsequent observations have confirmed his statement that the comma bacillus, as it is termed, occurs constantly in the true cholera, and in no other disease. It has the form of a slightly bent rod, which is thicker, but not more than about half the length of the tubercle bacillus, and sometimes occurs in corkscrew-like or S forms. The organisms grow upon a great variety of media and display distinctive and characteristic appearances. Koch found them in the water tanks in India, and they were isolated from the Elbe water during the Hamburg epidemic of 1892. During epidemics virulent bacilli may be found in the fæces of healthy persons. The bacilli are found in the intestine, in the stools from the earliest period of the disease, and very abundantly in the characteristic rice-water evacuations, in which they may be seen as an almost pure culture. They very rarely occur in the vomit. Post mortem, they are found in enormous numbers in the intestine. In acutely fatal cases they do not seem to invade the intestinal wall, but in those with a more protracted course they are found in the depths of the glands and in the still deeper tissues. Experimental animals are not susceptible to cholera germs administered per os. But if introduced after neutralization of the gastric contents, and if kept in contact with the intestinal mucosa by controlling peristalsis with opium, guinea-pigs succumb after showing cholera-like symptoms.

Cholera Toxin.—Koch in his studies of cholera failed to find the spirilla in the internal organs. He concluded that the constitutional symptoms of the disease resulted from the absorption of toxic bodies from the intestine. R. Pfeiffer has shown that the cholera toxin is intimately associated with the protein of the bacterial cells, and, being of a very labile nature, can not be separated. Dead cultures are toxic; and the symptoms produced by the introduction of even minimal amounts are often comparable with those of the algid stage of cholera asiatica. The symptoms occur very rapidly, and death often results in eight to twelve hours; in non-fatal cases recovery is often as rapid. The intracellular cholera toxin is poisonous to animals if introduced into the blood, peritoneal cavity, or subcutaneously. No absorption takes place from the intestine unless the epithelial layer is injured.

Immunity.—Animals may be immunized by repeated injections of non-fatal doses of the dead and later of the living organisms. The serum of an animal thus immunized has a protective power when injected into a guinea pig along with five or ten times the fatal dose. This serum has also agglutinative and other antibacterial properties. The blood serum of convalescent patients also possesses these properties, and for therapeutic purposes anti-serums have been introduced and used widely in India, the Philippines and in Russia.

Modes of Infection.—As in other diseases, individual peculiarities count for much, and during epidemics virulent cholera bacilli have been isolated from the normal stools of healthy men. Cholera cultures have also been swallowed with impunity.

The disease is not highly infectious; physicians, nurses, and others in close contact with patients are not often affected. On the other hand, washerwomen and those who are brought into very close contact with the linen of the cholera patients, or with their stools, are particularly prone to catch the disease. There have been several instances of so-called "laboratory cholera," in which students, having been accidentally infected while working with the cultures, have taken the disease, and at least one death has resulted.

Vegetables which have been washed in infected water, particularly lettuce and cress, may convey the disease. Milk may also be contaminated. The bacilli live on fresh bread, butter, and meat, for from six to eight days. In regions in which the disease prevails the possibility of the infection of food by flies should be borne in mind, since it has been shown that the bacilli may live for at least three days in their intestines.

The disease is propagated chiefly by contaminated water used for drinking, cooking, and washing. The virulence of an epidemic in any region is in direct proportion to the imperfection of its water-supply. In India the demonstration of the connection between drinking-water and cholera infection is complete. The Hamburg epidemic is a most remarkable illustration. The unfiltered water of the Elbe was the chief supply, although taken from the river in such a situation that it was directly contaminated by sewage. In August, 1892, there was a sudden explosive epidemic, and within three months nearly 18,000 persons were attacked, with a mortality of 42.3 per cent. The neighboring city of Altona, which also took its water from the Elbe, but which had a thoroughly well-equipped modern filtration system, had in the same period only 516 cases.

Two main types of epidemics are recognized: the first, in which many individuals are attacked simultaneously, as in the Hamburg outbreak, and in which no direct connection can be traced between the individual cases. In this type there is widespread contamination of the drinking-water. In the other the cases occur in groups, so-called cholera nests; individuals are not attacked simultaneously, but successively. A direct connection between the cases may be very difficult to trace. Both these types may be combined, and in an epidemic which has started in a widespread infection through water, there may be other outbreaks, examples of the second or chain-like type. The disease always follows the lines of human travel. In India it has, in many notable cases, been widely spread by pilgrims. It is carried also by caravans and in ships. It is not conveyed through the atmosphere.

Cholera "carriers" have an important influence. In Manila nearly 8 per cent. of 376 healthy persons harbored the bacilli. The perennial outbreaks in the Manila prison were due to carriers, 17 of whom were found among those who had to do with the preparation of the food and drink of 3,000 prisoners.

Places situated at the sea-level are more prone to the disease than inland towns. In high altitudes the disease does not prevail so extensively. A high temperature favors the development of cholera, but in Europe and America the epidemics have been chiefly in the late summer and in the autumn.

The disease affects persons of all ages. It is particularly prone to attack the intemperate and those debilitated by want of food and by bad surroundings. Depressing emotions, such as fear, undoubtedly have an influence. It is doubtful whether an attack furnishes immunity against a second one.

Morbid Anatomy.—A post mortem diagnosis can be made by any competent bacteriologist, as the organism is distinctive. The body has the appearances associated with profound collapse. There is often marked post mortem elevation of temperature. The *rigor mortis* sets in early and may produce displacement of the limbs. The lower jaw has been seen to move and the eyes to rotate. Various movements of the arms and legs have also been noted. The blood is thick and dark, and there is a remarkable diminution in the amount of its water and salts. The peritoneum is sticky, and the coils of intestines are congested and look thin and shrunken. The small intestine usually contains a turbid serum, similar to that passed in the stools. The mucosa is, as a rule, swollen, and in very acute cases slightly hyperæmic; later the congestion, which is not uniform, is more marked, especially about the Peyer's patches. Post mortem the epithelial lining is sometimes denuded, but this is probably not a change which takes place freely during life. The bacilli are found in the contents of the intestine and in the mucous membrane. The spleen is usually small. The liver and kidneys show cloudy swelling, and the latter extensive coagulation-necrosis and destruction of the epithelial cells.

Symptoms.—A period of incubation of uncertain length, probably not more than from two to five days, precedes the onset of the symptoms.

Three stages may be recognized in the attack: the preliminary diarrhœa, the collapse stage, and the period of reaction.

(*a*) The preliminary diarrhœa may set in abruptly without any previous indications. More commonly there are, for one or two days, colicky pains in the abdomen, with looseness of the bowels, perhaps vomiting, with headache and depression of spirits. There may be no fever.

(*b*) Collapse Stage.—The diarrhœa increases, or, without any of the preliminary symptoms, sets in with the greatest intensity, and profuse liquid evacuations succeed each other rapidly. There are in some instances griping pains and tenesmus. More commonly there is a sense of exhaustion and collapse. The thirst becomes extreme, the tongue is white; cramps of great severity occur in the legs and feet. Within a few hours vomiting sets in and becomes incessant. The patient rapidly sinks into a condition of collapse, the features are shrunken, the skin has an ashy-gray hue, the eyeballs sink in the sockets, the nose is pinched, the cheeks are hollow, the voice becomes husky, the extremities are cyanosed, and the skin is shriveled, wrinkled, and covered with a clammy perspiration. The temperature sinks. In the axilla or in the mouth it may be from five to ten degrees below normal, but in the rectum and in the internal parts it may be 103° or 104°. The blood pressure falls greatly and is often below 70 mm. Hg. The pulse becomes extremely feeble and flickering, and the patient gradually passes into a condition of coma, though consciousness is often retained until near the end.

The fæces are at first yellowish in color, from the bile pigment, but soon they become grayish-white and look like turbid whey or rice-water; whence the term "rice-water stools." Numerous small flakes of mucus and granular matter, and at times blood are found in them. The reaction is usually alkaline. The fluid contains albumin and the chief mineral ingredient is chloride of sodium. Microscopically, mucus and epithelial cells and innumerable bacteria are seen, the majority of the latter being the comma bacilli.

The condition of the patient is largely the result of the concentration of the blood consequent upon the loss of serum in the stools. Acidosis probably has some influence. The specific gravity of the blood rises to 1.060 to 1.072. There is almost complete arrest of secretion, particularly of the saliva and the urine. On the other hand, the sweat-glands increase in activity, and in nursing women it has been stated that the lacteal flow is unaffected. This stage sometimes lasts not more than two or three hours, but more commonly from twelve to twenty-four.

(*c*) Reaction Stage.—When the patient survives the collapse, the cyanosis gradually disappears, the warmth returns to the skin, which may have for a time a mottled color or present a definite erythematous rash. The heart's action becomes stronger, the urine increases in quantity, the irritability of the stomach disappears, the stools are at longer intervals, and there is no abdominal pain. In the reaction the temperature may not rise above normal. Not infrequently this is interrupted by a recurrence of severe diarrhœa and the patient is carried off in a relapse. Other cases pass into the condition of what has been called *cholera-typhoid,* in which the patient is delirious, the pulse rapid and feeble, and the tongue dry. Death finally occurs with coma. These symptoms have been attributed to uræmia and acidosis.

During epidemics attacks are found of all grades of severity. There are cases of diarrhœa with griping pains, liquid, copious stools, vomiting, and cramps, with slight collapse. They resemble the milder cases of *cholera nostras.* At the opposite end of the series there are the instances of *cholera sicca,* in which death may occur in a few hours after the onset, without diarrhœa. There are also cases in which the patients are overwhelmed with the poison and die comatose, without the preliminary stage of collapse.

Complications and Sequelæ.—The consecutive nephritis rarely induces dropsy. Diphtheritic colitis has been described. There is a special tendency to diphtheritic inflammation of the mucous membranes, particularly of the throat and genitals. Pneumonia and pleurisy may follow, and destructive abscesses may occur in different parts. Suppurative parotitis is not very uncommon. In rare instances local gangrene may occur. A troublesome symptom of convalescence is cramps in the muscles of the arms and legs.

Diagnosis.—The only affection with which Asiatic cholera could be confounded is the *cholera nostras,* the severe choleraic diarrhœa which occurs during the summer months in temperate climates. The clinical picture of the two affections is identical. The extreme collapse, vomiting, and rice-water stools, the cramps, the cyanosed appearance, are all seen in the worst forms of cholera nostras. In enfeebled persons death may occur within twelve hours. The diagnosis has to be made by bacteriological methods.

Attacks very similar to Asiatic cholera are produced in poisoning by arsenic, corrosive sublimate, and certain fungi; but a difficulty in diagnosis could scarcely arise.

The *prognosis* is always uncertain, as the mortality ranges in different epidemics from 30 to 80 per cent. Intemperance, debility, and old age are unfavorable conditions. The more rapidly the collapse sets in, the greater is the danger, and as Andral truly says of the malignant form, "It begins where other diseases end—in death." Patients with marked cyanosis and very low temperature rarely recover.

Prophylaxis.—Preventive measures are all-important, and isolation of the sick and thorough disinfection have effectually prevented the disease entering England or the United States since 1873. During epidemics the greatest care should be exercised in the disinfection of the stools and linen of the patients. When an epidemic prevails, persons should be warned not to drink water unless previously boiled. The milk should be boiled and all food and drinks carefully protected from flies. Errors in diet should be avoided. Uncooked vegetables and salads should not be eaten. As the disease is not more infectious than typhoid fever, the chance of a person passing safely through an epidemic depends very much upon how far he is able to carry out prophylactic measures thoroughly. Digestive disturbances are to be treated promptly, and particularly diarrhœa, which so often is a preliminary symptom. For this, opium and acetate of lead and large doses of bismuth should be given. Protective inoculation has been carried out extensively.

Treatment.—The patient should be at rest in bed, kept warm, and given boiled milk, whey and egg albumen. Water may be given freely. If vomiting occurs food should be withheld and the stomach washed with an alkaline solution. Hot applications to the abdomen should be used and hot baths given if they prove helpful. Early in the course the bowels should be moved by castor oil or calomel. During the initial stage, when the diarrhœa is not excessive but the abdominal pain is marked, opium is the most efficient remedy, and it should be given hypodermically as morphia. It is advisable to give a full dose at once which may be repeated on the return of the pain. It is best not to attempt to give remedies by the mouth, as they disturb the stomach. In the collapse stage, writers speak strongly against the use of opium. Undoubtedly it must be given with caution, but, judging from its effects in cholera nostras, it would seem that collapse *per se* was not a contraindication. Potassium permanganate (gr. ii, 0.13 gm. in keratin coated pills) is given every 15 minutes for two to four hours and then every half hour until the color of the stools is green or yellow. For collapse pituitary extract and caffeine are useful.

Owing to the profuse serous discharges the blood becomes concentrated, and absorption takes place rapidly from the lymph-spaces. To meet this, intravenous injections were introduced by Latta, of Leith, in the epidemic of 1832. Bovell first practised the intravenous injections of milk in Toronto, in the epidemic of 1854.

Saline injections, intravenous and into the bowel, have been much used and with great success by the method introduced by Leonard Rogers. The hypertonic solution is composed of sodium chloride, grains 120; potassium chloride, grains 6; calcium chloride, grains 4; water, 1 pint. If the blood pressure is below 70 or the specific gravity of the blood 1.063 or over the hypertonic solution is given intravenously (1500-3000 c. c.) and repeated as often as required to keep the blood pressure above 70 and the specific gravity below 1.063. Normal saline solution (500 c. c.) with glucose (5 per cent.) is given by the bowel every two hours and at longer intervals if the urine increases. If there is suppression of urine with the danger of acidosis, sodium chloride 4 gm. and sodium bicarbonate 10 gm. in 500 c. c. of water are given intravenously. This treatment has markedly reduced the mortality.

In the stage of reaction special pains should be taken to regulate the diet and to guard against recurrences of the severe diarrhœa.

XVI. THE PLAGUE

Definition.—A specific, infectious disease, caused by *Bacillus pestis,* and occurring in two chief forms: a bubonic, involving the lymphatic glands, and a pneumonic, causing an acute and rapidly fatal inflammation of the lungs.

History and Geographical Distribution.—The disease was probably not known to the classical Greek writers. The earliest positive account dates from the second century of our era. The plague of Athens and the pestilence of the reign of Marcus Aurelius were apparently not this disease (Payne). From the great plague in the days of Justinian (sixth century) to the middle of the seventeenth century epidemics of varying severity occurred in Europe. Among the most disastrous was the famous "black death" of the fourteenth century, which overran Europe and destroyed a fourth of the population. In the seventeenth century it raged virulently, and during the great plague of London, in 1665, about 70,000 people died. During the eighteenth and nineteenth centuries the ravages of the disease lessened.

The revival of the plague is the most important single fact in modern epidemiology. Throughout the nineteenth century it waned progressively, outbreaks of some extent occurring in Turkey and Asia Minor and Astrakan; but we had begun to place it with sweating sickness and typhus among the diseases of the past. We knew that it slumbered in parts of China, and in northwest India, but the outbreak in 1894 at Hong-Kong startled the world and showed that the "black death" was still virulent. Since then it has spread in an ominous manner, reaching India, China, French Indo-China, Japan, Formosa, Australia, the Philippine Islands, South America, the West Indies, the United States, Cape Colony, Madagascar, Egypt, Asia Minor, and Russia in Asia. In Europe, cases have been carried to Marseilles and other Mediterranean ports and to Hamburg and Glasgow. In the latter city there was a small outbreak in 1900, 36 cases. In the next year there were two cases and in 1907 two cases—this without fresh importation. There have been small outbreaks in the United States at intervals from 1907 to the present with infection of rats and ground squirrels.

In England there have been four sets of human cases in East Suffolk; at Shotley in 1906-07, 8 cases and 6 deaths; at Trimley, in December, 1909, and January, 1910, 8 cases and 5 deaths; at Freston in the autumn of 1910, 4 fatal cases; and a fourth case occurred in the autumn of 1911. The majority of these were of the pneumonic type. There was an infection of the rats in East Anglia, beginning in the region between Ipswich and the coast. The rats were entirely of the species *Mus decumanus* except in part of Ipswich. The infection was not very widespread as of 568 rats examined only 17 were found infected. The disease extended to rabbits, but not to any great extent. Some fleas from the rats were found to contain bacilli indistinguishable from plague. The disease was introduced into Suffolk by ship rats from plague infected countries. More serious is the fact that rats infected with the plague have been occasionally discovered at Wapping, but there does not seem to have been any widespread epidemic among them. The immunity of the human population seems to be due to the fact that 50 per cent. of the rat fleas are of the variety *Pulex cheopis,* which rarely bites man, and the other rat flea, the *Ceratophyllus fasciatus,* does not bite man very freely. The common brown rat is not a house resident to any extent, so that conditions in England are not favorable for an epidemic.

The distribution in India is remarkable, chiefly in the Punjab, Bombay, and the United Provinces, which have a combined population of about 100 millions. In these three provinces between 1896 and the middle of 1911, about five and a half million deaths from plague have occurred. In the remaining provinces of India, with a population of some 200 millions, only about two millions of plague deaths have occurred. In the Presidency of Madras the disease has not been very severe, while Eastern Bengal and Assam have remained free, though cases have been repeatedly imported. There have been recent outbreaks in China, a sharp outbreak in Hong-Kong, and the disease has been reported in Egypt, Japan, Straits Settlements, Java and Sumatra, Persia, Turkey in Asia, Astrakan, the Mauritius, and several of the South American countries. The Manchurian outbreak of pneumonic plague in the wrinter of 1910-11 was one of the most virulent on record, carrying off more than 45,000 persons in a few months.

Etiology.—The specific organism of the disease is a bacillus discovered by Kitasato. It resembles somewhat the bacillus of chicken cholera, and grows in a characteristic manner. *B. pestis* occurs in the blood, in the organs of the body and in the sputum, and has also been found in the dust and in the soil of houses in which the patients have lived, but outside the body the life of the bacillus is thought to be short. Bed-bugs may harbor it.

The disease prevails most frequently in hot seasons, though an outbreak may occur during the coldest weather. Persons of all ages are attacked. It spreads chiefly among the poor, in the slums of the great cities.

The following conclusions of the Plague Commission (1908) relate to bubonic plague: (*a*) Contagion occurs in less than 3 per cent. of the cases, playing a very small part in the general spread of the disease. (*b*) Bubonic plague in man is entirely dependent on the disease in the rat. (*c*) The infection is conveyed from rat to rat and from rat to man solely by means of fleas. (*d*) A case in man is not in itself infectious. (*e*) A large majority of cases occur singly in houses. When more than one case occurs in a house, the attacks are generally nearly simultaneous. (*f*) Plague is usually conveyed from place to place by imported fleas, which are carried by people on their persons or in their baggage. The human agent may himself escape infection. (*g*) Insanitary conditions have no relation to the occurrence of plague, except in so far as they favor infestation by rats. (*h*) The non-epidemic season is bridged over by acute plague in the rat, accompanied by a few cases among human beings.

In the pneumonic form personal infection from one person to another is the common way, as the bacilli are sprayed into the air by coughing. The possibility of the human flea as a carrier must be considered.

Clinical Forms.—PESTIS MINOR.—In this variety, also known as the ambulant, the patient has a few days of fever, with swelling of the glands of the groin, and possibly suppuration. He may not be ill enough to seek medical relief. These cases, often found at the beginning and end of an epidemic, are a very serious danger, as the urine and fæces contain bacilli.

BUBONIC PLAGUE.—This constitutes the common variety, 77.65 per cent. of 11,600 cases of plague treated in the Arthur Road Hospital, Bombay (N. H. Choksy). The stage of invasion is characterized by headache, backache, stiffness of the limbs, a feeling of anxiety and restlessness, and great depression of spirits. There is a steady rise in the fever until the third or fourth day, when there is a drop of two or three degrees. There is then a secondary fever, as some writers describe it, in which the temperature reaches a still higher point. The tongue becomes brown, collapse symptoms are apt to supervene, and in very severe infections the patient may die at this stage. In at least two-thirds of all cases there are glandular swellings or buboes. An analysis of 9,500 cases of buboes gave more than 54 per cent. with the glands of the groin affected. The swelling appears usually from the third to the fifth day. Resolution may occur, or suppuration, or in rare cases gangrene. Suppuration is a favorable feature, as noted by De Foe in his graphic account of the London plague. There is a high leucocytosis.

Petechiæ very commonly show themselves, and may be very extensive. These have been called the "plague spots," or the "tokens of the disease," and gave to it in the middle ages the name of the Black Death. Hæmorrhages from the mucous membranes may also occur; in some epidemics hæmoptysis has been especially frequent.

Septicæmic Plague.—In this, the most rapid form, the patient succumbs in three or four days with a virulent infection before the buboes appear. This form constituted 14.25 per cent. of the 11,600 cases. Hæmorrhages are common. The bacilli can be obtained from the blood.

Pneumonic Plague.—In the ordinary bubonic type, inflammation of the lungs is not an uncommon complication, but the true pneumonic plague begins abruptly with fever, shortness of breath, cough, and sometimes pain in the chest. The fever increases, the signs of the involvement of the lung occur early; there may be impaired resonance at both bases with harsh and tubular breathing; the sputum becomes bloody and stained and more fluid than in ordinary pneumonia. Cyanosis is an early feature; the pulse is small and rapid, the patient becomes profoundly prostrate; the spleen enlarges rapidly, as early as the second day, and a fatal result follows in from two to four days. Recovery is very rare.

In other varieties the chief manifestations may be in the skin and subcutaneous tissues, or in the intestines, causing diarrhœa and sometimes the features of typhoid fever.

Diagnosis.—At the early stage of an outbreak plague cases are easily overlooked, but if the suspicious cases are carefully studied by a competent bacteriologist, there is no disease which can be more positively identified. The San Francisco epidemic illustrates this. The nature of the cases was recognized by Kellog and by Kinyoun, but with an amazing stupidity (which was shared by not a few physicians, who should have known better) the Governor of the State refused to recognize the presence of plague, and the United States Government had to intervene and send a board of experts to settle the question. The widespread prevalence of the disease makes it the imperative duty of the health authorities to have on hand, in connection with large ports, skilled men who can promptly make the bacteriological diagnosis. There are dangers from the cultures in laboratories, but with proper precautions they may be reduced to a minimum. Acute, rapidly fatal pneumonia should arouse suspicion as in the Suffolk cases.

Prophylaxis.—Wherever plague exists an organized staff, an intelligent policy, and a long purse are needed. In India, where fifteenth-century conditions prevail, and where the scale of the epidemic is so enormous, the problem of prophylaxis looks hopeless. Simpson's recommendation of a specially trained plague service, organized on proper lines and on a liberal basis.

should be carried out. A careful watch should be kept on the mortality of rats. When found infected, energetic measures should be taken to stamp out the disease in them. Three things are necessary—the cleansing of premises, particularly stables and outhouses, so that the rats cannot find nesting places or food; systematic rat destruction; and making houses rat proof. Certain measures prevent the access of plague to healthy ports; fumigation of ships to destroy the rats, careful inspection of passengers and crew, and detention over a period which covers the incubation of the disease.

When a centre becomes infected, the sanitary organization should carry out the segregation of the sick in hospitals, the disinfection of infected rooms with sulphur, destruction of infected bedding, and thorough cleansing of the entire district; old, badly infected buildings should be destroyed.

Treatment.—In a disease the mortality of which may reach as high as 80 or 90 per cent. the question of treatment resolves itself into making the patient as comfortable as possible, and following out certain general principles such as guide us in the care of fever patients. Cantlie recommends purgation and stimulation from the outset, and the use of morphia for the pain. The local treatment of the buboes is important. Ice may be applied to them, and good results apparently follow the injection of the bichloride of mercury. The pyrexia of the disease is best treated by systematic hydrotherapy.

A plague serum, chiefly the Lustig and the Yersin-Roux, has been used. Choksy concludes that a reduction of 20-25 per cent. in the mortality may be obtained by its use.

Preventive Inoculation.—With Haffkine's serum in 12 districts of 224,228 persons inoculated, 3,399 took the disease; of 639,600 uninoculated, 49,430 were attacked. C. J. Martin concludes that the chances of infection are reduced four-fifths, and the chances of recovery are two and a half times as great as in the uninoculated. The reports from India are most favorable and in South America the value of this plan has been demonstrated. It is interesting to note that the laboratory staff at Bombay, 116 in number, have remained immune though in constant contact with plague infested rats.

XVII. TETANUS

(Lockjaw)

Definition.—An infectious malady characterized by tonic spasms of the muscles with marked exacerbations. The virus is produced by a bacillus, *B. tetani* of Nicolaier, which occurs in earth, in putrefying fluids, and manure, and is a normal inhabitant of the intestines of many ruminants.

Etiology.—In the United States, according to Anders and Morgan, it is most frequent in the Hudson valley, in Long Island and in the Atlantic States. In 1917 there were 1,329 deaths from tetanus in the registration area, of which 329 were in children under one year. An extraordinary number of cases have followed the accidents of the July 4th celebrations, but the propaganda of the Journal of the American Medical Association has succeeded in reducing these fatalities in a remarkable way.

In England the disease is not very common. There were 166 deaths in

1916. It is more prevalent in certain districts, e. g. the Thames valley. It is more frequent in the Radcliffe Infirmary, Oxford, than in any hospital with which the senior author was connected. It is more common in the summer months and males are more frequently attacked than females. In E. W. Hill's analysis of 3,038 cases in temperate climates 22.31 per cent. were in children under one year, 21 per cent. in the third and fourth decades.

In the tropics tetanus is a much more severe and common disease. In Jamaica and Cuba it is from five to six times more frequent as a cause of death than in the United States, and above 80 per cent of the deaths are in infants. In the Canal Zone the disease has not been common, only 25 cases have been admitted to the Ancon and Colon Hospital (E. W. Hill) to 1910. It is not only in the tropics that tetanus is a very fatal disease in infants. On an island near Iceland all the children born died; and for years the island of St. Kilda, one of the Western Hebrides, had been scourged by the "eight days sickness" among the new born. Of 125 children, 84 died within fourteen days of birth. Since the introduction of proper methods of treating the umbilical cord the disease has practically disappeared.

The tetanus bacillus has contaminated vaccines, and its presence in commercial gelatine is a grave danger. Outbreaks have occurred in general hospitals following the use of catgut. The disease has occurred after prolonged use of the hypodermic needle to inject morphia or quinine, and has followed the use of gelatine as a hæmostatic.

The disease usually follows an injury, often of a most trifling character, and particularly lacerated wounds of the hands which have been contaminated by dirt and splinters. It may occur without any recognizable wound, so-called idiopathic tetanus.

The Tetanus Bacillus.—The organism is widely diffused in nature, in garden mould, in and about stables and farmyards, and is a normal inhabitant of the intestines of many horses and of the herbivora. The disease has been produced by inoculating animals with garden earth. Living bacilli occur in the intestines of 5 per cent. of healthy men and up to 20 per cent. of hostlers and dairymen. It is a slender motile bacillus, one end of which is swollen and occupied by a spore. It is anaërobic and grows at ordinary temperatures. The spores are the most resistant known. From two steel nibs dipped in a tetanus culture in 1891 a growth of virulent bacilli was obtained from one in 1902 and from the other in 1909 (Semple). The toxin is perhaps the most virulent of known poisons. Whereas the fatal dose of strychnine for a man weighing 70 kilos is from 30 to 100 milligrammes, that of the tetanus toxin is estimated at 0.23 milligramme. Every feature of the disease can be produced by it experimentally without the presence of the bacilli. The symptoms do not arise immediately, but slowly, and it has been found to be absorbed by the end plates in the muscles and to pass up the motor nerves to the spinal cord. The bacilli have been found in a few cases. The period of incubation is the time required for the toxins to travel along the nerves to the centres. A high degree of antitoxic immunity can be conferred on animals, which then yield a protective serum. It is, however, difficult to cure animals with this serum on account of the combination of the toxin with nerve-cells by the time symptoms appear.

Morbid Anatomy.—No characteristic lesions have been found in the cord or in the brain. Congestions occur in different parts, and perivascular exudations and granular changes in the nerve-cells have been found. The condition of the wound is variable. The nerves are often found injured, reddened, and swollen. In tetanus neonatorum the umbilicus may be inflamed.

Symptoms.—The incubation period is from one to twenty days. Of 1,092 cases analyzed by E. W. Hill, in 17.49 per cent. it was from one to five days and in 55.06 per cent. from five to ten days. In only 8 cases was the incubation as long as twenty days. The patient complains at first of slight stiffness in the neck, or a feeling of tightness in the jaws, or difficulty in mastication. Occasionally chilly feelings or actual rigors may precede these symptoms. Gradually a tonic spasm of the muscles of these parts produces the condition of trismus or lockjaw. The eyebrows may be raised and the angles of the mouth drawn out, causing the so-called sardonic grin—*risus sardonicus*. In children the spasm may be confined to these parts. Sometimes the attack is associated with paralysis of the facial muscles and difficulty in swallowing —the head-tetanus of Rose, which has most commonly followed injuries in the neighborhood of the fifth nerve. Gradually the process extends and involves the muscles of the body. Those of the back are most affected, so that during the spasm the unfortunate victim may rest upon the head and heels—a position known as *opisthotonos*. The rectus abdominis muscle has been torn across in the spasm. The entire trunk and limbs may be perfectly rigid—*orthotonos*. Flexion to one side is less common—*pleurothotonos;* while spasm of the muscles of the abdomen may cause the body to be bent forward—*emprosthotonos*. In very violent attacks the thorax is compressed, the respirations are rapid, and spasm of the glottis may occur, causing asphyxia. The paroxysms last for a variable period, but even in the intervals the relaxation is not complete. The slightest irritation is sufficient to cause a spasm. The paroxysms are associated with agonizing pain, and the patient may be held as in a vise, unable to utter a word. Usually he is bathed in a profuse sweat. The temperature may remain normal throughout, or show only a slight elevation toward the close. In other cases the pyrexia is marked from the outset; the temperature reaches 105° or 106° F., and before death 109° or 110° F. In rare instances it may go still higher. The course is sometimes very rapid, with fever and general spasms; death may take place on the third day. Death either occurs during the paroxysm from heart-failure or asphyxia, or is due to exhaustion.

The cephalic tetanus (*Kopftetanus* of Rose) originates usually from a wound of the head, and is characterized by stiffness of the muscles of the jaw and paralysis of the facial muscles on the same side as the wound, with difficulty in swallowing. There may be no other symptoms. This form has been called hydrophobic because of the spasm of the throat. The prognosis is good in the chronic cases, which may show slight symptoms only. Tetanus of one extremity has been observed.

Tetanus neonatorum.—This is a common form, particularly in hot climates and in districts where the tetanus bacillus is very prevalent, as in the island of St. Kilda. The infection follows imperfect treatment of the navel. The symptoms may come on in a few days or be delayed for ten days. Trismus and difficulty in crying and taking food are the earliest symptoms, followed in a few days by more general spasms. It is a very fatal form. A form known as *visceral tetanus* is described by the French in which the disease originates in the intestines, and the possibility of this must be considered, as the spores have been found in human fæces. *Post-operative tetanus* occurs particularly after peritoneal operations. Paterson collected 150 cases in a large proportion of which catgut had been used. It is a very fatal form, with a short incubation and rapid course. Operation on an individual who has recovered from tetanus a short time before, may cause a relapse.

Diagnosis.—Well-marked cases following a trauma could not be mistaken for any other disease. The spasms are not unlike those of strychnia-poisoning, and in the celebrated Palmer murder trial this was the plea for the defence. The jaw-muscles, however, are never involved early, if at all, and between the paroxysms in strychnia-poisoning there is no rigidity. In tetany the distribution of the spasm at the extremities, the peculiar position, the greater involvement of the hands, and the condition under which it occurs are sufficient to make the diagnosis clear. In doubtful cases cultures should be made from the pus of the wound. A mild trismus may occur with throat infection and should not be mistaken for head-tetanus.

Escherich has described in children a form of generalized tonic contractures of the muscles of the jaw, neck, back, and limbs, usually a sequel of some acute infection, occasionally occurring as an independent malady. The contractures may be either intermittent or persistent. The condition may last from a week to a couple of months. The cases as a rule recover.

Prognosis.—Two of the Hippocratic aphorisms express tersely the general prognosis even at the present day: "The spasm supervening on a wound is fatal," and "such persons as are seized with tetanus die within four days, or if they pass these they recover." Of 1,264 cases analyzed by E. W. Hill only 414 recovered. If the disease lasts beyond the tenth day the patient has an even chance, and from this time the prognosis improves.

The mortality is greatest in children. Favorable indications are: late onset of the attack, localization of the spasms to the muscles of the neck and jaw, and an absence of fever.

Prophylaxis.—Suspicious wounds should be freely opened, thoroughly disinfected by hydrogen peroxide and cauterized with pure phenol. In districts where the disease prevails, special precautions should be taken with all injuries, and a prophylactic dose of anti-tetanic serum (500 to 1,500 units) administered. The experience in the United States with this treatment in the Fourth of July accidents has been most satisfactory. It should be carried out promptly in all street and infected injuries. As the serum is expensive, Boards of Health should arrange, if necessary, to provide it.

Treatment.—The patient should be kept in a darkened room, absolutely quiet, and attended by only one person. All possible sources of irritation should be avoided. Veterinarians appreciate the importance of this complete seclusion in treating horses.

When the lockjaw is extreme the patient may not be able to take food by the mouth, under which circumstances it is best to use rectal injections, or to feed by a catheter passed through the nose. The spasm should be controlled by chloroform, which may be repeatedly exhibited at intervals. It is more satisfactory to keep the patient thoroughly under the influence of morphia given hypodermically. Chloral hydrate, chloretone, bromide of potassium, and other drugs have been recommended, and recovery occasionally follows their use. Intraspinal injections of a solution of magnesium sulphate (25 per cent.) have been used (Meltzer); 1 c. c. is injected for every 25 pounds weight of the patient. Resection of the nerve and amputation of the limb have been advised. Although tetanus antitoxin of great strength can be obtained, its use in the treatment of human tetanus very often fails because it is given too late. Given at once and in sufficient doses, it should prove a specific. It may be given in various ways. The administration of 3,000 to 5,000 units intraspinally (repeated in 24 hours) and 10,000 units intravenously and 10,000 units subcutaneously three or four days later has given good results (Nicoll). Intramuscular injections about the site of the wound and intraneural into the large nerve trunk leading from the wounded area have seemed useful in some cases.

XVIII. GLANDERS

(Farcy).

Definition.—An infectious disease of the horse and ass, caused by *Bacillus mallei,* communicated occasionally to man. In the horse it is characterized by the formation of nodules, chiefly in the nares (glanders) and beneath the skin (farcy).

Etiology.—The disease belongs to the infective granulomata. The local manifestations in the nostrils and the skin of the horse are due to the same cause. The specific germ was discovered by Loeffler and Schutz. It is a short, non-motile bacillus, not unlike that of tubercle, but exhibits different staining reactions. It grows readily on the ordinary culture media. For the full recognition of glanders in man we are indebted to the labors of Rayer, whose monograph remains one of the best descriptions of the disease. Man becomes infected by contact with diseased animals, and usually by inoculation on an abraded surface of the skin. The contagion may also be received on the mucous membrane. In a Montreal case a gentleman was probably infected by the material expelled from the nostril of his horse, which was not suspected of having the disease. It is a rare disease. Only 3 deaths were registered from this cause in England and Wales in 1916 and none in 1915. Among laboratory workers the *Bacillus mallei* has caused more deaths than any other germ, and in working with it the greatest precautions should be taken.

Morbid Anatomy.—As in the horse, the disease may be localized in the nose (glanders) or beneath the skin (farcy). The essential lesion is the granulomatous tumor, characterized by the presence of numerous lymphoid and epithelioid cells, among and in which are seen the glanders bacilli. These nodular masses tend to break down rapidly, and on the mucous membrane result in ulcers, while beneath the skin they form abscesses. The glanders nodules may also occur in the internal organs.

Symptoms.—An acute and a chronic form of glanders may be recognized in man, and an acute and a chronic form of farcy.

Acute Glanders.—The period of incubation is rarely more than three or four days. There are signs of general febrile disturbance. At the site of infection there are swelling, redness, and lymphangitis. Within two or three days there is involvement of the mucous membrane of the nose, the nodules break down rapidly to ulcers, and there is a muco-purulent discharge. An eruption of papules, which rapidly become pustules, breaks out over the face and about the joints. It has been mistaken for variola. In a Montreal case this copious eruption led the attending physician to suspect smallpox, and the patient was isolated. There is a great swelling of the nose. There may be an eruption like erysipelas. The ulceration may go on to necrosis, in which case the discharge is very offensive. The lymph glands of the neck are usually much enlarged. Subacute pneumonia is very apt to occur. This form runs its course in about eight or ten days, and is invariably fatal. *Glanders pneumonia* may appear after subcutaneous infection (one case from infection with a hypodermic syringe stuck into the thumb). Grossly the lung appeared like a caseous pneumonia.

CHRONIC GLANDERS is rare and difficult to diagnose, as it is usually mistaken for a chronic coryza. There are ulcers in the nose and often laryngeal symptoms. It may last for months, or even longer, and recovery sometimes takes place. Tedeschi described a case of chronic osteomyelitis, due to the *Bacillus mallei*, which was followed by a fatal glanders meningitis. The diagnosis may be extremely difficult. In such cases a suspension of the secretion, or of cultures upon agar-agar made from the secretion, should be injected into the peritoneal cavity of a male guinea-pig. At the end of two days, in positive cases, the testicles are found to be swollen and the skin of the scrotum reddened. The testicles continue to increase in size, and finally suppurate. Death takes place after the lapse of two or three weeks, and generalized glanders nodules are found in the viscera. The use of mallein for diagnostic purposes is highly recommended. The principles and methods of application are the same as for tuberculin. McFadyean and others have shown that, while the glanders bacilli are agglutinated in a dilution of 1 to 200 by normal horse serum, that of a glanders horse will agglutinate at 1 to 1,000. The test must be made before mallein is given.

ACUTE FARCY in man results usually from the inoculation of the virus into the skin. There is an intense local reaction with a phlegmonous inflammation. The lymphatics are early affected, and along their course there are nodular subcutaneous enlargements, the so-called farcy buds, which may rapidly go on to suppuration. There are pains and swelling in the joints, and abscesses may form in the muscles. The symptoms are those of an acute infection, almost like an acute septicæmia. The nose is not involved and the superficial skin eruption is not common. The bacilli have been found in the urine in acute cases in man and animals.

The disease is fatal in a large proportion of the cases, usually in from twelve to fifteen days.

CHRONIC FARCY is characterized by the presence of localized tumors which break down into abscesses, and sometimes form deep ulcers, without much inflammatory reaction and without special involvement of the lymphatics. The disease may last for months or even years. Death may result from pyæmia, or occasionally acute glanders develops. The celebrated French veterinarian Bouley had it and recovered.

The disease is transmissible also from man to man. Washerwomen have been infected from the clothes of a patient. In the diagnosis the occupation is very important. In cases of doubt the inoculation should be made in animals or the complement fixation test used. Mallein, a product of the growth of the bacilli, is used for the purpose of diagnosing glanders in animals. Several instances of cured glanders have been reported in animals treated with small and repeated doses of mallein (Pilavios, Babes). In the acute cases there is very little hope. In the chronic cases recovery is possible, though often tedious. Vaccine treatment may be tried cautiously with doses from 10 to 100 millions given every two to four days. Increase in dosage must be governed by the reaction.

Treatment.—If seen early, the wound should be either cut out or thoroughly destroyed by caustics and an antiseptic dressing applied. The farcy buds should be early opened. Antiseptic solutions such as potassium permanganate and hydrogen peroxide should be used.

XIX. ANTHRAX

(*Splenic Fever; Charbon; Wool-sorter's Disease*)

Definition.—An acute infectious disease caused by *Bacillus anthracis,* occurring in three forms, cutaneous (malignant pustule), pulmonary, and intestinal. In animals, particularly in sheep and cattle, the disease has the character of an acute septicæmia with enlargement of the spleen—hence the name *splenic* fever. In man it occurs sporadically or as a result of accidental inoculations with the virus.

Etiology.—The infectious agent is a non-motile, rod-shaped organism, *Bacillus anthracis,* which has, by the researches of Pollender, Davaine, Koch, and Pasteur, become the best known perhaps of all pathogenic microbes. The bacillus has a length of from 2 to 25 μ; the rods are often united. The bacilli themselves are readily destroyed, but the spores are very resistant, and survive after prolonged immersion in a 5-per-cent. solution of carbolic acid, or withstand for some minutes a temperature of 212° F. They are capable also of resisting gastric digestion. Outside the body the spores are in all probability very durable.

In Animals.—Geographically and zoölogically the disease is the most widespread of all infections. It is much more prevalent in Europe and in Asia than in America. Its ravages among the herds of cattle in Russia and Siberia, and among sheep in certain parts of Europe, are not equalled by any other animal plague. In the United States anthrax is not very widespread. In France from 6 to 10 per cent. of the sheep and about 5 per cent. of the cattle formerly died of it.

The disease is conveyed sometimes by direct inoculation, as by the bites and stings of insects, by feeding on carcasses of animals which have died of the disease, but more commonly by grazing in pastures contaminated by the germs. Pasteur thought that the earthworm played an important part in bringing to the surface and distributing the bacilli from the buried carcass of an infected animal. Certain fields, or even farms, may thus be infected for an indefinite period. It seems probable that, if the carcass is not opened or the blood spilt, spores are not formed in the buried animal and the bacilli quickly die.

In man the disease does not occur spontaneously. It results always from infection, either through the skin or intestines, or in rare instances through the lungs. Workers in wool and hair, and persons whose occupations bring them into contact with animals or animal products, as stablemen, shepherds, tanners, and butchers, are specially liable to the disease. In the United States the disease is usually found in the workers in hides, in butchers, and in veterinarians. It is rare in general hospital work. In the United States there were 62 deaths from anthrax in 1917 in the registration area. In England and Wales in 1916 there were 28 deaths from this cause in man. Ponder states that 40 per cent. of all the cases of anthrax in British leather workers are due to handling Chinese or East Indian goods; 80 per cent. of the cases are malignant pustule from skin infection while handling hides at the docks or in the tanneries.

Various forms of the disease have been described, and two chief groups may be recognized: the external anthrax and the internal anthrax, of which there are pulmonary and intestinal forms.

Symptoms.—(*a*) External Anthrax.—(1) *Malignant Pustule.*—At the site of inoculation, usually on an exposed surface—the hands, arms, or face—there are, within a few hours, itching and uneasiness, and the gradual formation of a small papule, which soon becomes vesicular. Inflammatory induration extends around this, and within thirty-six hours at the site of inoculation there is a dark brownish eschar, at a little distance from which there may be a series of small vesicles. The brawny induration may be extreme. The œdema produces very great swelling of the parts. The inflammation extends along the lymphatics, and the neighboring lymph-glands are swollen and sore. The fever at first rises rapidly, and the concomitant phenomena are marked. Subsequently the temperature falls, and in many cases becomes subnormal. Death may take place in from three to five days. In cases which recover the constitutional symptoms are slighter, the eschar gradually sloughs out, and the wound heals. The cases vary much in severity. In the mildest form there may be only slight swelling. At the site of inoculation a papule is formed, which rapidly becomes vesicular and dries into a scab, which separates in the course of a few days.

(2) *Malignant Anthrax Œdema.*—This form occurs in the eyelid, and also in the head, hand, and arm, and is characterized by the absence of the papule and vesicle forms, and by the most extensive œdema, which may follow rather than precede the constitutional symptoms. The œdema reaches such a grade of intensity that gangrene results, and may involve a considerable surface. The constitutional symptoms then become extremely grave, and the cases invariably prove fatal. The greatest fatality is seen in cases of inoculation about the head and face, where the mortality, according to Nasarow, is 26 per cent.; the least in infection of the lower extremities, where it is 5 per cent.

In a case at the Johns Hopkins Hospital in 1895, in a hair-picker, there were most extensive enteritis, peritonitis, and endocarditis, which last lesion has been described by Eppinger.

A feature in both these forms of malignant pustule is the absence of feeling of distress or anxiety on the part of the patient, whose mental condition may be perfectly clear. He may be without any apprehension, even though the condition be most critical.

The *diagnosis* in most instances is readily made from the character of the lesion and the occupation of the patient. There is a remarkable freedom from pain which distinguishes anthrax from furuncle, carbuncle and cellulitis. When in doubt, the examination of the fluid from the pustule may show the presence of the anthrax bacilli. Cultures should be made, or a mouse or guinea-pig inoculated from the local lesion. The blood may not show the bacilli in numbers until shortly before death.

(*b*) Internal Anthrax.—(1) *Intestinal Form, Mycosis Intestinalis.*—In these cases the infection usually is through the stomach and intestines, and results from eating the flesh or drinking the milk of diseased animals; it may, however, follow an external infection if the germs are carried to the mouth. The symptoms are those of intense poisoning. The disease may set in with a chill, followed by vomiting, diarrhœa, moderate fever, and pains in the legs and back. It may be mistaken for intestinal obstruction. In acute cases there are dyspnœa, cyanosis, great anxiety and restlessness, and toward the end convulsions or spasms of the muscles. Hæmorrhage may occur from the mucous membranes. Occasionally there are small phlegmonous areas or petechiæ on the skin. The spleen is enlarged. The blood is dark and remains fluid for a long time after death. Late in the disease the bacilli may be found in the blood.

This is one of the forms of acute poisoning which may affect many individuals together. Butler and Huber described an epidemic in which twenty-five persons were attacked after eating the flesh of an animal which had had anthrax. Six died in from forty-eight hours to seven days.

(2) *Wool-sorter's Disease, Pulmonary Anthrax, Anthracœmia.*—This important form occurs in the large establishments in which wool or hair is sorted and cleansed. The hair and wool imported into Europe from Russia and South America appear to have induced the largest number of cases. Many of these show no external lesion. The infective material has been swallowed or inhaled with the dust. There are rarely premonitory symptoms. The patient is seized with a chill, becomes faint and prostrated, has pains in the back and legs, and the temperature rises to 102° or 103°. The breathing is rapid, and he complains of much pain in the chest. There may be a cough and signs of bronchitis. So prominent in some instances are these bronchial symptoms that a pulmonary form of the disease has been described. The pulse is feeble and very rapid. There may be vomiting, and death may occur within twenty-four hours with symptoms of profound collapse and prostration. Other cases are more protracted, and there may be diarrhœa, delirium, and unconsciousness. The cerebral symptoms may be most intense; in at least four cases the brain seems to have been chiefly affected, and its capillaries stuffed with bacilli (Merkel). The recognition of wool-sorter's disease as a form of anthrax is due to J. H. Bell, of Bradford.

In certain instances these profound constitutional symptoms of internal anthrax are associated with the external lesions of malignant pustule.

The *rag-picker's disease* has been made the subject of an exhaustive study by Eppinger (Die Hadernkrankheit, Jena, 1894), who has shown that it is a local anthrax of the lungs and pleura, with general infection.

Prophylaxis.—This is important, and should be carried out by a most rigid disinfection of the hides, hair, and rags before they are placed in the hands of the workmen. Those handling infected material should have the arms and neck covered, and wear gloves. Animals may be immunized against the disease and Pasteur's method of vaccination has been extensively employed in France with good results. The immunity is lost within a year in nearly 50 per cent. of the animals.

Treatment.—In malignant pustule the site of inoculation should be excised and, after the cautery or pure phenol is applied, powdered bichloride of mercury sprinkled over the exposed surface. The local development of the bacilli about the site of inoculation may be prevented by the subcutaneous injections of solutions of carbolic acid (3 per cent.) or bichloride of mercury (1 to 1,000). The injections should be made at various points around the pustule, and may be repeated two or three times a day. The internal treatment should be confined to the administration of stimulants and plenty of nutritious food. In malignant forms, particularly the intestinal cases, little can be done. Active purgatives may be given at the outset, so as to remove the infecting material. The anti-anthrax serum has given good results in some cases. An initial dose of 80 to 100 c. c. is given intravenously and 20 c. c. daily after this. The use of normal bovine serum (20-30 c. c. heated twice for half an hour) intravenously has been advised.

XX. LEPROSY

Definition.—A chronic infectious disease caused by *Bacillus lepræ,* characterized by the presence of tubercular nodules in the skin and mucous membranes (tubercular leprosy) or by changes in the nerves (anæsthetic leprosy). At first these forms may be separate, but ultimately both are combined, and in the characteristic tubercular form there are disturbances of sensation.

History.—The disease appears to have prevailed in Egypt even so far back as three or four thousand years before Christ. The Hebrew writers make many references to it, but, as is evident from the description in Leviticus, many different forms of skin disease were embraced under the term leprosy. Both in India and in China the affection was also known many centuries before the Christian era. The old Greek and Roman physicians were perfectly familiar with its manifestations. Evidence of a pre-Columbian existence of leprosy in America has been sought in the old pieces of Peruvian pottery representing deformities suggestive of this disease, but Ashmead denies their significance. Throughout the middle ages leprosy prevailed extensively in Europe, and the number of leper asylums has been estimated as at least 20,000. During the sixteenth century it gradually declined.

Geographical Distribution.—In Europe leprosy prevails in Iceland, Norway and Sweden, parts of Russia, particularly about Dorpat, Riga, and the Caucasus, and in certain provinces of Spain and Portugal. In Great Britain the cases are all imported. In the United States it is estimated that there are about 250 recognized cases. In Canada there are foci of leprosy in two or three counties of New Brunswick, settled by French Canadians, and in Cape Breton, Nova Scotia. The number has gradually lessened. The disease appears to have been imported from Normandy about the end of the 18th century.

Leprosy is endemic in the West India Islands and also occurs in Mexico. In the Sandwich Islands it spread rapidly after 1860, and strenuous attempts have been made to stamp it out by segregating all lepers on the island of Molokai. In the Philippine Islands, in a population of over six millions, there are about 5,000 lepers.

In British India, according to the Leprosy Commission, there are 100,000 lepers. This is probably a low estimate. In China leprosy prevails extensively. In South Africa it has increased rapidly. In Australia, New Zealand, and the Australasian islands it also prevails, chiefly among the Chinese. The essays of Ashburton Thompson and James Cantlie deal fully with leprosy in China, Australia, and the Pacific islands.

Etiology.—*Bacillus lepræ,* discovered by Hansen, of Bergen, in 1871, is universally recognized as the cause of the disease. It has many points of resemblance to the tubercle bacillus, but can be readily differentiated. It has been cultivated, but with difficulty, and is stated to have a pleomorphism of which the bacillus as seen in the tissues is only one phase.

Modes of Infection.—(*a*) *Inoculation.*—While it is highly probable that leprosy may be contracted by accidental inoculation, the experimental evidence is as yet inconclusive. With one possible exception, negative results have followed the attempts to reproduce the disease in man. The Hawaiian convict, under sentence of death, who was inoculated on September 30, 1884, by Arning, four weeks later had rheumatoid pains and gradual painful swelling of the ulnar and median nerves. The neuritis gradually subsided, but there developed a small lepra tubercle at the site of the inoculation. In 1887 the disease was manifest, and the man died of it six years after inoculation. The case is not regarded as conclusive, as he had leprous relatives and lived in a leprous country. The bed bug may take up the bacilli.

(*b*) *Heredity.*—For years it was thought that the disease was transmitted from parent to child, but the general opinion is now decidedly against this view. The possibility of its transmission cannot be denied, and in this respect leprosy and tuberculosis occupy very much the same position, though men with very wide experience have never seen a new-born leper. The youngest cases are rarely under three or four years of age.

(*c*) *By Contagion.*—The bacilli are given off from the open sores; they are found in the saliva and expectoration of the cases with leprous lesions in the mouth and throat, and occur in very large numbers in the nasal secretion. Sticker found in 153 lepers, subjects of both forms of the disease, bacilli in the nasal secretion in 128, and herein, he thinks, lies the chief source of danger. Schaffer collected lepra bacilli on clean slides placed on tables and floors near to lepers whom he had caused to read aloud. The bacilli have also been isolated from the urine and the milk of patients. It seems probable that they may enter the body in many ways through the mucous membranes and through the skin. Sticker believes that the initial lesion is in an ulcer above the cartilaginous part of the nasal septum. One of the most striking examples of the contagiousness of leprosy is the following: "In 1860, a girl who had hitherto lived at Holstfershof, where no leprosy existed, married and went to live at Tarwast with her mother-in-law, who was a leper. She remained healthy, but her three children (1, 2, 3) became leprous, as also her younger sister (4), who came on a visit to Tarwast and slept with the children. The younger sister developed leprosy after returning to Holstfershof. At the latter place a man (5), fifty-two years old, who married one of the 'younger sister's' children, acquired leprosy; also a relative (6), thirty-six years old, a tailor by occupation, who frequented the house, and his wife (7), who came from a place where no leprosy existed." There is evidence to show that the disease may be spread through infected clothing, and the high percentage of washerwomen among lepers is suggestive.

Conditions Influencing Infection.—The disease attacks persons of all ages. We do not yet understand all the conditions necessary. Evidently the closest and most intimate contact is essential. The doctors, nurses, and Sisters of Charity who care for the patients are very rarely attacked. In the lazaretto at Tracadie not one of the Sisters who for more than fifty years have so faithfully nursed the lepers has contracted the disease. Father Damian, in the Sandwich Islands, and Father Boblioli, in New Orleans, both fell victims in the discharge of their priestly duties.

Morbid Anatomy.—The leprosy tubercles consist of granulomatous tissue made up of cells of various sizes in a connective-tissue matrix. The bacilli in extraordinary numbers lie partly between and partly in the cells. The process gradually involves the skin, giving rise to tuberous outgrowths with intervening areas of ulceration or cicatrization, which in the face may gradually produce the so-called *facies leontina.* The mucous membranes, particularly the conjunctiva, the cornea, and the larynx, may gradually be involved. In many cases deep ulcers form which result in extensive loss of substance or loss of fingers or toes, the so-called *lepra mutilans.* In anæsthetic leprosy there is a peripheral neuritis due to the development of the bacilli in the nerve-fibres. Indeed, this involvement of the nerves plays a primary part in the etiology of many of the important features, particularly the trophic changes in the skin and the disturbances of sensation.

Clinical Forms.—(*a*) Tubercular Leprosy.—Prior to the appearance of the nodules there are areas of cutaneous erythema which may be sharply defined and often hyperæsthetic. This is sometimes known as *macular* leprosy. The affected spots in time become pigmented. In some instances this superficial change continues without the development of nodules, the areas become anæsthetic, the pigment gradually disappears, and the skin gets perfectly white—the *lepra alba.* Among the patients at Tracadie it was particularly interesting to see three or four in this early stage presenting on the face and forearms a patchy erythema with slight swelling of the skin. The diagnosis of the condition is perfectly clear, though it may be a long time before any other than sensory changes develop. The eyelashes and eyebrows and the hairs on the face fall out. The mucous membranes finally become involved, particularly of the mouth, throat, and larynx; the voice becomes harsh and finally aphonic. Death results not infrequently from the laryngeal complications and aspiration pneumonia. The conjunctivæ are frequently attacked, and the sight is lost by a leprous keratitis.

(*b*) Anæsthetic Leprosy.—This remarkable form has, in characteristic cases, no external resemblance whatever to the other variety. It usually begins with pains in the limbs and areas of hyperæsthesia or of numbness. Very early there may be trophic changes, seen in the formation of small bullæ (Hillis). Maculæ appear upon the trunk and extremities, and after persisting for a variable time gradually disappear, leaving areas of anæsthesia, but the loss of sensation may come on independently of the outbreak of maculæ. The nerve-trunks, where superficial, may be felt to be large and nodular. The trophic disturbances are usually marked. Pemphigus-like bullæ develop in the affected areas, which break and leave ulcers which may be very destructive. The fingers and toes are liable to contractures and to necrosis, so that in chronic cases the phalanges are lost. The course of anæsthetic leprosy is extraordinarily chronic and may persist for years without leading to much deformity. We knew a prominent clergyman who had anæsthetic leprosy for more than thirty years, which did not seriously interfere with his usefulness, and not in the slightest with his career.

Diagnosis.—Even in the early stage the dusky erythematous maculæ with hyperæsthesia or areas of anæsthesia are very characteristic. In an advanced grade neither the tubercular nor anæsthetic forms could possibly be mistaken for any other affection. In a doubtful case the microscopic examination of an excised nodule is decisive.

Treatment.—Vaccines have been prepared and good results are claimed by various observers. The Finsen light, X-rays, and radium do good to the local lesions. Chaulmoogra oil has been extensively used. Heiser advises chaulmoogra oil 60 c. c., camphorated oil 60 c. c., and resorcin 4 gm.; this is sterilised and 1 c. c. given subcutaneously once a week. The dose is gradually increased to 3 c. c. Rogers advises the intravenous injection of gynocardate of soda (prepared from the fatty acids of chaulmoogra oil) gr. 1/10 to 4/5 (0.006 to 0.05 gm.), in a 2 per cent. saline solution and 0.5 per cent. phenol.

Segregation should be compulsory in all cases except where the friends can show that they have ample provision in their own home for the complete isolation and proper care of the patient.

XXI. TUBERCULOSIS

I. GENERAL ETIOLOGY AND MORBID ANATOMY

Definition.—An infection caused by *Bacillus tuberculosis,* the lesions of which are characterized by nodular bodies, tubercles, and diffuse infiltrations, which either undergo caseation, necrosis, and ulceration, or heal with sclerosis and calcification.

The very varied clinical features depend upon the organ involved, the intensity of the infection, and the degree of resistance offered by the body.

History.—The Greek physicians made many observations upon the clinical features of pulmonary tuberculosis, and our description of the symptoms and of the consumptive "type" dates from Hippocrates. Galen recognized its contagious nature. In the 17th century F. Sylvius indicated the connection between the tuberculous nodule and phthisis, and Richard Morton, a friend and contemporary of Sydenham, wrote (1689) the first modern treatise on the subject, in which the clinical side of the disease was well considered. He regarded it as contagious. Pierre Desault, William Stark, and Matthew Baillie laid the foundation of our knowledge of the coarse characters of tubercle as the anatomical basis of tuberculosis. Our real knowledge of the disease is a 19th century contribution, beginning with the work of Bayle on the structure of the tubercle and on its identity in the widely distributed lesions. With the Traité d'Auscultation Médiate (1819) Laennec laid the foundation not only of our modern knowledge of tuberculosis, but of modern clinical medicine. This work (easily to be had in an English translation) should be read from cover to cover by every young doctor, and, when possible, by every senior student. The unity of the forms of the tubercle—the miliary granule, the infiltration, and the caseous mass—was recognized, and for the first time physical signs and anatomical features were correlated, and the course of the disease carefully studied. Virchow led a battle against the unity of tuberculous lesions, and held that the products of any simple inflammation might become caseous, and that the ordinary so-called catarrhal pneumonia might terminate in phthisis.

The contagiousness of the disease, a belief in which had all along been held by individuals, and was widely spread in certain countries—as in Italy—was emphasized and confirmed by the brilliant work of Villemin, who first placed the infective nature of the disease on a solid experimental basis. There is nothing more masterly in the literature of experimental medicine than his work. Then came the demonstration by Robert Koch (in 1882) of the *Bacillus tuberculosis*. The preliminary article in the Berliner klin. Wochenschrift (1882) and the more complete work (Mitteilungen a. d. k. Gesundheitsamte, Bd. 2) should be studied by all who wish to appreciate the value of scientific methods. The thoroughness of Koch's work is manifested by the fact that, in the years that have elapsed, the innumerable workers have amplified and extended, but in no way essentially modified his original position.

During the past thirty years we have been gradually getting accommodated to the new views, the most important single effect of which has been a world-wide crusade against tuberculosis as a preventable disease.

Distribution.—The disease is widely spread zoölogically.

(*a*) In Animals.—Of animals the cold-blooded are rarely affected. In birds the disease is not uncommon, particularly in fowls, but there are minor differences between the avian and mammalian forms. In the domestic animals tuberculosis is a common disease, particularly in cattle. In sheep, goats, and horses it is rare. In pigs it is not uncommon in certain parts of Europe. Cats and dogs are not prone to the disease. In monkeys in confinement it is very common. The most important single fact in the distribution of the disease in animals is its widespread prevalence in bovines, from which nearly all the milk and a large proportion of our meat are derived.

(b) In Man.—Tuberculosis is his most universal scourge, well deserving the epithet bestowed upon it by Bunyan of the "Captain of the Men of Death." It is estimated that at least one-eighth of all deaths are due to it. In England and Wales there were 53,858 deaths from tuberculosis in 1916. In the United States it is responsible for about one-tenth of all deaths. The rate in the registration areas was 201.9 per 100,000 in 1900 and 146.4 in 1917.

There has been a remarkable reduction in England in the death-rate within the past fifty years.

In London the death-rate from consumption declined 33 per cent. between 1901 and 1910, and other forms of tuberculosis show a similar fall. To a less striking degree, but practically everywhere in the civilized world, there has been a reduction in the death-rate—the most encouraging feature of modern sanitation. To what is this to be attributed? *First.* To the improved social condition of the people, better housing, better food, better habits. The falling death-rate began before the present campaign against the disease. *Secondly.* The education of the people, which has made great strides, and a larger proportion are striving to lead hygienic lives. There are less drunkenness, less overcrowding, better air, and better food. The habit of spitting in public has been checked and the seeds of the disease are not spread so broadcast. *Thirdly.* As Newsholme points out, segregation has done much to protect the healthy from the sick. In the year 1910, 20.5 per cent. of the deaths in England and Wales and 43.4 per cent. of the deaths in London occurred in public institutions for the sick. *Fourthly.* The cases are seen earlier and the condition is recognized before it is hopeless. In a larger number of persons with pulmonary disease the diagnosis is made at a stage when complete healing is possible. The two important elements then are, fewer seeds, more stony soil. The economic loss from tuberculosis has been estimated by various writers. Baldwin puts it for the United States at from 150 to 200 millions of dollars annually.

Etiology: the Bacillus tuberculosis.—(*a*) THE SEED.—The *Bacillus tuberculosis* is a minute rod-shaped organism slightly bent or curved, with an average length of from 3 to 4 μ. When stained it may present a beaded appearance; whether due to spores or vacuoles is doubtful. Aberrant forms are not uncommon, i. e., long filaments or branched forms. It stains in a characteristic way with aniline dyes, and in cultures the growth is distinctive.

Specific varieties are recognized. The avian form has well-marked peculiarities, but the great point of discussion has been the relation of the bacillus causing human to that which causes bovine tuberculosis. Differences in the character of the tubercles of these two classes had long been recognized, and Theobald Smith pointed out special differences between the human and the bovine bacilli. But the matter was brought to a focus in 1901 by Koch's statement that the bacilli of bovine tuberculosis did not cause human tuberculosis, and *vice versa.* The question has been submitted to the test and it is generally recognized that there are differences between the two forms. The report of the English commission confirms the view that the bovine organism is capable of producing the disease in man. in whom it may often be recognized as a special form.

The virulence of the individual strains varies, a factor of great importance in all specific infections.

In the Body.—The bacilli are found in all tuberculous lesions, particularly in those actively growing, but in the chronic disease of the lymph glands and of the joints they are scanty. In all caseous foci they are few in number. In the sputum in pulmonary tuberculosis they may be present in countless myriads. They are sometimes found in the blood, particularly in cases of miliary tuberculosis.

Outside the Body.—The tubercle bacilli are widely scattered and are found in varying numbers wherever human beings are crowded together. There are two chief sources—the expectoration of persons with advanced disease of the lungs and the milk of tuberculous cows.

From a patient in the Johns Hopkins Hospital, with moderately advanced disease, Nuttall estimated that from 1½ to 4 1-3 billions of bacilli were thrown off each twenty-four hours. Allowed to dry, the sputum becomes dust and is distributed far and wide. Experiments have shown the presence of the bacilli in dust samples from hospital wards, from public buildings, streets, railway carriages, and various localities. So widely spread are the bacilli that in cities at least few individuals pass a week without affording opportunity for their lodgment, usually in the throat or air passages, inhaled with dust. They may readily contaminate food. The hands of tuberculous subjects are almost always contaminated. From the street, tuberculous sputum may be brought into the house on shoes, on the long skirts of women, on the hair of dogs, etc. It is interesting to note that in some of the places most frequented by tuberculous subjects, e. g., the sanatoria, the dust (as shown by experiments at Saranac) may be free from bacilli.

Bovine bacilli are distributed by means of the milk, rarely by the flesh, and still more rarely by contact with the animals. A proportion of all cases of infection in childhood are with this variety. A study by Park and Krumwiede showed that bovine tuberculosis is practically negligible in adults but in young children causes about 10 per cent. of the deaths from tuberculosis.

So widely spread everywhere is the seed, that the soil, the conditions suitable for its growth, is practically of equal moment.

(*b*) THE SOIL.—Many years ago the senior author drew the parallel between infection in tuberculosis and the parable of the sower, which though now somewhat hackneyed illustrates in an effective way the importance of the nature of the ground upon which the seed falls. *"Some seeds fell by the wayside and the fowls of the air came and devoured them up."* These are the bacilli scattered broadcast outside the body, an immense majority of which die. *"Some fell upon stony places."* These are the bacilli that find lodgment in many of us, perhaps, with the production of a small focus, but nothing comes of it; they wither away "because they have no root." *"Some fell among thorns, and the thorns sprang up and choked them."* This represents the cases of tuberculosis, latent or active, in which the seed finds the soil suitable and grows, but the conditions are not favorable, as the thorns, representing the protecting force of the body, get the better in the struggle. *"But others fell on good ground and sprang up and bare fruit an hundredfold."* Of this fourth group were the 53,858 who died of the disease in 1916 in England—the soil suitable, the protecting forces feeble.

What makes a good soil? Fortunately the human body is not a very good culture medium for the tubercle bacillus. The adult human individual in normal health seems to be practically immune to natural infection (Baldwin). And yet about one-eighth of the human race dies of tuberculosis, but a large proportion of all individuals become infected before reaching adult life and never have the disease. The studies of Naegli, Burkhardt, and others show that in fully 90 per cent. of the bodies of city-dwellers who have died of disease other than tuberculosis small tuberculous lesions are present. This is probably too high an estimate for England or the United States. Franz has shown that over 60 per cent. of healthy young adults react to the subcutaneous tuberculin test. Using more delicate tuberculin tests, it is found that nearly all adults react, and according to Hamburger, who has employed the subcutaneous-local reaction, over 90 per cent. of children are infected before reaching the twelfth year of life. This means, of course, that in a very small proportion of those upon whom the seed falls is the soil suitable for active growth—only a natural immunity keeps the race alive.

What this suitable soil is has been the subject of much discussion. From the time of Hippocrates the profession has recognized a tuberculous habitus, which has been variously described as disposition, diathesis, dyscrasia, temperament, constitution, or by the German word "Anlage." These terms are not always regarded as interchangeable, but here for practical purposes Ribbert's definition suffices, that a disposition is "that peculiarity in the organism which allows of the effective working of the exciting causes of a disease." Manifestly, such a disposition or constitution of the body may be inherited or acquired. Pearson concludes that "the diathesis of pulmonary tuberculosis is certainly inherited, and the intensity of the inheritance is sensibly the same as that of any normal physical character yet investigated in man. Infection probably plays a necessary part, but in the artisan classes of the urban populations of this country (England) it is doubtful if their members can escape the risks of infection, except by the absence of diathesis—i. e., the inheritance of what amounts to a counter-disposition."

Hippocrates defines the *habitus phthisicus* in the following words: "The form of body peculiar to subjects of phthisical complaints was the smooth, the whitish, that resembled the lentil; the reddish, the blue-eyed, the leucophlegmatic, and that with the scapulæ having the appearance of wings." The so-called scrofulous type has broad coarse features, opaque skin, large thick bones, and heavy figure.

Acquired disposition may arise through a lowering of the resistance of the body forces. Dwellers in cities in the dark, close alleys, and tenement houses, workers in cellars and ill-ventilated rooms, persons addicted to drink, are much more prone to the disease. The influence of environment was never better demonstrated than in the well-known experiment of Trudeau, who found that rabbits inoculated with tuberculosis if confined in a dark, damp place, without sunlight and fresh air, rapidly succumbed, while others treated in the same way, but allowed to run wild, either recovered or showed very slight lesions. The occupants of prisons, asylums, and poorhouses, too often, indeed, in barracks and large workshops, are in the position of Trudeau's rabbits in the cellar, and under the conditions most favorable to foster the development of the bacilli which may have lodged in their tissues.

No *age* is exempt. The disease is met with in the suckling and in the octogenarian, but fatal tuberculosis is, as Hippocrates pointed out, more common between the eighteenth and thirty-fifth year. The influence of *sex* is very slight. On the other hand the influence of *race* is important. It is a very fatal disease in the negroes, particularly in the southern United States, and in the North American Indians, among whom in 1915, 35 per cent. of the deaths were due to tuberculosis. The Irish, both at home and in the United

States, are more prone to the disease than other European races. The Jews everywhere have a low mortality from tuberculosis.

Occupation has an influence, in so far as insanitary surroundings, exposure to dust, close confinement, long, irregular hours, and low rates of wages, favor the prevalence of the disease. The home conditions should be considered in estimating the influence of occupation. Certain local conditions influence the soil very greatly. Catarrh of the respiratory passages appears to lower the resistance and favor the conditions which enable the bacilli to enter the system, or to grow in the tissues. The specific fevers, particularly measles and whooping-cough, predispose to tuberculosis; and any lowering disease may do so, but in such cases it is very often not a fresh infection, but the blazing of a smouldering fire. The soil of diabetes is favorable to the growth of the tubercle bacilli. Many chronic affections lower the resistance and it is notorious in hospital practice how often the fatal event in arteriosclerosis, cirrhosis of the liver, etc., is a terminal acute tuberculosis.

Trauma, as for example a blow on the chest, injury to the knee, a blow upon the head, may be followed by local tuberculosis. The injured part for a time is a *locus minoris resistentiæ,* and the bacilli already present grow in the favorable conditions caused by the injury.

(*c*) Specific Reactions of the Bacilli.—In its growth the bacillus so far as we know does not form soluble toxins, at least not in the cultures. It causes (1) a local tissue reaction which results in the formation of a new growth, the tubercle; (2) changes in the metabolism of the body fluids. The local tissue reactions will be considered later; here we may speak of the phenomena grouped under the term immunity.

(1) *Tuberculin Reaction.*—An animal inoculated subcutaneously with tubercle bacilli, or with dead cultures, has a local reaction associated with the formation of a tubercle; the neighboring lymph glands become involved, and in susceptible animals the disease generalizes and causes death. Koch found that if to a guinea-pig with a subcutaneous focus of tuberculosis so caused a second injection of the bacillus was given, healing occurred in the primary nodule, and the animal did not die. Upon these facts his tuberculin treatment was based. Tuberculin consists of the dead and macerated bacilli together with any substances formed in the cultures. If into a healthy person .025 c. c. of original tuberculin is injected, there is a slight fever with a feeling of uneasiness which passes off in from twelve to twenty-four hours. If into an individual with a focus of tuberculosis doses of .015 c. c. of tuberculin are injected subcutaneously, there is an active *local* reaction about the tuberculous focus and a *constitutional* reaction (fever, general pains, etc.). This process, known as the "tuberculin reaction," is used extensively for purposes of diagnosis. The reaction may be local, focal or constitutional. The skin reactions are the safest because the reaction is local. The chief methods are the ophthalmo-reaction of Calmette and the cutaneous of von Pirquet. A drop of the solution, placed on the conjunctiva of a person with a focus of tuberculosis anywhere in the body, is followed in a few hours by deep injection of the blood-vessels, increased lachrymation, and a slight swelling of the membrane. This lasts for from twenty-four to thirty-six hours. This method is not without danger.

For the *skin* reaction of von Pirquet a couple of drops of tuberculin are placed on a disinfected region of the skin, and the epidermis is scarified through the drops without drawing blood. If positive, at the end of twenty-four hours there is an inflammatory reaction which reaches its maximum in from thirty-six to forty-eight hours. For clinical purposes the tuberculin reaction is to be relied on, but that it may be given by a small focus of latent disease in a healthy person and that it has been found to be positive in as large a proportion as 60 per cent. of apparently normal individuals are facts which diminish its practical value.

(2) *Immunity Changes.*—In an infected person certain changes occur in the blood serum, depending upon the development of so-called antibodies, the presence of which may be demonstrated by the method of complement fixation; and the serum also contains agglutinins which possess an agglutinating action on the tubercle bacilli. Either directly themselves or through the toxic products there are brought into play certain cellular and humoral reactions which are capable of destroying the infecting agents or of neutralizing their effects or of limiting their activities. Experimentally in animals, according to the virulence of the organism and the dose, all gradations of symptoms may be produced, from the slightest local reaction to the profoundest septicæmia with high fever and death. In a local tuberculous infection, such as happens to the great majority of us in some part of our bodies at some time in our lives, happily the protective mechanism suffices to localize and limit the invaders. It may amount only to a skirmish, such as is constantly going on at the frontiers of a great empire, but if the local infection is more virulent, or becomes wider spread, the products of the growth of the bacilli or the bacilli themselves enter the circulation, an auto-inoculation, in which case the general metabolism is disturbed, fever is produced, and antibodies are formed to counteract the infective products. The rationale of the use of tuberculin is to stimulate the fighting forces of the body—to mobilize them, so to speak—in the fight that is going on in an infected area.

Studies on anaphylaxis or hypersensitiveness to foreign proteins have an important bearing on the question of immunity in tuberculosis. Baldwin of Saranac Lake has demonstrated that sensitization to and subsequent intoxication by tubercle bacillus protein follow the general laws of anaphylaxis established for the parenteral introduction of horse serum. From his experiments we may reasonably interpret the tuberculin reaction as an anaphylactic phenomenon. Undoubtedly hypersensitiveness to the tubercle bacillus protein is directly responsible for the so-called toxic symptoms of tuberculous disease. Koch in his original experiments that led up to the introduction of tuberculin observed a marked difference in the reaction of healthy and tuberculous animals to cutaneous inoculation with tubercle bacilli. In healthy animals the wound closes and for a few days seems to heal, but in from ten to fourteen days a hard nodule appears, which soon breaks down. General infection occurs and the ulcer remains open to the time of the death of the animal. In tuberculous animals extensive ulceration occurs on the second or third day after vaccination, but the ulcer heals quickly and permanently, without even the neighboring lymph glands becoming infected. Roemer extended Koch's observations and demonstrated that tuberculous animals may react in one of three ways to injections of tubercle bacilli: (1) If a small dose be given, a dose, however, surely fatal for healthy animals, infection does not occur.

The animals are therefore highly resistant to re-infection. (2) If a large dose be given, the animals die promptly, with the symptoms of an intense intoxication. The condition is analogous to the anaphylactic shock. (3) If a moderate dose be given, the animals display the symptoms of a profound intoxication, but gradually recover, and, although infection follows, a mild and chronic form of the disease is produced. Upon the same principle depends the protective inoculation of calves, practised by v. Behring and Koch. The animals receive injections of human tubercle bacilli and, although anatomically disease does not follow their introduction, the calves become highly sensitive to tuberculin and at the same time immune to doses of bovine tubercle bacilli fatal to unprotected calves. At the end of a year the tuberculin hypersensitiveness disappears, and the calves again become susceptible to infection. While we are not in a position to state that protection depends upon the same mechanism that produces hypersensitiveness to the tubercle bacillus protein, the two phenomena are undoubtedly closely related.

(*d*) Modes of Infection.—(1) *Hereditary Transmission.*—In order that the disease could be transmitted by the sperm it would be necessary that the tubercle bacilli should lodge in the individual spermatozoön which fecundates an ovum. The chances that such a thing could occur are extremely small, looking at the subject from a numerical point of view, although we know that bacilli do occasionally exist in the semen; they become still smaller when we consider that the spermatozoön is made up of nuclear material, which the tubercle bacillus is never known to attack. The possibility of transmission by the ovum must be accepted. Baumgarten was able in one instance to detect the tubercle bacillus in the ovum of a female rabbit which had been artificially fecundated with tuberculous semen.

The almost constant method of transmission in congenital tuberculosis is through the blood current, the tubercle bacilli penetrating by way of the placenta. In these cases the placenta itself is usually the seat of tuberculosis; but there are undoubted instances in which, with an apparently sound placenta, both the placental blood and the fetal organs contained tubercle bacilli, although the organs appeared normal. The number of cases of congenital tuberculosis in man is very small (about 50); it is more common in cattle.

Latency of the Tubercle Germs.—Baumgarten and his followers assume that the tubercle bacilli, present in the new-born child, lie latent in the tissues and subsequently develop when, for some reason or other, the individual resistance is lowered. He likens such cases of latent tuberculosis to the late congenital forms of syphilis, and explains the lack of development of the germs by the greater resisting power of the tissues of children. The small number of congenital cases is against this view.

(2) *Inoculation.—Cutaneous.*—The infective nature of tuberculosis was first demonstrated by Villemin, who showed in 1865 that it could be transmitted to animals by inoculation. The experiments of Cohnheim and Salomonsen, who produced tuberculosis in the eyes of guinea-pigs and rabbits by inoculating fresh tubercle into the anterior chamber, confirmed and extended Villemin's original observations and paved the way for the reception of Koch's announcement. This mode of infection is seen in persons whose occupation brings them in contact with dead bodies or animal products. Demonstrators of morbid anatomy, butchers, and handlers of hides are subject to a local

tubercle of the skin, which forms a reddened mass of granulation tissue, usually capping the dorsal surface of the hand or a finger. This is the so-called post mortem wart, the *verruca necrogenica* of Wilks. The demonstration of its nature is shown by the presence of tubercle bacilli, and by inoculation experiments in animals.

In the performance of the rite of circumcision children have been accidentally inoculated. Infection in these cases is probably always associated with disease in the operator, and occurs in connection with the habit of cleansing the wound by suction. Other means of inoculation have been described: as the wearing of earrings, washing the clothes of tuberculous patients, the bite of a tuberculous subject, or inoculation from a cut by a broken spit-glass of a consumptive; and Czerny reported two cases of infection by transplantation of skin.

It has been urged by the opponents of vaccination that tuberculosis may be thus conveyed, but of this there is no evidence. Lymph of revaccinated consumptives is non-infective. Lupus has originated at the site of vaccination in a few cases (C. Fox, Graham Little). It may be said that inoculation in man plays a trifling rôle in the transmission of tuberculosis.

Mucous membrane inoculation is probably important in childhood through abrasions of the lips, tongue or gums, though a primary focus is not often seen. The open door in the mouth and throat is more often by loss of the protective epithelium due to catarrhal and ulcerative processes.

(3) *Infection in Childhood.*—The special points favoring this are: (*a*) The intimate contact between children and parents and other adults in households where tuberculosis exists. (*b*) The habit of playing about the floor and putting objects in the mouth. (*c*) The influence of certain infections, such as measles and whooping cough. (*d*) The large place which milk takes in the dietary. (*e*) The close contact with other children in school. The result may be: (*a*) Acute tuberculosis and death. (*b*) An infection of short duration with slight symptoms and recovery. (*c*) A more chronic condition. (*d*) Latency of the disease until adult life, when, as the result of lowered resistance by many factors, the infection becomes active. Present opinion places great stress on the importance of infection by ingestion early in life with the development of the clinical disease many years later. It is exceptional not to find a focus somewhere in the body of a child, no matter what disease caused death.

(4) *Infection by Inhalation.*—A belief in the contagiousness of pulmonary tuberculosis originated with the early Greek physicians, and has persisted among the Latin races. The investigations of Cornet afford conclusive proof that the dust of a room or other locality frequented by patients with pulmonary tuberculosis is infective. The bacilli attached to fine particles of dust are inhaled and gain entrance to the system through the lungs.

Flügge denies that the bacillus-containing dust is the dangerous element in infection. Experimentally he has only succeeded in producing the disease when there is some lesion in the respiratory tract. He thinks that the danger of infection by the dry sputum is very improbable. On the other hand, he thinks that the infection is chiefly conveyed by the free, finely divided particles of sputum produced in the act of coughing, and that these tiny fragments are suspended in the atmosphere. Those who cough very much and with the mouth open are most liable to infect the surrounding air.

It is well remarked by Cornet, "The consumptive in himself is almost harmless, and only becomes harmful through bad habits." It has been fully shown that the expired air of consumptives is not infective. The virus is contained in the sputum, which when dry is widely disseminated in the form of dust, and constitutes the great medium for the transmission of the disease. Among the points urged in favor of the inhalation view are:

(*i*) Primary tuberculous lesions are in a majority of all cases connected with the respiratory system. The frequency with which foci are met with in the lungs and in the bronchial glands is extraordinary, and the statistics of the Paris morgue show that a considerable proportion of all persons dying of accident or by suicide present evidences of the disease in these parts. The post mortem statistics of hospitals show the same widespread prevalence of infection through the air passages. Biggs reports that more than 60 per cent. of his post mortems showed lesions of pulmonary tuberculosis. In 125 autopsies at the Foundling Hospital, New York, the bronchial glands were tuberculous in every case. In adults the bronchial glands may be infected and the individual remain in good health.

(*ii*) The greater prevalence of tuberculosis in institutions in which the residents are confined and restricted in the matter of fresh air and a free open life—conditions which would favor, on the one hand, the presence of the bacilli in the atmosphere, and, on the other, lower the vital resistance of the individual. The investigations of Cornet upon the death-rate from consumption among certain religious orders devoted to nursing give some striking facts in illustration of this. In a review of 38 cloisters, embracing the average number of 4,028 residents, among 2,099 deaths in the course of twenty-five years, 1,320 (62.88 per cent.) were from tuberculosis. In some cloisters more than three-fourths of the deaths are from this disease, and the mortality in all the residents, up to the fortieth year, is greatly above the average, the increase being due entirely to tuberculosis. The more perfect the prophylaxis and hygienic arrangements of an institution, the lower the death-rate from tuberculosis. The mortality in prisons has been shown by Baer to be four times as great as outside. The death-rate from tuberculosis in prisons constitutes from 40 to 50 per cent., and in some countries, as Austria, over 60 per cent. of the total mortality. Flick studied the distribution of the deaths from tuberculosis in a single city ward in Philadelphia for twenty-five years. His researches go far to show that it is a house disease. About 33 per cent. of infected houses have had more than one case. There are, however, opposing facts. The statistics of the Brompton Consumption Hospital show that doctors, nurses, and attendants are rarely attacked. Dettweiler claims that no case of tuberculosis has been contracted among his nurses or attendants at Falkenstein. Among 174 previously healthy sanitarium physicians whose average term of service was three years only two became tuberculous (Sangmann). On the other hand, in the Paris hospitals tuberculosis decimates the attendants.

(*iii*) Special danger was believed to exist when the contact is very intimate, as between man and wife, but upon the figures of the late Ernest Pope, of Saranac, Karl Pearson bases the following conclusions: (*a*) There is some sensible but slight infection between married couples; (*b*) this is largely obscured or forestalled by the fact of infection from outside sources; (*c*) the liability to the infection depends on the presence of the necessary diathesis; (*d*) assortative mating probably accounts for at least two-thirds, and infective action not more than one-third of the whole correlation in these cases. There are cases in which this source of infection seems to play a rôle.

(5) *Infection by Ingestion.*—There are two other channels, the tonsils and the intestines, both of great importance.

(*i*) *Tonsillar Infection.*—The frequency of involvement of these glands has been shown by Schlenker, Arthur Latham, and Walsham. The bacilli pass to the glands of the neck and of the mediastinum, and reach the circulation through the lymph-channels. Or an infected bronchial gland becomes adherent to a branch of the pulmonary artery; if a large number of bacilli escape, miliary tuberculosis follows; if only a small number, they reach the lungs, at the apices of which they find conditions suitable for their growth. Through this tonsillar-cervical route bacilli may gain entrance without causing local disease at the portal of entry. It is a common method of infection in children, causing the "scrofulous" glands of the neck.

(*ii*) *Intestinal Infection.*—Behring announced in 1903 that pulmonary tuberculosis could be induced through intestinal infection, and he further maintained that milk fed to infants was the chief cause of consumption in adults, the infection remaining latent. Behring's first contention was supported by Ravenel and others, who produced pulmonary tuberculosis in animals by feeding experiments, and it was demonstrated that the intestinal surface itself might remain intact. This does away with the objection raised by Koch that, if infection through the milk of tuberculous cattle were common, primary intestinal tuberculosis should be more frequent, whereas in ten years among 3,104 cases of tuberculosis in children there were only 16 of primary bowel infection. Experiments have shown in a striking manner how the lungs act as filters for particles absorbed from the intestines. Vansteenberghe and Grysez produced anthracosis of the lungs by introducing china-ink emulsion directly into the stomach (see Anthracosis). They found a remarkable difference in young and adult guinea-pigs; in the former the carbon particles were filtered out by the mesenteric glands, while the lungs remained free; in the latter the glands were unaffected, but the lungs were carbonized. Calmette and Guérin have shown how easily the lungs may be infected through the intestinal route without leaving the slightest trace of disease of the bowel itself. Behring's view of the importance of infection through the intestinal route has thus received the strongest support, and many go so far as to maintain that a majority of all cases of tuberculosis originate in this manner. The truth is that this ubiquitous bacillus is not particular, and gains entrance through either portal, preferring the throat and intestines in childhood, the bronchi and lungs in adults. The important matter for the individual is the nature of the soil on which it falls.

Milk alone is a common source of intestinal infection, particularly in the large cities. In New York, Hess found tubercle bacilli in 16 per cent. of 107 specimens! The ordinary commercial pasteurization does not kill them.

The flesh of tuberculous animals is rarely dangerous.

(6) *Re-infection.*—This is a possibility in adult life but its frequency is difficult to state.

General Morbid Anatomy and Histology of Tuberculous Lesions.—(*a*) DISTRIBUTION OF THE TUBERCLES IN THE BODY.—The primary localization of the tubercle bacillus in the vast majority of cases, if not in all, is in the lymphatic structures; involvement of the lungs is secondary. Clinically in adults, the lungs may be regarded as the seat of election; in children, the lymph-nodes, bones, and joints. In 1,000 autopsies there were 275 cases with tuberculous lesions. With but two or three exceptions the lungs were affected. The distribution in the other organs was as follows: Pericardium, 7; peritoneum, 36; brain, 31; spleen, 23; liver, 12; kidneys, 32; intestines, 65; heart, 4; and generative organs, 8.

Among 8,873 surgical patients at the Würzburg clinic, 1,287 were tuberculous, with the following distribution of lesions: Bones and joints, 1,037; lymph-nodes, 196; skin and connective tissues, 77; mucous membranes, 10; genito-urinary organs, 20.

(*b*) THE CHANGES PRODUCED BY THE TUBERCLE BACILLI.—*The Nodular Tubercle.*—A "tubercle" *presents in its early formation nothing distinctive or peculiar, either in its components or in their arrangement.* Identical structures are produced by other parasites, such as the actinomyces, and by the strongylus in the lungs of sheep.

The following changes occur in the evolution of a tubercle:

(1) The tubercle bacilli multiply and disseminate in the surrounding tissues, partly by growth, partly in the lymph currents.

(2) The fixed cells, especially those of connective tissue and the endothelium of the capillaries, multiply and form rounded, cuboidal, or polygonal bodies with vesicular nuclei—the *epithelioid cells*—inside some of which the bacilli are soon seen.

(3) Leucocytes, chiefly polynuclear, migrate in numbers and accumulate about the focus of infection. They do not survive. Many undergo rapid destruction. Later, as the little tubercle grows, the leucocytes are chiefly of the mononuclear variety (lymphocytes), which do not undergo the rapid degeneration of the polynuclear forms.

(4) A reticulum of fibres is formed by the fibrillation and rarefaction of the connective-tissue matrix. This is most apparent, as a rule, at the margin of the growth.

(5) In some, but not all, tubercles *giant cells* are formed by an increase in the protoplasm and in the nuclei of an individual cell, or possibly by the fusion of several cells. The giant cells seem to be in inverse ratio to the number and virulence of the bacilli.

(*c*) THE DEGENERATION OF TUBERCLE.—(1) *Caseation.*—At the central part of the growth, owing to the direct action of the bacilli or their products, a process of coagulation necrosis goes on in the cells, which lose their outline, become irregular, no longer take stains, and are finally converted into a homogeneous, structureless substance. This may be due to the blood supply being cut off or to the toxins of the tubercle bacillus. Proceeding from the centre outward, the tubercle may be gradually converted into a yellowish-gray body, in which the bacilli are still abundant. No blood vessels are found in them.

Aggregated together these form cheesy masses which may undergo softening, fibroid limitation (encapsulation), or calcification.

(2) *Sclerosis.*—With the necrosis of the cell elements at the centre of the tubercle, hyaline transformation proceeds, together with great increase in the fibroid elements; so that the tubercle is converted into a firm, hard structure. Often the change is rather of a fibro-caseous nature; but the sclerosis predominates. In some situations, as in the peritoneum, this seems to be the natural transformation and it is by no means rare in the lungs.

In all tubercles two processes go on: the one—caseation—destructive and dangerous; and the other—sclerosis—conservative and healing. The ultimate result in a given case depends upon the capabilities of the body to fight the invaders. There are tissue-soils in which the bacilli are, in all probability, killed at once. There are others in which a lodgment is gained and more or less damage done, but finally the day is with the protecting forces. Thirdly, there are tissue-soils in which the bacilli grow luxuriantly, caseation and softening, not limitation and sclerosis, prevail, and the day is with the invaders.

The action of the bacilli injected directly into the blood-vessels illustrates many points in the histology and pathology of tuberculosis. If into the vein of a rabbit a pure culture of the bacilli is injected, the microbes accumulate chiefly in the liver and spleen. The animal dies usually within two weeks, and the organs apparently show no trace of tubercles. Microscopically, in both spleen and liver the young tubercles in process of formation are very numerous, and karyokinesis is going on in the liver-cells. After an injection of a more dilute culture, or one of less virulence, instead of dying within a fortnight the animal survives for five or six weeks, by which time the tubercles are apparent in the spleen and liver, and often in the other organs.

(d) THE DIFFUSED INFLAMMATORY TUBERCLE.—This is most frequently seen in the lungs and results from the fusion of many small foci of infection —so small indeed that they may not be visible to the naked eye, but which histologically are seen to be composed of scattered centres, surrounded by areas in which the air-cells are filled with the products of exudation and of the proliferation of the alveolar epithelium. Under the influence of the bacilli, caseation takes place, usually in small groups of lobules, occasionally in an entire lobe, or even the greater part of a lung. In the early stage of the process, the tissue has a gray gelatinous appearance, the *gray infiltration* of Laennec. The alveoli contain a sero-fibrinous fluid with cells, and the septa are also infiltrated. These cells accumulate and undergo coagulation necrosis, forming areas of caseation, the *infiltration tuberculeuse jaune* of Laennec, the scrofulous or cheesy pneumonia of later writers. There may also be a diffuse infiltration and caseation without any special foci, a widespread tuberculous pneumonia induced by the bacilli.

After all, the two processes are identical. As Baumgarten states: "There is no well-marked difference between miliary tubercle and chronic ceaseous pneumonia. Speaking histologically, miliary tuberculosis is nothing else than a chronic caseous miliary pneumonia, and chronic caseous pneumonia is nothing but a tuberculosis of the lungs."

(*e*) SECONDARY INFLAMMATORY PROCESSES.—(1) The irritation caused by the bacilli produces an inflammation which may, as has been described, be limited to exudation of leucocytes and serum, but may also be much more extensive, and vary with changing conditions. We find, for example, about the smaller tubercles in the lungs, pneumonia—either catarrhal or fibrinous—proliferation of the connective-tissue elements in the septa (which also become infiltrated with round cells), and changes in the blood and lymph-vessels.

(2) In processes of minor intensity the inflammation is of the slow reactive nature, which results in the production of a cicatricial connective tissue which limits and restricts the development of the tubercles and is the essential conservative element in the disease. It is to be remembered that in chronic pulmonary tuberculosis much of the fibroid tissue which is present is not in any way associated with the action of the bacilli.

(3) Suppuration. Do the bacilli themselves induce suppuration? In so-called cold tuberculous abscess the material is not histologically pus, but a *débris* consisting of broken-down cells and cheesy material. It is moreover sterile—that is, does not contain the usual pus organisms. The products of the tubercle bacilli are probably able to induce suppuration, as in joint and bone tuberculosis pus is frequently produced, although this may be due to a mixed infection. Tuberculin is one of the best agents for the production of experimental suppuration. In tuberculosis of the lungs the suppuration is largely the result of an infection with pus organisms.

II. ACUTE MILIARY TUBERCULOSIS

The modern knowledge of this remarkable form dates from the statement of Buhl (1856), that miliary tuberculosis is a specific infection dependent on the presence in the body of an unencapsulated yellow tubercle, or a tuberculous cavity in the lung; and that it bears the same relation to the primary lesion as pyæmia does to a focus of suppuration.

Carl Weigert established the truth of this brilliant conception by demonstrating the association of miliary tuberculosis with tuberculosis of the blood-vessels. There are two groups of vessel tubercle—the tuberculous periangitis in which there is invasion of the adventitia, and the endangitis in which the tubercles start in the intima. The parts most frequently affected are the pulmonary veins and the thoracic duct, less often the jugular vein, the suprarenal and the vena cava superior, and the sinuses of the dura mater, the aorta, and the endocardium. To the branches of the pulmonary veins it is not uncommon to find caseous glands adherent, penetrating the walls and showing a growth of miliary tubercles in the intima. A special interest belongs to tuberculosis of the thoracic duct, first accurately described by Sir Astley Cooper. Benda in a series of 19 cases of vessel tuberculosis found in many instances an enormous number of bacilli, particularly in the ceasous tubercles of the thoracic duct.

The bacilli do not increase in the blood, but settle in the different organs, producing a generalized tuberculosis, of which Weigert recognized three types or grades: I. The acute general miliary tuberculosis, in which the various organs of the body are stuffed with miliary and submiliary nodules. II. A second form characterized by a small number of tubercles in one or many organs. III. The occurrence of numerous tuberculous foci widely spread throughout the body, but in a more chronic form; the tubercles are larger and many are caseous. It is the chronic generalized tuberculosis of children.

Transitional forms between these groups occur. In the first variety, which we are here considering, there is an eruption into the circulation of an enormous number of bacilli. Benda suggests in explanation of the profound toxæmia seen in certain cases (the typhoid form) that in addition the blood is surcharged with toxins from a large caseous focus which has eroded the vessel.

Clinical Forms

The cases may be grouped into those with the symptoms of an *acute general infection*—the typhoid form; cases in which pulmonary symptoms predominate; and cases in which the *cerebral* or *cerebro-spinal* symptoms are marked—tuberculous meningitis. Other forms have been recognized, but this division covers a large majority of the cases. Taking any series of cases it will be found that the meningeal form of acute tuberculosis exceeds in numbers the cases with general or marked pulmonary symptoms.

General or Typhoid Form.—SYMPTOMS.—The patient presents the symptoms of a profound infection which simulates and is frequently mistaken for typhoid fever. After a period of failing health, with loss of appetite, he becomes feverish and weak. Occasionally the disease sets in more abruptly, but in many instances the anamnesis closely resembles that of typhoid fever. Nose-bleeding, however, is rare. The temperature increases, the pulse becomes rapid and feeble, the tongue dry; delirium becomes marked and the cheeks are flushed. The pulmonary symptoms may be very slight; usually bronchitis exists, but is not more severe than is common with typhoid fever. The pulse is seldom dicrotic, but is rapid in proportion to the pyrexia. Perhaps the most striking feature of the temperature is the irregularity; and if seen from the outset there is not the steady ascent noted in typhoid fever. There is usually an evening rise to 103° F., sometimes 104° F., and a morning remission of from two to three degrees. Sometimes the pyrexia is intermittent, and the thermometer may register below normal during the early morning hours. The inverse type of temperature, in which the rise takes place in the morning, is held by some writers to be more frequent in general tuberculosis than in other diseases. In rare instances there may be little or no fever. On three occasions we have had a patient admitted in a condition of profound debility, with a history of illness of from three to four weeks' duration, with rapid pulse, flushed cheeks, dry tongue, and very slight elevation in temperature, in whom (post mortem) the condition proved to be general tuberculosis. Reinhold, from Bäumler's clinic, called attention to these afebrile forms of acute tuberculosis. In 9 of 52 cases there was no fever, or only a transient rise.

In a considerable number of the cases the respirations are increased in frequency, particularly in the early stage, and there may be signs of diffuse bronchitis and slight cyanosis. Cheyne-Stokes breathing occurs toward the close. Active delirium is rare. More commonly there are torpor and dullness, gradually deepening into coma, in which the patient dies. In some cases the pulmonary symptoms become more marked; in others meningeal or cerebral features occur.

DIAGNOSIS.—The differential diagnosis between general miliary tuberculosis without local manifestations and typhoid fever is extremely difficult. A point of importance is the irregularity of the temperature curve. The greater frequency of the respirations and the tendency to slight cyanosis are much more common in tuberculosis. There are cases, however, of typhoid fever in which the initial bronchitis is severe and may lead to dyspnœa and disturbed oxygenation. The cough may be slight or absent. Diarrhœa is rare in tuberculosis; the bowels are usually constipated; but diarrhœa may occur and persist for days. In certain cases the diagnosis has been complicated still further by the occurrence of blood in the stools. Enlargement of the spleen occurs in general tuberculosis, but is neither so early nor so marked as in typhoid fever. In children, however, the enlargement may be considerable. The urine may show traces of albumin and contains tubercle bacilli in a considerable number of cases. The absence of the characteristic roseola is an important feature. Occasionally in acute tuberculosis reddish spots may occur and for a time cause difficulty, but they do not come out in crops, and rarely have the characters of the true typhoid eruption. Herpes is perhaps more common in tuberculosis. Toward the close, petechiæ may appear on the skin, particularly about the wrists. A rare event is jaundice, due possibly to the eruption of tubercles in the liver. It is to be remembered that the lesions of acute tuberculosis and of typhoid fever have been demonstrated in the same body.

A negative Widal test and the absence of typhoid bacilli in blood-cultures may be of decisive importance in these doubtful cases. In rare instances tubercle bacilli have been found in the blood. Leucocytosis is more common in miliary tuberculosis than in typhoid fever, in which leucopenia is the rule. Careful examination of the eyes may show choroidal tubercles, though we have never known a diagnosis made on their presence alone. In the fluid obtained by lumbar puncture the tubercle bacilli may be abundant, even when there is no active meningitis.

Pulmonary Form.—Symptoms.—From the outset the pulmonary symptoms are marked. The patient may have had a cough for months or for years without much impairment of health, or he may be known to be the subject of chronic pulmonary tuberculosis. In other instances, particularly in children, the affection follows measles or whooping cough, and is of a distinctly broncho-pneumonic type. The disease begins with the symptoms of diffuse bronchitis. The cough is marked, the expectoration muco-purulent, occasionally rusty. Hæmoptysis has been noted in a few instances. From the outset dyspnœa is a striking feature and may be out of proportion to the intensity of the physical signs. There is more or less cyanosis of the lips and finger-tips, and the cheeks are suffused. Apart from emphysema and the later stages of severe pneumonia, there is no other pulmonary condition in which the cyanosis is so marked. The physical signs are those of bronchitis. In children there may be defective resonance at the bases, from scattered areas of broncho-pneumonia; or, what is equally suggestive, areas of hyper-resonance. Indeed, the percussion note, particularly in the front of the chest, in some cases of miliary tuberculosis, is full and clear, and it will be noted (post mortem) that the lungs are unusually voluminous. This is probably the result of more or less widespread acute emphysema. On auscultation, the râles are either sibilant and sonorous or small, fine, and crepitant. There may be fine crepitation from the occurrence of tubercles on the pleura (Jürgensen). In children there may be high-pitched tubular breathing at the bases or toward the root of the lung. Toward the close the râles may be larger and more mucous. The temperature rises to 102° or 103° F., and may present the inverse type. The pulse is rapid and feeble. In the very acute cases the spleen is always enlarged. The disease may prove fatal in ten or twelve days, or may be protracted for weeks or even months.

Diagnosis.—The diagnosis of this form offers less difficulty and is more frequently made. There is often a history of previous cough, or the patient is known to be the subject of local disease of the lung, of the lymph glands, or of the bones. In children these symptoms following measles or whooping cough indicate in the majority of cases acute miliary tuberculosis, with or without broncho-pneumonia. Occasionally the sputum contains tubercle bacilli.

The choroidal tubercle occurs in a limited number of cases and may help the diagnosis. More important in an adult is the combination of dyspnœa with cyanosis and the signs of a diffuse bronchitis. In some instances the occurrence of cerebral symptoms at once gives a clew to the diagnosis.

Meningeal Form (*Tuberculous Meningitis*).—This affection, also known as acute hydrocephalus or "water on the brain," is essentially an acute tuberculosis in which the membranes of the brain, sometimes of the cord, bear the brunt of the attack. Our first accurate knowledge of it dates from the publication of Robert Whytt's Observations on the Dropsy of the Brain, Edinburgh, 1768. He studied 20 cases and divided the disease into three stages, according to the condition of the pulse.

Though Guersant had as early as 1827 used the name *granular meningitis* for this form of inflammation of the meninges, it was not until 1830 that Papavoine demonstrated the nature of the granules and noted their occurrence with tubercles in other parts. In 1832 and 1833, W. W. Gerhard, of Philadelphia, made a very careful study of the disease in the Children's Hospital at Paris, and his publications, more than those of any other author, served to place the disease on a firm anatomical and clinical basis.

There are several special *etiological* factors in connection with this form. It is much more common in children than in adults. It occurs during the first year of life, but is more frequent between the second and the fifth years. In a majority of the cases a focus of old tuberculous disease will be found, commonly in the bronchial or mesenteric glands. In a few instances the affection seems to be primary in the meninges. It is very difficult, however, in an ordinary post mortem to make an exhaustive search, and the lesion may be in the bones, sometimes in the middle ear, or in the genito-urinary organs. In cases in which no primary focus has been discovered it has been suggested that the bacilli reach the meninges through the cribriform plate of the ethmoid from the upper part of the nostrils, but this is not probable.

Morbid Anatomy.—The meninges at the base are most involved, hence the term basilar meningitis. The parts about the optic chiasm, the Sylvian fissures, and the interpeduncular space are affected. There may be only slight turbidity and matting of the membranes, and a certain stickiness with serous infiltration; but more commonly there is a turbid exudate, fibrino-purulent in character, which covers the structures at the base, surrounds the nerves, extends into the Sylvian fissures, and appears on the lateral, rarely on the upper, surfaces of the hemispheres. The tubercles may be very apparent, particularly in the Sylvian fissures, appearing as small, whitish nodules on the membranes. They vary much in number and size, and may be difficult to find. The amount of exudate bears no definite relation to the abundance of tubercles. The arteries of the anterior and posterior perforated spaces should be carefully withdrawn and searched, as upon them nodular tubercles may be found when not present elsewhere. In doubtful cases the middle cerebral arteries should be very carefully removed, spread on a glass plate with a black background, and examined with a lens. The tubercles are then seen as nodular enlargements on the smaller arteries. The lateral ventricles are dilated (acute hydrocephalus) and contain a turbid fluid; the ependyma may be softened, and the septum lucidum and fornix are usually broken down. The convolutions are often flattened and the sulci obliterated owing to the increased intra-ventricular pressure. The meninges are not alone involved, but the contiguous cerebral substance is more or less œdematous and infiltrated with leucocytes, so that anatomically the condition is in reality a *meningo-encephalitis.*

There are instances in which the acute process is associated with chronic meningeal tuberculosis; cases which may for months present the clinical picture of brain tumor. Although in a majority of instances the process is cerebral, the spinal meninges may also be involved, particularly those of the cervical cord. There are cases, indeed, in which the symptoms are chiefly spinal.

SYMPTOMS.—Tuberculous meningitis presents an extremely complex clinical picture. It will be best to describe the form found in children.

Prodromal symptoms are common. The child may have been in failing health for some weeks, or may be convalescent from measles or whooping cough. In many instances there is a history of a fall. The child gets thin, is restless, peevish, irritable, loses its appetite, and the disposition may completely change. Symptoms pointing to the disease may then set in, either quite suddenly with a convulsion, or more commonly with headache, vomiting, and fever, three essential symptoms of the onset which are rarely absent. The pain may be intense and agonizing. The child puts its hand to its head and occasionally, when the pain becomes worse, gives a short, sudden cry, the so-called hydrocephalic cry. Sometimes the child screams continuously until utterly exhausted. The vomiting is without apparent cause, and is independent of taking of food. Constipation is usually present. The fever is slight, but gradually rises to 102° to 103° F. The pulse is at first rapid, subsequently irregular and slow. The respirations are rarely altered. During sleep the child is restless and disturbed. There may be twitchings of the muscles, or sudden startings; or the child may wake up from sleep in great terror. In this early stage the pupils are usually contracted. These are the chief symptoms of the initial stage, or, as it is termed, the *stage of irritation.*

In the second period of the disease these irritative symptoms subside; vomiting is no longer marked, the abdomen becomes retracted, boat-shaped, or *carinated.* The bowels are obstinately constipated; the child no longer complains of headache, but is dull and apathetic, and when roused is more or less delirious. The head is often retracted and the child utters an occasional cry. The pupils are dilated or irregular, and a squint may develop. Sighing respiration is common. Convulsions may occur, or rigidity of the muscles of one side or of one limb. The temperature is variable, ranging from 100° to

102.5° F. A blotchy erythema is not uncommon on the skin. If the finger-nail is drawn across the skin of any region a red line comes out quickly, the so-called *tache cérébrale,* which, however, has no diagnostic significance.

In the final period, or stage of *paralysis,* the coma increases and the child can not be roused. Convulsions are not infrequent, and there are spasmodic contractions of the muscles of the back and neck. Spasms may occur in the limbs of one side. Optic neuritis and paralysis of the ocular muscles may be present. The pupils become dilated, the eyelids are only partially closed, and the eyeballs are rolled up so that the corneæ are only uncovered in part by the upper eyelids. Diarrhœa may occur, the pulse becomes rapid, and the child may sink into a typhoid state with dry tongue, low delirium, and involuntary passages of urine and fæces. The temperature often becomes subnormal, sinking in rare instances to 93° or 94° F. In some cases there is an ante-mortem elevation of temperature, the fever rising to 106° F. The entire duration of the disease is from a fortnight to several weeks. A leucocytosis is not infrequently present throughout the disease.

There are cases of tuberculous meningitis which pursue a more rapid course. They set in with great violence, often in persons apparently in good health, and may prove fatal within a few days. In these instances, more commonly seen in adults, the convex surface of the brain is usually involved. There are again instances which are essentially chronic and display symptoms of a limited meningitis, sometimes with pronounced psychical symptoms, and sometimes with those of cerebral tumor. The symptoms may vary from time to time; some are probably due to toxæmia rather than to the local lesion.

There are certain features which call for special comment.

The irregularity and slowness of the pulse in the early and middle stages of the disease are points upon which all authors agree. Toward the close, as the heart's action becomes weaker, the pulsations are more frequent. The temperature is usually elevated, but there are instances in which it does not rise in the whole course of the disease much above 100° F. It may be extremely irregular, and the oscillations are often as much as three or four degrees in the day. Toward the close the temperature may sink to 95° F., occasionally to 94° F., or there may be hyperpyrexia. In a case of Bäumler's the temperature rose before death to 43.7° C. (110.7° F.).

The *ocular* symptoms are of special importance. In the early stages narrowing of the pupils is the rule. Toward the close, with increase in the intra-cranial pressure, the pupils dilate and are irregular. There may be conjugate deviation of the eyes. Of ocular nerves the third is most frequently involved, sometimes with paralysis of the face, limbs, and hypoglossal nerve on the opposite side (syndrome of Weber), due to a lesion limited to the inferior and internal part of the crus. The changes in the retinæ are very important. Neuritis is the most common. According to Gowers, the disk at first becomes full colored and has hazy outlines, and the veins are dilated. Swelling and striation become pronounced, but the neuritis is rarely intense. Of 26 cases studied by Garlick, in 6 the condition was of diagnostic value. The tubercles in the choroid are rare and much less frequently seen during life than post mortem figures would indicate. Thus, Litten found them (post mortem) in 39 out of 52 cases. They were present in only 1 of the 26 cases of tuberculous meningitis examined by Garlick. Heinzel examined 41 cases with negative results.

Among the *motor* symptoms convulsions are most common, but there are other changes which deserve special mention. A tetanic contraction of one limb may persist for several days, or a cataleptic condition. Tremor and athetoid movements are sometimes seen. The paralyses are either hemiplegias or monoplegias. Hemiplegia may result from disturbance in the cortical branches of the middle cerebral artery, occasionally from softening in the internal capsule, due to involvement of the central branches. Of monoplegias, that of the face is perhaps most common, and if on the right side it may occur with aphasia. In two of our cases in adults aphasia occurred. Brachial monoplegia may be associated with it. In the more chronic cases the symptoms persist for months, and there may be a characteristic Jacksonian epilepsy. Kernig's sign may be present, but is not constant. The Babinski reflex is sometimes found.

The DIAGNOSIS of tuberculous meningitis is rarely difficult, and points upon which special stress is to be laid are the existence of a tuberculous focus in the body, the mode of onset and the symptoms, and the evidence obtained on lumbar puncture. The cerebro-spinal fluid is usually clear or slightly turbid, and after standing for 12 to 24 hours, a feathery clot of fibrin forms down the centre of the fluid, the presence of which indicates that it is not normal. In this clot the tubercle bacilli are usually found. By centrifugalization, careful staining, and long search, tubercle bacilli can be found in a large proportion of cases—in 135 of 137 in one series (Hemenway). The cells are usually much increased in number and a large percentage (over 90 per cent.) are small lymphocytes, though occasionally an excess of polymorphonuclear leucocytes is found.

The PROGNOSIS in this form of meningitis is always most serious. We have neither seen a case proved to be tuberculous recover, nor post mortem evidence of past disease of this nature. Cases of recovery have been reported by reliable authorities, but they are extremely rare. Pitfield collected 29 undoubted cases in 1913.

TREATMENT.—In a disease which is practically always fatal this does not offer much. The patients should be nourished as well as possible and given sedatives to control restlessness or pain. In the meningeal form, lumbar puncture should be done and repeated if it relieves the symptoms.

III. TUBERCULOSIS OF THE LYMPHATIC SYSTEM

1. *Tuberculosis of the Lymph-glands* (*Scrofula*)

Scrofula is tubercle, as it has been shown that the bacillus of Koch is the essential element. It is not definitely settled whether the organism which produces the chronic tuberculous adenitis differs from that which produces tuberculosis in other parts, or whether it is the local conditions in the glands which account for the slow development and milder course. The observations of Lingard are important as showing a variation in the virulence of the tubercle bacillus. Guinea-pigs inoculated with ordinary tubercle showed lymphatic infection within the first week and died within three months; infected with material from tuberculous glands, the lymphatic enlargement did not appear until the second or third week, and the animals survived for six or seven months. In 68 cases examined by A. S. Griffith, in 35 human and in 33 bovine, infection was found. The proportion is higher in children under five, but of 17 cases twenty years old and upwards 4 were bovine. The cases of bovine infection in cervical gland tuberculosis in different countries analysed by Griffith show that the proportion is lowest in Germany and highest in Scotland.

Tuberculous *adenitis*, met with at all ages, is more common in children than in adults, and may occur in old age.

Tubercle bacilli are ubiquitous; all are exposed to infection, and upon the local conditions, whether favorable or unfavorable, depends the fate of those organisms which find lodgment in our bodies. A special predisposing factor in lymphatic tuberculosis is catarrh of the mucous membranes, which in itself excites slight adenitis of the neighboring glands. In a child with constantly recurring naso-pharyngeal catarrh, the bacilli which lodge on the mucous membranes find in all probability the gateways less strictly guarded and are taken up by the lymphatics and passed to the nearest glands. The importance of the *tonsils* as an infection-atrium has been urged. In conditions of health the local resistance is active enough to deal with the invaders, but the irritation of a chronic catarrh weakens the resistance of the lymph-tissue, and the bacilli are enabled to grow and gradually to change a simple into a tuberculous adenitis. The frequent association of tuberculous adenitis of the bronchial glands with whooping cough and measles, and the association of tubercle in the mesenteric glands in children with intestinal catarrh, find in this way a rational explanation.

The following are some of the features of interest in tuberculous adenitis:

(*a*) The local character. Thus, the glands of the neck, or at the bifurcation of the bronchi, or those of the mesentery, may be alone involved.

(*b*) The tendency to spontaneous healing. In a large proportion of the cases the battle which ensues between the bacilli and the protective forces is long; but the latter are finally successful, and we find in the calcified remnants in the bronchial and mesenteric lymph-glands evidences of victory. Too often in the bronchial glands a truce only is declared and hostilities may break out afresh in the form of an acute tuberculosis.

(*c*) The tendency of tuberculous adenitis to pass on to suppuration. The frequency with which, particularly in the glands of the neck, we find the tuberculous processes associated with suppuration is a special feature of this form of adenitis. In nearly all instances the pus is sterile. Whether the suppuration is excited by the bacilli or by their products, or whether it is the result of a mixed infection with pus organisms, which are subsequently destroyed, has not been settled.

(*d*) The existence of an unhealed tuberculous adenitis is a constant menace to the organism. It is safe to say that in three-fourths of the instances of acute tuberculosis the infection is derived from this source. On the other hand, it has been urged that tuberculous adenitis in childhood gives immunity in adult life. There is evidence in favor of this. Only a small number of adults with pulmonary tuberculosis show scars from adenitis—3.2 per cent. of one series of 2,000 patients. Certain autopsy studies suggest that in the bodies of adults with mesenteric gland tuberculosis, pulmonary tuberculosis is less frequent.

Generalized Tuberculous Lymphadenitis.—In exceptional instances we find diffuse tuberculosis of nearly all the lymph-glands of the body with little or no involvement of other parts. The most extreme cases of it, which we have seen, have been in negro patients. Two well-marked cases occurred at the Philadelphia Hospital. In a woman, the chart from April, 1888, until March, 1889, showed persistent fever, ranging from 101° to 103° F., occasionally rising to 104° F. On December 16th the glands on the right side of the neck were removed. After an attack of erysipelas, on February 17th, she gradually sank and died March 5th. The lungs presented only one or two puckered spots at the apices. The bronchial, retro-peritoneal, and mesenteric glands were greatly enlarged and caseous. There was no intestinal, uterine, or bone disease. The continuous high fever in this case depended apparently upon the tuberculous adenitis. In these instances the enlargement is most marked in the retro-peritoneal, bronchial, and mesenteric glands, but may be also present in the groups of external glands. Occurring acutely, it presents a picture resembling Hodgkin's disease. In a case which died in the Montreal General Hospital this diagnosis was made. The cervical and axillary glands were enormously enlarged, and death was caused by infiltration of the larynx. In infants and children there is a form of general tuberculous adenitis in which the various groups of glands are successively, more rarely simultaneously, involved, and in which death is caused either by cachexia or by an acute infection of the meninges.

Local Tuberculous Adenitis.—(*a*) CERVICAL.—This is the most common form in children. It is seen particularly among the poor and those who live in the impure atmosphere of badly ventilated lodgings. Children in foundling hospitals and asylums are specially prone to the disease. In the United States it is most common in the negro race. It is often met with in catarrh of the nose and throat, or chronic enlargement of the tonsils; or the child may have had eczema of the scalp or a purulent otitis.

The submaxillary glands are first involved, and are popularly spoken of as enlarged *kernels.* They are usually larger on one side than on the other. As they increase in size, the individual tumors can be felt; the surface is smooth and the consistence firm. They may remain isolated, but more commonly they form large, knotted masses, over which the skin is, as a rule, freely movable. In many cases the skin ultimately becomes adherent, and inflammation and suppuration occur. An abscess points and, unless opened, bursts, leaving a sinus which heals slowly. The disease is frequently associated with coryza, with eczema of the scalp, ear, or lips, and with conjunctivitis or keratitis. When the glands are large and growing actively there is fever. The subjects are usually anæmic, particularly if suppuration has occurred. The progress of this form of adenitis is slow and tedious. Death, however, rarely follows, and many aggravated cases in children get well. Not only the submaxillary group, but the glands above the clavicle and in the posterior cervical triangle, may be involved. In other instances the cervical and axillary glands are involved together, forming a continuous chain which extends beneath the clavicle and the pectoral muscle. With them the bronchial glands may also be enlarged and caseous. Not infrequently the enlargement of the supra-clavicular and axillary group of glands on one side precedes a tuberculous pleurisy or pulmonary tuberculosis.

(*b*) Tracheo-bronchial.—The mediastinal lymph-glands constitute filters in which lodge the various foreign particles which escape the normal phagocytes of bronchi and lungs. Among these foreign particles, and probably attached to them, tubercle bacilli are not uncommon, and we find tubercles and caseous matter with great frequency in this group. Northrup found them involved in every one of 125 cases of tuberculosis at the New York Foundling Hospital. This tuberculous adenitis may, in the bronchial glands, attain the dimensions of a tumor of large size. In children the bronchial adenitis is apt to be associated with suppuration. The glands at the bifurcation of the trachea are first involved and chiefly on the right side—in 74 per cent. of Wollstein's cases. Irregular fever, failure of nutrition, loss of appetite, and lassitude may be caused by the absorption of toxins; pain is rare, though it is complained of sometimes in the mammary region. The cough is paroxysmal, often brassy, so that it has been mistaken for whooping cough. Stridor, when present, is more often expiratory. The physical signs are not very definite. Dilated veins over the anterior aspect of the thorax, absence of descent of the larynx during inspiration, and pain on pressure over the upper dorsal vertebræ are mentioned. Extension of the normal dulness over the upper four thoracic vertebræ to the fifth and sixth is of importance, and there may be para-vertebral dulness on delicate percussion. Some writers lay stress upon the whispered bronchophony over the upper thoracic vertebræ, and a venous hum may be heard sometimes over the manubrium. The X-ray pictures are regarded by experts as distinctive, showing the shadow extending from either side of the spine.

Some of the more uncommon effects are the following: Compression of the superior cava, of the pulmonary artery, and of the azygos vein. The trachea and bronchi, though often flattened, are rarely seriously compressed. The vagus nerve may be involved, particularly the recurrent laryngeal branch. More important are the perforations of the enlarged and softened glands into the bronchi or trachea, or a sort of secondary cyst may be formed between the lung and the trachea. Asphyxia has been caused by blocking of the larynx by a caseous gland which has ulcerated through the bronchus (Voelcker), and Cyril Ogle reported a case in which the ulcerated gland practically occluded both bronchi. Perforations of the vessels are much less common, but the pulmonary artery and the aorta have been opened. Perforation of the œsophagus has been described. One of the most serious effects is infection of the lung or pleura by the caseous glands situated deep along the bronchi. This may, as is often clearly seen, be by direct contact, and it may be difficult to determine in some sections where the caseous bronchial gland terminates and the pulmonary tissue begins. In other instances it takes place along the root of the lung and is subpleural. Among other sequences may be mentioned diverticulum of the œsophagus following adhesion of an enlarged gland and its subsequent retraction; and, in the case of the anterior mediastinal and aortic groups, the frequent production of pericarditis, either by contact or by rupture of a softened gland into the sac. A serious danger is systemic infection, which takes place through the vessels.

(*c*) Mesenteric; Tabes mesenterica.—In this affection, the abdominal scrofula of old writers, the glands of the mesentery and retro-peritoneum become enlarged and caseate; more rarely they suppurate or calcify. A slight tuberculous adenitis is extremely common in children, and is often accidentally found (post mortem) when they have died of other diseases. It may be a primary lesion associated with intestinal catarrh, or it may be secondary to tuberculous disease of the intestines.

The statistics of abdominal tuberculosis show a great variation in different localities. The small percentage in New York, less than one per cent. of all cases (Bovaird and Mt. Sinai Hospital figures), contrasts with the high figures given for Scotland by John Thomson, 3.57 for Edinburgh and 4.51 for Glasgow. "Scotland enjoys the unenviable distinction of having more abdominal tuberculosis than any other civilized country—twice as much at least as England generally, and more than ten times as much as Europe and North America. It accounts for one-half of the medical tuberculosis admissions." The general involvement of the glands interferes seriously with nutrition, and the patients are puny, wasted, and anæmic. The abdomen is enlarged and tympanitic; diarrhœa is a constant feature; the stools are thin and offensive. There is moderate fever, but the general wasting and debility are the most characteristic features. The enlarged glands can not often be felt, owing to the distended condition of the bowels. These cases are often spoken of as "consumption of the bowels," but in a majority of them the intestines do not present tuberculous lesions. In a considerable number of the cases of tabes mesenterica the peritoneum is also involved, and in such the abdomen is large and hard, and nodules may be felt.

In adults tuberculous disease of the mesenteric glands may occur as a primary affection, or in association with pulmonary disease. It may exist without tuberculous disease in the intestines or in any other part. The tumor mass is usually a little to the right of the umbilicus, freely movable. The general symptoms are loss of weight and slight fever; locally there is pain, sometimes diarrhœa, and appendicitis is often suspected.

2. *Tuberculosis of the Serous Membranes*

General Serous Membrane Tuberculosis (*Polyorrhomenitis*).—The serous membranes may be chiefly involved, simultaneously or consecutively, presenting a distinctive and readily recognizable clinical type of tuberculosis. There are three groups of cases. First, those in which an acute tuberculosis of the peritoneum and pleuræ occurs rapidly, caused by local disease of the tubes in women, or of the mediastinal or bronchial lymph-glands. Secondly, cases in which the disease is more chronic, with exudation into both peritoneum and pleuræ, the formation of cheesy masses, and the occurrence of ulcerative and suppurative processes. Thirdly, there are cases in which the pleuro-peritoneal affection is still more chronic, the tubercles hard and fibroid, the membranes much thickened, and with little or no exudate. In any one of these three forms the pericardium may be involved with the pleuræ and peritoneum. It is important to bear in mind that there may be no visceral tuberculosis in these cases.

Tuberculosis of the Pleura.—(*a*) ACUTE TUBERCULOUS PLEURISY.—It is difficult to estimate the proportion of instances of acute pleurisy due to tuberculosis (see Acute Pleurisy). The cases are rarely fatal. There are three groups of cases: (1) Acute tuberculous pleurisy with subsequent chronic course. (2) Secondary and terminal forms of acute pleurisy (these are not uncommon in hospital practice). And (3) a form of acute tuberculous suppurative pleurisy. A considerable number of the purulent pleurisies, designated as latent and chronic, are caused by tubercle bacilli, but the fact is not so widely recognized that there is an acute, ulcerative, and suppurative disease which may run a very rapid course. The pleurisy sets in abruptly, with pain in the side, fever, cough, and sometimes with a chill. There may be nothing to suggest a tuberculous process, and the subject may have a fine physique and come of healthy stock.

(*b*) The subacute and chronic tuberculous pleurisies are more common. The largest group of cases comprises those with sero-fibrinous effusion. The onset is insidious, the true character of the disease is frequently overlooked, and in almost every instance there are tuberculous foci in the lungs and in the bronchial glands. These are cases in which the termination is often in pulmonary tuberculosis or general miliary tuberculosis. In a few cases the exudate becomes purulent.

(*c*) And, lastly, there is a *chronic adhesive pleurisy,* a primary proliferative form which is of long standing, and may lead to very great thickening of the membrane, and sometimes to invasion of the lung.

Secondary tuberculous pleurisy is very common. The visceral layer is always involved in pulmonary tuberculosis. Adhesions usually form and a chronic pleurisy results, which may be simple, but usually tubercles are scattered through the adhesions. An acute tuberculous pleurisy may result from direct extension. The fluid may be sero-fibrinous or hæmorrhagic, or may become purulent. And, lastly, in pulmonary tuberculosis, a superficial spot of softening may perforate with the production of *pyo-pneumothorax.*

The general symptomatology of these forms will be considered under disease of the pleura.

Tuberculosis of the Pericardium.—Miliary tubercles may occur as a part of a general infection, but the term is properly limited to those cases in which, either as a primary or secondary process, there is extensive disease of the membrane. Tuberculosis is not so common in the pericardium as in the pleura and peritoneum, but it is certainly more common than the literature would lead us to suppose. George Norris found 82 instances among 1,780 post mortems in tuberculous subjects.

We may recognize four groups of cases: First, those in which the condition is entirely latent, and the disease is discovered accidentally in individuals who have died of other affections or of chronic pulmonary tuberculosis.

A second group, in which the symptoms are those of cardiac insufficiency following the dilatation and hypertrophy consequent upon a chronic adhesive pericarditis. The symptoms are those of cardiac dropsy, and suggest either idiopathic hypertrophy and dilatation, or, if there is a loud blowing systolic murmur at the apex, mitral valve disease, either insufficiency or stenosis. The condition of adherent pericardium is usually overlooked.

In a third group the clinical picture is that of an acute tuberculosis, either general or with cerebro-spinal manifestations, which has had its origin from the tuberculous pericardium or tuberculous mediastinal lymph-glands.

A fourth group, with symptoms of acute pericarditis, includes cases in which the affection is acute and accompanied with more or less exudation of a sero-fibrinous, hæmorrhagic, or purulent character. There may be no suspicion whatever of the tuberculous nature of the trouble.

Tuberculosis of the Peritoneum.—In connection with miliary and chronic pulmonary tuberculosis it is not uncommon to find the peritoneum studded with small gray granulations. They are constantly present on the serous surface of tuberculous ulcers of the intestines. Apart from these conditions the membrane is often the seat of extensive tuberculous disease, which occurs in the following forms:

(*a*) *Acute miliary tuberculosis* with sero-fibrinous or bloody exudation.

(*b*) *Chronic tuberculosis,* characterized by larger growths, which tend to caseate and ulcerate. The exudate is purulent or sero-purulent, and is often sacculated.

(*c*) *Chronic fibroid tuberculosis,* which may be subacute from the onset, or which may represent the final stage of an acute miliary eruption. The tubercles are hard and pigmented. There is little or no exudation, and the serous surfaces are matted together by adhesions.

The process may be primary and local, which was the case in 5 of 17 post mortems. In children the infection appears to pass from the intestines, and in adults this is the source in the cases associated with chronic tuberculosis. In women the disease extends commonly from the Fallopian tubes. In at least 30 or 40 per cent. of the instances of laparotomy in this affection the infection was from them. The prostate or the seminal vesicles may be the starting-point. In many cases the peritoneum is involved with the pleura and pericardium, particularly with the former membrane.

It is interesting to note that certain morbid conditions of the abdominal organs predispose to the development of the disease; thus patients with cirrhosis of the liver very often die of an acute tuberculous peritonitis. The frequency with which the condition is met with in operations upon ovarian tumors has been commented upon by gynæcologists. Many cases have followed trauma of the abdomen. An interesting feature is the occurrence of tuberculosis in hernial sacs which is not very uncommon. In a majority of the instances it is discovered accidentally during the operation for radical cure or for strangulation. In 7 instances the sac alone was involved.

It is generally stated that males are attacked oftener than females, but in the collected statistics the cases are twice as numerous in females as in males; in the ratio, indeed, of 131 to 60.

Tuberculous peritonitis occurs at all ages. It is common in children associated with intestinal and mesenteric disease. The incidence is most frequent between the ages of twenty and forty. It may occur in advanced life; one patient was eighty-two years of age. Of 357 cases collected from the literature, there were under ten years, 27; between ten and twenty, 75; from twenty to thirty, 87; between thirty and forty, 71; from forty to fifty, 61; from fifty to sixty, 19; from sixty to seventy, 4; above seventy, 2. In America it is more common in the negro than in the white race. More blacks than whites, 77 to 70, were admitted to the Johns Hopkins Hospital (Hamman).

Symptoms.—In certain special features the tuberculous varies considerably from other forms of peritonitis. It presents a symptom-complex of extraordinary diversity.

In the first place, the process may be *latent* and met with accidentally in the operation for hernia or for ovarian tumor. The *acute onset* is not uncommon. Four cases in our records were diagnosed appendicitis, two acute cholecystitis, and six had symptoms of intestinal obstruction, in two of these coming on with great abruptness (Hamman). The cases have been mistaken for strangulated hernia. Other cases set in acutely with fever, abdominal tenderness, and the symptoms of ordinary acute peritonitis. Cases with a slow onset, abdominal tenderness, tympanites, and low continuous fever are often mistaken for *typhoid fever.*

Ascites is frequent, but the effusion is rarely large. It is sometimes hæmorrhagic. In this form the diagnosis may rest between an acute miliary cancer, cirrhosis of the liver, and a chronic simple peritonitis—conditions which usually offer no special difficulties in differentiation. A most important point is the simultaneous presence of a pleurisy. The tuberculin test may be used. *Tympanites* may be present in the very acute cases, when it is due to loss of tone in the intestines owing to inflammatory infiltration; or it may occur in the old, long-standing cases when universal adhesion has taken place between the parietal and visceral layers. *Fever* is a marked symptom in the acute cases, and the temperature may reach 103° or 104°. In many instances the fever is slight. In the more chronic cases subnormal temperatures are common, and for days the temperature may not rise above 97°, and the morning record may be as low as 95.5°. An occasional symptom is pigmentation of the skin, which has led to the diagnosis of Addison's disease. A striking peculiarity of tuberculous peritonitis is the frequency with which it simulates or is associated with *tumor.* This may be:

(*a*) *Omental,* due to puckering and rolling of this membrane until it forms an elongated firm mass, attached to the transverse colon and lying athwart the upper part of the abdomen. This cord-like structure is found also with cancerous peritonitis, but is much more common in tuberculosis. Gairdner called special attention to this form of tumor, and in children saw it undergo gradual resolution. A resonant percussion note may sometimes be elicited above the mass. Though usually situated near the umbilicus, the omental mass may form a prominent tumor in the right iliac region.

(*b*) *Sacculated exudation,* in which the effusion is limited and confined by adhesions between the coils, the parietal peritoneum, the mesentery, and the abdominal or pelvic organs. This encysted exudate is most common in the middle zone, and has frequently been mistaken for ovarian tumor. It may occupy the entire anterior portion of the peritoneum, or there may be a more limited saccular exudate on one side or the other. Within the pelvis it is associated with disease of the Fallopian tubes. Eighteen cases in the gynæcological wards (J. H. H.) were operated upon for pyosalpinx (Hamman).

(*c*) In rare cases the tumor formations may be due to great retraction or thickening of the *intestinal coils.* The small intestine is found shortened, the walls enormously thickened, and the entire coil may form a firm knot close against the spine, giving on examination the idea of a solid mass. Not the small intestine only, but the entire bowel from the duodenum to the rectum, has been found forming such a hard nodular tumor.

(*d*) *Mesenteric glands,* which occasionally form very large, tumor-like masses, more commonly found in children than in adults. This condition may be confined to the abdominal glands. Ascites may coexist. The condition must be distinguished from that in children, in which, with ascites or tympanites—sometimes both—there can be felt irregular nodular masses, due to large caseous formations between the intestinal coils. No doubt in a considerable number of cases of the so-called tabes mesenterica, particularly in those with enlargement and hardness of the abdomen—the condition which the French call *carreau*—there is involvement also of the peritoneum.

The *diagnosis* of these peritoneal tumors is sometimes very difficult. The omental mass is a less frequent source of error than any other; but a similar condition may occur in cancer. The most important problem is the diagnosis of the saccular exudation from ovarian tumor. In fully one-third of the recorded cases of laparotomy in tuberculous peritonitis the diagnosis of cystic ovarian disease had been made. The most suggestive points for consideration are the history and the evidence of old tuberculous lesions. The physical condition is not of much help, as in many instances the patients have been robust and well nourished. Irregular febrile attacks, gastro-intestinal disturbance, and pains are more common in tuberculous disease. Unless inflamed there is usually not much fever with ovarian cysts. The local signs are very deceptive, and in certain cases have conformed in every particular to those of cystic disease. The outlines in saccular exudation are rarely so well defined. The position and form may be variable, owing to alterations in the size of the coils of which in parts the walls are composed. Nodular cheesy masses may sometimes be felt at the periphery. Depression of the vaginal wall is mentioned as occurring in encysted peritonitis; but it is also found in ovarian tumor. The condition of the Fallopian tubes, of the lungs and the pleuræ, should be thoroughly examined. The association of salpingitis with an ill-defined anomalous mass in the abdomen should arouse suspicion, as should also involvement of the pleura, the apex of one lung, or a testis or seminal vesicle in the male.

TREATMENT.—General measures should be carried out as in pulmonary tuberculosis. Direct exposure of the abdomen to sunlight and to the X-rays has proved useful in some cases. Surgical treatment is most helpful in the cases with ascites, but when there are tuberculous tumors and many adhesions the results are not satisfactory. In some cases the removal of a focus of infection, such as tuberculous mesenteric glands, a diseased appendix or a tuberculous Fallopian tube, has been of benefit.

IV. PULMONARY TUBERCULOSIS

(*Phthisis, Consumption*)

Three clinical groups may be recognized: (1) *acute pneumonic tuberculosis*—acute phthisis; (2) *chronic ulcerative tuberculosis;* and (3) *fibroid tuberculosis.*

According to the mode of infection there are two distinct types of lesions:

(*a*) When the bacilli reach the lungs through the blood-vessels or lymphatics the primary lesion is usually in the tissues of the alveolar walls, in the capillary vessels, the epithelium of the air-cells, and in the connective-tissue framework of the septa. The irritation of the bacilli produces, within a few days, the small, gray miliary nodules, involving several alveoli and consisting largely of round, cuboidal, uninuclear epithelioid cells. Depending upon the number of bacilli which reach the lung in this way, either a localized or a general tuberculosis is excited. The tubercles may be scattered through both lungs and form part of a general miliary tuberculosis, or be confined to the lungs, or even in great part to one lung. The further stages may be: (1) Arrest of the process of cell division, gradual sclerosis of the tubercle, and ultimately complete fibroid transformation. (2) Caseation of the centre of the tubercle, extension at the periphery by proliferation of the epithelioid and lymphoid cells, so that the individual tubercles or small groups become confluent and form diffuse areas which undergo caseation and softening. (3) Occasionally as a result of intense infection of a localized region through the blood-vessels the tubercles are thickly set. The intervening tissue becomes acutely inflamed, the air-cells are filled with the products of a desquamative pneumonia, and many lobules are involved.

(*b*) When the bacilli reach the lung through the bronchi—inhalation or aspiration tuberculosis—the picture differs. The smaller bronchi and bronchioles are more extensively affected; the process is not confined to single groups of alveoli, but has a more lobular arrangement, and the tuberculous masses from the onset are larger, more diffuse, and may in some cases involve an entire lobe or the greater part of a lung. It is in this mode of infection that we see the characteristic peri-bronchial granulations and the areas of the so-called nodular broncho-pneumonia. These broncho-pneumonic areas, with on the one hand caseation, ulceration, and cavity formation, and on the other sclerosis and limitation, make up the essential elements in the anatomical picture of pulmonary tuberculosis.

1. *Acute Pneumonic Tuberculosis of the Lungs*

This form, known also by the name of *galloping consumption,* is met with both in children and adults. In the former many of the cases are mistaken for simple broncho-pneumonia.

Two types may be recognized, the *pneumonic* and *broncho-pneumonic.*

The Pneumonic Form.—In the *pneumonic form* one lobe may be involved, or in some instances an entire lung. The organ is heavy, the affected portion airless; the pleura is usually covered with a thin exudate, and on section the picture resembles closely that of ordinary hepatization. The following is an extract from the post mortem report of a case in which death occurred twenty-nine days after the onset of the illness, having all the characters of an acute pneumonia: "Left lung weighs 1,500 grams (double the weight of the other organ) and is heavy and airless, crepitant only at the anterior margins. Section shows a small cavity the size of a walnut at the apex, about which are scattered tubercles in a consolidated tissue. The greater part of the lung presents a grayish-white appearance due to the aggregation of tubercles which in some places have a continuous, uniform appearance, in others are surrounded by an injected and consolidated lung-tissue. Toward the margins of the lower lobe strands of this firm reddish tissue separate anæmic, dry areas. There are in the right lung three or four small groups of tubercles but no caseous masses. The bronchial glands are not tuberculous." Here the intense local infection was due to the small focus at the apex of the lung, probably an aspiration process.

Only the most careful inspection may reveal the presence of miliary tubercles, or the attention may be arrested by the detection of tubercles in the other lung or in the bronchial glands. The process may involve only one lobe. There may be older areas which are of a peculiarly yellowish-white color and distinctly caseous. The most remarkable picture is presented by cases of this kind in which the disease lasts for some months. A lobe or an entire lung may be enlarged, firm, airless throughout, and converted into a dry, yellowish-white, cheesy substance. Cases are met with in which the entire lung from apex to base is in this condition, with perhaps only a small, narrow area of air-containing tissue on the margin. More commonly, if the disease has lasted for two or three months, rapid softening has taken place at the apex with extensive cavity formation.

Males are much more frequently attacked than females. Of a series of 15 cases, 11 were males. The onset was acute in 13, with a chill in 9. Bacilli were found in the sputum in one case as early as the fourth day. Fraenkel and Troje believe that the cases are of bronchogenous origin, due to infection from a small focus somewhere in the lung. Tendeloo regards the infection as sometimes hæmatogenous.

Symptoms.—The attack sets in abruptly with a chill, usually in an individual who has enjoyed good health, although in many cases the onset has been preceded by exposure to cold, or there have been debilitating circumstances. The temperature rises rapidly after the chill, there are pain in the side and cough, with at first mucoid, subsequently rusty-colored expectoration which may contain tubercle bacilli. The dyspnœa may become extreme and the patient may have suffocative attacks. The physical examination shows involvement of one lobe or of one lung, with signs of consolidation, dulness, increased fremitus, at first feeble or suppressed vesicular murmur, and subsequently well-marked bronchial breathing. The upper or lower lobe may be involved, or in some cases the entire lung.

At this time, as a rule, no suspicion enters the mind of the practitioner that the case is anything but one of frank lobar pneumonia. Occasionally there may be suspicious circumstances in the history of the patient or in his family; but, as a rule, no stress is laid upon them in view of the intense and characteristic mode of onset. Between the eighth and tenth day, instead of the expected crisis, the condition becomes aggravated, the temperature is irregular, and the pulse more rapid. There may be sweating, and the expectoration becomes muco-purulent and greenish in color—a point of special importance, to which Traube called attention. Even in the second or third week, with the persistence of these symptoms, the physician tries to console himself with the idea that the case is one of unresolved pneumonia, and that all will yet be well. Gradually, however, the severity of the symptoms, the presence of physical signs indicating softening, the existence of elastic tissue and tubercle bacilli in the sputum present the mournful proofs that the case is one of acute pneumonic tuberculosis. Death may occur on the sixth day, as in a case of Tendeloo's. The earliest death in our series was on the thirteenth day. A majority of the cases drag on, and death does not occur until the third month. In a few cases, even after a stormy onset and active course, the symptoms subside and the patient passes into the chronic stage.

Diagnosis.—Waters, of Liverpool, who gave an admirable description of these cases, called attention to the difficulty in distinguishing them from ordinary pneumonia. Certainly the mode of onset affords no criterion whatever. A healthy, robust-looking young Irishman, a cab-driver, who had been kept waiting on a cold, blustering night until three in the morning, was seized the next afternoon with a violent chill, and the following day was admitted to the University Hospital, Philadelphia. He was made the subject of a clinical lecture on the fifth day, when there was absent no single feature in history, symptoms, or physical signs of acute lobar pneumonia of the right upper lobe. It was not until ten days later, when bacilli were found in his expectoration, that we were made aware of the true nature of the case. There is no criterion by which cases of this kind can be distinguished in the early stage. A point to which Traube called attention, and which is also referred to as important by Hérard and Cornil, is the absence of breath-sounds in the consolidated region; but this does not hold good in all cases. The tubular breathing may be intense and marked as early as the fourth day; and again, how common it is to have, as one of the earliest and most suggestive symptoms of lobar pneumonia, suppression or enfeeblement of the vesicular murmur! In many cases, however, there are suspicious circumstances in the onset: the patient has been in bad health, or may have had previous pulmonary trouble, or there are recurring chills. Careful examination of the sputum and a study of the physical signs from day to day can alone determine the true nature of the case. A point of some moment is the character of the fever, which in true pneumonia is more continuous, particularly in severe cases, whereas in this form of tuberculosis remissions of 1.5° or 2° are not infrequent.

Acute Tuberculous Broncho-pneumonia.—Acute tuberculous broncho-pneumonia is more common, particularly in children, and forms a majority of the cases of *phthisis florida,* or "galloping consumption." It is an acute caseous broncho-pneumonia, starting in the smaller tubes, which become blocked with a cheesy substance, while the air-cells of the lobule are filled with the products of a catarrhal pneumonia. In the early stages the areas have a grayish red, later an opaque white, caseous appearance. By the fusion of contiguous masses an entire lobe may be rendered nearly solid, but areas of crepitant air tissue can usually be seen between the groups. This is not an uncommon picture in the acute tuberculosis of adults, but it is still more frequent in children. The following is an extract from the post mortem report of a case on a child aged four months, who died in the sixth week of illness: "On section, the right upper lobe is occupied with caseous masses from 5 to 12 mm. in diameter, separated from each other by an intervening tissue of a deep red color. The bronchi are filled with cheesy substance. The middle and lower lobes are studded with tubercles, many of which are becoming caseous. Toward the diaphragmatic surface of the lower lobe there is a small cavity the size of a marble. The left lung is more crepitant and uniformly studded with tubercles of all sizes, some as large as peas. The bronchial glands are very large, and one contains a tuberculous abscess."

There is a form of tuberculous aspiration pneumonia, to which Bäumler called attention, occurring as a sequence of hæmoptysis, and due to the aspiration of blood and the contents of pulmonary cavities into the finer tubes. There are fever, dyspnœa, and signs of a diffuse broncho-pneumonia. Some of these cases run a very rapid course. This accident may occur early in the disease, or follow hæmorrhage in a well-marked pulmonary tuberculosis..

In children the enlarged bronchial glands usually surround the root of the lung, and even pass deeply into the substance, and the lobules are often involved by direct contact.

In other cases the caseous broncho-pneumonia involves groups of alveoli or lobules in different portions of the lungs, more commonly at both apices, forming areas from 1 to 3 cm. in diameter. The size of the mass depends largely upon that of the bronchus involved. There are cases which probably should come in this category, in which, with a history of an acute illness of from four to eight weeks, the lungs are extensively studded with large gray tubercles, ranging in size from 5 to 10 mm. In some instances there are cheesy masses the size of a cherry. All of these are grayish-white in color, distinctly cheesy, and between the adjacent ones, particularly in the lower lobe, there may be recent pneumonia, or the condition of lung which has been termed splenization. In a case of this kind at the Philadelphia Hospital death took place about the eighth week from the abrupt onset of the illness with hæmorrhage. There were no extensive areas of consolidation, but the cheesy nodules were uniformly scattered throughout both lungs. No softening had taken place.

Secondary infections are not uncommon; but Prudden was able to show that the tubercle bacillus could produce not only distinct tubercle nodules, but also the various kinds of exudative pneumonia, the exudates varying in appearance in different cases, which phenomena occurred absolutely without the intervention of other organisms. The fact that these latter had not subsequently crept in was shown by cultures at the autopsy on the affected animal.

SYMPTOMS.—The symptoms of acute broncho-pneumonic tuberculosis are very variable. In adults the disease may attack persons in good health, but over-worked or "run down" from any cause. Hæmorrhage initiates the attack in a few cases. There may be repeated chills; the temperature is high, the pulse rapid, and the respirations are increased. The loss of flesh and strength is very striking.

The physical *signs* may at first be uncertain and indefinite, but finally there are areas of impaired resonance, usually at the apices; the breath sounds are harsh and tubular, with numerous râles. The sputum may early show elastic tissue and tubercle bacilli. In the acute cases, within three weeks, the patient may be in a marked typhoid state, with delirium, dry tongue, and high fever. Death may occur within three weeks. In other cases the onset is severe, with high fever, rapid loss of flesh and strength, and signs of extensive unilateral or bilateral disease. Softening takes place; there are sweats, chills, and progressive emaciation, and all the features of *phthisis florida*. Six or eight weeks later the patient may begin to improve, the fever lessens, the general symptoms abate, and a case which looked as if it would terminate fatally within a few weeks drags on and becomes chronic.

In *children* the disease most commonly follows the infectious diseases, particularly measles and whooping cough. At least *three groups* of these tuberculous broncho-pneumonias may be recognized. In the *first* the child is taken ill suddenly while teething or during convalescence from fever; the temperature rises rapidly, the cough is severe, and there may be signs of consolidation at one or both apices with râles. Death may occur within a few days, and the lung shows areas of broncho-pneumonia, with perhaps here and there scattered opaque grayish-yellow nodules. Macroscopically the affection does not look tuberculous, but histologically miliary granulations and bacilli may be found. Tubercles are usually present in the bronchial glands, but the appearance of the broncho-pneumonia may be exceedingly deceptive, and it may require careful microscopic examination to determine its tuberculous character. The *second group* is represented by the case of the child previously quoted, who died at the sixth week with the ordinary symptoms of severe broncho-pneumonia. And the *third group* is that in which, during the convalescence from an infectious disease, the child is taken ill with fever, cough, and shortness of breath. The severity of the symptoms abates within the first fortnight; but there is loss of flesh, the general condition is bad, and the physical examination shows the presence of scattered râles throughout the lungs, and here and there areas of defective resonance. The child has sweats, the fever becomes hectic in character, and in many cases the clinical picture gradually passes into that of chronic phthisis.

2. *Chronic Ulcerative Tuberculosis of the Lungs*

Under this heading may be grouped the great majority of cases of pulmonary tuberculosis, in which the lesions proceed to ulceration and softening.

Morbid Anatomy.—Inspection of the lungs shows a remarkable variety of lesions, comprising nodular tubercles, diffuse tuberculous infiltration, caseous masses, pneumonic areas, cavities of various sizes, with changes in the pleura, bronchi, and bronchial glands.

The Distribution of the Lesions.—For years it has been recognized that the most advanced lesions are at the apices, and that the disease progresses downward, usually more rapidly in one of the lungs. This general statement, which has passed current in the text-books ever since the masterly description of Laennec, has been carefully elaborated by Kingston Fowler, who finds that the disease in its onward progress through the lungs follows, in a majority of the cases, distinct routes. In the upper lobe the primary lesion is not, as a rule, at the extreme apex, but from an inch to an inch and a half below the summit of the lung, and nearer to the posterior and external borders. The lesion here tends to spread downward, probably from inhalation of the virus, and this accounts for the frequent circumstance that examination behind, in the supra-spinous fossa, will give indications of disease before any evidences exist at the apex in front. Anteriorly this initial focus corresponds to a spot just below the centre of the clavicle, and the direction of extension in front is along the anterior aspect of the upper lobe, along a line running about an inch and a half from the inner ends of the first, second, and third interspaces. A second less common site of the primary lesion in the apex "corresponds on the chest wall with the first and second interspaces below the outer third of the clavicle." The extension is downward, so that the outer part of the upper lobe is chiefly involved.

In the middle lobe of the right lung the affection usually follows disease of the upper lobe on the same side. In the involvement of the lower lobe the first secondary infiltration is about an inch to an inch and a half below the posterior extremity of its apex, and corresponds on the chest wall to a spot opposite the fifth dorsal spine. This involvement is of the greatest importance clinically, as "in the great majority of cases, when the physical signs of the disease at the apex are sufficiently definite to allow of the diagnosis of phthisis being made, the lower lobe is already affected." Examination, therefore, should be made carefully of this posterior apex in all suspicious cases. In this situation the lesion spreads downward and laterally along the line of the interlobular septa, a line which is marked by the vertebral border of the scapula, when the hand is placed on the opposite scapula and the elbow raised above the level of the shoulder. Once present in an apex, the disease usually extends in time to the opposite upper lobe; but not, as a rule, until the apex of the lower lobe of the lung first affected has been attacked. Of 427 cases, the right apex was involved in 172, the left in 130, both in 111.

Lesions of the base may be primary, though this is rare. Percy Kidd makes the proportion of basic to apical phthisis 1 to 500, a smaller number than existed in our series. In very chronic cases there may be arrested lesions at the apex and more recent lesions at the base.

Summary of the Lesions in Chronic Ulcerative Tuberculosis.—(*a*) *Miliary Tubercles.*—They have one of two distributions: (1) A dissemination due to aspiration of tuberculous material, the tubercles being situated in the air-cells or the walls of the smaller bronchi; (2) the distribution due to dissemination of tubercle bacilli by the lymph current, the tubercles being scattered about the old foci in a radial manner—the secondary crop of Laennec. Much more rarely there is a scattered dissemination from infection here and there of the smaller vessels, the tubercles then being situated in the vessel walls. Sometimes, in cases with cavity formation at the apex, the greater part of the lower lobes presents many groups of firm, sclerotic, miliary tubercles, which may indeed form the distinguishing anatomical feature—a chronic miliary tuberculosis.

(*b*) *Tuberculous Broncho-pneumonia.*—In a large proportion of cases of chronic tuberculosis the terminal bronchiole is the point of origin of the process, consequently we find the smaller bronchi and their alveolar territories blocked with the accumulated products of inflammation in all stages of *caseation.* At an early period a cross-section of an area of tuberculous broncho-pneumonia gives the most characteristic appearance. The central bronchiole is seen as a small orifice, or it is plugged with cheesy contents, while surrounding it is a caseous nodule, the so-called peribronchial tubercle. The longitudinal section has a somewhat dendritic or foliaceous appearance. The condition of the picture depends much upon the slowness or rapidity with which the process has advanced. The following changes may occur:

Ulceration.—When the caseation takes place rapidly or ulceration occurs in the bronchial wall, the mass may break down and form a small cavity.

Sclerosis.—In other instances the process is more chronic, and fibroid changes gradually produce a sclerosis of the affected area. This may be confined to the margin of the mass, forming a limiting capsule, within which is a uniform, firm, cheesy substance, in which lime salts are often deposited. This represents the healing of one of these areas of caseous broncho-pneumonia. It is only, however, when complete fibroid transformation or calcification has occurred that we can really speak of healing. In many instances the colonies of miliary tubercles about these masses show that the process is still active.

Subsequently, in ulcerative processes, these calcareous bodies—lung-stones, as they are sometimes called—may be expectorated.

(*c*) *Pneumonia.*—An important though secondary place is occupied by inflammation of the alveoli surrounding the tubercles, which become filled with epithelioid cells. The consolidation may extend for some distance about the tuberculous foci and unite them into areas of uniform consolidation. Although in some instances this inflammatory process may be simple, in others it is undoubtedly specific. It is excited by the tubercle bacilli and is a manifestation of their action. It may present a very varied appearance; in some instances resembling closely ordinary red hepatization, in others being more homogeneous and infiltrated, the so-called *infiltration tuberculeuse* of Laennec. In other cases the contents of the alveoli undergo fatty degeneration, and appear on the cut surface as opaque white or yellowish-white bodies. In early tuberculosis much of the consolidation is due to this pneumonic infiltration, which may surround the smaller foci for some distance.

(*d*) *Cavities.*—A vomica is a cavity in the lung tissue, produced by necrosis and ulceration. The process usually begins in the wall of the bronchus in a tuberculous area. Dilatation is produced by retained secretion, and necrosis and ulceration of the wall occur with gradual destruction of the contiguous tissues. By extension of the necrosis and ulceration the cavity increases, contiguous ones unite, and in an affected region there may be a series of small excavations communicating with a bronchus. In nearly all instances the process extends from the bronchi, though it is possible for necrosis and softening to take place in the centre of a caseous area without primary involvement of the bronchial wall. Three forms may be recognized.

The *fresh ulcerative,* seen in acute cases, in which there is no limiting membrane, but the walls are made up of softened, necrotic, and caseous masses. A small vomica of this sort, situated just beneath the pleura, may rupture and cause pneumothorax. In cases of acute pneumonic tuberculosis they may be large, occupying the greater portion of the upper lobe. In the chronic ulcerative form, cavities of this sort are invariably present in those portions of the lung in which the disease is advancing. At the apex there may be a large old cavity with well-defined walls, while at the anterior margin of the upper lobes, or in the apices of the lower lobes, there are recent ulcerating cavities communicating with the bronchi.

Cavities with well-defined Walls.—A majority of the cavities in the chronic cases have a well-defined limiting membrane, the inner surface of which constantly produces pus. The walls are crossed by trabeculæ which represent remnants of bronchi and blood-vessels. Even the cavities with the well-defined walls extend gradually by a slow necrosis and destruction of the contiguous lung tissue. The contents are usually purulent, similar in character to the grayish nummular sputa coughed up. Not infrequently the membrane is vascular or it may be hæmorrhagic. Occasionally, when gangrene has occurred in the wall, the contents are horribly fetid. These cavities may occupy the greater portion of the apex, forming an irregular series which communicate with each other and with the bronchi, or the entire upper lobe except the anterior margin may be excavated, forming a thin-walled cavity. In rare instances the process has proceeded to total excavation of the lung, not a remnant of which remains, except perhaps a narrow strip at the anterior margin. In a case of this kind, in a young girl, the cavity held 40 fluid ounces, in another 42 ounces.

Quiescent Cavities.—When quite small and surrounded by dense cicatricial tissue communicating with the bronchi they form the *cicatrices fistuleuses* of Laennec. Occasionally one apex may be represented by a series of these small cavities, surrounded by dense fibrous tissue. The lining membrane of these old cavities may be quite smooth, almost like a mucous membrane. Cavities of any size do not heal completely. Cases are often seen in which it has been supposed that a cavity has healed; but the signs of excavation are notoriously uncertain, and there may be pectoriloquy and cavernous sounds with gurgling resonant râles in an area of consolidation close to a large bronchus.

In the formation of cavities the blood-vessels gradually become closed by an obliterating inflammation. They are the last structures to yield and may be completely exposed in a cavity, even when the circulation is still going on in them. Unfortunately, the erosion of a large vessel which has not yet been obliterated is by no means infrequent, and causes profuse and often fatal hæmorrhage. Another common event is the formation of aneurisms on the arteries running in the walls of cavities. These may be small, bunch-like dilatations, or they may form sacs the size of a walnut or even larger. They are important with regard to hæmoptysis.

And, finally, about cavities of all sorts, the connective tissue grows, tending to limit their extent. The thickening is particularly marked beneath the pleura, and in chronic cases an entire apex may be converted into a mass of fibrous tissue, inclosing a few small cavities.

(*e*) *Pleura.*—Practically, in all cases of chronic tuberculosis the pleura is involved. Adhesions take place which may be thin and readily torn, or dense and firm, uniting layers of from 2 to 5 mm. in thickness. This pleurisy may be simple, but in many cases it is tuberculous, and miliary tubercles or caseous masses are seen in the thickened membrane. Effusion is not at all infrequent, either serous, purulent, or hæmorrhagic. Pneumothorax is a common accident.

(*f*) Changes in the *smaller bronchi* control the situation in the early stages of pulmonary tuberculosis, and play an important rôle throughout. The process very often begins in the walls of the smaller tubes and leads to caseation, distention with products of inflammation, and broncho-pneumonia of the lobules. In many cases the visible implication of the bronchus is an extension upward of a process which has begun in the smallest bronchiole. This involvement weakens the wall, leading to bronchiectasis, not an uncommon event. The mucous membrane of the larger bronchi, which is usually involved in a chronic catarrh, is more or less swollen, and in some instances ulcerated. Besides these specific lesions, they may be the seat, especially in children, of inflammation due to secondary invasion, most frequently by the *pneumococcus* with the production of a broncho-pneumonia.

(*g*) The *bronchial glands,* in the more acute cases, are swollen and œdematous. Miliary tubercles and caseous foci are usually present. In cases of chronic tuberculosis the caseous areas are common, calcification may occur, and not infrequently purulent softening.

(*h*) *Changes in the Other Organs.*—Of these, tuberculosis is the most common. In 275 autopsies the brain presented tuberculous lesions in 31, the spleen in 33, the liver in 12, the kidneys in 32, the intestines in 65, and the pericardium in 7. Other groups of lymphatic glands besides the bronchial may be affected.

Amyloid change may occur in the liver, spleen, kidneys, and mucous membrane of the intestines. The *liver* is often the seat of extensive fatty infiltration, which may cause marked enlargement. The *intestinal tuberculosis* occurs in advanced cases and is responsible in great part for the diarrhœa.

Endocarditis is not very common, and was present in 12 of 275 post mortems and in 27 of Percy Kidd's 500 cases. Tubercle bacilli have been found in the vegetations. Tubercles may be present on the endocardium, particularly of the right ventricle.

The *larynx* is frequently involved, and ulceration of the vocal cords and destruction of the epiglottis are not at all uncommon.

Modes of Onset.—We have already seen that tuberculosis of the lungs may occur as the chief part of a general infection, or may set in with symptoms which closely simulate acute pneumonia. In the ordinary type of pulmonary tuberculosis the invasion is gradual and less striking, but presents an extraordinarily diverse picture, so that the practitioner is often led into error. Among the most characteristic modes of onset are the following:

(*a*) Latent Types.—Many such cases are found in the routine examination of large groups of people. It is probable that many slight, ill-defined ailments are due to unrecognized tuberculosis. In the history of patients with tuberculosis such attacks are not infrequently mentioned.

The disease makes considerable progress before there are serious symptoms to arouse the attention of the patient. In workingmen the disease may even advance to excavation of an apex before they seek advice. It is not a little remarkable how slight the lung symptoms may have been.

The symptoms may be masked by the existence of serious disease in other organs, as in the peritoneum, intestines, or bones.

(*b*) With Symptoms of Dyspepsia and Anæmia.—The gastric mode of onset is very common, and the early manifestations may be great irritability of the stomach with vomiting or a type of acid dyspepsia with eructations. In young girls (and in children) with this dyspepsia there is very frequently a pronounced chloro-anæmia, and the patient complains of palpitation of the heart, increasing weakness, slight afternoon fever, and amenorrhœa.

(*c*) Malarial Symptoms.—In a considerable number of cases the onset of pulmonary tuberculosis is with symptoms which suggest malarial fever. The patient has repeated paroxysms of chills, fevers, and sweats, which may recur with great regularity. In districts in which malaria prevails there is no more common mistake than to confound the initial rigors of pulmonary tuberculosis with it.

(*d*) Onset with Pleurisy.—The first symptoms may be a dry pleurisy over an apex, with persistent friction murmur. In other instances the pulmonary symptoms have followed an attack of pleurisy with effusion. The exudate gradually disappears, but the cough persists and the patient becomes feverish, and signs of disease at one apex gradually become manifest. About one-third of all cases of pleurisy with effusion subsequently have pulmonary tuberculosis.

(*e*) With Laryngeal Symptoms.—The primary localization may be in the larynx, though in a majority of the instances in which huskiness and laryngeal symptoms are the first noticeable features of the disease there are doubtless foci already existing in the lung. The group of cases in which for many months throat and larynx symptoms precede the manifestations of pulmonary tuberculosis is a very important one.

(*f*) Onset with Hæmoptysis.—Frequently the very first symptom is a brisk hæmorrhage from the lungs, following which the pulmonary symptoms may come on with great rapidity. In other cases the hæmoptysis recurs, and it may be months before the symptoms become well established. In a majority of these cases the local tuberculous lesion exists at the date of the hæmoptysis. Blood-streaked sputum may have the same significance.

(*g*) With Tuberculosis of the Cervico-axillary Glands.—Preceding the onset of pulmonary disease for months, or even for years, the lymph-glands of the neck or of the neck and axilla of one side may be enlarged. These cases are of importance because of the latency of the pulmonary lesions and it is well to bear in mind that in such patients the corresponding apex of the lung may be extensively involved.

(*h*) With Nervous Symptoms.—Malaise, fatigue and indefinite nervous disturbances with loss of weight may be the marked features and suggest neurasthenia.

(*i*) Bronchial Symptoms.—In by far the largest number of all cases the onset is with a *bronchitis,* or, as the patient expresses it, a neglected cold. There has been, perhaps, a liability to catch cold easily or the patient has been subject to naso-pharyngeal catarrh; then, following some unusual exposure, a cough begins, which may be frequent and irritating. The examination of the lungs may reveal localized moist sounds at one apex and perhaps wheezing bronchitic râles in other parts. In a few cases the early symptoms are often suggestive of asthma with marked wheezing and diffuse piping râles.

(*j*) *Miscellaneous Group.* (1) Following acute infections, such as influenza. (2) With or after pregnancy. (3) After an operation in which ether anæsthesia was used. (4) In association with ischio-rectal abscess and fistula-in-ano. In all of these an inactive process may be rendered active.

Symptoms.—In discussing the symptoms it is usual to divide the disease into three periods: the first embracing the time of the growth and development of the tubercles; the second, when they soften; and the third, when there is a formation of cavities. Unfortunately, these anatomical stages can not be satisfactorily correlated with corresponding clinical periods, and we often find that a patient in the third stage with a well-marked cavity is in a far better condition and has greater prospects of recovery than a patient in the first stage with diffuse consolidation. It is therefore better perhaps to disregard them altogether.

Local Symptoms.—*Pain* in the chest may be early and troublesome or absent throughout. It is usually associated with pleurisy, and may be sharp and stabbing in character, and either constant or felt only during coughing. Perhaps the commonest situation is in the lower thoracic zone, though in some instances it is beneath the scapula or referred to the apex. The attacks may recur at long intervals. Intercostal neuralgia occasionally occurs in the course of ordinary pulmonary tuberculosis.

Cough is one of the earliest symptoms, and is present in the majority of cases from beginning to end. There is nothing peculiar or distinctive about it. At first dry and hacking, and perhaps scarcely exciting the attention of the patient, it subsequently becomes looser, more constant, and associated with a glairy, muco-purulent expectoration. In the early stages the cough is bronchial in its origin. When cavities have formed it becomes more paroxysmal, and is most marked in the morning or after a sleep. Cough is not a constant symptom, however, and a patient may present himself with well-marked excavation at one apex who declares that he has had little or no cough. So, too, there may be well-marked physical signs, dulness and moist sounds, without either expectoration or cough. In well-established cases the nocturnal paroxysms are most distressing and prevent sleep. The cough may be of such persistence and severity as to cause vomiting, and the patient becomes rapidly emaciated from loss of food—Morton's cough (Phthisiologia, 1689, p. 101). The laryngeal complications give a peculiarly husky quality to the cough, and when erosion and ulceration have proceeded far in the vocal cords the coughing becomes much less effective.

Sputum.—This varies greatly in amount and character with the different stages. There are patients with well-marked local signs at one apex, with slight cough and moderately high fever, without a trace of expectoration. So, also, there are instances with the most extensive consolidation (caseous pneumonia) and high fever, but without enough expectoration to enable an examination for bacilli to be made. In the early stage of pulmonary tuberculosis the sputum is chiefly catarrhal and has a glairy, sago-like appearance, due to the presence of alveolar cells which have undergone the myeline degeneration. There is nothing distinctive or peculiar in this form of expectoration, which may persist for months without indicating serious trouble. The earliest trace of characteristic sputum may show the presence of small grayish or greenish-gray purulent masses. These, when coughed up, are always suggestive and should be the portions picked out for microscopic examination. As softening comes on, the expectoration becomes more profuse and purulent, but may still contain a considerable quantity of alveolar epithelium. Finally, when cavities exist, the sputum assumes the so-called nummular form; each mass is isolated, flattened, greenish-gray in color, quite airless, and, when spat into water, sinks to the bottom.

By the microscopic examination of the sputum we determine whether the process is tuberculous, and whether softening has occurred. The bacilli in stained preparations are seen as elongated, slightly curved, red rods, sometimes presenting a beaded appearance. They are frequently in groups of three or four, but the number varies considerably. Only one or two may be found in a preparation, or, in some instances, they are so abundant that the entire field is occupied. Repeated examinations may be necessary.

The continued presence of tubercle bacilli in the sputum is an infallible indication of the existence of tuberculosis. One or two may possibly be due to accidental inhalation. A number may come from a spot of softening 3 by 3 cm. In the nummular sputa of later stages the bacilli are very abundant.

Elastic tissue may be derived from the bronchi, the alveoli, or from the arterial coats; and naturally the appearance of the tissue will vary with the locality from which it comes. In the examination for this it is not necessary to boil the sputum with caustic potash. In almost all instances if the sputum is spread in a sufficiently thin layer the fragments of elastic tissue can be seen with the naked eye. The thick, purulent portions are placed upon a glass plate 15 × 15 cm. and flattened into a thin layer by a second glass plate 10 × 10 cm. In this compressed grayish layer between the glass slips any fragments of elastic tissue show on a black background as grayish-yellow spots and can either be examined at once under a low power or the uppermost piece of glass is slid along until the fragment is exposed, when it is picked out and placed upon the ordinary microscopic slide. Fragments of bread and collections of milk-globules may also present an opaque white appearance, but with a little practice they can readily be recognized. Fragments of epithelium from the tongue, infiltrated with micrococci, are still more deceptive, but the miscroscope at once shows the difference.

The bronchial elastic tissue forms an elongated network, or two or three long, narrow fibres are found close together. From the blood-vessels a somewhat similar form may be seen and occasionally a distinct sheeting is found as if it had come from the intima of a good-sized artery. The elastic tissue of the alveolar wall is quite distinctive; the fibres are branched and often show the outline of the arrangement of the air-cells. The elastic tissue from bronchi or alveoli indicates extensive erosion of a tube and softening of the lung-tissue.

Another occasional constituent of the sputum is blood, which may be present as the chief characteristic of the expectoration in hæmoptysis or may simply tinge the sputum. In chronic cases with large cavities, in addition to bacteria, various forms of fungi may be found, of which the aspergillus is the most important. Sarcinæ may also occur.

Calcareous Fragments.—Formerly a good deal of stress was laid upon their presence in the sputum, and Morton described a phthisis *a calculis in pulmonibus generatis*. Bayle also described a separate form of *phthisis calculeuse*. The size of the fragments varies from a small pea to a large cherry. As a rule, a single one is ejected; sometimes large numbers are coughed up in the course of the disease. They are formed in the lung by the calcification of caseous masses, and it is said also occasionally in obstructed bronchi. They may come from the bronchial glands by ulceration into the bronchi, and there is a case on record of suffocation in a child from this cause.

The daily amount of expectoration varies. In rapidly advancing cases, with much cough, it may reach as high as 500 c. c. in the day. In cases with large cavities the chief amount is brought up in the morning. The expectoration of tuberculous patients usually has a heavy, sweetish odor, and occasionally it is fetid, owing to decomposition in the cavities.

Hæmoptysis.—One of the most famous of the Hippocratic axioms says, "From a spitting of blood there is a spitting of pus." The older writers thought that the phthisis was directly due to the inflammatory or putrefactive changes caused by the hæmorrhage into the lung. Morton, however, in his interesting section, *Phithisis ab Hæmoptöe,* rather doubted this sequence. Laennec and Louis, and later in the century Traube, regarded the hæmoptysis as an evidence of existing disease of the lung. From the accurate views of Laennec and Louis the profession was led away by Graves, and particularly by Niemeyer, who held that the blood in the air-cells set up an inflammatory process, a common termination of which was caseation. Since Koch's discovery we have learned that many cases in which the physical examination is negative show, either during the period of hæmorrhage or immediately after it, tubercle bacilli in the sputum, so that opinion has veered to the older view, and we now regard the appearance of hæmoptysis as an indication of existing disease. In young, apparently healthy, persons cases of hæmoptysis may be divided into three groups. In the first the bleeding has come on without premonition, without overexertion or injury, and there is no family history of tuberculosis. The physical examination is negative, and the examination of the expectoraton at the time of the hæmorrhage and subsequently shows no tubercle bacilli. Such instances are not uncommon, and, though one may suspect strongly the presence of some focus of tuberculosis, yet the individuals may retain good health for many years, and have no further trouble. Of the 386 cases of hæmoptysis noted by Ware in private practice 62 recovered, and pulmonary disease did not subsequently occur.

In a second group individuals in apparently perfect health are suddenly attacked, perhaps after a slight exertion or during some athletic exercises. The physical examination is also negative, but tubercle bacilli are found sometimes in the bloody sputum, more frequently a few days later.

In a third set of cases the individuals have been in failing health for a month or two, but the symptoms have not been urgent and perhaps not noticed. Physical examination shows the presence of well-marked tucerculous disease, and there are both tubercle bacilli and elastic tissue in the sputum.

A very interesting study of the subject of hæmoptysis, particularly in its relation to tuberculosis, was made in the Prussian army by Stricker. During the five years 1890-'95 there were 900 cases admitted to the hospitals; in 480 the hæmorrhage came on without recognizable cause. Of these, 417 cases, 86 per cent., were certainly or probably tuberculous. In only 221, however, was the evidence conclusive. In a second group of 213 cases the hæmorrhage came on during the military exercise, and of these 75 patients were shown to be tuberculous. In 118 cases the hæmorrhage followed special exercises, as in the gymnasium or riding or swimming. In 24 cases it occurred during the exercise of the voice in singing or in giving command or in the use of wind instruments. A group of 24 cases is reported in which the hæmorrhage followed trauma, either a fall or a blow upon the thorax. In 7 of these tuberculosis was positively present, and in 6 other cases there was a strong probability of its existence.

Among the conclusions which Stricker draws the following are the most important: namely, that soldiers attacked with hæmoptysis without special cause are in at least 86.8 per cent. tuberculous. In the cases in which the hæmoptysis follows the special exercises, etc., of military service at least 74.4 per cent. are tuberculous. In the cases which come on during swimming or as a consequence of direct injury to the thorax about one-half are not associated with tuberculosis.

Hæmoptysis occurs in from 60 to 80 per cent. of all cases of pulmonary tuberculosis. It is more frequent in males than in females.

In a majority of all cases the bleeding recurs. Sometimes it is a special feature throughout the disease, so that a hæmorrhagic form has been recognized. The amount of blood brought up varies from a couple of drams to a pint or more. In 69 per cent. of 4,125 cases of hæmoptysis at the Brompton Hospital the amount brought up was under half an ounce.

A distinction may be drawn between the hæmoptysis early in the disease and that which occurs in the later periods. In the former the bleeding is usually slight, is apt to recur, and fatal hæmorrhage is very rare. In these cases the bleeding is usually from small areas of softening or from early erosions in the bronchial mucosa. In the later periods, after cavities have formed, the bleeding is, as a rule, more profuse and is more apt to be fatal. Single large hæmorrhages, proving quickly fatal, are very rare, except in the advanced stages of the disease. In these cases the bleeding comes either from an erosion of a good-sized vessel in the wall of a cavity or from the rupture of an aneurism of the pulmonary artery.

The bleeding, as a rule, sets in suddenly. Without any warning the patient may notice a warm salt taste and the mouth fills with blood. It may come up with a slight cough. The total amount may not be more than a few drams, and for a day or two the patient may spit up small quantities. When a large vessel is eroded or an aneurism bursts, the amount of blood brought up is large, and in the course of a short time a pint or two may be expectorated. Fatal hæmorrhage may occur into a very large cavity without any blood being coughed up. The character of the blood is, as a rule, distinctive. It is frothy, mixed with mucus, generally bright red in color, except when large amounts are expectorated, and then it may be dark. The sputum may remain blood-tinged for some days, or there are brownish-black streaks in it, or friable nodules consisting entirely of blood-corpuscles may be coughed up. Blood moulds of the smaller bronchi are sometimes expectorated.

The microscopic examination of the sputum in hæmorrhage cases is most important. If carefully spread out, there may be noted, even in an apparently pure hæmorrhagic mass, little portions of mucus from which bacilli or elastic tissue may be obtained. Flick and others have called attention to the frequency with which hæmoptysis is associated with the appearance or an increase of pneumococci and influenza bacilli in the sputum.

Dyspnœa is not a common accompaniment of ordinary tuberculosis. The greater part of one lung may be diseased and local trouble exist at the other apex without any shortness of breath. Even in the paroxysms of very high fever the respirations may not be much increased. Dyspnœa occurs (*a*) with the rapid extension in both lungs of a broncho-pneumonia; (*b*) with the occurrence of miliary tuberculosis; (*c*) sometimes with pneumothorax; (*d*) in old cases with much emphysema, and it may be associated with cyanosis; (*e*) in cases with marked adhesions to the diaphragm interfering with its action; (*f*) and, lastly, in long-standing cases, with contracted apices or great thickening of the pleura, the right heart is enlarged, and the dyspnœa may be cardiac.

General Symptoms.—*Fever.*—It is well to bear in mind that the temperature varies slightly in normal individuals, and the afternoon range may be 99°, 99.5° or even 100° F. The difference between the mouth and rectal temperature may be a full degree, and in young full-blooded persons, in the nervous, and after exercise the normal rectal temperature may be 100.5° or even 101° F. To get a correct idea of the temperature range in pulmonary tuberculosis it is necessary to make observations every two hours at first. The usual 8 A. M. and 8 P. M. record is, in a majority of the cases, very deceptive, giving neither the minimum nor maximum. The former usually occurs between 2 and 6 A. M., and the latter between 2 and 6 P. M.

Fever, one of the earliest and most important symptoms, is due to the effect on the heat centres of the toxins or materials absorbed from the tuberculous focus. Later in the disease the hectic fever is caused in part by the absorption of the bacterial products of other organisms. From a small spot of disease not a sufficient amount of toxin may be produced to disturb the body metabolism, but in the lymph glands, lungs, and bones, from progressing areas of infection sufficient absorption takes place to cause fever. It is an auto-inoculation comparable with the fever produced by an injection of tuberculin. Anything that stimulates the local lymph and blood flow favors the discharge of the toxins and causes fever. A patient at rest may be afebrile; after exercise the temperature may be 102.5°, due to an auto-inoculation. In acute cases the fever is more or less continuous, resembling that of typhoid fever or pneumonia, with slight morning remissions. It may set in with a chill and be followed by sweats, and there are cases with a marked intermittent pyrexia from the onset. As a rule, the degree of activity of the local process may be gauged by the persistency and the range of the fever; and favorable cases are those in which the temperature yields rapidly to rest. In a few cases progress of the local disease continues and may even be rapid without fever. The temperature of consumptives is easily influenced by trivial causes which would not affect a normal person, such as mental excitement, exercise, constipation, etc. The patient is usually aware when fever is present and may feel more comfortable with a temperature of 101°. Except the sweating, there are rarely any unpleasant feelings connected with it.

With breaking down of the lung-tissue and formation of cavities, associated as these processes always are with suppuration and mixed infection, the fever assumes a characteristically intermittent or hectic type. For a large part of the day the patient is not only afebrile, but the temperature is subnormal. In the annexed two-hourly chart, from a case of chronic tuberculosis of the lungs, it will be seen that, from 10 P. M. to 8 A. M. or noon, the temperature continuously fell and went as low as 95°. A slow rise then took place through the late morning and early afternoon hours and reached its maximum between 6 and 10 P. M. As shown in the chart, there were in the three days about forty-three hours of pyrexia and twenty-nine hours of apyrexia. The rapid fall of the temperature in the early morning hours is usually associated with sweating. This hectic, as it is called, which is a typical fever of septic infection, is met with when the process of cavity formation and softening is advanced and extending.

Sweating—Drenching perspirations are common and are one of the most distressing features of the disease. They occur usually with the drop in the fever in the early morning, or at any time in the day when the patient sleeps. They may come on early in the disease, but are more persistent and frequent after cavities have formed. Some patients escape altogether.

The *pulse* is increased in frequency and usually in proportion to the height of the fever. Even when at rest and afebrile the pulse may be rapid, but the excitement of counting it may increase the rate 20 to 30 beats. The pulse is often remarkably full, soft and compressible; even after recovery it may remain rapid. Pulsation may sometimes be seen in the capillaries and in the veins on the back of the hand.

Emaciation is a pronounced feature, from which the two common names of the disease have been derived. The loss of weight is gradual and, if the disease is extending, progressive. The scales give one of the best indications of the progress of the patient. It is most rapid early in the disease, when the patient may lose at the rate of five or six pounds a week; and usually is in direct relation to the intensity and duration of the fever. With the arrest of the progress and the fall in temperaure the patient usually begins to regain

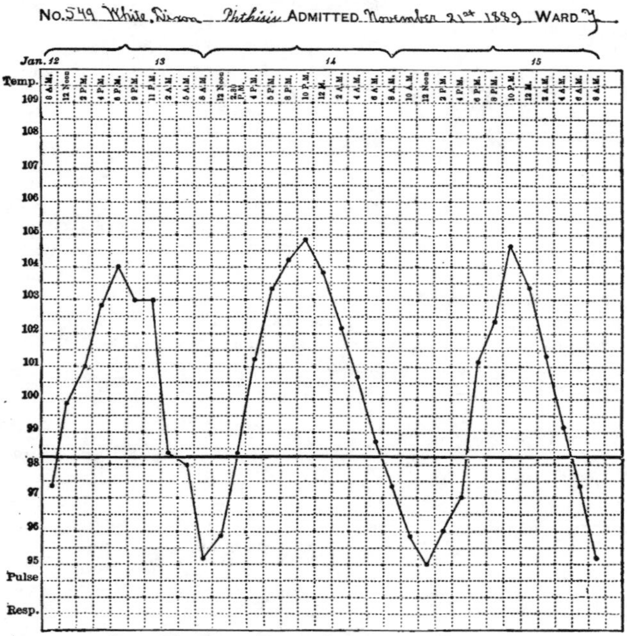

CHART V.—THREE DAYS. CHRONIC TUBERCULOSIS.

weight. The average gain in weight of 901 patients at the Adirondack Sanatorium was fourteen pounds (L. Brown). A gain of two pounds a week is satisfactory. Loss of strength may be out of proportion to and quite independent of loss of weight. Early debility may be a marked feature.

PHYSICAL SIGNS.—(*a*) *Inspection.*—The shape of the chest is often suggestive, though it is to be remembered that the disease may be met with in chests of any build. Practically, however, in a considerable proportion of cases the thorax is long and narrow, with very wide intercostal spaces, the ribs more vertical in direction, and the costal angle very narrow. The scapulæ are "winged," a point noted by Hippocrates. Another type of chest which is very common is that which is flattened in the antero-posterior diameter. The costal cartilages may be prominent and the sternum depressed. Occasionally the lower sternum forms a deep concavity, the so-called funnel breast (*Trichter-Brust*). Special examination should be made of the clavicular regions to see if one clavicle stands out more distinctly than the other, or if the spaces above or below it are more marked. Defective expansion at one apex is an early and important sign. The condition of expansion of the lower zone of the thorax may be well estimated by inspection. The condition of the præcordia should also be noted, as a wide area of impulse, particularly in the second, third, and fourth interspaces, often results from disease of the left apex. From a point behind the patient, looking over the shoulders, one can often better estimate the relative expansion of the apices. Atrophy of the muscles of the shoulder-girdle on the affected side is not uncommon, and a slight scoliosis may be present. Movement may be restricted on the affected side, particularly at the apex. Pleurisy with adhesions or with effusion, fibrosis, and pneumonic consolidation may limit the movement of one side. The Litten phenomenon (seen best on the right side) may be restricted in extent or absent. The chest expansion may be much reduced. It should be recorded carefully at the first examination.

(*b*) *Palpation.*—Deficiency in expansion at the apices or bases is perhaps best gauged by placing the hands in the subclavicular spaces and then in the lateral regions of the chest and asking the patient to draw slowly a full breath. Standing behind the patient and placing the thumbs in the supraclavicular and the fingers in the infraclavicular spaces one can judge accurately as to the relative mobility of the two sides. Disease at an apex, though early and before dulness is at all marked, may be indicated by deficient expansion. The tactile fremitus is increased wherever there is local growth of tubercle or extensive caseation. In comparing the apices it is important to bear in mind that normally the fremitus is stronger over the right than the left. In the later stages, when cavities form, the tactile fremitus is usually much exaggerated over them. When the pleura is greatly thickened the fremitus may be diminished.

(*c*) *Percussion.*—Tubercles, inflammatory products, fibroid changes, and cavities produce important changes in the pulmonary resonance. There may be localized disease, even of some extent, without inducing much alteration, as when the tubercles are scattered there is air-containing tissue between them. In incipient cases percussion may be negative, 28 out of 201 in L. Brown's series. It requires a fair-sized area of infiltration to cause a change in the percussion note, 4 x 6 cm., according to Cornet. One of the earliest and most valuable signs is defective resonance upon and above a clavicle. In a considerable proportion of all cases the dulness is first noted in these regions. The comparison between the two sides should be made also when the breath is held after a full inspiration, as the defective resonance may then be more clearly marked. In the early stages the percussion note is usually higher in pitch, and it may require an experienced ear to detect the difference. In recent consolidation from caseous pneumonia the percussion note often has a tympanitic quality. A wooden dulness is rarely heard except in old cases with extensive fibroid change at the apex or base. Over large, thin-walled cavities at the apex the so-called cracked-pot sound may be obtained. Percussion should be carefully done in the supraspinous fossæ and the interscapular space, as they correspond to very important areas early involved in the disease. By light percussion along the border of the trapezius and in the supraclavicular and supraspinous fossæ, areas of apical resonance may be mapped out (Kronig's apical resonance zones). Under normal conditions the areas are equal on the two sides. Consolidation or retraction of an apex causes definite narrowing of the zone on the affected side. The procedure requires considerable skill. It gives valuable information in the early stage of infiltration. Goldscheider uses a special pleximeter and percusses out the borders of the apex of the lung projecting above the clavicle. The method is less satisfactory than that of Kronig. In cases with numerous isolated cavities at the apex, without much fibroid tissue or thickening of the pleura, the percussion note may show little change, and the contrast between the signs obtained on auscultation and percussion is most marked. In the direct percussion of the chest, particularly in thin patients over the pectorals, one frequently sees the phenomenon known as *myoidema,* a local contraction of the muscle causing bulging, which persists for a variable period and gradually subsides. It has no special significance.

(*d*) *Auscultation.*—Feeble breath-sounds are among the most characteristic early signs, since not as much air enters the tubes and vesicles of the affected area. It is well at first always to compare carefully the corresponding points on the two sides of the chest without asking the patient either to draw a deep breath or to cough. With early apical disease the inspiration on quiet breathing may be scarcely audible. Expiration is usually prolonged. On the other hand, there are cases in which the earliest sign is a harsh, rude, respiratory murmur. On deep breathing it is frequently to be noted that inspiration is jerking or wavy, the so-called "cog-wheel" rhythm; which, however, is by no means confined to tuberculosis. With extension of the disease the inspiratory murmur is harsh, and, when consolidation occurs, whiffing and bronchial. With these changes in the character of the murmur there are râles. The patient should first breathe quietly, then take a full breath, and then cough. When heard with quiet breathing, if they persist and are present in one area only, they are of great importance. The fine rustling crepitus at one or both apices which is heard when the patient first takes a deep breath is of no moment. It may also be present at the bases. Râles at the end of deep inspiration which disappear on repeated breathing may also be disregarded. Râles which are brought out by coughing (most useful during expiration), which persist, and are repeatedly heard at the same spot are of the greatest importance. It is of equal import when moist, clicking râles are present with change in the percussion note. Attention to these rules will save many of the unnecessary diagnoses of pulmonary tuberculosis made on auscultatory signs alone.

When softening occurs the râles are louder and have a bubbling, sometimes a characteristic clicking quality. These "moist sounds," as they are called, when associated with change in the percussion resonance are extremely suggestive. When cavities form the râles are louder, more gurgling, and resonant in quality. When there is consolidation of any extent the breath sounds are tubular, and in the large excavations loud and cavernous, or have an amphoric quality. In the unaffected portions of the lobe and in the opposite lung the breath sounds may be harsh and even puerile. The vocal resonance is usually increased in all stages of the process, and bronchophony and pectoriloquy are met with in the regions of consolidation and over cavities. Pleuritic friction may be present at any stage and, as mentioned before, occurs very early. There are cases in which it is a marked feature throughout. When the lappet of lung over the heart is involved there may be a pleuro-pericardial friction, and when this area is consolidated there may be curious clicking râles synchronous with the heart-beat, due to the compression by the heart of this portion with expulsion of air from it. An interesting auscultatory sign met with in thin-chested persons, in nervous patients, and often in early pulmonary tuberculosis is the so-called cardio-respiratory murmur, a whiffing systolic bruit due to the propulsion of air out of the tubes by the impulse of the heart. It is best heard during inspiration and in the antero-lateral regions of the chest.

A systolic murmur is frequently heard in the subclavian artery on either side, the pulsation of which may be very visible. The murmur is in all probability due to pressure on the vessels by the thickened pleura.

The signs of cavity may be here briefly enumerated.

(1) When there is not much thickening of the pleura or condensation of the surrounding lung-tissue, the percussion sound may be full and clear, resembling the normal note. More commonly there is defective resonance or a tympanitic quality which may at times be purely amphoric. The pitch of the percussion note changes over a cavity when the mouth is opened or closed (Wintrich's sign), or it may be brought out more clearly on change of position. The cracked-pot sound is obtainable over tolerably large cavities with thin walls or when one cavity is above another. It is best elicited by a firm, quick stroke, the patient at the time having the mouth open. In those rare instances of almost total excavation of one lung the percussion note may be amphoric in quality. (2) On auscultation the so-called cavernous sounds are heard: (i) Various grades of modified breathing—blowing or tubular, cavernous or amphoric. There may be a curiously sharp hissing sound, as if the air was passing from a narrow opening into a wide space. In very large cavities both inspiration and expiration may be typically amphoric. (ii) There are coarse bubbling râles which have a resonant quality, and on coughing may have a metallic or ringing character. On coughing they are often loud and gurgling. In very large thin-walled cavities, and more rarely in medium-sized cavities, surrounded by recent consolidation, the râles may have a distinctly amphoric echo, simulating those of pneumothorax. There are dry cavities in which no râles are heard. (iii) The vocal resonance is greatly intensified, and whispered bronchophony is clearly heard. In large apical cavities the heart-sounds are well heard, and occasionally there may be an intense systolic murmur, probably always transmitted to, and not produced, as has been supposed, in the cavity itself. In large excavations of the left apex the heart impulse may cause gurgling sounds or clicks synchronous with the systole. They may even be loud enough to be heard at a little distance from the chest wall. A large cavity with smooth walls and thin fluid contents may give the succussion sound when the trunk is abruptly shaken (Walshe), and even the coin sound may be obtained.

Pseudo-cavernous signs may be caused by an area of consolidation near a large bronchus. The condition may be most deceptive—the high-pitched or tympanitic percussion note, the tubular or cavernous breathing, and the resonant râles simulate closely the signs of cavity.

3. *Fibroid Tuberculosis*

In their monograph on Fibroid Diseases of the Lung, Clark, Hadley, and Chaplin make the following classification: 1. Pure fibroid—a condition in which there is no tubercle. 2. Tuberculo-fibroid disease—a condition primarily tuberculous, but which has run a fibroid course. 3. Fibro-tuberculous disease—a condition primarily fibroid, but which has become tuberculous. The tuberculo-fibroid form may come on gradually as a sequence of a chronic tuberculous broncho-pneumonia or follow a chronic tuberculous pleurisy. In other instances the process supervenes upon ordinary ulcerative tuberculosis. The disease becomes limited to one apex, the cavity is surrounded by layers of dense fibrous tissue, the pleura is thickened, and the lower lobe is gradually invaded by the sclerotic change. Ultimately a picture is produced little if at all different from the condition known as cirrhosis of the lungs. It may even be difficult to say that the process is tuberculous, but in advanced cases the bacilli are usually present in the walls of the cavity at the apex, or old, encapsulated caseous areas are present, or there may be tubercles at the apex of the other lung and in the bronchial glands. Dilatation of the bronchi is present; the right ventricle, sometimes the entire heart, is hypertrophied.

The disease is chronic, lasting from ten to twenty or more years, during which time the patient may have fair health. The chief symptoms are cough, often paroxysmal in character and most marked in the morning, and dyspnœa on exertion. The expectoration is purulent, and in some instances, when the bronchiectasis is extensive, fetid. There is rarely any fever.

The physical signs are very characteristic. The chest is sunken and the shoulder lower on the affected side; the heart is often drawn over and displaced. If the left lung is involved there may be an unusually large area of cardiac pulsation in the third, fourth, and fifth interspaces. Heart murmurs are common. There are dulness and deficient tactile fremitus over the affected side, except over cavities where fremitus is increased. At the apex there may be well-marked cavernous sounds; at the base, distant bronchial breathing. In some cases the other lung becomes involved, or the patient has repeated attacks of hæmoptysis, in one of which he dies. As a result of the chronic suppuration, amyloid degeneration may take place; dropsy frequently supervenes from failure of the right heart.

A more detailed account is found under Cirrhosis of the Lung, with which this form is clinically identical.

Complications of Pulmonary Tuberculosis

In the Respiratory System.—The larynx is rarely spared in chronic pulmonary tuberculosis. The first symptom may be huskiness of the voice. There are pain, particularly in swallowing, and a cough which is often wheezing, and in the later stages very ineffectual. Aphonia and dysphagia are the two most distressing symptoms of the laryngeal involvement. When the epiglottis is seriously diseased and the ulceration extends to the lateral wall of the pharynx, the pain in swallowing may be very intense, or, owing to the imperfect closure of the glottis, there may be coughing spells and regurgitation of food through the nostrils. Bronchitis and tracheitis are almost invariable accompaniments.

Pneumonia is a not infrequent complication of pulmonary tuberculosis. It may run a perfectly normal course, while in other instances resolution may be delayed, and one is in doubt, in spite of the abruptness of the onset, as to the presence of a simple or a tuberculous pneumonia. In some cases a pneumonia is a terminal complication.

Emphysema of the uninvolved portions of the lung is common, rarely producing any special symptoms. There are, however, cases of chronic tuberculosis in which emphysema dominates the picture, and in which the condition comes on slowly during a period of many years. General subcutaneous emphysema, met with in a few rare cases, is due either to perforation of the trachea or to the rupture of a cavity adherent to the chest wall.

Gangrene of the lung is an occasional event, due in almost all instances to sphacelus in the walls of the cavity, rarely in the lung-tissue itself.

Complications in the Pleura.—A dry pleurisy is a very common accompaniment of the early stages of tuberculosis. It is always a conservative, useful process. In some cases it is very extensive, and friction murmurs may be heard over the sides and back. The cases with dry pleurisy and adhesions are, of course, much less liable to the dangers of pneumothorax. Pleurisy with effusion more commonly precedes than occurs in the course of pulmonary tuberculosis. Still, it is common enough to meet with cases in which a serofibrinous effusion arises in the course of the chronic disease. There are cases in which it is a special feature, and it seems to favor chronicity. A patient may during a period of four or five years have signs of local disease at one apex with recurring effusion in the same side. Owing to adhesions in different parts of the pleura, the effusion may be encapsulated. Hæmorrhagic effusions, not uncommon in connection with tuberculous pleurisy, are comparatively rare in pulmonary tuberculosis. Chyliform or milky exudates are sometimes found. Purulent effusions are not frequent apart from pneumothorax. An empyema, however, may occur in the course of the disease or as a sequence of a serofibrinous exudate. *Pneumothorax* is an extremely common complication. Of 49 cases at the Johns Hopkins Hospital, 23 were tuberculous (Emerson). It may prove fatal in twenty-four hours. In other instances a pyo-pneumothorax follows and the patient lingers for weeks or months. In a third group of cases it seems to have a beneficial effect and is sometimes produced for the therapeutic effect.

Symptoms Referable to the Other Organs.—(*a*) *Cardio-vascular.*—The retraction of the left upper lobe exposes a large area of the heart. In thin-chested subjects there may be pulsation in the second, third, and fourth interspaces close to the sternum. Sometimes with much retraction of the left upper lobe the heart is drawn up. A systolic murmur over the pulmonary area and in the subclavian arteries is common in all stages. Apical murmurs are not infrequent and may be extremely rough and harsh without necessarily indicating that endocarditis is present. The association of heart disease with tuberculosis is not, however, very uncommon. There were 12 instances of endocarditis in 216 autopsies. The arterial tension is usually low and the capillary resistance lessened so that the pulse is often full and soft even in the later stages. The capillary pulse is not infrequently found, and pulsation of the veins in the back of the hand is occasionally seen.

(*b*) *Blood.*—The early anæmia is often more apparent than real, and the blood-count rarely sinks below two millions per c. mm. The blood-plates are, as a rule, enormously increased and are seen in the withdrawn blood as the so-called Schultze's granule masses. Without any significance, they are of interest chiefly from the fact that every few years some tyro announces their discovery as a new diagnostic sign of tuberculosis. The leucocytes are greatly increased, particularly in the later stages.

(*c*) *Gastro-intestinal System.*—The tongue is usually furred, but may be clean and red. Small aphthous ulcers are sometimes distressing. A red line on the gums, a symptom to which at one time much attention was paid as a special feature of tuberculosis, occurs in other cachectic states. Extensive tuberculous disease of the pharynx, associated with a similar affection of the larynx, may interfere seriously with deglutition and prove a very distressing and intractable symptom. The saliva has full digestive powers.

Tuberculosis of the stomach is rare. Ulceration may occur as an accidental complication and multiple catarrhal ulcers are not uncommon. Interstitial and parenchymatous changes in the mucosa are common (possibly associated with the venous stasis) and lead to atrophy, but these cannot always be connected with the symptoms, and they may be found when not expected. On the other hand, when the gastric symptoms have been most persistent the mucosa may show very little change. It is impossible always to refer the anorexia, nausea, and vomiting of consumption to local conditions. The hectic fever and the neurotic influences must be taken into account, as they play an important rôle. There is interference with both the secretory and motor functions early in the course. Hyperacidity is rare (Mohler and Funk).

Anorexia is often a marked symptom at the onset; there may be positive loathing for food, and even small quantities cause nausea. Sometimes, without any nausea or distress after eating, the feeding of the patient is a daily battle. When practicable, forced alimentation is of great benefit in such cases. Nausea and vomiting, though occasionally troublesome at an early period, are more marked in the later stages. The latter may be caused by the severe attacks of coughing. S. H. Habershon refers to four causes of vomiting: (1) central, as from tuberculous meningitis; (2) pressure on the vagi by caseous glands; (3) stimulation from the peripheral branches of the vagus, either pulmonary, pharyngeal, or gastric; and (4) mechanical causes.

Of the *intestinal* symptoms diarrhœa is the most serious. It may come on early, but is more usually a symptom of the later stages, and is associated with ulceration, particularly of the large bowel. Extensive ulceration of the ileum may exist without any diarrhœa. The associated catarrhal condition may account in part for it, and in some instances the amyloid degeneration of the mucous membrane. Perforation occurred in 13 of 475 autopsies in chronic pulmonary tuberculosis.

(*d*) *Nervous System.*—(1) *Focal lesions* due to the development of coarse tubercles and areas of tuberculous meningo-encephalitis. Aphasia, for instance, may result from the growth of meningeal tubercles in the fissure of Sylvius, or even hemiplegia may occur. The solitary tubercles are more common in the chronic tuberculosis of children. (2) *Basilar meningitis* is an occasional complication. It may be confined to the brain, though more commonly it is a (3) *cerebro-spinal meningitis,* which may come on in persons without well-marked local signs in the chest so that the existence of pulmonary disease is not discovered until the post mortem. (4) *Peripheral neuritis,* which is not common, may cause an extensor paralysis of the arm or leg, more commonly the latter, with foot-drop. It is usually a late manifestation. (5) The *brachial plexus,* close to the pleuro-pulmonary apex, is sometimes involved, either by adhesion to the tuberculous glands in the neighborhood or in the thickening of the tissues about the pleura itself. There may be pains in the arm, trophic disturbances and occasionally paralysis, particularly in the distribution of the lower cord in the plexus. (6) Mental symptoms. It was noted, even by the older writers, that consumptives had a peculiarly hopeful temperament, and the *spes phthisica* forms a curious characteristic of the disease. Patients with extensive cavities, high fever, and too weak to move will often make plans for the future and confidently expect to recover.

Apart from tuberculosis of the brain, there is sometimes in chronic tuberculosis a form of insanity not unlike that which occurs in the convalescence from acute affections.

(*e*) *Eyes.*—The conjunctiva is rarely involved. Iritis may occur and not always of the tuberculous variety. The pupils are often unduly dilated. With the common apical pleurisy, irregularity of the pupils may be present. Myosis with narrowing of the palpebral fissure and retraction of the eye or mydriasis with associated vaso-motor features may be found with small lesions of the apex with pleural involvement.

(*f*) *Hypertrophy of the mammary gland* may occur in pulmonary tuberculosis, most commonly in males. It may be only on the affected side. It is a chronic interstitial, non-tuberculous mammitis (Allot). Mastitis adolescentium, not very uncommon, is not necessarily suggestive of pulmonary tuberculosis.

(*g*) *Genito-urinary System.*—The urine presents no special peculiarities in amount or constituents. Fever, however, has a marked influence upon it. Albumin is met with frequently and may be associated with the fever, or is the result of definite changes in the kidneys. Tubercle bacilli may be present without any disease of the kidney. Amyloid disease of the kidneys is not uncommon. Its presence is shown by albumin and tube casts, and sometimes by a great increase in the amount of urine. In other instances there is dropsy, and the patients have all the characteristic features of chronic nephritis.

Pus in the urine may be due to disease of the bladder or of the pelves of the kidneys. In some instances the entire urinary tract is involved. In pulmonary tuberculosis, however, extensive tuberculous disease is rarely found in the urinary organs. Bacilli may occasionally be detected in the urine. Hæmaturia is not a very common symptom. It may occur occasionally as a result of congestion of the kidneys, and pass off, leaving the urine albuminous. In other instances it results from disease of the pelvis or of the bladder, and is associated either with early tuberculosis of the mucous membranes or more commonly with ulceration. In a medical clinic the routine inspection of the testes for tubercle will save two or three mistakes a year.

(*h*) *Cutaneous System.*—The skin is often dry and harsh. Local tubercles occasionally occur on the hands. There may be pigmentary staining, the *chloasma phthisicorum,* which is more common when the peritoneum is involved. Upon the chest and the back the brown stains of *pityriasis versicolor* are very frequent. The hair of the head and beard may become dry and lanky. The terminal phalanges, in chronic cases, become clubbed and the nails incurvated—the Hippocratic fingers. Landouzy called attention to a curious bending, usually of the ring and little fingers, which permits of flexion, but not of extension—a condition which he calls camptodactaly. A remarkable and unusual complication is general emphysema, which may result from ulceration of an adherent lung or perforation of the larynx.

Diagnosis of Pulmonary Tuberculosis

With fever, well-marked physical signs and bacilli in the sputum, no disease is more easily diagnosed. Successful treatment depends largely upon early diagnosis, and special attention must be paid to the obscure, variable, and uncertain symptoms and signs of the initial stage. The active crusade against the disease has made both the public and the profession more alert, and we have, as so often happens, gone to an extreme, and are apt to see early tuberculosis in trivial complaints. This is based on the experience of cases seen in consultation, and is borne out by the records of institutions. Hamman, in charge of the Phipps Tuberculosis Dispensary of the Johns Hopkins Hospital, makes the interesting confession that in the early days, when they depended on slight physical signs and the tuberculin reaction, there were innumerable early cases, but with a wider experience and greater confidence in clinical symptoms the outlook on these borderland cases has changed completely, and they are found to keep well under the ordinary conditions of life, in spite of the persistence of slight abnormal signs. How important this feature of tuberculosis work has become is also indicated by the figures for the first year at the Tuberculosis Dispensary of the Radcliffe Infirmary. Of the 580 cases, all sent by physicians, 243 were found not to be tuberculous! One lesson from the work of the past few years is that we should pay more attention to symptoms than to physical signs. The following are the points of special importance in the diagnosis of early cases:

History.—Tuberculosis in the family, "Phthisical habitus," unusual exposure to infection, special debilitating circumstances, as worry, grief, dissipation, or a chronic illness.

Symptoms.—Loss of weight, loss of strength, marked nervous and physical exhaustion, and anæmia, if progressive and not otherwise accounted for, are of first importance. Fever is at once a most trustworthy and the most fallacious symptom. The thermometer has needlessly condemned many patients to the sanatorium. Regard should be had to the points already mentioned in speaking of the fever. In nervous persons, particularly in stout, flabby young girls, a temperature from 99.5° to 100.5° may mean nothing, and the rectal temperature is often very deceptive: if taken after exercise or excitement it may be a degree and a half above normal. In the case of a flabby, fat girl of ten, with an anxious mother, a foolish nurse, and an alarmist doctor, for months the rectal temperature was taken hourly during the day; the child had been in bed; there was no cough, and the only physical sign a few rustling râles at one apex. The *cure* followed rapidly on the breaking of the thermometer and getting rid of the nurse. In a suspicious case a two-hour temperature record should be taken during the day for ten days and the influence of exercise upon it carefully estimated.

A *cough* is always suspicious in the young, more in the winter than in the summer, and more in the morning than at other times in the day. Throat and sinus conditions should be carefully excluded, particularly the irritation from cigarette smoking. The spitting of blood has been considered and its importance in the diagnosis of tuberculosis is universally recognised. A brisk, early hæmoptysis is often helpful, not only for the positive information it gives us, but for its useful moral effect on the patient. The greater the care with which the bloody sputum is examined the more likely will it be that bacilli are found.

Sputum.—The patient should be instructed to collect what is expectorated, particularly early in the morning, and everything brought up should be sent. The difficulty in private practice is that it requires a long series of examinations to exclude positively the presence of tubercle bacilli. Time and again with suspicious cases, or in pleurisy with effusion, the clinical clerk has been asked day by day "Any bacilli yet?", and in one instance there were none found until the twentieth examination! Of course, in private practice this is impossible, but it is well to bear in mind that one or two negative examinations are not sufficient. Various methods of digesting the sputum and examining the centrifugalized sediment are important when few bacilli are present. The antiformin method introduced by Uhlenhuth is simple and often reveals tubercle bacilli missed by an ordinary examination.

Physical Signs.—These raise the difficulty. At present, so far as the lungs are concerned, the position resembles that of twenty-five years ago in respect to the heart, when any murmur was regarded as serious. Now, if we see the apex beat within the nipple line and there is no shortness of breath, and the pulse is regular, we discount physical signs and tell the patient to live a rational life. This is what we should do with many cases of suspected early tuberculosis. If the symptoms above dealt with are not present, "discount" the physical signs. These have already been considered: change in the character of the respiratory murmur and the presence of râles are the two most important, as dulness is rarely present in early cases. Altogether too much stress has been laid upon roughened or impure inspiration associated with a few dry râles. Only upon repeated examination should a decision be reached. Practically, in these early cases, we have two groups—the one with symptoms and no physical signs, and the other with physical signs and no symptoms. Of the two, the former is of the greater importance.

In regard to the extent of disease in the lung, caution is advisable in patients seen for the first time with fever and acute symptoms. Signs may be found over a large area, but these may be due principally to an acute intercurrent infection and lessen materially in a few days.

Certain conditions may be *wrongly diagnosed as tuberculous.* Foreign bodies in the bronchi may be a cause of error. In patients with infection of the mouth or throat, tonsillitis, sinusitis, and adenoids, there may be a persistent cough with bronchitis and fever. Recognition and proper treatment of the cause may result in the prompt disappearance of the pulmonary signs. In some cases these non-tuberculous infections may cause some fibroid change. There are certain non-tuberculous chronic bronchial and pulmonary diseases which may be mistaken for tuberculosis. Actinomycosis, streptothrix infection, syphilis, chronic bronchitis, and bronchiectasis are in this group. It is a good rule that with signs of advanced chronic disease in the lungs and no tubercle bacilli in the sputum, the condition is not likely to be tuberculous. A diagnosis of tuberculosis based on *marked* lung changes without finding tubercle bacilli in the sputum is often wrong. Atypical forms of pneumonia, disease of the pleura, especially apical, cardiac disease and aneurism may lead one astray.

Specific Reaction.—*Tuberculin Test.*—The experience of observers in different parts of the world testifies to its value. But we must remember the reaction simply means that the organism has developed a responsive activity to tuberculous infection, and by no means indicates that an individual has tuberculous disease, in the ordinary sense of the term "disease." From the studies made at the Phipps Dispensary, the conjunctival test was found of greater value in indicating the presence of an active lesion. The following conclusions reached by Hamman and his colleagues appear to be sane: "When a patient fails to react to either test, and there are no striking symptoms or physical signs of pulmonary disease, we feel that the negative diagnosis has received a valuable confirmation. If the eye reaction is positive, this is a strong indication that the patient has an active tuberculous focus; if symptoms and signs are present it is an important aid in excluding other pulmonary conditions; if they are absent it marks the patient as a suspect. * * * None of these tests can replace in the slightest degree a carefully taken history and a well-made examination. They can never stand censor over these; rather their value must ultimately be adjudged by them. They are aids and nothing more."

While the cutaneous and conjunctival are the more important as a routine procedure, still in special instances in which it is desired to elicit a focal reaction the subcutaneous tuberculin test is invaluable.

Complement fixation Test.—This may be of much value in doubtful cases as it is usually positive in active tuberculosis. Several negative tests are important and it is useful in deciding as to the arrest of the disease.

X-ray Diagnosis.—In skilful hands the study of cases with the Röntgen rays is of great value. In a normal case the radiogram shows a shadow beneath and extending beyond the sternum due to the contents of the mediastinum. Extending from the mediastinum and radiating out into the various lobes is a series of shadows which may be likened to the branches of a tree, the thickest shadow being at the hilus and thinning toward the periphery of the lungs. In diseased conditions changes are seen in the hilus, shadows due to enlarged or calcified glands and to the increase in the fibrous and lymphatic tissues in the mediastinum. The pulmonary vessels with their contained blood play an important part in the production of the shadow. The X-rays undoubtedly show very early changes in the lungs, but they can not always determine the etiological factor. In the majority of cases the X-rays tell no more than a careful clinical examination, and they do not differentiate an active from a healed lesion. More than any others, radiographers need the salutary lessons of the dead house to correct their visionary interpretations of shadows, particularly of those radiating from the roots of the lungs.

Concurrent Infections and Diseases Associated with Pulmonary Tuberculosis

Concurrent Infections in Pulmonary Tuberculosis.—It has long been known that in pulmonary tuberculosis organisms other than the specific bacilli are present, particularly the pneumococcus, *Streptococcus pyogenes,* the influenza bacillus, *Micrococcus catarrhalis,* and *Staphylococcus aureus;* less frequently *Bacillus pyocyaneus.*

Many cases of pulmonary tuberculosis are combined infections; streptococci and pneumococci may be found in the sputum, and the former have been isolated from the blood. Prudden arrives at the following conclusions: The pulmonary lesions of tuberculosis are subject to variations depending largely on the different modes of distribution of the bacilli, whether by the blood vessels or through the bronchi, and also whether a concurrent infection with other organisms has taken place. The pneumonia complicating tuberculosis may be the direct result of the tubercle bacillus or its toxins, or it may follow secondary infection with other germs, particularly the *Streptococcus pyogenes,* the *Micrococcus lanceolatus,* and the *Staphylococcus pyogenes.* An infection with the influenza bacillus or *Micrococcus catarrhalis* may be followed by increased fever and an aggravation of the general symptoms. The frequency of these secondary infections and the relative significance of their germs are not fully decided. It is probable that in man the effect of contamination with the pus organisms is important in hastening necrosis and softening, and also in the chronic cases they doubtless produce in large amounts the toxins which are responsible for many of the symptoms. The work of Hastings indicates that secondary infections are not so important as we had thought, and a study by Radcliffe at the King Edward Sanatorium points in this direction.

Diseases Associated with Pulmonary Tuberculosis.—*Lobar pneumonia* is a not uncommon cause of death. It is met with as a terminal event in the chronic cases or may occur early, and be difficult to distinguish from an acute caseous pneumonia. The sputum in the latter is rarely rusty, while the fever in the former is more continuous and higher, but in many cases it is impossible to differentiate between the two conditions.

The association of tuberculosis and *typhoid fever* has been discussed.

Erysipelas not infrequently attacks old *poitrinaires* in hospital wards and almshouses. There are instances in which the attack seems to be beneficial, as the cough lessens and the symptoms ameliorate. It may prove fatal.

Erythema nodosum.—Some regard it as a symptom of the disease, a "tuberculide" as the French call it. Guinea pigs have been successfully inoculated from the lesions but clinically we rarely see any definite association.

The *eruptive fevers,* particularly measles, frequently precede but rarely occur in the course of pulmonary tuberculosis. In the revaccination of a tuberculous subject the vesicles run a normal course.

Fistula in ano, so often associated with pulmonary tuberculosis, in a majority of such cases is a tuberculous process. The general affection may progress rapidly after an operation.

Heart Disease.—Cardiac hypoplasia seems uncommon in tuberculosis, though it was much referred to by the older writers. It was present in only 3 cases in 1,764 autopsies on tuberculous patients (Norris). Rokitansky taught that there was an antagonism between valvular lesions and aneurisms and tuberculosis. All forms of congenital heart disease predispose to it, particularly stenosis of the pulmonary artery. Mitral stenosis, on the other hand, has a distinctly inhibitory influence. The two conditions are rarely found associated. Endocarditis has already been mentioned. A terminal acute tuberculosis, particularly of the serous membranes, is not at all uncommon in cardio-vascular diseases.

In chronic and arrested tuberculosis *arterio-sclerosis* and *phlebo-sclerosis* are not uncommon. Ormerod noted 30 cases of chronic renal disease in 100 post mortems.

Diabetes mellitus.—Among 31,834 cases of tuberculosis there were 151 with glycosuria, and in 1047 autopsies there were 6 cases of diabetes mellitus. The association means an unfavorable prognosis.

Cancer—Not often associated with active tuberculosis, many persons dying of cancer show foci of old tuberculosis. There does not seem to be any active antagonism between the diseases.

Peculiarities of Pulmonary Tuberculosis at the Extremes of Life

Old Age.—It is remarkable how common tuberculosis is in the aged, particularly in institutions. McLachlan noted 145 cases in which tuberculosis was the cause of death in old persons in Chelsea Hospital. All were over sixty years of age. The experience at the Salpêtrière is the same. Laennec met with a case in a person over ninety-nine years of age.

At the Philadelphia Hospital, in the bodies of aged persons sent over from the almshouse, it was extremely common to find either old or recent tuberculosis. One patient died at the age of eighty-two with extensive peritoneal tuberculosis. Pulmonary tuberculosis in the aged is usually latent and runs a slow course. The physical signs are often masked by emphysema and by the coëxisting chronic bronchitis. The diagnosis may depend entirely upon the discovery of the bacilli and elastic tissue. Contrary to the opinion which was held some years ago, tuberculosis is by no means uncommon with senile emphysema. Some of the cases of tuberculosis in the aged are instances of quiescent disease which may have dated from an early period.

Infancy.—The occurrence of acute tuberculosis in children has been mentioned, and also that the disease is occasionally congenital. The incidence is variable, from 13 to 42 per cent. in collected statistics. In Wollstein's study from the New York Babies' Hospital, among 1,131 autopsies in children under four years of age, in 192 tuberculosis was present; the percentage was: first year 1.8 per cent., second year 11 per cent., third year 16 per cent., and fourth year 23 per cent. Chronic ulcerative tuberculosis of the lungs is much more rare than in adults. In Parrot's series of 219 cases in children under three years of age, in only 57 were cavities found in the lungs.

Modes of Death in Pulmonary Tuberculosis

(a) By asthenia, a gradual failure of the strength. The end is usually peaceable and quiet, occasionally disturbed by paroxysms of cough. Consciousness is often retained until near the close.

(b) By asphyxia, as in some cases of acute miliary tuberculosis and in acute pneumonic tuberculosis. In chronic pulmonary tuberculosis it is rarely seen, even when pneumothorax develops.

(c) By syncope. This is not common but may happen in patients who insist upon going about when in the advanced stages. There may be, but not necessarily, fatty degeneration of the heart. Rapid syncope may follow hæmorrhage or may be due to thrombosis or embolism of the pulmonary artery, or to pneumothorax.

(d) From hæmorrhage. The fatal bleeding in chronic tuberculosis is due to erosion of a large vessel or rupture of an aneurism in a pulmonary cavity, most commonly the latter. Of 26 cases analyzed by S. West, in 11 the fatal hæmoptysis was due to aneurism, and, of 35 cases collected by Percy Kidd, aneurism was present in 30. In a case of Curtin's, at the Philadelphia Hospital, the bleeding proved fatal before hæmoptysis occurred, as the eroded vessel opened into a capacious cavity.

(e) With cerebral symptoms. Coma may be due to meningitis, less often to uræmia. Death in convulsions is rare. The hæmorrhagic pachy-meningitis which occurs in some cases occasionally causes loss of consciousness, but is rarely a direct cause of death. In one of our cases death resulted from thrombosis of the cerebral sinuses with symptoms of meningitis.

V. TUBERCULOSIS OF THE ALIMENTARY CANAL

(a) Lips.—Tuberculosis of the lip is very rare. It occurs occasionally in the form of an ulcer, either alone or more commonly with laryngeal or pulmonary disease. The ulcer is usually very sensitive and may be mistaken for a chancre or an epithelioma. The diagnosis may be made in cases of doubt by inoculation or the examination of a portion for tubercle bacilli.

(b) Tongue.—The disease begins by an aggregation of small granular bodies on the edge or dorsum. Ulceration proceeds, leaving an irregular sore with a distinct but uneven margin, and a rough, often caseous base. The disease extends slowly and may form an ulcer of considerable size. It may be mistaken for epithelioma and the tongue excised. It is rarely met with except when other organs are involved. The glands of the angle of the jaw are not enlarged and the sore does not yield to iodide of potassium, which are points of distinction between the tuberculous and the syphilitic ulcer. In doubtful cases the inoculation test should be made, or a portion excised for microscopic examination.

(c) Salivary Glands.—The salivary glands belong to that small group of organs of the body which seem to possess an immunity; a very few cases have been reported.

(d) Palate.—Tubercles of the hard or soft palate nearly always follow extension of the disease from neighboring parts.

(e) Tuberculosis of the Tonsils.—In 7 of 45 consecutive cases in children from three months to fifteen years, A. Latham demonstrated, by inoculation, the presence of tuberculosis of the tonsils either in organs removed by operation or post mortem. The observation is of interest in connection with the views of Schlenker, who claims that the majority of the cases of tuberculous cervical glands result from infection with tubercle bacilli which gain admission by way of the tonsil. A large number of his cases of tuberculous cervical adenitis were definitely of a descending variety and associated with tuberculosis of these glands. The majority also had pulmonary tuberculosis, and he regards surface infection of the tonsil by tuberculous food and sputum far more common than infection by way of the circulation. The disease may occur as a superficial ulceration. More commonly there is an infiltration of the tonsil with miliary tubercles, which produces a greater or less hypertrophy which it is practically impossible to distinguish from an ordinary enlargement of the tonsil without a microscopic examination.

(f) **Pharynx.**—In extensive laryngeal tuberculosis an eruption of miliary granules on the posterior wall of the pharynx is not very uncommon. In chronic tuberculosis an ulcerative pharyngitis, due to extension of the disease from the epiglottis and larynx, is a most distressing complication, rendering deglutition acutely painful. Adenoids of the naso-pharynx may be tuberculous, as shown by Lermoyez. Macroscopically, they do not differ from the ordinary vegetations found in this situation.

(g) **Œsophagus.**—A few instances occur in the literature of tuberculosis of the œsophagus. The condition is a pathological curiosity, except in the slight extension from the larynx, which is not infrequent; but in a case described by Flexner, the ulcer perforated and caused purulent pleurisy. The condition has been considered by Claribel Cone, who described a second case from the Johns Hopkins Hospital (Bulletin, Nov., 1897).

(h) **Stomach.**—Many cases are reported which are doubtful. In 2,501 gastric operations at the Mayo Clinic in four years only one instance was found. Broders, in a study of the literature (1917), accepts 49 proved cases, not one of which was primary. Ulcer is the most common lesion and occurred in about 80 per cent. of the cases. Miliary tubercles, pyloric stenosis and the occurrence of a nodule are the other lesions. Perforation of the stomach occurred six times in the 12 cases collected by Marfan, thrice by a tuberculous gland. Three cases were described from the Hopkins clinic by Alice Hamilton (J. H. H. Bulletin, April, 1897).

(i) **Intestines.**—The tubercles may be (1) primary in the mucous membrane, or more commonly (2) secondary to disease of the lungs, or in rare cases the affection may (3) pass from the peritoneum.

(1) Primary intestinal tuberculosis occurs most frequently in children, in whom it may be associated with enlargement and caseation of the mesenteric glands, or with peritonitis. There is great discrepancy in the statistics on this point, and the question needs careful study. Biedert gives 16 cases in 3,104 instances of tuberculosis in children. In adults primary intestinal tuberculosis is rare, occurring in but 1 instance in 1,000 autopsies upon tuberculous adults at the Munich Pathological Institute; but now and then cases occur in which the disease sets in with irregular diarrhœa, moderate fever, and colicky pains. In a few cases hæmorrhage has been the initial symptom. Regarded at first as a chronic catarrh, it is not until the emaciation becomes marked or the signs of disease appear in the lungs that the true nature is apparent. Still more deceptive are the cases in which the tuberculosis begins in the *cæcum* and there are symptoms of appendicitis—tenderness in the right iliac fossa, constipation, or an irregular diarrhœa and fever. These signs may gradually disappear, to recur in a few weeks and still further complicate the diagnosis. Fatal hæmorrhage has occurred. Perforation into the peritoneum

may take place, a pericæcal abscess may form, or in very rare instances there is partial healing with great thickening of the walls and narrowing of the lumen. Tuberculosis of the *appendix* is found in about one per cent. but often can only be diagnosed microscopically. The symptoms are those of a suppurative appendicitis.

(2) Secondary involvement of the bowels is very common in chronic pulmonary tuberculosis, *e. g.*, in 566 of the 1,000 Munich autopsies in tuberculosis. In only three of these cases were the lungs not involved. The lesions are chiefly in the ileum, cæcum, and colon. The affection begins in the solitary and agminated glands, or on the surface of or within the mucosa. The caseation and necrosis lead to ulceration, which may be very extensive and involve the greater portion of the mucosa of the large and small bowels. In the ileum the Peyer's patches are chiefly involved and the ulcers may be ovoid, but in the jejunum and colon they are usually round or transverse to the long axis. The tuberculous ulcer has the following characters: (*a*) It is irregular, rarely ovoid or in the long axis, more frequently girdling the bowel; (*b*) the edges and base are infiltrated, often caseous; (*c*) the submucosa and muscularis are usually involved; and (*d*) on the serosa may be seen colonies of young tubercles or a well-marked tuberculous lymphangitis. Perforation and peritonitis are not uncommon events in the secondary ulceration. Stenosis of the bowel from cicatrization may occur; the strictures may be multiple.

Localized chronic tuberculosis of the *ileo-cæcal region* is of great importance. The cæcum may present a chronic hyperplastic tuberculosis, which not uncommonly extends into the appendix. As a consequence of the changes produced a definite tumor-like mass is formed in the right iliac fossa. This varies in size, is usually elongated in a vertical direction, hard, slightly movable, or bound down by adhesions and very sensitive to pressure. The tumor simulates more or less closely a true neoplasm of this region, particularly carcinoma. The condition is characterized by gradual constriction of the lumen of the bowel, periodic attacks of severe pain, and alternating diarrhœa and constipation. The extremely localized character of the disease warrants an exploratory operation, as the results of enterectomy are favorable. Of 11 cases reported by F. M. Caird, 7 recovered. In a second form of this disease, occurring less frequently, there is no definite tumor mass, but a general induration and thickening in the right iliac fossa similar to the local changes produced by a recurring appendicitis. In this variety a fistula discharging fæcal matter occasionally results. Both forms may be distinguished from the diseases they simulate by the finding of tubercle bacilli in the stools or in the discharge from the fistula when such exists.

Tuberculosis of the *rectum* has a special interest in connection with *fistula in ano*, which occurs in about 3.5 per cent. of cases of pulmonary disease. In many instances the lesion has been shown to be tuberculous. It is very rarely primary, but if the tissue on removal contains bacilli and is infective the lungs are almost invariably involved. It is a common opinion that the pulmonary symptoms progress rapidly after the fistula is cut. This may have some basis if the operation consists in laying the tract open, and not in a free excision.

(3) Extension from the peritoneum may excite tuberculous disease in the bowels. The affection may be primary in the peritoneum or extend from the

tubes in women or the mesenteric glands in children. The coils of intestines become matted together, caseous and suppurating foci develop between the folds, and perforation may take place between the coils.

VI. TUBERCULOSIS OF THE LIVER

This organ is very constantly involved in (*a*) *Miliary tuberculosis.* This is seen in acute generalized tuberculosis, though the granules may be small and have to be looked for very carefully. In chronic tuberculosis miliary tubercles are not at all uncommon in the liver. (*b*) *Solitary tubercle.* Occasionally large tuberculous masses are found, sometimes associated with perihepatitis, sometimes with tuberculous peritonitis, and in children with tuberculous adenitis. In a few cases the masses are large, though it is only in exceptional cases that the tumor can be felt through the abdominal wall. The organ may be enlarged by numerous caseous masses and present the clinical picture of an enlarged rough tender liver with jaundice, as in a case reported by Thayer. The solitary tubercles become infected with pus organisms, soften, and form an abscess. (*c*) *Tuberculosis of the bile ducts.* This is the most characteristic tuberculous change in the organ, and is not uncommon. It was well described by Bristowe in 1858. The liver is enlarged, and section shows numerous small cavities, which look at first like multiple abscesses in suppurative pylephlebitis, but the pus is bile-stained and the whole process is a local tuberculous cholangitis. (*d*) *Tuberculous cirrhosis.* With the eruption of miliary tubercles there may be slight increase in the connective tissue, which is overshadowed by the fatty change. In all the chronic forms of tubercle in this organ there may be fibrous overgrowth. Hanot, who described several varieties, states that the condition may be primary. Practically it is very rare, except in connection with chronic tuberculous peritonitis and perihepatitis, when the organ may be much deformed by a sclerosis involving the portal canals and the capsule, which may be greatly involved in a polyserositis.

Jaundice is not common. It is usually due to some form of tuberculosis of the liver, either solitary tubercles or larger nodules. It is important to note its frequency in acute general miliary tuberculosis.

VII. TUBERCULOSIS OF THE BRAIN AND CORD

Tuberculosis of the *brain* occurs as (*a*) an acute miliary infection causing meningitis and acute hydrocephalus; (*b*) as a chronic meningo-encephalitis, usually localized, and containing small nodular tubercles; and (*c*) as the so-called solitary tubercle. Between the last two forms there are all gradations, and it is rare to see the meninges uninvolved. The acute variety has already been considered. The *chronic* form, which comes on slowly and has the clinical characters of a tumor, is more common in the young. Of 148 cases collected by Pribram 118 were under fifteen years of age. Other organs are usually involved, particularly the lungs, the bronchial glands, or the bones. In rare instances no tubercles are found elsewhere. They occur most frequently in the cerebellum; next in the cerebrum, and then in the pons. The growths are often multiple, in 100 out of 183 cases (Gowers). They range in size from a pea to a walnut; large tumors occasionally occur, and sometimes an entire lobe of the cerebellum is affected. On section the tubercle presents a grayish-yellow, caseous appearance, usually firm and hard, and encircled by a translucent, softer tissue. The centre of the growth may be semi-diffluent. As in other localities the tubercle may calcify. The tumors are as a rule attached to the meninges, often to the pia at the bottom of a sulcus so that they look imbedded in the brain-substance. About the longitudinal fissure there may be an aggregation of the growths, with compression of the sinus, and the formation of a thrombus. The tuberculous tumor not infrequently excites acute meningitis. In localized meningo-encephalitis the pia is thickened, tubercles are adherent to the under surface and grow about the arteries. It is often combined with cerebral softening from interference with the circulation. Several of the most characteristic instances are on the meninges covering the insula. This form may occur in pulmonary tuberculosis, causing hemiplegia or aphasia which may persist for months.

The symptoms of tuberculous growths in the brain are those of tumor, and will be considered in the section on the brain.

In the *spinal cord* the same forms are found. The acute tuberculous meningitis is almost always cerebro-spinal. The solitary tubercle of the cord is rare and usually secondary. Herter reported 3 cases and collected 24 from the literature. The symptoms are those of spinal tumor or meningitis.

VIII. TUBERCULOSIS OF THE GENITO-URINARY SYSTEM

Recent studies, and particularly the work of surgeons and gynæcologists, have taught as the great importance of tuberculosis of this tract. Any part of the genito-urinary system may be invaded. The successive involvement of the organs may be so rapid that unless the case has been seen early it may be impossible to state with any degree of certainty which has been the primary seat of infection. There may be simultaneous involvement of various portions of the tract. In tuberculosis of the genito-urinary system one always has to bear in mind the possibility of latent disease elsewhere. As Bollinger says, tubercle bacilli may gain admission at some part of the respiratory tract without producing any lesion at the point of entrance, and finally reach a bronchial gland, where they set up a tuberculous process of extremely slow development without producing any symptoms. From this point bacilli may enter the blood stream and lodge in the epididymis, and produce nodules which are readily discovered owing to the ease with which this part is examined. Such a case might be easily mistaken for one of primary genital tuberculosis, whereas the true primary tuberculous focus is far distant.

Infection of the genito-urinary tract occurs in various ways:

(*a*) By Hereditary Transmission.—It has been met with in the fetus. The comparative frequency of tuberculosis of the testicle in very young children suggests very strongly that the uro-genital organs may be involved as a result of direct transmission of the disease.

(*b*) By Infection from Areas of Tuberculosis Already Existing.—(1) *Hæmatogenous.*—In many cases uro-genital tuberculosis is found at autopsy associated with disease of some distant organ, particularly the lungs, and it would appear most probable that in them infection has been through the blood-vessels. Jani's observations, published by Weigert after the author's death, strongly support this theory. In studying sections of the genital organs of patients who died of pulmonary tuberculosis, he found tubercle bacilli in 5 out of 8 cases in the testicle, and in 4 out of 6 cases in the prostate, without in any instance finding microscopic evidences of tubercles in these organs. The bacilli lay, in the testis, partly within and partly close beside the cellular and granular contents of the seminal tubules, while in the prostate they were always situated in the neighborhood of the glandular epithelium.

(2) *Infection from the Peritoneum.*—This source of infection, in both men and women, is much more frequent than is commonly supposed. The intimate relationship between the peritoneum and bladder in both sexes, and with the vesiculæ seminales and vasa deferentia in the male, allows a ready way of invasion of these organs by direct extension of the disease. The peritoneum is a frequent source of genital tuberculosis in the female. No doubt many cases of tuberculosis of the Fallopian tubes originate from this source. The fact that the fimbriated extremity of the tube is often most seriously involved points in this direction, although the fact might be taken as a point in favor of blood infection, favored by its greater vascularity. Various observations go to show that the action of the cilia lining the lumina of the Fallopian tubes tends to attract particles introduced into the peritoneal cavity. Jani's observation is interesting in this connection, as showing the possibility of tubercle bacilli entering the tubes from the peritoneal cavity without there being any tuberculous peritonitis. He found typical tubercle bacilli in the lumen, in sections of a normal Fallopian tube, in a woman who died of pulmonary and intestinal tuberculosis. The explanation advanced was that the bacilli made their way through the thin peritoneal coat from one of the intestinal ulcers, thus reaching the peritoneal cavity, and thence were attracted into the Fallopian tube by the current produced by the action of the cilia lining the lumen. The intimate relationship between tuberculous peritonitis and tuberculosis of the Fallopian tubes is shown in the fact that the latter are affected in from 30 to 40 per cent. of the cases.

(3) *Infection from Other Organs by Direct Extension.*—The occurrence of direct extension from the peritoneum has already been mentioned. In tuberculous ulceration of the intestine or rectum adhesions to the bladder in the male or to the uterus and vagina in the female may occur, with resulting fistulæ and a direct extension of the disease. Perirectal tuberculous abscesses may lead to secondary involvement of some portion of the genito-urinary tract. Tuberculosis of the vertebræ may be followed by tuberculosis of the kidney as a result of direct extension of the disease.

(*c*) BY INFECTION FROM WITHOUT.—Whether uro-genital tuberculosis may occur as a result of the entrance of tubercle bacilli into the urethra or vagina is a disputed question. That bacilli gain admission to these passages during coitus with a person the subject of uro-genital tuberculosis, or by the use of foul instruments, seems quite probable. The possibility of genital tuberculosis occurring in the female as a result of coitus with a male the subject of tuberculosis in some portion of the genito-urinary system was first suggested by Cohnheim, who stated, however, that it rarely, if ever, occurred. In a patient with intestinal tuberculosis the tubercle bacilli might accidentally reach the urethra or vagina from the rectum.

Uro-genital tuberculosis is commonest between the ages of twenty and forty years—that is, during the period of greatest sexual activity. Males are affected much more frequently than females, the proportion being 3 to 1. This great difference is no doubt partly due to the more intimate relationship between the urinary and genital systems in the former than in the latter.

Once the uro-genital tract has been invaded the disease is likely to spread rapidly, and the method of extension is an important one. Frequently there is direct extension, as when the bladder is involved secondarily to the kidney by passage of the disease along the ureter, or where the tuberculous process extends along the vas deferens to the vesiculæ seminales. No doubt surface inoculation occurs in some instances, and to this cause may be attributed a certain percentage of cases of vesical and prostatic disease following tuberculosis of the kidney. Although this probability is acknowledged, there is an element of doubt as to the possibility of the kidney becoming affected secondarily to the bladder or prostate by the direct passage of the bacilli up the lumen of one ureter; for in such a case we have to suppose that a non-motile bacillus ascends against an almost constant current of urine flowing in the opposite direction. The lymphatics may afford a means for the spreading of the disease, but in the majority of cases the infection is hæmatogenous. Cystoscopic examinations of the bladder not infrequently show the presence of tubercles beneath the mucous membrane before there is any evidence of superficial ulceration—a fact suggesting strongly a blood infection.

The discovery of tubercle bacilli in the urine and the obtaining of tuberculous lesions in animals as a result of inoculation with the urinary sediment afford us the only positive evidence of genito-urinary tuberculosis. So far there are no authentic accounts of tubercle bacilli having been found in the semen of men with tuberculosis of the testicle or vesiculæ seminales. Owing to the fact that the smegma bacillus has the same staining reaction as the tubercle bacillus, and, morphologically is practically indistinguishable from it, the greatest care must be used in obtaining the specimen of urine for examination, to eliminate, if possible, all chances of contamination. One or more guinea-pigs should be inoculated with some of the suspected urine. If tubercle bacilli be present the animals will manifest tuberculous lesions in from three to five weeks.

Tuberculosis of the Kidneys.—In general tuberculosis the kidneys frequently present scattered miliary tubercles. In pulmonary tuberculosis it is common to find a few nodules in the substance of the organ, or there may be pyelitis. In the first 17,000 admissions to the medical wards of the Johns Hopkins Hospital there were 1,085 cases of tuberculous infection. In 17 of these a clinical diagnosis of renal tuberculosis was made. Walker analyzed the first 1,369 autopsies in the same hospital and found that 784 had tuberculosis in some part of the body. In all there were 61 cases of renal tuberculosis. Of 482 cases of pulmonary tuberculosis showing symptoms during life, one or both kidneys were involved in 23. There were 36 cases of acute general miliary tuberculosis, and in every instance the kidney was affected. The 2 other cases of renal tuberculosis occurred in patients with latent disease. Primary tuberculosis of the kidneys is not very rare, but in no instance in the above series did Walker demonstrate a primary infection in the kidney. The tuberculous process was primary in some other part of the genito-urinary tract in 6 cases. In a majority of the cases the process involves the pelvis and the ureter as well, sometimes the bladder and prostate. It may be difficult to say in advanced cases whether the disease has started in the bladder, prostate, or vesicles, or whether it started in the kidneys and proceeded downward. In a majority of cases the infection is through the blood. Walker thinks that a hæmatogenous infection takes place in 90 per cent. of the cases, and that this is the channel of infection in the majority of instances where renal follows vesical tuberculosis rather than along the ureter. One kidney alone may be involved, and the disease creeps down the ureter and may only extend a few millimetres on the vesical mucosa. A man with aortic insufficiency, who had no lesions in the lungs, presented a localized patch in the pelvis of the kidney, involving a pyramid, while the ureter, 5 cm. from the bladder and at its orifice, was thickened and tuberculous. The prostate showed an area of caseation. The process is most common between twenty and thirty years of age, but it may occur at the extremes of age. In a series of 386 cases collected by Walker in which the sex was stated 182 of the patients were males and 204 females. In the earliest stage, which may be met with accidentally, the disease is seen to begin in the pyramids and calyces. Necrosis and caseation proceed rapidly, and the colonies of tubercles start throughout the pyramids and extend upon the mucous membrane of the pelvis. As a rule, from the outset it is a tuberculous pyo-nephrosis. It may be confined to one kidney, or progress more extensively in one than in the other. At autopsy both organs are usually found enlarged. In only 3 of the 61 autopsies previously referred to was the disease unilateral. One kidney may be completely destroyed and converted into a series of cysts containing cheesy substance—a form of kidney which the older writers called scrofulous. In the putty-like contents of these cysts lime salts may be deposited. In other instances the walls of the pelvis are thickened and cheesy, the pyramids eroded, and caseous nodules are scattered through the organ, even to the capsule, which may be thickened and adherent. The other organ is usually less affected, and shows only pyelitis or a superficial necrosis of one or two pyramids. The ureters are usually thickened and the mucous membrane ulcerated and caseous. Involvement of the bladder, vesiculæ seminales, and testes is not uncommon in males.

The SYMPTOMS are those of pyelitis. The urine may be purulent for years, and there may be little or no distress. Even before the bladder becomes involved micturition is frequent, and many instances are mistaken for cystitis. The frequent micturition is in part due to an initial polyuria, in part to reflex irritation, but chiefly to a non-tuberculous inflammation over the trigone of the bladder. It is usually the earliest and most constant symptom. *Hæmaturia,* of a mild grade, occurs at some time during the course in the majority of cases. Dull, aching pain in the lumbar region on one side is frequently complained of and may be the first symptom. The condition is for many years compatible with fair health. The curability is shown by the accidental discovery of the so-called scrofulous kidney, converted into cysts containing a putty-like substance. In cases in which the disease becomes advanced and both organs are affected constitutional symptoms are more marked. There is irregular fever, with chills and loss of weight and strength. General tuberculosis is common and the lungs are usually involved.

In a case at the Montreal General Hospital a cyst perforated and caused fatal peritonitis.

Examination may detect special tenderness on one side, or the kidney may be palpable in front on deep pressure; but tuberculous pyelo-nephritis seldom causes a large tumor. Occasionally the pelvis becomes enormously distended; but this is rare in comparison with its frequency in calculous pyelitis. The urine presents changes similar to those of ordinary calculous pyelitis—pus-cells, epithelium, and occasionally definite caseous masses. It is nearly always acid in reaction. Albumin is present but casts are rare. Tubercle bacilli may be demonstrated and should be searched for when there are any unusual sensations. There may be "showers" of bacilli at these times.

DIAGNOSIS.—To distinguish the condition from calculous pyelitis is often difficult. Hæmorrhage may be present in both, though not nearly so frequently in the tuberculous disease. The appearance of the ureteral orifices on cystoscopic examination is often characteristic. The diagnosis rests on: (1) The detection of some focus of tuberculosis, as in the testis; (2) the presence of tubercle bacilli in the sediment; (3) the use of tuberculin; and (4) cystoscopic examination and catheterization of the ureters.

Tuberculosis of the suprarenal glands will be considered under Addison's Disease.

Tuberculosis of the Ureter and Bladder.—This rarely occurs as a primary affection, but is nearly always secondary to involvement of other parts, particularly the pelvis of the kidney. Protracted cystitis which has come on without apparent cause is always suggestive of tuberculosis. The renal regions, the testes, the seminal vesicles, and the prostate should be examined with care. It may follow a pyelo-nephritis, or be associated with primary disease of the prostate or vesiculæ seminales. Primary tuberculosis of the posterior wall of the bladder may simulate stone.

Tuberculosis of the Prostate and Vesiculæ Seminales.—The prostate is frequently involved in tuberculosis of the uro-genital tract. In Krzyincki's cases, of 15 males the prostate was involved in 14 and the vesiculæ seminales in 11. In Orth's cases the prostate was involved in 18 of the 37 cases in males. These parts are much more frequently involved than ordinary post mortem statistics indicate. The prostatic lobes are felt to be occupied by hard nodules varying in size from a pea to a bean. There is great irritability of the bladder, and agonizing pain in catheterization. An extremely rare lesion is primary urethral tuberculosis, which may simulate stricture.

Tuberculosis of the Testes.—This somewhat common affection may be primary, or, more frequently, is secondary to tuberculous disease elsewhere. Many cases occur before the second year, and it is stated to have been met with in the fetus. In infants it is serious and usually associated with tuberculous disease in other parts. In 9 cases reported by Hutinel and Deschamps, in every one there was a general affection. In 20 cases reported by Jullien, 6 were under one year, and 6 between one and two years old. In 5 of the cases both testicles were affected. Koplik holds that most of the instances of this kind are congenital, in Baumgarten's sense. In the adult the tubercles begin within the substance of the gland, but in children the tunica albuginea is first affected. The tubercle does not always undergo caseation, but it may present a number of embryonic cells, not unlike a sarcoma.

Tubercle of the testes is most likely to be confounded with syphilis. In the latter the body of the organ is most often affected, there is less pain, and the outlines of the growth are more nodular and irregular. In obscure peritoneal disease the detection of tubercle in a testis has not infrequently led to a correct diagnosis. The association of the two conditions is not uncommon. The lesion in the testis may heal completely or the disease may become generalized. General infection has followed operation. Too much stress can not be laid on the importance of a routine examination of the testes.

Tuberculosis of the Fallopian Tubes, Ovaries, and Uterus.—The *Fallopian tubes* are by far the most frequent seat of genital tuberculosis. The disease may be primary and produce a most characteristic form of salpingitis, in which the tubes are enlarged, the walls thickened and infiltrated, and the contents cheesy. Adhesion takes place between the fimbriæ and the ovaries, or the uterus may be invaded. The condition is usually bilateral. It may occur in young children. Although, as a rule, very evident to the naked eye, there are specimens resembling ordinary salpingitis, which show on microscopic examination numerous miliary tubercles (Welch and Williams). Tuberculous salpingitis may cause serious local disease with abscess formation, and it may be the starting-point of peritonitis. Tuberculosis of the *ovary* is always secondary. There may be an eruption of tubercles over the surface in an extensive involvement of the stroma with abscess formation.

Tuberculosis of the *uterus* is very rare. Only four examples have come under our observation, all in connection with pulmonary tuberculosis. It may be primary. The mucosa of the fundus is thickened and caseous, and tubercles may be seen in the muscular tissue. Occasionally the process extends to the vagina. Tuberculosis of the *placenta* is more common than has been supposed. Of 20 placentas from tuberculous women, 9 were affected; 5 of these were from cases of advanced disease of the lung. The lesions are easily overlooked.

IX. TUBERCULOSIS OF THE MAMMARY GLAND

There may be solitary or disseminated nodules, a sclerosing mastitis or caseation with abscess formation. The disease is most common between the fortieth and sixtieth years. The breast is frequently fistulous, unevenly indurated, and the nipple is retracted. The fistulæ and ulcers present a characteristic tuberculous aspect. There is also a cold tuberculous abscess of the breast. The axillary glands are affected in about two-thirds of the cases. The disease runs a chronic course of months or years. The diagnosis can be made by the general appearance of the fistulæ and ulcers, and by the existence of tubercle bacilli. The prognosis is not serious, if total eradication of the disease be possible.

In 1836 Bedor described an hypertrophy of the breast in the subjects of pulmonary tuberculosis. As a rule, if one gland is involved, usually on the side of the affected lung, as already mentioned, the condition is one of chronic interstitial mammitis and is not tuberculous.

X. TUBERCULOSIS OF THE CIRCULATORY SYSTEM

Myocardium.—Scattered miliary tubercles are sometimes met with in the acute disease. Larger caseous tubercles are excessively rare. A. Moser found 46 cases on record. There is also a sclerotic tuberculous myocarditis. The infection often passes from a mediastinal gland.

Endocardium.—In 216 autopsies in cases of chronic tuberculosis endocarditis was found in 12. It was present in only 151 among more than 11,000 autopsies on tuberculous cases (G. W. Norris). As a rule, it is a secondary form, the result of a mixed infection, so common in pulmonary tuberculosis. A true tuberculous endocarditis does, however, occur, directly dependent upon infection with the bacillus of Koch. As a rule, it is a vegetative endocarditis, not to be distinguished from that caused by a streptococcus or staphylococcus. In rare cases, however, caseous tubercles develop.

Arteries.—Primary tuberculosis of the larger blood-vessels is very rare and is usually the result of invasion from without. The disease may, however, occur in a large artery and not result from external invasion. In a case of chronic tuberculosis Flexner found a fresh tuberculous growth in the aorta, which had no connection with cheesy masses outside the vessel. Simmitsky collected 18 cases of tuberculosis of the aorta.

In the lungs and other organs attacked by tuberculosis the *arteries* are involved in an acute infiltration which usually leads to thrombosis, or tubercles may develop in the walls and proceed to caseation and softening, frequently with a resulting hæmorrhage. By extension into vessels, particularly veins, the bacilli are widely distributed with the production of miliary tuberculosis.

XI. THE PROGNOSIS IN TUBERCULOSIS

The parable of the sower already referred to expresses better than in any other way the question of individual predisposition. There are five groups of cases of tuberculous infection. 1. Those who become infected and recover spontaneously without knowing they have been infected. 2. Mild infections which produce slight symptoms, recovery following after a few months of change of air or special treatment. 3. Cases with well-marked signs of lung disease in which thorough treatment is followed by complete recovery. 4. Cases with extensive local disease and cavity formation in which arrest takes place and the patients live for many years. 5. The cases in which the infection is of such a type that death follows no matter what is done. The late Austin Flint, *facile princeps* among American students of the disease, called attention to the self-limitation and intrinsic tendency to recovery in pulmonary tuberculosis. This natural tendency to cure is still more strikingly shown in lymphatic and bone tuberculosis.

The following may be considered favorable circumstances in the prognosis of pulmonary tuberculosis: An early diagnosis, a good family history, previous good health, a strong digestion, a suitable environment, and an insidious onset, without high fever, and without extensive pneumonic consolidation. Cases beginning with pleurisy seem to run a more protracted and more favorable course. Repeated attacks of hæmoptysis are unfavorable. When well established the course of tuberculosis in any organ is marked by intervals of weeks or months in which the fever lessens, the symptoms subside, and there is improvement in the general health.

In pulmonary cases the duration is extremely variable. Laennec placed the average duration at two years, and for the majority of cases this is perhaps a correct estimate. Pollock's large statistics of over 3,500 cases show a mean duration of the disease of over two years and a half. Williams's analysis of 1,000 cases in private practice shows a much more protracted course, as the average duration was over seven years.

Tuberculosis and Marriage.—Under the subject of prognosis comes the question of the marriage of persons who have had tuberculosis, or in whose family the disease prevails. The following brief statements may be made:

(*a*) Subjects with healed lymphatic or bone tuberculosis marry with personal impunity and may beget healthy children. In such families adenitis, caries of the bone, arthritis, cerebral and pulmonary tuberculosis are more common. The risks, however, are such as may properly be taken.

(*b*) The question of marriage of a person who has arrested or cured lung tuberculosis is more difficult to decide. In a male the personal risk is not so great; and when the health and strength are good, the external environment favorable, and the family history not extremely bad, the experiment—for it is such—is often successful, and many healthy and happy families are begotten under these circumstances. In women the question is complicated with that of child-bearing, which increases the risks enormously. With a localized lesion, absence of hereditary taint, good physique, and favorable environment marriage might be permitted. When tuberculosis has existed in a girl whose family history is bad, and whose physique is below the standard, the physician should, if possible, place his veto upon marriage.

(*c*) With existing disease, fever, bacilli, etc., marriage should be prohibited. Pregnancy usually hastens the process, though it may be held in abeyance. After parturition the disease advances rapidly. There is much truth, indeed, in the remark of Dubois: "If a woman threatened with phthisis marries, she may bear the first accouchement well; a second, with difficulty; a third, never." Conception may occur in an advanced stage of the disease.

XII. PROPHYLAXIS IN TUBERCULOSIS

General.—Among the more important measures may be mentioned the following: *First,* education of the public. Much has been done in this direction by the antituberculosis crusade, which has resulted in the formation of many active societies, and has stimulated widespread interest in the disease. *Secondly,* the placing of pulmonary tuberculosis on the list of reportable diseases. This gives the board of health control of the situation, and, as the New York experience has demonstrated, is perhaps the most helpful measure in the prophylaxis. *Thirdly,* the improved sanitary condition of the poor, particularly with reference to housing. *Fourthly,* direct preventive measures, such as the enactment of laws against spitting in public, the proper disinfection and cleaning of the rooms and houses which have been occupied by tuberculous patients, and the careful inspection of dairies and abattoirs. *Fifthly,* in the large cities, *organization* of sanatoria and hospitals for early curable and late incurable cases, and the establishment of separate dispensaries with a system of visiting the patients at their homes by specially assigned nurses. *Lastly,* the care of the sputum of the tuberculous. Thorough boiling or putting it into the fire is sufficient. In hospitals it is well to have printed directions as to the care of the sputum, and also printed cards for out-patients, giving the most important rules. It should be explained to the patient that the only risk, practically, is from this source.

Individual.—Individual prophylaxis in the case of delicate children is most important. An infant born of tuberculous parents, or of a family in which tuberculosis prevails, should be brought up with the greatest care and guarded most particularly against infections of all kinds. Special attention should be given to the throat and nose, and on the first indication of mouth-breathing, or any obstruction of the naso-pharynx, a careful examination should be made for adenoid vegetations. The child should be clad in flannel and live in the open air as much as possible, avoiding close rooms. It is a good practice to sponge the throat and chest night and morning with cold water. Special attention should be paid to diet and to the mode of feeding. The meals should be at regular hours and the food plain and substantial. From the outset the child should be encouraged to drink freely of milk. Unfortunately, in these cases there seems to be an aversion to fats of all kinds. As the child grows older, systematically regulated exercise or a course of pulmonary gymnastics may be taken. In the choice of an occupation preference should be given to an out-of-door life. Families with a marked predisposition to tuberculosis should, if possible, reside in an equable climate.

The examination of children who have been in contact with tuberculous individuals is important. Four groups of suspects come to tuberculosis dispensaries: (1) The under-fed, anæmic, badly developed child, without local lesions; the question is one of malnutrition. (2) Cases of thymo-lymphatism usually having adenoids and enlarged tonsils. These children may not be anæmic, but they have stunted, badly formed chests, and the superficial lymph glands may be enlarged. (3) Children with obviously enlarged lymph glands, usually cervical; it may not be easy to determine whether the adenopathy is due to throat infection or bad teeth, or whether it is actually tuberculosis. (4) Children with physical signs in the chest pointing to definite local lesion, the tuberculous nature of which may not at first be easy to determine.

The trifling ailments of children should be carefully watched. In the convalescence from the fevers which so frequently prove dangerous the greatest caution should be exercised to prevent catching cold. An open air life, a generous diet, especially in fats, and iron or arsenic if there is anæmia, are important aids. Care of the throat in these children is important; enlarged tonsils and adenoids should be removed.

XIII. TREATMENT OF TUBERCULOSIS

The Natural or Spontaneous Cure.—The spontaneous healing of local tuberculosis is an every-day affair. A majority of those infected never have the disease, *i. e.,* they recover without symptoms, without the slight lesion having disturbed the health. Many cases of adenitis and disease of the bone or of the joints terminate favorably. The healing of pulmonary tuberculosis is shown clinically by the recovery of patients in whose sputum elastic tissue and bacilli have been found; anatomically, by the presence of lesions in all stages of repair. In the granulation products and associated pneumonia a scar-tissue is formed, while the smaller caseous areas become impregnated with lime salts. To such conditions alone should the term healing be applied. When the fibroid change encapsulates but does not involve the entire tuberculous tissue, the tubercle may be termed involuted or quiescent, but is not destroyed. When cavities of any size have formed, healing, in the proper sense of the term, does not occur. We have yet to see a specimen which would indicate that a vomica had cicatrized. Cavities may be greatly reduced in size—indeed, an entire series of them may be so contracted by sclerosis of the tissue about them that an upper lobe, in which this process most frequently occurs, may be reduced to a third of its ordinary dimensions. Laennec understood thoroughly this natural process of cure in tuberculosis, and recognized the frequency with which old tuberculous lesions occurred in the lungs. He described *cicatrices complètes* and *cicatrices fistuleuses,* the latter being the shrunken cavities communicating with the bronchi; and remarked that, as tubercles growing in the glands, which are called scrofula, often heal, why should not the same take place in the lungs?

There is an old German axiom, *Jedermann hat am Ende ein bischen Tuberculose,* a statement partly borne out by the statistics showing the proportions of cases in persons dying of all disease in whom quiescent or tuberculous lesions are found in the lungs. We find at the apices the following conditions, which have been held to signify healed tuberculous processes: (*a*) Thickening of the pleura, usually at the posterior surface of the apex, with subadjacent induration for a distance of a few millimetres. This has, perhaps, no greater significance than the milky patch on the pericardium. (*b*) Puckered cicatrices at the apex, depressing the pleura, and on section showing a large pigmented, fibrous scar. The bronchioles in the neighborhood may be dilated, but there are neither tubercles nor cheesy masses. This may sometimes, but not always, indicate a healed tuberculous lesion. (*c*) Puckered cicatrices with cheesy or cretaceous nodules, and with scattered tubercles in the vicinity. (*d*) The *cicatrices fistuleuses* of Laennec, in which the fibroid puckering has reduced the size of one or more cavities which communicate directly with the bronchi.

General Measures.—The cure of tuberculosis is a question of nutrition; digestion and assimilation control the situation; as a rule, make a patient grow fat and strong, and the local disease may be left to take care of itself. There are three indications: First, to place the patient in surroundings most favorable for the maintenance of a maximum degree of nutrition; second, to take such measures as, in a local or general way, influence the tuberculous processes; third, to alleviate symptoms. The importance of rest must always be kept in mind and the amount of exertion allowed carefully ordered.

Open-air Treatment.—The value of fresh air and out-of-door life is well illustrated by an experiment of Trudeau. Inoculated rabbits confined in a dark, damp place rapidly succumbed, while others, allowed to run wild, either recovered or show slight lesions. It is the same in human tuberculosis. A patient confined to the house—particularly in the close, overheated, stuffy dwellings of the poor, or treated in a hospital ward—is in a position analogous to that of the rabbit confined to a hutch in the cellar; whereas a patient living in the fresh air or sunshine for the greater part of the day has chances comparable to those of the rabbit running wild.

The open-air treatment of tuberculosis may be carried out at home, by change of residence to a suitable climate, or in a sanatorium.

(*a*) *At Home.*—In a majority of all cases the patient has to be cared for in his own home, and, if in the city, under very disadvantageous circumstances. Much, however, may be done even in cities to promote arrest by insisting upon systematic treatment. How much may be done by care and instruction is shown by the success of J. H. Pratt's *tuberculosis classes.* As not five per cent. of the patients can be dealt with in sanatoria, it is surprising and gratifying to see how successful the home treatment may be. Even in cities the patients may be trained to sleep out of doors, and the results obtained by Pratt, Millett, and others are as good as any that have been published. *While there is fever the patient should be at rest in bed,* and night and day the windows should be open, so that he may be exposed freely to the fresh air. Low temperature is not a contra-indication. If there is a balcony or a suitable yard or garden, on the brighter days the patient may be wrapped up and put in a reclining chair or on a sofa. The important thing is for the physician to emphasize the fact that neither the cough, fever, night sweats, and not even hæmoptysis contra-indicate a full exposure to the fresh air. In country places this can be carried out much more effectively. In the summer the patient should be out of doors for at least eleven or twelve hours, and in winter six or eight hours. At night the room should be cool and thoroughly well ventilated. It may require several months of this rest treatment in the open air before the temperature falls to normal.

(*b*) *Treatment in Sanatoria.*—Perhaps the most important advance in the treatment of tuberculosis has been in the establishment of institutions in which patients are made to live according to strict rules. To Brehmer, of Göbersdorf, we owe the successful execution of this plan, which has been followed with most gratifying results. In the United States the zeal, energy, and scientific devotion of Edward L. Trudeau demonstrated its feasibility, and the Saranac institution has become a model of its kind. The results at hundreds of institutions demonstrate the great importance of system and rigid discipline in carrying out a successful treatment. Much has been done to promote the sanatorium treatment and the good results have quite justified the heavy expenditure of money. In many places it has been demonstrated that with an inexpensive plant excellent results may be obtained. A reaction has naturally followed the "stuffing" plan of feeding, and more reasonable methods are now employed. The "absolute rest" plan has been modified to meet individual cases. The all-important matter is the establishment near to the large cities of public sanatoria for the treatment of cases in the early stages. The large general hospitals should have special out-patient departments for tuberculous patients, from which suitable cases could be sent to the sanatoria. Much discussion has taken place as to the result of sanatorium treatment. There is no doubt of its extraordinary benefits in suitable cases. To pay a visit with Dr. Bardwell to the King Edward Sanatorium at Midhurst and see nearly every one of 100 patients looking in good condition with fresh air, judicious rest, proper exercise and diet, without drugs and without tuberculin, impresses one immensely with the value of the method. Statistics are notoriously uncertain, but there is perhaps no institution of the English-speaking world in which greater care has been taken to trace the after-history of the patients than at the Adirondack Sanatorium. The total number of patients from the years 1885 to 1919 inclusive was 4,976. It has been impossible to trace 263 of these. Of the remaining 4,713, 2,892 were living (1919) and 1,821 dead.

(*c*) *Climatic Treatment.*—This, after all, is only a modification of the open-air method. The first question to be decided is whether the patient is fit to be sent from home. In many instances it is a positive hardship. A patient with well-marked cavities, hectic fever, night sweats, and emaciation is much better at home, and the physician should not be too much influenced by the importunities of the sick man or his friends. The requirements of a suitable climate are a *pure atmosphere,* an *equable temperature* not subject to rapid variations, and a *maximum amount of sunshine.* Given these three factors, it makes little difference *where* a patient goes, so long as he lives *an outdoor life.* Woodruff believes that sunshine may be hurtful, and collected statistics to show that tuberculosis is more prevalent and more fatal among the dark races, who live where the sun shines the brightest. The different climates may be grouped into the high altitudes, the dry, warm climates, and the moist, warm climates. Among high altitudes in the United States, the Colorado resorts are the most important. Of others, those in Arizona and New Mexico have been growing rapidly. The rarefaction of the air in high altitudes is of benefit in increasing the respiratory movements, but brings about in time a condition of dilatation of the air-vesicles and a permanent increase in the size of the chest which is a marked disadvantage when such persons attempt subsequently to reside at the sea-level. The great advantage of these western resorts is that they are in progressive, prosperous countries, in which a man may find means of livelihood and live in comfort. In Europe the chief resorts at high altitudes are Davos, Les Avants, and St. Moritz. Of resorts at a moderate altitude, Asheville and the Adirondacks are the best known in America. The Adirondack cure has become quite famous. One decided advantage is that after arrest of the disease the patient can return to the sea-level without any special risk. The cases most suitable for high altitudes are those in which the disease is limited, without much cavity formation, and without much emaciation. The thin, irritable patients with chronic tuberculosis and a good deal of emphysema are better at the sea-level. The cold winter climate seems to be of decided advantage in tuberculosis, and in the Adirondacks, where the temperature falls sometimes to 20° or even more below zero, the patients are able to lead an out-of-door life throughout the entire winter.

Of the moist, warm climates, in America Florida and the Bermudas, in Europe the Madeira Islands, and in Great Britain Eastbourne, Bournemouth, Torquay, and Falmouth are the best known. Of the dry, warm climates, Southern California in the United States is the most satisfactory. Many of the health resorts in the Southern States are delightful winter climates for tuberculous cases. Egypt, Algiers, and the Riviera are the most satisfactory resorts for patients from Europe.

Other considerations which should influence the choice of a locality are good accommodations and good food. It is also important to be under the care of a competent physician. Very much is said concerning the choice of locality in the different stages of pulmonary tuberculosis, but when the disease is limited to an apex, in a man of fairly good personal and family history, the chances are that he may fight a winning battle if he lives out of doors in any climate, whether high, dry, and cold, or low, moist, and warm. With bilateral disease and cavity formation there is but little hope of permanent cure, and the mild or warm climates are preferable.

Measures which, by their Local or General Action, Influence the Tuberculous Process.—Under this heading we may consider the specific, the dietetic, and the general medicinal treatment of tuberculosis.

(*a*) Specific Treatment.—Introduced by Koch in 1890, the tuberculin treatment soon fell into disfavor, but, in spite of the bad results that naturally followed its injudicious use, certain men (among them, particularly, Trudeau) continued to use it. Of late years there has been a reaction in its favor, and tuberculin is again lauded by some fanatics as the one and only means of cure. Unquestionably in suitable cases it has a very beneficial influence; the difficulty is to decide which they are. At present so indiscriminate is its use that an estimation of the results is very difficult. The preliminary question arises as to what justifies the diagnosis of tuberculosis, and it is impossible to compare the results obtained by different observers. Anybody, by any method, can secure 100 per cent. of cures in the so-called "closed" pulmonary tuberculosis. As Hamman states very sensibly: "If in the case of every patient who presents himself for examination and shows some trifling deviation from the normal physical signs a diagnosis of tuberculosis is made, or if tuberculin is made the ultimate test of a correct diagnosis, similar results may be obtained with any or with no method." A variety of preparations come under the name Tuberculin: O. T. and T. R., which are Koch's old and new preparations; Denys' tuberculin, *bouillon filtré,* known as B. F., and a bacillary emulsion of Koch, B. E. The smallest dose which will bring out a response should be used, 1/2000 or 1/1000 mgm., and re-inoculations are made at intervals of from one to two weeks. The amount is gradually increased when it is found that the dose previously given ceases to bring out a sufficient response. It is administered to afebrile patients. It is not thought desirable—quite the contrary, in fact—to get a severe general reaction, particularly as this may be associated with marked focal reactions. The aim striven for is to get as high a grade of tuberculin tolerance as possible. Trudeau, who had probably the longest individual experience of anyone using tuberculin, began with doses so small that no reaction is produced; then the dose is cautiously raised, avoiding the slightest reaction. On the other hand, Wilkinson begins with a very high dose, and uses the tuberculin in a much wider range of cases.

(*b*) Dietetic Treatment.—The outlook in tuberculosis depends much upon the digestion. It is rare to see recovery in a patient in whom there is persistent gastric trouble, and the physician should ever bear in mind the fact that in this disease the *primæ viæ* control the position. The early nausea and loss of appetite in many cases are serious obstacles. Many patients loathe food of all kinds. A change of air or a sea voyage may promptly restore the appetite. When either of these is impossible, and if, as is almost always the case, fever is present, the patient should be placed at rest, kept in the open air nearly all day, and fed at stated intervals with small quantities either of milk, buttermilk, or koumyss, alternating if necessary with meat juice and egg albumen. Some patients who are disturbed by eggs and milk do well on koumyss. It may be necessary to resort to Débove's method of over-alimentation or forced feeding. The stomach is washed out with cold water, and then, through the tube, a mixture is given containing a litre of milk, an egg, and 100 grams of very finely powdered meat. This is given three times a day. Sometimes the patients will take this mixture without the necessity of the stomach-tube, in which case a smaller amount may be given. Raw eggs are suitable for the purpose of over-feeding, and may be taken between meals. Beginning with one three times a day, the number may be increased to two, three, or even four at a time. In the German sanatoria a special feature is this over-feeding, even when fever is present. R. W. Philip advises a raw meat diet, half a pound three times a day, either minced or as a soup.

In many cases the digestion is not at all disturbed and the patient can take an ordinary diet. It is remarkable how rapidly the appetite and digestion improve with the fresh-air treatment, even in patients who have to remain in the city. Care should be taken that the medicines do not disturb the stomach. Not infrequently the sweet syrups used in cough mixtures, cod-liver oil, creosote, and the hypophosphites produce irritation, and by interfering with digestion do more harm than good. On the other hand, the bitter tonics, with acids, and the various malt preparations are often most satisfactory. A routine administration of alcohol is not advisable, and there is no evidence that its persistent use promotes fibroid processes in the tuberculous areas. In the advanced stages, particularly when the temperature is low between eight and ten in the morning, whisky and milk, or whisky, egg, and milk may be given with advantage.

(*c*) Exercise.—The patient with fever does best at absolute rest, and exercise should only be taken after an afebrile period, and then very gradually. It has long been known that following exercise the temperature is raised, and Paterson, of Frimly, has adopted a method of graded exercises which have yielded excellent results. The plan is based upon the view that physical exercise induces auto-inoculation, the extent of which may be controlled by the amount of muscular effort. By a study of the fever-chart, the body weight, the amount of sputum, and the appetite the rate of progress may be estimated. The febrile patient is regarded as one in whom auto-inoculation is excessive. To overcome this the patient is immobilized in bed so far as possible, and not allowed to make any movements whatever. The effect of this is often remarkable in reducing the fever. Once afebrile, the principal element in the treatment is the induction of an auto-inoculation by exercises, which Paterson believes has much the same effect as a dose of tuberculin. A scheme of graded labor has been devised, which has many advantages in sanatorium life, and the results at Frimly are very gratifying.

(*d*) Immobilizing the Lung by Induction of Pneumothorax.—Years ago Cayley induced pneumothorax in a case of hæmoptysis. The method never came into general use; but, on the principle of keeping an inflamed organ at rest, this method was advocated in pulmonary tuberculosis by Forlanini and by J. B. Murphy. Sterile nitrogen is introduced into the pleural cavity. It is best to use a special apparatus with a water-manometer, so that measured quantities may be injected. At first from 200 to 300 c. c.; later as much as 500 c. c. are introduced, at intervals of a day or every other day, until the lung is completely collapsed, and until there is a positive interpleural pressure of from 5 to 10 cm. of water. The method has been widely practised with excellent results in certain cases; but there are dangers, as hæmoptysis, serous effusion, and empyema, and a serious objection is the duration of the treatment, as the pleural cavity requires to be refilled every month or two.

(*e*) General Medical Treatment.—No medicinal agents have any special or peculiar action upon tuberculous processes. The influence which they exert is upon the general nutrition, increasing the physiological resistance, and rendering the tissues less susceptible to invasion. The following are the most important remedies which seem to act in this manner:

Creosote, which may be administered in capsules, in increasing doses, beginning with 1 minim three times a day and, if well borne, increasing the dose to 8 or 10 minims. It may also be given in solution with tincture of cardamon and alcohol. It is an old remedy, strongly recommended by Addison, and the reports of Jaccoud, Fraentzel, and many others show that it has a positive value. It may be used as an inhalation. Guaiacol may be given as a substitute, either internally or hypodermically.

Cod-liver Oil.—In glandular and bone tuberculosis this remedy is undoubtedly beneficial in improving the nutrition. In pulmonary tuberculosis its action is less certain, and it is scarcely worthy of the unbounded confidence which it enjoyed for so many years. It should be given in small doses, not more than a teaspoonful three times a day after meals. It seems to act better in children than in adults. Fever and gastric irritation are contra-indications to its use. Rich cream is an excellent substitute; the clotted or Devonshire cream is preferable.

Arsenic.—There is no general tonic more satisfactory in cases of tuberculosis of all kinds than Fowler's solution. It may be given in 5-minim doses three times a day and gradually increased, stopping its use whenever unpleasant symptoms arise, and in any case intermitting it every third or fourth week. Intramuscular injections of the salts of cacodylic acid have been used to combat the anæmia so commonly present in tuberculous infections with, it is claimed, unusual success.

Treatment of Special Symptoms.—(*a*) The Fever.—There is no more difficult problem than the treatment of the pyrexia of tuberculosis. The patient should be at absolute rest, and *in the open air night and day for some weeks.* Fever does not contra-indicate an out-of-door life, but it is well for patients with a temperature above 100.5° F. to be at rest. For the continuous pyrexia or the remittent type of the early stages, quinine and the salicylates may be tried; but they are uncertain and rarely reliable. In large doses quinine has a moderate antipyretic action, but it is just in these efficient doses that it is so apt to disturb the stomach. It is better, when the fever rises above 103° F. to rely upon cold sponging or the tepid bath, gradually cooled. When softening has taken place and the fever assumes the characteristic septic type, the problem becomes still more difficult. As shown by Chart V (which is not by any means an exceptional one), the pyrexia, at this stage, lasts only for twelve or fifteen hours. As a rule there are not more than from eight to ten hours in which the fever is high enough to demand antipyretic treatment. Sometimes phenacetine, given in 2-grain (0.13 gm.) doses every hour for three or four hours before the rise in temperature takes place, either prevents entirely or limits the paroxysm. It answers better in this way than given in the single doses. Careful sponging of the extremities for from half an hour to an hour during the height of the fever is useful.

(*b*) SWEATING.—Atropine, in doses of gr. $\frac{1}{120}$-$\frac{1}{60}$ (0.0005-0.001 gm.), and the aromatic sulphuric acid in large doses are the best remedies. When there are cough and nocturnal restlessness, morphia (gr. 1/8, 0.008 gm.) may be given with the atropine. Camphoric acid (gr. x, 0.65 gm.) at bedtime may be tried. The patient should use light flannel night-dresses, as the cotton night-shirts, when soaked with perspiration, have a very unpleasant cold, clammy feeling.

(*c*) COUGH.—The *cough* is a troublesome, though necessary, feature in pulmonary tuberculosis. Unless very worrying and disturbing sleep at night, or so severe as to produce vomiting, it is not well to attempt to restrict it. When irritative and bronchial in character, inhalations are useful, particularly the tincture of benzoin or preparations of menthol, creosote, or turpentine. The throat should be carefully examined, as some of the most irritable and distressing forms of cough result from laryngeal erosions. The distressing nocturnal cough, which begins just as the patient gets into bed and is preparing to fall asleep, requires, as a rule, preparations of opium. Codein (gr. 1/4-1/2, 0.016-0.03 gm.) may be given. An excellent combination for the nocturnal cough is morphia (gr. $\frac{1}{8}$, 0.008 gm.), dilute hydrocyanic acid (♏ iij, 0.2 c. c.), and syrup of wild cherry (ʒ j, 4 c. c.). The spirit of chloroform, or a mixture of chloroform and sedatives or Hoffman's anodyne, given in whisky before going to sleep, is efficacious. Mild counter-irritation, or the application of a hot poultice, will sometimes promptly relieve the cough. The morning cough is often much relieved by taking immediately after getting up a glass of hot milk or a cup of hot water, to which 15 grains of bicarbonate of soda have been added. In the later stages, when cavities have formed, the accumulated secretion must be expectorated and the paroxysms of coughing are most exhausting. The sedatives, such as morphia and hydrocyanic acid, should be given cautiously. The aromatic spirit of ammonia in full doses helps to allay the paroxysm. When the expectoration is profuse, creosote internally, or inhalations of turpentine and iodine, or oil of eucalyptus, are useful. For the troublesome dysphagia a strong solution of cocaine (gr. x, 0.6 gm.) with boric acid (gr. v, 0.3 gm.) in glycerine and water (℥ j, 30 c. c.) may be used locally.

(*d*) DIARRHŒA.—For the diarrhœa large doses of bismuth, combined with Dover's powder, and small starch enemata, with or without opium, may be given. The acetate of lead and opium pill often acts promptly, and the acid diarrhœa mixture, dilute acetic acid (♏ x-xv, 1 c. c.), morphia (gr. 1/8, 0.008 gm.), and acetate of lead (gr. j-ij, 0.1 gm.), may be tried.

In some cases, 5 c. c. of a 5 per cent. solution of calcium chloride injected intravenously is useful.

(*e*) The treatment of the hæmoptysis will be considered in the section on hæmorrhage from the lungs. Dyspnœa is rarely a prominent symptom except in the advanced stages, when it may be very troublesome and distressing. Ammonia and morphia, cautiously administered, may be used.

If the pleuritic pains are severe, the side may be strapped, or painted with tincture of iodine. The dyspeptic symptoms require careful treatment, as the outlook in individual cases depends much upon the condition of the stomach. Small doses of calomel and soda often allay the distressing nausea.

The treatment of lesions such as of the kidney, epididymis, etc., is surgical if the condition is recognized early enough. Disease elsewhere, as in the lungs, is not a necessary contra-indication. The possible harm resulting from ether anæsthesia must always be kept in mind.

A last word on the subject of tuberculosis to the general practitioner. *The leadership of the battle against this scourge is in your hands. Much has been done, much remains to do. By early diagnosis and prompt, systematic treatment of individual cases, by striving in every possible way to improve the social condition of the poor, by joining actively in the work of the local and national antituberculosis societies you can help in the most important and the most hopeful campaign ever undertaken by the profession.*

B. NON-BACTERIAL FUNGUS INFECTIONS—THE MYCOSES

Much attention has been paid to the local and general infections caused by the group of fungoid organisms variously classed as Streptothrix, Actinomyces, Cladothrix and Leptothrix. The French workers group the various diseases caused by these organisms under the term Mycoses, which is a convenient and useful designation. Four or five of these diseases are of sufficient importance to be considered in a work of this scope.

I. ACTINOMYCOSIS

Definition.—A chronic infective disorder produced by the actinomyces or ray-fungus, *Streptothrix actinomyces.*

Etiology.—The disease is widespread among cattle, and occurs also in the pig. It was first described by Bollinger in the ox, in which it forms the affection known in America as "big-jaw." The first accurate description of the disease in man was given by James Israel, and subsequently Ponfick insisted upon the identity of the disease in man and cattle.

In the United States and England the disease is less common than in Germany. It is nearly three times as common in men as in women.

The *parasite* belongs probably to the *Streptothrix* group. In both man and cattle it can be seen in the pus from the affected region as yellowish or opaque granules from one-half to two millimetres in diameter, which are made up of cocci and radiating threads, presenting bulbous, club-like terminations. The youngest granules are gray in color and semi-translucent; in these the bulbous extremities are wanting. The parasite has been successfully cultivated, and in a few instances the disease has been inoculated both with the natural and artificially grown organism.

The Mode of Infection.—There is no evidence of direct infection with the flesh or milk of diseased animals. The streptothrix has not been detected outside the body. It seems highly probable that it is taken in with the food. The site of infection in a majority of cases in man and animals is in the mouth or neighboring passages. In the cow, possibly also in man, barley, oats, and rye have been carriers of the germ.

Morbid Anatomy.—As in tubercle, the first effect is the destruction of adjacent cells and the attraction of leucocytes—later the surrounding cells begin to proliferate. After the tumor reaches a certain size there is great proliferation of the surrounding connective tissue, and the growth may, particularly in the jaw, look like, and was long mistaken for, osteo-sarcoma. Finally suppuration occurs, which in man, according to Israel, may be produced directly by the streptothrix itself.

Clinical Forms.—(*a*) Digestive Tract.—Israel is said to have found the fungus in the cavities of carious teeth. The jaw has been affected in a number of cases in man. The patient comes under observation with swelling of one side of the face, or with a chronic enlargement of the jaw which may simulate sarcoma.

The *tongue* has been involved in several cases, showing small growths, either primary or following disease of the jaw. In the *intestines* the disease may occur either as a primary or secondary affection. The most common seat is the region of the cæcum and appendix. An actinomycotic appendicitis has been described; primary actinomycosis of the large intestine with metastases has also been found. Ransom has found the actinomyces in the stools. Actinomycotic *peritonitis* due to infection through a gastrostomy wound has been described. Actinomycosis of the *liver* is rare. Auvray in 1903 could only collect 31 cases (Rolleston). It forms a most characteristic lesion, an alveolar honey-combed abscess—like a sponge soaked in pus. It is usually secondary to an intestinal lesion, but in a few cases no other focus has been found.

(*b*) Pulmonary Actinomycosis.—In September, 1878, James Israel described a remarkable mycotic disease of the lungs, which subsequent observation showed to be the affection described the year before by Bollinger in cattle. Since that date many instances have been reported in which the lungs were affected. It is a chronic infectious pulmonary disorder, characterized by cough, fever, wasting, and a muco-purulent, sometimes fetid, expectoration. The lesions are unilateral in a majority of the cases. Hodenpyl classifies them in three groups: (1) Lesions of chronic bronchitis; the diagnosis has been made by the presence of the actinomyces in the sputum. (2) Miliary actinomycosis, closely resembling miliary tubercle, but the nodules are seen to be made up of groups of fungi, surrounded by granulation tissue. This form of pulmonary actinomycosis is not infrequent in oxen with advanced disease of the jaw or adjacent structures. (3) The cases in which there is more extensive destructive disease of the lungs, broncho-pneumonia, interstitial changes, and abscesses, the latter forming cavities large enough to be diagnosed during life. Actinomycotic lesions of other organs are often present in connection with the pulmonary disease; erosion of the vertebræ, necrosis of the ribs and sternum, with node-like formations, subcutaneous abscesses, and occasionally metastases in all parts of the body.

Symptoms.—The fever is of an irregular type and depends largely on the existence of suppuration. The cough is an important symptom, and the diagnosis in 18 of the cases was made during life by the discovery of the actino-

myces. Death results usually with septic symptoms. Occasionally there is a condition simulating typhoid fever. The average duration of the disease was ten months. Recovery is not very rare. Clinically the disease closely resembles certain forms of pulmonary tuberculosis and of fetid bronchitis. It is not to be forgotten in the examination of the sputum that, as Bizzozero mentions, certain degenerated epithelial cells may be mistaken for the organism. The radiating leptothrix threads about the epithelium of the mouth sometimes present a striking resemblance. Streptothrix organisms, non-acid fast, are relatively common in the sputum and apparently have little pathological significance.

(*c*) Cutaneous Actinomycosis.—In more than half of the recorded cases the disease has involved the skin of the head and neck; the buccal, lingual and pharyngeal structures may be involved also. It is a very chronic affection resembling tuberculosis of the skin, associated with the growth of tumors which suppurate and leave open sores, which may remain for years.

(*d*) Cerebral Actinomycosis.—Bollinger has reported an instance of primary disease of the brain with the symptoms of tumor. A second case was reported by Gamgee and Delepine. The patient was admitted to St. George's Hospital with left-sided pleural effusion. At the post mortem three pints of purulent fluid were found in the left pleura; there was an actinomycotic abscess of the liver, and in the brain there were abscesses in the frontal, parietal, and temporo-sphenoidal lobes which contained the mycelium, but no clubs. A third case, reported by O. B. Keller, had *empyema necessitatis,* which was opened and actinomycetes were found in the pus. Subsequently she had Jacksonian epilepsy, for which she was trephined twice and abscesses opened, which contained actinomyces grains. Death occurred after the second operation.

Diagnosis.—The disease is in reality a chronic pyæmia. The only test is the presence of the actinomyces in the pus. Metastases may occur as in pyæmia and in tumors. The tendency, however, is rather to the production of a local purulent affection which erodes the bones and is very destructive.

Treatment.—This is largely surgical and is practically that of pyæmia. Incision of the abscess, removal of the dead tissue, and thorough irrigation are appropriate measures. Thomassen recommended potassium iodide, which, in doses of from 40 to 60 grains (2.5 to 4 gm.) daily, has proved curative in a number of cases. The X-rays and radium have been successful.

II. THE SPOROTRICHOSES

Definition.—A chronic infection characterized by cutaneous and internal lesions due to the growth of various forms of parasitic fungi of the sporotrichosis group.

History.—In November, 1896, a patient presented himself at Finney's outpatient clinic at the Johns Hopkins Hospital with an infection of the right arm, which had lasted for several weeks. There were ulcerations on the hand and indurations on the forearm. The condition was recognized as unusual and Schenck, who undertook its study, found on culture a branched mycelium with numerous spores or conidia. Its identification was made by the well-known expert, Erwin F. Smith, and it was named *Sporotrichum schenckii.* Since then, the disease has been widely recognized, owing chiefly to the studies of Beurmann and Gougerot, and it is now evident that it is widely distributed and one of the most clearly defined of the mycoses.

The Parasite.—In the tissues and in the pus the parasite is a large short rod from 3 to 5 μ long and from 2 to 3 μ in breadth. In cultures it grows in filaments of about 2 μ in diameter and forms characteristic ovoid spores. The points of differentiation between the forms are due largely to variation in the modes of sporulation. The parasite is introduced chiefly by accidental inoculation, and possibly through grains and fruit. The fungi have an identical action with the pathogenic bacteria, producing toxins towards which there are active humoral reactions. Widal and Abrami determined the agglutinating and fixation properties of the serum in individuals affected, and specific reactions have been determined. There are minor differences between the form described by Schenck and that described by Beurmann.

Clinical Forms.—Beurmann and Gougerot recognize three groups: First, the disseminated gummatous form in which in the subcutaneous tissues in various parts of the body there are small, firm, solid nodules, which break down and form small abscesses, ulcerating the skin. In the second, ulcerative, type the lesions are not unlike those of cutaneous tuberculosis, occurring commonly on the hands and arms, though they may appear on the legs or on the body. They may be single or in groups of two or three, and in several cases seen in Paris they resembled very much eroded syphilitic gummata. In the third form there is a localized lesion, a hard chancroid body, eroded on the surface. Dissemination occurs through the lymphatics, the regional glands become involved and there may be a group of open sores along the arm or on the side of the head. Fourthly, there are certain extra-cutaneous forms—ulcerous lesions of the mucous membranes, gummata of the muscles and an ulcerative osteo-myelitis. The disease rarely generalizes in the internal organs but the parasite has been found in connection with a pyelonephrosis.

The disease is essentially chronic, lasting often for a year or two; sometimes disturbing the health very slightly, and other times leading to anæmia. There may be no fever, but instances of acute attacks have been reported.

Diagnosis.—This has to be made from tuberculosis, syphilis, and actinomycosis, which may be done by cultures (as the parasites grow in a very specific way) and by sporo-agglutination and the fixation reaction, the full details of which are given in Beurmann's and Gougerot's manual.

Treatment.—As a rule this is surgical, but the iodide of potassium has a most beneficial effect.

III. NOCARDIOSIS

J. H. Wright of Boston separated this group from the actinomycoses and the streptothrix infections. On the one hand the parasites resemble bacteria, on the other hand the hypomycetes or moulds, in forming branching, thread-like filaments and in the production of fine conidia. They represent a transition between the bacteria and the lower fungi. The majority of reported cases have had the signs and symptoms of pulmonary tuberculosis or of multiple abscesses. In the lungs nodules, caseous masses and lesions not unlike tubercle have been found. In three cases there was abscess of the brain. The parasite may be recognized by the typically branched filaments and by the growth in cultures.

IV. OÏDIOMYCOSIS

Under this term is described a form of infective dermatitis, of which the majority of the reported cases have been in the United States. It has been called blastomycosis and saccharomycosis. The parasite grows as a spherical or oval budding cell which is capable of producing a mycelium with aerial hyphæ.

The essential lesion is a granuloma, resembling tuberculosis and involving the skin of the face as a rule, but sometimes the lesions are multiple and there is extensive ulceration from the breaking down of the nodules. In some cases the lungs and other parts have been affected. A secondary meningitis has been described, and grayish nodular infiltrations have been found in the liver, spleen, lymph glands and other organs. The disease is chronic, lasting for many years. The *diagnosis* is easily made by the microscopic examination of material from the small abscesses, or a fragment of the tissue.

When localized, recovery may take place, but when the lungs or internal organs are involved, or if the skin lesions are very extensive, death follows. For *treatment*, the actual cautery, excision, the X-rays and the internal administration of iodide of potassium may be tried.

The coccidioidal granuloma, which occurs in California, is a separate disease much like oïdiomycosis but the organism belongs to the yeast group. The initial lesion is on the skin. The features of the lung infection are much like tuberculosis. It is almost always fatal.

V. MYCETOMA

(Madura Disease)

Vandyke Carter of Bombay, a pioneer in the study of tropical diseases, gave an admirable description of this affection, which prevails largely in certain districts of India, and sporadically in other parts of the world.

The disease, usually involving the foot, is characterized by great swelling, nodular growths and the formation of multiple abscesses. There are remarkable granules 1 mm. in diameter, usually of a black color, which occur in the discharges; in other cases the granules are yellow or brownish in color. In the pale variety a streptothrix has been found, which morphologically closely resembles actinomyces. It is held by most observers that this streptothrix maduræ and actinomyces are distinct species. From the black variety of granules a hypomycete has been grown, an organism closely allied to aspergillus.

The disease begins as a granuloma, with swelling of the foot, generally on the sole. The tumors gradually soften, others form, the foot increases enormously in bulk, becomes much deformed, numerous sinuses pass between the bones, the discharges are muco-purulent and contain the characteristic granules. *Treatment* by the use of the X-rays and the intravenous injection of antimony has been helpful. Sometimes early excision or, in later stages, amputation of the foot is necessary.

VI. ASPERGILLOSIS

Bennett in 1842 described the parasite from the lungs, the *Aspergillus fumigatus,* a fungus widely distributed as a harmless parasite, having been found in the auditory canal, nose and throat. In birds, in cattle, more rarely in dogs, the aspergillus may cause lesions of the lungs resembling tuberculosis, and there have of late years been a good many cases reported in man, particularly in pigeon keepers and hair sorters. In the majority of cases the infection is secondary to some long-standing affection of the lungs, but it has been met with as a primary disease with lesions resembling broncho-pneumonia, which undergo necrosis and softening and the clinical picture is that of ordinary tuberculosis.

The *symptoms* are those of chronic pulmonary disease, cough, fever, and expectoration, in which the aspergillus is found. It is readily recognized by the character of its spores. In the case reported by the senior author, at intervals of two or three months for twelve years the patient coughed up, usually with a good deal of difficulty, a grayish-brown mass the size of a small bean, which was made up entirely of the mycelium and spores of the aspergillus. The interesting point was that the patient had no symptoms, other than the cough, and was in excellent health.

In the majority of cases the outlook is bad, and the treatment is that of chronic tuberculosis.

C. PROTOZOAN INFECTIONS

I. PSOROSPERMIASIS

Though widely spread in invertebrates, pathogenic psorosperms are not common in mammals, and in man serious disease is very rarely caused by them. One of the commonest and most readily studied forms of psorosperm is the so-called Rainey's tube, an ovoid body found in the muscle of the pig, within the sarcolemma, filled with small sickle-shaped unicellular organisms, *Sarcocystis miescheri.* In a few instances similar structures have been found in the muscles of man. The only human parasite of this group which has caused serious disease belongs to the *coccidia.*

Coccidiosis.—In a majority of the cases of this group the psorosperms have been found in the liver, producing a disease similar to that which occurs in rabbits. In Guebler's case there were tumors which could be felt during life, and they were determined by Leuckart to be due to coccidia. A patient of W. B. Haddon's was admitted to St. Thomas's Hospital with slight fever and drowsiness, and gradually became unconscious—death occurring on the fourteenth day of observation. Whitish neoplasms were found upon the peritoneum, omentum, and on the layers of the pericardium; and a few were found in the liver, spleen, and kidneys. A somewhat similar case, though more remarkable, as it ran a very acute course, is reported by Silcott. A woman, aged fifty-three, admitted to St. Mary's Hospital, was thought to be suffering from typhoid fever. She had had a chill six weeks before admission. There were fever of an intermittent type, slight diarrhœa, nausea, tenderness over the liver and spleen, and a dry tongue; death occurred from heart-failure. The liver was enlarged, weighed 83 ounces, and in its substance there were caseous foci, around each of which was a ring of congestion. The spleen weighed 16 ounces and contained similar bodies. The ileum presented six papule-like elevations. The masses resembled tubercles, but on examination coccidia were found.

The parasites are also found in the kidneys and ureters. Cases of this kind have been recorded by Bland Sutton and Paul Eve. In Eve's case the symptoms were hæmaturia and frequent micturition, and death took place on the seventeenth day. The nodules throughout the pelvis and ureters have been regarded as mucous cysts.

II. AMŒBIASIS

(Amœbic Dysentery, Amœbic Hepatitis)

Definition.—A colitis, acute or chronic, caused by *Entamœba histolytica* with a special liability to the formation of abscesses of the liver.

Distribution.—The disease is widely prevalent in Egypt, in India and in tropical countries. In Europe sporadic cases occur, rarely small epidemics. It is uncommon in Great Britain. It is common throughout the United States, particularly in the South, where it is endemic, increasing sometimes to epidemic proportions. Sporadic cases occur in all temperate regions. The relative frequency of this form of dysentery in the tropics is illustrated by the Manila statistics given by Strong; of 1,328 cases in the United States Army, 561 were of the amœbic variety. The cases of acute and chronic dysentery in the Johns Hopkins Hospital have been almost exclusively amœbic. To 1908 of 182 cases, 123 came from the State of Maryland.

Age.—It is not uncommon in children but the greatest number of cases occur between the ages of 20 and 35.

Sex.—Males are much more frequently affected. Of 182 cases at the Johns Hopkins Hospital 171 were males (Futcher).

Race.—The white race is more susceptible, 163 whites to 19 blacks in the Johns Hopkins Hospital series. In the Philippines the whites are more often attacked. In India the disease is common in the native races.

The Amœba.—The organism *Entamœba histolytica* was first described by Lambl in 1859 and subsequently by Lösch in 1875. Kartulis in 1886 found them in the stools of the endemic dysentery in Egypt and in the liver abscesses. In 1890 the senior author found them in a case of dysentery with abscess of the liver originating in Panama. Subsequently from his wards a series of cases was described by Councilman and Lafleur. The studies of Quincke and Roos, of Dock, Harris and others in the United States, of Strong and Musgrave in the Philippines, of Kruse and Pasquale in Egypt and of Leonard Rogers in India have put our knowledge of the disease on a firm basis. To find the amœbæ the little flakes of mucus or pus in the stools should be selected for examination or the mucus obtained by passing a soft rubber tube. It is sometimes necessary to give the patient a saline cathartic and then examine the fluid portion of the stool.

Entamœba histolytica is from 15 to 20 μ in diameter, has a clear outer zone (ectosarc) and a granular inner zone (endosarc). The nucleus is seen with difficulty and contains little chromatin. The movements are similar to those of the ordinary pond amœba, consisting of slight protrusions of the protoplasm. They vary a good deal, and usually may be intensified by having the slide heated. Not infrequently the amœbæ contain red blood corpuscles. In the tissues they are very readily recognized by suitable stains. They may be in enormous numbers, and sometimes the field of the microscope is completely occupied. In the pus of a liver abscess they may be very abundant, though in large, long standing abscesses they may not be found until after a few days, when the pus begins to discharge from the wall. In the sputum in the cases of pulmono-hepatic abscess they are readily recognized.

Amœbæ are frequently found in the stools of healthy persons, as Cunningham and Lewis pointed out. Schaudinn found them in from 20 to 60 per cent. in Germany, but they vary greatly in different localities. Among 300 persons in Manila, Musgrave found 101 infected with amœbæ; 61 of these had dysentery, the remaining 40 had no diarrhœa. In the next two months 8 of the 40 cases died and showed amœbic infection of the bowel. Within the next three months the remaining 32 had dysentery. Schaudinn described two distinct forms—a non-pathogenic *Ent. coli,* and a pathogenic larger form, the *Ent. histolytica,* with a strongly refractile hyaline ectoplasm. The amœbæ can be cultivated, but with difficulty. The encysted forms are apparently the chief factor in the spread of the disease. They are found in the stools of convalescents and healthy carriers. Infection occurs through food or water, the common source being a carrier. Flies may convey the infection.

Morbid Anatomy.—Intestines.—The lesions consist of ulceration, produced by preceding infiltration, general or local, of the submucosa, due to an œdematous condition and to multiplication of the fixed cells of the tissue. In the earliest stage these local infiltrations appear as hemispherical elevations above the general level of the mucosa. The mucous membrane over these becomes necrotic and is cast off, exposing the infiltrated submucous tissue as a grayish yellow gelatinous mass, which at first forms the floor of the ulcer, but is subsequently cast off as a slough. The individual ulcers are round, oval, or irregular, with infiltrated, undermined edges. The visible aperture is often small compared to the loss of tissue beneath it, the ulcers undermining the mucosa, coalescing, and forming sinuous tracts bridged over by apparently normal mucous membrane. According to the stage, the floor of the ulcer may be formed by the submucous, the muscular, or the serous coat of the intestine. The ulceration may affect the whole or some portion only of the large intestine, particularly the cæcum, the hepatic and sigmoid flexures, and the rectum. In severe cases the whole of the intestine is much thickened and riddled with ulcers, with only here and there islands of intact mucous membrane. In 100 autopsies on this disease in Manila the appendix was involved in 7; perforation of the colon took place in 19.

The disease advances by progressive infiltration of the connective tissue layers of the intestine, which produces necrosis of the overlying structures. Thus, in severe cases there may be in different parts of the bowel sloughing *en masse* of the mucosa or of the muscularis, and the same process is observed, but not so conspicuously, in the less severe forms. In some cases a secondary diphtheritic inflammation occurs. Healing takes place by the gradual formation of fibrous tissue in the floor and at the edges of the ulcers, which may result in partial and irregular strictures of the bowel.

Microscopic examination shows a notable absence of the products of purulent inflammation. In the infiltrated tissues polynuclear leucocytes are seldom found, and never constitute purulent collections. On the other hand, there is proliferation of the fixed connective tissue cells. Amœbæ are found more or less abundantly in the tissues at the base of and around the ulcers, in the lymphatic spaces, and occasionally in the blood vessels. The portal capillaries occasionally contain them, and this fact seems to afford the best explanation for the mode of infection of the liver.

Liver.—The lesions are of two kinds: first, local necroses of the parenchyma, scattered throughout the organ, and possibly due to the action of chemical products of the amœbæ; and, secondly, abscesses. These may be single or multiple. There were 37 cases of hepatic abscess among the 182 cases of amœbic dysentery in the Hopkins Hospital. Of these, 18 came to autopsy. In 10 the abscess was single and in 8 multiple. When single they are generally in the right lobe, either toward the convex surface near its diaphragmatic attachment or on the concave surface in proximity to the bowel. Multiple abscesses are small and generally superficial. There may be innumerable miliary abscesses containing amœbæ scattered throughout the organ. Although the hepatic abscess usually occurs within the first two months from the onset of the dysentery, in one of our cases the latter had lasted one and in another six years. In 5 cases the intestinal symptoms had been so slight that dysentery had never been complained of. In 2 fatal cases there were only scars of old ulcers and in 2 others the mucosa appeared normal. In an early stage the abscesses are grayish yellow, with sharply defined contours, and contain a spongy necrotic material, with more or less fluid in its interstices. The larger abscesses have ragged necrotic walls, and contain a more or less viscid, greenish yellow or reddish yellow purulent material mixed with blood and shreds of liver tissue. The older abscesses have fibrous walls of a dense, almost cartilaginous toughness. There is the same absence of purulent inflammation as in the intestine, except in those cases in which a secondary infection with pyogenic organisms has taken place.

Lesions in the Lungs are seen when an abscess of the liver—as so frequently happens—points toward the diaphragm and extends by continuity through it into the lower lobe of the right lung. This is the commonest situation for rupture to occur. Nine of our cases ruptured into the lung. In 3 cases rupture into the right pleura occurred, causing an empyema. In one the lung abscess ruptured into the pleura, producing a pyo-pneumothorax. Perforation may occur into *adjacent structures.* In 3 of the cases perforation took place into the inferior vena cava and in another the upper pole of the right kidney was invaded. The abscess may rupture into the pericardium, peritoneum, stomach, intestine, portal and hepatic veins, or externally.

Symptoms.—Three groups of cases may be recognized:

Mild Form.—Infection may be present for a month or two before the individual is aware of it. There may be vague symptoms—headache, lassitude, weakness, slight abdominal pains and occasional diarrhœa, features common enough in the tropics. Latency is the feature in a large number of cases. The amœbæ may be present without exciting symptoms, or there may be slight transient attacks of diarrhœa, and yet these are the very cases in which hepatic abscess may follow. Herrick found in the Canal zone that 20 per cent. of his cases gave no previous history of dysentery.

Acute Amœbic Dysentery.—Many cases have an acute onset. Pain and tenesmus are common. The stools are bloody, or mucus and blood occur together. In very severe cases there may be constant tenesmus, with pain of the greatest intensity, and the passage every few minutes of a little blood and mucus. In some cases large sloughs are passed. The temperature as a rule is not high. The patient may become rapidly emaciated; the heart's action becomes feeble, and death may occur within a week of the onset. Among other symptoms are hæmorrhage from the bowels, which occurred in three cases, and perforation of an ulcer with general peritonitis, which occurred in three cases. A majority of the patients recover; in others the disease drags on and becomes chronic, the symptoms often showing a periodicity. In a few cases, after the separation of the sloughs, there is extensive ulceration remaining, with thickening and induration of the colon, and the patient has constant diarrhœa, loses weight, and ultimately dies exhausted, usually within three months of the onset. With the exception of cancer of the œsophagus and anorexia nervosa, no such extreme emaciation is seen. Extensive ulceration of the cornea may occur.

Chronic Amœbic Dysentery.—The disease may be subacute from the onset, and gradually passes into a chronic stage, the special characteristic of which is alternating periods of constipation and of diarrhœa. These may occur over a period of from six months to a year or more. Some of our patients have been admitted to the hospital five or six times within a period of two years. During the exacerbations there are pain, frequent passages of mucus and blood, and a slight rise of temperature. Many patients do not feel very ill, and retain their nutrition in a remarkable way; indeed, in the United States it is rare to see the extreme emaciation so common in the chronic cases from the tropics. Alternating periods of improvement with attacks of diarrhœa are the rule. The appetite is capricious, the digestion disordered, and slight errors in diet are apt to be followed at once by an increase in the number of stools. The tongue is often red, glazed, and beefy.

Complications and Sequelæ.—Liver Abscess.—A pre-suppurative stage lasting for several weeks or months is recognized by Rogers, characterized by fever of an intermittent type, moderate leucocytosis, and an enlarged and tender liver. Suppuration in the liver is the most serious and frequent complication. Abscess of the brain has occurred.

Perforation of the intestine and peritonitis occurred in three of our cases. *Intestinal hæmorrhage* occurred three times. The infrequency of this complication is probably due to the thrombosis of the vessels about the areas of infiltration. Occasionally an *arthritis*, probably toxic in origin, may occur. There was one case in our series. Five cases were complicated by malaria; 1 by typhoid fever; 1 by pulmonary tuberculosis; and 1 by a strongyloides intestinalis infection.

Urinary Amœbiasis.—Macfie reports a case and states that there are about a dozen instances in the literature. In the majority the infection has been with the organism *Ent. histolytica* (*tetragena*). The infection may be of the kidney, bladder, seminal vesicles or urethra. The process may be a primary infection or secondary to amœbic dysentery.

Diagnosis.—From the other forms of dysentery the disease is recognized by the finding of amœbæ in the stools. Unless one sees undoubted amœboid movement a suspected body should not be considered an amœba. A non-motile body containing one or more red cells is most probably an amœba, but should lead to further search for motile organisms. Swollen epithelial cells are confusing, but the hyaline periphery is not amœboid in its action as is the ectosarc of the amœba. The trichomonads and cercomonads so frequently associated with amœbæ are not likely to give trouble. The *Ent. histolytica* is distinguished from non-pathogenic forms by its larger size, distinct refractile ectoplasm, faint nucleus, marked mobility, vacuoles, contained red blood cells, and scanty chromatin in the nucleus. The cysts are small and do not contain more than four nuclei. In the cysts of *Ent. coli* the nuclei are eight or more. Various stains are an aid in differentiation. The extent of liver dulness should be watched throughout the course, and any increase upward or downward should lead to the suspicion of a liver abscess. Hepatic abscess is usually accompanied by fever, sweats, or chills and local pain, but may be entirely latent. Exploratory puncture is safe as a rule but severe hæmorrhage into the peritoneum, six cases of which were recorded by Hatch in India, may occur. A varying leucocytosis occurs in the abscess cases. The highest count in our series was 53,000, the average being 18,350. The average leucocyte count in the uncomplicated dysentery cases was 10,600. Hepato-pulmonary abscess is attended by local lung signs and the expectoration of "anchovy sauce" sputum in which amœbæ are almost invariably found.

Prognosis.—In many cases the disease yields to treatment but the tendency to relapse of the dysenteric symptoms is one of the striking characteristics. One of our patients was admitted to the hospital five times in nine months.

Treatment.—Rest in bed is very important, even in mild attacks, and materially hastens recovery. The diet should be governed by the severity of the intestinal manifestations. In the very acute cases the patient should be given a liquid diet, consisting of milk, whey, and broths.

A return to the use of ipecacuanha is the most important event of late years in the treatment of this form of dysentery. It should always be tried, even in chronic cases. It must be given in salol-coated pills or keratin capsules so that it is not dissolved in the stomach. The patient should be on milk diet and without anything by mouth for three hours before the drug is given, the best time being at bedtime. One dose is given each night; the first may be 60 to 90 grains (4 to 6 gm.), which is reduced by five grains each night until it is down to ten grains (0.6 gm.). This course should be repeated in a week if amœbæ remain in the stools. Emetine hydrochloride hypodermically is generally preferable to ipecac by mouth. An average dose is ½ grain (0.03 gm.) three times a day for three to six days, and this repeated if necessary. Emetine sometimes causes diarrhœa which may be mistaken for the original dysentery. Rogers advises ipecac to prevent liver abscess when there is a suspicion of hepatitis. Doses of 20 to 30 grains (1.3 to 2 gm.) are given daily and continued for two weeks after the temperature is normal.

Bismuth probably does more harm than good, owing to the fact that it coats the surface of the ulcers. It is well in the chronic forms to give an occasional dose of saline or castor oil. Large injections of quinine solution in the strength of 1 to 5,000, gradually increasing to 1 to 500, have given the most satisfactory results of all the local remedies. The amœbæ are rapidly destroyed by the drug. The success of the treatment depends largely on the care with which the injections are given. The failures are undoubtedly, in many instances, due to the fact that sufficient care is not used to insure the solution reaching the cæcum and ascending colon, where the ulceration is often most severe. From a litre to two litres should be allowed to flow into the colon. The patient's hips should be elevated and he should change his position so as to allow the fluid to flow into all parts of the colon. The solution should be retained, if possible, for fifteen minutes. One or two injections may be given daily. Injections of silver nitrate solution (1 to 2,000, increased to 1 to 500) are useful in chronic cases, given in the same way. When there is much tenesmus a small injection of thin starch and half a drachm to a drachm of laudanum gives great relief. Local applications to the abdomen, in the form of light poultices, or turpentine stupes, are very grateful.

When medical treatment fails, cæcostomy may be tried or irrigations given through the appendix.

The treatment of *carriers* is a different problem. The use of emetine bismuth iodide has proved of value. It is given in capsules in daily doses of gr. ii-iv (0.12-0.24 gm.) to a total amount of about gr. xxx (2 gm.). Others advise the oil of chenopodium given after free purgation. An ounce of epsom salts is given at 6 A. M., oil of chenopodium in capsules (♏ xv, 1 c. c.) at 8 and 10 A. M., and noon; castor oil ℥i (30 c. c.) with 50 minims of chloroform at 2 P. M.

Hepatic abscess should be drained at once and the cavity irrigated by quinine solution (1 to 1,000). Emetine should be given persistently, as advised for the dysentery.

III. MALARIAL FEVER

Definition.—A protozoal disease with: (*a*) paroxysms of intermittent fever of quotidian, tertian, or quartan type; (*b*) a continued fever with marked remissions; (*c*) certain pernicious, rapidly fatal forms; and (*d*) a chronic cachexia, with anæmia and enlarged spleen.

The hæmosporidia described by Laveran, which are transmitted to man by the bite of the mosquito, are invariably associated with the disease. Malaria occurs as an endemic and epidemic disease, the latter prevailing in the tropics under favoring conditions. No infection except, perhaps, tuberculosis compares with it in the extent of its distribution or its importance as a killing and disabling disease.

Geographical Distribution.—In Europe, southern Russia and certain parts of Italy are now the chief seats of the disease. It is rare in Germany, France, and England, and the foci of epidemics are becoming yearly more restricted. In the United States malaria has progressively diminished in extent and severity during the past fifty years. From New England, where it once prevailed extensively, it has gradually disappeared, but there has of late years been a slight return in some places. In the city of New York even the milder forms of the disease are very rare. In Philadelphia and along the valleys of the Delaware and Schuylkill Rivers, formerly hot-beds of malaria, the disease has become much restricted. In Baltimore a few cases occur in the autumn, but a majority of the patients are from the outlying districts and some of the inlets of Chesapeake Bay. Throughout the Southern States there are many regions in which malaria prevails; but here, too, the disease has diminished in prevalence and intensity. In temperate regions, like the Central Atlantic States, there are only a few cases in the spring, usually in the month of May, and a large number of cases in September and October, and sometimes in November. In the Northwestern States malaria is almost unknown. The St. Lawrence basin remains free from the disease.

In India the disease is very prevalent, particularly in the great river basins. Terrible epidemics occur. In the Punjab in 1908 there were more than three million deaths from fever, a large proportion of which were from malaria. In the months of October and November there were 307,317 deaths from the disease. In Burma and Assam severe types are met with. In Africa the malarial fevers form the great obstacle to European settlements on the coast and along the river basins. The *black-water* or West African fever of the Gold Coast is a very fatal type of malarial hæmoglobinuria. The Atlantic coast line of Central America is severely infected, and the Isthmus of Panama for centuries was known as the "white man's grave." In the tropics there are minimal and maximal periods, the former corresponding to the summer and winter, the latter to the spring and autumn months.

Etiology: The Parasite.—History.—Parasites of the red blood corpuscles —hæmocytozoa—are very widespread throughout the animal series. They are met with in the blood of frogs, fish, birds, and among mammals in monkeys, bats, cattle, and man. In birds and in frogs the parasites appear to do no harm except when present in very large numbers.

In 1880 Laveran, a French army surgeon stationed at Algiers, noted in the blood of patients with malarial fever pigmented bodies, which he regarded as parasites, and as the cause of the disease. Richard, another French army surgeon, confirmed these observations. In 1885 Marchiafava and Celli described the parasites with great accuracy, and in the same year Golgi made the all-important observation that the paroxysm of fever invariably coincided with the sporulation or segmentation of a group of the parasites. In the following year (1886) Laveran's observations were brought before the profession of the United States by Sternberg. Councilman and Abbott had already, in the previous year, described the remarkable pigmented bodies in the red blood corpuscles in the blood vessels of the brain in a fatal case, and in 1886 Councilman confirmed the observations of Laveran in clinical cases. Stimulated by his work, the senior author began studying the malarial cases in the Philadelphia Hospital, and soon became convinced of the truth of Laveran's discovery, and was able to confirm Golgi's statement as to the coincidence of the sporulation with the paroxysm. The work was taken up actively in the United States by Walter James, Dock, Koplik, Thayer, Hewetson, and others, and in a number of subsequent communications the extraordinary clinical importance of Laveran's discovery was emphasized.*

Among British observers, Vandyke Carter alone, in India, seems to have appreciated at an early date the profound significance of Laveran's work.

The next important observation was the discovery by Golgi that the parasite of quartan malarial fever differed from the tertian. From this time on the Italian observers took up the work with great energy, and in 1889 Marchiafava and Celli determined that the organism of the severer forms of malarial fever differed from the parasite of the tertian and quartan varieties.

The connection of insects with the disease is an old story suggested in Roman times and revived by John Crawford, of Baltimore (1807), King of Washington, and settled finally by Ross.

The idea that fever was transmitted by the bite of the mosquito prevailed widely in the West Indies and in the Southern States. The important rôle played by insects as an intermediate host had been shown in the case of the Texas cattle fever, in which Theobald Smith demonstrated that the hæmatozoa developed in, and the disease was transmitted by, ticks; but it remained for Manson to formulate in a clear and scientific way the theory of infection in malaria by the mosquito. Impressed with the truth of this, Ross studied the problem in India, and showed that the parasites developed in the bodies of the mosquitoes, demonstrating conclusively that the infection in birds was transmitted by the mosquito. W. G. MacCallum suggested that the flagella were sexual elements, and observed the process of fertilization by them. Studies by Grassi, Bastianelli and Bignami, and many others, confirmed the observations of Ross and demonstrated the fact that the malarial parasites of human beings develop only in mosquitoes of the genus anopheles.

Then came the practical demonstration by Italian observers, and by the interesting experiments on Manson, Jr., of the direct transmission of the disease to man by the bite of infected mosquitoes. And lastly, as a practical conclusion of the whole matter, the anti-malarial campaigns so energetically advocated and carried out by Ross have shown that by protecting the individual from the bites of mosquitoes, by exterminating the insects, or by carefully treating all patients so that no opportunity may be offered for the parasite to enter the mosquito, malaria may be eradicated from any locality.

THE PARASITE.—Belonging to the sporozoa, it has received a large number of names. The term *Plasmodium,* inapt though it may be, must, according to the rules of zoological nomenclature, be applied to the human parasite. There are three well-marked varieties which exist in two separate phases or

* The following references to work on malaria which has been done in connection with the Hopkins clinic, chiefly under the supervision of Professor Thayer, may be of interest: Phila. Med. Times, 1886; British Med. Jour., March, 1887; Med. News, 1889, vol. i; Johns Hopkins Hosp. Bull., 1889; the first edition of this Text-Book of Medicine, 1892; Thayer and Hewetson, Johns Hopkins Hosp. Rep., 1895; Thayer, Lectures on Malarial Fever, 1897; W. G. MacCallum, Hæmatozoa of Birds, Jour. of Exp. Med., 1898; Opie, on the Hæmatozoa of Birds, 1898; Barker, on Fatal Cases of Malaria, Johns Hopkins Hosp. Rep., 1899; MacCallum, on the Significance of the Flagella, Lancet, 1897; Thayer, Trans. Am. Med. Con., vol. iv, 1900; Lazear, Structure of the Malarial Parasites, Johns Hopkins Hosp. Rep., 1902.

stages: (*a*) the parasite in man, who acts as the intermediate host, and in whom, in the cycle (asexual) of its development, it causes symptoms of malaria; and (*b*) an extracorporeal cycle (sexual), in which it lives and develops in the body of the mosquito, which is its definitive host. The parasites have been grown in artificial media (Bass).

(*a*) *The Parasite in Man.*—(1) The Parasite of Tertian Fever (*Plasmodium vivax*).—The earliest form seen in the red blood corpuscle is round or irregular in shape, about 2 μ in diameter and unpigmented. It corresponds very much in appearance with the segments of the rosettes formed during the chill. A few hours later the body has increased in size, is still ring-shaped, and there is pigment in the form of fine grains. It has a relatively large nuclear body, consisting of a well-defined, clear area, in part almost transparent, in part consisting of a milk-white substance, in which there lies a small, deeply staining chromatin mass. At this period it usually shows active amœboid movements, with tongue-like protrusions. The pigment increases in amount and the corpuscle becomes larger and paler, owing to a progressive diminution of its hæmoglobin. There is a gradual growth of the parasite, which, toward the end of forty-eight hours, occupies almost all of the swollen red corpuscle. It is now much pigmented, and is in the stage of what is often called the full-grown parasite. Between the fortieth and forty-eighth hours many of the parasites are seen to have undergone the change known as segmentation, in which the pigment becomes collected into a single mass or block, and the protoplasm divides into a series of from fifteen to twenty spores, often showing a radial arrangement. Certain full-grown tertian parasites, however, do not undergo segmentation. These forms, which are larger than the sporulating bodies, and contain very actively dancing pigment granules, represent the sexually differentiated form of the parasite—gametocytes.

(2) The Parasite of Quartan Fever (*Plasmodium malariæ*).—The earliest form is very like the tertian in appearance, but as it increases in size the earlier granules are coarser and darker and the movement is not nearly so marked. By the second day the parasite is still larger, rounded in shape, scarcely at all amœboid, and the pigment is more often arranged at the periphery of the parasite. The rim of protoplasm about it is often of a deep yellowish-green color or of a dark brassy tint. On the third day the segmenting bodies become abundant, the pigment flowing in toward the centre of the parasite in radial lines so as to give a star-shaped appearance. The parasites finally break up into from six to twelve segments. Here also, as in the case of the tertian parasite, some full-grown bodies persist without sporulating, representing the gametocytes.

(3) The Parasite of the Æstivo-Autumnal Fever (*Plasmodium falciparum*).—This parasite is considerably smaller than the other varieties; at full development it is often less than one-half the size of a red blood corpuscle. The pigment is much scantier, often consisting of a few minute granules. At first only the earlier stages of development, small, hyaline bodies, sometimes with one or two pigment granules, are to be found in the peripheral circulation; the later stages are ordinarily to be seen only in the blood of certain internal organs, the spleen and bone marrow particularly. Some workers believe that there are two varieties of this form, tertian and quotidian. The corpuscles containing the parasites become not infrequently shrunken, cre-

nated, and brassy-colored. After the process has existed for about a week, larger, refractive, crescentic, ovoid, and round bodies, with central clumps of coarse pigment granules, begin to appear. These bodies are characteristic of æstivo-autumnal fever. The crescentic and ovoid forms are incapable of sporulation; they are analogous to the large, full-grown, non-sporulating bodies of the tertian and quartan parasites which have been mentioned above, and represent sexually differentiated forms—gametocytes. Within the human host they are incapable of further development, but upon the slide, or within the stomach of the normal intermediate host, the mosquito, the male elements (micro-gametocytes) give rise to a number of long, actively motile flagella (micro-gametes) which break loose, penetrating and fecundating the female forms—macro-gametes (W. G. MacCallum). The fecundated female form enters into the stomach wall of the intermediate host, the mosquito, where it undergoes a definite cycle of existence.

(b) *The Parasite within the Body of the Mosquito.*—The brilliant researches of Ross, followed by the work of Grassi, Bastianelli, Bignami, Stephens, Christophers, and Daniels, have proved that a certain genus of mosquito—anopheles—is not only the intermediate host of the malarial parasite, but also the sole source of infection. The more common genera of mosquito in temperate climates are culex and anopheles. The different species of culex form the great majority of our ordinary house mosquitoes, and are apparently incapable of acting as hosts of the malarial parasite. All malarial regions, however, which have been investigated contain anopheles. Although this is apparently a positive rule, anopheles may, however, be present without the existence of malaria under two circumstances: first, when the climate is too cold for the development of the malarial parasite; and secondly, in a region which has not yet been infected. So far as is known, the parasite exists only in the mosquito and in man.

A large number of species of anopheles have been described in different parts of the world. In North America, the commonest variety, and that which in all probability is most concerned in the spread of the disease, is *A. maculipennis,* which is, also, the most important agent in the spread of the disease in Europe. The culex lays its eggs in sinks, tanks, cisterns, and any collection of water about or in houses, while the anopheles lays its eggs in small, shallow puddles or slowly running streams, especially those in which certain forms of algæ exist. The culex is essentially a city mosquito, the anopheles a country insect.

Evolution in the Body of the Mosquito.—When a mosquito of the genus anopheles bites an individual whose blood contains sex-ripe forms (gametocytes) of the malarial parasite, flagellation and fecundation of the female element occur within the stomach of the insect. The fecundated element then penetrates the wall of the mosquito's stomach and begins a definite cycle of development in the muscular coat. Two days after biting there begin to appear small, round, refractive, granular bodies in the stomach wall of the mosquito, which contain pigment granules clearly identical with those previously contained in the malarial parasite. These develop until at the end of seven days they have reached a diameter of from 60 to 70 μ. At this period they may be observed to show a delicate radial striation due to the presence of great numbers of small sporoblasts. The mother oöcyst (zygote) then bursts, setting free into the body cavity of the mosquito an enormous number of delicate spindle-shaped sporozoids. These accumulate in the cells of the veneno-salivary glands of the mosquito, and, escaping into the ducts, are inoculated with subsequent bites of the insect. These little spindle-shaped sporozoids develop, after inoculation into the warm-blooded host, into fresh young parasites. The sporozoid which has developed in the oöcyst in the stomach wall of the mosquito is then the equivalent of the spore resulting from the asexual segmentation of the full-grown parasite in the circulation. Either one, on entering a red blood corpuscle, may give rise to the asexual or sexual cycle. As a rule the first several generations of parasites in the human body pursue the asexual cycle, the sexual forms developing later. These sexual forms, sterile while in the human host, serve as the means of preserving the life of the parasite and spreading infection when the individual is subjected to bites of anopheles.

Morbid Anatomy.—The changes result from the disintegration of the red blood corpuscles, accumulation of the pigment thereby formed, and possibly the influence of toxic materials produced by the parasite. Cases of simple malarial infection are rarely fatal, and our knowledge of the morbid anatomy is drawn from the pernicious malaria or the chronic cachexia. Rupture of the enlarged spleen may occur spontaneously, but more commonly from trauma. Fatal hæmorrhage has followed the exploratory puncture of an enlarged malarial spleen.

Pernicious Malaria.—The blood is hydræmic and the serum may even be tinged with hæmoglobin. The red blood corpuscles present the endoglobular forms of the parasite and are in all stages of destruction. The capillaries of the brain may be filled by masses of red cells and parasites, often forming thrombi. The *spleen* is enlarged, often only moderately; thus, of two fatal cases the spleens measured 13×8 cm. and 14×8 cm. respectively. In a fresh infection the spleen is usually very soft, and the pulp lake-colored and turbid. The *liver* is swollen and turbid.

In some acute pernicious cases with choleraic symptoms the capillaries of the gastro-intestinal mucosa may be packed with parasites.

Malarial Cachexia.—In fatal cases of chronic paludism death occurs usually from anæmia or the hæmorrhage associated with it. The anæmia is profound, particularly if the patient has died of fever.

The spleen may weigh from five to ten pounds. The liver may be greatly enlarged, and presents to the naked eye a grayish-brown or slate color, due to the large amount of pigment. In the portal canals and beneath the capsule the connective tissue is impregnated with melanin. The pigment is seen in the Kupffer's cells and the perivascular tissue. The kidneys may be enlarged and present a grayish-red color, or areas of pigmentation may be seen. The peritoneum is usually of a deep slate color. The mucous membrane of the stomach and intestines may have the same hue, due to the pigment in and about the blood-vessels. In some cases this is confined to the lymph nodules of Peyer's patches, causing the shaven-beard appearance.

The Accidental and Late Lesions of Malarial Fever.—(*a*) *The Liver.*—Paludal hepatitis plays a very important rôle in the history of malaria, as described by French writers. Only those cases in which the history of chronic malaria is definite, and in which the melanosis of both liver and spleen coexist, should be regarded as of paludal origin.

(*b*) *Pneumonia* is believed by many authors to be common in malaria, and even to depend directly upon the malarial parasite, occurring either in the acute or in the chronic forms of the disease.

(*c*) *Nephritis.*—Moderate albuminuria is a frequent occurrence, having occurred in 46.4 per cent. of the cases in the Hopkins Hospital. Acute nephritis is relatively frequent in æstivo-autumnal infections, having occurred in over 4.5 per cent. of our cases. Chronic nephritis occasionally follows long-continued or frequently repeated infections.

Clinical Forms of Malarial Fever.—The relative frequency of the different forms varies in different regions. The tertian is the most common in temperate regions, the æstivo-autumnal in the tropics, the quartan is everywhere rare except in certain parts of India. In the Canal Zone the relative frequency of the different forms from 1904 to January 1st, 1910, was as follows: æstivo-autumnal, 22,089; tertian, 8,013; mixed infections, 677, and quartan, 20 cases. The quartan is relatively much more frequent in Baltimore; of 1,618 cases of malaria, there were 15 instances (Thayer).

I. The Regularly Intermittent Fevers.—(*a*) Tertian fever; (*b*) quartan fever. These forms are characterized by recurring paroxysms, in which, as a rule, chill, fever, and sweat follow each other in orderly sequence. The stage of *incubation* is not definitely known; it probably varies much according to the amount of the infectious material absorbed. Experimentally the period of incubation varies from thirty-six hours to fifteen days, being a trifle longer in quartan than in tertian infections. Attacks have been reported within a very short time after the apparent exposure. On the other hand, the infection may be, as is said, "in the system," and the patient may have a paroxysm months after he has removed from a malarial region, though of course this can not be the case unless he has had the disease when living there.

Description of the Paroxysm.—The patient generally knows he is going to have a chill a few hours before its advent by unpleasant feelings and uneasy sensations, sometimes by headache. The paroxysm is divided into three stages—cold, hot, and sweating.

Cold Stage.—The onset is indicated by a feeling of lassitude and a desire to yawn and stretch, by headache, uneasy sensations in the epigastrium, sometimes by nausea and vomiting. Even before the chill begins the thermometer indicates a rise in temperature. Gradually the patient begins to shiver, the face looks cold, and in the fully developed rigor the whole body shakes, the teeth chatter, and the movements may often be violent enough to shake the bed. Not only does the patient look cold and blue, but a surface thermometer will indicate a reduction of the skin temperature. On the other hand, the axillary or rectal temperature may, during the chill, be greatly increased, and, as shown in the chart, the fever may rise meanwhile even to 105° or 106°. Of symptoms associated with the chill, nausea and vomiting are common. There may be intense headache. The pulse is quick, small, and hard. The urine is increased in quantity. The chill lasts for a variable time, from ten or twelve minutes to an hour, or even longer.

The *hot stage* is ushered in by transient flushes of heat; gradually the coldness of the surface disappears and the skin becomes intensely hot. The contrast in the patient's appearance is striking: the face is flushed, the hands congested, the skin reddened, the pulse full and bounding, the heart's action forcible, and the patient may complain of a throbbing headache. There may be active delirium. One patient in this stage jumped through

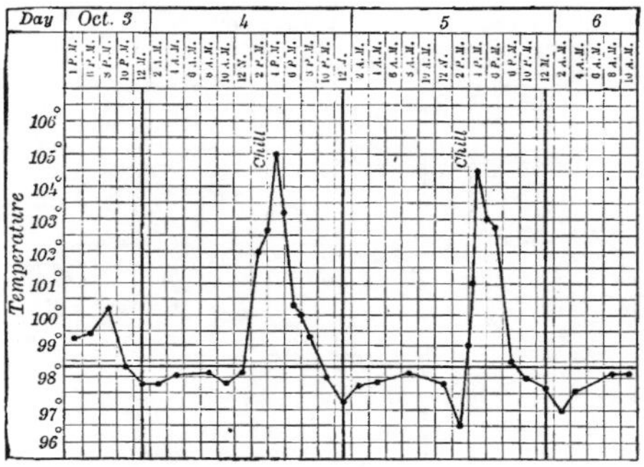

CHART VI*a*.—DOUBLE TERTIAN INFECTION.—QUOTIDIAN FEVER.

a window and sustained fatal injuries. The rectal temperature may not increase much during this stage; in fact, by the termination of the chill the fever may have reached its maximum. The duration of the hot stage varies from half an hour to three or four hours. The patient is intensely thirsty and drinks eagerly of cold water.

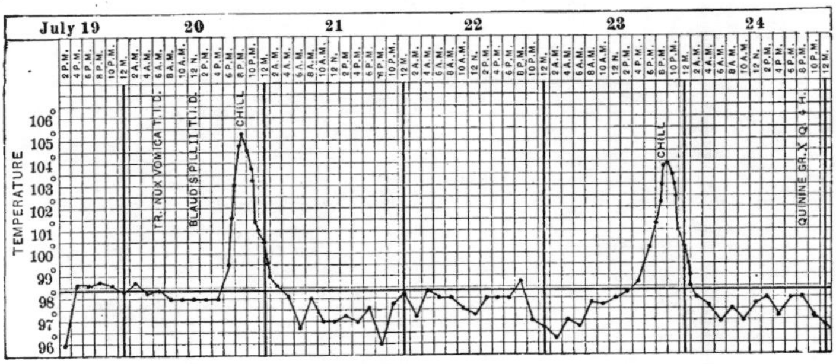

CHART VI*b*.—QUARTAN FEVER.

Sweating Stage.—Beads of perspiration appear upon the face and gradually the entire body is bathed in a copious sweat. The uncomfortable feeling associated with the fever disappears, the headache is relieved, and within an hour or two the paroxysm is over and the patient usually sinks into a refreshing sleep. The sweating varies much. It may be drenching in character or it may be slight.

Chart VI*a* is from a case of double tertian infection with resulting quotidian paroxysms. Chart VI*b* shows a quartan ague. Charts VI*c* and VI*d* give temperature curves in æstivo-autumnal forms.

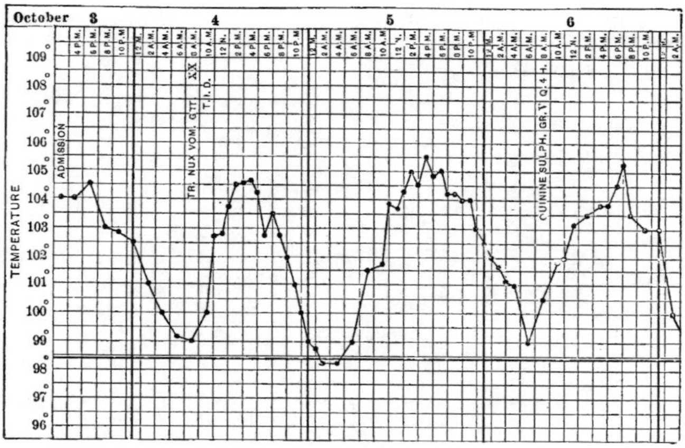

CHART VI*c*.—ÆSTIVO-AUTUMNAL FEVER.—QUOTIDIAN PAROXYSMS.

The total duration of the paroxysm averages from ten to twelve hours, but may be shorter. Variations in the paroxysm are common. Thus the pa-

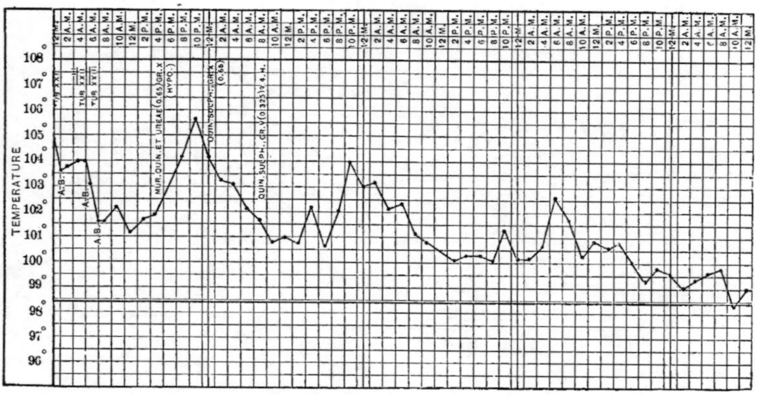

CHART VI*d*.—ÆSTIVO-AUTUMNAL INFECTION.—REMITTENT FEVER.

The case was treated for a week as one of typhoid fever.

tient may, instead of a chill, experience only a slight feeling of coldness. The most common variation is the occurrence of a hot stage alone, or with very slight sweating. During the paroxysm the spleen is enlarged and the edge can usually be felt below the costal margin. In the interval or intermission of the paroxysm the patient feels very well, and, unless the disease is unusually severe, he is able to be up. Bronchitis is a common symptom. Herpes, usually labial, is almost as frequent in malaria as in pneumonia.

Types of the Regularly Intermittent Fevers.—Two distinct types of the regularly intermittent fevers have been separated. These are (*a*) tertian fever and (*b*) quartan fever.

(*a*) Tertian Fever.—This type of fever depends upon the presence in the blood of the tertian parasite, an organism which is usually present in sharply defined groups, whose cycle of development lasts approximately forty-eight hours, segmentation occurring every third day. In infections with one group of tertian parasite the paroxysms occur synchronously with segmentation at remarkably regular intervals of about forty-eight hours, every third day—hence the name *tertian*. Very commonly, however, there may be two groups of parasites which reach maturity on alternate days, resulting thus in daily (*quotidian*) paroxysms—*double tertian infection.*

(*b*) Quartan Fever.—The symptoms resemble those of the tertian infection, but as a rule are milder. Paroxysms appear on the fourth day and correspond with the evolution of a parasitic cycle of seventy-two hours. In recent infections the recurrence of the paroxysm may be almost precisely the same hour every fourth day. The infection may be double, in which case there are two paroxysms followed by a day of intermission, or triple, in which there is a daily paroxysm. As pointed out by the old Greek physicians, the quartan infection is very difficult to cure. Disappearing for a time spontaneously, or yielding promptly to quinine, it has a singular proneness to relapse, even after the most energetic treatment.

Thus a quotidian intermittent fever may be due to infection with either the tertian or quartan parasites.

Course.—After a few paroxysms, or after the disease has persisted for ten days or two weeks, the patient may get well without any special medication. The chills may stop spontaneously. Relapses are common. The infection may persist for years, and an attack may follow an accident, an acute fever, or a surgical operation. A resting stage of the parasite has been suggested in explanation of these long intervals. Persistence of the fever leads to anæmia and hæmatogenous jaundice, owing to the destruction of blood cells. Ultimately the condition may become chronic—malarial cachexia.

II. The More Irregular, Remittent, or Continued Fevers.—(*a*) *Æstivo-autumnal Fever.*—This type of fever occurs in temperate climates, chiefly in the later summer and autumn; hence the term given to it by Marchiafava and Celli, *æstivo-autumnal* fever. The severer forms of it prevail in the Southern States and in tropical countries.

This type of fever is associated with the presence in the blood of the æstivo-autumnal parasite, an organism the length of whose cycle of development, ordinarily about forty-eight hours, is probably subject to considerable variations, while the existence of multiple groups of the parasite, or the absence of arrangement into definite groups, is not infrequent.

The *symptoms* are therefore, as might be expected, often irregular. In some instances there may be regular intermittent fever occurring at uncertain intervals of from twenty-four to forty-eight hours, or even more. In the cases with longer remissions the paroxysms are longer. Some of the quotidian intermittent cases may closely resemble the quotidian fever depending upon double tertian or triple quartan infection. Commonly, however, the paroxysms show material differences; their length averages over twenty hours, instead of from ten to twelve; the onset occurs often without chills and even without chilly sensations. The rise in temperature is frequently gradual and slow, instead of sudden, while the fall may occur by lysis instead of by crisis. There may be a marked tendency toward anticipation in the paroxysms, while frequently, from the anticipation of one paroxysm or the retardation of another, more or less continuous fever may result. Sometimes there is continuous fever without sharp paroxysms. In these cases of continuous and remittent fever the patient, seen fairly early in the disease, has a flushed face and looks ill. The tongue is furred, the pulse is full and bounding, but rarely dicrotic. The temperature may range from 102° to 103°, or is in some instances higher. The general appearance of the patient is strongly suggestive of typhoid fever—a suggestion still further borne out by the existence of acute splenic enlargement of moderate grade. As in intermittent fever, an initial bronchitis may be present. The course of these cases is variable. The fever may be continuous, with remissions more or less marked; definite paroxysms with or without chills may occur, in which the temperature rises to 105° or 106° F. Intestinal symptoms are usually absent. A slight hæmatogenous jaundice may arise early. Delirium of a mild type may occur. The cases vary very greatly in severity. In some the fever subsides at the end of the week, and the practitioner is in doubt whether he has had to do with a mild typhoid or a simple febricula. In other instances the fever persists for from ten days to two weeks; there are marked remissions, perhaps chills, with a furred tongue and low delirium. Jaundice is not infrequent. These are the cases to which the terms *bilious remittent* and *typho-malarial* fevers are applied. In other instances the symptoms become grave and assume the character of the pernicious type. It is in this form of malarial fever that so much confusion exists. The similarity of the cases to typhoid fever is striking, more particularly the appearance of the facies; the patient *looks* very ill. The cases occur, too, in the autumn, at the very time when typhoid fever occurs. The fever yields, as a rule, promptly to quinine, though cases are met with—rarely indeed in our experience—which are refractory. Several of the charts in Thayer and Hewetson's monograph show how closely, in some instances, the disease may simulate typhoid fever.

The *diagnosis* may be definitely made by the examination of the blood. Repeated examinations at short intervals may be required before the parasites are found. The small, actively motile, hyaline forms of the æstivo-autumnal parasite are to be found, while, if the course has been over a week, the larger crescentic and ovoid bodies are often seen. In many cases one is unable to distinguish between typhoid and continued malarial fever without a blood examination.

(*b*) *Pernicious Malarial Fever.*—This is fortunately rare in temperate climates, and the number of cases which now occur, for example, in Philadelphia and Baltimore, is very much less than it was thirty or forty years ago. Pernicious fever is always associated with the æstivo-autumnal parasite. The following are the most important types:

(1) Comatose Form.—In this the patient is struck down with symptoms of the most intense cerebral disturbance, either acute delirium or, more frequently, a rapidly developing coma. A chill may or may not precede the attack. The fever is usually high, and the skin hot and dry. The unconsciousness may persist for from twelve to twenty-four hours, or the patient may sink and die. After regaining consciousness a second attack may come on and prove fatal. In these instances the special localization of the infection is in the brain, where actual thrombi of parasites with marked secondary changes in the surrounding tissues have been found.

(2) Algid Form.—In this the attack sets in usually with gastric symptoms; there are vomiting, intense prostration, and feebleness out of all proportion to the local disturbance. The patient complains of feeling cold, although there may be no actual chill. The temperature may be normal, or even subnormal; consciousness may be retained. The pulse is feeble and small, and the respirations are increased. There may be most severe diarrhœa, the attack assuming a choleriform nature. The urine is often diminished, or even suppressed. This condition may persist with slight exacerbations of fever for several days and the patient may die in a condition of profound asthenia. This is essentially the same as described as the *asthenic* or *adynamic* form of the disease. In the cases with vomiting and diarrhœa the gastro-intestinal mucosa is often the seat of a special invasion by the parasites, actual thrombosis of the small vessels with superficial ulceration and necrosis occurring.

(3) Hæmorrhagic Forms—Black-water Fever—Hæmoglobinuric Fever—Malarial Hæmoglobinuria.—There are two types of hæmoglobinuria in malaria, the one associated with any severe pernicious malaria, in which an enormous number of red blood corpuscles are directly destroyed by parasites. Not very uncommon, we had a number of cases of this type at the Johns Hopkins Hospital. But in the true *black-water fever* there is a solution of red blood corpuscles by an unknown hæmolysin, not directly by the malarial parasites themselves.

The figures at Panama, based on five years' work at the Ancon Hospital, given by Deeks and James, show 230 cases in more than 40,000 cases of malaria. Their studies strongly favor the association of black-water fever with malaria, holding that there are three causes superadded to the previous malarial infection: (i) A renewed malarial attack with production of toxins sufficient to destroy many red blood corpuscles; (ii) a lowering of the bodily resistance; (iii) quinine, which appears to be the *tertium quid* necessary to produce the hæmolysin. The general experience at Panama is in favor of withholding quinine in the true erytholytic hæmoglobinuria.

(*c*) *Malarial Cachexia.*—The general symptoms are those of secondary anæmia—breathlessness on exertion, œdema of the ankles, and hæmorrhages, particularly into the retina. Occasionally the bleeding is severe, and fatal hæmatemesis may occur in association with the enlarged spleen. The fever is variable. The temperature may be low for days, not going above 99.5°. In other instances there may be irregular fever, and the temperature rises gradually to 102.5° or 103° F.

With careful treatment the outlook is good, and a majority of cases recover. The spleen is gradually reduced in size, but it may take several months, or, indeed, years, before the "ague-cake" entirely disappears.

Latent Malarial Infection.—There may be parasites in the body without any clinical manifestations of the disease. The parasites are present in the spleen in all the stages of the human cycle.

Rarer Complications.—Paraplegia may be due to a peripheral neuritis or to changes in the cord, and hemiplegia may occur in the pernicious comatose form, or occasionally at the very height of a paroxysm. Acute ataxia has been described, and there are remarkable cases with the symptoms of disseminated sclerosis (Spiller). Multiple gangrene may occur. *Orchitis* has been described by Charvot in Algiers and Fedeli in Rome.

Relapse.—It is not easy to explain the relapse. Some think there is a resting stage of the parasite which remains in the spleen or the bone marrow. Schaudinn believed that there is a special parthenogenetic form which may remain latent for an indefinite period. This seems most likely, as there can be no question that months or even years may elapse between the primary infection and a relapse occurring under conditions that preclude the possibility of re-infection.

Diagnosis.—The endemic index of a country may be determined by the "parasite rate" or by the "spleen rate." It is best sought for in children, in whom, as is well known, the infection may occur without much disturbance of the health. To determine the index by examining the blood for the parasites is a laborious and almost impossible task; on the other hand, as the work of Ross in Greece and Mauritius has shown, the index may be readily gauged by an examination of the spleen. Thus, in the last-named island, of 31,022 children, 34.1 per cent. had enlarged spleen. In Bombay, among 50,000 children examined, the spleen index varied from 5.3 per cent. in the Hindoos to 23.2 per cent. in the Parsees (Bentley).

The individual forms of malarial infection are readily recognized by examination of the fresh or stained film, but it requires a long and careful training to become an expert in blood examination. Great progress has been made and a diagnosis of malaria is no longer a refuge for our ignorance. One lesson it is hard for the practitioner to learn—namely, that an intermittent fever which resists quinine is not malarial.

The malarial poison is supposed to influence many affections in a remarkable way, giving to them a paroxysmal character. A whole series of minor ailments and some more severe ones, such as neuralgia, are attributed to certain occult effects of paludism. The more closely such cases are investigated the less definite appears the connection with malaria.

Prophylaxis.—In the discovery of Laveran there lay the promise of benefits more potent than any gift science had ever offered to mankind—viz., the possibility of the extermination of malaria. By the persistent missionary efforts of Ross this promise has reached the stage of practical fulfilment, and one of the greatest scourges of the race is now under our command. The story of the Canal Zone, Panama, under Colonel Gorgas is a triumph of the application of scientific methods. Between 1881 and 1904 among the employees of the French Canal Company (a maximum in 1887 of 17,995, of whom 15,726 were negroes) the monthly mortality ranged from 60 to 70, and on seven occasions was above 100, once reaching the enormous figure of 176.97 per 1,000. With the measures given below, the mortality has fallen below that of temperate regions. For the year 1910 the death rate among 50,802 employees was, total deaths 558, from disease 381, from violence 177; the death rate from disease was 7.5 per 1,000.

This most successful campaign has been carried out on the following lines: (1) The eradication of mosquito propagation areas by drainage, and the filling of places where the larvæ exist. This has been done in large districts.

(2) The control of propagation areas that are allowed to exist, or that cannot be economically and permanently treated. On small areas the larvæ are prevented from arriving at the adult stage by the use of crude oil or kerosene, and in large bodies of water by treating the edges where alone the mosquito larvæ exist. A concentrated larvacide of carbolic acid, resin, and caustic soda, so made as to form an emulsion with the water into which it is placed, has been found effective, when applied to the edges of large pools, ditches, wet areas and streams. A barrel of oil with an automatic drip at the head of a stream has been found to work satisfactorily.

(3) Protection by screening of houses. On the Zone all the houses occupied by Americans are protected by copper-bronze screens of 18 mesh to the inch. Cotton bar treated with wax is also recommended as inexpensive. Screened vestibules decrease the chance of access of mosquitoes. Mosquito nets over the beds are found, as a rule, to be a failure, chiefly because few persons sleep through a whole night without an arm or leg coming in contact with the netting on which the anopheles settle.

(4) The destruction of adult anopheles. In two sets of barracks not far apart, with many anopheles, in one all the adult mosquitoes were killed daily, in the other they were not; in the latter during a period of several months there was forty-two times as much malaria. The mosquitoes are easily caught; they are usually in the corners, and very often within a foot of the floor.

Of the enormous importance of these anti-malarial measures there can be no question. It requires system, organization, energy and perseverance. But the story of Havana, the story of Ismalia, and, above all, the story of the Panama Canal Zone show what can be done. The following chart, taken from an article of Le Prince, the chief sanitary inspector of the Zone, gives a good idea of the results. The objection offered on the score of cost in the tropics has been shown by Gorgas to be fallacious.

Every patient with malaria should be regarded as a centre of infection (a carrier), and in a systematic warfare reported to the health authorities. In the tropics segregation of Europeans may do much to lessen the chances of infection. Every patient should receive thorough and prolonged treatment with quinine. There is far too much carelessness on this point in the profession. Malarial infection is a difficult one to eradicate. Quinine is the only known drug which is an effective parasiticide. Patients should be told to resume the treatment in the spring and autumn for several years after the primary infection. In very malarial districts, as many persons harbor the parasites who do not show any (or at the most very few) signs, a systematic treatment with quinine should be instituted, particularly of the young children.

Patients with the disease should be protected from mosquitoes as far as possible. As a rule, anopheles are more likely to bite after sundown, so that in regions in which the disease prevails extensively mosquito netting should be used. Persons going to a malarial region should take 5 grains (0.3 gm.) of quinine daily and a double dose once a week.

Treatment.—The patient should be in bed and given liquid or soft diet. The bowels should be moved freely, for which a calomel and saline purge is best. In quinine we possess a specific remedy against malarial infection. Experiment has shown that the parasites are most easily destroyed by quinine at the stage when they are free in the circulation—that is, during and just after segmentation. While in most instances the parasites of the regularly intermittent fevers may be destroyed, even in the intra-corpuscular stage, in æstivo-autumnal fever this is much more difficult. It should, then, be our

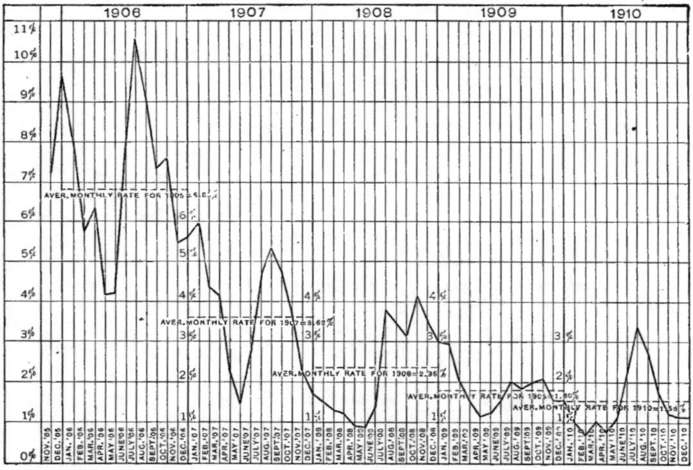

CHART VII.—MALARIA CASES AMONG THE EMPLOYEES OF THE ISTHMIAN CANAL COMMISSION, 1906-1910.

object to have as much quinine in circulation at the time of the paroxysm and shortly before as is possible, for this is the period at which segmentation occurs. In the regularly intermittent fevers from 10 to 30 grains (0.6 to 2 gm.) in divided doses throughout the day will in many instances prevent any fresh paroxysms. If the patient comes under observation shortly before an expected paroxysm, the administration of quinine just before its onset may be advisable to obtain a maximum effect upon the group of parasites. The quinine will not prevent the paroxysm, but will destroy the greater part of the group of organisms and prevent its recurrence. It is safer to give at least 20 to 30 grains (1.3 to 2 gm.) daily for the first three days, and then to continue the remedy in smaller doses for the next two or three weeks. In æstivo-autumnal fever larger doses may be necessary, though in relatively few instances is it necessary to give more than 30 grains (2 gm.) in the twenty-four hours. As to the length of time during which quinine should be taken, after the acute features are over, there is much difference of opinion. Small doses (gr. v-x, 0.3-0.6 gm.) daily for six weeks are usually efficient. It is wise to take a course of quinine twice a year for three years after. During the paroxysm the patient should, in the cold stage, be wrapped in blankets and given hot drinks. The reactionary fever is rarely dangerous even if it reaches a high grade. The body may, however, be sponged.

The quinine should be given in solution or capsules. Pills and compressed tablets are uncertain, as they may not be dissolved. Euquinine, in the same dosage, or quinine tannate, double the amount, may be given to patients with whom quinine disagrees.

A question of interest is the efficient dose of quinine necessary to cure the disease. Grain doses three times a day will in many cases prevent the paroxysm, but not with the certainty of larger doses. In cases of æstivo-autumnal fever with pernicious symptoms it is necessary to get the system under the influence of quinine as rapidly as possible. In these instances the drug should be administered by injection into the muscles, as the dihydrochloride in ten-grain (0.6 gm.) doses, in a freshly prepared solution (1 to 2) in sterile water and repeated in two hours. Further administration must be decided by the condition. The muriate of quinine and urea is also a good form in which to administer the drug intramuscularly; 10-grain (0.6 gm.) doses may be given. In the most severe instances some observers advise the intravenous administration of quinine, for which the very soluble bimuriate is well adapted. Fifteen grains (1 gm.) with 40 grains (2.6 gm.) of sodium chloride may be injected in ten ounces (300 c. c.) of freshly distilled water, or the same amount of the dihydrochloride in 500 c. c. of saline solution. The intravenous administration is not without danger. For extreme restlessness in these cases opium is indicated, and cardiac stimulants may be necessary. If in the comatose form the internal temperature is raised, the patient should be sponged or given a tub bath. For malarial anæmia iron and arsenic are indicated.

An interesting question is much discussed, whether quinine does not cause, or at any rate aggravate, hæmoglobinuria. We have not seen a case in which this condition has occurred as a result of the use of the drug, and Bastianelli states that it is not seen in the Roman malarial fevers. In any case of hæmoglobinuria if the blood shows parasites quinine should be administered cautiously. In the post-malarial forms quinine aggravates the attack. In an active malarial infection the patient runs less risk with the quinine.

In malarial cachexia the patient should have a change of climate, be given a liberal diet, and take quinine in small doses with iron and arsenic for some time.

IV. TRYPANOSOMIASIS

Definition.—A chronic disorder characterized by fever, lassitude, weakness, wasting, and often a protracted lethargy—sleeping sickness. *Trypanosoma gambiense* and *T. rhodesiense* are the active agents in the disease.

Trypanosomes are flagellate infusoria, parasitic in a great many invertebrate and vertebrates. The life history is in two stages, a flagellate monadine phase, in which they live in the blood stream of vertebrates and in some of which they cause serious disease; the other is a gregarine non-flagellate phase which may also be parasitic and which is met with in forms of Kala-Azar.

History.—In 1843 Gruby found a blood parasite in the frog which he called *Trypanosoma sanguinis.* Subsequently it was found to be a very common blood parasite in fishes and birds. In 1878 Lewis found it in the rat—*T. lewisi*—in which it apparently does no harm. The pathological significance of the protozoa was first suggested in 1880 by Griffith Evans, who discovered *trypanosomes*—*T. evansi*—in the disease of horses and cattle in India known as *surra.* In 1895 Bruce made the important announcement that the tsetze fly disease or *nagana* of South Africa, which made whole districts impassable for cattle and horses, was really due to a trypanosome—*T. brucei.* Normally present in the blood of the big-game animals of the districts, it was conveyed by the tsetze fly to the non-immune horses and cattle imported into what were called the fly-belts. Other trypanosomes are *T. cruzi* (Brazil), the Philippine surra, studied by Musgrave, the *mal de caderas*—*T. equinum*—of South America and a harmless infection in cattle in the Transvaal caused by *T. theileri.*

Human Trypanosomiasis.—In 1901 Dutton found a trypanosome in the blood of a West Indian. In 1903 Castellani found trypanosomes in the cerebro-spinal fluid and in the blood of five cases of African sleeping sickness. The Royal Society Commission (Bruce and Nabarro) demonstrated the frequency of the parasites in the cerebro-spinal fluid and in the blood in sleeping sickness, and suggested that it was a sort of human tsetze fly infection.

Distribution.—For many years it had been known that the West African natives were subject to a remarkable malady known as the lethargy or sleeping sickness. It was also met with among the slaves imported into America. The demonstration of the association of the trypanosomes with the terrible sleeping sickness has been the most important recent "find" in tropical medicine. The disease prevails in Gambia, Sierra Leone, and Liberia, and is spreading rapidly in the Congo basin, Uganda, and Rhodesia. The opening up of equatorial Africa has led to intercommunication between districts which were formerly isolated, and the seriousness of the disease may be appreciated from the fact that within three years after its introduction 100,000 negroes died of it in Uganda. In the infected regions a large number of natives, not apparently suffering from the disease, harbor the parasites in the blood and suffer only with occasional attacks of fever, during which the trypanosomes are also found in the cerebro-spinal fluid.

The disease is not confined to negroes, and Europeans may be attacked. Persons particularly prone are those who live on the wooded shores of the lakes and rivers, such as fishermen and canoe men.

The parasite is introduced by the bite of a fly, the *Glossina palpalis,* and where this insect exists the disease is liable to prevail. The fly lives on the bushes on the lake shores or river banks, and feeds on the blood of crocodiles, antelopes, etc. The trypanosomes undergo changes in the body of the fly and the infectivity does not appear until the thirty-second day, but continues for at least 75 days (Bruce).

Symptoms.—There is stated to be a long latent period. The Uganda Commissioners divide the course of the disease into three stages: first, of fever with rapid pulse, dulling of the mind, and loss of weight; secondly, the stage of tremors in which the gait becomes shuffling, the speech slow, and there are tremors of the tongue and of the hands and feet; lastly, a stage in which the patient becomes lethargic with low temperature and presents the typical picture of the dreaded sleeping sickness. The parasites are found in the cerebrospinal fluid, less constantly in the blood. In the early stages the glands of the neck are involved, and Todd and Dutton recommend puncture of these glands for the purpose of diagnosis. Death is usually caused by some intercurrent infection, as purulent meningitis or suppuration of the lymph glands. The duration is seldom longer than eighteen months. To stay the ravages and prevent the spread of the disease will tax the energies of the nations interested in the settlement of tropical Africa. The hope appears to be in the extermination of the animals upon which the *Glossina palpalis* feeds, just as the killing off of the big game in other parts of Africa has saved the cattle from the ravages of the tsetze fly. Though a colossal task, the examination of natives of infected districts should be undertaken, isolation villages established, and the cases kept under observation and treatment.

Prognosis.—A few cases in Europeans have been cured, and some of these have been without symptoms for a number of years. The criteria of cure are the absence of symptoms, failure to find the trypanosomes, and negative inoculation of the blood into susceptible animals. The outlook is hopeless in the stage of sleeping sickness.

Treatment.—Atoxyl introduced by Wolferstan Thomas and Breinl appears to have given the most satisfactory results. The parasites seem to vary in their resistance to arsenic. In some places the arsenophenylglycin seems to have acted almost as a specific. Antimony has been used a good deal and Kerandel, a member of the French Commission, cured himself with it, injecting intravenously on successive days a solution of tartar emetic in seventeen 10-centigram doses. Arsphenamine has been used without much benefit.

V. LEISHMANIASIS

(*Kala-Azar*)

Definition.—Leishmaniasis is an affection caused by parasites of the Leishmania group, of which there are three chief forms: the *Indian kala-azar*, the *infantile kala-azar*, and *tropical sore*.

Indian Kala-Azar.—An affection characterized by enlarged spleen, anæmia and irregularly remittent fever. Leishman in 1900 discovered the parasite, which was subsequently studied by Donovan (*Leishmania donovani*). It is a protozoon of very constant form, living in the spleen and bone-marrow. It has been successfully cultivated by Rogers and others, and develops into a flagellate form.

Distribution.—The disease is widely spread in Asia, particularly in Assam, many parts of India, Burma, Indo-China, Ceylon and Syria. Europeans contract it rarely.

Etiology.—Rogers believes the bedbug of India is the chief agent in transmitting it, a view which Patton shares, as he found the ingested parasite in the bedbug underwent development into flagellate forms. Donovan suggests that the disease is transmitted by the plant-feeding bug, the conorrhinus, which is an occasional blood-sucker.

SYMPTOMS.—Enlargement of the spleen is almost constant; there is irregular fever, which lasts for months and is sometimes characterized by a double rise in the twenty-four hours. The other features are those of a progressive anæmia of a secondary type with marked emaciation. Recovery is possible, but the mortality is above 80 per cent.

Infantile Kala-Azar.—This form, separated by Nicole and his associates at Tunis, is the infantile splenic anæmia long recognized in the countries of the Mediterranean basin. It differs from the Indian form in attacking children almost exclusively, and in the presence of a parasite known as the *L. infantum.* Another special feature is that the disease may be reproduced in dogs and monkeys and a spontaneous infection of dogs exists in the endemic areas of infantile Kala-Azar. Observations strongly suggest that the disease is transmitted to children through the dog flea, or through the human flea having bitten an infected dog.

Tropical Sore.—Under the various names Aleppo boil, Delhi boil, Bagdad sore, Nile sore and many others, has been described a form of disease characterized by ulcerating and non-ulcerating lesions, almost always on the exposed parts of the body. The parasite discovered by Homer Wright and known as *Leishmania tropica* has very much the same characters as the other forms, but there are slight differences, morphological and cultural. The mode of transmission has not been definitely determined.

Treatment.—For Indian kala-azar not much can be done. Quinine given in the ordinary way seems useless, but from hypodermic injections into the muscles good results are reported. Atoxyl has been freely used. Both for this and the infantile form arsphenamine has been used, but with doubtful benefit. Tartar emetic (1 per cent. solution) has been given intravenously, 5 c. c. for the first dose, and, if well borne, 10 c. c. in subsequent doses. For the tropical sore dusting with potassium permanganate, and a few days later applying a 10 per cent. solution of Prussian blue, has been found useful.

VI. RELAPSING FEVER

(*Febris recurrens, Tick Fever*)

Definition.—A group of specific infections caused by spirochætes, characterized by febrile paroxysms which usually last five or six days with remissions of about the same length of time. The paroxysms may be repeated three or even four times, whence the name relapsing, or recurring, fever. European, Indian, American and African forms are described presenting clinically much the same features, but the parasites differ in certain peculiarities.

Etiology.—The European form, which has also the name "famine fever" and "seven-day fever," has been known since the early part of the eighteenth century, and has from time to time extensively prevailed, especially in Ireland. It is a very rare disease in England. In the United States the disease appeared in 1844, when cases were admitted to the Philadelphia Hospital, which are described by Meredith Clymer in his work on Fevers. Flint saw cases in 1850-'51. In 1869 it prevailed extensively in epidemic form in New York and Philadelphia; since when it has not reappeared. While clinically the same as the European form, the organism is different and has been called *S. novyi.* In India, where the disease is very prevalent, the parasite called after Vandyke Carter differs from the spirochæte of Obermeier. Possibly it may be transmitted by mosquitoes as well as bugs.

The *African relapsing fever,* known as *tick fever,* is a very serious and widespread affection, the parasite of which, *S. duttoni,* is distinct from the other forms. It is transmitted by the tick *Ornithodoros moubata,* but as Leishman has shown, not by direct inoculation with the salivary secretion, but from other secretions voided in the act of gorging. The symptoms are very similar to those of European relapsing fever, and as many as from five to seven relapses may take place. The mortality is not very high.

The *Spirillum* or spirochæte, described by Obermeier in 1873, was one of the first micro-organisms shown to be definitely associated with a specific fever. It is from 15 to 40 μ in length, spirally arranged like a corkscrew, sometimes curved and twisted. The ends are tapering; whether furnished with flagella or not is doubtful. It is actively motile, and it is present in the blood during the febrile paroxysm, disappearing at intervals. Plotz reported the cultivation of the spirochætes directly from the blood.

The mode of transmission is probably through lice and bed bugs. The disease has been reproduced by injecting into a healthy monkey blood sucked by a bug from an infected animal. The special conditions under which it occurs are similar to those of typhus fever. Neither age, sex, nor season seems to have any special influence. One attack does not confer immunity.

Morbid Anatomy.—There are no characteristic anatomical appearances in relapsing fever. If death takes place during the paroxysm the spleen is large and soft, and the liver, kidneys and heart show cloudy swelling. There may be infarcts in the kidneys and spleen. The bone-marrow has been found in a condition of hyperplasia. Ecchymoses are not uncommon.

Symptoms.—The *incubation* appears to be short; in some instances the attack occurs within twelve hours after exposure; more frequently, however, from five to seven days elapse.

The *invasion* is abrupt, with chill, fever, and intense pain in the back and limbs. In young persons there may be nausea, vomiting, and convulsions. The temperature rises rapidly and may reach 104° on the evening of the first day. Sweats are common. The pulse is rapid, ranging from 110 to 130. There may be delirium if the fever is high. Swelling of the spleen can be detected early. Jaundice is common in some epidemics. The gastric symptoms may be severe, but there are seldom intestinal symptoms. Cough may be present. Occasionally herpes is noted, and there may be miliary vesicles and petechiæ. During the paroxysm the blood invariably shows the spirochæte, and there is usually a leucocytosis. After the fever has persisted with severity or even with an increasing intensity for five or six days the crisis occurs. In the course of a few hours, accompanied by profuse sweating, sometimes by diarrhœa, the temperature falls to normal or even subnormal, and the period of apyrexia begins.

The crisis may occur as early as the third day, or it may be delayed to the tenth; it usually comes, however, about the end of the first week. In delicate and elderly persons there may be collapse. The convalescence is rapid, and in a few days the patient is up and about. Then in a week, usually on the fourteenth day, he again has a rigor, or a series of chills; the fever returns and the attack is repeated. A second crisis occurs from the twentieth to the twenty-third day, and again the patient recovers rapidly. As a rule, the relapse is shorter than the original attack. A second and a third may occur, and there are instances on record of even a fourth and a fifth. In epidemics there are cases which terminate by crisis on the seventh or eighth day without the occurrence of relapse. In protracted cases the convalescence is very tedious, as the patient is much exhausted.

Relapsing fever is not a very fatal disease. Murchison states that the mortality is about 4 per cent., but it has been as high as 30 per cent. in India. In the enfeebled and old, death may occur at the height of the first paroxysm.

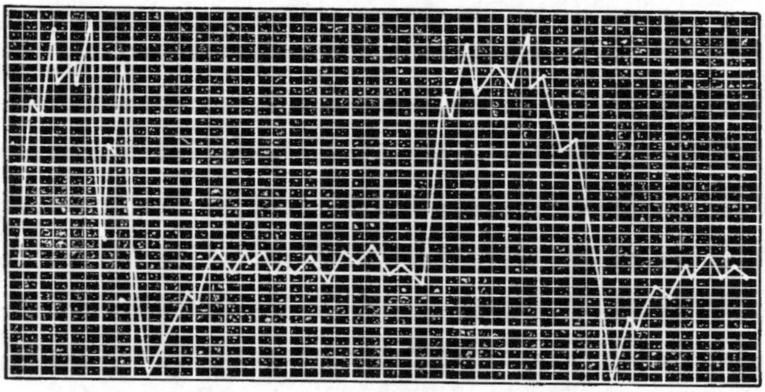

CHART VIII.—RELAPSING FEVER (Murchison).

Complications are not frequent. In some epidemics hæmatemesis and hæmaturia have occurred. Pneumonia is not infrequent. The acute enlargement of the spleen may end in rupture. Post-febrile paralyses may occur. Ophthalmia has followed in certain epidemics, and may prove a very tedious and serious complication. In pregnant women abortion usually takes place. Convulsions occasionally follow. Dutton, the well-known worker on tropical diseases, died in *status epilepticus* some weeks after the attack.

Diagnosis.—The onset and general symptoms may not at first be distinctive. At the beginning of an epidemic the cases are usually regarded as anomalous typhoid; but once the typical course is followed in a case the diagnosis is clear. The blood examination is distinctive.

Prophylaxis.—As overcrowding is an important element in the transmission, the patient should be isolated. The bedding, clothing, and dwellings of infected persons should be thoroughly disinfected and care taken that all cracks and crevices in woodwork which may harbor bedbugs are treated with disinfectants.

Treatment.—The disease should be treated like any other continued fever, by careful nursing, a regular diet, and ordinary hygienic measures. Arsphenamine has proved very efficient. Pain in the back, limbs and joints may require sedatives. In enfeebled persons the collapse at the crisis may be serious, and ammonia and digitalis should be given freely.

VII. YELLOW FEVER

Definition.—A fever of tropical and subtropical countries, characterized by a toxæmia of varying intensity, with jaundice, albuminuria, and a marked tendency to hæmorrhage, especially from the stomach, causing the "black vomit." The disease is transmitted through the bite of a mosquito, the *Stegomyia calopus.*

Etiology.—The disease prevails endemically in certain sections of the Spanish Main. Until recently it has existed in Cuba. From these regions it occasionally extended and, under suitable conditions, prevailed epidemically in the Southern States. Now and then it was brought to the large seaports of the Atlantic coast. Formerly it occurred extensively in the United States. In the latter part of the eighteenth century and the beginning of the nineteenth frightful epidemics prevailed in Philadelphia and other Northern cities. The epidemic of 1793, in Philadelphia, so graphically described by Matthew Carey, was the most serious that has ever visited any city of the Middle States. The mortality, as given by Carey, during the months of August, September, October, and November, was 4,041, of whom 3,435 died in the months of September and October. The population of the city at the time was only 40,000. Epidemics occurred in the United States in 1797, 1798, 1799, and in 1802, when the disease prevailed slightly in Boston and extensively in Baltimore. In 1803 and 1805 it again appeared; then for many years the outbreaks were slight and localized. In 1853 the disease raged throughout the Southern States. There were moderately severe epidemics in 1867, 1873, and 1878, and still milder ones in 1897, 1898, and 1899. In July, 1899, a local outbreak occurred in the Soldiers' Home at Hampton, Va. There were 45 cases, with 13 deaths. In September, 1903, yellow fever became epidemic along the Mexican side of the Rio Grande. It crossed into Texas and prevailed in several of the border towns. In Laredo there were 1,014 cases, with 107 deaths. The efficient work of the public health service is shown by the differences between New Laredo on the Mexican border, just across the river, where 50 per cent. of the population contracted the disease, and Laredo, Texas, in which only 10 per cent. out of a population of 10,000 were attacked. In Europe it has occasionally gained a foothold, but there have been no widespread epidemics in the Spanish ports. The disease has existed on the west coast of Africa, and the late Rubert Boyce claimed that it is still widely prevalent. It is sometimes carried to ports in Great Britain and France, but it has never extended into these countries. As Ross points out, yellow fever is a disease in which the parasites live a very short time in the human host, unlike malaria. The infective period in a case lasts only about three days, so that, unless the stegomyia index is high, the disease has no chance to reach epidemic form.

The epidemics in the United States have always been in the summer and autumn months, disappearing rapidly with the onset of cold weather.

Guitéras recognizes three areas of infection: (1) The local zone in which the disease is never absent, including Vera Cruz, Rio, and other Spanish-American ports. (2) The perifocal zone or regions of periodic epidemics, including the ports of the tropical Atlantic in America and Africa. (3) The zone of accidental epidemics, lying between the 35th and 15th parallels of north latitude.

Mode of Transmission.—No belief has been more strong among the laity than that the disease is transmitted by infected clothing, and quarantine efforts were chiefly directed to the disinfection of fomites of all sorts shipped from infected ports. The remarkable series of experiments carried out by the Yellow Fever Commission of the United States Army, consisting of Drs. Walter Reed, Carroll, Lazear, and Agramonte, demonstrated conclusively that the disease cannot be conveyed in this way. At Camp Lazear, Cuba, a frame house was so constructed as to shut out the sunlight and fresh air, and the vestibule was thoroughly screened. The average temperature for sixty-three days was kept about 76° F. Boxes filled with sheets, pillow-slips, blankets, etc., contaminated by contact with cases of yellow fever and the discharges, were placed in the house. Dr. R. P. Cooke and two privates of the hospital corps, all non-immunes, entered this building and for a period of twenty days occupied the room, each morning packing the infected articles in the boxes, and at night unpacking them. In their experiments with the fomites, seven non-immune subjects during the period of sixty-three days lived in contact with the fomites and remained perfectly well. These experiments, conducted in the most rigid and scientific manner, completely discredit the belief in the transmission of the disease by fomites.

We must bear testimony to the heroism of the young soldiers who voluntarily, without compensation and purely in the interests of humanity, submitted to the experiments, and also to the zeal with which members of our profession, at great personal risk, attempted to solve the riddle of this most serious disease. The deaths of Dr. Lazear, of the American Commission, and of Dr. Myers, of the Liverpool Commission, add two more names to the already long roll of the martyrs of science.

Carlos Finlay, of Havana, in 1881 suggested that the disease was transmitted by mosquitoes. Stimulated by the work of Ross on malaria, the American Commission demonstrated conclusively that yellow fever is transferred by a mosquito, *Stegomyia calopus,* previously fed on the blood of infected persons. The Commission showed also that in non-immunes the disease could be produced by either the subcutaneous or the intravenous injection of blood taken from patients suffering with the disease.

An interval of about twelve days or more after contamination appears to be necessary before the mosquito is capable of transmitting the disease. The bite at an early period after contamination does not confer immunity against a subsequent attack. As Reed pointed out, the mosquito theory fits in with well-recognized facts in connection with the epidemics. After the importation of a case into an uninfected region, a definite period elapses, rarely less than two weeks, before a second case occurs. The disease prevails most during the mosquito season, and disappears with the appearance of frost. Probably, too, as in very malarious districts, the disease is kept up by its prevalence in a very mild form among children. As Guitéras remarks, "the foci of endemicity are essentially maintained by the creole infant population, which is subject to the disease in a very mild form." In all probability the immunity which is acquired by prolonged residence in a locality in which the disease is endemic is due to the occurrence of very slight attacks.

One attack does not always confer immunity. Rosenau reports two attacks within eight years, and Libby two attacks within a period of two years.

Noguchi discovered an organism, which he termed *Leptospira icteroides*, belonging to the general order of spirochætes. It was obtained from the blood of patients and produced characteristic symptoms and lesions in guinea pigs from the blood of which the organism was obtained in pure culture. These cultures were virulent for susceptible animals. The organism is an actively motile delicate filament, 4 to 9 μ in length and 0.2 μ in breadth. A positive Pfeiffer phenomenon was observed in 15 of 18 convalescent cases studied.

Morbid Anatomy.—The skin is more or less jaundiced, even though the patient did not appear yellow before death. Cutaneous hæmorrhages may be present. No specific or distinctive internal lesions have been found. The blood-serum may contain hæmoglobin, owing to destruction of the red cells, just as in pernicious malaria. The heart sometimes, not invariably, shows fatty change; the stomach presents more or less hyperæmia of the mucosa with catarrhal swelling. It contains the material which, ejected during life, is known as the *black vomit*. The essential ingredient in this is transformed blood-pigment. There is often general glandular enlargement; the cervical, axillary and mesenteric groups are most involved. The liver is usually of a pale yellow or brownish-yellow color, and the cells are in various stages of a fatty degeneration. From the date of Louis' observations at Gibraltar in 1828, the appearances of this organ have been very carefully studied, and some have thought the changes in it to be characteristic. Hæmorrhagic and necrotic areas are common. The kidneys show acute parenchymatous inflammation. The epithelium of the convoluted tubules is swollen and very granular; there may also be necrotic changes.

Symptoms.—The incubation is usually three or four days; in 13 experimental cases it ranged from forty-one hours to five days, seventeen hours. The onset is sudden, as a rule, without premonitory symptoms, and in the early hours of the morning. Chilly feelings are common, and are usually associated with headache and very severe pains in the back and limbs. The fever rises rapidly and the skin feels very hot and dry. The tongue is furred, but moist; the throat sore. Nausea and vomiting are not constant, and become more intense on the second or third day. The bowels are usually constipated. The following in detail, are the more important characteristics:

Facies.—Even as early as the first morning the patient may present a characteristic facies, one of the three distinguishing features of the disease, which Guitéras describes as follows: The face is flushed, more so than in any other acute infectious disease at such an early period. The eyes are injected, the color is a bright red, and there may be a slight tumefaction of the eyelids and of the lips. Even at this early date there is to be noticed in connection with the injection of the superficial capillaries of the face and conjunctivæ a slight icteroid tint, and "the early manifestation of jaundice is undoubtedly the most characteristic feature of the facies of yellow fever."

The Fever.—On the morning of the first day the temperature may range from 100° to 106° F., usually it is between 102° and 103° F. During the evening of the first day and the morning of the second day the temperature keeps about the same. There is a slight diurnal variation on the second and third day. In very mild cases the fever may fall on the evening of the second or on the morning of the third day, or in abortive cases even at the end of twenty-four hours. In cases that are to terminate favorably the defervescence takes place by lysis during a period of two or three days. The remission or stage of *calm*, as it has been called, is succeeded by a febrile reaction or secondary fever, which lasts one, two, or three days, and in favorable cases falls by a short lysis. On the other hand, in fatal cases the temperature is continuous, becomes higher than in the initial fever, and death follows shortly.

THE PULSE.—On the first day the pulse is rarely more than 100 or 110. On the second or third day, while the fever still keeps up, the pulse begins to fall, as much perhaps as 20 beats, while the temperature has risen 1.5° or 2°. On the evening of the third day there may be a temperature range of 103° and a pulse of only 75, or "a temperature between 103° and 104° with a pulse running from 70 to 80." This important diagnostic feature was first described by Faget, of New Orleans. During defervescence the pulse may become still lower, down to 50, 48, or 45, or even as low as 30; a slow pulse at this period is not the special circulatory feature of the disease, but *the slowing of the pulse with a steady or even rising temperature.*

ALBUMINURIA.—This, the third characteristic symptom of the disease, occurs as early as the evening of the third day. Guitéras says very truly that it is very rare so early in other fevers except those of an unusually severe type. "Even in the mild cases that do not go to bed—cases of 'walking yellow fever'—on the second, third, or fourth day of the disease albuminuria will show itself." It may be quite transient. In the severer cases the amount of albumin is very large, and there may be numerous tube casts and all the signs of an acute nephritis; or complete suppression may supervene, and death occurs in uræmic convulsions or coma within twenty-four or thirty-six hours.

GASTRIC FEATURES.—*"Black Vomit."*—Irritability of the stomach is present from the very outset, and the vomited matter consists of the contents of the stomach, and subsequently of mucus and a grayish fluid. In the third stage of the disease the vomiting becomes more pronounced and in the severe cases is characterized by the presence of blood. It may be copious and forcible, producing much pain in the abdomen and along the gullet. There is nothing specific in this "black vomit," which consists of altered blood, and it is not necessarily a fatal symptom, though occurring only in the severer forms of the disease. Other hæmorrhagic features may be present—petechiæ on the skin and bleeding from the gums or from other mucous membranes. The bowels are usually constipated, the stools not clay-colored, except late in the disease. They are sometimes tarry from the presence of altered blood.

MENTAL FEATURES.—In very severe cases the onset may be with active delirium. "As a rule, in a majority of cases, even when there is black vomit, there is a peculiar alertness; the patient watches everything going on about him with a peculiar intensity and liveliness. This may be due in part to the terror the disease inspires" (Guitéras).

Relapses occasionally occur. Among the varieties of the disease it is important to recognize the mild cases, characterized by slight fever, continuing for one or two days, and succeeded by a rapid convalescence. In the absence of a prevailing epidemic they would scarcely be recognized as yellow fever. Cases of greater severity have high fever and the features of the disease are well marked—vomiting, extreme prostration, and hæmorrhages. And, lastly, in the malignant form the patient is overwhelmed by the intensity of the fever, and death takes place in two or three days.

In severe cases convalescence may be complicated by parotitis, abscesses in various parts of the body, and diarrhœa.

Diagnosis.—(*a*) FROM DENGUE.—The difficulty in the differential diagnosis of these two diseases lies in their frequent coexistence, as during the epidemic of 1897 in parts of the Southern States. During the autumn of 1897 the profession of Texas was divided on the question of the existence of yellow fever in the State, some claiming that the disease was dengue, others, including Guitéras and West, that yellow fever also existed. In a majority of the cases the three diagnostic points upon which Guitéras lays stress—the facies, the albuminuria, and the slowing of the pulse with maintenance or elevation of the fever—are sufficient for the diagnosis. He states, too, that jaundice, which does sometimes occur in dengue, rarely appears as early as the second or third day of the disease, and on this much stress should be laid. Hæmorrhages are much less common in dengue, but that they do occur has been recognized by authorities ever since the time of Rush.

(*b*) FROM MALARIAL FEVER.—In the early stages of an epidemic cases are very apt to be mistaken for malarial fever. In the Southern States the outbreaks have usually been in the late summer months, the season in which æstivo-autumnal fever prevails. Among the points to be specially noted is the absence of early jaundice. Even in the most intense types of malarial infection the color of the skin is rarely changed within four or five days. To the experienced eye the facies would be of considerable help if the case was seen from the outset. Albumin is rarely present in the urine so early as the second day in a malarial infection. Other important points are the marked swelling of the spleen in malaria, while in yellow fever it is not much enlarged. Hæmorrhages, and particularly the black vomit, epistaxis, and bleeding gums are very rare in malarial infection. In the so-called hæmorrhagic malarial fever the patient has usually had previous attacks of malaria. Hæmaturia is a prominent feature, while in yellow fever it is by no means frequent. The point of greatest importance is the examination of the blood for malarial parasites.

Prognosis.—In its graver forms yellow fever is one of the most fatal of epidemic diseases. The mortality has ranged, in various epidemics, from 15 to 85 per cent. In heavy drinkers and those who have been exposed to hardships the death-rate is much higher than among the better classes. In the epidemic of 1878, in New Orleans, while the mortality in hospitals was over 50 per cent. of the white and 21 per cent. of the colored patients, in private practice it was not more than 10 per cent. among the white patients. The death-rate was very low in the epidemic of 1897.

Prophylaxis.—The clearing of Havana by Gorgas was a direct outcome of the work of Reed and his colleagues. The city, with 250,000 people, had been infected continuously for 130 years. Non-immunes came in at the rate of 20,000 a year, and there were 6,000 children born. The city was divided into districts, each under the charge of an inspector, whose work was arranged under three heads: (1) To prevent the breeding of stegomyia mosquitoes. (2) To destroy those that had become infected. (3) To prevent mosquitoes becoming infected by protecting the sick so that they could not be bitten by mosquitoes. The work was begun in February, 1901, and the last case of yellow fever occurred in September of that year, since which date, with the exception of a slight return, the city has been free.

At Panama in 1904, the date of the American occupation, the serious problem was how to fight yellow fever. Conditions were such that it took sixteen months before the disease disappeared. There has been no return. It is interesting to note that in the yellow fever wards at Ancon during 1905 all the physicians and nurses were non-immune, but not one of them contracted the disease, as the wards were so screened that no stegomyia mosquitoes could get at the patients to become infected.

Treatment.—Careful nursing and a symptomatic plan of treatment probably give the best results. The patient should be at rest in bed and for the first few days the diet should consist of very simple fluids. Elimination is an important part of treatment. Water should be given as freely as possible, best in the form of cold carbonated alkaline water. The bowels should be opened by a calomel and saline purge and enemata used if necessary. If there is vomiting, fluid should be given by the bowel or by infusion. Ice in small quantities or cocaine (gr. ¼, 0.016 gm.) may be tried. The fever should be treated by hydrotherapy, sponges, packs or baths being used. The alkaline treatment is favorably regarded, sodium bicarbonate in full doses being given at short intervals and as much alkaline water as possible. For gastric and intestinal hæmorrhage the perchloride of iron or oil of turpentine may be given in doses of 15 minims (1 c.c.). Uræmic symptoms are best treated by the hot baths or packs, the free administration of fluid and hot bowel irrigations. Stimulants, especially strychnine, should be used during the second stage when the heart becomes feeble and rapid.

VIII. SYPHILIS

I. HISTORY, ETIOLOGY AND MORBID ANATOMY

Definition.—A specific disease of slow evolution caused by *Treponema pallidum* (spirochæta pallida) propagated by inoculation (acquired syphilis) or transmission through the mother (congenital syphilis).

History.—Whether the disease was known in Europe before 1493 is still discussed. Block, in the System of Syphilis, Vol. I, 1908, insists that there is no evidence of pre-Columbian syphilis in the Eastern hemisphere before the return of the Spanish sailors from Hayti, from whom it spread among the inhabitants of Barcelona. In 1493 it reached Italy with the army of Charles VIII. His soldiers syphilized Naples; the disease spread throughout Italy, and in a few years Europe was aflame. On the other hand, writers who contend for the antiquity of the disease in Asia and Europe rely on certain old Chinese records, on references in the Bible and in old medical writers to diseases resembling syphilis and on suggestive bone lesions in very old skeletons. The balance of evidence, according to the best syphilographers, is in favor of the American origin. At first it was called the Neapolitan disease, the French pox, or Morbus Gallicus; and in 1530 Fracastorius, in a poem entitled "Syphilis sive Morbus Gallicus," gave it the name by which it is now commonly known. The etymology of the name is uncertain.

At first the disease was thought to be transmitted like any other epidemic, but gradually the venereal nature was recognized, and Fernel, a famous Paris physician of the 16th century, insisted on the necessity of a primary inoculation. Paracelsus observed its congenital character. Throughout the 16th century the symptoms were well described. The disease appears to have been of much greater severity then than at present. Mercury and guaiacum were introduced as the important remedies. In the 18th century Lancisi recognized the relations existing between syphilis and aneurism, and Morgagni described many of the visceral lesions. Hunter, misled by inoculations made on his own person, decided in favor of the unity of the venereal poisons, gonorrhœa, soft chancre and syphilis. Ricord clearly differentiated the soft and hard chancre, and throughout the 19th century the clinical and pathological lesions were so thoroughly studied that scarcely a feature of the disease remained unknown. But all efforts at discovering the cause had failed, until in 1905 Schaudinn demonstrated the presence of a spirochæte in the lesions. Since then his work has been amply verified, and in 1910 Ehrlich announced the discovery of a compound which would destroy the parasite and not damage the individual.

Etiology: The Parasite.—The treponema is a spiral, curved organism from 5 to 15 μ in length, showing active movements in fresh specimens. It is present in the primary sore, in the regional lymph glands, in the secondary lesions, in many gummata, and in special abundance in the congenital lesions, particularly in the liver. It may live in the body as long as the host is alive. It is inoculable into monkeys, with the production of a disease resembling in most particulars that of man. The parasite has been cultivated by Noguchi.

There are apparently various strains of the treponema and this may explain some of the clinical differences. Workers in the United States Army Medical School have grown spirochætes showing different results in the primary and secondary lesions produced by them. The spirochætes from cases of general paresis take 60 to 80 days for propagation and 60 days for lesions to be produced in rabbits, whereas in the case of organisms from early lesions three or four weeks is sufficient. The spirochætes cause the production of antibodies in the tissues and it seems possible that with time a strain of spirochætes may result with greater resistance but perhaps less power of reproduction. The infection then does not cause any active symptoms, but may persist indefinitely in a latent form to resume activity after a long interval of quiescence. In some cases the tissues, so to speak, become accustomed to the spirochætes, antibodies are not produced, and in the absence of these the Wassermann reaction is negative. The infection must be active to cause the production of antibodies. In many cases a resistance to the usual remedies is apparently established.

One of the most important results of the discovery of the parasite has been the application of the methods of serum diagnosis. What is called the Wassermann reaction is a special way of determining the presence of immune bodies in the blood of a patient suffering from syphilitic infection. An enormous amount of work has been done upon it with the general result of confirming its value. A positive result has been obtained in from 90 to 95 per cent. of all cases. It appears from the end of the second to the end of the fourth week, becomes more marked and may continue for an indefinite period. During active treatment it may be absent, to reappear again. Its intensity bears some relation to the activity of the lesions.

Modes of Infection.—(*a*) In a majority of all cases the disease is transmitted by *sexual congress,* but the designation *venereal* disease (*lues venerea*) is not always correct, as there are many other modes of inoculation. In the St. Louis Hospital collection there are illustrations of 26 varieties of extra-genital chancres.

(*b*) *Accidental Infection.*—In surgical and in midwifery practice physicians are not infrequently inoculated. Infection may occur without a characteristic local sore. Midwifery chancres are usually on the fingers, but may be on the back of the hand. The lip chancre is the most common of these extra-genital forms, and may be acquired in many ways apart from direct infection. Mouth and tonsillar sores result as a rule from improper practices. Wet-nurses are sometimes infected on the nipple, and it occasionally happens that relatives of a syphilitic child are accidentally contaminated.

(*c*) *Congenital Transmission.*—The disease is not inherited, but the fetus is infected through the placenta. It is a question entirely of intra-uterine infection. The mother herself may be, and often is, apparently quite healthy, but the Wassermann reaction is present and it is through her and not directly from the father that the disease is transmitted. We can now understand what is known as Beaumès' or Colles' law, which was thus stated by the distinguished Dublin surgeon: "That a child born of a mother who is without obvious venereal symptoms, and which, without being exposed to any infection subsequent to its birth, shows this disease when a few weeks old, this child will infect the most healthy nurse, whether she suckle it, or merely handle and dress it; and yet this child is never known to infect its own mother, even though she suckle it while it has venereal ulcers of the lips and tongue." So, too, a child showing no taint, but born of a woman suffering with syphilis, may with impunity be suckled by its mother (Profeta's law).

Morbid Anatomy.—The typical *primary lesion,* or chancre, shows: (*a*) A diffuse infiltration of the connective tissue with small, round cells. (*b*) Larger epithelioid cells. (*c*) Giant cells. (*d*) Changes in the small arteries and veins, chiefly thickening of the intima, and alterations in the nerve fibres going to the part. The sclerosis is due in part to this acute obliterative endarteritis. Associated with the initial lesions are changes in the adjacent lymph glands, which undergo hyperplasia, and finally become indurated.

The *secondary lesions* of syphilis are too varied for description here. They consist of condylomata, skin eruptions, affections of the eye, etc.

The *tertiary lesions* consist of circumscribed tumors known as gummata, various skin lesions, and a special type of arteritis.

Gummata.—Syphilomata occur in the bones or periosteum—here they are called nodes—in the muscles, skin, brain, lungs, liver, kidneys, heart, testes, and adrenals. They vary in size from small, almost microscopic bodies to large solid tumors from 3 to 5 cm. in diameter. They are usually firm and hard, but in the skin and on the mucous membranes they tend to break down rapidly and ulcerate. On cross-section a medium-sized gumma has a grayish-white, homogeneous appearance, presenting in the centre a firm, caseous substance, and at the periphery a translucent, fibrous tissue. Often there are groups of three or more surrounded by dense sclerotic tissue.

The arteritis will be considered in a separate section.

II. ACQUIRED SYPHILIS

Primary Stage.—This extends from the appearance of the initial sore until the onset of the constitutional symptoms, and has a variable duration of from six to twelve weeks. The initial sore appears within a month after inoculation, and it first shows itself as a small red papule, which gradually enlarges and breaks in the centre, leaving a small ulcer. The tissue about this becomes indurated so that it ultimately has a gristly, cartilaginous consistence—hence the name, hard or indurated chancre. The size attained is variable, and when small the sore may be overlooked, particularly if it is just within the urethra. The initial lesion has no invariable characteristic and may not be indurated. It must be emphasized that infection may occur without any marked primary lesion. A negative history as to the occurrence of a chancre is of no value in excluding the possibility of infection. There are a considerable number of extragenital infections. Syphilitic infection may occur with a chancroid. The glands in the lymph-district of the chancre enlarge and become hard. Suppuration both in the initial lesion and in the glands may occur as a secondary change. The general condition of the patient in this stage is good. There may be no fever and no impairment of health.

Secondary Stage.—The first constitutional symptoms are usually manifested within three months of the appearance of the primary sore. They rarely occur earlier than the sixth or later than the twelfth week:

(*a*) *Fever,* slight or intense, and very variable in character, may occur early before the skin rash; more frequently it is the "fever of invasion" with the secondary symptoms, or the fever may occur at any period. It may be a mild continuous pyrexia, or in other instances with marked remissions, but the most remarkable form is the intermittent, often mistaken for malaria. The fever may reach 105° and the paroxysms persist for months. We have had several cases in which typhoid fever or tuberculosis was suspected.

(*b*) *Anæmia.*—In many cases the syphilitic poison causes a pronounced anæmia which gives to the face a muddy pallor, and there may even be a light-yellow tinging of the conjunctivæ or of the skin, a hæmatogenous icterus. This syphilitic cachexia may in some instances be extreme. The red blood corpuscles do not show any special alterations. The blood count may fall to three millions per cubic millimetre, or even lower. The anæmia may come on suddenly. In a case of syphilitic arthritis in a young girl, following three or four inunctions of mercury, the blood-count fell below two millions per cubic millimetre in a few days.

(*c*) *Cutaneous Lesions.*—The earliest and most common is a *macular syphilide* or *syphilitic roseola,* which occurs on the trunk, and on the front of the arms. The face is often exempt. The spots, which are reddish-brown and symmetrically arranged, persist for a week or two. There may be multiple relapses of roseola, sometimes at long intervals, even eleven years (Fournier). The *papular syphilide,* which forms acne-like indurations about the face and trunk, is often arranged in groups. Other forms are the *pustular rash,* which may closely simulate variola. A *squamous syphilide* occurs, not unlike ordinary psoriasis, except that the scales are less abundant. The rash is more copper-colored and not specially confined to the extensor surfaces.

In the moist regions of the skin, such as the perineum and groins, and at the angles of the mouth, the so-called *mucous patches* occur, which are flat, warty outgrowths, with well-defined margins and surfaces covered with a grayish secretion. They are among the most distinctive lesions of syphilis.

Frequently the hair falls out (alopecia), either in patches or by a general thinning. Occasionally the nails become affected (syphilitic onychia).

(*d*) *Mucous Lesions.*—With the fever and the roseolous rash the throat and mouth become sore. The pharyngeal mucosa is hyperæmic, the tonsils are swollen and often present small, kidney-shaped ulcers with grayish-white borders. Mucous patches are seen on the inner surfaces of the cheeks and on the tongue and lips. Hypertrophy of the papillæ in various portions of the mucous membrane produces the syphilitic warts or condylomata which are most frequent about the vulva and anus.

(*e*) *Adenitis.*—This is often general. The glands are hard, painless and not much enlarged. Involvement of the epitrochlear and posterior cervical glands is specially significant.

(*f*) *Arthritis* and pains in the limbs are common secondary symptoms. Occasionally the joint affection is severe and rheumatic fever is suspected.

(*g*) *Other Lesions.*—An increase of the cells in the *spinal fluid* is found in 30 to 40 per cent. of cases. *Iritis* is common, and usually affects one eye before the other. It comes on from three to six months after the chancre. There may be only slight ciliary congestion in mild cases, but in severer forms there is great pain, and the condition is serious and demands careful management. *Choroiditis* and *retinitis* are rare secondary symptoms. Pupillary changes are not uncommon in the early stages. Ear affections are not common in the secondary stage, but instances are found in which sudden deafness occurs, which may be due to labyrinthine disease; more commonly the impaired hearing is due to the extension of inflammation from the throat to the middle ear. Epididymitis and parotitis are rare. Jaundice may occur, the *icterus syphiliticus præcox.* The acute nephritis will be referred to later.

Tertiary Stage.—No hard and fast line can be drawn between the lesions of the secondary and those of the tertiary period; and, indeed, in exceptional cases, manifestations which usually appear late may set in even before the primary sore has properly healed. The special affections of this stage are certain skin eruptions, visceral gummata, and amyloid degenerations.

(*a*) The late *syphilides* show a greater tendency to ulceration and destruction of the deeper layers of the skin, so that in healing scars are left. They are also more scattered and seldom symmetrical. One of the most characteristic of the syphilides is *rupia,* the dry stratified crusts of which cover an ulcer which involves the deeper layers of the skin and in healing leaves a scar.

(*b*) *Gummata.*—These may occur in the skin, subcutaneous tissue, muscles, or internal organs. In the skin they tend to break down and ulcerate, leaving ugly sores which heal with difficulty. In the solid organs they undergo fibroid transformation and produce puckering and deformity. On the mucous membranes these tertiary lesions lead to ulceration, in the healing of which cicatrices are formed; thus, in the larynx great narrowing may result, and in the rectum ulceration with fibroid thickening and retraction may lead to stricture. Gummatous ulcers may be infective.

(c) *Amyloid Degeneration.*—Syphilis plays a most important rôle in the production of this affection. Of 244 instances analyzed by Fagge, 76 had syphilis, and of these 42 had no bone lesions. It follows the acquired form and is very common in association with rectal syphilis in women. In congenital lues amyloid degeneration is rare.

(d) *Syphilis of the Bones.*—This is by no means uncommon and should be searched for by radiography in doubtful cases. The commonest lesions are periostitis and osteo-periostitis which may exist without any symptoms. Occasionally a gumma is found. The bone lesions occur both in the acquired and congenital form. Pain is common, often nocturnal and relieved by exercise. It may occur only on pressure over small areas. Involvement of the *spine* is not unusual. There may be periostitis, osteomyelitis with necrosis, and sometimes the formation of exostoses, which may be felt. The cervical region is most often involved and the process is generally limited to a small number of vertebræ. The main features are pain, tenderness, rigidity, and sometimes deformity. In a number of patients neural symptoms are present and root pains may be marked. The degree of deformity varies. There is often marked muscle spasm in the region involved and hypotonicity in other parts of the spine. Involvement of the cord itself is comparatively common. The diagnosis of involvement of the spine may not be easy. Careful search should be made for luetic lesions elsewhere; for example, ulceration of the larynx has been found in a certain number of cases of involvement of the cervical region.

Quaternary Stage.—Long years it may be from the primary sore and from any active manifestations, certain forms of syphilis may appear, the chief of which are tabes dorsalis and general paresis.

Latent Syphilis.—In many cases there is a persistence of the spirochætal infection without evident clinical signs of the disease, proved by the presence of the spirochætes in certain tissues, especially the heart, aorta and testicles. Warthin has drawn especial attention to this and has demonstrated the organisms in about one-third of autopsies on adults. Careful examination will often show clinical evidence in the form of myocarditis, aortitis, or induration of the testicle. Warthin suggests that latent syphilis is the chief factor in causing myocardial insufficiency and the cardiovascular-renal complex. The Wassermann reaction and examination of the spinal fluid are useful in the recognition of these cases.

III. CONGENITAL SYPHILIS

With the exception of the primary sore, every feature of the acquired disease may be seen in the congenital form.

The intra-uterine conditions leading to the death of the fetus do not here concern us. The child may be born healthy-looking or with well-marked evidences of the disease. In the majority of instances the former is the case and within the first month or two the signs of the disease appear.

Symptoms.—(a) *At Birth.*—When the disease exists at birth the child is feebly developed and wasted, and a skin eruption is usually present, commonly in the form of bullæ about the hands and feet (pemphigus neonatorum syphiliticus). The child snuffles, the lips are ulcerated, the angles of the mouth fissured, and there is enlargement of the liver and spleen. The bone symptoms may be marked, and the epiphyses may even be separated. In such cases the children rarely survive long.

(*b*) *Early Manifestations.*—When born healthy the child thrives, is fat and plump, and shows no abnormity whatever; then from the fourth to the eighth week, rarely later, a nasal catarrh occurs, *syphilitic rhinitis,* which impedes respiration, and produces the characteristic symptom which has given the name *snuffles* to the disease. The discharge may be sero-purulent or bloody. The child nurses with great difficulty. In severe cases ulceration takes place with necrosis of the bone, leading to a depression at the root of the nose and a deformity characteristic of congenital syphilis. This coryza may be mistaken at first for an ordinary catarrh, but the coexistence of other manifestations usually makes the diagnosis clear. The disease may extend into the Eustachian tubes and middle ears and lead to deafness.

The *cutaneous* lesions arise with or shortly after the onset of the snuffles. The skin often has a sallow, earthy hue. The eruptions are first noticed about the nates. There may be an erythema or an eczematous condition, but more commonly there are irregular reddish-brown patches with well-defined edges. A papular syphilide in this region is by no means uncommon. A desquamative dermatitis of the palms of the hands and soles of the feet may occur. Fissures occur about the lips, either at the angles of the mouth or in the median line. These *rhagades,* as they are called, are very characteristic. There may be marked ulceration of the muco-cutaneous surfaces. The secretions from these mouth lesions are very virulent, and it is from this source that the wet-nurse is usually infected. Not only the nurse, but members of the family, may be contaminated. There are instances in which other children have been accidentally inoculated from a syphilitic infant. The hair of the head or of the eyebrows may fall out. The syphilitic *onychia* is not uncommon. Enlargement of the glands is not so frequent in the congenital as in the acquired disease. When the cutaneous lesions are marked the contiguous glands can usually be felt. As pointed out by Gee, the spleen is enlarged in many cases. The condition may persist for a long time. Enlargement of the liver, though often present, is less significant, since in infants it may be due to various causes. These are among the most constant symptoms of congenital syphilis, and usually arise between the third and twelfth weeks. Frequently they are preceded by a period of restlessness and wakefulness, particularly at night. Some authors have described a peculiar syphilitic cry, high-pitched and harsh. Among rarer manifestations are hæmorrhages—the *syphilis hæmorrhagica neonatorum.* The bleeding may be subcutaneous, from the mucous surfaces, or, when early, from the umbilicus. All of such cases, however, are not syphilitic, and the disease must not be confounded with the acute hæmoglobinuria of new-born infants. E. Fournier described a remarkable enlargement of the subcutaneous veins.

(*c*) *Late Manifestations.*—Children with congenital syphilis rarely thrive. Usually they present a wizened, wasted appearance, and a prematurely aged face. In the patients who recover the general nutrition may remain good and the child may show no further manifestations; commonly, however, at the period of second dentition or at puberty the disease reappears. Although the child may have recovered from the early lesions, it does not develop like other children. Growth is slow, development tardy, and there are facial and cranial characteristics which often render the disease recognizable at a glance. A young man of nineteen or twenty may neither look older nor be more developed than a boy of ten or twelve—infantilism. The forehead is prominent, the frontal eminences are marked, and the skull may be very asymmetrical. The bridge of the rose is depressed, the tip *retroussé*. The lips are often prominent, and there are striated lines running from the corners of the mouth. The *teeth* are deformed and may present appearances which Jonathan Hutchinson claimed are specific and peculiar. The upper central incisors of the permanent set are peg-shaped, stunted in length and breadth, and narrower at the cutting edge than at the root. On the anterior surface the enamel is well formed, and not eroded or honeycombed. At the cutting edge there is a single notch, usually shallow, sometimes deep, in which the dentine is exposed. The upper first large molar may have a supernumerary cusp on the inner side which forms a protuberance.

Among late manifestations, particularly apt to appear about puberty, is the interstitial *keratitis,* which usually begins as a slight steaminess of the corneæ, which present a ground-glass appearance. It affects both eyes, though one is attacked before the other. It may persist for months, and usually clears completely, though it may leave opacities, which prevent clear vision. *Iritis* and *choroiditis* may occur. Of *ear affections,* apart from those which follow the pharyngeal disease, a form occurs, about the time of puberty or earlier, in which deafness comes on rapidly and persists in spite of treatment. It is unassociated with obvious lesions, and is probably labyrinthine in character. *Bone lesions,* occurring oftenest after the sixth year, are not rare among the late manifestations of congenital syphilis. The tibiæ are most frequently attacked. It is really a chronic gummatous periostitis, which gradually leads to great thickening of the bone. The nodes of congenital syphilis, which are often mistaken for rickets, are more commonly diffuse and affect the bones of the upper and lower extremities. They are generally symmetrical and rarely painful. They may occur late, even after the twenty-first year.

Joint lesions are rare. Clutton has described a symmetrical synovitis of the knee in hereditary syphilis. Enlargement of the spleen, sometimes with the lymph-glands, may be one of the late manifestations, and may occur either alone or in connection with disease of the liver.

The central nervous system is often affected. This may show itself in various degrees of lack of mental development or general paresis may result. Certain patients show symptoms much like the ordinary chorea. It is a safe rule to consider syphilis in any abnormality in a child.

Gummata of the liver, brain, and kidneys have been found in late congenital syphilis.

Is syphilis transmitted to the third generation? The discovery of the treponema answers this question. The disease can be carried through as many generations as are able to reproduce. This makes a thorough study of the family for several generations an important aid in the diagnosis of congenital syphilis.

IV. VISCERAL SYPHILIS

1. *Cerebro-spinal Syphilis*

The nervous system is frequently involved in the primary and secondary stages as shown by changes in the cerebro-spinal fluid. In the great majority there are no later manifestations. Mattauschek and Pilcz followed 4,143 cases of syphilis for from twenty to thirty years with special reference to this point: 4.7 per cent. developed paresis, 3.2 per cent. had cerebro-spinal syphilis and 2.7 per cent. tabes dorsalis. The figures were highest in those who had little or no treatment.

Pathology.—The process may involve (*a*) the meninges, (*b*) the arteries and (*c*) the parenchyma. In the majority of cases the lesions are not limited to one of these structures. Involvement of one alone is probably most common in the arteries—endarteritis. With this the cerebro-spinal fluid shows little if any change and the symptoms are due to the vascular disease. In all forms marked perivascular changes are common. The exudate due to these interferes with the lymphatic circulation. This with the endarteritis often results in marked interference with the blood supply. In general the lesions may be classified as (1) parenchymatous, which includes tabes and paresis, and (2) interstitial, which comprises the forms usually termed cerebro-spinal syphilis.

The parenchymatous lesions appear much later than the interstitial, but there is often a history of earlier nervous symptoms which responded quickly to treatment. These are usually due to a basilar meningitis. The interval suggests that there has been a slow process gradually advancing which gives time for degenerative processes to develop. The majority of the cases of the interstitial type appear within five years of infection.

(*a*) *Meninges.*—Meningitis is a common manifestation and occurs particularly at the base, about the chiasm and along the Sylvian fissures. *Gummata* form, attached to the pia mater, sometimes to the dura; they are most common in the cerebrum. They form definite tumors varying in size from a pea to a walnut and are usually multiple. They are rarely found unassociated with the meninges. When small they have a uniform, translucent appearance, but when large the centre undergoes a fibrocaseous change with a firm grayish tissue at the periphery. They may resemble tuberculous tumors. Occasionally they undergo cystic degeneration. Large growths are not so common in the cord. Intense encephalitis or myelitis may occur in the neighborhood of a gumma.

In the brain, gummatous arteritis is a common cause of softening, which may be extensive, as when the middle cerebral artery is involved, or when there is a large patch of meningitis. In such cases the process is really a meningo-encephalitis and the symptoms are due to the secondary changes.

(*b*) *Arteries.*—A common lesion is the typical progressive endarteritis. Perivascular changes are common. There may be a marked inflammatory reaction with œdema and resulting interference with the lymphatics or small nodular tumors on the vessels which may break down or lead to rupture. Arterial disease is often combined with lesions in the meninges.

(*c*) *Parenchyma.*—The changes here are largely degenerative and are due partly to interference with nutrition by the vascular lesions and partly to the direct action of toxins from spirochætes in the tissues (especially in paresis). It is evident that lesions of the meninges and vessels offer much more hope of benefit from treatment than those of the parenchyma.

Cerebro-spinal Fluid.—The examination of this is of great value in diagnosis and in estimating the effect of treatment. The special points in cerebro-spinal syphilis are:

(*a*) *Cell Content.*—A lymphocytosis occurs in 85-90 per cent. of cases. The cells are often over 100 and may reach 1,000 per c.mm., the number being some guide to the intensity of the meningitis. With endarteritis alone the cells may be normal.

(*b*) *Globulin.*—An increase is present in 90-95 per cent. of cases. It probably represents abnormal transudation from damaged vessels and may occur in a great variety of conditions. An increase in globulin may be the only change in the fluid in the early secondary periods.

(*c*) *Wassermann Reaction.*—This is positive in 85-90 per cent., and indicates some active process in the cerebro-spinal tissues. In the early secondary period it may be absent even with increase in cells and globulin.

(*d*) *Colloidal Gold Reaction.*—This is present in 75-80 per cent. of cases. The type of curve is useful in distinguishing paresis from tabes and cerebro-spinal syphilis.

Symptoms.—The chief features are as follows:

(*a*) Psychical features. A sudden and violent onset of delirium may be the first symptom. In other instances prior to the occurrence of delirium there may have been headache, alteration of character, and loss of memory. The condition may be accompanied by convulsions. There may be no neuritis, no palsy, and no localizing symptoms.

(*b*) More commonly following headache, giddiness, or an excited state which may amount to delirium, the patient has an epileptic seizure or a hemiplegic attack, or there is involvement of the nerves of the base. Some of these cases display a prolonged torpor, a special feature of brain syphilis to which both Buzzard and Huebner have referred, which may persist for a month.

(*c*) In some cases the clinical picture is that of general paresis.

(*d*) Many cases of cerebral syphilis display the symptoms of brain tumor —headache, optic neuritis, vomiting, and convulsions. Of these symptoms convulsions are the most important, and both Fournier and Wood have laid great stress on the value of this symptom in persons over thirty. The first symptoms may, however, rather resemble those of embolism or thrombosis; thus there may be sudden hemiplegia, with or without loss of consciousness.

The symptoms of *spinal syphilis* are extremely varied and may be caused by large gummatous growths attached to the meninges, in which case the features are those of tumor, by gummatous arteritis with secondary softening, by meningitis with secondary cord changes, or by late scleroses. Syphilitic myelitis will be considered under affections of the spinal cord.

Diagnosis.—The history is of the first importance, but it may be extremely difficult to get a trustworthy account. Careful examination should be made for traces of the primary sore, for the cicatrices of bubo, for scars of the skin eruption or throat ulcers, and for bone lesions. The oculo-cardiac reflex may be absent. The character of the symptoms is often of great assistance. They are multiform, variable, and often such as could not be explained by a single lesion; thus there may be anomalous spinal symptoms or involvement of the nerves of the brain on both sides. The study of the spinal fluid and the Wassermann reaction in it and in the blood are of the greatest aid. The result of treatment has a bearing on the diagnosis, as the symptoms may disappear with the use of anti-syphilitic remedies.

2. *Syphilis of the Respiratory Organs*

Syphilis of the Trachea and Bronchi.—L. A. Conner has analyzed 128 recorded cases of syphilis of the trachea and bronchi. In 52 per cent. of the cases the trachea was alone involved. In only 10 per cent. were characteristic lesions of syphilis found in the lungs. Bronchial dilatation below the lesion was found in 15 per cent. of the cases. In ten of the cases the lesion occurred in congenital syphilis.

Syphilis of the Lung.—This is a rare disease. In 2,800 post mortems at the Johns Hopkins Hospital there were 12 cases with syphilitic disease in the lungs; in 8 of these the lesions were in congenital syphilis. In 11 cases there were definite gummata. Clinically the presence of syphilis of the lung was suspected in three cases. Fowler visited the museums of the London hospitals and the Royal College of Surgeons, and could find only twelve specimens illustrating syphilitic lesions of the lungs, two of which are doubtful. For a consideration of pulmonary syphilis, the reader is referred to chapter xxxvii of Fowler and Godlee's work on Diseases of the Lungs.

It occurs under the following forms:

(*a*) *The white pneumonia of the fetus.*—This may affect large areas or an entire lung, which then is firm, heavy, and airless, even though the child may have been alive. On section it has a grayish-white appearance—the so-called white hepatization of Virchow. The chief change is in the alveolar walls, which are greatly thickened and infiltrated, and the section is like one of the pancreas—"pancreatization" of the lung. In the early stages, for example, in a seven or eight months' fetus, there may be scattered miliary foci of this induration chiefly about the arteries. The air-cells are filled with desquamated and swollen epithelium.

(*b*) In the form of definite *gummata,* which vary in size from a pea to a goose-egg. They occur irregularly scattered through the lung, but, as a rule, are more numerous toward the root. They present a grayish-yellow caseous appearance, are dry and usually imbedded in a translucent, more or less firm, connective tissue. In a case described by Councilman there was extensive involvement of the root of the lungs. Bands of connective tissue passed inward from the thickened pleura, and between these strands and surrounding the gummata there was in places a mottled red pneumonic consolidation. In the caseous nodules there is typical hyaline degeneration. In a few rare instances there are most extensive caseous gummata with softening and formation of *bronchiectatic* cavities, and clinically a picture of pulmonary tuberculosis without the presence of tubercle bacilli. Bronchiectasis in children may be due to syphilis.

(*c*) *A form suggesting tuberculosis.*—Areas may be involved either at the root, or at the apex or base of the lung. The physical signs are much as in tuberculosis. There may be cough, possibly with a good deal of sputum, sometimes blood-streaked, loss of weight and fever, with signs at one apex or base. The picture may suggest tuberculosis but tubercle bacilli are not found. The condition may persist for a considerable time without very marked change. The differential diagnosis is difficult. It is important to look for lesions elsewhere, particularly in the larynx, and to try the Wassermann test. In some cases the results of treatment are very suggestive. The signs may suggest advanced tuberculosis. In one case, a man aged twenty-seven had cough and bloody expectoration for a year and died of severe hæmoptysis. Bacilli were never found in the sputum. There were extensive caseous gummata throughout both lungs, with much fibrous thickening, and in the lower lobe of the right lung a cavity 3 by 5 cm. in diameter, on the wall of which a branch of the pulmonary artery was eroded. This is the only instance among our cases in which there was an extensive destruction of the lung tissue with the clinical picture simulating pulmonary tuberculosis.

(*d*) A majority of authors follow Virchow in recognizing the fibrous interstitial pneumonia at the root of the lung and passing along the bronchi and vessels as probably syphilitic. This much may be said, that in certain cases gummata are associated with these fibroid changes. Again, this condition alone is found in persons with well-marked syphilitic history or with other visceral lesions. It seems in many instances to be a purely sclerotic process, advancing sometimes from the pleura, more commonly from the root of the lung, and invading the interlobular tissue, gradually producing a more or less extensive fibroid change. It rarely involves more than a portion of a lobe or portions of the lobes at the root of the lung. The bronchi are often dilated.

Diagnosis.—It is to be borne in mind, in the first place, that hospital physicians and pathologists the world over bear witness to the extreme rarity of lung syphilis. In the second place, the therapeutic test upon which so much reliance is placed is by no means conclusive. With pulmonary tuberculosis there should be no confusion, owing to the readiness with which the presence of bacilli is determined. Bronchiectasis in the lower lobe of a lung, dependent upon an interstitial pneumonia of syphilitic origin, could not be distinguished from any other form of the disease. So far as our experience goes, tuberculosis in a syphilitic subject has no special peculiarities. The lesions of syphilis and tuberculosis can coexist in a lung. The Wassermann reaction is helpful in a doubtful case.

3. *Syphilis of the Liver*

Varieties.—(*a*) *Congenital.*—Gubler in 1852 described the diffuse hepatitis which occurs in a large percentage of all deaths in congenital lues. While there may be little or no macroscopic change, the liver preserves its form and is usually enlarged, hard and resistant, and has a yellowish color, compared by Trousseau to sole-leather. Small grayish nodules may be seen on the section. In other cases there are definite gummata with extensive sclerosis. The spirochætes are present in extraordinary numbers.

The child may be still-born, die shortly after birth, or may be healthy when born and the liver enlarges within a few weeks. The organ is firm; the edge may be readily felt, usually far below the navel. The spleen is also enlarged. The features are those of cirrhosis, but jaundice and ascites are not common. Hochsinger states that of 45 cases recovery took place in 30.

(*b*) *Delayed Congenital Syphilis.*—The condition is by no means rare. Of 132 cases of syphilis hereditaria tarda collected by Forbes, in 34 the liver was involved. The children are nearly always ill-developed, sometimes with marked clubbing of the fingers and showing signs of infantilism. Jaundice is rare. The liver is usually enlarged, or it may show nodular masses.

ACQUIRED SYPHILIS.—(*a*) In the *secondary stage* the liver is not often involved, but may be slightly enlarged. Jaundice may occur coincident with the rash and with the enlargement of the superficial glands. Rolleston thinks it is probably due to a catarrhal condition of the smaller ducts, part of a general syphilitic hepatitis. There are cases in which it has passed on to a state of acute yellow atrophy. The prognosis is generally good.

(*b*) *Tertiary Lesions.*—The frequency with which the liver is involved in syphilis in adults is very variously estimated. J. L. Allen, quoted by Rolleston, found 37 cases of hepatic gummata among 11,629 autopsies at St. George's Hospital; in 27 cases cicatrices alone were present. Flexner at the Philadelphia Hospital found 88 cases of hepatic syphilis among 5,088 autopsies. Among 2,300 autopsies at the Johns Hopkins Hospital there were 47 cases of syphilis of the liver, gummata in 19, scars in 16, cirrhosis in 21 cases; 6 of the cases were congenital. In our experience the disease is by no means uncommon in the United States.

Anatomically the lesions may be either gummata or scars or a syphilitic sclerosis. The gummata range in size from a pea to an orange. When small they are pale and gray; the larger ones present yellowish centres; but later there is a "pale, yellowish, cheese-like nodule of irregular outline, surrounded by a fibrous zone, the outer edge of which loses itself in the lobular tissue, the lobules dwindling gradually in its grasp. This fibrous zone is never very broad; the cheesy centre varies in consistence from a gristle-like toughness to a pulpy softness; it is sometimes mortar-like, from cretaceous change" (Wilks). They may form enormous tumors, as in the remarkable one figured in Rolleston's work on Diseases of the Liver. They may be felt as large as an orange beneath the skin in the epigastrium and they may disappear with the same extraordinary rapidity as the subcutaneous or periosteal gumma. Macroscopically they may at first look like a massive cancer. Extensive caseation, softening and calcification may occur. The syphilitic scars are usually linear or star-shaped. They may be very numerous and divide the liver into small sections—the so-called botyroid organ, of which a remarkable example is figured in the *Lectures on Abdominal Tumors.*

Symptoms.—In the first place, the clinical picture may be that of cirrhosis—slight jaundice, fever, portal obstruction, ascites. There may not be the slightest suspicion of the syphilitic nature of the case. One of our patients had been tapped thirteen times before admission to the hospital. The diagnosis was made by finding gummata on the shins. She recovered promptly.

In a second group of cases the patient is anæmic, passes large quantities of pale urine containing albumin and tube-casts; the liver is enlarged, perhaps irregular, and the spleen also is enlarged. Dropsical symptoms may supervene, or the patient may be carried off by some intercurrent disease. Extensive amyloid degeneration of the spleen, the intestinal mucosa, and of the liver, with gummata, is found.

Thirdly, in a very important group the symptoms are those of tumor of the liver, causing pain and distress, and on examination an irregular or nodular mass is discovered. The tumor may be large, causing a prominent bulging in the epigastrium. Naturally carcinoma is thought of, as there may be nothing to suggest syphilis. In other cases the history or the presence of gummata elsewhere should aid in the diagnosis. In other instances the rapid disappearance under treatment even of a large visible tumor makes the syphilitic nature quite positive. Lastly, in a few cases the irregular fever with enlargement and irregularity of the liver may suggest suppuration, or the uniform great enlargement of the organ hypertrophic biliary cirrhosis, while there are some cases in which the spleen is so greatly enlarged, the anæmia so pronounced, and the liver so small and contracted that the diagnosis of splenic anæmia is made.

4. *Syphilis of the Digestive Tract*

The base of the *tongue* may show obliteration of the usual surface markings with smoothness of the surface and induration of the tissues due to fibroid change. The *œsophagus* is very rarely affected. Stenosis is the usual result. The frequency of syphilis of the *stomach* is difficult to estimate but it is not rare. There is no definite clinical picture, the symptoms depending on the site and extent of the lesion. There may be the usual features of dyspepsia or ulcer, or the findings may suggest carcinoma. A positive Wassermann test and rapid improvement under specific treatment are suggestive, but gastric disease and ulcer in patients with syphilis are not necessarily due to it. Syphilitic ulceration has been found in the small intestine and in the cæcum.

Syphilis of the *rectum* is found most commonly in women, and results from the growth of gummata in the submucosa above the internal sphincter. The process is slow and tedious, and may last for years before it finally induces stricture. The symptoms are usually those of narrowing of the lower bowel. The condition is readily recognized by rectal examination. The history of gradual on-coming stricture, the state of the patient, and the fact that there is a hard, fibrous narrowing, not an elevated crater-like ulcer, usually render easy the diagnosis from malignant disease. In medical practice these cases come under observation for other symptoms, particularly amyloid degeneration; and the rectal disease may be entirely overlooked, and only discovered post mortem.

5. *Circulatory System*

Syphilis of the Heart.—A fresh, warty *endocarditis* due to syphilis is not recognized, though occasionally in persons dead of the disease this form is present, as is not uncommon in conditions of debility.

The frequency of the association of syphilis with myocarditis, anæmic necrosis, and coronary artery disease has long been known. It is only since the introduction of newer methods that we have been able to determine how frequently this organ is the seat of syphilitic infection. Warthin made a study of 200 hearts, 50 from congenital and 150 from acquired syphilis, from which he groups the primary lesions of cardiac syphilis as follows: Large colonies of spirochætes may be found in the myocardium in congenital and in the active stages of acquired syphilis without definite changes in the heart muscle.

An œdema with loss of striation is not uncommon. A focal fatty degeneration may be the only lesion, or there may be areas of necrosis 5 mm. in diameter; a very striking feature is the presence of myxoma-like translucent areas which contain the spirochætes in large numbers. Interstitial changes are common, œdema associated with the presence of numerous spirochætes and leukocytes. Interstitial proliferation, usually perivascular, may be the earliest recognizable lesion. A transition is found between focal œdema and small, sharply localized non-caseating gummata. It is interesting to note that spirochætes may be found in great numbers in the myocardium when no others can be found elsewhere in the body.

Involvement of the *myocardium* may occur in the secondary stage but is usually more marked later. There may be fatty degeneration, sometimes secondary to coronary artery disease, or fibroid changes. Epicardial changes, with peri-arteritis, are common. The *symptoms* are those of slight cardiac insufficiency with a varying amount of precordial pain, sometimes vague, sometimes severe and localized. There may be increase in rate and some irregularity with a soft apex systolic murmur, not transmitted, and increased by exercise. Later the signs are those of myocarditis with pain and precordial tenderness; the pain may suggest angina pectoris. The association of pain with signs of myocarditis in a young adult should suggest the possibility of syphilis. The pain differs in position from that of acute aortitis which may be associated with it. Dyspnœa is often marked. The giving of mercury often results in rapid improvement. Rupture or sudden death may take place; indeed, sudden death is frequent, occurring in 21 of 63 cases (Mracek).

Syphilis of the Arteries.—Syphilis plays an important rôle in arteriosclerosis and aneurism. Its connection with these processes will be considered later; here we shall refer only to the syphilitic affection of the smaller vessels, which occurs in two forms:

(*a*) An *obliterating endarteritis,* characterized by a proliferation of the subendothelial tissue. The new growth lies within the elastic lamina, and may gradually fill the entire lumen; hence the term obliterating. The media and adventitia are also infiltrated with small cells. This form of endarteritis is not characteristic of syphilis, and its presence alone in an artery could not be considered pathognomonic. If, however, there are gummata in other parts, or if the condition about to be described exists in adjacent arteries, the process may be regarded as syphilitic.

(*b*) *Gummatous Periarteritis.*—With or without involvement of the intima, nodular gummata may develop in the adventitia of the artery, producing globular or ovoid swellings, which may attain considerable size. They are not infrequent in the cerebral arteries, which seem to be specially prone to this affection. This form is specific and distinctive of syphilis. Many observers have found *Treponema pallidum* in the syphilitic aortitis, and also in gummatous arteritis of the cerebral vessels.

6. *Syphilis of the Urinary Tract*

Acute Syphilitic Nephritis.—This condition has been carefully studied by the French writers and by Lafleur of Montreal. It is estimated to occur in the secondary stage in about 3.8 per cent., and may occur in from three to six months, sometimes later, from the initial lesion. The outlook is good, though often the albuminuria may persist for months; more rarely chronic nephritis follows. In a few instances syphilitic nephritis has proved rapidly fatal in a fortnight or three weeks. The lesions are not specific, but are similar to those in other acute infections.

Gummata.—Gummata occasionally are found in the kidneys, particularly in cases in which there is extensive gummatous hepatitis. They are rarely numerous, and occasionally lead to scattered cicatrices. Clinically the affection is not recognizable.

Bladder.—This is not common, but should be considered in cases of unexplained frequency of urination with hæmaturia. Papilloma may be simulated and a gumma may suggest carcinoma.

7. *Syphilitic Orchitis*

This affection is of special significance, as its detection may clinch the diagnosis in obscure disorders. Syphilis occurs in the testes in two forms:

(*a*) The gummatous growth, forming an indurated mass or group of masses in the substance of the organ, and sometimes difficult to distinguish from tuberculous disease. The area of induration is harder and it affects the body of the testes, while tubercle more commonly involves the epididymis. It rarely tends to invade the skin, or to break down, soften, and suppurate, and is usually painless.

(*b*) An *interstitial orchitis* which leads to fibroid induration. It is a slow, progressive change, coming on without pain, and usually involving one organ more than the other.

V. DIAGNOSIS, TREATMENT, ETC.

Diagnosis.—General Diagnosis.—There is seldom any doubt concerning the recognition of syphilitic lesions; but the number of persons, without any evident sign of the disease, in whom a positive Wassermann reaction is found proves that a negative diagnosis cannot be based on the absence of history and clinical manifestations. Syphilis is common in the community, and is no respecter of age, sex, or station in life. The primary sore may have been of trifling extent, or urethral and masked by a gonorrhœa, and the patient may not have had severe secondary symptoms, or the infection may occur without any chancre and the secondary lesions may be so slight that they are not noticed. Inquiries should be made into the history to ascertain if the patient has had skin rashes, sore throat, or if the hair has fallen out. Careful inspection should be made of the throat and skin for signs of old lesions. Skin lesions with induration or scarring and a crescentic shape should excite suspicion. Scars in the groins, the result of buboes, are uncertain evidences of syphilitic infection. The cicatrices on the legs are often copper-colored, though this cannot be regarded as peculiar to syphilis. The bones should be examined for nodes. In doubtful cases the scar of the primary sore may be found, or there may be signs of atrophy or of hardening of the testes. In women the occurrence of miscarriages and the bearing of stillborn children are always suggestive. In doubtful cases the study of the spinal fluid is important.

In the congenital disease, the occurrence within the first three months of snuffles and skin rash is conclusive. Later, the characters of the syphilitic facies often give a clew to the nature of some obscure visceral lesion. Other distinctive features are the symmetrical development of nodes on the bones and the interstitial keratitis.

The *Treponema pallidum* may be found in the fresh lesion. After cleaning carefully, serum is sucked out and the living spirochætes may be seen in the special "dark field" apparatus.

Serum Diagnosis.—The complement fixation test in good hands may be accepted as a most valuable aid in diagnosis. It is obtained in from 80 to 90 per cent. of all cases of syphilis with manifestations. The results in tabes and general paresis are very constant.

Cutaneous Reaction.—An emulsion or extract of pure cultures of *Treponema pallidum*—termed *luetin*—has been employed by Noguchi to obtain a skin reaction. The skin is sterilized and 0.05 c. c. injected intradermically. The local reaction is usually papular, and surrounded by a zone of redness, but may become pustular. There is very slight constitutional effect. The reaction is most constant and marked in tertiary and congenital cases; it is infrequent, and, if present, mild in the primary and secondary stages, in which the complement fixation test is more constant. Treatment affects the latter more than the cutaneous reaction which may be given by non-syphilitics who have been taking iodide recently.

Therapeutic Test.—In a doubtful case, as, for example, an obstinate skin rash or an obscure tumor in the abdomen, antisyphilitic treatment may prove successful, but this cannot always be relied upon.

Prophylaxis.—Irregular intercourse has existed from the beginning of recorded history, and unless man's nature wholly changes—and of this we can have no hope—will continue. Resisting all attempts at solution, the social evil remains the great blot upon our civilization, and inextricably blended with it is the question of the prevention of syphilis. Two measures are available—the one personal, the other administrative.

Personal purity is the prophylaxis which we, as physicians, are especially bound to advocate. Continence may be a hard condition (to some harder than to others), but it can be borne, and it is our duty to urge this lesson upon young and old who seek our advice in matters sexual. Certainly it is better, as St. Paul says, to marry than to burn, but if the former is not feasible there are other altars than those of Venus upon which a young man may light fires. He may practise at least two of the five means by which, as the physician Rondibilis counseled Panurge, carnal concupiscence may be cooled and quelled—hard work of body and hard work of mind. Idleness is the mother of lechery; and a young man will find that absorption in any pursuit will do much to cool passions which, though natural and proper, cannot in the exigencies of our civilization always obtain natural and proper gratification.

To carry out successfully any administrative measures seems hopeless, at any rate in our Anglo-Saxon civilization. The state accepts the responsibility of guarding citizens against small-pox or cholera, but in dealing with syphilis the problem has been too complex and has hitherto baffled solution. Inspection, segregation, and regulation are difficult, if not impossible, to carry out, and public sentiment is bitterly opposed to this plan. The compulsory registration of every case of gonorrhœa and syphilis, with greatly increased facilities for thorough treatment, offers a more acceptable alternative.

The patient should be warned of the various ways in which he may spread the disease and given directions regarding this. Measures for the prevention of infection after exposure can be carried out in the military and naval services more readily than in civil life. The most successful is the application of mercurial ointment mixed with lanolin soon after exposure.

Treatment.—That the later stages which come under the charge of the physician are so common results, in great part, from the carelessness of the patient, who, wearied with treatment, cannot understand why he should continue to take medicine after all the symptoms have disappeared; but, in part, the profession also is to blame for not insisting more urgently that acquired syphilis is not cured in a few months, but takes at least three years, during which time the patient should be under careful supervision.

The patient should lead a regular life, avoiding excess of all kinds. If there is fever rest in bed is advisable. The usual diet can be taken and the patient should drink large quantities of water. The use of alcohol and tobacco should be forbidden during active treatment. When mercury is being taken special care must be given to the mouth. A mouth wash and a potassium chlorate tooth paste should be used frequently. Treatment to rid the body of spirochætes consists in the use of two remedies, mercury and arsenic; iodide of potassium influences certain of the tissue changes resulting from the infection.

Energetic treatment in the acute stages should be started as soon as the diagnosis is made. The object is to kill the spirochætes as rapidly as possible and the treatment should be intensive in the hope of completely ridding the body of the infection. Mild treatment may result in the production of a resistant strain of spirochætes and mercury by mouth alone is not a proper method. There is no agreement as to the best method and many variations are employed; it is advisable to use both arsenic and mercury. Some give them alternately; others use the arsenic preparations at short intervals for a time and then a full course of mercury. The main thing is to carry on active treatment.

Arsenic.—The arsenic preparation (dioxydiamido-arsenobenzol) is given various names and the terms arsphenamine and neo-arsphenamine are employed here. If treatment is begun with arsphenamine an initial full dose is 0.5 or 0.6 gm. intravenously. It should be given well diluted (50 c. c. for each 0.1 gm. of the drug) and always in a freshly prepared solution. It is usually injected into one of the veins at the elbow, care being taken to be sure that the needle is in the vein and some salt solution being run in first. It is well to keep the patient in bed until the following morning. The frequency of repetition varies. A second similar dose may be given in five to ten days and then the same or smaller doses (0.2-0.3 gm.) at the same or shorter intervals until six or eight doses are given. After this a complete course of mercury is given by inunction or injection. Another method is to give a full dose of arsphenamine, then a vigorous course of mercury for two or three weeks, then another full dose of arsphenamine, and mercury again, this being carried on for a period of three or four months. Whichever method is chosen, after a period of vigorous treatment an interval of four weeks may pass without any treatment and then the complement fixation test is tried. If this is negative it should be taken every three months for a year, and if all are negative, the infection is probably cured. If the reaction is positive, the treatment should be resumed until it is negative. The complement fixation test should be used as a guide to treatment throughout.

Many things influence the dose of arsphenamine. In general the weight of the patient is a good guide. For young children doses of 0.1 to 0.15 gm. are used and for infants 0.02 to 0.1 gm. Changes in the eye grounds and severe circulatory and renal lesions always suggest caution and may be contra-indications. In such cases doses of 0.2 gm. are the usual maximum. In general the dose of neo-arsphenamine may be considered as slightly less than double that of arsphenamine. Many prefer to use the neo-arsphenamine throughout.

The conditions in which arsphenamine is especially useful are: (1) at the onset when an early diagnosis is made, (2) in patients with severe skin or mucous membrane lesions, (3) in intractable cases in those resistent to or unable to take mercury, (4) in malignant cases, (5) in congenital syphilis, and (6) in latent cases, in which without any signs of syphilis a Wassermann reaction is present. In visceral syphilis the drug is less useful. Its value in tabes dorsalis and paresis is not settled, but some patients are undoubtedly benefited. The earlier in the course of syphilis the drug is given the better the effect. Mercury should always be given after arsphenamine which, except in a few cases given early, can not be regarded as a complete remedy in itself.

MERCURY.—It is well to push its administration so that the patient is brought under its influence as rapidly as possible; salivation is to be avoided. *Inunction* is the most effective means of administration. One-half to a dram (2-4 gm.) of mercurial ointment or oleate of mercury is thoroughly rubbed into the skin, on areas free from hair, daily for six days; on the seventh a warm bath is taken. It is well to apply the ointment to different places on successive days. The sides of the chest and abdomen and the inner surfaces of the arms and thighs are the best positions. Thirty inunctions is an average number for each course. *Intramuscular* injection is also satisfactory, care being taken to avoid infection and to give the injections deeply. Mercury salicylate (gr. i-ii, 0.06-0.12 gm.) in a 10 per cent. solution is probably the best, an injection being given every five to seven days. Bichloride of mercury (gr. 1/20-1/10, 0.003-0.006 gm.) in olive oil, biniodide of mercury (gr. 1/6, 0.01 gm.), the "gray oil," calomel (gr. i, 0.065 gm.) in equal parts of glycerine and water (1 of calomel to 10 of this mixture) are also used. A course of twenty to thirty injections should be given. *Intravenous* injections are sometimes given, usually of the bichloride (♏ xv, 1 c. c. of a 0.1 to 0.2 per cent. solution in sterile salt solution). By *mouth* the gray powder, hydrargyrum cum cretâ in one grain (0.065 gm.) doses with a grain of Dover's powder, may be given. The bichloride (gr. 1/16-1/8, 0.004-0.008 gm.), the biniodide (gr. 1/16, 0.004 gm.) and the protoiodide (gr. 1/4, 0.016 gm.) may also be used. It is well for the profession not to forget that mercury is still in existence; some men seem to have forgotten it.

The Wassermann reaction should be tried twice a year for three years and active treatment resumed if it is positive. No one can be regarded as free of the disease from a negative blood test alone; the spinal fluid should be studied also. In the later stages it is well to follow much the same general course, as a rule giving treatment intensively for certain periods, with a rest between. While the Wassermann reaction is a helpful guide in treatment it is not always possible to secure a negative reaction. If mercury by mouth and the "mixed" treatment are used, it should be only after a thorough administration by inunction or injection.

In CONGENITAL SYPHILIS the treatment of patients born with bullæ and other signs of the disease is not satisfactory, and the infants usually die within a few days or weeks. The child should be nursed by the mother alone, or, if this is not feasible, should be hand-fed, but under no circumstances should a wet-nurse be employed. Arsphenamine is generally useful. The child is most rapidly and thoroughly brought under the influence of mercury by inunction. The mercurial ointment may be smeared on the flannel binder. This is not a very cleanly method, and sometimes rouses the suspicion of the mother. The drug may be given by mouth, in the form of gray powder, half a grain (0.03 gm.) three times a day. In the late manifestations associated with bone lesions the combination of mercury and iodide of potassium is most suitable and is well given in the form of Gilbert's syrup, which consists of the biniodide of mercury (gr. j, 0.065 gm.), of potassium iodide (℥ss, 15 gm.), and water (℥ij, 60 c. c.). Of this the dose for a child under three is from five to ten drops three times a day, gradually increased. Under these measures the cases of congenital syphilis usually improve with great rapidity. The medication should be continued at intervals for many months, and it is well to watch these patients carefully during the period of second dentition and at puberty, and if necessary to place them on specific treatment.

In the treatment of the VISCERAL LESIONS, iodide of potassium is of equal or even greater value than mercury. The iodide saturates the unsaturated fatty acid radicals which inhibit autolysis. The ferments then become active, autolysis follows and the necrotic tissue is absorbed. Under its use ulcers rapidly heal, gummatous tumors melt away, and we have an illustration of a specific action only equaled by that of mercury or arsenic in the secondary stages, by iron in certain forms of anæmia, and by quinine in malaria. It is as a rule well borne in an initial dose of 10 grains (0.6 gm.); given in milk the patient does not notice the taste. It should be gradually increased to 30 or more grains three times a day. In syphilis of the nervous system it may be used in still larger doses. Arsphenamine or mercury should also be given.

For syphilitic hepatitis the combination of mercury and iodide of potassium is most satisfactory. If there is ascites, Addison's or Guy's pill (as it is often called) of mercury, digitalis, and squill will be found very useful. Occasionally the iodide of sodium is more satisfactory than the potassium salt. It is less depressing and agrees better with the stomach.

Syphilis and Marriage.—Upon this question the family physician is often called to decide. He should insist upon the necessity of two full years elapsing between the date of infection and the contracting of marriage. This, it should be borne in mind, is the earliest possible limit, and marriage should be allowed only if the treatment has been thorough, at least a year has passed without any manifestation of the disease, and the Wassermann test is negative.

Syphilis and Life Insurance.—An individual with syphilis can not be regarded as a first-class risk unless he can furnish evidence of prolonged and thorough treatment and of immunity for two or three years from all manifestations. Even then, when we consider the extraordinary frequency of the cerebral and other complications in persons who have had this disease and who may even have undergone thorough treatment, the risk to the company is certainly increased (see Bramwell, Clinical Studies, vol. i).

Yaws.—(*Frambœsia*).—This is a disease much like syphilis, prevalent in Africa, parts of Asia, the West Indies and tropical America, caused by *Spirochœta pertenuis* (v. *pallidula*). Wood brings up the possibility that the disease has been present unrecognized in the Southern States. It is particularly a disease of children and is readily communicated from one to another. The primary lesion is a papule which later shows a fungoid appearance; in the secondary stage similar lesions develop generally. The skin lesions consist of raspberry-like growths from which a sero-purulent fluid exudes, or they are covered by a yellow crust. The secondary general eruption has the same character and is widespread. The mucous membranes are not involved. There may be fever, headache and general malaise. The course is from a few months to three years. The mortality is low. Arsphenamine is specific and its use results in a rapid cure.

IX. DISEASES DUE TO PARASITIC INFUSORIA

Several flagellates are parasitic in man. *Trichomonas vaginalis,* which measures 15 μ to 25 μ in length and has four flagella, as long as or longer than the body, is by no means uncommon in the acid vaginal mucus.

Trichomonas or *Cercomonas hominis* lives in the intestines, and is met with in the stools under all sorts of conditions. Freund from Dock's clinic reported a series of cases which show that the parasite may cause acute and chronic diarrhœa with severe abdominal pain, and anatomically an acute enteritis. In one of Dock's cases the parasites were associated with a hæmorrhagic cystitis without bacteria.

Lamblia intestinalis was a frequent cause of enteritis during the recent war. The onset was often insidious and the condition tended to become chronic. The general condition of the patient was markedly affected. Flagellates have been found in the expectoration in cases of gangrene of the lung and of bronchiectasis, and in the exudate of pleurisy.

Balantidium coli, oval in form, 70 μ to 100 μ long and 50 μ to 70 μ broad, may be pathogenic. It is common in pigs, and has been known to produce an epidemic dysentery in apes (Harlow Brooks). The pathological significance of this parasite has been demonstrated by Strong and Musgrave in the Philippines, where it is a cause of dysentery. It has not only been found in the stools and on the mucous membrane of the intestine, but the parasites have occurred in the mucosa itself and in the submucosa. Apparently they do not extend beyond the wall of the bowel.

D. DISEASES DUE TO METAZOAN PARASITES

I. DISEASES DUE TO FLUKES—DISTOMIASIS

The Trematoda or flukes are parasitic platyhelminths, usually with flattened or leaf-shaped bodies. The term *Distomiasis* is based upon Distoma, the term being used to designate the trematodes.

The following are the important clinical forms:

1. **Pulmonary Distomiasis; Parasitic Hæmoptysis.**—*Paragonimus* (Distoma) *westermanii*, the Asiatic lung or bronchial fluke, is from 8 to 16 mm. in length by 4 to 8 mm. broad, and of a pinkish or reddish-brown color.

It is found extensively in China and Japan, Formosa, and the Philippines, and cases are occasionally imported into Europe and America, and have been met with in the oriental population of the Pacific coast. It has been found in the United States in the cat, in the dog, and in the hog. One instance of pulmonary distomiasis has been reported caused by the giant liver fluke.

Clinically the disease, as described by Manson and Ringer, is characterized by a chronic cough, with rusty-brown sputum, and occasional attacks of hæmoptysis, usually trifling, but sometimes very severe. The disease is very apt to be mistaken for tuberculosis, but the diagnosis is easily made by microscopic examination of the sputum. The ova, which are abundant in the sputum, are oval, smooth, and measure from 80 μ to 100 μ in length by 40 μ to 60 μ in breadth. The parasites may affect other organs—the liver, the brain, and eyelid.

2. **Hepatic Distomiasis.**—Six species of liver flukes are known to occur in man. More specifically these are: (1) The common liver fluke—*Fasciola hepatica*—which is a very common parasite in the ruminants. It is a rare and accidental parasite in man, but in Syria a strange disease called *Halzoun* is caused by eating raw goat-liver infected with the parasite. (2) The lancet fluke—*Dicrocœlium lanceatum.* (3) *Opisthorchis felineus,* which is found in Prussia and Siberia, and by Ward in cats in Nebraska. (4) *Opisthorchis noverca*—the Indian liver fluke described in man by McConnell. (5) *Clonorchis sinensis* and *C. endemicus,* the most important of the liver flukes which occur extensively in Japan, China, and India. The eggs are oval, 27 μ to 30 μ by 15 μ to 17 μ, dark brown, with sharply defined operculum. Imported cases have been found in Canada and the United States. White found 18 cases in San Francisco.

The *symptoms* of hepatic distomiasis are best described in connection with the last form. The following account is abstracted from Wallace Taylor. Young children are the chief sufferers. Many members of a family are usually affected. In some villages a large proportion of the inhabitants are attacked. Among important symptoms is an irregular, intermittent diarrhœa; at first there may or may not be blood. The liver enlarges and a condition of cirrhosis gradually comes on. There may be pain and an intermittent jaundice. There is not much fever. After lasting for two or three years dropsy comes on, with anasarca and ascites. Even then transient recovery may take place, but as a rule there is a recurrence, and the patient dies after many years of illness. The ova of the parasite are readily found in the stools.

3. Intestinal Distomiasis.—In India the *Fasciolopsis buskii* has been found in a number of cases in the small intestines.

The *Asiatic Amphistome—Gastrodiscus* (*Amphistoma*) *hominis*—a not uncommon parasite in India—is easily recognized by its large posterior sucker.

4. Hæmic Distomiasis; Bilharziasis.—One of the most important of parasitic diseases, caused by the blood fluke, *Schistosoma hæmatobium* (*Bilharzia hæmatobia*). Endemic hæmaturia has been known for many years, particularly in Egypt, where in 1851 Bilharz discovered the parasite of the disease. It prevails in South and North Africa, particularly the latter, in Arabia, Persia, and the west coast of India. Imported cases are not very uncommon in Europe, and an occasional instance is met with in the United States. In Egypt, among 11,698 patients admitted to the Cairo Hospital, 1,270 were infected, practically 10 per cent. (Madden). Of 500 autopsies at the same hospital, in 8 per cent. death was due to the effects of Bilharzial disease. The seriousness of the condition in Egypt is well illustrated by the fact that in 7.5 per cent. of army recruits the ova are found in the urine.

A lateral spined form—*S. mansoni*—is found only in the fæces. This enters a snail and ultimately the human host. It occurs in the West Indies and Brazil.

The *parasite* is singular among flukes in having the sexes separate, and the male usually carries the female in a gynæcophorous canal. The eggs are characteristic, oval in shape, 0.16 mm. by 0.06 mm., and one end has a terminal spine. The eggs hatch in water, and emerging from the terminal spined egg the miracidium enters the liver of a fresh water mollusc, common in the canals of Egypt, and becomes transformed into sporocysts and daughter sporocysts, in which numbers of cercariæ develop. These escape into the water, penetrate the skin of man, travel to the portal veins and liver, where in six to ten weeks they mature to adult trematodes. They travel to various parts of the body, particularly to the veins of the bladder and rectum, and produce the terminal spined eggs which escape with the urine. A majority of the parasites remain in the tissues and cause irritation, fibroid changes, and papillomata in the bladder and rectum. Collecting in the bladder as foreign bodies they form the nuclei of calculi.

Symptoms.—As is so often the case with animal parasites, they may cause no inconvenience. Irritability of the bladder, dull pain in the perineum, and hæmaturia are the most frequent symptoms. A chronic cystitis follows when the walls of the bladder are much thickened by the irritation caused by the ova. The anæmia caused by the hæmorrhage is slight in comparison with that of uncinariasis. When the rectum is involved there are straining and tenesmus, with the passage of mucus and blood; in severe cases large papillomata form and a chronic ulcerative proctitis. There may be a chronic vaginitis. Of the complications, calculi in kidney and bladder are the most important. Milton, Madden, and others of the Cairo School of Medicine have studied carefully the surgical aspects. Periurethral abscess and perineal fistulæ are common in the chronic cases.

Few symptoms are caused by the presence of the parasites in the portal veins, but there may be an advanced cirrhosis of a Glissonian type due to an enormous thickening of the periportal tissues (Symmers). This author has also reported an instance of the Bilharzia in the pulmonary blood in a case of Bilharzial colitis, and the worms were found living in the pulmonary circulation. The *diagnosis* is readily made by finding the characteristic ova in the bloody urine or in the blood and mucus from the rectum. The Bilharzia may be present in the body for years without producing serious damage, and in slight infections the symptoms may disappear (Sandwith), particularly in children.

Schistosoma japonicum.—In China, Japan and the Philippines there is a disease characterized by cirrhosis of the liver, splenomegaly, ascites, dysentery, progressive anæmia, and sometimes by focalized epilepsy. Dermatitis and angio-neurotic œdema may occur. It occurs extensively in one district of Japan, and is known as the "Katayama" disease. Woolley met with it in the Philippines, and Catto in China. It seems that the so-called urticarial fever, which is not very uncommon in China and Japan, is associated with the presence of this parasite, and an eosinophilia with fever and urticaria should lead to a careful examination of the stools for its eggs. The parasite lives in the vessels of the alimentary canal; the ova are smaller than those of *S. hæmatobium*, and have not the characteristic spine. The parasite develops in a snail and the disease is acquired by working in wet rice fields.

Treatment.—We know of nothing which can kill the parasites in the blood. Extract of male fern is recommended for the hæmaturia. Tartar emetic has been used with good results.

II. DISEASES CAUSED BY CESTODES—TÆNIASIS

Man harbors the adult parasites in the small intestine, the larval forms in the muscles and solid organs.

1. INTESTINAL CESTODES; TAPEWORMS

Tænia solium (Pork Tapeworm).—This is not a common form in the United States and is more frequent in parts of Europe and Asia. When mature it is from 6 to 12 feet in length. The head is small, round, not so large as the head of a pin, and provided with four sucking disks and a double row of hooklets; hence it is called, in contradistinction to the other form in man, the *armed* tapeworm. To the head succeeds a narrow, thread-like neck, then the segments, or proglottides, as they are called. The segments possess both male and female generative organs, and at about the four-hundred-and-fiftieth they become mature and contain ripe ova. The worm attains its full growth in from three to three and a half months, after which time the segments are continuously shed and appear in the stools. The segments are about 1 cm. in length and from 7 to 8 mm. in breadth. Pressed between glass plates the uterus is seen as a median stem with about eight to fourteen lateral branches. There are many thousands of ova in each ripe segment, and each ovum consists of a firm shell, inside of which is a little embryo, provided with six hooklets. The segments are continuously passed, and if the ova are to attain further development they must be taken into the stomach, either of a pig, or of man himself. The egg-shells are digested, the six-hooked embryos become free, and passing from the stomach reach various parts of the body (the liver, muscles, brain, or eye), where they develop into the larvæ or cysticerci. A hog under these circumstances is said to be *measled,* and the cysticerci are spoken of as measles or bladder worms.

Tænia solium received its name because it was thought to exist as a solitary parasite in the bowel, but two or three or even more worms may occur.

Tænia saginata or Mediocanellata (Unarmed, Fat, or Beef Tapeworm).—This is a longer and larger parasite than *Tænia solium.* It is certainly the common tapeworm of North America. According to Bérenger-Féraud it has spread rapidly in western Europe, owing probably to the importation of beef and live-stock from the Mediterranean basin. It may attain a length of 15 or 20 feet, or more. The head is large in comparison with that of *Tænia solium,* and measures over 2 mm. in breadth. It is square-shaped and provided with four large sucking disks, but there are no hooklets. The ripe segments are from 17 to 18 mm. in length and from 8 to 10 mm. in breadth. The uterus consists of a median stem with from fifteen to thirty-five lateral branches, which are given off more dichotomously than in *Tænia solium.* The ova are somewhat larger, and the shell is thicker, but the two forms can scarcely be distinguished by their ova. The ripe segments are passed as in *Tænia solium,* and are ingested by cattle, in the flesh or organs of which the eggs develop into the bladder worms or cysticerci.

Of other forms of tapeworm may be mentioned:

Dipylidium caninum.—A small parasite common in the dog and occasionally found in man; the larvæ develop in the lice and fleas of the dog.

Hymenolepis diminuta.—This small cestode was found in the intestine of a child in Boston, and has since been met with in twelve cases (Ransom). It is common in rats. The larvæ develop in moths and beetles.

Hymenolepis nana occurs not infrequently in Italy. It is not very uncommon in the United States (Stiles). The *Davainea madagascariensis* is a rare form.

Tænia confusa, a new species described by Ward.

Dibothriocephalus latus.—A cestode worm found in certain districts bordering on the Baltic Sea, in parts of Switzerland, and in Japan. Nickerson has shown that it is common in the Northwestern States, especially among the Finns, and it seems probable that the fish in the Great Lakes have become infected, as cases have increased of late years. The parasite is large and long, measuring from 25 to 30 feet or more. Its head is different from that of the tænia, as it possesses two lateral grooves or pits and has no hooklets. The larvæ develop in the peritoneum and muscles of the pike and other fish, and grow into the adult worm when eaten by man.

Symptoms of Tapeworm Infection.—These parasites are found at all ages. They are not uncommon in children and are occasionally found in sucklings. W. T. Plant refers to a number of cases in children under two years, and there is one in the literature in which it is stated that the tapeworm was found in an infant five days old!

The parasites may cause no disturbance and are rarely dangerous. A knowledge of the existence of the worm is generally a source of worry and anxiety; the patient may have considerable distress and complain of abdominal pains, nausea, diarrhœa, and sometimes anæmia. Occasionally the appetite is ravenous. In women and in nervous patients the constitutional disturbance may be considerable, and we not infrequently see great mental depression and even hypochondria. Various nervous phenomena, such as chorea, convulsions, or epilepsy, are believed to be caused by the parasites. Such effects, however, are very rare. The *Dibothriocephalus* may cause a severe and even fatal form of anæmia, which has been described fully in the monograph of Schaumann, of Helsingfors. It has been suggested that the metabolic products of the worm may have in some cases a hæmolytic action. Eosinophilia may occur.

Diagnosis.—The diagnosis is never doubtful. The presence of the segments is distinctive and the ova may be recognized in the stools. As regards the variety the ripe segments of *Tænia saginata* are larger and broader, and show differences in the generative system as already mentioned.

Prophylaxis.—This is most important and careful attention should be given to three points. First, all tapeworm segments should be burned; they should never be thrown into the water-closet or outside; secondly, careful inspection of meat at the abattoirs; and, thirdly, cooking the meat sufficiently to kill the parasites.

In the case of the beef measles, the distribution of the parasites, as given by Ostertag, shows that the muscles of the jaw are much more frequently affected than other parts—360 times—while other organs were infected but 55 times. Sometimes there are instances of general infection. Cold storage kills the cysticercus usually within three weeks. The measles are more readily overlooked in beef than in pork, as they do not present such an opaque white color.

In the examination of hogs for cysticerci "particular stress should be laid upon the tongue, the muscles of mastication, and the muscles of the shoulder, neck, and diaphragm" (Stiles). They may be seen very easily on the under surface of the tongue. American hogs are comparatively free. In Prussia one hog is infected in about every 637. Specimens have been found alive twenty-nine days after slaughtering. In the examination of 1,000 hogs in Montreal, 76 instances of cysticerci were found.

Treatment.—Three days should be given to preparation for treatment, whatever drug is employed. For two days the patient should take soft food and the third day liquids only. The bowels should be well moved by castor oil taken each evening and a saline in the morning if necessary. Unless the bowels have moved freely an enema should be given. On the third night a laxative, such as cascara, should be taken. There are many drugs, but male fern is usually the most reliable, given in the form of the oleoresin. This is taken early in the morning of the fourth day before any food is taken. The usual dose is ʒi (4 c. c.), which is repeated in an hour. It may be given in capsules or in glycerine (℥ ss, 15 c. c.). If there is fear of nausea a cup of coffee may be taken before the drug. The drug may be given by the duodenal tube. After taking the male fern the patient should remain quiet and resist any desire to vomit. One hour after the second dose of male fern a full dose of saline is taken (magnesium or sodium sulphate, or magnesium citrate), and an hour later a second dose if the bowels have not moved. Great care should be taken during the expulsion of the worm, which should be passed into a chamber containing water at about the body temperature, a practice recommended by Celsus.

The pomegranate root is a very efficient remedy, and may be given as an infusion of the bark, 3 ounces of which may be macerated in 10 ounces of water and reduced to one-half by evaporation. The entire quantity is taken in divided doses. It occasionally produces colic, but is very effective. The active principle, pelletierine, is employed as the tannate, given in doses of 6 to 8 or even 10 grains (0.4 to 0.6 gm.), and followed in an hour by a purge.

Pumpkin seeds are sometimes efficient. Three or four ounces should be carefully bruised, macerated for twelve or fourteen hours, the entire quantity taken and followed in an hour by a purge. Of other remedies, cusso, naphthalein (gr. v, 0.3 gm.), and thymol (gr. v, 0.3 gm. daily for a week) may be mentioned. Sometimes a combination of remedies is effectual when one fails. In children the use of pumpkin seeds or pelletierine is generally best. One cause of failure is the use of drugs which are old and inert.

Unless the head is brought away, the parasite continues to grow, and within a few months the segments again appear. Some cases are extraordinarily obstinate. Doubtless almost everything depends upon the exposure of the worm. The head and neck may be thoroughly protected beneath the valvulæ conniventes, in which case the remedies may not act. Owing to its armature *Tænia solium* is more difficult to expel. It is probable that no degree of peristalsis can dislodge the head, and unless the worm is killed it does not let go its firm hold. Owing to the danger of cysticercosis, treatment should not be delayed in case of infection with *Tænia solium.*

2. SOMATIC TÆNIASIS

Whereas adult tænia may give rise to little or no disturbance, and rarely, if ever, prove directly fatal, the affections caused by the larvæ or immature forms in the solid organs are serious. There are two chief cestode larvæ known to frequent man: (*a*) the *Cysticercus cellulosæ,* the larva of *Tænia solium,* and (*b*) the *Echinococcus,* the larva of *Tænia echinococcus.* The *Cysticercus tæniæ saginatæ* has been found very rarely in man.

Cysticercus cellulosæ.—When man accidentally takes into his stomach the ripe ova of *Tænia solium* he is liable to become the intermediate host, a part usually played for this tapeworm by the pig. This may occur in an individual the subject of *Tænia solium,* in which case the mature proglottides either themselves wander into the stomach or are forced into the organ in attacks of prolonged vomiting. The accidental ingestion from the outside of a few ova is quite possible, and the liability of infection should always be borne in mind in handling the segments of the worm.

The *symptoms* depend entirely upon the number of ova ingested and the localities reached. In the hog the cysticerci produce very little disturbance. The muscles, the connective tissue, and the brain may be swarming with the "measles," as they are called, and yet the nutrition is maintained and the animal does not appear to be seriously incommoded. In the invasion period, if large numbers of the parasites are taken, there is, in all probability, constitutional disturbance; certainly this is seen in the calf, when fed with the ripe segments of *Tænia saginata.*

In man a few cysticerci lodged beneath the skin or in the muscles give no trouble, and in time the larvæ die and become calcified. They are occasionally found in dissection subjects or in post mortems as ovoid white bodies in the muscles or subcutaneous tissue. In America they are very rare. We have seen but two instances in post mortem experience. Depending on the number and the locality specially affected, the symptoms may be grouped into general, cerebro-spinal, and ocular. In 155 cases compiled by Stiles, the parasite in 117 was found in the brain, in 32 in the muscles, in 9 in the heart, in 3 in the lungs, subcutaneously in 5, in the liver in 2.

1. General.—As a rule the invasion of the larvæ in man, unless in very large numbers, does not cause very definite symptoms. It occasionally happens, however, that a striking picture is produced. A patient was admitted very stiff and helpless, so much so that he had to be assisted upstairs and into bed. He complained of numbness and tingling in the extremities and general weakness, so that at first he was thought to have a peripheral neuritis. At the examination, however, a number of painful subcutaneous nodules were discovered, which proved on excision to be the cysticerci. Altogether 75 could be felt subcutaneously, and from the soreness and stiffness they probably existed in large numbers in the muscles. There were none in his eyes, and he had no brain symptoms.

2. Cerebro-spinal.—Remarkable symptoms may result from the presence of the cysticerci in the brain and cord. In the silent region they may be abundant without producing any symptoms. In the ventricles of the brain the cysticerci may attain a considerable size, owing to the fact that in regions in which they are unrestrained in their growth, as in the peritoneum, the bladder-like body grows freely. When in the fourth ventricle remarkable irritative symptoms may be produced. In 1884 the senior author saw with Friedländer in Berlin a case from Riess's wards in which during life there had been symptoms of diabetes and anomalous nervous symptoms. Post mortem, the cysticercus was found beneath the valve of Vieussens, pressing upon the floor of the fourth ventricle.

3. Ocular.—Since von Graefe demonstrated the presence of the cysticercus in the vitreous humor many cases have been placed on record, as it is a condition easily recognized.

Except in the eye, the diagnosis can rarely be made; when the cysticerci are subcutaneous one may be excised. It is possible that when numerous throughout the muscles they may be seen under the tongue, in which situation they may exist in the pig in numbers.

Echinococcus or Hydatid Disease.—The hydatid worms or echinococci are the larvæ of *Tænia echinococcus* of the dog. This is a tiny cestode not more than 4 or 5 mm. in length, consisting of only three or four segments, of which the terminal one alone is mature, and has a length of about 2 mm. and a breadth of 0.6 mm. The head is small and provided with four sucking disks and a rostellum with a double row of hooklets. This is an exceedingly rare parasite in the dog. Cobbold states that he has never met with a natural specimen in England. Leidy had not one in his large collection; Curtice, of Washington, found it once in an American dog. The worms are so small that they may be readily overlooked, since they form small, white, thread-like bodies closely adherent among the villi of the small intestines. The ripe segment contains about 5,000 eggs, which attain their development in the solid organs of various animals, particularly the hog and ox, more rarely the horse and the sheep. In some countries man is an intermediate host, owing to accidental ingestion of the ova.

DEVELOPMENT.—The little six-hooked embryo, freed from the egg-shell by digestion, burrows through the intestinal wall and reaches the peritoneal cavity or the muscles; it may enter the portal vessels and be carried to the liver. It may enter the systemic vessels, and, passing the pulmonary capillaries, as it is protoplasmic and elastic, may reach the brain or other parts. Once having reached its destination, it undergoes the following changes: The hooklets disappear and the little embryo is gradually converted into a small cyst which presents two distinct layers—an external, laminated, cuticular membrane or capsule, and an internal, granular, parenchymatous layer, the endocyst. The little cyst or vesicle contains a clear fluid. There is more or less reaction in the neighboring tissues, and the cyst in time has a fibrous investment. When this primary cyst or vesicle has attained a certain size, buds develop from the parenchymatous layer, which are gradually converted into cysts, presenting a structure identical with that of the original cyst, namely, an elastic chitinous membrane lined with a granular parenchymatous layer. These secondary or daughter cysts are at first connected with the lining membrane of the primary cyst, but are soon set free. In this way the parent cyst as it grows may contain a dozen or more daughter cysts. Inside these daughter cysts a similar process may occur, and from buds in the walls granddaughter cysts are developed. From the granular layer of the parent and daughter cysts buds arise which develop into brood capsules. From the lining membrane the little outgrowths arise and gradually develop into bodies known as scolices, which represent in reality the head of the *T. echinococcus* and present four sucking disks and a circle of hooklets. Each scolex is capable when transferred to the intestines of a dog of developing into an adult tapeworm. The difference between the ovum of an ordinary tapeworm, such as *T. solium,* and *T. echinococcus* is in this way very striking. In the former case the ovum develops into a single larva—*Cysticercus cullulosæ*—whereas the egg of *T. echinococcus* develops into a cyst which is capable of multiplying enormously and from the lining membrane of which millions of larval tapeworms develop. Ordinarily in man the development of the echinococcus takes place as above mentioned and by an endogenous form in which the secondary and tertiary cysts are contained within the primary; but in animals the formation may be different, as the buds from the primary cyst penetrate between the layers and develop externally, forming the exogenous variety. A third form is the multilocular echinococcus, in which form the primary cyst buds develop which are cut off completely and are surrounded by thick capsules of a connective tissue, which join together and ultimately form a hard mass represented by strands of connective tissue inclosing alveolar spaces about the size of peas or a little larger. In these spaces are found the remnants of the echinococcus cyst, occasionally the scolices or hooklets, but they are often sterile.

The fluid is limpid, non-albuminous; specific gravity 1.005 to 1.009, occasionally higher. It may contain sugar and succinic acid, and, after repeated tapping of the cyst, albumin. When not degenerated the hydatid heads or the characteristic hooklets are found in the contents of the cyst.

CHANGES IN THE CYST.—It is not known definitely how long the echinococcus remains alive, probably many years, possibly as long as twenty years.

The most common change is death and the gradual inspissation of the contents and conversion of the cyst into a mass containing putty-like granular material which may be partially calcified. Remnants of the chitinous cyst wall or hooklets may be found. These obsolete hydatid cysts are not infrequently found in the liver. A more serious termination is rupture, which may take place into a serous sac, or perforation may take place externally when the cysts are discharged, as into the bronchi or alimentary canal or urinary passages. More unfavorable are the instances in which rupture occurs into the bile-passages or into the inferior cava. Recovery may follow the rupture and discharge of the hydatids externally. Sudden death has been known to follow the rupture. A third and very serious mode of termination is suppuration, which may occur spontaneously or follow rupture and is found most frequently in the liver.

Geographical Distribution.—The disease prevails most extensively in those countries in which man is brought into close contact with the dog, particularly when, as in Australia, the dogs are used for herding sheep, the animal in which the larval form of *T. echinococcus* is most often found. In Iceland the cases are numerous. In Europe the disease is not uncommon. In Great Britain and in North America it is rare, and a majority of the cases are in foreigners. Statistics of the prevalence of the disease in America have been published by Osler (1882), Sommer (1895-'96), and Lyon (1902), who collected 241 cases. Of these, 136 cases were in foreigners; in 92 the nationality was not stated; 10 were negroes; 2 Canadians, and only 1 a native American. Fifty-six cases occurred in Manitoba, where there is a settlement of Icelanders, who brought the disease with them. Only one instance is known in a Canadian-born offspring of an Icelandic emigrant.

Distribution in the Body.—Of 1,634 cases in the statistics of Davaine, Böcker, Finsen, and Neisser, the parasite existed in the liver in 820; in the lung or pleura in 137; in the abdominal organs, including the kidneys, bladder, and genitalia, in 334; in the nervous system in 122; in the circulatory system in 42; in other organs 179. Of the 241 cases in Lyon's series in America the liver was the seat in 177, and the omentum, peritoneal cavity, and mesentery in 26. In 11 cases cysts were passed per rectum, in 7 cases cysts or hooklets were expectorated, and in 2 cases passed per urethram.

Symptoms.—1. *Hydatids of the Liver.*—Small cysts may cause no disturbance; large and growing cysts produce signs of tumor of the liver with great increase in the size of the organ. Naturally the physical signs depend much upon the situation of the growth. Near the anterior surface in the epigastric region the tumor may form a distinct prominence and have a tense, firm feeling, sometimes with fluctuation. A not infrequent situation is to the left of the suspensory ligament, the resulting tumor pushing up the heart and causing an extensive area of dulness in the lower sternal and left hypochondriac regions. In the right lobe, if the tumor is on the posterior surface, the enlargement of the organ is chiefly upward into the pleura and the vertical area of dulness in the posterior axillary line is increased. Superficial cysts may give what is known as the hydatid fremitus. If the tumor is palpated lightly with the fingers of the left hand and percussed at the same time with those of the right, there is felt a vibration or trembling movement which persists for a certain time. It is not always present, and it is doubtful whether it is peculiar to the hydatid tumors or due to the collision of the daughter cysts. Very large cysts are accompanied by feelings of pressure or dragging in the hepatic region, sometimes actual pain. The general condition of the patient is at first good and the nutrition little, if at all, interfered with. Unless some of the accidents already referred to occur, the symptoms may be trifling and due only to the pressure or weight of the tumor.

Historically, one of the most interesting cases is that of the first Lord Shaftesbury (Achitopel), who had a tumor below the costal border for many years. It suppurated and was opened by the philosopher John Locke, his physician, who describes with great detail the escape of the bladder-like bodies. Among the Shaftesbury papers in the Record Office are several other cases collected by Locke; the disease may have been more common in England at that period.

Suppuration of the cyst changes the picture into one of pyæmia. There are rigors, sweats, more or less jaundice, and rapid loss of weight. Perforation may occur into the stomach, colon, pleura, bronchi, or externally, and in some instances recovery has taken place. Perforation has occurred into the pericardium and inferior vena cava; in the latter case the daughter cysts have been found in the heart, plugging the tricuspid orifice and pulmonary artery. Perforation of the bile-passages causes intense jaundice, and may lead to suppurative cholangitis.

An interesting symptom connected with the rupture of hydatid cysts is the occurrence of urticaria, which may also follow aspiration of the cysts. Brieger separated a highly toxic material from the fluid, and to it the symptoms of poisoning may be due.

Diagnosis.—Cysts of moderate size may exist without producing symptoms. Large multiple echinococci may cause great enlargement with irregularity of the outline, and such a condition persisting for any time with retention of the health and strength suggests hydatid disease. An irregular, painless enlargement, particularly in the left lobe, or the presence of a large, smooth, fluctuating tumor in the epigastric region is suggestive, and in this situation, when accessible to palpation, it gives a sensation of a smooth elastic growth and possibly also the hydatid tremor. When suppuration occurs the clinical picture is really that of abscess, and only the existence of previous enlargement of the liver with good health would point to the fact that the suppuration was associated with hydatids. *Syphilis* may produce irregular enlargement without much disturbance in the health, sometimes also a very definite tumor in the epigastric region, but this is usually firm and not fluctuating. The clinical features may simulate *cancer* very closely. In one case the liver was greatly enlarged and there were many nodular tumors in the abdomen. The post mortem showed enormous suppurating hydatid cysts in the left lobe of the liver which had perforated the stomach in two places and also the duodenum. The omentum, mesentery, and pelvis also contained numerous cysts. As a rule, the clinical course suffices to separate it clearly from cancer. Dilatation of the gall-bladder and hydronephrosis have been mistaken for hydatid disease. In the former the mobility of the tumor, its shape, and the mucoid character of the contents suffice for the diagnosis. In some instances of hydronephrosis only the exploratory puncture could distinguish between the conditions. More frequent is the mistake of confounding a hydatid cyst of the right lobe pushing up the pleura with pleural effusion of the right side. The heart may be dislocated, the liver depressed, and dulness, feeble breathing, and diminished fremitus are present in both conditions. Frerichs lays stress upon the different character of the line of dulness; in the echinococcus cyst the upper limit presents a curved line, the maximum of which is usually in the scapular region. Suppurative pleurisy may be caused by the perforation of the cyst. If adhesions result, the perforation takes place into the lung, and fragments of the cysts or small daughter cysts may be coughed up. For diagnostic purposes the exploratory puncture should be used. The fluid is usually perfectly clear or slightly opalescent, the reaction is neutral, and the specific gravity varies from 1.005 to 1.009. It is non-albuminous, but contains chlorides and sometimes traces of sugar. Hooklets may be found in the clear fluid or in the suppurating cysts. They are sometimes absent, however, as the cyst may be sterile.

2. *Echinococcus of the Respiratory System.*—Of 809 cases of single hydatid cyst collected by Thomas in Australia, the lung was affected in 134 cases. Of 241 American cases, in 16 the pleura or lung was affected. The larvæ may develop primarily in the pleura and attain a large size. The symptoms are at first those of compression of the lung and dislocation of the heart. The physical signs are those of fluid in the pleura. The line of dulness may be quite irregular. As in the echinococcus of the liver, the general condition of the patient may be excellent in spite of the existence of extensive disease. Pleurisy is rarely excited. The cysts may become inflamed and perforate the chest wall. Cary and Lyon analyzed 40 cases of primary echinococcus cyst of the pleura; death results in a majority of the cases from the toxæmia following the rupture and the absorption of the fluid or from the sepsis following suppuration.

Echinococci occur more frequently in the lung than in the pleura. If small, they may exist for some time without causing serious symptoms. In their growth they compress the lung and sooner or later lead to inflammatory processes, often to gangrene, and the formation of cavities which connect with the bronchi. Fragments of membrane or small cysts may be expectorated. Hæmorrhage is not infrequent. Perforation into the pleura with empyema is common. A majority of the cases are regarded during life as tuberculosis or gangrene, and it is only the detection of the characteristic membranes or the hooklets which leads to the diagnosis. Of a series of 21 cases, 17 recovered; 5 of the cases suppurated (C. H. Fleming, Victoria).

3. *Echinococcus of the Kidneys.*—In the collected statistics referred to above the genito-urinary system comes second as the seat of hydatid disease, though here the affection is rare in comparison with that of the liver. Of the 241 American cases, there were 17 in which the kidneys or bladder were involved. The kidney may be converted into an enormous cyst resembling a hydronephrosis. The *diagnosis* is only possible by puncture and examination of the fluid. The cyst may perforate into the pelvis of the kidney, and portions of the membrane or cysts may be discharged with the urine, sometimes producing renal colic. In one case for many months the patient passed at intervals numbers of small cysts with the urine. The general health was little if at all disturbed, except by the attacks of colic during the passage of the parasites.

4. *Echinococcus of the Nervous System.*—The common cystic disease of the choroidal plexuses has been mistaken for hydatids. Davies Thomas, of Australia, tabulated 97 cases, including some of the *Cysticercus cellulosæ.* According to his statistics, the cyst is more common on the right than on the left side, and is more frequent in the cerebrum.

The symptoms, very indefinite, as a rule are those of tumor. Persistent headache, convulsions, either limited or general, and gradually developing blindness have been prominent features in many cases.

Multilocular Echinococcus.—This form merits a brief description, as it differs so remarkably from the usual type. It has been met with only in Bavaria, Württemberg, the adjacent districts of Switzerland, and in the Tyrol. Possett reported 13 cases from von Rokitansky's clinic at Innsbruck. In the United States a few cases have been described, chiefly in Germans. Delafield and Prudden's patient had lived there five years, and for a year before his death had been jaundiced. A fluctuating tumor was found in the right flank, apparently connected with the liver. This was opened, and death followed from hæmorrhage. In Oertel's case the patient had lived there ten years. He was deeply jaundiced, and had a tumor mass at the right border of the liver, which was enlarged. Bacon resected a cyst from the left lobe of the liver. The primary tumor presents irregularly formed cavities separated from each other by strands of connective tissue, and lined with the echinococcus membrane. The cavities are filled with a gelatinous material, so that the tumor has very much the appearance of an alveolar colloid cancer. It is possible that a special form of tænia echinococcus represents the adult type of this peculiar parasite. This form is almost exclusively confined to the liver, and the symptoms resemble more those of tumor or cirrhosis. The liver is, as a rule, enlarged and smooth, not irregular as in the ordinary echinococcus. Jaundice is common and the spleen is usually enlarged; there is progressive emaciation and toward the close hæmorrhages are common.

Treatment of Echinococcus Disease.—Medicines are of no avail. Post mortem reports show that in a considerable number of cases the parasite dies and the cyst becomes harmless. Operative measures should be resorted to when the cyst is large or troublesome. The simple aspiration of the contents has been successful in a number of cases, and may be tried before the more radical procedure of incision and evacuation of the cysts. Suppuration has occasionally followed the puncture. Injections into the sac should not be practised. Surgeons open and evacuate the echinococcus cysts with great boldness, and the Australian records, which are the most numerous and important on this subject, show that recovery is the rule in a large proportion of the cases. Suppurative cysts in the liver should be treated as abscess. The treatment of hydatid disease has been greatly advanced by Australian surgeons. The works of the Australian physicians, James Graham and Thomas, may be consulted for details in diagnosis and treatment.

Sparganum mansoni is a larval bothriocephalus met with in Japan and China, usually in the subcutaneous tissues, the adult form of which is not known.

III. DISEASES CAUSED BY NEMATODES

1. ASCARIASIS

Ascaris lumbricoides, the most common human parasite, is found chiefly in children. The female is from 7 to 12 inches in length, the male from 4 to 8 inches. In form it is cylindrical, pointed at both ends, with a yellowish-brown, sometimes a slightly reddish color. Four longitudinal bands can be seen, and it is striated transversely. The ova, which are sometimes found in large numbers in the fæces, are small, brownish-red in color, elliptical, and have a very thick covering. They measure 0.075 mm. in length and 0.058 mm. in width. The life history has been demonstrated to be "direct"—*i. e.,* without intermediate host. The larvæ enter the tissues, migrate through the lungs and return to the alimentary tract. The parasite occupies the upper portion of the small intestine. Usually not more than one or two are present, but occasionally they occur in enormous numbers. The migrations are peculiar. They may pass into the stomach, whence they may be ejected by vomiting, or they may crawl up the œsophagus and enter the pharynx, from which they may be withdrawn. A child in the smallpox department of the Montreal General Hospital, during convalescence, withdrew in this way more than thirty round worms within a few weeks. In other instances the worm reaches the larynx, and has been known to produce fatal asphyxia, or, passing into the trachea, to cause gangrene of the lung. They may go through the Eustachian tube and appear at the external meatus. The worms have been found in extraordinary numbers in the bile-ducts. Remarkable specimens exist in the Dupuytren, the Wistar-Horner (Philadelphia), and the Netley Museums. Chalmers (Ceylon) and Leys (U. S. N.) have called attention to their importance in causing abscess of the liver. Ebstein reported certain markings, strangulations, on the round worms, as if they had been nipped in the bile-ducts! The bowel may be blocked, or in rare instances an ulcer may be perforated. Even the healthy bowel wall may be penetrated.

A peculiarly irritating substance, often evident to the sense of smell in handling specimens, is formed by the round worms. Peiper and others suggest that the nervous symptoms, sometimes resembling those of meningitis, are due to this poison. Chauffard, Marie, and Tauchon report a remarkable condition of fever, intestinal symptoms, foul breath, and intermittent diarrhœa in connection with the presence of lumbricoides. They call it typho-lumbricosis. The febrile condition may continue for a month or more. There may be eosinophilia to 25 to 30 per cent., and in some cases a marked anæmia. The question of the toxins produced by these parasites is an open one.

A few parasites may cause no disturbance. In children irritative symptoms of many kinds are attributed to worms, such as restlessness, irritability, picking at the nose, grinding of the teeth, twitchings, or convulsions. The *diagnosis* is made by finding the worms or eggs in the stools.

Treatment.—Care should be taken to avoid auto-infection by thorough washing after defecation, and those infected should not be allowed to prepare food or serve it to others. It is well to give soft diet on the day previous and a dose of castor oil the night before treatment. *Santonin* is usually efficient given in the morning in doses of one grain (0.065 gm.) for a small child, and three to five grains (0.2 to 0.3 gm.) for an adult. One to two grains of calomel should be given with it. Three hours later a good dose of saline should be given. This should be done two mornings in succession and repeated in a week if worms or eggs are again passed. The occasional effects of santonin (yellow vision, vertigo) should be explained beforehand. Oil of chenopodium is useful in doses of 10 to 15 drops in an ounce of castor oil, followed in an hour by a second dose of castor oil. If these are not effectual male fern or thymol may be given.

Oxyuris vermicularis (Thread-worm; Pin-worm).—This common parasite occupies the rectum and colon. The male measures about 4 mm. in length, the female about 10 mm. They produce great irritation and itching, particularly at night, symptoms which become intensely aggravated by the nocturnal migration of the parasites. The oxyuris may traverse the intestinal wall, and has been found in the peritoneal cavity, where they may form verminous tubercles in Douglas's fossa or peri-rectal abscesses.

The patients become extremely restless and irritable, the sleep is often disturbed, and there may be loss of appetite and anæmia. Though most common in children, the parasite occurs at all ages.

The worm is readily detected in the fæces. Infection probably takes place through the water, or possibly through salads, such as lettuce and cresses. A person the subject of the worms passes ova in large numbers in the fæces, and the possibility of re-infection must be scrupulously guarded against.

Treatment.—Every care should be taken to avoid auto-infection or the infection of others, by care in cleansing the anus and perineum, and thorough washing of the hands after defecation. Auto-infection is often responsible for the persistence of the disease. Treatment must be directed to the removal of the worms both from the small intestine and rectum. Santonin and calomel are useful, given as in ascaris infection for several days. Thymol and naphthalein are also used. To remove the worms from the rectum injections are required which should be retained as long as possible; it is well to wash out the bowel before giving them and the injection need not be over six ounces. Cold solutions of salt and water, ice water, glycerine, infusion of quassia (one ounce of quassia chips to a pint of water), or lime water may be employed and should be used daily for two weeks. For the itching, carbolated vaseline, gall and opium ointment, or menthol (5 per cent.) in vaseline may be employed.

2. TRICHINIASIS

The *Trichina or Trichinella spiralis* in its adult condition lives in the small intestine. The disease is produced by the embryos, which pass from the intestines and reach the voluntary muscles, where they finally become encapsulated larvæ—muscle trichinæ. It is in the migration of the embryos (possibly from poisons produced by them) that the group of symptoms known as trichiniasis is produced.

The ovoid cysts were described in human muscle by Tiedemann in 1822, and by Hilton in 1832; the parasite was figured and named by Richard Owen. Leidy in 1845 described it in the pig. For a long time the trichina was looked upon as a pathological curiosity; but in 1860 Zenker discovered in a girl in the Dresden Hospital, who had symptoms of typhoid fever, both the intestinal and muscle forms, and established their connection with a serious and often fatal disease.

Description of the Parasites.—(*a*) Adult or intestinal form. The female measures from 3 to 4 mm.; the male, 1.5 mm., and has two little projections from the hinder end. (*b*) The larva or muscle trichina is from 0.6 to 1 mm. in length and lies coiled in an ovoid capsule, which is at first translucent, but subsequently opaque and infiltrated with lime salts. The worm presents a pointed head and a somewhat rounded tail.

When flesh containing the trichinæ is eaten by man or by any animal in which the development can take place, the capsules are digested and the trichinæ set free. They pass into the small intestine, and about the third day attain their full growth and become sexually mature. On the sixth or seventh day the embryos are fully developed. The young produced by each female trichina have been estimated at several hundred. Leuckart thought that various broods are developed in succession, and that as many as a thousand embryos may be produced by a single worm. The time from the ingestion of the flesh containing the muscle trichinæ to the development of the brood of embryos in the intestines is from seven to nine days. The female worm penetrates the intestinal wall and the embryos are probably discharged directly into the lymph spaces, thence into the venous system, and by the blood stream to the muscles, which constitute their seat of election. J. Y. Graham gives strong arguments in favor of the transmission through the blood stream. They have been found in the *blood* early in the infection and since the demonstration of their presence by Herrick and Janeway have been seen by a number of observers. They are found also in the *spinal fluid* in some cases. They have been reported as occurring in the fluid of a pleural exudate, in the milk of a nursing woman and in the pus from a furuncle. After a preliminary migration in the inter-muscular connective tissue they penetrate the primitive muscle-fibres, and in about two weeks develop into the full-grown muscle form. In this process an interstitial myositis is excited and gradually an ovoid capsule develops about the parasite. Two, occasionally three or four, worms may be seen within a single capsule. This process of encapsulation has been estimated to take about six weeks. Within the muscles the parasites do not undergo further change. Gradually the capsule becomes thicker, and ultimately lime salts are deposited within it. This change may take place in man within four or five months. In the hog it may be deferred for many years. The calcification renders the cyst visible, and these small, opaque, oat-shaped bodies are familiar objects to demonstrators of normal and morbid anatomy. The trichinæ may live within the muscles for an indefinite period. They have been found alive and capable of developing as late as twenty or even twenty-five years after their entrance into the system. In many instances, however, the worms are completely calcified. The trichina has been found or "raised" in twenty-six different species of animals (Stiles). Medical literature abounds in references to its presence in fish, earthworms, etc., but these parasites belong to other genera. In fæcal examinations for the parasite it is well to remember that the "cell body" of the anterior portion of the intestine is a diagnostic criterion of the *T. spiralis*. Experimentally, guinea-pigs and rabbits are readily infected by feeding them with muscle containing the larval form. Dogs are infected with difficulty; cats more readily. Experimentally, animals sometimes die of the disease if large numbers of the parasites have been eaten. In the hog the trichinæ, like the cysticerci, cause few if any symptoms. An important point is the fact that in the hog the capsule does not readily become calcified, so that the parasites are not visible as in the human muscles.

The *anatomical* changes are chiefly in the voluntary muscles. The trichinæ enter the primitive muscle bundles, which undergo granular degeneration with marked nuclear proliferation. There is a local myositis, and gradually about the parasite a cyst wall is formed. These changes, as well as the remarkable alterations in the blood, have been described by Brown. Cohnheim described a fatty degeneration of the liver and enlargement of the mesenteric glands. At the time of death, in the fourth or fifth week or later, the adult trichinæ are still found in the intestines.

Incidence.—Man is infected by eating the flesh of trichinous hogs. In Germany, where a systematic microscopic examination of all swine flesh is made, the proportion of trichinous hogs is about 1 in 1,852. Statistics are not available in England. In America inspections have been made since 1892. The percentage of animals found infected has ranged from 1.04 to 1.95. In 1883, with A. W. Clement, the senior author examined 1,000 hogs at the Montreal abattoir, and found only 4 infected.

Modes of Infection.—The danger of infection depends entirely upon the mode of preparation of the flesh. Thorough cooking, so that all parts of the meat reach the boiling point, destroys the parasites; but in large joints the central portions are often not raised to this temperature. The frequency of the disease in different countries depends largely upon the habits of the people in the preparation of pork. In North Germany, where raw ham and *Wurst* are freely eaten, the greatest number of instances have occurred. In South Germany, France, and England cases are rare. In the United States the greatest number of persons attacked have been Germans. Salting and smoking the flesh are not always sufficient, and the Havre experiments showed that animals are readily infected when fed with portions of the pickled or the smoked meat as prepared in America. Carl Fraenkel, however, states that the experiments on this point have been negative, and that it is very doubtful if any cases of trichiniasis in Germany have been caused by American pork. Germany has yet to show a single case of trichiniasis due to pork of unquestioned American origin.

Frequency of Infection.—H. U. Williams, of Buffalo, made a thorough study of the muscle from 505 unselected autopsies, and found 27 cases of trichiniasis, 5.3 per cent. The subjects had all died of causes other than trichiniasis. This important study shows how widespread is the disease, and that in reality we frequently overlook the sporadic form.

The disease occurs in groups or outbreaks in which from a dozen to several hundred individuals are attacked, and in sporadic cases which have been shown of late years to be not infrequent. In the epidemics a large number of persons are infected from one source; in the two famous outbreaks of Hedersleben and Emersleben 337 and 250 individuals were attacked. In the United States Stiles estimates that there have been more than 1,000 small outbreaks. The discovery in the wards at the Johns Hopkins Hospital by T. R. Brown of the eosinophilia in the disease has led to the much more frequent detection of the sporadic cases, and this form of the disease is not at all uncommon in the United States.

Symptoms.—The ingestion of trichinous flesh is not necessarily followed by the disease. When a limited number are eaten only a few embryos pass to the muscles and may cause no symptoms. Well-characterized cases present a gastro-intestinal period and a period of general infection.

In the course of a few days after eating the infected meat there are signs of gastro-intestinal disturbance—pain in the abdomen, loss of appetite, vomiting, and sometimes diarrhœa. The preliminary symptoms, however, are by no means constant, and in some of the large epidemics cases have been observed in which they have been absent. In other instances the gastro-intestinal features have been marked from the outset, and the attack has resembled cholera nostras. Pain in different parts of the body, general debility, and weakness have been noted in some of the epidemics.

The invasion symptoms occur between the seventh and the tenth day, sometimes not until the end of the second week. There is fever, except in very mild cases. Chills are not common. The thermometer may register 102° or 104° F., and the fever is usually remittent or intermittent. The migration of the parasites into the muscles excites a more or less intense myositis, which is characterized by pain on pressure and movement, and by swelling and tension of the muscles, over which the skin may be œdematous. The limbs are placed in the positions in which the muscles are in least tension. The involvement of the muscles of mastication and of the larynx may cause difficulty in chewing and swallowing. In severe cases the involvement of the diaphragm and intercostal muscles may lead to intense dyspnœa, which sometimes proves fatal. Œdema, a feature of great importance, may be early in the face, particularly about the eyes. Later it occurs in the extremities when the swelling and stiffness of the muscles are at their height. Profuse sweats, tingling and itching of the skin, and in some instances urticaria, have been described. Kernig's sign is usually present and the leg reflexes may be absent.

Blood.—A marked leucocytosis, which may reach above 30,000, is usually present. A special feature is the extraordinary increase in the number of eosinophilic cells, which may comprise more than 50 per cent. of all the leucocytes. There were in four years, in the Johns Hopkins Hospital, 7 cases in which the eosinophilia was most pronounced. In 4 of them the diagnosis was actually suggested by the great increase in the eosinophiles; in 1 case they reached 68 per cent. of the total number of leucocytes.

The general nutrition is much disturbed and the patient becomes emaciated and often anæmic, particularly in the protracted cases. The patients are usually conscious, except in cases of very intense infection, in which the toxæmia, dry tongue, and tremor give a picture suggesting typhoid fever. In addition to the dyspnœa present in the severer infections, there may be bronchitis, and in the fatal cases pneumonia or pleurisy. In some epidemics polyuria has been a common symptom. Albuminuria is frequent.

The intensity and duration of the symptoms depend entirely upon the grade of infection. In the mild cases recovery is complete in from ten to fourteen days. In the severe forms convalescence is not established for six or eight weeks, and it may be months before the patient recovers the muscular strength. One patient in the Hedersleben epidemic was weak eight years after the attack.

Of 72 fatal cases in the Hedersleben epidemic, the greatest mortality occurred in the fourth and fifth and sixth weeks; namely, 52 cases. Two died in the second week with severe choleraic symptoms. The mortality has ranged in different outbreaks from 1 or 2 per cent. to 30 per cent. Among 456 cases reported in the United States there were 122 deaths.

The **prognosis** depends much upon the quantity of infected meat eaten and the number of trichinæ which mature in the intestines. In children the outlook is more favorable. Early diarrhœa and moderately intense gastro-intestinal symptoms are, as a rule, more favorable than constipation.

Diagnosis.—The disease should always be suspected when a large party among Germans is followed by cases of apparent typhoid fever. The parasites may be found in the remnants of the ham or sausages used on the occasion. The worms may be discovered in the stools or found in the duodenal contents. The stools should be spread on a glass plate or black background and examined with a low-power lens, when the trichinæ are seen as small, glistening, silvery threads. In doubtful cases the diagnosis may be made by the removal of a piece of muscle. The disease may be mistaken for rheumatic fever, particularly as the pains are so severe on movement, but there is no special swelling of the joints. The great increase of the eosinophiles in the blood is a most suggestive point in diagnosis. The tenderness is in the muscles both on pressure and on movement. The intensity of the gastro-intestinal symptoms has led to the diagnosis of cholera. Many of the former epidemics were described as typhoid fever, which the severer cases, owing to the prolonged fever, the sweats, the delirium, dry tongue, and gastro-intestinal symptoms, somewhat resemble. The pains in the muscles, with tension and swelling, œdema, particularly about the eyes, and shortness of breath, are the most important diagnostic points.

Prophylaxis.—It is not definitely known how swine become diseased. It has been thought that they are infected from rats about slaughter-houses, but it is just as reasonable to believe that the rats are infected by eating the trichinous flesh of swine. The swine should, so far as possible, be grain-fed, and not allowed to eat offal. The most satisfactory prophylaxis is the complete cooking of pork and sausages, and to this custom in England, France, South Germany, and the United States immunity is largely due.

Treatment.—If it has been discovered within twenty-four or thirty-six hours that a large number of persons have eaten infected meat, the indications are to thoroughly evacuate the gastro-intestinal canal. Calomel (gr. ii, 0.13 gm.) should be given at once and repeated in two hours. Four hours after the second dose half an ounce of castor oil or magnesium sulphate should be given and repeated if necessary. An enema should be given unless the bowels move freely. Glycerine has been recommended in large doses, in order that by passing into the intestines it may by its hygroscopic properties destroy the worm. Male fern, kamala, santonin, and thymol have all been recommended in this stage. Turpentine may be tried in full doses. There is no doubt that diarrhœa in the first week or ten days of the infection is distinctly favorable. The indications in the stage of invasion are to relieve the pains, to secure sleep, and to support the patient's strength. There are no medicines which have any influence upon the embryos in their migration through the muscles. The use of arsphenamine has been advised but proof of its value is lacking.

3. UNCINARIASIS

(*Hookworm Disease, Ankylostomiasis*)

Synonyms.—One of the most important, widespread of all metazoan infections, variously known as anæmia of miners, bricklayers, tunnel-workers; tropical and Egyptian chlorosis.

History.—For three centuries the disease, but not its nature, was recognized in the tropics under various names. Dubini, in 1838, first described the worms, and gave the name from the curved or bent appearance of the mouth. In 1853 and 1854 Bilhartz and Griesinger recognized the relation of the parasites to the anæmia and dropsy. In South America in 1866 Wucherer called attention to the frequency of the disease in negro slaves. In the "seventies" and "eighties" of the last century the anæmia of brick-workers in Italy and of miners and tunnel diggers was shown to be due to this parasite. Occasional statements were made as to the occurrence of the disease in the United States, but it was not until the extensive investigations of Stiles in 1901, and later, that it was shown that the hookworm was widely prevalent, that it was responsible for an enormous amount of ill health and anæmia, and that it was directly connected with the old and long-ago described practice of dirt-eating. It was gradually realised how widespread the disease was in the Southern States. Ashford and King studied the disease in Porto Rico, and carried out one of the most successful of modern sanitary campaigns. In 1898 Looss discovered the cardinal fact of the penetration of the skin by the larvæ, and of the route by which they reach the intestine. Special monographs have been published by Dock and Bass, by Ashford and Igaravidez, and by Boycott (all in 1911).

Distribution.—The parasite exists in most parts of the world, and there is scarcely a tropical country in which it does not prevail. In India the infection is from 60 to 80 per cent., in Porto Rico 90 per cent., in the Philippines about 15 per cent. In Europe it is chiefly an affection of miners in Germany, Hungary, France, and Belgium. In England there was a small outbreak in Cornwall, but the disease has not extended. Stiles showed that more than 12 per cent. of cotton-mill employees in the Southern United States were infected, and the examination of recruits, college students, and school children in different parts of the country gave a percentage of infection of from 20 to 70 or even 80. Among 18,390 white troops examined, hook-worm was found in 13.7 per cent. In the West Indies the Rockefeller Commission found 97,632 infected among 165,866 examined.

Parasites.—There are two chief forms, the *Ancylostoma duodenale,* the old world species, and the *Necator americanus,* the new world species. The Ancylostoma is a small cylindrical nematode, the male about 10 mm. and the female from 8 to 18 mm. in length. The mouth has chitinous plates, and is provided with two pairs of sharp, hook-shaped teeth, with which they pierce the mucosa of the bowel. The male has a prominent, umbrella-like caudal expansion. The new world worm has much the same characters, only it is more slender, the mouth globular, and the arrangement of the teeth quite different. The eggs are from 52 μ to 60 μ by about 34 μ in width in the European form, and from 64 μ to 76 μ by about 36 μ in breadth in the American form. They are very characteristic bodies in the fæces of infected individuals. When laid they are already in process of segmentation. Complete desiccation, and direct sunlight, or much water in the fæces kills the eggs; but they are sometimes very resistant, and may survive freezing followed by a gentle thawing. The rapidity of development depends upon favoring conditions and temperature, and the larvæ after escaping from the eggs may live for months in the mud or water of the mines, and they pass through a series of moults before they reach what is called the ripe stage. They then show a remarkable tenacity of life, and may live in water or slime for many months; and in this, which is the infective stage, they have a great tendency to wander.

Modes of Infection.—An extraordinary number of eggs are passed with each stool of a badly infected person, as many it has been estimated as four millions. They develop most readily in fæces mixed with sand or earth at a temperature of from 70° to 90°. The larvæ become infective when about 4 or 5 days old. Infection takes place either by the mouth directly, which is rare, or by the skin. Looss showed experimentally that the larvæ entering the skin are carried by the veins to the heart, and thence to the lungs, in which they escape from the pulmonary vessels, pass up the bronchi and trachea, and so to the gullet, stomach and intestines. These remarkable observations of Looss have been abundantly confirmed. As C. A. Smith's work has shown, it takes about seven weeks before the ova appear in the stools, and in the process of infection there may be sore throat and fever. It would appear that the skin is the common channel of entrance, and usually shows signs of irritation—*ground itch*. Larvæ accidentally swallowed may pass through the stomach, and develop in the intestines.

The careless disposition of fæces permits the pollution of the soil, and in tropical and sub-tropical districts, and in mines, it is easy to understand how children and others are infected through the skin. Ashford and King give a history of ground-itch in more than 90 per cent. of their cases.

Morbid Anatomy and Pathology.—The worms are chiefly in the jejunum; Sandwith found 1,353 out of 1,524 worms in the first six feet of the bowel. They are also occasionally found in the stomach. A variable number of worms are found attached to the mucosa. Very characteristic lesions are the ecchymoses and small erosions of the mucosa, in the centre of which may be a pale area, slightly raised, to which the worm is attached; it may be almost buried in the mucosa. There are usually more bites or holes than worms. Blood cysts occur in the sub-mucosa, in which, occasionally, worms are found (Whipple). The contents of the bowel are often blood-stained. In long-standing cases the mucosa may show many areas of pigmentation. Other lesions are those of chronic anæmia with fatty degeneration. Much discussion has taken place as to whether the worms live on blood or not. They are certainly built for blood-sucking, and, as Whipple states, when the mucosa is normal the worms feed chiefly on blood, when it is thickened and infiltrated they have to be content with the epithelium and mucosa. The loss of blood is largely direct, but it has been shown by Loeb and A. J. Smith that the head-glands of the worm secrete a substance which retards coagulation, probably a hæmolytic poison, the presence of which Whipple has demonstrated. Another feature of importance is the liability to infection through the bites; and the anæmia may in part, at any rate, be due to poisonous products absorbed through the bowel lesions.

Symptoms.—Hookworm disease presents a very variable picture, nor does the severity of the symptoms seem to depend always upon the number of worms. There have been fatal cases in which only ten or twelve worms were found, while recovery has followed after more than 4,000 worms have been expelled (Dock). In infected districts, as in the Southern States, the hookworm disease causes a widespread degeneration in the community, the children and young adults showing a pallor, under-development, and failure of nutrition. With the infection, too, are associated apathy and lack of energy, so that the common opinion in the South is that the hookworm is the cause of laziness. There is no question that, as Stiles and others have shown, the widespread infection is responsible for a great deal of ill health and physical incapacity, often without any actual illness. In more severe cases the anæmia is pronounced, the hæmoglobin being from 40 to 50 per cent.; the child is stunted and puberty is long delayed, and the patient may belong to the group of dirt-eaters. The retardation of growth is remarkable, and the individual may continue to grow until he is 25 or 26 years of age. In the severest type of all the anæmia is still more pronounced; the hæmoglobin below 25 or 20 per cent.; œdema occurs, the patient is bedridden, and death occurs from exhaustion, diarrhœa, or some intercurrent affection. The *anæmia* is of a secondary type, averaging from 50 to 60 per cent. of the corpuscles, with, as a rule, a low color index. Leucocytosis is not often present, and the differential count shows nothing unusual except the great increase in the eosinophiles, ranging from 15 to 26 or even 30 per cent. The eosinophilia bears no relation to the severity of the infection.

"Ground-itch," the local lesion through which the parasites enter the system, is most commonly on the feet and legs in children, or on the arms and hands in gardeners and miners. The most common region is between and beneath the toes. The eruption is vesicular at first, and then pustules form with a sticky exudate, and sometimes with much swelling of the skin. The vesicles and pustules gradually dry, and in about eight or ten days heal with exfoliation.

Other general features are the well known circulatory and respiratory features of anæmia. The digestive symptoms are remarkable. In the mild cases there are slight epigastric pain and discomfort; in the severer ones there are anorexia and remarkable perversion of appetite; the patients eat earth, paper, chalk, starch, hair and clay. The dirt-eaters of the Southern States are all subject to hookworm disease. With the apathetic, listless expression there is dilatation of the pupils, and Stiles has remarked upon the "dull, blank, almost fish-like or cadaveric stare," which gives a very characteristic appearance to the expression.

Diagnosis.—In tropical and sub-tropical regions slight anæmia and ill health should lead to the examination of the stools, from which a certain diagnosis may be made by finding the eggs. "The combination of anæmia with under-development, weakness, dilated heart, and the history of ground-itch is not likely to be confused with anything else" (Stiles). In badly infected regions a fairly accurate diagnosis may be made on inspection alone, and this may be confirmed by the examination of the fæces and by the rapid improvement after the administration of thymol. Two or three drachms of fæces suffice; they should be collected in a wide-mouthed bottle. A little practice may be required at first, but the necessary technique is easily acquired. The eggs are characteristic structures, usually containing 4 or 8 segments, sometimes the complete embryo nearly ready to burst its shell. Various estimates have been made of the number of worms based on the number of eggs found. It is to be remembered that the eggs vary greatly in number, and the stools may be negative one day and contain many a few days later. Grassi states that 150 eggs per centigram of fæces represent about 1,000 worms. For special methods of examining the stools the student is referred to the monograph of Dock and Bass. The presence of eosinophilia is an important diagnostic aid. Boycott and Haldane found that 94 per cent. of infected persons had over 8 per cent. of eosinophiles.

Prophylaxis.—Destruction of the adult worms, removing conditions suitable to the growth of the embryos, and a campaign of sanitary education are the three essentials. The proper disposal of fæces, obtaining a pure water supply, and decreasing the chance of infection by wearing shoes and stockings are important points. The work of the Porto Rico commission shows what can be done in the tropics, even in the most unfavorable surroundings. More than 300,000 persons have received specific treatment for the disease since the commission began its work. That the mortality in the island has fallen from 42 per 1,000 in 1899-1900 to 20.9 in 1910 is in great part due to the devoted work of the medical staff and the nurses in dealing with hookworm cases.

The International Health Board of the Rockefeller Foundation is continuing its active campaign, and has introduced what is called the intensive method, which is an attempt as nearly as possible to relieve and control hookworm disease within a given area by sanitary and therapeutic measures. A census of the population is taken, a microscopic examination made of the stools, all infected persons are treated, and the treatment continued until microscopic examination shows that a cure has resulted. The people are educated both as to the method of cure and the dangers of soil pollution.

In mines care should be taken to prevent local conditions favoring the growth of the embryos. Oliver has found that cinder and slag are destructive of the larvæ. New workers should be examined and proved not to have the disease before being admitted.

Treatment.—The following directions are given by the Porto Rican commission:

Take one of the two purgatives to-night in water.
Take at 6 o'clock to-morrow morning half of the capsules (thymol).
Take the other half at 8 o'clock the same morning.
Take the other purgative at 10 o'clock.
You should neither drink wine nor any alcoholic liquor during the time you are taking these medicines.
Have a privy in your house. Do not defecate on the surface of the ground, but in the privy.
Do not walk barefooted, so that you may avoid contracting the disease in your feet. Wear shoes and you will never suffer from anæmia.

The purgative preferred is an ordinary saline, and the dose of the thymol is graduated according to the age of the patient, seven grains (0.5 gm.) for children under five, and increasing the dose according to age and strength to sixty grains (4 gm.) for adults. Very few ill effects follow its use, but it sometimes is irritating to the bowels, and occasionally it has been toxic. This treatment should be carried out on one day of each week until the patient is cured. No alcohol or oil should be given at the time of administration of thymol.

Oil of chenopodium (wormseed oil) is often efficient, given in doses of 15 drops in castor oil every two hours for two or three doses. Two hours later a full dose of castor oil is given. The anæmia should receive the usual treatment.

4. FILARIASIS

For a full discussion of the zoölogical relations of this important group see Stiles' article in our "System of Medicine," Second Edition, Vol. II.

The important species are:

Filaria bancrofti (Cobbold, 1877).—This is the ordinary blood filaria. The embryos are found in the peripheral circulation only during sleep or at night. The mosquito is the intermediate host. The embryos measure 270 to 340 μ long by 7 to 11 μ broad; tail pointed. The adult male measures 83 mm. long by 0.407 mm. broad; the tail forms two turns of a spiral. The adult female measures 155 mm. long by 0.715 mm. broad; vulva 2.56 mm. from anterior extremity; eggs 38 μ by 14 μ. This is the species to which the hæmatochyluria and elephantiasis are attributed.

Filaria loa (Cobbold, 1864).—This is the eye-worm of tropical West Africa which causes "Calabar swellings." It occurs in the peripheral circulation during the day. The adults move about in the subcutaneous tissues.

Filaria perstans (Manson, 1891).—The adult is found in the retroperitoneal tissues and the embryo is present in the blood both by day and night.

The most important of these is the *Filaria bancrofti,* which produces the hæmatochyluria and the lymph-scrotum.

The female produces an extraordinary number of embryos, which enter the blood current through the lymphatics. Each embryo is within its shell, which is elongated, scarcely perceptible, and in no way impedes the movements. They are about the ninetieth part of an inch in length and the diameter of a red blood-corpuscle in thickness, so that they readily pass through the capillaries. They move with the greatest activity, and form very striking and readily recognized objects in a blood-drop under the microscope. A remarkable feature is the periodicity in the occurrence of the embryos in the blood. In the daytime they are almost or entirely absent, whereas at night, in typical cases, they are present in large numbers. This does not occur in the Pacific islands, one reason given being that there a day-feeding stegomyia mosquito is the common intermediary. The night-feeding *Culex fatigans* is not the usual carrier in these islands as it is in Asia, Africa and America. If, however, as Stephen Mackenzie has shown, the patient, reversing his habits, sleeps during the day, the periodicity is reversed. Lynch suggests that the periodicity is largely dependent on the difficulty of passage through the peripheral capillaries during periodic tonicity. In the case reported by Lothrop and Pratt the number of embryos per cubic centimetre of blood was calculated hourly during the night; it rose steadily from four o'clock in the afternoon till midnight, when 2,100 per c. c. were present, then fell, none being found at ten o'clock the following morning. The further development of the embryos is associated with the mosquito, which sucks the blood and in this way frees them from the body. They develop in the mosquito and reach the proboscis from which they pass to the human host. The filariæ may be present in the body without causing any symptoms. In the blood of animals filariæ are very common and rarely cause inconvenience. It is only when the adult worms or the ova block the lymph channels that certain definite symptoms occur. Manson suggests that it is the ova (prematurely discharged), which are considerably shorter and thicker than the full-grown embryos, which block the lymph channels and produce the conditions of hæmatochyluria, elephantiasis, and lymph-scrotum.

The parasite is widely distributed, particularly in tropical and sub-tropical countries. Guitéras has shown that the disease prevails extensively in the Southern States, and, since his paper, contributions have been made by Matas, of New Orleans, Mastin, of Mobile, De Saussure, of Charleston, and Opie.

The effects produced may be described under the following conditions:

1. Hæmatochyluria.—Without any external manifestations, and in many cases without special disturbance of health, the subject from time to time passes urine of an opaque white, milky appearance, or bloody, or a chylous fluid which on settling shows a slightly reddish clot. The condition indicates dilatation and rupture of dilated lymphatics in some part of the urinary tract and obstruction of the thoracic duct. The urine may be normal in quantity or increased. The condition is usually intermittent, and the patient may pass normal urine for weeks or months at a time. Microscopically, the chylous urine contains minute molecular fat granules, and usually red blood cells in various amounts. The embryos were first discovered by Demarquay at Paris (1863), and in the urine by Wucherer, at Bahia, in 1866. It is remarkable for how long the condition may persist without serious impairment of the health. A patient, sent by Dawson, of Charleston, had hæmatochyluria intermittently for eighteen years. The only inconvenience had been in the passage of blood-clots which collected in the bladder. At times he had uneasy sensations in the lumbar region. The embryos were present in his blood at night in large numbers. Chyluria is not always due to filaria. There is a non-parasitic form of the disease.

Opportunities for studying the anatomical condition of these cases rarely occur. In the case described by Stephen Mackenzie the renal and peritoneal lymph plexuses were enormously enlarged, extending from the diaphragm to the pelvis. The thoracic duct above the diaphragm was impervious.

2. Elephantiasis is common in all countries in which the filariæ prevail. The parasites are not always found in the blood. The condition is more common in the legs, one or both, beginning below the knee, but gradually involving the entire limb. Next in frequency is *lymph-scrotum* and other forms involving the genitalia. The *scrotal* tumor may reach an enormous size, and 40 to 50 pounds in weight. The onset may be painless and slow, or it may be sudden, with fever and rapid swelling and redness of the

part. There may be a series of such attacks, each one leaving the part more swollen. The so-called "elephantoid fever" may occur in all forms of the infection.

Sporadic Elephantiasis.—A non-parasitic type may be mentioned here, which is not very uncommon in temperate regions, characterized by progressive enlargement of a limb or portion of the body, with a hyperplasia of the skin and subcutaneous tissues, due apparently to an obstructive inflammation of the lymph-vessels. It may arise spontaneously without any obvious cause, or follow an inflammation of the skin of the part, occasionally removal of the lymph-glands. The legs are most frequently involved, beginning usually in one leg, about the foot or ankle, and gradually extending until the whole leg is greatly enlarged. The skin is usually smooth, but it may be hard and indurated or warty and nodular. Most of the cases are in young women, in whom the affection has come on without any obvious cause and progressed slowly until the leg was greatly enlarged. In one case eight years elapsed before the other leg became involved, and in another case more than ten years passed with the disease still confined to one leg.

Diagnosis.—The filaria larva may be found in the blood, urine or chylous fluid. A negative finding does not exclude filarial infection. Adult worms may be found in lymph glands or in abscesses. Eosinophilia is present.

Treatment.—So far as known, no drug destroys the embryos in the blood with certainty. In infected districts the drinking-water should be boiled or filtered. In cases of chyluria the patients should use a dry diet and avoid all excess of fat. The chyle may disappear quite rapidly from the urine under these measures, but it does not necessarily indicate that the case is cured. So long as clots and albumin are present the leak in the lymphoid varix is not healed, although the fat, not being supplied to the chyle, may not be present. A single tumblerful of milk will at once give ocular proof of the patency or otherwise of the rupture in the varix (Manson).

Elephantoid fever demands rest, liquid diet, free purgation and sedative applications to painful areas. In *elephantiasis* during periods with acute symptoms the patient should be at rest and the legs firmly bandaged. Good results are reported from the use of fibrolysin.

The surgical treatment of some of these cases is most successful, particularly in the removal of the adult filariæ from the enlarged lymph-glands, especially in the groin. Surgical measures may be advisable in elephantiasis.

Infected individuals should be protected from mosquitoes.

5. DRACONTIASIS

(*Guinea-worm Disease*)

Dracunculus medinensis is a widely spread parasite in parts of Africa and the East Indies. In the United States instances occasionally occur. Jarvis reported a case in a post chaplain who had lived at Fortress Monroe, Va., for thirty years. Van Harlingen's patient, a man aged forty-seven, had never lived out of Philadelphia, so that the worm must be included among the parasites of the United States. A majority of the cases reported in American journals have been imported.

The female develops in the subcutaneous and intermuscular connective tissues and produces vesicles and abscesses. In the large majority of the cases the parasite is found in the leg. Of 181 cases, in 124 the worm was found in the feet, 33 times in the leg, and 11 times in the thigh. It is usually solitary, though there are cases on record in which six or more have been present. It is cylindrical in form, about 2 mm. in diameter, and from 50 to 80 cm. in length. The male has been found by Leiper in a monkey, a very small worm only 22 mm. in length.

In water the embryos develop in a cyclops—a small crustacean—and it seems likely that man is infected by drinking the water containing these developed larvæ. It is probable that both male and female are ingested; but the former dies and is discharged, while the latter after impregnation penetrates the intestine and attains its full development in the subcutaneous tissues, where it may remain quiescent for a long time and can be felt beneath the skin like a bundle of string. The worm contains an enormous number of living embryos, and to enable them to escape she travels slowly downward head first, and usually reaches the foot or ankle. The head then penetrates the skin and the epidermis, forms a little vesicle, which ruptures, and a small ulcer is left, at the bottom of which the head often protrudes. The distended uterus ruptures and the embryos are discharged in a whitish fluid. After getting rid of them the worm will spontaneously leave her host.

When the worm first appears it should not be disturbed, as after parturition it may leave spontaneously. When the worm begins to come out a common procedure is to roll it round a portion of smooth wood and in this way prevent the retraction, and each day wind a little more until the entire worm is withdrawn. It is stated that special care must be taken to prevent tearing of the worm, as disastrous consequences sometimes follow, probably from the irritation caused by the migration of the embryos.

The parasite may be excised entire, or killed by injections of bichloride of mercury (1 to 1,000). It is stated that the leaves of the plant called *amarpattee* are almost a specific in the disease. Asafetida in full doses is said to kill the worm.

6. OTHER NEMATODES

Filariæ.—Among less important filarian worms parasitic in man the following may be mentioned: *Filaria volvulus* occurs on the West Coast of Africa. It causes masses in the axillæ which are easily removed. *F. immitis*—the common *F. sanguinis* of the dog—of which Bowlby described two cases in man. In one case with hæmaturia female worms were found in the portal vein, and the ova were present in the thickened bladder wall and in the ureters. *F. equina* has rarely infected man.

Trichocephaliasis.—*Trichuris trichiura* (whipworm) is not infrequently found in the cæcum and large intestine of man. It measures from 4 to 5 cm. in length, the male being somewhat shorter than the female. The worm is readily recognized by the remarkable difference between the anterior and posterior portions. The former, which forms at least three-fifths of the body, is extremely thin and hair-like in contrast to the thick hinder portion of the body, which in the female is conical and pointed, and in the male more obtuse and usually rolled like a spring. The eggs are oval, lemon-shaped, 0.05 mm. in length, and provided with a button-like projection.

The number of the worms found is variable, as many as a thousand having been counted. It is a widely spread parasite. In parts of Europe it occurs in from 10 to 30 per cent. of all bodies examined, but in the United States it is not so common. In 285 West Indian workers at Panama Darling found 46 per cent. infected. It is possible, he thinks, that these parasites play a rôle in amœbic dysentery, the lesions of which begin at the exact location of the points of their attachment. The whipworm rarely causes symptoms. French and Boycott found ova in 40 of 500 Guy's Hospital patients. They found no etiological relationship of the parasite to appendicitis. Several cases have been reported in which profound anæmia has occurred in connection with this parasite, usually with diarrhœa. Enormous numbers may be present, as in Rudolph's case, without producing any symptoms.

The *diagnosis* is readily made by the examination of the fæces, which contain the characteristic lemon-shaped, hard, dark-brown eggs.

Dioctophyme renale (*Eustrongylus gigas*).—This enormous nematode, the male of which measures about a foot in length and the female about three feet, occurs in many animals and has occasionally been found in man. It is usually found in the renal region and may entirely destroy the kidney.

Anguillula aceti.—The Anguillula aceti, or vinegar eel, is sometimes present in urine (in one case it is said from the bladder). It is probably a contamination from a dirty bottle in which the urine is collected.

Strongyloides stercoralis.—The parasite was discovered in 1876 by Normand, and was formerly described as *Anguillula intestinalis*. It is a common parasite in tropical diarrhœa, particularly in Cochin China. It is found in about 3 per cent. of the medical patients in the Isthmus of Panama, and in from 20 to 30 per cent. of the patients in the insane division. When in large numbers they cause diarrhœa, but Darling concludes that they are not the cause of severe diarrhœa, though they may produce moderate anæmia. The mother worm burrows in the mucous membrane and deposits ova. The parasite is found in the upper parts of the small intestines. They are met with occasionally in the temperate regions. Three cases were reported from the Hopkins clinic by Thayer. Thymol and sulphur are useful in treatment.

Acanthocephali (*Thorn-headed Worms*).—The *Gigantorhynchus* or *Echinorhynchus gigas* is a common parasite in the intestine of the hog and attains a large size. The larvæ develop in cockchafer grubs. The American intermediate host is the June bug (Stiles). A case of *Echinorhynchus moniliformis* has been described in Italy by Grassi and Calandruccio.

IV. PARASITIC ARACHNIDA AND TICKS

Pentastomes.—1. Linguatula rhinaria (*Pentastoma tænioides*) has a somewhat lancet-shaped body, the female being from 3 to 4 inches in length, the male about an inch in length. The body is tapering and marked by numerous rings. The adult worm infests the frontal sinuses and nostrils of the dog, more rarely of the horse. The larval form, known as *Linguatula serrata* (*Pentastomum denticulatum*), is seen in the internal organs, particularly the liver, but has also been found in the kidney. The adult worm has been found in the nostril of man, but is very rare and seldom occasions any inconvenience. The larvæ are by no means uncommon, particularly in parts of Germany. The parasite is very rare. Flint refers to a Missouri case in which from 75 to 100 of the parasites were expectorated. The liver was enlarged and the parasites probably occupied this region.

2. The Porocephalus armillatus (*Pentastomum constrictum*) has the length of half an inch, with twenty-three rings on the abdomen. It is found in the Congo district and in parts of Asia. The larvæ, found in cysts in the lungs and liver, cause disease as they wander. The adult form lives in the nasal cavities and lungs of pythons and other snakes and man is infected probably through the drinking water.

Demodex (Acarus) folliculorum (var. hominis).—A minute parasite, from 0.3 mm. to 0.4 mm. in length, which lives in the sebaceous follicles, particularly of the face. It is doubtful whether it produces any symptoms. Possibly when in large numbers they may excite inflammation of the follicles, leading to acne.

Sarcoptes (Acarus) scabiei (*Itch Insect*).—This is the most important of the arachnid parasites. The male is 0.23 mm. in length and 0.19 mm. in breadth; the female is 0.45 mm. in length and 0.35 mm. in width. The female can be seen readily with the naked eye and has a pearly-white color. It is not so common in the United States and Canada as in Europe.

The insect lives in a small burrow, about 1 cm. in length, which it makes for itself in the epidermis. At the end of this burrow the female lives. The male is seldom found. The chief seat of the parasite is in the folds where the skin is most delicate, as in the web between the fingers and toes, the backs of the hands, the axilla, and the front of the abdomen. The head and face are rarely involved. The lesions which result from the presence of the itch insect are very numerous and result largely from the irritation of the scratching. The commonest is a papular and vesicular rash, or, in children, an ecthymatous eruption. The irritation and pustulation which follow the scratching may completely destroy the burrows, but in typical cases there is rarely doubt as to the diagnosis.

The *treatment* is simple. It should consist of warm baths with a thorough use of a soft soap, after which the skin should be anointed with sulphur ointment, which in the case of children should be diluted. An ointment of naphthol (drachm to the ounce) is very efficacious.

Leptus autumnalis (*Harvest Bug*).—This reddish-colored parasite, about half a millimetre in size, is often found in large numbers in fields and in gardens. They attach themselves to animals and man with their sharp proboscides, and the hooklets of their legs produce a great deal of irritation. They are most frequently found on the legs. They are readily destroyed by sulphur ointment or corrosive-sublimate lotions.

Ixodiasis (*Tick-fever*).—In South Africa, particularly in the western provinces of the Uganda Protectorate, the western districts of German East Africa and the eastern regions of the Congo Free State, there is a disease known by this name, believed to be transmitted by a tick—the *Ornithodorus* or *Argas moubata*. The ticks live in old houses, and their habits are very much like those of the common bedbug. This tick transmits the *Spirochœta duttoni*, the cause of the African form of relapsing fever.

The *Dermacentor occidentalis* is present in the Northwestern States from California to Montana. The bites may cause severe lymphangitis. It appears to be the medium of transmission of the Rocky Mountain spotted fever.

In Arizona and other parts of the Southwestern States a tick—*Ornithodorus megnini*—is occasionally found in the ear and in the nose, causing suppuration and intense suffering. Several other varieties of ticks are occasionally found on man—the *Ixodes ricinus* and the *Dermacentor americanus*, which are met with in horses and oxen.

Tick paralysis.—In connection with the bites of ticks of the genus Ixodes and the genus Dermacentor a flaccid paralysis of the legs has been described, particularly in British Columbia, Wyoming, Montana, and possibly in Australia. Children are usually affected, and, curiously enough, if the tick is found and removed promptly, the child gets well within twenty-four hours, but if not, the paralysis may spread to the arms, stupor may come on, and the child may die of a widespread paralysis. In adults sometimes there are pain, an erythematous rash, and vertigo. It appears to be a toxic effect of the parasite and not an infection.

V. PARASITIC INSECTS

Pediculi (*Phthiriasis; Pediculosis*).—There are three varieties:

PEDICULUS HUMANUS (*Head Louse*).—The male is from 1 to 1.5 mm. in length and the female nearly 2 mm. The color varies somewhat with the different races of men. It is light gray with a black margin in the European, and very much darker in the negro and Chinese. They are oviparous, and the female lays about sixty eggs, which mature in a week. The ova are attached to the hairs, and are known popularly as nits. The symptoms are irritation and itching of the scalp. When numerous, the insects may excite an eczema or a pustular dermatitis, which causes crusts and scabs, particularly at the back of the head. In extreme cases the hair becomes tangled in these crusts and matted together, forming a firm mass which is known as *plica polonica*, as it was not infrequent among the Jewish inhabitants of Poland.

PEDICULUS CORPORIS (*vestimentorum*).—This is considerably larger than the head louse. It lives on the clothing, and in sucking the blood causes minute hæmorrhagic specks, which are very common about the neck, back, and abdomen. The irritation of the bites may cause urticaria, and the scratching is usually in linear lines. In long-standing cases, particularly in old dissipated characters, the skin becomes rough and greatly pigmented, a condition which has been termed the vagabond's disease—*morbus errorum*—which may be mistaken for the bronzing of Addison's disease. The pigmentation may be extreme and extend to the face and buccal mucosa.

PHTHIRIUS PUBIS (*crab louse*) differs somewhat from the other forms, and is found in the parts of the body covered with short hairs, as the pubes; more rarely the axilla and eyebrows.

The *taches bleuâtres, maculæ ceruleæ*, or peliomata, excited by the irritation of pediculi, are peculiar subcuticular bluish or slate-colored spots from

5 to 10 mm. in diameter seen about the abdomen and thighs, particularly in febrile cases. The spots are more marked on white thin skins. They are stains caused by a pigment in the secretion of the salivary glands of the louse.

TREATMENT.—For the *Pediculus humanus,* when the condition is very bad, the hair should be cut short, as it is very difficult to destroy all the nits. Repeated saturations of the hair in coal-oil or in turpentine are usually efficacious, or with lotions of carbolic acid, 1 to 50. The application of a mixture of equal parts of xylene, alcohol and ether is useful. Scrupulous cleanliness and care are sufficient to prevent recurrence. In the case of the *Pediculus corporis,* the clothing should be placed for hours in a disinfecting oven. To allay the itching a warm bath containing 4 or 5 ounces of bicarbonate of soda is useful. For the *Phthirius pubis* white precipitate or ordinary mercurial ointment should be used, and the parts should be thoroughly washed two or three times a day with soft soap and water.

Cimex lectularius (*Common Bedbugs*).—The tropical and sub-tropical variety is *Cimex rotundalius* (W. S. Patton). It lives in the crevices of the bedstead and in the cracks in the floor and in the walls. It is nocturnal in its habits. The peculiar odor of the insect is caused by the secretion of a special gland. The parasite possesses a long proboscis, with which it sucks the blood. Individuals differ remarkably in the reaction to the bite of this insect; some are not disturbed in the slightest by them, in others the irritation causes hyperæmia and often intense urticaria. Fumigation with sulphur or scouring with corrosive-sublimate solution or kerosene destroys them. Iron bedsteads should be used.

Pulex irritans (*Common Flea*).—The male is from 2 to 2.5 mm. in length, the female from 3 to 4 mm. The flea is a transient parasite on man. The bite causes a circular red spot of hyperæmia in the centre of which is a little speck where the boring apparatus has entered. The amount of irritation caused by the bite is variable. Many persons suffer intensely and a diffuse erythema or an irritable urticaria develops; others suffer no inconvenience whatever.

The *Pulex penetrans* (*sand-flea, jigger*) is found in tropical countries, particularly in the West Indies and South America. It is much smaller than the common flea, and not only penetrates the skin, but burrows and produces an inflammation with pustular or vesicular swelling. It most frequently attacks the feet. It is readily removed with a needle. Where they exist in large numbers the essential oils are used on the feet as a preventive.

VI. PARASITIC FLIES

(*Myiasis, Myiosis*)

The accidental invasion of the body cavities and of the skin by the larvæ of the diptera is known as myiasis.

The larvæ of the *Compsomyia macellaria,* the so-called screw-worm, have been found in the nose, in wounds, and in the vagina after delivery. They can be removed readily with forceps; if there is any difficulty, thorough cleansing and the application of an antiseptic bandage are sufficient to kill them. The ova of the blue-bottle fly may be deposited in the nostrils, the ears, or the conjunctiva—the myiasis narium, aurium, conjunctivæ. This invasion rarely takes place unless these regions are the seat of disease. In the nose and in the ear the larvæ may cause serious inflammation. Even the urethra has not been spared in these dipterous invasions.

Gastro-intestinal myiasis may result from the swallowing of the larvæ of the common house-fly or of species of the genus *Anthomyia*. There are many cases on record in which the larvæ of the *Musca domestica* have been discharged by vomiting. Instances in which dipterous larvæ have been passed in the fæces are less common. Finlayson, of Glasgow, has reported an interesting case in a physician, who, after protracted constipation and pain in the back and sides, passed large numbers of the larvæ of the flower-fly—*Anthomyia canicularis*. Among other forms of larvæ or gentles, as they are sometimes called, which have been found in the fæces are those of the common house-fly, the blue-bottle fly, and the *Techomyza fusca*. The larvæ of other insects are extremely rare. It is stated that the caterpillar of the taby moth has been found in the fæces.

A specimen of the *Homalomyia scalaris,* one of the privy flies, was sent by Dr. Hartin, of Kaslo City, British Columbia, the larvæ of which were passed in large numbers in the stools of a man aged twenty-four, a native of Louisiana. They were present in the stools from May 1 to July 15, 1897. There are cases in which the larvæ have been passed for years.

Although no grave results necessarily follow the invasion of the alimentary tract by these larvæ, yet they may be the cause of serious intestinal ulceration manifesting itself by a dysenteric disease with fatal result. Cockayne, who studied the question, states that there are four deaths on record.

Cutaneous Myiasis.—The most common form is that in which an external wound becomes "living," as it is called. This is caused by the larvæ of either the blue-bottle or the common flesh-fly. The skin may also be infected by the larvæ of the *Musca vomitoria*; but more commonly by the bot-flies of the ox and sheep which occasionally attack man. This is rare in temperate climates. Matas described a case in which œstrus larvæ were found in the gluteal region. In parts of Central America the eggs of another bot-fly, the *Dermatobia,* are not infrequently deposited in the skin and produce a swelling very like the ordinary boil.

Dermamyiasis linearis migrans œstrosa is a remarkable cutaneous condition, observed particularly in Russia and occasionally in other countries, in which the larva of *Gastrophilus equi* (Samson), the horse bot-fly, makes a slightly raised pale red "line" which travels over the body surface, sometimes with great rapidity. It has been referred to as Larva migrans and as Creeping Eruption. (See Hamburger, Journal of Cutaneous Diseases, 1904.)

In Africa the larvæ of the Cayor fly are not uncommonly found beneath the skin in little boils. In the Congo region Dutton, Todd, and Christy found a troublesome blood-sucking dipterous larva, known as the floor maggot, the fly of which is the *Anchmeromyia luteola.*

Phlebotomous Fever.—In Herzegovina, Malta and Crete and other parts of the Mediterranean there is a fever of two or three days' duration, caused by the bite of the sand-fly, *Phlebotomus papatasii.* The manifestations are those of fever alone, and may be mistaken for abortive typhoid, febricula or mild Malta fever. The disease is known as pappataci fever and sand fly fever. The experiments of Doerr and of Birt show that the disease is readily caused by the bite of infected sand-flies.

Caterpillar Rash.—In some districts in Europe the hairs of the procession caterpillar, particularly of the species *Cnethocampa,* cause an intense urticaria, the so-called *U. epidemica.* There are districts in Switzerland which have been rendered uninhabitable in consequence of the skin rashes caused by the caterpillars. Of late years in New England and some other parts of the United States the caterpillar of the brown-tailed moth has caused much discomfort. The hairs are widely distributed by the wind, and the barbs are so arranged that they readily work into the skin. Whole families have been affected by an intense eruption which has been mistaken for that of small-pox. In England, Thresh called attention to the frequency of these caterpillar rashes due to the yellow-tailed moth, *Porthesia similis.*

Harvest Rash (*Erythema Autumnale*).—In parts of England during the autumn many people are attacked by the harvest bug or harvesters, which may cause a very obstinate and distressing malady. Usually attributed to the harvest spider, it is in reality caused by a mite, parasitic upon it, the hexapod larva of the silky trombidian. It is so small as to be scarcely visible and is brick-red in color. They chiefly attack persons with delicate skins on the ankles and legs, but they may also attack the arms and the neck. The mite attaches itself to the skin by its claws, sucks the blood, and the swollen red abdomen may sometimes be seen as a bright-red dot. A papulo-vesicular, sometimes a pustular, eruption with an intolerable itching is caused by it. So intense may the eruption be, with perhaps an entire family attacked at once, that suspicion of poisoning may be aroused. The parasite is readily killed by benzine.

E. INFECTIOUS DISEASES OF DOUBTFUL OR UNKNOWN ETIOLOGY

I. SMALL-POX (Variola)

Definition.—An acute infectious disease characterized by a cutaneous eruption which passes through the stages of papule, vesicle, pustule, and crust.

History.—The existence of the disease in ancient Egypt is suggested by the eruption on the skin of a mummy of the 20th dynasty—1,200 to 1,100 B. C. (Rüffer and Ferguson). The disease existed in China many centuries before Christ. The *pesta magna* described by Galen (of which Marcus Aurelius died) is believed to have been small-pox. In the sixth century it prevailed, and subsequently, at the time of the Crusades, became widespread. It was brought to America by the Spaniards early in the sixteenth century. The first accurate account was given by Rhazes, an Arabian physician who lived in the ninth century, and whose admirable description is available in Greenhill's translation for the Sydenham Society. In the seventeenth century the illustrious Sydenham differentiated measles from small-pox. Special events in the history of the disease are the introduction of inoculation into

Europe, by Lady Mary Wortley Montagu, in 1718, and the discovery of vaccination by Jenner, in 1796.

Etiology.—Small-pox is one of the most virulent of contagious diseases, and persons exposed, if unprotected by vaccination, are almost invariably attacked. Instances of natural immunity are rare. It is said that Diemerbroeck, a celebrated Utrecht professor in the seventeenth century, was not only himself exempt, but likewise many members of his family. An attack may not protect for life. There are undoubted cases of a second, reputed instances, indeed, of a third attack. Louis XV of France died of a second attack of small-pox.

Age.—Small-pox is common at all ages, but is particularly fatal to young children. Of 3,164 deaths in the Montreal epidemic of 1885-'86, 2,717 were of children under ten years of age. The *fetus in utero* may be attacked, but only if the mother herself is the subject of the disease. The child may be born with the rash out or with the scars. In the case of twins, only one may be attacked; Kaltenbach records an instance of triplets, only two of which were affected (Comby). Children born in a small-pox hospital, if vaccinated immediately, may escape the disease; usually, however, they die early.

Sex.—Males and females are equally affected.

Race.—Among aboriginal races small-pox is terribly fatal. When the disease was first introduced into America the Mexicans died by thousands, and the North American Indians have also been frequently decimated by this plague. It is stated that the negro is especially susceptible, and the mortality is greater—about 42 per cent. in the black, against 29 per cent. in the white (W. M. Welch).

It is claimed that isolation hospitals increase the incidence of the disease in a locality. J. Glaister, who considered the question very carefully, concludes that as a centre of traffic such an institution, through the channels of human intercourse, naturally favors the spread of the disease locally, but decides against its aerial conveyance, in spite of the strong evidence.

The disease smoulders here and there and when conditions are favorable becomes epidemic. This was well illustrated by the Montreal outbreak of 1885. For several years there had been no small-pox in the city, and a large unprotected population grew up among the French-Canadians, many of whom were opposed to vaccination. On February 28 a Pullman-car conductor, who had traveled from Chicago, was admitted into the Hôtel-Dieu, the civic small-pox hospital being closed at the time. Isolation was not carried out, and on the 1st of April a servant in the hospital died of small-pox. Following her decease, the authorities of the hospital dismissed all patients presenting no symptoms of contagion who could go home. The disease spread like fire in dry grass, and in nine months 3,164 persons died in the city of small-pox.

Variations in the Virulence of Epidemics.—Sydenham states that "small-pox also has its peculiar kinds, which take one form during one series of years, and another during another"; and not only does what he called the epidemic constitution vary greatly, but one sometimes sees the most extraordinary variations in the intensity of the disease in members of a family all exposed to the same infection. A striking illustration of this variability has been given in recent epidemics, which have been of so mild a character that in many localities it has been mistaken for chicken-pox; in others, particularly in the United States, the belief prevailed that a new disease had arisen, to which the name "Cuban itch" or "Philippine itch" was given. Very often a correct diagnosis is not reached until a fatal case has occurred. A small outbreak occurred in one of the Hopkins wards for colored patients, which we mistook at first for chicken-pox. The same peculiarities have been observed in the Leicester, Nottingham, and Cambridge outbreaks. Even in unvaccinated children the disease has been exceedingly mild. Some of the Leicester cases had only a few pocks (Allan Warner); but this is an old story in the history of the disease. John Mason Good, in commenting on this very point, refers to the great variability in the epidemics, and states that he himself as a child of six (1770) passed through small-pox with "scarcely any disturbance and not more than twenty scattered pustules"!

The disease described in some Brazilian states as Alastrin amas, or varioloid varicella, seen also in the West Indies, is probably mild small-pox.

Recent Prevalence.—In the United States in 1917 there were 204 deaths in the registration area. The mild type of the disease continues, but in places there have been virulent outbreaks. In England and Wales there were 18 deaths from the disease in 1916.

NATURE OF CONTAGION.—Protozoön-like bodies were described in the skin lesions by Guarnieri—*the cytoryctes variolæ.* Councilman and his colleagues describe a protozoön with a double cycle and cytoplasmic stage, with small structureless bodies in the lower layer of the epithelial cells. Infection occurs probably by the nasal secretion and sputum. The dried scales are also an important element, and as a dust-like powder are distributed everywhere in the room during convalescence, becoming attached to clothing and various articles of furniture. The disease is probably infectious from a very early stage, though it has not been determined whether the contagion is active before the eruption develops. The poison is of unusual tenacity and clings to infected localities. It is conveyed by persons who have been in contact with the sick and by fomites. During epidemics it is no doubt widely spread in street-cars and public conveyances. An unprotected person may contract a very virulent form of the disease from a patient with a mild attack.

Morbid Anatomy.—The pustules may be seen upon the tongue and the buccal mucosa, and on the palate; sometimes also in the pharynx and the upper part of the œsophagus. In exceptionally rare cases the rash extends down the œsophagus and even into the stomach. Swelling of the Peyer's follicles is not uncommon; the pustules have been seen in the rectum.

In the larynx the eruption may be associated with a fibrinous exudate and sometimes with œdema. Occasionally the inflammation penetrates deeply and involves the cartilages. In the trachea and bronchi there may be ulcerative erosions, but true pocks, such as are seen on the skin, do not occur.

The heart occasionally shows myocardial changes, parenchymatous and fatty; endocarditis and pericarditis are uncommon. French writers have described an endarteritis of the coronary vessels. The spleen is markedly enlarged. Apart from the cloudy swelling and areas of coagulation-necrosis, lesions of the kidneys are not common. Nephritis may occur.

In the hæmorrhagic form extravasations are found on the serous and mucous surfaces, in the parenchyma of organs, in the connective tissues, about the nerve-sheaths and in the muscles. In one instance the entire retroperitoneal tissue was infiltrated with a large coagulum, and there were also extensive extravasations in the course of the thoracic aorta. Hæmorrhages in the bone-marrow have been described. The spleen is firm and hard in hæmorrhagic small-pox. In these rapidly fatal forms the liver has been described as fatty, but in 5 of 7 cases it was of normal size, dense, and firm.

Symptoms.—Three forms of small-pox are described, but they only represent various degrees of severity.

(*a*) *Variola vera;* (1) Discrete, (2) Confluent.

(*b*) *Variola hæmorrhagica;* (1) Purpura variolosa or black small-pox; (2) Hæmorrhagic pustular form, variola hæmorrhagica pustulosa.

(*c*) *Varioloid,* or small-pox modified by vaccination.

(*a*) VARIOLA VERA.—The affection may be conveniently described under various stages: *Incubation.*—"From nine to fifteen days; oftenest twelve." The senior author saw it as early as the eighth day after exposure, and there

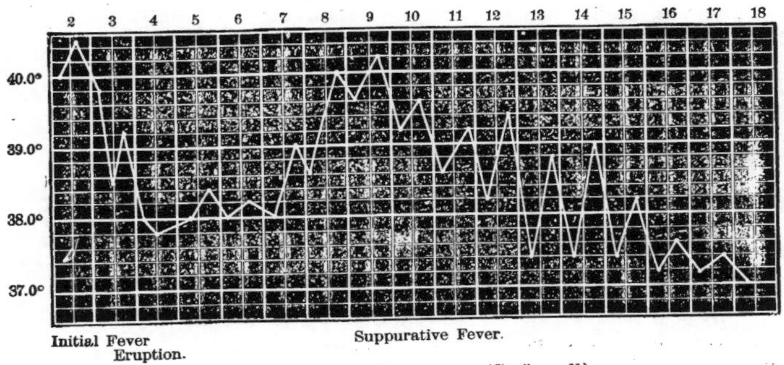

CHART IX.—TRUE SMALL-POX (Strümpell).

are authenticated instances in which this stage has been prolonged to twenty days. It is unusual for patients to complain of any symptoms.

Invasion.—In adults a chill and in children a convulsion are common initial symptoms. There may be repeated chills within the first twenty-four hours. Intense frontal headache, severe lumbar pains, and vomiting are very constant features. The pains in the back and in the limbs are more severe in the initial stage of this than of any other eruptive fever, and their combination with headache and vomiting is so suggestive that precautionary measures may often be taken several days before the eruption appears. The temperature rises quickly, and may on the first day be 103° or 104°. The pulse is rapid and full, not often dicrotic. In severe cases there may be marked delirium, particularly if the fever is high. The patient is restless and distressed, the face flushed, and the eyes bright and clear. The skin is usually dry, though occasionally there are profuse sweats. One cannot judge from the initial symptoms whether a case is likely to be discrete or confluent, as convulsions, severe headache, and high fever may precede a mild attack.

Initial Rashes.—Two forms can be distinguished: the diffuse, scarlatinal, and the macular or measly form; either of which may be associated with petechiæ and occupy a variable extent of surface. In some instances they are general, but as a rule are limited either to the lower abdominal areas, to the inner surfaces of the thighs, and to the lateral thoracic region, or to the axillæ. Occasionally they are found over the extensor surfaces, particularly in the neighborhood of the knees and elbows. These rashes, usually purpuric, are often associated with an erythematous or erysipelatous blush. The scarlatinal rash may come out as early as the second day, and be as diffuse and vivid as in a true scarlatina. The measly rash may also be diffuse and resemble closely that of measles. Urticaria is seen only occasionally. It was present once in the Montreal cases. The initial rashes are more abundant in some epidemics than in others. They occur in from 10 to 16 per cent. of cases.

Eruption.—(1) In the *discrete form*, usually on the fourth day, macules appear on the forehead, preceded sometimes by an erythematous flush, and on the anterior surfaces of the wrists. Within the first twenty-four hours from their appearance they occur on other parts of the face and on the extremities, and a few are seen on the trunk. The spots are from 2-3 millimetres in diameter, of a bright red color, and disappear completely on pressure. As the rash comes out the temperature falls, the general symptoms subside, and the patient feels comfortable. On the fifth or sixth day the papules change into vesicles with clear summits. Each one is elevated, circular, and presents a little depression or umbilication in the centre. About the eighth day the vesicles change into pustules, the umbilication disappears, the flat top assumes a globular form and becomes grayish-yellow in color, owing to the contained pus. There is an areola of injection about the pustules and the skin between them is swollen. This maturation first takes place on the face, and follows the order of the appearance of the eruption. The temperature now rises—secondary fever—and the general symptoms return. The swelling about the pustules is attended with a good deal of tension and pain in the face; the eyelids become swollen and closed. In the discrete form the temperature of maturation does not usually remain high for more than twenty-four or twenty-six hours, so that on the tenth or eleventh day the fever disappears and the stage of convalescence begins. The pustules rapidly dry, first on the face and then on the other parts, and by the fourteenth or fifteenth day desquamation may be far advanced on the face. The march and distribution of the rash are often most characteristic. The abdomen and groins and the legs are the parts least affected. The rash is often copious on the upper part of the back, scanty on the lower. Vesicles in the mouth, pharynx, and larynx cause soreness and swelling in these parts, with loss of voice. Whether pitting takes place depends a good deal upon the severity of the disease. In a majority of cases Sydenham's statement holds good, that "it is very rarely the case that the distinct small-pox leaves its mark." The odor of a small-pox patient is very distinctive even in the early stages, and has been a help in the diagnosis of a doubtful case.

(2) *The Confluent Form.*—With the same initial symptoms, though usually of greater severity, the rash appears on the fourth, or, according to Sydenham, on the third day. The more the eruption shows itself before the fourth day the more sure it is to become confluent (Sydenham). The papules at first may be isolated, and it is only later in the stage of maturation that the eruption is confluent. But in severer cases the skin is swollen and hyperæmic and the papules are very close together. On the feet and hands, too, the

papules are thickly set; more scattered on the limbs; and quite discrete on the trunk. With the appearance of the eruption the symptoms subside and the fever remits, but not to the same extent as in the discrete form. Occasionally the temperature falls to normal and the patient may be very comfortable. Then, usually on the eighth day, the fever again rises, the vesicles change to pustules, the hyperæmia becomes intense, the swelling of the face and hands increases, and by the tenth day the pustules have fully maturated, many of them have coalesced, and the entire skin of the head and extremities is a superficial abscess. The fever rises to 103° or 105°, the pulse is from 110 to 120, and there is often delirium. As pointed out by Sydenham, salivation in adults and diarrhœa in children are common symptoms of this stage. There is usually much thirst. The eruption may also be present in the mouth, and usually the pharynx and larynx are involved and the voice is husky. Great swelling of the cervical lymphatic glands occurs. At this stage the patient presents a terrible picture, unequaled in any other disease and one which fully justifies the horror and fright with which small-pox is associated in the public mind. Even when the rash is confluent on the face, hands, and feet, the pustules remain discrete on the trunk. The danger, as pointed out by Sydenham, is in proportion to the number upon the face. "If upon the face they are as thick as sand, it is no advantage to have them few and far between on the rest of the body." In fatal cases by the tenth or eleventh day the pulse gets feebler and more rapid, the delirium is marked, there is subsultus, sometimes diarrhœa, and with these symptoms the patient dies. In other instances between the eighth and eleventh day hæmorrhagic features occur. When recovery takes place, the patient enters on the eleventh or twelfth day the period of desiccation.

Desiccation.—The pustules break and the pus exudes or they dry and form crusts. Throughout the third week the desiccation proceeds and in cases of moderate severity the secondary fever subsides; but in others it may persist until the fourth week. The crusts in confluent small-pox adhere for a long time and the process of scarring may take three or four weeks. On the face they fall off singly, but the tough epidermis of the hands and feet may be shed entire.

(*b*) HÆMORRHAGIC SMALL-POX occurs in two forms. In one, the petechial or black small-pox—*purpura variolosa*—the special symptoms appear early and death follows in from two to six days. In the other form the case progresses as one of ordinary variola, and in the vesicular or pustular stage hæmorrhages take place into the pocks or from the mucous membranes—*variola hœmorrhagica pustulosa.*

Purpura variolosa is more common in some epidemics than in others. It is less frequent in children than in adults. Young and vigorous persons seem more liable to this form. Men are more frequently affected than women; thus in one series there were 21 males and only 6 females. The influence of vaccination is shown in the fact that of the cases 14 were unvaccinated, while not one of the 13 who had scars had been revaccinated. The illness starts with the usual symptoms, but with more intense constitutional disturbance. On the second or the third day there is a diffuse hyperæmic rash, particularly in the groins, with small punctiform hæmorrhages. The rash extends, becomes more distinctly hæmorrhagic, and the spots increase in size. Ecchymoses appear on the conjunctivæ, and as early as the third day there may be hæmorrhages from the mucous membranes. Death may take place before the papules appear. In this truly terrible affection the patient may present a frightful appearance. The skin may have a uniformly purplish hue and the unfortunate victim may even look plum-colored. The face is swollen and large conjunctival hæmorrhages with the deeply sunken corneæ give a ghastly appearance. The mind may remain clear to the end. Death occurs from the third to the sixth day; thus in thirteen of the series it took place between these dates. The earliest death was on the third day and there were no traces of papules. There may be no mucous hæmorrhages; thus in one case of a most virulent character death occurred without bleeding early on the fourth day. Hæmaturia is perhaps most common, next hæmatemesis, and melæna was noticed in a third of the cases. Metrorrhagia was present in only one of the six females. The pulse in this form is rapid and often hard and small. The respirations are greatly increased in frequency and out of all proportion to the intensity of the fever.

In *variola pustulosa hæmorrhagica* the disease progresses as a severe case, and the hæmorrhages do not occur until the vesicular or pustular stage. The first indication is hæmorrhage into the areolæ of the pocks, and later the maturated pustules fill with blood. The earlier the hæmorrhage the greater is the danger. Bleeding from the mucous membranes is also common in this form, and the great majority of the cases prove fatal, usually on the seventh, eighth, or ninth day, but a few cases recover. In patients with the discrete form, if allowed to get up early, hæmorrhage may take place into the pocks on the legs.

Leucocytes.—In variola vera there is a marked leucocytosis, 12-16 thousand, about the eighth day, then a slight decline and a rise again about the twelfth or fourteenth day, sometimes to 18,000 or 20,000. There is an increase in the mononuclear elements, which may be the only marked feature of the mild cases (Magrath, Brinckerhoff, and Bancroft).

(*c*) VARIOLOID.—This term is applied to the modified form which affects persons who have been vaccinated. It may set in with abruptness and severity, the temperature reaching 103°. More commonly it is in every respect milder in its initial symptoms, though the headache and backache may be very distressing. The papules appear on the evening of the third or on the fourth day. They are few in number and may be confined to the face and hands. The fever drops at once and the patient feels perfectly comfortable. The vesiculation and maturation of the pocks take place rapidly, and there is no secondary fever. There is rarely any scarring. As a rule, when small-pox attacks a person who has been vaccinated within five or six years the disease is mild, but it may prove severe, even fatal.

Abortive Types.—Recent epidemics have been characterized by the large number of mild cases. Even in unvaccinated children only a few pustules may appear, and the disease is over in a few days. Even with a thickly set eruption the vesicles at the fifth or sixth day, instead of filling, dry and abort, forming the so-called horn-, crystalline-, or wart-pox. *Variola sine eruptione* is described. It seems to have been not uncommon in the recent epidemics. Bancroft observed twelve cases in the Boston outbreak, all among physicians and attendants. The symptoms are headache, pain in the back, fever, and vomiting. As already mentioned, the pocks may be very scanty and easily overlooked, even in unvaccinated persons. One of Bancroft's cases was of special interest—a pregnant woman who had slight symptoms after exposure, but no rash. Her child showed a typical eruption when two days old.

Complications.—Considering the severity of many of the cases and the character of the disease, associated with multiple foci of suppuration, the complications in small-pox are remarkably few.

Laryngitis is serious in three ways: it may produce a fatal œdema of the glottis; it is liable to extend and involve the cartilages, producing necrosis; and by diminishing the sensibility of the larynx it may allow irritating particles to reach the lower air-passages, where they excite bronchitis or broncho-pneumonia. *Broncho-pneumonia* is almost invariably present in fatal cases. *Lobar pneumonia* is rare. *Pleurisy* is common in some epidemics.

The *cardiac* complications are also rare. In the height of the fever a systolic murmur at the apex is not uncommon; but endocarditis, either simple or malignant, is rarely met with. Pericarditis, too, is very uncommon. Myocarditis seems to be more frequent, and may be associated with endarteritis of the coronary vessels.

Of complications in the *digestive* system, parotitis is rare. In severe cases there is extensive pseudo-diphtheritic angina. Vomiting, which is so marked a symptom in the early stage, is rarely persistent. Diarrhœa is not uncommon, as noted by Sydenham, and particularly in children.

Albuminuria is frequent, but true *nephritis* is rare. Inflammation of the testes and of the ovaries may occur.

Among the most interesting and serious complications are those pertaining to the *nervous* system. In children convulsions are common. In adults the delirium of the early stage may persist and become violent, and finally subside into a fatal coma. Post-febrile insanity is occasionally met with during convalescence, and very rarely epilepsy. Many of the old writers spoke of paraplegia in connection with the intense backache of the early stage, but it is probably associated with the severe agonizing lumbar and crural pains and is not a true paraplegia. It must be distinguished from the form occurring in convalescence, which may be due to peripheral neuritis or to a diffuse myelitis (Westphal). The neuritis may, as in diphtheria, involve the pharynx alone, or it may be multiple. Of this nature, in all probability, is the so-called pseudo-tabes, or *ataxie variolique*. Hemiplegia and aphasia have been met with in a few instances, the result of encephalitis.

Among the most constant and troublesome complications are those involving the *skin*. During convalescence boils are very frequent and may be severe. Acne and ecthyma are also met with. Local gangrene in various parts may occur. A remarkable secondary eruption (recurrent small-pox) occasionally occurs after desquamation.

Arthritis may occur, usually in the period of desquamation, and may pass on to suppuration. Acute necrosis of the bone is sometimes met with.

Special Senses.—The eye affections which were formerly so common and serious are not now so frequent, owing to the care which is given to keeping the conjunctivæ clean. A catarrhal and purulent conjunctivitis is common in severe cases. The secretions cause adhesions of the eyelids, and unless great care is taken a diffuse keratitis is excited, which may go on to ulceration and perforation. Iritis is not very uncommon. Otitis media may result from an extension of the disease through the Eustachian tubes.

Prognosis.—In unprotected persons small-pox is a very fatal disease, the death-rate ranging from 25 to 35 per cent. In Japan the mortality among unprotected persons has been even higher. In the recent mild epidemics in the United States the mortality has been very slight, often less than 1 per cent. At the Municipal Hospital, Philadelphia, of 2,831 cases of variola, 1,534—i. e., 54.18 per cent.—died, while of 2,169 cases of varioloid only 28—i. e., 1.29 per cent.—died (W. M. Welch). Purpura variolosa is invariably fatal, and a majority of those attacked with the severer confluent forms die. The intemperate and debilitated succumb more readily to the disease. As Sydenham observed, the danger is directly proportionate to the intensity of the disease on the face and hands. "When the fever increases after the appearance of the pustules, it is a bad sign; but if it is lessened on their appearance, that is a good sign" (Rhazes). Very high fever, delirium and subsultus are symptoms of ill omen. The disease is particularly fatal in pregnant women and abortion usually takes place. It is not, however, uniformly so, and severe cases may recover after miscarriage. Moreover, abortion is not inevitable. Very severe pharyngitis and laryngitis are fatal complications.

Death results in the early stage from the action of the poison upon the nervous system. In the later stages it usually occurs about the eleventh or twelfth day, at the height of the eruption. In children, and occasionally in adults, the laryngeal and pulmonary complications prove fatal.

Diagnosis.—During an epidemic the initial chill, the headache and backache, and the vomiting at once put the physician on his guard.

The initial rashes may lead to error. The scarlatinal rash has rarely the extent and never the persistence of the rash in true scarlet fever. The rash of measles has been mistaken for the initial rash of small-pox. The general condition of the patient, the presence of coryza, conjunctivitis and Koplik's sign, may be better guides than the rash itself.

Malignant hæmorrhagic small-pox may prove fatal before the characteristic rash appears. Of 27 cases of purpura variolosa, in only one, in which death occurred on the third day, did inspection fail to show the papules. In 3 cases dying on the fourth day the characteristic papular rash was noticed. It may be difficult or impossible to recognize this form of hæmorrhagic small-pox from *hæmorrhagic scarlet fever* or *hæmorrhagic measles,* though in the latter there is rarely so constant involvement of the mucous membranes.

Naturally enough, as they are allied affections, *varicella* is the disease which most frequently leads to error. Particularly has this been the case in the mild epidemics which have prevailed during the past few years. The following points are to be borne in mind: first, very mild epidemics of true small-pox may occur; secondly, any large number of cases of a contagious disease with a pustular eruption occurring in adults is strongly in favor of small-pox. The characters of the rash are of less value. Its abundance on the trunk in varicella is important. At the outset the papules have rarely the shotty, hard feel of small-pox. The vesicles are more superficial, the infiltrated areola is not so intense nor so constant, and as a rule the pocks may be seen in the same patient in all stages of development. The longer period of invasion, the prodromal rashes, the great intensity of the onset are also important points in small-pox. But there are mild epidemics in which it must be confessed that the diagnosis is only confirmed by the appearance of a severe case of the confluent or hæmorrhagic form.

The disease may be mistaken for *cerebro-spinal fever,* in which purpuric symptoms are not uncommon. A four-year-old child was taken suddenly ill with fever, pains in the back and head, and on the second or third day petechiæ appeared. There were retraction of the head and marked rigidity of the limbs. The hæmorrhages became more abundant; and finally hæmatemesis occurred and the child died on the sixth day. At the post mortem there were no lesions of cerebro-spinal fever, and in the deeply hæmorrhagic skin the papules could be readily seen. The post mortem diagnosis of small-pox was confirmed by the mother taking the disease and dying of it.

Pustular Syphilides.—A copious pustular rash may resemble variola, particularly if accompanied by fever, but the history and distribution, particularly the slight amount on the face, leave no question as to the diagnosis.

Pustular glanders has been mistaken for small-pox. In an instance in Montreal there was a widespread pustular eruption, which we thought at first was small-pox, but the course and the fact that there was glanders among the horses in the stable led to the correct diagnosis. The eruption resembled exactly that described in Rayer's monograph (De la Morve, 1837).

Impetigo contagiosa is stated to have been mistaken for variola.

Specific Test.—Rabbits sensitized to vaccine virus give a marked reaction in 24 to 48 hours after the intradermic injection of small-pox vesicle contents. The result of inoculation of material from the pocks in the cornea of the rabbit is helpful when positive.

Prophylaxis.—Thorough vaccination and re-vaccination are the most important preventive measures. All those exposed to infection should be vaccinated at once, as four days after exposure a successful vaccination may protect from the disease. During epidemics general vaccination of the community should be done and special care taken to recognize mild cases. Those who have been exposed should be isolated for sixteen days. Isolation of those with the disease should be rigid and, if possible, they should be placed in a special hospital. The attendants should wear gowns and caps; rubber gloves are an advantage. The linen should be placed in phenol solution (2 per cent.) and boiled afterwards. Dressings should be burned. The patient should not be discharged until all the crusts are removed; a thorough sponging with phenol solution (2 per cent.) is advisable.

Treatment.—General Considerations.—Segregation in special hospitals is imperative. In the case of local outbreaks temporary barracks or tents may be constructed.

We have no specific treatment. There should be abundance of fresh air; the diet should be liquid and large amounts of water and cold drinks given. A calomel and saline purge is advisable at the onset and later the bowels should be kept open by salines. In the early stages two symptoms call for treatment: the pain in the back, which, if not relieved by phenacetine (gr. v, 0.3 gm.), requires opium in some form, as advised by Sydenham; and the vomiting, which is very difficult to check and may be uncontrollable. Nothing should be given except a little ice, and it usually stops with the appearance of the eruption.

For the fever, cold sponging or the tub bath may be used; when there is much delirium with high fever the latter or the cold pack is preferable. In some cases, particularly with severe toxæmia and marked eruption, the continuous warm bath is advisable.

The treatment of the *eruption* is important. After trying all sorts of remedies, such as puncturing the pustules with nitrate of silver, or treating them with iodine and various ointments, Sydenham's conclusion that in guarding the face against being disfigured "the only effect of oils, liniments, and the like was to make the white scurfs slower in coming off seems correct." The constant application on the face and hands of lint soaked in cold water, to which antiseptics such as phenol (2 per cent.) or bichloride of mercury (1 to 5,000) may be added, is perhaps the most suitable local treatment. It is pleasant to the patient, and for the face it is well to make a mask of lint, which can be covered with oiled silk. When the crusts begin to form, the chief point is to keep them thoroughly moist with oil or glycerine. This prevents the desiccation and diffusion of the flakes of epidermis. Vaseline is particularly useful, and at this stage may be freely used upon the face. Phenol (3 to 5 per cent.) in oil or vaseline may be used. It also relieves the itching. For the odor, which is sometimes so disagreeable, the dilute phenol solutions are best. If the eruption is abundant on the scalp, the hair should be cut short to prevent matting and decomposition of the crusts. When suppuration is marked the continuous warm bath (95°) is useful. Boric acid, alum or potassium permanganate may be added to the water.

The papules do not maturate so well when protected from the light, and for centuries attempts have been made to modify the course of the pustules by either excluding the light or by changing its character. In the Middle Ages John of Gaddesden recommended wrapping the patient in red flannel, and treated in this way the son of Edward I. It was an old practice of the Egyptians and Arabians to cover the exposed parts of small-pox patients with gold-leaf. Lutzenberg, a distinguished New Orleans physician, in 1832 treated patients by exclusion of the sunlight. The red-light treatment of the disease has been advocated by Finsen, but the statements do not agree as to its value. Nash states that the course of the rash may be modified by the treatment, but Ricketts and Byles could see no influence whatever, even in cases taken at the earliest possible date.

Complications.—If the diarrhœa is severe, paregoric may be given. When the pulse becomes feeble and rapid, stimulants may be freely given. The maniacal delirium may require chloroform or morphia, but for less intense nervous symptoms the bath or cold pack is the best. For the severe hæmorrhages of the malignant cases nothing can be done, and it is only cruel to drench the patient with iron, ergot, and other drugs. Symptoms of obstruction in the larynx, usually from œdema, may call for tracheotomy. In the late stages, if the patient is debilitated and the subject of abscesses and bed-sores, he may be placed on a water-bed or treated in the continuous bath.

The care of the *eyes* is most important. The lids should be thoroughly cleansed and the conjunctivæ washed with a warm solution of salt or boracic acid. In the confluent cases the eyelids are swollen and glued together, and only constant watchfulness prevents keratitis. The edges of the lids should be smeared with vaseline. The mouth and throat should be kept clean, a potassium permanganate mouth wash and gargle used, and the treatment of the nose with glycerin or oil should be begun early, as it prevents the formation of hard crusts. Douching the nose with a warm alkaline solution is helpful.

The treatment in the stage of convalescence is important. Frequent bathing helps to soften the crusts, and the skin may be oiled daily. Convalescence should not be considered established until the skin is perfectly smooth and clean and free from any trace of scabs.

II. VACCINIA (Cow-pox)—VACCINATION

Definition.—An eruptive disease of the cow, the virus of which, inoculated into man (vaccination), produces a local pock with constitutional disturbance, which affords protection, more or less permanent, against small-pox.

History.—For centuries it had been a popular belief among farmer folk that cow-pox protected against small-pox. The notorious Duchess of Cleveland, replying to some joker who suggested that she would lose her occupation if she was disfigured with small-pox, said that she was not afraid of the disease, as she had had a disease that protected her against small-pox. Jesty, a Dorsetshire farmer, had had cow-pox, and in 1774 vaccinated successfully his wife and two sons. Plett, in Holstein, in 1791, also successfully vaccinated three children. When Jenner was a student at Sodbury, a young girl, who came for advice, when small-pox was mentioned, exclaimed, "I cannot take that disease, for I have had cow-pox." Jenner subsequently mentioned the subject to Hunter, who in reply gave the famous advice: "Do not think, but try; be patient, be accurate." As early as 1780 the idea of the protective power of vaccination was firmly impressed on Jenner's mind. The problem which occupied his attention for many years was brought to a practical issue when, on May 14, 1796, he took matter from the hand of a dairy-maid, Sarah Nelmes, who had cow-pox, and inoculated a boy names James Phipps, aged eight years. On July 1st, matter was taken from a small-pox pustule and inserted into the boy, but no disease followed. In 1798 appeared An Inquiry into the Causes and Effects of the Variola Vaccinæ, a Disease discovered in some of the Western Counties of England, particularly Gloucestershire, and known by the Name of Cow-pox (pp. iv, 75, four plates, 4to. London, 1798).

In the United States cow-pox was introduced by Benjamin Waterhouse, Professor of Physic at Harvard, who on July 8, 1800, vaccinated seven of his children. In Boston on August 16, 1802, nineteen boys were inoculated with the cow-pox. On November 9th twelve of them were inoculated with small-pox; nothing followed. A control experiment was made by inoculating two unvaccinated boys with the same small-pox virus; both took the disease. The nineteen children of August 16th were again unsuccessfully inoculated with fresh virus from these two boys. This is one of the most crucial experiments in the history of vaccination, and fully justified the conclusion of the Board of Health—*cow-pox is a complete security against the small-pox.*

Practitioners should familiarize themselves with the literature on vaccination. The centenary number of the British Medical Journal is particularly valuable (1896). The report of the Royal Commission on vaccination (1897), the exhaustive articles in Allbutt and Rolleston's System by T. D. Acland, Copeman and McVail, and Cory's monograph on the subject afford a large body of material. To public health officials who wish for distribution in handy shape Facts about Small-pox and Vaccination leaflets issued by the British Medical Association will be of the greatest value. The *Vaccination Law* of the German Empire, printed in English (Berlin, B. Paul, 1904), contains important information and statistics.

Nature of Vaccinia.—Is cow-pox a separate independent disease, or is it only small-pox modified by passing through the cow? In spite of a host of observations, this is not yet settled. The experiments may be divided into two groups. First, those in which the inoculation of the small-pox matter in the heifer produced pocks corresponding in all respects to the vaccine vesicles. Lymph from the first calf inoculated into a second or third produced the characteristic lesions of cow-pox, and from the first, second, or third animal lymph used to vaccinate a child produced a typical localized vaccine vesicle without any of the generalized features of small-pox. The experiments of Ceely, of Babcock, and many other workers seem to leave no question whatever that typical vaccinia may be produced in the calf by the inoculation of variolous matter. A great deal of the vaccine material at one time in use in England was obtained in this way. Secondly, against this are urged Chauveau's Lyons experiments. Seventeen young animals were inoculated with the virus of small-pox. Small reddish papules occurred which disappeared rapidly, but the animals did not acquire cow-pox. Fifteen of the seventeen animals were also vaccinated. Of these only one showed a typical cow-pox eruption. To determine the nature of the original papules one was excised and inoculated into a non-vaccinated child, which developed as a result generalized confluent small-pox. A second child inoculated from the primary pustule of the first child developed discrete small-pox. The French hold to the Lyons experiments as demonstrating the duality of the diseases.

The weight of evidence favors the view that cow-pox and horse-pox are variola modified by transmission; or "small-pox and vaccinia are both of them descended from a common stock—from an ancestor, for instance—which resembled vaccinia far more than it resembled small-pox" (Copeman).

The bodies described by Guarnieri have been very thoroughly studied by Councilman and his colleagues, who regard them as forms of a protozoön—*Cytoryctes vacciniæ*—with a well-characterized development cycle, increasing in size until they undergo segmentation.

Normal Vaccination.—Period of Incubation.—At first there may be a little irritation at the site of inoculation, which subsides.

Period of Eruption.—On the third day, as a rule, a papule is seen surrounded by a reddish zone. This gradually increases, and on the fifth or sixth day shows a definite vesicle, the margins of which are raised while the centre is depressed. By the eighth day the vesicle has attained its maximum size. It is round and distended with a limpid fluid, the margin hard and prominent, and the umbilication is more distinct. By the tenth day the vesicle is still large and is surrounded by an extensive areola. The contents have now become purulent. The skin is also swollen, indurated, and often painful. On the eleventh or twelfth day the hyperæmia diminishes, the lymph becomes more opaque and begins to dry. By the end of the second week the vesicle is converted into a brownish scab, which gradually becomes dry and hard, and in about a week (that is, about the twenty-first or twenty-fifth day from the vaccination) separates and leaves a circular pitted scar. If the points of inoculation have been close together, the vesicles fuse and may form a large combined vesicle. Constitutional symptoms of a more or less marked degree follow the vaccination. Usually on the third or fourth day the temperature rises, and may persist, increasing until the eighth or ninth day. There is a marked leucocytosis. In children it is common to have with the fever restlessness, particularly at night, and irritability; but as a rule these symptoms are trivial. If the inoculation is made on the arm, the axillary glands become large and sore; if on the leg, the inguinal glands. Immunity is not necessarily complete at once after vaccination; it may take as long as three weeks; on the other hand, a person exposed to small-pox and successfully vaccinated at once may escape entirely, or the two diseases may run concurrently, with the small-pox much modified. The duration of the immunity is extremely variable, differing in different individuals. In some instances it is permanent, but a majority of persons within ten or twelve years again become susceptible.

Revaccination should be performed about the ninth or tenth year, and whenever small-pox is epidemic. The susceptibility to revaccination is very general. In 1891-'92 vaccination pustules developed in 88.7 per cent. of the newly enrolled troops of the German army, most of whom had been vaccinated twice in their lives before. The vesicle in revaccination is usually smaller, has less induration and hyperæmia, and the resulting scar is less perfect. Particular care should be taken to watch the vesicle of revaccination, as it not infrequently happens that a spurious pock is formed, which reaches its height early and dries to a scab by the eighth or ninth day.

Irregular Vaccination.—(*a*) Local Variations.—We occasionally meet with instances in which the vesicle develops rapidly with much itching, has not the characteristic flattened appearance, the lymph early becomes opaque, and the crust forms by the seventh or eighth day. The evolution of the pocks may be abnormally slow. In such cases the operation should again be performed with fresh lymph. The contents of the vesicles may be watery and bloody. In the involution the bruising or irritation of the pocks may lead to ulceration and inflammation. A very rare event is the recurrence of the pock in the same place. Sutton reports four such recurrences within six months.

(*b*) Generalized Vaccinia.—It is not uncommon to see vesicles in the vicinity of the primary sore. Less common is a true generalized pustular rash, developing in different parts of the body, often beginning about the wrists and on the back. The secondary pocks may continue to make their appearance for five or six weeks after vaccination. In children the disease may prove fatal. They may be most abundant on the vaccinated limb, and occur usually about the eighth to the tenth day.

(*c*) Complications.—In unhealthy subjects, or as a result of uncleanliness, or sometimes injury, the vesicles inflame and deep excavated ulcers result. Sloughing and deep cellulitis may follow. In debilitated children there may be a purpuric rash with this. Acland thus arranges the dates at which the possible eruptions and complications may be looked for:

1. During the first three days: Erythema; urticaria; vesicular and bullous eruptions; invaccinated erysipelas.

2. After the third day and until the pock reaches maturity: Urticaria; lichen urticatus, erythema multiforme; accidental erysipelas.

3. About the end of the first week: Generalized vaccinia; impetigo; vaccinal ulceration; glandular abscess; septic infections; gangrene.

(*d*) Transmission of Diseases by Vaccination.—Syphilis has undoubtedly been transmitted by vaccination, but such instances are very rare, and a large number of the cases of alleged vaccino-syphilis must be thrown out. The question is now of no importance since the general use of animal lymph. Dr. Cory's sad experiment may be referred to. He vaccinated himself four times from syphilitic children. With the first vaccination followed, but no syphilis. Two other attempts (negative) were made. The fourth time he was vaccinated from a child the subject of congenital syphilis. The lymph was taken from the child's arm with care, avoiding any contamination with blood. At two of the points of insertion red papules appeared on the twenty-first day. On the thirty-eighth day a little ulcer was found, which Sir Jonathan Hutchinson decided was syphilitic. The diseased parts were then removed. By the fiftieth day the constitutional symptoms were well marked.

Tuberculosis.—"No undoubted case of invaccinated tubercle was brought before the Royal Commission on Vaccination" (Acland). The risk of transmitting tuberculosis from the calf is so slight that it need not be considered. The transmission of leprosy by vaccination is doubtful.

The observations on the presence of actinomyces in vaccine virus have been confirmed by W. T. Howard, Jr., who found it 24 times in 95 cultures from the virus of five producers in the United States.

Tetanus.—McFarland collected 95 cases, practically all American. Sixty-three occurred in 1901, a majority of which could be traced to one source of supply, in which R. W. Wilson demonstrated the tetanus bacillus. Most of the cases occurred about Philadelphia. Since that date very few cases have been reported. The occurrence of this complication emphasizes the necessity of the most scrupulous care in the preparation of the virus, as the tetanus bacillus is almost constantly present in the intestines of cattle.

(*e*) Influence of Vaccination upon Other Diseases.—A quiescent malady may be lighted into activity by vaccination. This has happened with congenital syphilis, occasionally with tuberculosis. An old idea was prevalent that vaccination had a beneficial influence upon existing diseases. Thomas Archer, the first medical graduate in the United States, recommended it in whooping-cough, and said that it had cured six or eight cases in his hands.

Technique.—That part of the arm about the insertion of the deltoid is usually selected for the operation. Mothers "in society" prefer to have girl babies vaccinated on the leg. The skin should be cleansed and put upon the stretch. Then, with a scalpel, needle, or the ivory point, superficial incisions should be made in one or more places. Four points of insertion, an inch apart, or two incisions, each about half an inch long and a little less than an inch apart, may be made. The incision should not be deep enough to draw blood in large drops. The virus is rubbed gently into the incisions and allowed to dry. When glycerin lymph is used the drops may be placed on the skin first and the incisions then made. When the lymph has dried on the points it is best to moisten it in sterile water. The clothing should not be adjusted until the spot has dried, and it should be protected for a day or two with lint or a soft handkerchief. Another method is by *acupuncture.* In doing this the vaccine is deposited on the cleaned skin, which is then drawn tight. An ordinary needle is used with the point slanting and nearly parallel with the skin. It is pressed against the skin through the drop of vaccine and a very slight puncture made. Six of these are made in a small space. When the vesicle forms it can be protected by sterile gauze held in place by strapping. Vaccination is usually performed between the fourth and sixth month. If unsuccessful, it should be repeated from time to time. It should be postponed if the child has any ailment or suffers from syphilis or a skin disease. Revaccination should be done at the age of nine years. A person exposed to the contagion of small-pox should always be revaccinated. This, if successful, will usually protect; but not always. The cases in which small-pox is taken within a few years after vaccination are probably instances of spurious vaccination.

The Value of Vaccination.—Sanitation cannot account for the diminution in small-pox and for the low rate of mortality. Isolation is a useful auxiliary, but it is no substitute. Vaccination is not claimed to be an invariable and permanent preventive of small-pox, but in an immense majority of cases successful inoculation renders the person for many years insusceptible. Communities in which vaccination and revaccination are thoroughly and systematically carried out are those in which small-pox has the fewest victims. On the other hand, communities in which vaccination and revaccination are persistently neglected are those in which epidemics are most prevalent. Owing to a widespread prejudice against vaccination in Montreal, there grew up, between the years 1876 and 1884, a considerable unprotected population, and the materials were ripe for an extensive epidemic. The soil had been prepared and it only needed the introduction of the seed, which in due time came with the Pullman-car conductor from Chicago, on the 28th of February, 1885. Within the next ten months thousands of persons were stricken with the disease, and 3,164 died. The statistics from Japan, published by Kitasato (1911), show strikingly the efficacy of vaccination in that country. In the Japanese army of more than a million men in a war waged in a country in which small-pox was then epidemic there were only 362 cases and 35 deaths. He shows with great clearness the gradual lessening of the intensity of the epidemics in Japan as the system of vaccination has been perfected.

Although the effects of a single vaccination may wear out, as we say, and the individual again becomes susceptible to small-pox, yet the mortality in such cases is very much lower than in persons who have never been vaccinated. There is evidence that the greater the number of marks the greater the protection in relation to small-pox; thus, the English Vaccination Report states that out of 4,754 cases the death-rate with one mark was 7.6 per cent.; with two marks, 7 per cent.; with three marks, 4.2 per cent.; with four marks, 2.4 per cent. W. M. Welch's statistics of 5,000 cases on this point give with good cicatrices 8 per cent.; with fair cicatrices, 14 per cent.; with poor cicatrices, 27 per cent.; postvaccinal cases, 16 per cent.; unvaccinated cases, 58 per cent.

III. VARICELLA (Chicken-pox)

Definition.—An acute contagious disease, characterized by an eruption of vesicles on the skin.

History.—Ingrassias, a distinguished Neapolitan professor, first recognized the disease as differing from small-pox (1553). Heberden gave it the name chicken-pox (1767).

Etiology.—The disease occurs in epidemics, but sporadic cases are also met with. It may prevail at the same time as small-pox or may follow or precede epidemics of this disease. It is a disease of childhood; a majority of the cases occur between the second and sixth years. Adults who have not had the disease in childhood are very liable to be attacked. The specific germ has not been discovered. There are many reports of an association with herpes zoster.

Varicella is an affection distinct from variola and without any relation to it. An attack of the one does not confer immunity from an attack of the other. A boy, aged five, was admitted to St. Thomas' Hospital with a vesicular eruption, and isolated in a ward on the same floor as the small-pox ward. The disease was pronounced chicken-pox by Risdon Bennett and Bristowe. The patient was then removed and vaccinated, with a result of four vesicles which ran a pretty normal course. On the eighth day from the vaccination the child became feverish. On the following day the papules appeared and the child had a well-developed attack of small-pox with secondary fever (Sharkey).

Symptoms.—After a period of incubation of ten or fifteen days the child becomes feverish and in some instances has a slight chill. There may be vomiting, and pains in the back and legs. Convulsions are rare. The eruption usually occurs within twenty-four hours. It is first seen upon the trunk, either on the back or on the chest. It may begin on the forehead and face. At first in the form of raised red papules, these are in a few hours transformed into hemispherical vesicles containing a clear or turbid fluid. As a rule there is no umbilication, but in rare instances the pocks are flattened, and a few may even be umbilicated. They are often ovoid in shape and look more superficial than the variolous vesicles. The skin in the neighborhood is not often infiltrated or hyperæmic. At the end of thirty-six or forty-eight hours the contents of the vesicles are purulent. They begin to shrivel, and during the third and fourth days are converted into dark brownish crusts, which fall off and as a rule leave no scar. Fresh crops appear during the first two or three days of the illness, so that on the fourth day one can usually see pocks in all stages of development and decay. They are always discrete, and the number may vary from eight or ten to several hundreds. As in variola, a scarlatinal rash occasionally precedes the development of the eruption. The eruption may occur on the mucous membrane of the mouth, and occasionally in the larynx. In adults the disease may be much more severe, the initial fever high, the rash very widespread, and the constitutional symptoms comparatively severe, so that the diagnosis of variola may be made—the so-called varicella variolaformes. The fever in varicella is slight, but it does not as a rule disappear with the appearance of the rash. The course of the disease is in a large majority of the cases favorable, and no ill effects follow. The disease may recur in the same individual. There are instances in which a person has had three attacks.

There are one or two modifications of the rash which are interesting. The vesicles may become very large and develop into regular bullæ, looking not unlike ecthyma or pemphigus (varicella bullosa). The irritation of the rash may be excessive, and if the child scratches the pocks ulcerating sores may form, which leave scars on healing. Cicatrices after chicken-pox are more common than after varioloid.

In delicate children, particularly the tuberculous, gangrene (varicella escharotica) may occur about the vesicles, or in other parts, as the scrotum.

Cases of hæmorrhagic varicella have been described with cutaneous ecchymoses and bleeding from the mucous membranes.

Nephritis may occur. Infantile hemiplegia has occurred during an attack of the disease. Death has followed in an uncomplicated case from extensive involvement of the skin.

Diagnosis.—The diagnosis is as a rule easy, particularly if the patient has been seen from the onset. When a case comes under observation for the first time with the rash well out, there may be considerable difficulty. The abundance of the rash on the trunk in varicella is most important. The pocks in varicella are more superficial, more bleb-like, have not so deeply an infiltrated areola about them, and may usually be seen in all stages of development. They rarely at the outset have the hard, shotty feeling of those of small-pox. The general symptoms, the greater intensity of the onset, the prolonged period of invasion, and the more frequent occurrence of prodromal rashes in small-pox are important points in the diagnosis.

Death is very rare, and, unless from the complications, raises a suspicion of the correctness of the diagnosis. Thus of the 123 deaths in England and Wales in 1916 ascribed to chicken-pox, it is probable, as Tatham suggests, that many of these were from unrecognized small-pox.

Vaccination from the vesicles has been tried as a preventive and seems to have decreased the incidence in those exposed to infection.

No special *treatment* is required. If the rash is abundant on the face, care should be taken to prevent the child from scratching the pustules. A soothing lotion or phenol (3 to 5 per cent.) in vaseline should be applied.

IV. SCARLET FEVER

Definition.—An infectious disease characterized by a diffuse exanthem and an angina of variable intensity.

History.—In the sixteenth century Ingrassias of Naples and Coyttarus of Poitiers recognized the disease; but Sydenham in 1675 gave a full account of it under the name febris scarlatina.

Etiology.—No one of the acute infections varies so greatly in the intensity of the outbreaks, a point to which both Sydenham and Bretonneau called attention. In some years it is mild; in others, with equally widespread epidemics, it is fearfully malignant. It is a widespread affection, occurring in nearly all parts of the globe and attacking all races.

Sporadic cases occur from time to time. The epidemics are most intense in the autumn and winter. There is an extraordinary variability in the severity of the outbreaks, which on the whole appear to be lessening in severity; thus, in Boston from 1894 to 1903 the ratio of cases per ten thousand has ranged from 45.80 to 16.18, and the mortality from 3.94 to 0.60. In England and Wales the disease is declining. In 1883 there were over 12,000 deaths; in 1903, 4,158; in 1909, 3,215, and in 1916, 1,381 deaths. Newsholme attributes this in part to the general improvement in sanitation in the home and to hospital isolation, and in part to the decline in the severity of the disease.

Seibert's studies in New York show that the disease increases steadily from week to week until the middle of May; the frequency diminishes gradually until the end of June, and gradually increases through October, November, and December. He associates the remarkable drop in July, August, and September with the closure of the schools and the cessation of the daily congregation of infectious material in small areas—school-houses and playgrounds—for so many hours each day.

AGE is the most important predisposing factor. Ninety per cent. of the fatal cases are under the tenth year. Sucklings are rarely attacked. The general liability to the disease in childhood is less widespread than in measles. Many escape in childhood; others escape until adult life; some never take it.

FAMILY SUSCEPTIBILITY is not infrequently illustrated by the death in rapid succession of four or five members. On the other hand, individual resistance is common, and many physicians constantly exposed escape. An attack as a rule confers subsequent immunity. In rare instances there have been one or even two recurrences.

The natives of India are said to enjoy comparative immunity.

INFECTIVITY.—It is not yet accurately known where in the body the poison is formed. It is probably given off with the secretions of the nose, throat, and respiratory tract. The mild angina of the ambulatory cases may convey the disease, and in this way it is spread in schools, and the "return cases" may find in this way their explanation. More attention has been paid to this aspect of the scarlatinal infection, and it has been suggested that the skin is only infective by contamination with the secretions. The general opinion, however, is that the poison is given off chiefly from the skin, particularly when desquamating. Unlike measles, the germ is very resistant and clings tenaciously to clothing, to bedding, the furniture of the room, etc. Even after the most complete disinfection, children who have been removed from an infected house may catch the disease on their return. The possibility of throat and nose infection must be considered. The intractable character of the nasal discharge after scarlet fever is well recognized and this secretion appears to be highly infectious. The chief organisms in it are streptococci. A third person may convey the disease, but undoubted instances are rare.

The disease is stated to have been conveyed by *milk*. Of 99 epidemics studied by Kober the disease prevailed in 68 either at the dairy or the milk farm. There appear to be two groups of cases: first, genuine scarlet fever, in which the infection is conveyed through the milk having come in contact with infected persons; and, secondly, outbreaks of an infection resembling scarlet fever, due to disease of the udder of the cows.

By SURGICAL SCARLATINA, first brought to the attention of the profession by Sir James Paget in 1864, is understood an erythematous eruption following an operation or occurring during septic infection. It differs from scarlet fever in the large number of adults attacked, the shorter incubation, the mildness of the throat symptoms, the starting of the eruption at the wound, and the precocious desquamation. Alice Hamilton, after analyzing 174 cases reported in the literature, concludes that the eruption is most frequently due to septic infection and is not truly scarlatinal, and that in those cases in which the disease was undoubtedly scarlet fever there is no convincing evidence that the relation between the wound and the scarlet fever was anything more than coincidence.

The SPECIFIC GERM is not known. The relation of the streptococcus is under discussion and the trend of work indicates that it is only a secondary invader, and that there is not a specific streptococcus, though some have gone so far as to use streptococcic immunization as a prophylactic. The question of experimental scarlet fever is still uncertain.

Morbid Anatomy.—Except in the hæmorrhagic form, the skin after death shows no traces of the rash. There are no specific lesions. Those which occur in the internal organs are due partly to the fever and partly to infection with pus-organisms.

The anatomical changes in the throat are those of simple inflammation, follicular tonsillitis, and, in extreme grades, of diphtheroid angina. In severe cases there are intense lymphadenitis and much inflammatory œdema of the tissues of the neck, which may go on to suppuration, or even to gangrene. Streptococci are found abundantly in the glands and in the foci of suppuration. The lymph glands and the lymphoid tissue may show hyperplasia and the spleen, liver, and other organs may be the seat of widespread focal necroses. Endocarditis and pericarditis are not infrequent. Myocardial changes are less common. The renal changes will be considered with the diseases of the kidney. Affections of the respiratory organs are not frequent. When death results from the pseudo-membranous angina, broncho-pneumonia is not uncommon. Cerebro-spinal changes are rare.

Symptoms.—INCUBATION.—"From one to seven days, oftenest two to four." McCollom considered the usual period to be ten to fourteen days.

INVASION.—The onset is as a rule sudden. It may be preceded by a slight, scarcely noticeable, indisposition. An actual chill is rare. Vomiting is one of the most constant initial symptoms; convulsions are common. The fever is intense; rising rapidly, it may on the first day reach 104° or even 105°. The skin is unusually dry and to the touch gives a sensation of very pungent heat. The tongue is furred, and as early as the first day there may be complaint of dryness of the throat. Cough and catarrhal symptoms are uncommon. The face is often flushed and the patient has all the objective features of an acute fever.

ERUPTION.—Usually on the second day, in some instances within the first twenty-four hours, the rash appears in the form of scattered red points on a deep subcuticular flush; at first on the neck and chest, and spreading so rapidly that by the evening of the second day it may have invaded the entire skin. After persisting for two or three days it gradually fades. At its height the rash has a vivid scarlet hue, quite distinctive and unlike that seen in any other eruptive disease. It is an intense hyperæmia, and the anæmia produced by pressure instantly disappears. There may be fine punctiform hæmorrhages, which do not disappear on pressure. In some cases the rash does not become uniform but remains patchy, and intervals of normal skin separate large hyperæmic areas. Tiny papular elevations may sometimes be seen, but they are not so common as in measles. With each day the rash becomes of a darker color, and there may be in parts even a bluish-red shade. Smooth at the beginning, the skin gradually becomes rougher, and to the touch feels like "goose skin." At the height of the eruption sudaminal vesicles may develop, the fluid of which may become turbid. The entire skin may at the same time be covered with small yellow vesicles on a deep red background—*scarlatina miliaris.* McCollom laid stress upon the appearance of a punctate eruption in the arm-pits, groins, and on the roof of the mouth as proof of scarlet fever. Marked transverse lines at the bend of the elbow may occur early. Occasionally there are *petechiæ,* which in the malignant type of the disease become widespread and large. Small skin hæmorrhages are not uncommon. They are sometimes produced by the pressure of the cuff of the blood-pressure apparatus.

The eruption does not always appear upon the face. There may be a good deal of swelling of the skin, which feels uncomfortable and tense. The itching is variable; not as a rule intense at the height of the eruption. By the seventh or eighth day the rash has disappeared. The mucous membrane of the palate, the cheeks, and the tonsils present a vivid red, punctiform appearance. The tongue at first is red at the tip and edges, furred in the centre; and through the white fur are often seen the swollen red papillæ, which give the so-called "strawberry" appearance to the tongue, particularly if the child puts out the tip of the tongue between the lips. In a few days the "fur" desquamates and leaves the surface red and rough, and it is this condition which some writers call the "strawberry," or, better, the "raspberry" tongue. Enlargement of the papillæ was the only constant sign in 1,000 cases (McCollom). The breath often has a very heavy, sweet odor.

The pharyngeal symptoms are: 1. Slight redness, with swelling of the pillars of the fauces and of the tonsils. 2. A more intense grade of swelling and infiltration of these parts with a follicular tonsillitis. 3. Diphtheroid angina with intense inflammation of all the pharyngeal structures and swelling of the glands below the jaw, and in very severe cases a thick brawny induration of all the tissues of the neck.

The *fever,* which sets in with such suddenness and intensity, may reach 105° or even 106° F. It persists with slight morning remissions, gradually declining with the disappearance of the rash. In mild cases the temperature may not reach 103° F.; on the other hand, in very severe cases there may be hyperpyrexia, 108° F., or before death even 109° F.

The *pulse* ranges from 120 to 150; in severe cases with very high fever from 190 to 200. The respirations show an increase proportionate to the intensity of the fever. Leucocytosis is usually present and inclusion bodies may be seen in the leucocytes. The gastro-intestinal symptoms are not marked after the initial vomiting, and food is usually well taken. In some instances there are abdominal pains. The edge of the spleen may be palpable. The liver is not often enlarged. With the initial fever nervous symptoms are present in a majority of the cases; but as the rash comes out the headache and the slight nocturnal wandering disappear. The urine has the ordinary febrile characters, being scanty and high colored. Slight albuminuria is by no means infrequent during the stage of eruption. Careful examination of the urine should be made every day. There is no cause for alarm in the trace of albumin which is so often present, not even if it is associated with a few tube casts.

Desquamation.—With the disappearance of the rash and the fever the skin looks somewhat stained, is dry, a little rough, and gradually the upper layer of the cuticle begins to separate. The process usually begins about the neck and chest, and flakes are gradually detached. The degree and character of the desquamation bear some relation to the intensity of the eruption. When the latter has been very vivid and of long standing large flakes may be thrown off. In rare instances the hair and even the nails have been shed. It must

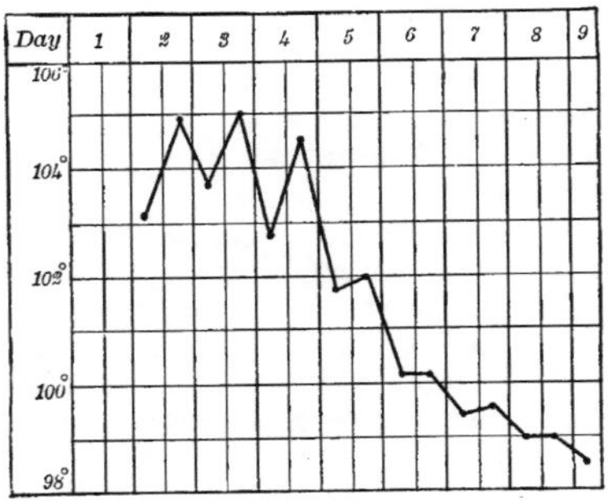

Chart X.—Scarlet Fever.

not be forgotten that there are cases in which the desquamation has been prolonged, according to Trousseau, even to the seventh or eighth week. The entire process lasts from ten to fifteen or even twenty days.

Atypical Scarlet Fever.—Mild and Abortive Forms.—In cases of exceptional mildness the rash may be scarcely perceptible. During epidemics, when several children of a household are affected, one child sickens as if with scarlet fever, and has a sore throat and the "strawberry tongue," but the rash does not appear—*scarlatina sine eruptione*. In school epidemics a third or more of the cases may be without the rash. Desquamation, however, may follow, and in these very mild forms nephritis may occur.

Malignant Scarlet Fever.—*Fulminant Toxic Variety*.—With all the characteristics of an acute intoxication, the patient is overwhelmed by the intensity of the poison and may die within twenty-four or thirty-six hours. The disease sets in with great severity—high fever, extreme restlessness, headache, and delirium. The temperature may rise to 107° or even 108°, in rare cases even higher. Convulsions may occur and the initial delirium rapidly gives place to coma. The dyspnœa may be urgent; the pulse is very rapid and feeble.

Hæmorrhagic Form.—Hæmorrhages occur into the skin, and there are hæmaturia and epistaxis. In the erythematous rash scattered petechiæ appear, which gradually become more extensive, and ultimately the skin may be universally involved. Death may take place on the second or on the third day. While this form is perhaps more common in enfeebled children, it may attack adults apparently in full health.

ANGINOSE FORM.—The throat symptoms appear early and progress rapidly; the fauces and tonsils swell and are covered with a thick membranous exudate, which may extend to the posterior wall of the pharynx, forward into the mouth, and upward into the nostrils. The glands of the neck rapidly enlarge. Necrosis occurs in the tissues of the throat, the fetor is extreme, the constitutional disturbance profound, and the child dies with the clinical picture of a malignant diphtheria. Occasionally the membrane extends into the trachea and the bronchi. The Eustachian tubes and the middle ear are usually involved. When death does not take place rapidly from toxæmia there may be extensive abscess formation in the tissues of the neck and sloughing. In the separation of deep sloughs about the tonsils the carotid artery may be opened, causing fatal hæmorrhage.

SEPTICÆMIC FORM.—In this there is a marked secondary infection and death occurs in the second or third week from severe toxæmia.

Complications and Sequelæ.—ALBUMINURIA.—At the height of the fever there is often a slight trace of albumin in the urine, which is not of special significance. In a majority of cases the kidneys escape without greater damage than occurs in other acute febrile affections.

NEPHRITIS is most common in the second or third week and may follow a very mild attack. It may be delayed until the third or fourth week. As a rule, the earlier it occurs the more severe the attack. It occurs in from 10 to 20 per cent. of the cases. Three grades of cases may be recognized:

1. Acute hæmorrhagic nephritis. There may be suppression of urine or only a small quantity of bloody fluid laden with albumin and tube casts. Vomiting is constant, there are convulsions, and the child dies with the symptoms of acute uræmia. In severe epidemics there may be many cases of this sort, and an acute, rapidly fatal, nephritis due to the scarlet fever poison may occur without an exanthem.

2. Less severe cases without serious acute symptoms. There is a puffy appearance of the eyelids, with slight œdema of the feet; the urine is diminished in quantity, smoky, and contains albumin and tube casts. The kidney symptoms then dominate the entire case, the dropsy persists, and there may be effusion into the serous sacs. The condition may drag on and become chronic, or the patient may succumb to uræmic accidents. Fortunately, in a majority of the cases recovery takes place.

3. Cases so mild that they can scarcely be termed nephritis. The urine contains albumin and a few tube casts, but rarely blood. The œdema is extremely slight or transient, and the convalescence is scarcely interrupted. Occasionally, however, serious symptoms may supervene. Œdema of the glottis may prove rapidly fatal, and in one case of the kind the child died of acute effusion into the pleural sacs.

In other cases the œdema disappears and the child improves, though he remains pale, and a slight amount of albumin persists in the urine for months or even for years. Recovery may take place or a chronic nephritis may follow. Occasionally œdema occurs without albuminuria or signs of nephritis. Possibly it may be due to the anæmia; but there are instances in which marked changes have been found in the kidney after death, when the urine did not show the features characteristic of nephritis.

Arthritis.—There are two forms: first, the severe scarlatinal pyæmia, with suppuration of one or more joints—part of a widespread streptococcus infection. This is an extremely serious and fatal form. Secondly, scarlatinal arthritis, analogous to that in gonorrhœa and other infections. It occurs in the second or third week; many joints are attacked, particularly the small joints of the hands. The heart may be involved. Chorea, subcutaneous nodules, purpura, and pleurisy may be complications. The outlook is usually good.

Cardiac Complications.—In the severe septic cases a malignant endocarditis, sometimes with purulent pericarditis, closes the scene. Simple endocarditis is not uncommon. It may not be easy to say whether the apex systolic murmur, so often heard, signifies a valvular lesion. The persistence after convalescence, with signs of slight enlargement of the heart, may alone decide that the murmur indicated an organic change. As is the rule, such cases give no symptoms. And, lastly, there may be a severe toxic myocarditis, sometimes leading to acute dilatation and sudden death. It is to be borne in mind that the cardiac complications of the disease are often latent.

Acute bronchitis and broncho-pneumonia are not common. *Empyema* is an insidious and serious complication.

Ear Complications.—Common and serious, due to extension of the inflammation from the throat through the Eustachian tubes, they rank among the most frequent causes of deafness in children. The severe forms of membranous angina are almost always associated with otitis, which goes on to suppuration and to perforation of the drum. The process may extend to the labyrinth and rapidly produce deafness. In other instances there is suppuration in the mastoid cells. In the necrosis which follows the middle-ear disease the facial nerve may be involved and paralysis follow. Later, still more serious complications may follow, such as thrombosis of the lateral sinus, meningitis, or abscess of the brain.

Adenitis.—In comparatively mild cases of scarlet fever the submaxillary lymph-glands may be swollen. In severer cases the swelling of the neck becomes extreme and extends beyond the limits of the glands. Acute phlegmonous inflammations may occur, leading to widespread destruction of tissue, in which vessels may be eroded and fatal hæmorrhage ensue. The suppurative processes may also involve the retro-pharyngeal tissues.

The swelling of the lymph-glands usually subsides, and within a few weeks even the most extensive enlargement gradually disappears. There are rare instances, however, in which the lymphadenitis becomes chronic, and the neck remains with a glandular collar which almost obliterates its outline. This may prove intractable to all ordinary measures of treatment. A case came under observation in which, two years after scarlet fever, the neck was enormously enlarged and surrounded by a mass of firm brawny glands.

Nervous Complications.—Chorea occasionally complicates the arthritis and endocarditis. Sudden convulsions followed by hemiplegia may occur. In seven of a series of 120 cases of infantile hemiplegia the trouble came on during scarlet fever. Progressive paralysis of the limbs with wasting may present the features of a subacute ascending spinal paralysis. Thrombosis of the cerebral veins may occur. Mental symptoms, mania, and melancholia have been described. Vagotonia may be marked in convalescence.

Other rare complications and sequelæ are œdema of the eyelids, without nephritis, symmetrical gangrene, enteritis, noma, and perforation of the soft palate.

The fever may persist for several weeks after the disappearance of the rash, and the child may remain in a septic or typhoid state. This so-called scarlatinal typhoid is usually the result of some chronic suppurative process about the throat or the nose, occasionally the result of a chronic adenitis, and in a few cases nothing whatever can be found to account for the fever.

Measles may be concurrent or follow in the stage of convalescence.

Relapse is rare. It was noted in 7 per cent. of 12,000 (Caiger), in 1 per cent. of 1,520 cases (Newsholme), and in 3 per cent. of 5,000 cases (McCollom).

Diagnosis.—The diagnosis of scarlet fever is not difficult, but there are cases in which the true nature of the disease is for a time doubtful. The following are the most common conditions with which it may be confounded:

Acute Exfoliating Dermatitis.—This pseudo-exanthem simulates scarlet fever very closely. It has a sudden onset, with fever. The eruption spreads rapidly, is uniform, and after persisting for five or six days begins to fade. Even before it has entirely gone desquamation usually begins. Some of these cases cannot be distinguished from scarlet fever in the stage of eruption. The throat symptoms, however, are usually absent, and the tongue rarely shows the changes which are so marked in scarlet fever. In the desquamation of this affection the hair and nails are commonly affected. It is, too, a disease liable to recur. Some of the instances of second and third attacks of scarlet fever have been cases of this form of dermatitis.

Measles, which is distinguished by the longer period of invasion, the characteristic nature of the prodromes, and the later appearance of the rash. The greater intensity of the measly rash upon the face, the more papular character and the irregular crescentic distribution are distinguishing features in a majority of the cases. Other points are the absence in measles of the sore throat, the peculiar character of the desquamation, the absence of leucocytosis, and the presence of Koplik's sign.

Rötheln.—The rash of rubella is sometimes strikingly like that of scarlet fever, but in the great majority of cases the mistake could not arise. In cases of doubt the general symptoms are our best guide.

Sepicæmia.—The so-called puerperal or surgical scarlatina shows an eruption which may be identical in appearance with that of scarlet fever.

Diphtheria.—The practitioner may be in doubt whether he is dealing with a case of scarlet fever with intense membranous angina, a true diphtheria with an erythematous rash, or coexisting scarlet fever and diphtheria. In the angina occurring early in and during the course of scarlet fever, though the clinical features may be those of true diphtheria, Löffler's bacilli are rarely found. On the other hand, in the membranous angina occurring during convalescence the bacilli are usually present. The rash in diphtheria is, after all, not so common, is limited usually to the trunk, is not so persistent, and is generally darker than the scarlatinal rash.

Scarlet fever and diphtheria may coexist, but in a case presenting widespread erythema and extensive membranous angina with Löffler's bacilli it would puzzle Hippocrates to say whether the two diseases coexisted, or whether it was only an intense rash in diphtheria. Desquamation occurs in either case. The streptococcus angina is not so apt to extend to the larynx, nor are recurrences so common; but it is well to bear in mind that general infection may occur, that the membrane may spread downward with great rapidity, and, lastly, that all the nervous sequelæ of diphtheria may follow the streptococcus form.

Drug Rashes.—These are partial, and seldom more than a transient hyperæmia of the skin. Occasionally they are diffuse and intense, and in such cases very deceptive. They are not associated, however, with the characteristic symptoms of invasion. There is no fever, and with care the distinction can usually be made. They are most apt to follow the use of belladonna, quinine, and iodide of potassium. The antitoxin erythema is a frequent cause of doubt, particularly in hospitals for infectious diseases.

Coexistence of other Diseases.—Of 48,366 cases of scarlet fever in the Metropolitan Asylum Board Hospitals which were complicated by some other disease, in 1,094 cases the secondary infection was diphtheria, in 899 cases chicken-pox, in 703 measles, in 404 whooping-cough, in 55 erysipelas, in 11 typhoid fever, and in 1 typhus fever (F. F. Caiger). Farnarier (1904) could collect only 39 undoubted cases of the coexistence of typhoid and scarlet fever.

How Long Is a Child Infective?—Usually, after desquamation is complete, in four or five weeks the danger is thought to be over, but the occurrence of so-called "return cases" shows that patients remain infective even at this stage. In 1894, with 2,593 patients from the Glasgow fever hospitals sent to their homes convalescent, fresh cases appeared in 70 of the houses (Chalmers). With 15,000 cases submitted to an average period of isolation of forty-nine days or under, the percentage of return cases was 1.86; with an average period of fifty to fifty-six days the percentage was 1.12; where the isolation extended to between fifty-seven and sixty-five days the percentage of return cases was 1 (Neech). This author suggests eight weeks as a minimum and thirteen weeks as a maximum. Special care should be taken of cases with rhinorrhœa and otorrhœa and throat trouble, as the secretions from these parts are of great importance in the conveyance of the disease.

Prognosis.—As stated, the death-rate has been falling of late years. Epidemics differ remarkably in severity and the mortality is extremely variable. Among the better classes the death-rate is much lower than in hospital practice. There are physicians who have treated consecutively a hundred or more cases without a death. On the other hand, in hospitals and among the poorer classes the death-rate is considerable, ranging from 5 to 10 per cent. in mild epidemics to 20 or 30 per cent. in the very severe. In 1,000 cases reported from the Boston City Hospital by McCollom the death-rate was 9.8 per cent. There is a curious variability in the local mortality from this disease. In England, for example, in some years, certain counties enjoy almost immunity from fatal scarlet fever. The younger the child the greater the danger. In infants under one year the death-rate is very high. The great proportion of fatal cases occurs in children under six years of age. The unfavorable symptoms are very high fever, early mental disturbance with great jactitation, the occurrence of hæmorrhages (cutaneous or visceral), intense diphtheroid angina with cervical bubo, and signs of laryngeal obstruction. Nephritis is always a serious complication, and when setting in with suppression of the urine may quickly prove fatal; a large majority of the cases recover.

Prophylaxis.—Much may be done to prevent the spread of the disease if the physician exercises scrupulous care in each case. Much is to be expected from a rigid system of school inspection, and from the more general recognition of the importance of the latent cases and the persistence of the infection in the secretions of the nose and throat. The attendant in a case of scarlet fever should take the most careful precautions against the conveyance of the disease, wearing a gown in the room and thoroughly washing the hands and face after leaving the room. To the busy practitioner the minutiæ of proper disinfection are irksome, but it is his duty to carry out the most rigid disinfection possible, and intelligent people expect it. The duration of quarantine varies with the attack: six to eight weeks is the average period. Patients with discharge from the ear or nose require longer isolation.

Treatment.—The patient may be treated at home or sent to an isolation hospital. The difficulty in *home treatment* is in securing complete isolation. The risks are well illustrated by the careful studies of Chapin, of Providence, who found that during eight years 26.1 per cent. of the 4,412 persons under twenty-one years of age in infected families took the disease. When practicable, it is better to send the other children out of the house. Chapin's experience on this point is most interesting. In seventeen years, from 652 families infected with scarlet fever, 1,051 children, none of whom had had the disease, were removed. Only 5 per cent. were attacked while away from home. Nineteen who had been sent away from the infected houses were attacked on their return. In Great Britain a very considerable proportion of all patients are removed from their homes. In the segregation hospital groups of patients, from ten to twenty, are treated in separate wards.

The disease cannot be cut short. In the presence of the severer forms we are too often helpless. There is no disease in which the successful issue and the avoidance of complications depend more upon the skilled judgment of the physician and the care with which his instructions are carried out.

The child should be isolated and placed in charge of a competent nurse. The temperature of the room should be constant and the ventilation thorough. The child should wear a light flannel nightgown, and the bedclothing should not be too heavy. The mouth should be kept clean and rinsed freely with a mild antiseptic solution. The diet should consist of milk, buttermilk, whey, and ice cream; water and fruit juices should be freely given. Cream and lactose may be added to the milk. With the fall of the temperature the diet may be increased and the child may gradually return to ordinary fare. When desquamation begins the child should be thoroughly rubbed every day, or every second day, with sweet oil, or carbolated vaseline, or a 5-per-cent. hydronaphthol soap, which prevents the drying and the diffusion of the scales. An occasional warm bath may then be given. At any time during the attack the skin may be sponged with warm water. The patient may be allowed to get up after the temperature has been normal for ten days, but for at least three weeks from this time great care should be exercised to prevent exposure to cold. It must not be forgotten that the renal complications are very apt to occur during convalescence, and after all danger is apparently past. Ordinary cases may be given a simple fever mixture, and during convalescence a bitter tonic. The bowels should be carefully regulated.

When the fever is above 103° F. the extremities may be sponged with tepid water. In severe cases, with the temperature rapidly rising, this will not suffice, and more thorough measures of hydrotherapy should be practised. With pronounced delirium and nervous symptoms the cold pack should be used. When the fever is rising rapidly but the child is not delirious, he should be placed in a warm bath, the temperature of which can be gradually lowered. The bath with the water at 80° is beneficial. In giving the cold pack a rubber sheet and a thick layer of blankets should be spread upon a sofa or a bed, and over them a sheet wrung out of cold water. The naked child is then laid upon it and wrapped in the blankets. An intense glow of heat quickly follows the preliminary chilling, and from time to time the blankets may be unfolded and the child sprinkled with cold water. The good effects which follow this treatment are often striking, particularly in allaying the delirium and jactitation, and procuring quiet sleep. Parents will object less, as a rule, to the warm bath gradually cooled than to any other form of hydrotherapy. The child may be removed from the warm bath, placed upon a sheet wrung out of tolerably cold water, and then folded in blankets. The ice-cap is useful and may be kept constantly applied in cases in which there is high fever. Medicinal antipyretics are not of much service in comparison with cold water. If the child is restless or sleepless, hydrotherapy is usually effectual. If not moderate doses of bromide may be given.

The throat symptoms, if mild, do not require much treatment. If severe, the local measures mentioned under diphtheria should be used. The nose should be kept clean, for which a simple alkaline douche, given gently, is best. Cold applications to the neck are to be preferred to hot, though it is sometimes difficult to get a child to submit to them. If cervical adenitis occurs, an ice bag should be applied, and with the first signs of suppuration an incision made. In connection with the throat, the ears should be specially looked after, and a careful disinfection of the mouth and fauces by suitable antiseptic solutions should be practised. When the inflammation extends through the tubes to the middle ear, the practitioner should examine daily the condition of the drum, or, when available, a specialist should be called in to assist. The careful watching of this membrane day by day and the puncturing of it if the tension becomes too great may save the hearing of the child. With the aid of cocaine the drum is readily punctured. The operation may be repeated at intervals if the pain and distention return. No complication of the disease is more serious than this extension of the inflammatory process to the ear.

The nephritis should be dealt with as in ordinary cases; indications for treatment will be found under the appropriate section. It is worth mentioning, however, that Jaccoud insists upon the great value of milk diet in scarlet fever as a preventive of nephritis.

Among other indications for treatment in the disease is cardiac weakness, for which digitalis, or if urgent strophanthin intramuscularly may be given. Camphor (gr. ii, 0.12 gm.) should also be given intramuscularly and repeated as necessary.

SERUM TREATMENT.—As a streptococcus infection frequently complicates scarlet fever and is responsible for the secondary infections, the use of antistreptococcus serum seems rational, but it has not proved of great value in the acute stages. More is to be expected from it in the more chronic infections, in which an autogenous vaccine may be useful. The dosage should be small at first and increased gradually.

V. MEASLES

(Morbilli)

Definition.—An acute, highly contagious fever with specific localization in the upper air passages and in the skin.

As a cause of death measles ranks high among the acute fevers of children. In 1915 there were 16,445 deaths from this disease in England and Wales, but only 5,413 deaths in 1916. In the U. S. registration area there were 10,745 deaths in 1917. The death rate is highest in the second year.

History.—Rhazes, an Arabian physician, in the ninth century described the disease with small-pox, of which it was believed to be a mild form until Sydenham separated them in the seventeenth century.

Etiology.—The liability to infection is almost universal in persons unprotected by a previous attack. It is a disease of childhood, but, as shown in the widespread epidemics in the Faroe Islands and in the Fiji Islands, unprotected adults of all ages are attacked. Within the first three months of life there is a relative immunity. Occasionally infants of a month or six weeks take the disease. Intra-uterine cases have been described, and a mother with measles may give birth to a child with the eruption, or the rash may appear in a few days.

The disease is endemic in cities, and becomes epidemic at intervals, prevailing most extensively in the cooler months, though this is by no means a fixed rule.

The germ of the disease is unknown. J. F. Anderson has shown that the blood of a patient inoculated into the Rhesus monkey produces after eight days a fever of short duration with a well-marked slight exanthem. The contagion is present in the blood, the secretions of the mouth and nose, and in the skin. In the eighteenth century Monro and others demonstrated the inoculability of the disease. Direct contagion is the most common. The poison is probably not in the expired air, but in the particles of mucus and in the sputum and the secretions of the mouth and nose, which, dried, are conveyed with the dust. An important point is the contagiousness of the disease in the pre-eruptive stage. A child with only the catarrhal symptoms may be at school and a source of active infection. Indirect contagion by means of fomites is very common. Measles may be thus conveyed by a third person, by clothes, and by infected toys. The germ soon loses its virulence.

Recurrence is rare. Many cases of supposed second and third attacks represent mistakes in diagnosis. Relapse is occasionally seen, the symptoms recurring at intervals from ten to forty days; but it is not always easy to say whether there may not have been new infection from without.

Morbid Anatomy.—The catarrhal and inflammatory appearances seen post mortem have nothing characteristic. Fatal cases show, as a rule, bronchopneumonia and an intense bronchial catarrh. The lymphatic elements all over the body are swollen, the tonsils, the lymph-glands, and the solitary and agminated follicles of the intestines. The spleen is rarely much enlarged. During convalescence latent tuberculous foci are very apt to become active.

Symptoms.—INCUBATION.—"From seven to eighteen days; oftenest fourteen." The child shows no special changes, but coryza and swelling of the cervical lymph-glands may be present. A leucocytosis has been observed, and the pulse is said to be slow.

INVASION.—In this period, lasting from three to four days, very rarely five or six, the child presents the symptoms of a feverish cold. The onset may be insidious, or it may start with great abruptness, even with a convulsion. There is not often a definite chill. Headache, nausea, and vomiting may usher in the severe cases. The common catarrhal symptoms are sneezing and running at the nose, redness of the eyes and lids, and cough. The fever is slight at first, but gradually there is pungent heat of the skin with turgescence of the face. Prodromal rashes precede the eruption in a few cases, usually a blotchy erythema or scattered macules. The tongue is furred and the mucous membranes of the mouth and throat are hyperæmic, and frequently show a distinct punctiform rash. The fever of the stage of invasion may rise abruptly; more frequently it takes twenty-four or forty-eight hours to reach the fastigium. The pulse-rate increases with the fever, and may reach 140 or 160 per minute, gradually falling with defervescence.

ERUPTION.—"The symptoms increase till the fourth day. At that period (although sometimes a day later) little red spots, just like flea-bites, begin to come out on the forehead and the rest of the face. These increase both in size and number, group themselves in clusters, and mark the face with largish red spots of different figures. These red spots are formed by small red papules, thick set, and just raised above the level of the skin. The fact that they really protrude can scarcely be determined by the eye. It can, however, be ascertained by feeling the surface with the fingers. From the face—where they first appear—these spots spread downward to the breast and belly; afterward to the thighs and legs" (Sydenham). The papules may feel quite shotty, but do not extend deeply. On the trunk and extremities the swelling of the skin is not so noticeable, the color of the rash not so intense and often less uniform. The mottled, blotchy character is seen most clearly on the chest and the abdomen. It is hyperæmic and disappears on pressure, but in the malignant cases it may become of a deep rose, inclining to purple. These general symptoms do not abate with the occurrence of the eruption, but persist until the end of the fifth or the sixth day, when they lessen. Among peculiarities of the rash may be mentioned the development of numerous miliary vesicles and the occurrence of petechiæ, which are seen occasionally even in cases of moderate severity. Recession of the rash, so much dwelt upon by older writers, is rarely seen. When the "measles sink in suddenly after they have begun to come out, and then the patient is seized with anxiety and a swooning comes on, it is a sign of speedy death" (Rhazes). In reality it is the failing circulation which causes the rash to fade.

BUCCAL SPOTS were described by Filatow in 1895, and by Koplik in 1896.

They are seen on a level with the bases of the lower milk molars on either side, or at the line of junction of the molars when the jaws are closed. They are white or bluish-white specks, surrounded by red areolæ. Their importance depends upon their early appearance and remarkable constancy in the disease —six-sevenths of all cases (Heubner), 97.7 per cent. of 214 cases (Balme).

The fauces may be injected, and there is sometimes an eruption of scattered spots over the entire mucous membrane of the mouth. Ringer called attention to opaque white spots on the mucous membrane of the lips.

Desquamation.—After the rash fades desquamation begins, usually in the form of fine scales, more rarely in large flakes. It bears a definite relationship to the extent and intensity of the rash. In mild cases desquamation may take only a few days, in severe cases several weeks.

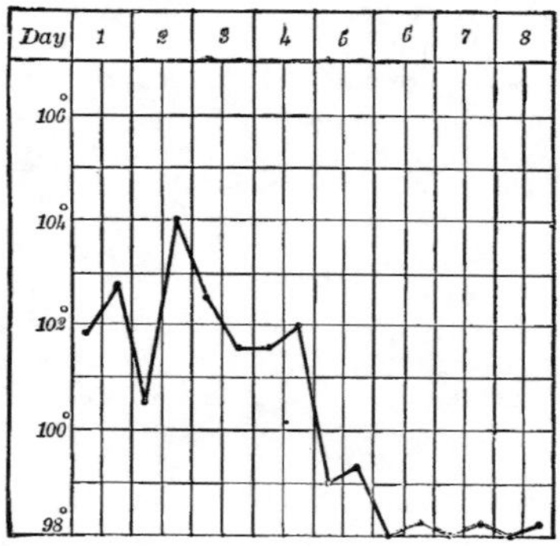

Chart XI.—Measles.

The tonsils and the cervical lymph glands may be slightly swollen and sore; sometimes there is a polyadenitis.

During the course leucocytosis is absent. Its presence generally points to a complication. Myelocytes are often present in small numbers during the eruption (Tileston).

Atypical Measles.—Variations in the course of the disease are not common. There is an *attenuated* form, in which the child may be well by the fourth or fifth day, and an *abortive* form, in which the initial symptoms may be present, but no eruption appears—*morbilli sine morbillis.*

Malignant or *black measles* is seen most frequently in the widespread epidemics, but it is also met with in institutions, and occasionally in general practice among children, more rarely in adults. Hæmorrhages occur into the skin and from the mucous membranes, there is very high fever, and all the features of a profound toxæmia, often with cyanosis, dyspnœa, and extreme cardiac weakness. Death may occur from the second to the sixth day.

Complications.—Those of the air passages are the most serious. The *coryza* may become chronic and lead to irritation of the lymphoid tissues of the naso-pharynx, causing enlarged tonsils and adenoids, and probably leaving these parts less able to resist tuberculous invasion. *Epistaxis* is sometimes serious. *Laryngitis* is not uncommon: the voice becomes husky and the cough croupy in character. Œdema of the glottis and pseudo-membranous inflammation are rare. Ulceration, abscess, and perichondritis may occur.

Bronchitis and Broncho-pneumonia.—In every case of severe measles the possibility of the existing bronchitis extending to the small tubes and causing broncho-pneumonia has to be considered. It is more apt to occur at the height of the eruption or as desquamation begins. The high mortality in institutions is due to this complication, which, as Sydenham remarked, kills more than the small-pox. (For the symptoms, see the section on the subject.)

Lobar pneumonia is less common. *Thrombosis* in veins has been described.

Severe *stomatitis* may follow the slight catarrhal form. In institutions *cancrum oris* or *gangrenous stomatitis* is a terrible complication, attacking sometimes many children. *Parotitis* occasionally occurs. *Intestinal catarrh* and *acute colitis* are special complications of some epidemics.

Nephritis is less rare than is stated. It is not very uncommon to see cases of chronic nephritis which date from an attack of measles. Vulvitis may be present as part of the general catarrhal condition.

Endocarditis is rare. *Arthritis* may follow the fever or come on at its height. It may be general and severe, and in one instance anchylosis of the jaw followed an attack of measles in a child of four years. The conjunctivitis may be followed by *keratitis*. *Otitis media* is not at all uncommon and may lead to perforation of the drum or mastoid disease. *Hemiplegia* is a most serious complication. In 4 of a series of 120 cases the hemiplegia came on during measles. It usually persists. *Paraplegia* due to acute myelitis has been described. *Polyneuritis* may occur with widespread atrophy. Acute mania, *meningitis, abscess of the brain,* and *multiple sclerosis* are among the rare complications or sequelæ. *Scarlet fever* may occur with measles. *Whooping-cough* not infrequently follows measles.

Diagnosis.—During the prevalence of an epidemic the disease is easily recognized. Physicians to isolation hospitals appreciate the practical difficulties and patients with measles may be sent to the small-pox hospital; it is well to bear in mind that in adults the beginning of the eruption on the face, its nodular character, and the isolation of the spots may be suggestive of variola. From scarlet fever measles is distinguished by the longer initial stage with characteristic symptoms, and the blotchy irregular character of the rash, so unlike the diffuse uniform erythema. In measles the mouth (with the early Koplik sign), in scarlet fever the throat, is chiefly affected. Occasionally in measles, when the throat is very sore and the eruption pretty diffuse, there may at first be difficulty in determining which disease is present, but a few days should suffice to make the diagnosis clear. As a rule there is no leucocytosis. It may be extremely difficult to distinguish from rötheln. The shorter prodromal stage, the absence of oculo-nasal catarrh, and the slighter fever in many cases are perhaps the most important features. It is difficult to speak definitely about the distinctions in the rash, though perhaps the more uniform distribution and the absence of the crescentic arrangement are more constant in rötheln. In Africans the disease is easily recognized; the papules stand out with great plainness, often in groups; the hyperæmia is to be seen on all but the very black skins. The distribution of the rash, the coryza, and the rash in the mouth are important points. Of drug eruptions, that induced by copaiba is very like measles, but is readily distinguished by the absence of fever and catarrh. Antipyrin, chloral, and quinine rashes rarely cause any difficulty in diagnosis. The serum exanthem of a diphtheria antitoxin may be difficult to recognize. In adults the acute malignant measles may resemble typhus fever. Occasionally erythema multiforme may simulate measles.

Prognosis.—The mortality from the disease itself is not high, but the pulmonary complications render it one of the most serious of the diseases of children. In some epidemics, particularly in institutions and in armies, the death-rate may be high, not so much from the fever itself as from the extension of the catarrhal symptoms to the finer bronchial tubes. Imported in 1875 from Sydney by H. M. S. Dido to the Fiji Islands, 40,000 out of 150,000 of the inhabitants died in four months. Panum, the distinguished Danish physician, described the widespread and fatal epidemic which decimated the inhabitants of the Faroe Islands in 1846. In private practice the mortality is from 2 to 3 per cent.; in hospitals from 6 to 8 or 10 per cent.

Prophylaxis.—The difficulty is inherent in the prolonged incubation and the four days of invasion, during which the catarrhal symptoms are marked, and the disease is contagious, and one often finds that the quarantine which has been carried out has been in vain. From contact with cases in the stage of invasion and mild cases with scarcely any fever the disease is readily disseminated through schools and conveyed to healthy children in the every-day contact with each other on the streets, in the squares and playgrounds. Once manifested, the child should be carefully quarantined and all possible precautions taken against the spread of the disease in the house. Some health authorities quarantine only for five days after the appearance of the rash, unless there is cough or discharge from the nose or ears.

Treatment.—Confinement to bed in a well-ventilated room, a light diet with abundance of water and a simple fever mixture are the only measures necessary in cases of uncomplicated measles. The fever rarely reaches a dangerous height. If it does it may be lowered by sponging or by the tepid bath gradually reduced. If the rash does not come out well, warm drinks and a hot bath will hasten its maturation. The bowels should be freely opened. If the cough is distressing compresses should be applied to the chest and inhalations of the compound tincture of benzoin or small doses of paregoric or codein given. The patient should be kept in bed for a few days after the fever subsides. During desquamation the skin should be oiled daily, and warm baths given to facilitate the process. The mouth and nostrils should be carefully cleansed, even in mild cases. The convalescence from measles is the most important stage and watchfulness and care may prevent serious pulmonary complications. The frequency with which the mothers of children with simple or tuberculous broncho-pneumonia tell us that "the child caught cold after measles," and the contemplation of the mortality bills, should make us extremely careful in our management of this affection.

VI. RUBELLA

(Rötheln, German Measles)

This exanthem has also the names of *rubeola notha,* or epidemic roseola, and, as it is supposed to present features common to both, has been also known as hybrid measles or hybrid scarlet fever. It is generally regarded, however, as a separate and distinct affection.

Etiology.—It is propagated by contagion and spreads with great rapidity. It frequently attacks adults, and the occurrence of either measles or scarlet fever in childhood is no protection against it. The epidemics of it are often very extensive. The causal organism is not known.

Symptoms.—These are usually mild, and it is altogether a less serious affection than measles. Very exceptionally, as in the epidemics studied by Cheadle, the symptoms are severe.

The stage of incubation is two weeks or even longer.

In the stage of invasion there are chilliness, headache, pains in the back and legs, and coryza. A macular, rose-red eruption on the throat is a constant symptom, and, indeed, it was on this account that it was originally regarded as a hybrid, having the sore throat of scarlet fever and the rash of measles. There may be very slight fever. In 30 per cent. of Edwards's cases the temperature did not rise above 100°. The duration of this stage is somewhat variable. The *rash* usually appears on the first day, some writers say on the second, and others again give the duration of the stage of invasion as three days. Griffith places it at two days. The eruption comes out first on the face, then on the chest, and gradually extends so that within twenty-four hours it is scattered over the whole body. It may be the first symptom noted by the mother. The eruption consists of a number of round or oval, slightly raised spots, pinkish-red in color, usually discrete, but sometimes confluent.

The color of the rash is somewhat brighter than in measles. The patches are less distinctly crescentic. After persisting for two or three days (sometimes longer), it gradually fades and there is a slight furfuraceous desquamation. The rash persists as a rule longer than in scarlet fever or measles, and the skin is slightly stained after it. In some cases the rash is scarlatiniform, which may even follow a measly eruption. The lymphatic glands of the neck are frequently swollen, and, when the eruption is very intense and diffuse, the lymph-glands in the other parts of the body.

There are no special complications. The disease usually progresses favorably; but in rare instances the symptoms are of greater severity. Albuminuria, arthritis, or even nephritis may occur. Pneumonia and colitis have been present in some epidemics. Icterus has been seen.

Diagnosis.—The slightness of the prodromal symptoms, the mildness or the absence of the fever, the more diffuse character of the rash, its rose-red color, and the early enlargement of the cervical glands, are the chief points of distinction between rötheln and measles.

The treatment is that of a simple febrile affection.

"Fourth Disease."—Clement Dukes, in a paper on the confusion of two different diseases under the name rubella, describes what he calls a "fourth disease," in which the body is covered in a few hours with a diffuse exanthem of a bright red color, almost scarlatiniform in appearance. The face may remain quite free. The desquamation is more marked than in rötheln.

Erythema Infectiosum.—Under this term there has been described in Germany, particularly by Escherich, a feebly contagious disease, characterized by a rose-red, maculo-papular rash, appearing chiefly between the ages of four and twelve. It has occurred in epidemic form in the spring and summer. It has followed outbreaks of measles or of rötheln. The most characteristic feature is the morbilliform eruption on the extremities, chiefly on the extensor surfaces. The trunk as a rule remains free.

VII. EPIDEMIC PAROTITIS

(Mumps)

Definition.—A specific infectious disease, characterized by swelling of the salivary glands and a special liability to orchitis in males.

Hippocrates described the disease and its peculiarities—an affection of children and young male adults, the absence of suppuration, and the orchitis.

Etiology.—The nature of the virus is unknown.

It is endemic in large centres of population, and at certain seasons, particularly spring and autumn, the cases increase rapidly. It is met most frequently in childhood and adolescence. Very young infants and adults are seldom attacked. Males are somewhat more frequently affected than females. In institutions, barracks, and schools the disease has been known to attack over 90 per cent. of the residents. It may be curiously localized in a city or district, or even in one part of a school or barrack. The disease is infectious and spreads from patient to patient. The infection may persist for as long as six weeks. It may be congenital, and Hale White has reported a case in which the mother and her new-born child were attacked at the same time.

A remarkable idiopathic, non-specific parotitis may follow injury or disease of the abdominal or pelvic organs (see Diseases of the Salivary Glands).

Foci of acute interstitial inflammation have been found post-mortem.

Symptoms.—The period of incubation is from two to three weeks, and there are rarely any symptoms during this stage. The invasion is marked by fever, which is usually slight, rarely rising above 101°, but in exceptionally severe cases reaches 103° or 104°. The child complains of pain just below the ear on one side, where a slight swelling is noticed, which increases gradually, and within forty-eight hours there is great enlargement of the neck and side of the cheek. The swelling passes forward in front of the ear, the lobe of which is lifted, and back beneath the sterno-mastoid muscle. The other side usually becomes affected within a day or two, and the whole neck is surrounded by a collar of doughy infiltration. Only one gland may be involved, or an interval of four or five days may elapse before the other side is involved. The submaxillary and sublingual glands become swollen, though not always; in a few cases they may be alone attacked. The lachrymal glands may be involved. The greatest inconvenience is experienced in taking food, for the patient is unable to open the mouth, and even speech and deglutition become difficult. There may be an increase in the secretion of the saliva, but the reverse is sometimes the case. The mucous membrane of the mouth and throat may be slightly inflamed. There is seldom great pain, but an unpleasant feeling of tension and tightness. There may be earache, even otitis media, and slight impairment of hearing.

After persisting for from seven to ten days, the swelling gradually subsides and the child rapidly regains his strength and health and is none the worse for the attack. Occasionally the disease is very severe and characterized by high fever, delirium, and great prostration. The patient may even lapse into a typhoid condition.

Relapse is rare, but there may be two or three slight recurrences within a few weeks, in which the cervical glands may enlarge. A second or even a third attack may occur.

Orchitis.—Excessively rare before puberty, it occurs usually about the eighth day, and more particularly if the boy is allowed to leave his bed. One or both testicles may be involved. The swelling may be great, and occasionally effusion takes place into the tunica vaginalis. The orchitis may occur before the parotitis, or in rare instances may be the only manifestation of the infection (*orchitis parotidea*). The inflammation increases for three or four days, and resolution takes place gradually. There may be a muco-purulent discharge from the urethra. In severe cases atrophy may follow, fortunately as a rule only in one organ; occurring in both before puberty, the natural development is usually checked. Even when both testicles are atrophied and small, sexual vigor may be retained. The proportion of cases of orchitis varies in different epidemics; 211 cases occurred in 699 cases, and 103 cases of atrophy followed 163 instances of orchitis (Comby). No satisfactory explanation of this metastasis has been given. Military surgeons, who see much of the disease in young recruits, have suggested the transference of the virus to the penis with the fingers and its transmission along the urethra.

A vulvo-vaginitis sometimes occurs in girls, and the breasts may become enlarged and tender. Mastitis has been seen in boys. Involvement of the ovaries is rare. The thyroid gland may enlarge in the attack, and there have been features suggestive of acute pancreatitis.

Complications and Sequelæ.—Of these the cerebral affections are perhaps the most serious. There may be delirium and signs of meningeal irritation but actual meningitis is rare. Hemiplegia and aphasia may also occur. A majority of the fatal cases are associated with meningeal symptoms which are very rare in comparison with the frequency of the disease. Acute mania has occurred, and there are instances on record of insanity following the disease.

Arthritis, albuminuria, nephritis, with acute uræmia and convulsions, endocarditis, pleurisy, facial paralysis, hemiplegia, and peripheral neuritis are occasional complications. Suppuration of the gland is extremely rare. Gangrene has occasionally occurred. The special senses may be seriously involved. Deafness may occur, and may be permanent. Affections of the eye are rare, but optic neuritis with atrophy has been described.

Chronic hypertrophy of the gland may follow.

Diagnosis.—The diagnosis of the disease is usually easy. The position of the swelling in front of and below the ear and the elevation of the lobe on the affected side definitely fix the locality of the swelling. In children inflammation of the parotid, apart from ordinary mumps, is excessively rare.

Treatment.—It is well to keep the patient in bed during the height of the disease. Special care should be given to the mouth by cleaning after feeding and the use of akaline antiseptic solutions. The bowels should be freely opened, and the patient given a light liquid diet. No medicine is required unless the fever is high, in which case aconite may be given. Cold compresses may be placed on the gland, but children, as a rule, prefer hot applications. Belladonna or ichthyol ointment is sometimes useful. Suppuration is hardly ever to be dreaded, even though the gland become very tense. With delirium and head symptoms the ice-cap may be applied. For the orchitis, rest, with support and protection of the swollen gland with cotton-wool, is usually sufficient.

VIII. DENGUE

Definition.—An acute infectious disease of tropical and subtropical regions, characterized by febrile paroxysms, pains in the joints and muscles, an initial erythematous and a terminal polymorphous eruption. It is known as *break-bone* fever from the atrocious character of the pain, and *dandy fever* from the stiff, dandified gait. The word dengue is supposed to be derived from a Spanish, or possibly Hindostanee, equivalent of the word dandy.

History and Geographical Distribution.—The disease was first recognized in 1779 in Cairo and in Java, where Bylon described the outbreak in Batavia. There have been widespread epidemics in India and China. The description by Benjamin Rush of the epidemic in Philadelphia in 1780 is one of the first and one of the very best accounts of the disease. Between 1824 and 1828 it was prevalent at intervals in India and in the Southern States. S. H. Dickson gives a graphic description of the disease as it appeared in Charleston in 1828. Since that date there have been four or five widespread epidemics in tropical countries and in North America along the Gulf States, the last in 1897. None of the recent epidemics extended into the Northern States, but in 1888 it prevailed as far north as Virginia.

Etiology.—The rapidity of diffusion and the pandemic character are the two most important features of dengue. There is no disease, not even influenza, which attacks so large a proportion of the population. In Galveston, in 1897, 20,000 people were attacked within two months. The specific cause is not determined but it is a filterable virus. The disease is transmitted by mosquitoes (*Stegomyia calopus, Culex fatigans?*). Epidemics in Australia corresponded with the distribution of the *Stegomyia calopus* but there was no evidence that *Culex fatigans* transmitted the disease. Biting experiments were successful and it was transmitted by injecting the blood subcutaneously. The virus was present in the whole blood, the serum, and the fluid part of citrated blood.

As the disease is rarely fatal, no observations have been made upon its pathological anatomy.

Symptoms.—The period of incubation is from three to five days, during which the patient feels well. The attack sets in suddenly with headache, chilly feelings, and intense aching pains in the joints and muscles. The temperature rises gradually, and may reach 106° or 107°. The pulse is rapid, and there are the other phenomena associated with acute fever—loss of appetite, coated tongue, slight nocturnal delirium, and concentrated urine. The face has a suffused, bloated appearance, the eyes are injected, and the visible mucous membranes are flushed. There is a congested erythematous state of the skin. Rush's description of the pains is worth quoting, as in it the epithet break-bone occurs in the literature for the first time. "The pains which accompanied this fever were exquisitely severe in the head, back, and limbs. The pains in the head were sometimes in the back parts of it, and at other times they occupied only the eyeballs. In some people the pains were so acute in their backs and hips that they could not lie in bed. In others the pains affected the neck and arms, so as to produce in one instance a difficulty of moving the fingers of the right hand. They all complained more or less of a soreness in the seats of these pains, particularly when they occupied the head and eyeballs. A few complained of their flesh being sore to the touch in every part of the body. From these circumstances the disease was sometimes believed to be a rheumatism, but its more general name among all classes of people was the break-bone fever." The large and small joints are affected, sometimes in succession, and become swollen, red, and painful. In some cases cutaneous hyperæsthesia has been noted. Hæmorrhage from the mucous membranes was noted by Rush, and black vomit has also been described.

The fever gradually reaches its maximum by the third or fourth day; the patient then enters upon the apyretic period, which may last from two to four days, and in which he feels prostrated and stiff. A second paroxysm of fever then occurs, and the pains return. In a large number of cases an eruption is common, which, judging from the description, has nothing distinctive, being sometimes macular, like that of measles, sometimes diffuse and scarlatiniform, or papular, or lichen-like. In other instances the rash has been described as urticarial, or even vesicular. The rash may persist for a month after the symptoms have disappeared. Certain writers describe inflammation and hyperæmia of the mucous membrane of the nose, mouth and pharynx. Enlargement of the lymph-glands is not uncommon, and may persist for weeks after the disappearance of the fever. Convalescence is often protracted, and there is a degree of mental and physical prostration out of all proportion to the severity of the primary attack. The pains in the joints or muscles, sometimes very local, may persist for weeks. Rush refers to the former, stating that a young lady after recovery said it should be called break-heart, not break-bone, fever. The average duration of a moderate attack is from seven to eight days. Dengue is very seldom fatal. Dickson saw three deaths in the Charleston epidemic.

Complications are rare. Insomnia and occasionally delirium, resembling somewhat the alcoholic form, have been observed, and convulsions in children. Atrophy of the muscles may occur after the attack. A relapse may occur even as late as two weeks.

Diagnosis.—The diagnosis of the disease, prevailing as it does in epidemic form and attacking all classes indiscriminately, rarely offers any special difficulty. Isolated cases might be mistaken at first for rheumatic fever. The seven-day fever of East Indian ports is believed to be dengue. It is a sporadic fever of the hot weather, attacking a large proportion of Europeans within the first year or two of their arrival. Possibly, as Rogers thinks, it may be a distinct disease, and it is variously known in India as ephemeral fever, mild malaria, or simple continued fever. It is characterized by early and severe pains in the back and limbs, and a fever of six to seven days' duration.

Treatment.—The patients should be protected from mosquitoes during the febrile period. The treatment is entirely symptomatic. Hydrotherapy may be employed to reduce the fever. The salicylates or antipyrin may be tried for the pains, which usually, however, require opium. During convalescence iodide of potassium is recommended for the arthritic pains, and tonics are indicated.

IX. HYDROPHOBIA

(*Lyssa; Rabies*)

Definition.—An acute disease of warm-blooded animals, dependent upon a virus which is communicated by inoculation to man.

Distribution.—Rabies is very variously distributed. In Russia it is common. In North Germany it is relatively rare, owing to the wise provision that all dogs must be muzzled. In France it is much more common. In England the muzzling order has been followed by an almost complete disappearance of the disease and there were only 4 deaths from 1901-1916. In the decennium ending with 1890 the deaths averaged 29 annually (Tatham). In the United States there were 66 deaths in the registration area in 1917.

Etiology.—Dogs are especially liable to the disease. It also occurs in the wolf, fox, skunk, cat, horse and cow. Most animals are susceptible; and it is communicable by inoculation to the rabbit and pig. The disease is propagated chiefly by the dog. The nature of the poison is as yet unknown. It is contained chiefly in the nervous system and in some of the secretions, particularly in the saliva. Bartarelli has shown that the virus reaches the dog's salivary glands by way of the nerves and not through the blood-vessels.

A variable time elapses between the introduction of the virus and the appearance of the symptoms. Horsley stated that this depends upon the following factors: "(*a*) Age. The incubation is shorter in children than in adults. For obvious reasons the former are more frequently attacked. (*b*) Part infected. The rapidity of onset of the symptoms is greatly determined by the part of the body which may happen to have been bitten. Wounds about the face and head are especially dangerous; next in order in degrees of mortality come bites on the hands, then injuries on the other parts of the body. This relative order is, no doubt, greatly dependent upon the fact that the face, head, and hands are usually naked, while the other parts are clothed; it would also appear to depend somewhat upon the richness in nerves of the part. (*c*) The extent and severity of the wound. Puncture wounds are the most dangerous; the lacerations are fatal in proportion to the extent of the surface afforded for absorption of the virus. (*d*) The animal conveying the infection. In order of decreasing severity come: first, the wolf; second, the cat; third, the dog; and fourth, other animals." Only a limited number of those bitten by rabid dogs become affected by the disease; according to Horsley, not more than 15 per cent. On the other hand, the death-rate of those persons bitten by wolves is higher, not less than 40 per cent. Babes gives the mortality as from 60 to 80 per cent.

The incubation period in man is extremely variable. The average is from six weeks to two months. In a few cases it has been under two weeks. It may be prolonged to three months. It is stated that the incubation may be prolonged for a year or even two years, but this has not been definitely settled.

Morbid Anatomy.—The important lesions consist in the accumulation of leucocytes around the blood-vessels and the nerve-cells, particularly the motor ganglion cells, of the central nervous system (rabic tubercles of Babes). Especial importance in the rapid diagnosis of rabies is attached by van Gehuchten and Nelis to the accumulation of lymphoid and endothelioid cells around nerve-cells of the sympathetic and cerebro-spinal ganglia. Negri described in the central nervous system irregular bodies varying from 4 to 10 microns in size, widespread, frequently in the cells of the cerebellum, cerebral cortex and pons, and in the spinal cord. They are probably protozoa, and it is stated that they furnish a rapid and trustworthy means of diagnosis. The inoculation experiments show that the virus is not present in the liver, spleen, or kidneys, but is abundant in the spinal cord, brain, and peripheral nerves.

Symptoms.—Three stages of the disease are recognized:

(*a*) Premonitory stage, in which there may be irritation about the bite, pain, or numbness. The patient is depressed and melancholy; and complains of headache and loss of appetite. He is irritable and sleepless, and has a sense of impending danger. There is often greatly increased sensibility. A bright light or a loud voice is distressing. The larynx may be injected, the voice becoming husky, and the first symptoms of difficulty in swallowing are experienced. There is a slight rise in the temperature and pulse.

(*b*) Stage of Excitement.—This is characterized by great excitability and restlessness, and an extreme degree of hyperæsthesia. "Any afferent stimulant—i. e., a sound or a draught of air, or the mere association of a verbal suggestion—will cause a violent reflex spasm. In man this symptom constitutes the most distressing feature of the malady. The spasms, which affect particularly the muscles of the larynx and mouth, are exceedingly painful and are accompanied by an intense sense of dyspnœa, even when the glottis is widely opened or tracheotomy has been performed" (Horsley). Any attempt to take water is followed by an intensely painful spasm of the muscles of larynx and of the elevators of the hyoid bone. It is this which makes the patient dread the very sight of water and gives the name *hydrophobia* to the disease. These spasmodic attacks may be associated with maniacal symptoms. In the intervals the patient is quiet and the mind unclouded. The temperature in this stage is usually elevated and may reach from 100° to 103°. In some instances the disease is afebrile. The patient rarely attempts to injure his attendants, and in the intense spasms may be particularly anxious to avoid hurting any one. There are, however, occasional fits of furious mania, and the patient may, in the contractions of the muscles of the larynx and pharynx, give utterance to odd sounds. This stage lasts from a day and a half to three days and gradually passes into the—

(*c*) Paralytic Stage.—In rodents the preliminary and furious stages are absent, as a rule, and the paralytic stage may be marked from the outset —the so-called dumb rabies. This stage rarely lasts longer than from six to eighteen hours. The patient then becomes quiet; the spasms no longer occur; unconsciousness gradually supervenes; the heart's action becomes more and more enfeebled, and death occurs by syncope.

Diagnosis.—In man this offers no special difficulties. It is advisable, in cases with any doubts, as soon as possible after the injury, to secure the brain of the supposed rabid animal for examination. The recognition of the Negri bodies in smears of brain substance enables the diagnosis to be made promptly.

Treatment.—Prophylaxis is of the greatest importance, and by a systematic muzzling of dogs the disease can be practically eradicated.

In case of a bite from a suspicious animal, bleeding should be encouraged, the wound freely opened and washed with bichloride of mercury solution (1 to 1,000). Thorough cauterization should be done as soon as possible, for which pure carbolic or nitric acid should be used, being applied to every part of the wound. The wound is washed with a saturated solution of bicarbonate of soda and then with alcohol. When once established the disease is hopelessly incurable. No measures have been found of the slightest avail, consequently the treatment must be palliative. The patient should be kept in a darkened room, in charge of not more than two attendants. To allay the spasm, chloroform may be administered and morphia given hypodermically. It is best to use these powerful remedies from the outset, and not to temporize with chloral, bromide of potassium, and other less potent drugs. By the local application of cocaine, the sensitiveness of the throat may be diminished sufficiently to enable the patient to take liquid nourishment. Sometimes he can swallow readily. Fluid can be given by the bowel.

Preventive Inoculation.—Pasteur found that the virus, when propagated through a series of rabbits, increases in its virulence; so that whereas subdural inoculation of the brain of a mad dog takes from fifteen to twenty days to produce the disease, in successive inoculation in a series of rabbits the incubation period is gradually reduced to seven days (*virus fixe*). The spinal cords of these rabbits contain the virus in great intensity, but when they are preserved in dry air this gradually diminishes. If now dogs are inoculated from cords preserved for from twelve to fifteen days, and then from cords preserved for a shorter period, i. e., with a progressively stronger virus, they gradually acquire immunity against the disease. Relying upon these experiments, Pasteur began inoculations in the human subject, using, on successive days, material from cords in which the virus was of varying degrees of intensity.

In 1910, 410 patients were treated at the Pasteur Institute of Paris without a death; in 1908 and 1909, 991 cases with 2 deaths. There has been a progressive decline in the number of cases and in the mortality.

Pseudo-hydrophobia (*Lyssophobia*).—This may closely resemble hydrophobia, but is nothing more than a neurotic or hysterical manifestation. A nervous person bitten by a dog, either rabid or supposed to be rabid, has within a few months, or even later, symptoms somewhat resembling the true disease. He is irritable and depressed. He constantly declares his condition to be serious and that he will inevitably become mad. He may have paroxysms in which he says he is unable to drink, grasps at his throat, and becomes emotional. The temperature is not elevated and the disease does not progress. It lasts much longer than the true rabies, and is amenable to treatment. It is not improbable that a majority of the cases of alleged recovery in this disease have been of this hysterical form. Certain cases of acute bulbar paralysis may resemble hydrophobia, and, as already mentioned, there is a form of tetanus with hydrophobic symptoms.

X. RHEUMATIC FEVER

Definition.—An acute infection, dependent upon an unknown infective agent, and characterized by arthritis, myocarditis, and a marked tendency to inflammation of the endocardium of the valves of the heart.

Etiology.—Distribution and Prevalence.—It prevails in temperate and humid climates, and is apparently very rare in the tropics. In the Registrar General's report for England and Wales for 1916 there were 1,886 deaths from the disease and 2,276 deaths under the age of twenty years from acute endocarditis and pericarditis. The disease prevails more in the northern latitudes. In the Montreal General Hospital there were, for the twelve years ending 1903, 2 deaths in 482 cases among 12,044 admissions; at the Royal Victoria Hospital, Montreal, for ten years ending 1903, 3 deaths in 285 cases among 9,286 admissions (John McCrae). At the Johns Hopkins Hospital for the fifteen years ending 1904 there were 360 admissions (330 patients) and 9 deaths. The general impression is that the disease prevails more in the British Isles than elsewhere; but the returns are very imperfect (this holds good everywhere).

Season.—In London the cases reach the maximum in the months of September and October. Bell's statistics of 456 cases in Montreal show that the largest number was admitted in February, March, and April. And the same is true in Baltimore; 55 per cent. of our cases were admitted in the first four months of the year. The disease prevails most in dry years or a succession of such, and is specially prevalent when the subsoil water is abnormally low and the temperature of the earth high (Newsholme).

Age.—Young adults are frequently affected, but the disease is common in children. In England the incidence in children is very high. In 2,556 examined by Langmead, 133 were definitely rheumatic and in all but 18 the heart was involved. In 43 per cent. of these cases there was some abnormality of the tonsils or pharyngeal mucosa. Sucklings are rarely attacked. Milton Miller analyzed 19 undoubted cases. They have to be distinguished from a totally different affection, the pyogenic arthritis of infants. Of 456 cases admitted to the Montreal General Hospital there were, under fifteen years, 4.38 per cent.; from fifteen to twenty-five years, 48.68 per cent.; from twenty-five to thirty-five years, 25.87 per cent.; from thirty-five to forty-five years, 13.6 per cent.; above forty-five years, 7.4 per cent. Of our 360 admissions, 110 were in the third decade and 65 per cent. below the thirtieth year of age. Ten per cent. of the cases had the first attack in the first decade. Of 655 cases analyzed by Whipham, only 32 cases occurred under the tenth year and 80 per cent. between the twentieth and fortieth years. These figures do not give the ratio of cases in children, in whom the milder types of arthritis are very common.

Sex.—If all ages are taken, males are affected oftener than females. Of our patients, 239 were males, 91 females. In the Collective Investigation Report there were 375 males and 279 females. Up to the age of twenty, however, females predominate. Between the ages of ten and fifteen girls are more prone to the disease.

HEREDITY.—It is a deeply grounded belief that this is a family disease, but the evidence is imperfect. The not rare occurrence in several members of the same family is used by those who believe in the infectious origin as an argument in favor of its being a house disease.

CHILL.—Exposure to cold, a wetting, and a sudden change of temperature are among the factors in determining the onset of an attack, but they were present in only 12 per cent. of our cases.

Not only does an attack not confer *immunity,* but, as in pneumonia, predisposes the subject to the disease.

Rheumatic Fever as an Acute Infectious Disease.—Rheumatic fever, as Newsholme has shown, has epidemic prevalence with irregular periodicity, recurring at intervals of three, four, or six years, and varying much in intensity. A severe epidemic is usually followed by two or three years of slight prevalence. The disease has features suggestive of septic infection. In the character of the fever, the arthritis, the tendency to relapse, the sweats, the anæmia, the leucocytosis, and, above all, in the great liability to endocarditis, and to involvement of the serous membranes, the disease resembles pyæmia.

The tonsils are culture centres for many septic organisms, particularly of the streptococcus type. The association of rheumatic fever and arthritic affections generally with infected tonsils is a prevailing view, but it is an old story insisted on by Lasague and other French writers years ago. A not inconsiderable number of cases of rheumatic fever begin with tonsillitis. With organisms isolated from the tonsils experimental arthritis and endocarditis have been caused. The removal of the tonsils has been followed by a complete recovery of sub-acute and chronic forms of arthritis. This is as far as the evidence goes.

There is no agreement as to the causal organism. On the one hand are those who claim to have isolated a specific organism which can be found in many of the lesions of the disease, e. g., pericarditis and endocarditis, and sometimes obtained from the blood. To this the name of *Micrococcus rheumaticus* has been given. On the other hand many observers consider that a variety of streptococci, usually of the milder types, are concerned. Many organisms, especially those obtained from the tonsils, cause arthritis, endocarditis, etc., when injected into the blood of animals, but this does not prove them to be the causal agent in rheumatic fever. The question can not be regarded as settled but the view that a specific causal organism is responsible has much to support it and is in agreement with the etiology of acute infectious diseases generally. There is considerable evidence against the view that it is simply a mild pyogenic infection. Salicylates have no effect on the ordinary streptococcus infections, and the clinical course in the streptococcus arthritis is very different; rheumatic joints never suppurate. The isolation of streptococci may simply indicate the presence of secondary invaders such as occur in scarlet fever and small-pox.

Morbid Anatomy.—The affected joints show hyperæmia and swelling of the synovial membranes and of the ligamentous tissues. The fluid in the joint is turbid, albuminous, and contains leucocytes and a few fibrin flakes. Rheumatic fever rarely proves fatal, except when there are serious complications, such as pericarditis, endocarditis, myocarditis, pleurisy, or pneumonia. The changes in the myocardium are regarded as characteristic by many workers. Klotz has drawn attention to the frequency of arterial lesions, especially in the aorta, which involve particularly the outer portion of the media and the adventitia. Changes in the coronary arteries, an inflammatory fibrosis, are common.

Symptoms.—As a rule, the disease sets in abruptly, but it may be preceded by irregular pains in the joints, slight *malaise,* sore throat, and particularly by tonsillitis. A definite rigor is uncommon; more often there is slight chilliness. The fever rises quickly, and with it one or more of the joints become painful. Within twenty-four hours from the onset the disease is fully manifest. The temperature range is from 102° to 104°. The pulse is frequent, soft, and usually above 100. The tongue is moist, and rapidly becomes covered with a white fur. There are the ordinary symptoms associated with an acute fever, such as loss of appetite, thirst, constipation, and a scanty, highly acid, highly colored urine. In a majority of the cases there are profuse, very acid sweats, of a peculiar sour odor. Sudaminal and miliary vesicles are abundant, the latter usually surrounded by a minute ring of hyperæmia. The mind is clear, except in the cases with hyperpyrexia. The affected joints are painful to move, soon become swollen and hot, and present a reddish flush. The order of frequency of involvement of the joints in our series was knee, ankle, shoulder, wrist, elbow, hip, hand, foot. The joints are not attacked together, but successively. For example, if the knee is first affected, the redness may disappear from it as the wrists become painful and hot. The disease is seldom limited to a single articulation. The amount of swelling is variable. Extensive effusion into a joint is rare, and much of the enlargement is due to the infiltration of the periarticular tissues with serum. The swelling may be limited to the joint proper, but in the wrists and ankles it sometimes involves the sheaths of the tendons and produces great enlargement of the hands and feet. Corresponding joints are often affected. In attacks of great severity every one of the larger joints may be involved. The vertebral, sterno-clavicular, and phalangeal articulations are less often inflamed than in gonorrhœal arthritis. Perhaps no disease is more painful; the inability to change the posture without agonizing pain, the drenching sweats, the prostration and helplessness, combine to make it a most distressing affection. A special feature is the tendency of the inflammation to subside in one joint while increasing in another.

The temperature range in an ordinary attack is between 102° and 104° F. In only 18 of our cases did the temperature rise above 104° F. In 100 it reached 103° F. or over. It is peculiarly irregular, with marked remissions and exacerbations, and defervescence is usually gradual. The profuse sweats materially influence the temperature curve. If a two-hourly chart is made and observations upon the sweats are noted, the remissions will usually be found coincident with them. The perspiration is sour-smelling and acid at first; but, when persistent, becomes neutral or even alkaline.

The blood is profoundly altered and there is no acute febrile disease in which an anæmia occurs with greater rapidity. The average leucocyte count in our cases was about 12,000 per c. mm.

With the high fever a murmur may often be heard at the apex region. Endocarditis is also a common cause of an apex *bruit.* The heart should be carefully examined at the first visit and subsequently each day.

The urine is, as a rule, reduced in amount, of high density and high color. It is very acid, and, on cooling, deposits urates. The chlorides may be greatly diminished or even absent. Formic acid is present (Walker). Febrile albuminuria is not uncommon.

The so-called *subacute rheumatism* represents a milder form of the disease, in which all the symptoms are less pronounced. The fever rarely rises above 101°; fewer joints are involved; and the arthritis is less intense. The cases may drag on for weeks or months. It should not be forgotten that this mild or subacute form may be associated with endocarditis or pericarditis.

The influence of age on the manifestations of the disease is marked. While the usual description applies to the disease as seen in adults, in young children there may not be any pronounced arthritis, and the discovery of endocarditis often suggests the diagnosis. Endocarditis and myocarditis are the prominent features in children as arthritis is in adults.

Complications.—These are important and serious.

(*a*) Hyperpyrexia.—The temperature may rise rapidly a few days after the onset, and be associated with delirium; but not necessarily, for the temperature may rise to 108° or, as in one of Da Costa's cases, 110°, without cerebral symptoms. Hyperpyrexia is most common in first attacks, 57 of 107 cases (Church). It is most apt to occur during the second week. Delirium may precede or follow its onset. As a rule, with the high fever, the pulse is feeble and frequent, the prostration is extreme, and finally stupor supervenes. In our series there was no instance of hyperpyrexia, which seems rare in the United States.

(*b*) Cardiac Affections.—(1) *Endocarditis* occurs in a considerable percentage of all cases. Of 889 cases, 494 had signs of old or recent endocarditis (Church). The liability to endocarditis diminishes as age advances. Its incidence in our cases was more than double in patients who had their first attack before the age of twenty years, compared with those with the first attack after twenty years of age. It increases directly with the number of attacks. Of 116 cases, in the first attack 58.1 per cent. had endocarditis, 63 per cent. in the second attack, and 71 per cent. in the third attack (Stephen Mackenzie). Thirty-five per cent. of our cases showed organic valve lesions, in 96 per cent. the mitral was involved, in 27 per cent. the aortic, and in 23 per cent. the lesions were combined. The mitral segments are most frequently involved and the affection is usually of the simple, verrucose variety. Ulcerative endocarditis is very rare. The valvulitis in itself is rarely dangerous, producing few symptoms, and often overlooked. Unhappily, though the valve at the time may not be seriously damaged, the inflammation starts changes which lead to sclerosis and retraction of the segments, and so to chronic valvular disease. Venous thrombosis is an occasional complication.

(2) *Pericarditis* may occur independently of or together with endocarditis. It may be simple fibrinous, sero-fibrinous, or in children purulent. Clinically we meet it more frequently in connection with this disease than

in any other acute affection. It was present in 20 cases of our series—6 per cent.—in only four of which did effusion occur. The physical signs are very characteristic. The condition is described under its appropriate section. A peculiar form of delirium may accompany rheumatic pericarditis.

(3) *Myocarditis* is probably always present in some degree and is especially marked in connection with endopericardial changes. As Sturges insisted, the term *carditis* is applicable to many cases. The anatomical condition is a granular or fatty degeneration of the heart-muscle, which leads to weakening of the walls and dilatation. There is dilatation of the heart in the majority of cases during the acute period.

(*c*) Aortitis.—This is especially common in children and particularly with aortic endocarditis. The enlargement of the aorta may be marked. In some cases the acute condition results in permanent dilatation.

(*d*) Pulmonary Affections.—Pneumonia and pleurisy occurred in 9.94 per cent. of 3,433 cases (Stephen Mackenzie). They frequently accompany the cases of endo-pericarditis. According to Howard's analysis of a large number of cases, there were pulmonary complications in only 10.5 per cent. of cases of rheumatic endocarditis; in 58 per cent. of cases of pericarditis; and in 71 per cent. of cases of endo-pericarditis. Congestion of the lung is occasionally found, and in several cases has proved rapidly fatal.

(*e*) Nervous Complications.—These are due, in part, to the hyperpyrexia and in part to the special action of the toxic agent. They may be grouped as follows: (*i*) *Cerebral rheumatism,* as it is called, which is characterized by (α) *Delirium,* associated with the hyperpyrexia or the toxæmia, may be active and noisy in character; more rarely it is a low, muttering delirium, passing into stupor and coma. It may be excited by the salicylate of soda, either shortly after its administration, or more commonly a few days later. It was present in only 5 of our 360 cases, and in 4 of these we thought the salicylates at fault. A peculiar delirium occurs in connection with rheumatic pericarditis. (β) *Coma,* which is more serious, may occur without preliminary delirium or convulsions, and prove rapidly fatal. Certain of these cases occur with hyperpyrexia, but others are associated with renal changes and are evidently uræmic. The coma may supervene during the attack, or after convalescence has set in. (γ) *Convulsions* are less common, though they may precede the coma. Of 127 observations cited by Besnier, there were 37 of delirium, only 7 of convulsions, 17 of coma and convulsions, 54 of delirium, coma, and convulsions, and 3 of other varieties (Howard). "Cerebral rheumatism" is a very serious complication; among 107 cases collected by the Clinical Society of London there were 57 deaths. (*ii*) *Chorea.* The relations of this disease and rheumatic fever will be subsequently discussed. It is sufficient here to say that in only 88 out of 554 cases analyzed from the Infirmary for Diseases of the Nervous System, Philadelphia, were chorea and rheumatism associated. It is most apt to develop in the slighter attacks in childhood. (*iii*) *Meningitis* is extremely rare, though undoubtedly it does occur. (*iv*) *Polyneuritis* has been described and may follow hyperpyrexia. In one case free venesection saved the patient's life. After many months the patient recovered, but with ataxia.

(*f*) Cutaneous Affections.—Sweat-vesicles are extremely common and a red miliary rash may also develop. Scarlatiniform eruptions are occasionally seen. Purpura, with or without urticaria, and various forms of erythema may occur. It is doubtful whether the cases of extensive purpura with urticaria and arthritis—peliosis rheumatica—belong to rheumatic fever.

(*g*) RHEUMATIC NODULES.—These curious structures, described originally by Meynet, occur in the form of small subcutaneous nodules. Barlow and Warner, in England, and T. B. Futcher, in the United States, have paid special attention to their varieties and importance. They vary in size from a small shot to a large pea, and are most numerous on the fingers, hands, and wrists. They also occur about the elbows, knees, the spines of the vertebræ, and the scapulæ. They are not often tender. They are more common after the decline of the fever and in the children with mitral valve disease. In only 5 of our patients were they present during the acute attack. The nodules may grow with great rapidity and usually last for weeks or months. They are more common in children than in adults, and in the former their presence may be regarded as a positive indication of rheumatic fever. They have been noted particularly in association with rheumatic endocarditis. Subcutaneous nodules occur also in migraine, gout, and arthritis deformans. Histologically they are made up of round and spindle-shaped cells. In addition to these firm, hard nodules, there occur in rheumatism and in chronic vegetative endocarditis remarkable bodies, which have been called by Féréol "nodosités cutanées éphémères."

(*h*) Swelling or tenderness of the thyroid gland may be present.

Course.—The *course* is extremely variable. It is, as Austin Flint first showed, a self-limited disease, and it is not probable that drugs have any special influence upon its *duration* or *course.* Gull and Sutton, who studied a series of 62 cases without special treatment, arrived at the same conclusion.

Prognosis.—Rheumatic fever is the most serious of all diseases with a low death-rate. The mortality is rarely above 2 or 3 per cent. Only 9 of our 330 patients died, 2.7 per cent., all with endocarditis and 6 with pericarditis.

Sudden death in rheumatic fever is due most frequently to myocarditis. Herringham has reported a case in which on the fourteenth day there was fatty degeneration and acute inflammation of the myocardium. In a few rare cases it results from embolism. Alarming symptoms of depression sometimes follow excessive doses of the salicylate of soda.

Diagnosis.—Practically, the recognition of rheumatic fever is usually easy; but there are several affections which, in some particulars, closely resemble it.

(*a*) MULTIPLE SECONDARY ARTHRITIS.—Under this term may be embraced the forms of arthritis which occur with or follow gonorrhœa, tonsillitis, scarlet fever, dysentery, cerebro-spinal meningitis, etc.

(*b*) SEPTIC ARTHRITIS, which occurs in the course of pyæmia from any cause, and particularly in puerperal fever. No hard and fast line can be drawn between these and the cases in the first group: but the inflammation rapidly passes on to suppuration and there is more or less destruction of the joints. The conditions under which the arthritis occurs give a clue to the nature of the case. Under this section may be mentioned:

(1) *Acute necrosis* or *acute osteo-myelitis* may be mistaken for rheumatic fever. Sometimes it is multiple. The greater intensity of the local symptoms, the involvement of the epiphyses rather than the joints, and the more serious constitutional disturbances are points to be considered. The condition is

unfortunately often mistaken for acute arthritis, and, as the treatment is essentially surgical, the error may cost the life of the patient.

(2) *The acute arthritis of infants* is usually confined to one joint (the hip or knee), the effusion in which rapidly becomes purulent. The affection is most common in sucklings and undoubtedly pyæmic in character. It may also occur with the gonorrhœal ophthalmia or vaginitis of the new-born.

(*c*) Gonococcus Arthritis.—This may give difficulty at the onset, but there is not the rapid shifting from joint to joint and there is usually some thickening about the most affected joints in a short time. A careful search for gonococci is important and the complement fixation test may aid.

(*d*) Gout.—While the localization in a single, usually a small, joint, the age, the history, and the mode of onset are features which enable us to recognize acute gout, there are everywhere cases of acute arthritis, called rheumatic fever, which are in reality gout. The involvement of several of the larger joints is not so infrequent in gout, and unless tophi are present or bursitis occurs, the diagnosis may be difficult.

(*e*) Acute Arthritis Deformans.—This may easily be mistaken for rheumatic fever. It may come on with fever and multiple arthritis, and for weeks there may be no suspicion of the true nature of the disease. Gradually the fever subsides, but the periarticular thickening persists. As a rule, however, in the acute febrile cases the involvement of the smaller joints, the persistence and the early changes in the articulations suggest arthritis deformans.

In *children* the diagnosis may be very difficult, as arthritis may be slight or entirely absent. The possibility of rheumatic fever should be considered in all febrile attacks in children for which no definite cause can be found. Special care should be given to the examination of the heart, particularly for any signs of dilatation or endocarditis.

Treatment.—The main object should be to bring the patient through the attack with an undamaged heart or with as little injury as possible. The first essential is complete rest, which should be begun at once and insisted upon for as long as is necessary. This is especially important for children. The bed should have a smooth, soft, yet elastic, mattress. The patient should wear a flannel nightgown, which may be opened all the way down the front and slit along the outer margin of the sleeves. Three or four of these should be made, so as to facilitate the frequent changes required after the sweats. He may wear also a light flannel cape about the shoulders. He should sleep in blankets, not in sheets, so as to reduce the chance of being chilled.

Milk is the most suitable diet and may be diluted with alkaline mineral waters. Fruit juices, lemonade and oatmeal or barley water should be freely given. The thirst is usually great and may be fully satisfied. There is no objection to soups if the milk is not well borne. As convalescence is established a fuller diet may be allowed, but meat should be used sparingly.

Local treatment is usually necessary. It often suffices to wrap the affected joints in cotton. If the pain is severe, hot cloths may be applied, saturated with Fuller's lotion (carbonate of soda, 6 drams, 24 gm.; laudanum, 1 oz., 30 c. c.; glycerine, 2 oz., 60 c. c.; and water, 9 oz., 270 c. c.) or the lead and opium lotion. Oil of wintergreen is useful, the joint being gently rubbed with it or small amounts sprinkled over flannel, which is then applied. Chloroform liniment is also a good application. Fixation of the joints is of great service in allaying the pain. Splints, padded and bandaged with moderate firmness, will often give comfort. Friction is rarely well borne in an acutely inflamed joint. Cold compresses are sometimes useful. The application of blisters above and below the joint often relieves the pain. This is not to be compared with the light application of the Paquelin cautery. If there is much effusion, aspiration of the joint is useful.

The drug treatment is still far from satisfactory, though the introduction of the salicyl compounds has been a great boon.

THE SALICYL COMPOUNDS.—Salicin, introduced in 1876 by Maclagan, may be used in doses of 20 grains (1.3 gm.) every hour or two until the pain is relieved. It has the advantage of being less depressing than the salicylate of soda. It is also perhaps the best drug to use for children. Salicylate of soda, 15 grain (1 gm.) doses every three hours, is perhaps the best for general use in adults. After the pain has been relieved, the drug should be given every four or five hours until the temperature begins to fall. Potassium or solium bicarbonate may be given with it. If sodium salicylate causes gastric disturbance it can be given by rectum in thin starch solution. Large doses can be administered in this way. Oil of wintergreen, 20 minims (1.25 c. c.) every two hours in milk, or acetyl-salicylic acid (gr. xv, 1 gm.), may be used if the salicylate of soda disagrees. There are other salicyl compounds, but the best results are obtained from the use of one or the other of the above-named preparations. There can be no question as to their efficacy in relieving the pain. Some observers consider that they also protect the heart, shorten the course, and render relapse less likely.

THE ALKALINE TREATMENT.—The urine should be rendered alkaline as soon as possible. Potassium acetate and citrate in doses of 15 grains (1 gm.) each are given every three hours until the urine is alkaline and then often enough to keep it so. Potassium or sodium bicarbonate may be given with the sodium salicylate. Fuller's plan was to give 90 grains (6 gm.) of sodium bicarbonate with 30 grains (2 gm.) of potassium acetate in water, rendered effervescent at the time of administration by citric acid or lemon-juice.

A widespread popular belief attributes marvelous efficacy to bee-stings in all sorts of "rheumatism," and a formic-acid treatment has been introduced. A 2½ per cent. solution is injected in the neighborhood of the painful joints. Ainley Walker collected (B. M. J., October 10, 1908) an interesting literature on the subject.

To allay the *pain* opium may be given in the form of Dover's powder, or morphia hypodermically. The coal tar products are useful sometimes for the purpose. During convalescence iron is indicated in full doses. Of the complications, hyperpyrexia should be treated by the bath or the cold pack. The treatment of endocarditis and pericarditis and the pulmonary complications will be considered under their respective sections. In all the cardiac complications the importance of prolonged rest must be remembered.

To prevent and arrest endocarditis Caton urges the use of a series of small blisters along the course of the third, fourth, fifth, and sixth intercostal nerves of the left side, applied one at a time and repeated at different points. Potassium or sodium iodide is given in addition to the salicylates. The patients are kept in bed for about six weeks.

TONSILS.—With disease of these and the possibility that they are the portals of entry for the infective agent, the question arises as to their removal. In patients with diseased tonsils in whom rheumatic fever has occurred removal is advisable and should be complete. In patients with endocarditis and fever this may be done apparently without risk. It is comparable to the removal of any local focus of infection which is causing general symptoms.

XI. ACUTE TONSILLITIS

Definition.—An acute infection, sporadic or epidemic, involving the structures of the tonsillar ring, usually due to organisms of the streptococcus class.

Etiology.—Acute tonsillitis occurs in sporadic and epidemic forms. The *sporadic* variety, a common disease, is met with in young persons particularly at the school age. Infants are rarely attacked. Chronic enlargement of the lymphatic structures of the throat is an important predisposing cause. Exposure to cold and wet may bring on an attack. It is directly communicated from one child to another. A not infrequent precursor of rheumatic fever, Cheadle described it as one link in the rheumatic chain. It may be directly followed by endocarditis, erythema nodosum, chorea, and acute nephritis. In Great Britain it prevails in the autumn months, in the United States in the spring. An old notion held that there was a close relation between the tonsils and the testes and ovaries, and F. J. Shepherd called attention to the frequency of acute tonsillitis in newly married persons.

Epidemic tonsillitis is not infrequent, the cases increasing in the community to epidemic proportions. As a rule it is impossible to trace it to any special cause. There are remarkable localized outbreaks, sometimes in institutions, which have been traced to milk infection. The one in Boston in 1911 was exceptionally severe, involving more than 1,000 persons, and the connection with the use of the milk from one dairy seems to have been clearly traced. More females than males were attacked, and a large proportion of the cases were adults.

The bacteriology has been carefully studied. The tonsils, swarming with saprophytic and pathogenic germs, are the main gates through which the invaders try to storm the town. Normally the protecting forces suffice to keep them at bay, but now and again a fiercer battle than usual rages, barricades have to be set up in the shape of exudates and necroses—and a local tonsillitis is the outward and visible sign of the struggle. Too often the enemy gains entrance, and streptococci, staphylococci, pneumococci, etc., pass to distant parts and excite arthritis, endocarditis, and serous membrane inflammations. In the Boston epidemic the streptococcus was the common germ, and the same holds good in the sporadic cases.

Morbid Anatomy.—The lacunæ of the tonsils become filled with exudation products, which form cheesy-looking masses, projecting from the orifices of the crypts. Not infrequently the exudations from contiguous lacunæ coalesce. The intervening mucosa is usually swollen, deep red in color, and may present herpetic vesicles, or, in some instances, even membranous exudation, in which case it may be difficult to distinguish the condition from diphtheria. The contents of the crypt are made up of micrococci and epithelial débris.

Symptoms.—Chilly feelings, or even a definite chill, and aching pains in the back and limbs may precede the onset. The fever rises rapidly and in the case of a young child may reach 105° F. on the evening of the first day. The patient complains of soreness of the throat and difficulty in swallowing. On examination the tonsils are seen to be swollen and the crypts present the characteristic exudate. The tongue is furred, the breath is heavy and foul, and the urine is highly colored and loaded with urates. In children the respirations are usually hurried and the pulse increased in rapidity. Swallowing is painful and the voice often becomes nasal. Slight swelling of the cervical glands is present.

In epidemic cases the fever may be very high, the secondary enlargement of the glands considerable, and even the deeper tissues may be involved. The complications are very serious: endocarditis, pericarditis, pneumococcic peritonitis, and pneumonia. In the Boston epidemic the clinical sequence was not unlike that seen in rheumatic fever—sore throat, adenitis, multiple arthritis, endocarditis, and pneumonia. Febrile albuminuria is common and acute nephritis may follow. A diffuse erythema may simulate scarlet fever. Acute otitis media is a frequent complication in children. Relapses are not uncommon and the tonsils may remain enlarged. Occasionally paralyses follow the streptococcus tonsillitis which are identical with those of diphtheria.

In the sporadic and mild epidemic form it is rare to see a fatal case, but in severe outbreaks the mortality from complications may be three or four per cent. There were about 50 deaths in the Boston epidemic.

Diagnosis.—It may be difficult to distinguish tonsillitis from diphtheria. In the follicular form, the individual yellowish-gray masses, separated by the reddish tonsillar tissue, are very characteristic; whereas in diphtheria the membrane is ashy-gray and uniform, not patchy. A point of the greatest importance in diphtheria is that the membrane is not limited to the tonsils, but creeps up the pillars of the fauces and appears on the uvula. The diphtheritic membrane, when removed, leaves a bleeding, eroded surface; whereas the exudation of lacunar tonsillitis is easily separated, and usually there is no erosion beneath it. In all doubtful cases cultures should be made to determine the presence or absence of the diphtheria bacillus.

Treatment.—The patient should be in bed and stay there until the attack is over. The diet should be liquid with soft foods added if desired. Water should be taken in large amounts. The bowels should be moved freely by a calomel and saline purge and kept open by daily doses of saline if required. Aconite in full doses often acts beneficially in children. The combination of salol and phenacetine (of each, gr. iii-v, 0.2-0.3 gm.) can be given every three hours. Acetylsalicylic acid (gr. v, 0.3 gm.) is often useful in relieving symptoms. Ten grains (0.6 gm.) of Dover's powder or codein (gr. ½, 0.03 gm.) may be given at night. One of the best applications to the throat is a 10 per cent. solution of silver nitrate. Gargles should only be used if they do not cause pain. Solutions of iron, iodine, phenol (1 per cent.), hydrogen peroxide (25 per cent.) or an alkaline antiseptic mixture may be employed. The application of sodium bicarbonate directly to the tonsils sometimes gives relief. An ice bag to the neck is usually an advantage. In convalescence abundant nourishment and a tonic, such as the tincture of nux vomica (♏ xv, 1 c. c.), are useful.

XII. ACUTE CATARRHAL FEVER

(*Acute Coryza*)

Definition.—An acute infection of the mucous membrane of the upper air passages associated with the presence of the *Micrococcus catarrhalis* alone, or with other organisms.

Etiology.—The micrococcus described by R. Pfeiffer is a diplococcus with close resemblance to the meningococcus and the pneumococcus. It is a normal habitant of the throat and bronchial secretions of many persons. In acute inflammatory conditions of the upper air passages it is found, sometimes in almost pure culture, in the sputum. It is readily cultivated.

Prevailing most extensively in the changeable weather of the spring and early winter, coryza may occur in epidemic form, many cases arising in a community within a few weeks, outbreaks which are very like though less intense than the epidemic influenza. More often it is a local outbreak among the members of a house or of a school.

Symptoms.—The patient feels indisposed, perhaps chilly, has slight headache, and sneezes frequently. In severe cases there are pains in the back and limbs. There is usually slight fever, the temperature rising to 101° F. The pulse is quick, the skin is dry, and there are all the features of a feverish attack. At first the mucous membrane of the nose is swollen, "stuffed up," and the patient has to breathe through the mouth. A thin, clear, irritating secretion flows, and makes the edges of the nostrils sore. The mucous membrane of the tear-ducts is swollen, so that the eyes weep and the conjunctivæ are injected. The sense of smell and, in part, the sense of taste are lost. With the nasal catarrh there is slight soreness of the throat and stiffness of the neck; the pharynx looks red and swollen, and sometimes the act of swallowing is painful. The larynx also may be involved and the voice becomes husky or is even lost. If the inflammation extends to the Eustachian tubes the hearing may be impaired. In more severe cases there are bronchial irritation and cough. Occasionally there is an outbreak of labial or nasal herpes. Usually within thirty-six hours the nasal secretion becomes turbid and more profuse, the swelling of the mucosa subsides, the patient gradually becomes able to breathe through the nostrils, and within four or five days the symptoms disappear, with the exception of the increased discharge from the nose and upper pharynx. There are rarely any bad effects from a simple coryza. When the attacks are frequently repeated the disease may become chronic.

Diagnosis.—This is always easy, but caution must be exercised lest the initial catarrh of measles or influenza be mistaken for the simple coryza.

Treatment.—Many attacks are so mild that the patients are able to be about and attend to their work. If there are fever and constitutional disturbance, the patient should be kept in bed and take a simple fever mixture, and at night a drink of hot lemonade and a full dose of Dover's powder. Many persons find great benefit from the Turkish bath. For the distressing sense of tightness and pain over the frontal sinuses, cocaine is useful and sometimes gives immediate relief. The 4-per-cent. solution may be injected into the nostrils or cotton wool soaked in it may be inserted into them. Ointments containing menthol and camphor may be applied locally. When the secretion is profuse atropine can be given in doses sufficient to lessen this. Simple saline or oily sprays are often employed but should be used very gently.

The vaccine treatment may be tried in persons subject to recurring colds, especially as a preventive.

XIII. FEBRICULA—EPHEMERAL FEVER

Definition.—Fever of slight duration, probably depending upon a variety of causes, some autogenous, others extrinsic and bacterial.

A febrile paroxysm lasting for twenty-four hours and disappearing completely is spoken of as ephemeral fever. If it persists for three, four, or more days without local affection it is referred to as febricula.

The cases may be divided into several groups:

(*a*) Those which represent mild or abortive types of the infectious diseases. It is not very unusual, during an epidemic of typhoid, scarlet fever, or measles, to see patients with some of the prodromal symptoms and slight fever, which persist for two or three days without any distinctive features. Possibly some of the cases are due to mild streptococcus infections.

(*b*) In a larger group of cases the symptoms develop with dyspepsia. In children indigestion and gastro-intestinal catarrh are often accompanied by fever. Possibly some instances of longer duration may be due to the absorption of toxic substances. Slight fever has been known to follow the eating of decomposing substances; but the gastric juice has remarkable antiseptic properties, and the frequency with which persons take from choice articles which are "high" shows that poisoning is not likely to occur unless there is existing gastro-intestinal disturbance.

(*c*) Cases which follow exposure to foul odors or sewer gas. That a febrile paroxysm may follow a prolonged exposure to noxious odors has been suggested. The cases described under this heading are of two kinds: an acute, severe form with nausea, vomiting, colic, and fever, followed perhaps by a condition of collapse or coma; secondly, a form of low fever with or without chills. A good deal of doubt exists about these cases of so-called sewer-gas poisoning. Workers in sewers are remarkably free from disease, and in many of the reported cases the illness may have been only a coincidence. There are instances in which persons have been taken ill with vomiting and slight fever after exposure to the odor of a very offensive post mortem. Whether true or not, the idea is firmly implanted in the minds of the laity that very powerful odors from decomposing matters may produce sickness.

(*d*) Many cases doubtless depend upon slight unrecognized lesions, such as tonsillitis or occasionally an abortive or larval pneumonia. Children are much more frequently affected than adults.

The *symptoms* set in, as a rule, abruptly, though in some instances there may have been preliminary *malaise* and indisposition. Headache, loss of appetite, and furred tongue are present. The urine is scanty and high-colored, the fever ranges from 101° to 103°, sometimes in children it rises higher. The cheeks may be flushed and the patient has the outward manifestations of fever. In children there may be bronchial catarrh with slight cough. Herpes on the lips is a common symptom. Occasionally in children the cerebral symptoms are marked at the outset, and there may be irritation, restlessness, and nocturnal delirium. The fever terminates abruptly by crisis from the second to the fourth day; in some instances it may continue for a week.

The *diagnosis* generally rests upon the absence of local manifestations, particularly the characteristic skin rashes of the eruptive fevers, and, most important of all, the rapid disappearance of the pyrexia. The cases most readily recognized are those with acute gastro-intestinal disturbance.

The *treatment* is that of mild pyrexia—rest in bed, a laxative, and a fever mixture containing nitrate of potassium and sweet spirits of nitre.

XIV. INFECTIOUS JAUNDICE

(*Epidemic Jaundice; Spirochætosis Ictero-Hæmorrhagica; Weil's Disease*)

There are several forms of infectious jaundice which may occur in epidemic form, due to a variety of organisms, some of which can be definitely determined. Outbreaks of the disease have occurred in many parts of the world and it was common in the recent war. Certain forms may be separated.

(1) *Epidemic catarrhal jaundice.*—This seems to be a definite entity, the cause of which is obscure but due to a common source rather than to infection from one to another. No proved etiological organism has been found. The early features are abdominal discomfort, gastric symptoms, diarrhœa or constipation, fever for two to four days, and malaise. Jaundice appears about the fourth day with pale stools and bile in the urine. The jaundice reaches a maximum in about ten days. There is enlargement of the liver and spleen, with tenderness of the former. Dilatation of the right heart is not uncommon but usually is present for a few days only. The mortality in a large series in soldiers was only 0.4 per cent. In some cases severe toxæmia or icterus gravis occurred.

(2) *Spirochætosis ictero-hæmorrhagica.*—Discovered in Japan in 1914, the *Spirochæta ictero-hæmorrhagica* has been found to be widely distributed. The infection in rats has been found in many countries. The onset is often acute. but may be gradual, with a chill, vertigo, headache and general pains, vomiting, diarrhœa and prostration. The temperature rises to 102° or over. Jaundice appears about the fourth day, reaching the maximum about the tenth day. Hæmorrhage is common, from the nose, gums, lungs, stomach and bowel. Herpes is common and often becomes hæmorrhagic. Purpura occurs in some cases. The liver may be enlarged and tender but the spleen is not enlarged. Myositis is common, the muscles being very tender and sometimes swollen. Nephritis may occur. Moderate leucocytosis is common. The course varies with the severity of the attack. The fever usually lasts for about ten days.

The spirochætes are in the blood in the first week. They may be found on examination or the infection may be conveyed to a guinea-pig by intraperitoneal injection of blood. The spirochætes are found in the urine in the later stages and are agglutinated by the patient's blood after the second week of the attack.' The mortality has varied greatly: in Japan it has been 30 per cent. but in some of the army series was only 4 to 6 per cent.

(3) *Weil's Disease.*—This term is applied to a disease described in 1886 with features much like the preceding, with a high mortality and marked splenic enlargement.

Treatment.—Rest, liquid diet, water freely, alkalies and open bowels, by salines and enemata, are indicated.

XV. MILK-SICKNESS

This remarkable disease prevails in certain districts of the United States, west of the Alleghany Mountains, and is connected with the affection in cattle known as the *trembles.* It prevailed extensively in the early settlements in certain of the Western States and proved very fatal. The general opinion is that it is communicated to man only by eating the flesh or drinking the milk of diseased animals. The butter and cheese are also poisonous. In animals, cattle and the young of horses and sheep are most susceptible. It is stated that cows giving milk do not themselves show marked symptoms unless driven rapidly, and, according to Graff, the secretion may be infective when the disease is latent. When a cow is very ill, food is refused, the eyes are injected, the animal staggers, the entire muscular system trembles, and death occurs in convulsions, sometimes with great suddenness. The disease is most frequent in new settlements.

In man the symptoms are those of a more or less acute intoxication. After a few days of uneasiness and distress the patient is seized with pains in the stomach, nausea and vomiting, fever and intense thirst. There is usually obstinate constipation. The tongue is swollen and tremulous, the breath is extremely foul, and, according to Graff, is as characteristic of the disease as is the odor in small-pox. Cerebral symptoms—restlessness, irritability, coma, and convulsions—are sometimes marked, and a typhoid state may gradually be produced in which the patient dies.

The duration is variable. In the most acute form death occurs within two or three days. It may last for ten days, or even for three or four weeks. Graff states that insanity occurred in one case. The poisonous nature of the flesh and milk has been demonstrated. An ounce of butter or cheese, or four ounces of the beef, raw or boiled, given three times a day, will kill a dog within six days. Fortunately, the disease has become rare. No definite pathological lesions are known. Jordan and Harris studied a New Mexico epidemic (1908) and found a bacillus (*B. lactimorbi*) with cultures of which the disease may be reproduced in other animals.

XVI. GLANDULAR FEVER

Definition.—An infectious disease of children, developing, as a rule, without premonitory signs, and characterized by slight redness of the throat, high fever, swelling and tenderness of the lymph-glands of the neck, particularly those behind the sterno-cleido-mastoid muscles. The fever is of short duration but the enlargement of the glands persists for ten days to three weeks.

In children acute adenitis of the cervical and other glands with fever had been noted by many observers, but Pfeiffer in 1889 called special attention to it under the name of *Druesenfieber.* He described it as an infectious disease of young children between the ages of five and eight years, characterized by the above-mentioned symptoms. A good deal of work has been done in connection with the subject, and in the United States West and Hamill, and in England Dawson Williams, have particularly emphasized the condition.

Etiology.—It may occur in epidemic form. West, of Bellaire, Ohio, described an epidemic of 96 cases in children between the ages of seven months and thirteen years. Bilateral swelling of the carotid lymph-glands was a most marked feature. In three-fourths of the cases the post-cervical, inguinal, and axillary glands were involved. The mesenteric glands were felt in 37 cases, the spleen was enlarged in 57, and the liver in 87 cases. Coryza was not present, and there were no bronchial or pulmonary symptoms. The nature of the infection has not been determined.

Symptoms.—The onset is sudden and the first complaint is of pain on moving the head and neck. There may be nausea and vomiting and abdominal pain. The temperature ranges from 101° to 103°. The tonsils may be a little red and the lymphatic tissues swollen, but the throat symptoms are quite transient and unimportant. On the second or third day the enlarged glands appear, and during the course they vary in size from a pea to a goose-egg. They are painful to the touch, but there is rarely any redness or swelling of the skin, though at times there is some puffiness of the subcutaneous tissues of the neck, and there may be a little difficulty in swallowing. In some instances there has been discomfort in the chest and a paroxysmal cough, indicating involvement of the tracheal and bronchial glands. The swelling of the glands persists for from two to three weeks. Among the serious features are the termination of the adenitis in suppuration, which seems rare (though Neumann met with it in 13 cases), and hæmorrhagic nephritis. Acute otitis media and retro-pharyngeal abscess have also been reported.

The outlook is favorable. West suggests the use of small doses of calomel during the height of the trouble.

XVII. MILIARY FEVER—SWEATING SICKNESS

The disease is characterized by fever, profuse sweats, and an eruption of miliary vesicles. It prevailed and was very fatal in England in the fifteenth and sixteenth centuries, and was made the subject of an important memoir by Johannes Caius, 1552. Of late years it has been confined entirely to certain districts in France (Picardy) and Italy. An epidemic of some extent occurred in France in 1887. Hirsch gives a chronological account of 194 epidemics between 1718 and 1879, many of which were limited to a single village or to a few localities. Occasionally the disease has become widely spread. Slight epidemics have occurred in Germany, Austria and Switzerland. They are usually of short duration, lasting only for three or four weeks—sometimes not more than seven or eight days. As in influenza, a large number of persons are attacked in rapid succession. In the mild cases there is only slight fever, with loss of appetite, and erythematous eruption, profuse perspiration, and an outbreak of miliary vesicles. The severe cases present the symptoms of intense infection—delirium, high fever, profound prostration, and hæmorrhage. The death-rate at the outset of the disease is usually high, and, as is so graphically described in the account of some of the epidemics of the middle ages, death may occur in a few hours.

XVIII. FOOT-AND-MOUTH DISEASE—EPIDEMIC STOMATITIS—APHTHOUS FEVER

Foot-and-mouth disease is an acute infectious disorder met with chiefly in cattle, sheep, and pigs, but attacking other domestic animals. It is of extraordinary activity, and spreads with "lightning rapidity" over vast territories. The nature of the ultra-microscopic virus has not been determined. In cattle, after a period of incubation of three or five days, the animal becomes feverish, the mucous membrane of the mouth swells, and little grayish vesicles the size of a hemp seed begin to develop on the edges and lower portion of the tongue, on the gums, and on the mucous membrane of the lips. They contain at first a clear fluid, which becomes turbid, and then they enlarge and gradually become converted into superficial ulcers. There is ptyalism, and the animals lose flesh rapidly. In the cow the disease is also frequently seen about the udder and teats, and the milk becomes yellowish-white in color and of a mucoid consistency.

The transmission to man is by no means uncommon, and several important epidemics have been studied in the neighborhood of Berlin. In Friedberger and Fröhner's Pathology and Therapeutics of Domestic Animals the disease is thus described: "In man the symptoms are: fever, digestive troubles, and vesicular eruption upon the lips, the buccal and pharyngeal mucous membranes (angina)." The disease is apparently transmitted by contact and by drinking the milk.

In widespread epidemics there has been sometimes a marked tendency to hæmorrhages. The disease runs, as a rule, a favorable course, but in Siegel's report of an epidemic the mortality was 8 per cent.

When epidemics are prevailing in cattle the milk should be boiled, and measures taken to isolate both the cattle and individuals who come in contact with them. The treatment is local, a mouth wash of potassium permanganate solution and the application of silver nitrate to the affected areas.

XIX. PSITTACOSIS

A disease in birds, characterized by loss of appetite, weakness, diarrhœa, convulsions, and death. In Germany, France, and Italy a disease in man characterized by an atypical pneumonia, great weakness and depression, and signs of a profound infection has been ascribed to contagion from birds, particularly parrots. There have usually been house epidemics with a very high rate of mortality. A few cases have been reported in England, and Vickery, of Boston, reported three probable cases. The bacteriology is doubtful.

XX. ROCKY MOUNTAIN SPOTTED FEVER; TICK FEVER

In the Bitter-root Valley of Montana and in the mountains of Idaho, Nevada, and Wyoming there is an acute infection characterized by chill, fever, pains in back and bones, and a macular rash, becoming hæmorrhagic. It was reported upon occasionally by army surgeons—e. g., Wood—but nothing definite was known until the studies of Wilson and Chowning (1902), who believed the disease to be transmitted by ticks. The studies of King and Ricketts demonstrated the transmission of the disease by the tick, *Dermacentor venustus.* Wolbach considers that the cause of the disease is a minute parasite which he thinks is probably a new organism. The lesions are endothelial cell proliferation, local necrosis of endothelium, and thrombosis. Perivascular accumulations of endothelial cells are common. The disease is readily given to the guinea-pig and monkey, and is transmissible from one animal to another by the bite of the tick. Immunity is given by an attack, and in animals this is transmitted to the young. After an incubation of from three to ten days the disease begins with a chill, fever, and severe pains in the limbs. The *rash* appears from the second to the seventh day, is macular, dark, and becomes hæmorrhagic. Illustrations of it show a rash not unlike that of typhus. The skin is often swollen. Hæmorrhages from the mucous membranes are not uncommon. The temperature range is from 103° to 105° F., and at the height of the disease there are delirium and stupor. Convalescence begins in the fourth week. The death-rate is high for an eruptive fever, reaching 70 per cent. in Montana, but in Idaho it is not more than 2 or 3 per cent. As a prophylactic measure, destruction of the ticks by dipping or scouring the horses and cattle should be carried out. The treatment is that of an acute infection.

XXI. SWINE FEVER

A few cases have been described from accidental inoculation in the preparation of cultures and in making post mortems upon pigs. In the course of from twelve hours to three days there is swelling of the fingers of the affected hand, which have a blue-red color, and small nodules form. In some of the instances the course has been like that of a painful erythema migrans, with swelling of the lymph-glands. A specific serum has been used with success in several cases.

XXII. RAT-BITE FEVER

A remarkable infection, following rat-bite, characterized by brief febrile paroxysms which may recur at intervals for months.

The disease has been known in China and Japan for several centuries. The features are very unusual. There is a prolonged period of incubation, lasting in some cases for many months. The wound, which has run the ordinary course and perhaps healed, becomes swollen, red, and eroded; an ulcer forms and the regional lymph-glands are involved. The fever sets in suddenly with a chill and lasts three or four days. With its onset there is a skin rash, either erythema or a blotchy eruption somewhat resembling measles. The patient feels very ill, there may be pains in the muscles and joints and sometimes delirium. After persisting for a few days, the temperature falls and the patient feels well. After a varying interval of from a few days to a couple of weeks the attack is repeated, and this may go on for several months or, according to the Japanese reports, for several years. The outlook is favorable; among 49 Japanese cases only 1 died.

In Horder's last case the boy was bitten on September 15th. From October 6th to 11th, on the 13th, 14th, 17th, 18th, 19th, 23d, 24th, 25th, 28th to 30th, and November 4th, 5th, and 6th, he had attacks of fever, the temperature rising to between 104° and 105° F., and once reaching nearly 106°. Each attack was associated with a rash.

Various organisms have been described. In one of Horder's cases spirilla were seen. Ogata describes a sporozoan parasite, and Proescher a bacillus. Japanese observers have reported spirochætes and suggested the name *Spirochæta morsus-muris*. Patients recovered after treatment by mercury or arsphenamine. Schotmüller, Blake and Tileston each found a streptothrix in their cases. In Tileston's case the organisms were found in fresh smears by dark-field illumination. Blake isolated a streptothrix in a case which at autopsy showed endocarditis, in the vegetations of which the same organism was found.

Treatment.—The wound should be cauterized, arsphenamine given intravenously, and the febrile paroxysms treated symptomatically.

XXIII. TRENCH FEVER

Definition.—An acute infection, with a short period of fever, followed by a second rise or by two or three or more paroxysms of one or two days' duration. The organism, as yet unknown, is transmitted through the louse.

History.—The disease was first recognized in 1915 during the War. As it is not likely to be prevalent in civil life only a brief description is necessary.

Symptoms.—The disease usually sets in acutely with chilliness, headache, and general pains, the latter sometimes of great severity. The fever is usually not high and of two or three days' duration. After an afebrile period one or more recurrences lasting for one or two days are very characteristic. In some instances the fever lasted for four or five days. The greatest complaint was of *tender shins*. As a rule there was no swelling or redness, and the pain was usually most marked at night. The course of the fever and the tender shins are the two most important aids in diagnosis. Many cases were regarded at first as influenza. There is no specific treatment. Complete rest is important and acetylsalicylic acid sometimes relieved the pain. A local application of a saturated solution of magnesium sulphate sometimes gave relief.

XXIV. ACUTE ULCERATIVE CONJUNCTIVITIS TRANSMITTED FROM RABBITS

In the United States there is a disease of rodents, particularly in rabbits, the ground squirrels, guinea-pigs and rats, characterized by enlargement of the lymph glands, and features suggestive of plague; but the organism was isolated by McCoy and Chapin and shown to be the *Bacterium tularense*, which is possibly transmitted by flies. Man is sometimes affected, and Wherrey reported two cases characterized by acute ulcerative conjunctivitis, enlargement of the pre-auricular and cervical glands, fever and great debility. Both of the patients had been cutting up wild rabbits in preparation for cooking.

XXV. SIX (SEVEN) DAY FEVER

This is described by Rogers as occurring in the seaports in India; it is uncommon in the tropics and is regarded by many as a variety of dengue. An organism of the colon group has been isolated from the blood. The disease begins suddenly, the temperature shows marked remissions, skin rashes are common, usually a blotchy erythema, sometimes with petechiæ. It terminates on the sixth or seventh day by crisis, and when the date of onset is known the defervescence may be predicted within a few hours. Rogers shows that the disease is common in India, and it was described by Deakes in 1911-12 in the Canal Zone.

SECTION II

DISEASES DUE TO PHYSICAL AGENTS

I. SUNSTROKE; HEAT EXHAUSTION

(*Insolation, Thermic Fever, Siriasis*)

Definition.—Under these terms are comprised certain manifestations following exposure to excessive heat, of which thermic fever or sunstroke, heat exhaustion, and heat cramps are the common forms.

History.—It is one of the oldest of recognized diseases. The case of the son of the Shunammite woman (2 Kings, IV) is perhaps the oldest on record. The Arabians called the symptoms due to excessive heat "Siriasis," after Sirius the Dog Star. Cardan recognized it in the sixteenth century and thought it was apoplexy due to heat—morbus attonitus. In the eighteenth century Boerhaave regarded it as phrenitis. It was not until the nineteenth century that the Anglo-Indian surgeons and the physicians of the United States gave us a full knowledge of the different affections due to excessive heat. Various classifications have been suggested, but two chief forms are everywhere recognized—heat exhaustion and thermic fever or sunstroke—to which Edsall added the remarkable heat cramps which occur in persons working under very high external temperatures.

Distribution.—Sunstroke occurs in the tropics and in temperate regions during protracted heat waves. It is very common in the Atlantic Coast cities of the United States during the hot spells of summer. Heat exhaustion is frequently met with in conditions similar to those in which sunstroke takes place, and it is not infrequent in the engine-rooms of large steamships, less often in foundries. In the U. S. Navy in 35 years (to 1913) there were 20 deaths and 33 invalided on account of heat prostration (Fiske).

Heat Exhaustion.—In the tropics and in temperate regions during protracted heat waves many persons become depressed physically and are unable to work or take nourishment. In children the condition is very often associated with gastro-intestinal disturbances and fever. The true heat syncope is specially seen in persons who have not been in good health or who are intemperate. The heat may be that of the sun or artificial heat, as in the engine-rooms of steamers. The symptoms begin with giddiness, nausea, an uncertain, staggering gait; there is pallor, the pulse is small, the heart's action weak, the respirations rapid, and the patient may quickly become unconscious. Muscular spasms, often painful, are common. Externally the body may be clammy, with sweat, but as a rule the rectal temperature is decreased. In the axilla it may be as low as 95° or 96° F. From slight attacks, such as are seen in steamships, the patients recover rapidly when brought on deck; in other cases the unconsciousness may end in deep coma and death.

Thermic Fever.—This is more common in men than in women and children, and is principally seen in persons who work in very high external temperatures, and who are too heavily clad, or who are addicted to alcohol. In India regiments on the march are not infrequently attacked. It is more common in Europeans than in the dark races, but in the United States negroes are often attacked.

Morbid Anatomy.—Rigor mortis occurs early. Putrefactive changes may come on with great rapidity. The venous engorgement is extreme, particularly in the cerebrum. The left ventricle is contracted (Wood) and the right chamber dilated. The blood is usually fluid; the lungs are intensely congested. Parenchymatous changes occur in the liver and kidneys.

Symptoms.—The patient may be struck down and die within an hour, with symptoms of heart-failure, dyspnœa, and coma. This form, sometimes known as the asphyxial, occurs chiefly in soldiers and is graphically described by Parkes. Death indeed may be almost instantaneous, the victims falling as if struck upon the head. The more usual form comes on during exposure, with pain in the head, dizziness, a feeling of oppression, and sometimes nausea and vomiting. Visual disturbances are common, and a patient may have colored vision. Diarrhœa or frequent micturition may supervene. Insensibility follows, which may be transient or which deepens into a profound coma. The patients are usually admitted to hospital in an unconscious state, with the face flushed, the skin hot, the pulse rapid and full, and the temperature ranging from 107° to 110° F., or even higher. The breathing is labored and deep, sometimes stertorous. Usually there is complete relaxation of the muscles, but twitchings, jactitation, or very rarely convulsions may occur. The pupils may at first be dilated, but by the time the patients are admitted to hospital they are (in a majority) extremely contracted. Petechiæ may be present upon the skin. In the fatal cases the coma deepens, the cardiac pulsations become more rapid and feeble, the breathing becomes hurried and shallow and of the Cheyne-Stokes type. The fatal termination may occur within twenty-four or thirty-six hours. Favorable indications are the return of consciousness and a fall in the fever. The recovery in these cases may be complete. In other instances there are remarkable after-effects, the most constant of which is a permanent inability to bear high temperatures. Such patients become very uneasy when the thermometer reaches 80° F. in the shade. Loss of the power of mental concentration and failure of memory are troublesome sequelæ. Such patients are always worse in the hot weather. Occasionally there are convulsions, followed by marked mental disturbance. Dercum has described peripheral neuritis as a sequence.

Many observers have called attention to a fever in the tropics which lasts for a few days, with no special symptoms other than those of pyrexia and weakness. This may be simply heat exhaustion. It is not uncommon in the Southern States, where it may be mistaken for malaria or mild typhoid fever. John Guitéras, who has unrivalled knowledge of tropical affections, regards these conditions as directly due to prolonged high external temperatures.

Diagnosis.—It is rarely difficult to distinguish thermic fever from the malignant types of malaria and from the various other forms of coma. The diagnosis in heat exhaustion or thermic fever is readily made. In the one the skin is moist, pale, and cool, the pulse small and soft, and consciousness may remain till near the end; whereas in the other there is high fever with early unconsciousness.

Prognosis.—In the old, the infirm, and alcoholic subjects the mortality during a very hot wave may be as high as 30 or 40 per cent. In New York and Philadelphia the death-rate varies very much in different seasons.

Treatment.—In heat exhaustion stimulants should be given freely, and if the temperature is below normal the hot bath should be used. Ammonia may be given if necessary. In thermic fever the indications are to reduce

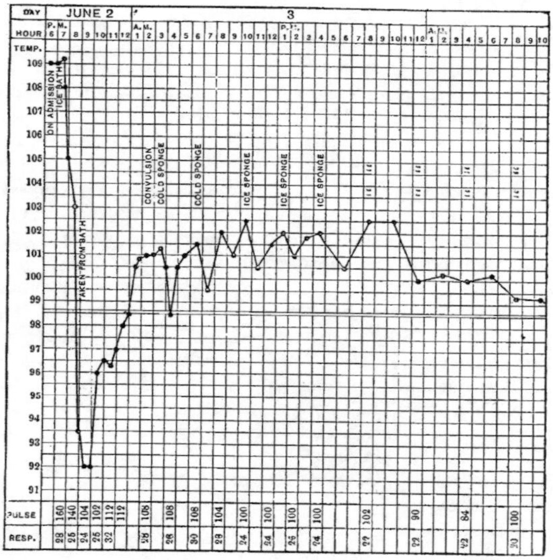

Chart XII.—Case of Sunstroke Treated by the Ice-bath; Recovery.

the temperature as rapidly as possible. Rubbing the body with ice was practised at the New York Hospital by Darrach in 1857, and is an excellent procedure to lower the temperature rapidly. The wet or ice pack or the bath may be used. Ice-water enemata may also be employed. In the cases in which the symptoms are those of intense asphyxia, and in which death may take place in a few minutes, free bleeding should be practised, a procedure which saved Weir Mitchell when a young man. For the convulsions, chloroform should be given at once. Of other remedies, the antipyretics have been employed, and may be given when there is any special objection to hydrotherapy, for which, however, they cannot be substituted.

Heat Cramps.—Persons who use the muscles while exposed to a very high temperature are liable to attacks of severe cramp. The condition, which has been described very thoroughly by Edsall, occurs principally in stokers in the furnace-rooms of steamships and in workers in iron foundries. The spasms occur spontaneously, chiefly in the muscles of the calves, the arms, and sometimes in the abdomen; they are often of great intensity and very painful. A movement, pressure, or any stimulus, as electricity, may send the muscle into spasm at once. In addition to ordinary cramps there are sometimes fibrillary contractions. The attacks may last for from 12 to 34 hours and are followed by muscular soreness and sometimes by great weakness.

II. CAISSON DISEASE

(*Compressed Air Disease; Diver's Paralysis*)

Definition.—A disease of caisson workers and divers, due to a saturation of the tissues with nitrogen under the increased pressure. If the decompression takes place quickly, a too-rapid escape of the nitrogen as bubbles into the blood causes air embolism.

History.—The French writers, Bucquoy, Foley, and Bert, first studied the disease. Leyden recognized the anatomical changes. A. H. Smith and others in the United States contributed important papers, and the studies of Haldane, Leonard Hill, and Boycott have thrown light upon the etiology and means of prevention.

Etiology.—The cases are met with chiefly in workers in caissons and tunnels and in divers. "The higher the pressure and the shorter the period of decompression the greater is the risk" (Hill). In caissons the pressure is rarely 30 to 35 pounds, but in the St. Louis bridge the pressure reached as high as 45 to 50 pounds. Divers go down to 20 fathoms with a pressure of 53 pounds; the record depth attained by divers is 210 feet (Hill). The disease may also occur in very deep mines.

In building the St. Louis bridge across the Mississippi, among 352 workers there were 50 cases of paralysis and 14 deaths. In constructing the East River tunnels in New York, among 10,000 men employed there were 3,692 cases. Twenty fatal cases occurred, with symptoms of nausea, vomiting, rapid prostration and paralysis.

Pathology.—To Hoppe-Seyler, Bucquoy, and Paul Bert we owe a rational explanation of the disease. During compression the blood passing through the lungs becomes saturated with nitrogen, which is carried to the tissues until the whole body is saturated. "The mass of blood is about 5 per cent. of the body, and the capacity of the tissues to dissolve N is estimated by Boycott as 35 times that of the blood—in a fat man considerably more" (Hill). With active work it does not take long to effect complete saturation. During decompression the process is just the reverse. "The blood gives up N to the alveolar air and returns to the tissues for more. Those organs in which the circulation is rapid will yield up their N quickly, and those with a sluggish circulation slowly . . . . . and at the end of decompression a condition may be set up in which the slow tissues still hold, say 3 per cent. of N, while the blood can dissolve only 1 per cent. Herein we have a danger of bubbles forming" (Hill). The nitrogen in the body fluids begins to dissolve out as soon as the pressure is lowered. This is only harmful if the nitrogen separates in the form of bubbles. These may form in the blood, in the synovial fluid of the joints, and in the nervous system. As a rule a very rapid reduction in pressure must occur before the formation of the bubbles follows. Experimentally all the symptoms can be produced in goats, and the spinal cord may contain numerous air emboli. This was the anatomical lesion determined by Leyden, who found fissuring and laceration of the cord, which explains the paraplegia. Pulmonary air embolism also occurs and is responsible for certain features. In an analysis of gas from the right heart, Erdman found 80 per cent. of N and 20 per cent. of CO_2.

Symptoms.—Within from half an hour to one hour after leaving the caisson, the patient may have headache, giddiness and feel faint, symptoms which may pass off and leave no further trouble. In other instances the patients have severe pains in the extremities, usually the legs and the abdomen, sometimes associated with nausea and vomiting—attacks which the workmen usually speak of as "the bends." The pains may be of the greatest intensity and associated with giddiness and vomiting. The paralysis, usually of the legs, comes on rapidly, and varies in degree from a slight paralysis to complete loss both of motion and sensation. This occurred in 15 per cent. of A. H. Smith's cases and in 61 per cent. of the St. Louis cases. Monoplegia and hemiplegia are rare. In extreme instances the attacks resemble apoplexy; the patient rapidly becomes comatose and death occurs in a few hours. The paraplegia may be permanent, but in slight cases it gradually disappears and recovery may be complete. Late resulting features are spinal cord changes, chronic arthritis and deafness.

Prophylaxis.—The only safeguard is a gradual decompression, which obviates the risk of rapidly setting free the nitrogen from the tissues. Haldane and his colleagues introduced what they call the "Stage Method," which is now widely adopted with the most beneficial results. For work in very high pressures the shifts should be short, not more than two hours.

Treatment.—The caisson workers found very early that the best remedy for "the bends" was immediate recompression, and Andrew H. Smith of New York introduced a medical air-lock for the Brooklyn bridge workers. The workers should live and sleep not far from the works, where such an air-lock should be provided for immediate treatment. Cases with severe symptoms may be saved by recompression. Hot fomentations, massage and hypodermics of morphia may be necessary for the extreme pains.

III. MOUNTAIN SICKNESS

Definition.—An illness associated with adaptation to low atmospheric pressures, characterized by cyanosis, nausea, headache, intestinal disturbances, hyperpnœa and sometimes fainting.

Pathology.—The symptoms are directly referable to want of oxygen produced by the diminished pressure of the atmosphere. Haldane, Douglas and Henderson made an exhaustive study of the process of accommodation in a five weeks' residence at the top of Pike's Peak. After acclimatization the symptoms above mentioned disappeared, but dyspnœa, blueness and periodic breathing are apt to follow exertion. The alveolar carbon dioxide pressure was reduced from about 40 mm. to about 27 mm. during rest, which corresponded to an increase of about 50 per cent. in the ventilation of the lung alveoli.. This process of accommodation is associated with a remarkable increase in the red blood corpuscles and hæmoglobin to 120 to 150 per cent. These authors conclude that the acclimatization is largely due to increased secretory activity of the alveolar epithelium, to the greater lung ventilation and to the increased hæmoglobin production.

The disturbance known as "Aviators' Sickness" also involves the problem of a low barometric pressure. The pressure of the oxygen in the arterial blood in high altitudes may be higher than in the alveolar air. Active secretion of oxygen occurs in the lungs; that is the passage of oxygen is accelerated and this apparently has a selective action. There is a tendency to bradycardia in aviators after a sudden descent, which is probably a part of a vagobulbar syndrome.

Symptoms.—The symptoms just given, which are the most important, pass away gradually, but may return on exertion. In feeble persons the heart's action may be weak and intermittent, and syncope may follow any effort. Whymper in the ascent of Chimborazo at a height of 16,000 feet had headache, fever, gasping respiration and great weakness. Nausea, vomiting, bleeding at the nose, ringing in the ears and palpitation are not infrequent symptoms.

IV. GAS POISONING

Carbon Monoxide.—Acute cases of poisoning with illuminating gas are comparatively common. The frequency of chronic gas poisoning is difficult to state. In occupations about furnaces in many trades and in mining (carbon monoxide derived from the explosive) there are possibilities of poisoning. The chief effect of the carbon monoxide is to displace the oxygen from the oxyhæmoglobin and so reduce the oxygen-carrying function.

The main *symptoms* are a general feeling of illness, headache, vertigo, nausea and vomiting, and marked muscular weakness. If the dose is large the subject becomes drowsy and then unconscious. Muscular twitchings and convulsions often occur. At this stage the respiration is usually rapid, the pulse is rapid also, and usually weak. Cyanosis is marked, accompanied by a peculiar redness of the skin. The blood has a bright red color. Pulmonary complications are important, particularly broncho-pneumonia, and any of them may appear some time after the poisoning. A great variety of nervous sequels have resulted, neuritis, tremor, paralyses, etc.

In chronic poisoning, headache, vertigo, nausea, weakness and sometimes mental disturbance are common. The diagnosis is rarely in doubt in the acute cases. The odor of the breath may be characteristic and the spectroscopic test is positive.

The *treatment* consists in removal from the poisoned atmosphere, free use of oxygen with artificial respiration in some form, free venesection with transfusion of blood or the administration of salt solution subcutaneously. Active stimulation should be given when necessary.

Carbon Bisulphide.—This is used to treat india rubber and poisoning may occur. Headache, vertigo, insomnia and depression are common. Subsequently areas of anæsthesia may occur and paræsthesias of various kinds. Vision and taste may both show changes. A great variety of symptoms from disturbance of the nervous system results and organic nervous diseases may be closely simulated. Prophylactic measures are usually successful and the treatment is symptomatic.

Gas-poisoning in War.—Our interest is now concerned with the after-effects in those who were gassed. Several possibilities exist. (1) The psychical result is a factor in some cases, but time should help the majority of them. (2) Actual damage to the respiratory tract. Some show this but the exact effects are difficult to estimate; chronic bronchitis and emphysema are the most important. (3) Changes in the respiratory exchange which may be a permanent result. (4) There is no evidence that there is any increased liability to tuberculosis.

SECTION III

THE INTOXICATIONS

I. ALCOHOLISM

(a) Acute Alcoholism.—When a large quantity of alcohol is taken, the influence is chiefly on the nervous system, and is manifested in muscular incoordination, mental disturbance, and, finally, narcosis. The individual presents a flushed, sometimes slightly cyanosed face, the pulse is full, respirations deep but rarely stertorous. The pupils are dilated. The temperature is frequently below normal, particularly if the patient has been exposed to cold. Perhaps the lowest reported temperatures have been in cases of this sort. An instance is on record in which the patient on admission to hospital had a temperature of 24° C. (ca. 75° F.), and ten hours later the temperature had not risen to 91° F. The unconsciousness is rarely so deep that the patient cannot be roused to some extent, and in reply to questions he mutters incoherently. Muscular twitchings may occur, but rarely convulsions. The breath has a heavy alcoholic odor. The respirations may be slow; in one case they were only six in the minute.

The diagnosis is not difficult, yet mistakes are frequently made. Persons are brought to a hospital by the police supposed to be drunk when in reality they are dying from apoplexy. Too great care cannot be exercised, and the patient should receive the benefit of the doubt. In some instances the mistake has arisen from the fact that a person who has been drinking heavily has been stricken with apoplexy. In this condition the coma is usually deeper, stertor is present, and there may be evidence of hemiplegia in the greater flaccidity of the limbs on one side. The diagnosis will be considered in the section upon uræmic coma.

Dipsomania is a form of acute alcoholism seen in persons with a strong hereditary tendency to drink. Periodically the victims go "on a spree," but in the intervals they are entirely free from any craving for alcohol.

(b) Chronic Alcoholism.—In moderation, wine, beer, and spirits may be taken throughout a long life without impairing the general health.

The poisonous effects of alcohol are manifested (1) as a functional poison, as in acute narcosis; (2) as a tissue poison, in which its effects are seen on the parenchymatous elements, particularly epithelium and nerve, producing a slow degeneration, and on the blood vessels, causing thickening and ultimately fibroid changes; and (3) as a checker of tissue oxidation, since the alcohol is consumed in place of the fat. This leads to fatty changes and sometimes to a condition of general steatosis.

The chief effects of chronic alcohol poisoning may be thus summarized:

Nervous System.—Functional disturbance is common. Unsteadiness of the muscles in performing any action is a constant feature. The tremor is best seen in the hands and in the tongue. The mental processes may be dull, particularly in the early morning hours, and the patient is unable to transact any business until he has had his accustomed stimulant. Irritability of temper, forgetfulness, and a change in the moral character of the individual gradually come on. The judgment is seriously impaired, the will enfeebled, and in the final stages dementia may supervene. An interesting combination of symptoms in chronic alcoholics is characterized by peripheral neuritis, loss of memory, and pseudo-reminiscences—that is, false notions as to the patient's position in time and space, and fabulous explanations of real occurrences. The peripheral neuritis is not always present; there may be only tremor and jactitation of the lips, and thickness of the speech, with visual hallucinations. The mental condition was described by Jackson and by Wilks. Korsakoff speaks of it as a *psychosis polyneuritica,* and the symptom-complex is sometimes called by his name. The relation of chronic alcoholism to insanity has been much discussed. It is one of the important elements in the strain which leads to mental breakdown. Epilepsy may result directly from chronic drinking. It is a hopeful form, and may disappear entirely with a return to habits of temperance.

There is a remarkable condition in chronic alcoholism termed *"wet brain,"* in which a heavy drinker, who may perhaps have had attacks of delirium tremens, begins to get drowsy or a little more befuddled than usual; gradually the stupor deepens until he becomes comatose, in which state he may remain for weeks. There may be slight fever, but there are no signs of paralysis, and no optic neuritis. The urine may be normal. The lumbar puncture yields a clear fluid, but under high pressure. In one patient who died at the end of six weeks, there were the anatomical features of a serous meningitis.

No characteristic changes are found in the nervous system. Hæmorrhagic pachymeningitis is not very uncommon. There are opacity and thickening of the pia-arachnoid membranes, with more or less wasting of the convolutions. These are in no way peculiar to chronic alcoholism, but are found in old persons and in chronic wasting diseases. In the very protracted cases there may be chronic encephalo-meningitis with adhesions of the membranes. Finer changes in the nerve-cells, their processes, and the neuroglia have been described. The alcoholic neuritis will be considered later.

Digestive System.—Catarrh of the stomach is the most common symptom. The toper has a furred tongue, heavy breath, and in the morning a sensation of sinking at the stomach until he has had his dram. The appetite is usually impaired and the bowels are constipated. In beer-drinkers dilatation of the stomach is common.

Alcohol produces definite changes in the liver, leading ultimately to the various forms of cirrhosis. In Welch's laboratory J. Friedenwald caused typical cirrhosis in rabbits by the administration of alcohol. The effect is a primary degenerative change in the liver-cells. A special vulnerability of the liver-cells is necessary in the etiology of alcoholic cirrhosis. There are cases in which comparatively moderate drinking for a few years has been followed by cirrhosis; on the other hand, the livers of persons who have been steady drinkers for thirty or forty years may show only a moderate grade of sclerosis. For years before cirrhosis develops heavy drinkers may present an enlarged and tender liver, with at times swelling of the spleen. With the gastric and hepatic disorders the facies often becomes very characteristic. The venules of the cheeks and nose are dilated; the latter becomes enlarged, red, and may present the condition known as *acne rosacea*. The eyes are watery, and conjunctivæ hyperæmic and sometimes bile-tinged.

The *heart and arteries* in chronic topers show degenerative changes, and alcoholism is a factor in causing arterio-sclerosis. Steell pointed out the frequency of cardiac dilatation in these cases.

Kidneys.—The influence of chronic alcoholism upon these organs is by no means so marked. According to Dickinson the total of renal disease is not greater in the drinking class, and he holds that the effect of alcohol on the kidneys has been much overrated. Formad directed attention to the fact that in a large proportion of chronic alcoholics the kidneys are increased in size. The Guy's Hospital statistics support this statement, and Pitt notes that in 43 per cent. of the bodies of hard drinkers the kidneys were hypertrophied without showing morbid change. A granular kidney may result indirectly through the arterial changes.

It was formerly thought that alcohol was in some way antagonistic to tuberculous disease, but the reverse is the case and chronic drinkers are much more liable to both acute and pulmonary tuberculosis. It is probably altogether a question of altered tissue-soil, the alcohol lowering the vitality and enabling the bacilli to develop and grow more readily.

(c) Delirium tremens, an incident in chronic alcoholism, results from the long-continued action of the poison. The condition was first accurately described early in the 19th century by Sutton, of Greenwich, who had numerous opportunities for studying the different forms among sailors. One of the most careful studies of the disease was made by Ware, of Boston. A spree in a temperate person, no matter how prolonged, is rarely if ever followed by delirium tremens; but in the case of an habitual drinker a temporary excess may bring on an attack or it follows the sudden withdrawal of alcohol. An accident, a sudden shock, or an acute inflammation, particularly pneumonia, may determine the onset. It is especially apt to occur in drinkers admitted to hospitals for injuries, especially fractures, and, as this seems most likely to occur when alcohol is withdrawn, it is well to give such patients a moderate amount of alcohol. At the outset of the attack the patient is restless and depressed and sleeps badly; after a day or two the characteristic delirium sets in. The patient talks constantly and incoherently; he is incessantly in motion, and desires to go out and attend to some imaginary business. Hallucinations of sight and hearing develop. He sees objects in the room, such as rats or mice, and fancies that they are crawling over his body. The terror inspired by these imaginary objects is great and the patients need to be watched constantly, for in their delusions they may jump out of the window or escape. Auditory hallucinations are not so common, but the patient may complain of hearing animals or the threats of imaginary enemies. There is much muscular tremor; the tongue is covered with a thick white fur and is tremulous. The pulse is soft, rapid, and readily compressed. There is usually fever, but the temperature rarely registers above 102° or 103°. In fatal cases it may be higher. Insomnia is a constant feature. On the third or fourth day in favorable cases the restlessness abates, the patient sleeps, and improvement gradually sets in. The tremor persists for some days, the hallucinations gradually disappear, and the appetite returns. In more serious cases the insomnia persists, the delirium is incessant, the pulse becomes more frequent and feeble, the tongue dry, the prostration extreme, and death takes place from gradual heart-failure.

Some regard *mania a potu* as a distinct form in which the onset is sudden and the patients are very violent, but hallucinations and terror are rare.

There is a condition termed *acute hallucinosis,* in which auditory hallucinations are marked, orientation is retained, and the mental disturbances are fixed. Ideas of persecution are common. There are intermediate forms between this and the ordinary delirium tremens.

Diagnosis.—The clinical picture can scarcely be confounded with any other. Cases with fever may be mistaken for meningitis. The most common error is to overlook some local disease, such as pneumonia, or an injury, as a fractured rib, which in a chronic drinker may precipitate an attack of delirium tremens. In every instance a careful examination should be made, particularly of the lungs. It is to be remembered that in the severer forms, particularly the febrile cases, congestion of the bases of the lungs is by no means uncommon. Another point to be borne in mind is the fact that pneumonia of the apex may be accompanied by similar delirium.

Prognosis.—Recovery takes place in a large proportion of the cases in private practice. In hospital practice, particularly in large city hospitals to which debilitated patients are taken, the death-rate is higher. Gerhard states that of 1,241 cases admitted to the Philadelphia Hospital 121 proved fatal. Recurrence is frequent, indeed, the rule, if the drinking is kept up.

Treatment.—Acute alcoholism rarely requires any special measures, as the patient sleeps off the effects of the debauch. In the case of profound alcoholic coma it may be advisable to wash out the stomach, and if collapse symptoms occur the limbs should be rubbed and hot applications made to the body. Should convulsions supervene, chloroform may be carefully administered. In the acute, violent alcoholic mania the hypodermic injection of apomorphia, one-eighth of a grain (0.008 gm.), is usually very effectual, causing nausea and vomiting, and rapid disappearance of the maniacal symptoms.

Chronic alcoholism is a condition very difficult to treat, and once fully established the habit is rarely abandoned. The most obstinate cases are those with marked hereditary tendency. Withdrawal of the alcohol is the first essential. This is most effectually accomplished by placing the patient in an institution, in which he can be carefully watched. The absence of temptation in institution life is of special advantage. For the sleeplessness the bromides or hyoscine may be employed. Quinine and strychnine in tonic doses may be given. Prolonged seclusion in a suitable institution is in reality the only effectual means of cure. When an hereditary tendency exists a lapse into the drinking habit is almost inevitable.

In *delirium tremens* the patient should be confined to bed and carefully watched night and day. The danger of escape in these cases is very great, as the patient imagines himself pursued by enemies or demons. Flint mentions the case of a man who escaped in his nightclothes and ran barefooted for fifteen miles on the frozen ground before he was overtaken. The patient should not be strapped in bed, as this aggravates the delirium; sometimes, however, it may be necessary, in which case a sheet tied across the bed may be sufficient, and this is certainly better than violent restraint by three or four men. Alcohol should be withdrawn at once unless the pulse is feeble.

Delirium tremens is a disease which, in a large majority of cases, runs a course very slightly influenced by medicine. The indications for treatment are to procure sleep and to support the strength. In mild cases half a dram (2 gm.) of bromide of potassium combined with tincture of capsicum may be given every three hours. Chloral is often of great service, and may be given without hesitation unless the heart's action is feeble. Good results sometimes follow the hypodermic use of hyoscine (gr. 1/100, 0.00065 gm.). Opium must be used cautiously. A special merit of Ware's work was the demonstration that on an expectant plan of treatment the percentage of recoveries was greater than with the indiscriminate use of sedatives, which had been in vogue for many years. When opium is indicated it should be given as morphia, hypodermically. The effect should be carefully watched, and, if after three or four quarter-grain doses have been given the patient is still restless and excited, it is best not to push it farther. Repeated doses of trional (grs. xv, 1 gm.) every four hours may be tried. Lambert advises ergotin hypodermically in both the acute and chronic alcoholism. With acidosis alkalies and water should be given freely. When fever is present the tranquilizing effects of a douche or bath may be tried, or the cold or warm packs. The large doses of digitalis formerly employed are not advisable.

Careful feeding is the most important element in the treatment of these cases. Milk and concentrated food should be given at stated intervals. If the pulse becomes rapid and shows signs of flagging, alcohol may be given in combination with the aromatic spirit of ammonia.

II. MORPHIA HABIT

Taken at first to allay pain, a craving for the drug is gradually engendered, and the habit in this way acquired. The effects of the constant use of opium vary very much. In the East, where opium-smoking is as common as tobacco-smoking with us, the ill effects are, according to good observers, not very striking. Taken as morphia and hypodermically, as is the rule, it is very injurious, but a moderate amount may be taken for years without serious damage.

The habit is particularly prevalent among women and physicians who use the hypodermic syringe for the alleviation of pain, as in neuralgia or sciatica. The acquisition of the habit as a pure luxury is rare.

Symptoms.—The symptoms at first are slight and for months there may be no disturbance of health. There are exceptional instances in which for a period of years excessive amounts have been taken without deterioration of the mental or bodily functions. As a rule, the dose necessary to obtain the desired sensation has gradually to be increased. As the effects wear off the victim experiences sensations of lassitude and mental depression, accompanied often with slight nausea and epigastric distress, or even recurring colic, which may be mistaken for appendicitis. The confirmed opium-eater usually has a sallow, pasty complexion, is emaciated, and becomes prematurely gray. He is restless, irritable, and unable to remain quiet for any time. Itching is a common symptom. The sleep is disturbed, the appetite and digestion are deranged, and except when directly under the influence of the drug the mental condition is one of depression. Occasionally there are profuse sweats, which may be preceded by chills. The pupils, except when under the direct influence of the drug, are dilated, sometimes unequal. In one case there was a persistent œdema of the legs without sufficient renal changes or anæmia to account for it. Persons addicted to morphia are inveterate liars, and no reliance whatever can be placed upon their statements. In many instances this is not confined to matters relating to the vice. In women the symptoms may be associated with those of pronounced hysteria or neurasthenia. The practice may be continued for an indefinite time, usually requiring increase in the dose until ultimately enormous quantities may be needed to obtain the desired effect. Finally a condition of asthenia is induced, in which the victim takes little or no food and dies from the extreme bodily debility. An increase in the dose is not always necessary, and there are *habitués* who reach the point of satisfaction with a daily amount of 2 or 3 grains of morphia, and who are able to carry on successfully for many years the ordinary business of life. They may remain in good physical condition, and indeed often look ruddy.

Treatment.—The treatment is extremely difficult, and can rarely be successfully carried out by the general practitioner. Isolation, systematic feeding, and gradual withdrawal of the drug are the essential elements. As a rule, the patients must be under control in an institution and should be in bed for the first ten days. It is best in a majority of cases to reduce the morphia gradually. The sufferings of the patients are usually very great, more particularly the abdominal pains, sometimes nausea and vomiting, and the distressing restlessness. Usually within a week or ten days the opium may be entirely withdrawn. In all cases the pulse should be carefully watched and, if feeble, the aromatic spirit of ammonia and digitalis should be given. For the extreme restlessness a hot bath is serviceable. The sleeplessness is the most distressing symptom, and various drugs may have to be resorted to, particularly hyoscine and sulphonal and sometimes, if the insomnia persists, morphia itself.

It is essential in the treatment of a case to be certain that the patient has no means of obtaining morphia. Even under the favorable circumstances of seclusion in an institution and constant watching, patients may practise deception. After an apparent cure the patients are only too apt to lapse into the habit.

The condition is one which has become so common, and is so much on the increase, that physicians should exercise the utmost caution in prescribing morphia, particularly to female patients. Under no circumstances should a patient be allowed to use the hypodermic syringe, and it is even safer not to intrust this dangerous instrument to the hands of the nurse.

Heroin.—Of recent years the use of heroin has increased in the United States. This addiction seems less serious than morphinism; it requires the same treatment.

III. LEAD POISONING

(Plumbism, Saturnism)

Etiology.—The disease is widespread, particularly in the lead industries and among plumbers, painters, and glaziers. In 1916 there were 60 deaths in England and Wales, of which 55 were due to occupational poisoning. In the United States it is not easy to get accurate statistics. In the registration area there were 147 deaths in 1917. Alice Hamilton reports 358 cases with 16 deaths in 23 white lead factories during the 16 months to May 1, 1911. The metal is introduced into the system in many forms. Miners usually escape, but those engaged in the smelting of lead-ores are often attacked. Animals in the neighborhood of smelting furnaces have suffered with the disease, and even the birds that feed on the berries in the neighborhood may be affected. Men engaged in the white-lead factories are particularly prone to plumbism. Accidental poisoning may come in many ways; most commonly by drinking water which has passed through lead pipes or been stored in lead-lined cisterns. Wines and cider which contain acids quickly become contaminated in contact with lead. It was the frequency of colic in certain of the cider districts of Devonshire which gave the name of Devonshire colic, as the frequency of it in Poitou gave the name *colica Pictonum*. Among the innumerable sources of accidental poisoning may be mentioned milk, various sorts of beverages, hair dyes, false teeth, and thread. A few cases have followed the retention of lead bullets in gun-shot wounds. Given medicinally, lead rarely causes poisoning, but we had in the Johns Hopkins Hospital four cases following the use of lead and opium pills for dysentery, of which cause Miller collected many cases from the literature. It has followed the use of Emplastrum Diachylon to produce abortion, and there is a case reported in an infant from the application of lead-water on the mother's nipples. One grain every three hours for three days, and two grains every three hours for one day, have caused signs of poisoning. A serious outbreak of lead-poisoning occurred in Philadelphia, owing to adulteration of a baking-powder with chromate of lead, used to give a yellow tint to the cakes.

All ages are attacked, but children are relatively less liable. The largest number of cases occur between thirty and forty. According to Oliver, females are more susceptible than males. They are much more quickly brought under its influence, and in an epidemic in which a thousand cases were involved the proportion of females to males was four to one. Miscarriage is common, and it is rare for a woman working in lead to carry a child to term. It also destroys the reproductive power in man.

The lead gains entrance through the lungs, the digestive organs, or the skin. Poisoning may follow the use of cosmetics containing lead. Through the lungs it is freely absorbed. The chief channel, according to Oliver, is the digestive system. It is rapidly eliminated by the kidneys and skin, and is present in the urine of lead-workers. The susceptibility is remarkably varied. The symptoms may be manifest within a month of exposure. On the other hand, Tanquerel (des Planches) met with a case in a man who had been a lead-worker for fifty-two years. E. R. Hayhurst examined 100 painters, in not one of whom were there symptoms of acute plumbism but 70 showed in varying degrees symptoms, signs, or after-effects of chronic plumbism; a lead-line on the gums was present in 19 cases.

Morbid Anatomy.—Small quantities of lead occur in the body in health. J. J. Putnam's reports show that of 150 persons not presenting symptoms of lead-poisoning traces of lead occurred in the urine of 25 per cent. Of 264 deaths in persons subjects of plumbism 32 were due to an encephalopathy, 43 to nephritis, 47 to cerebral hæmorrhage, 43 to paralysis, 44 to lead poisoning, 38 to tuberculosis, and 40 to various maladies, pneumonia, heart disease, aneurism, etc. (Legge).

In chronic poisoning lead is found in the various organs. The affected muscles are yellow, fatty, and fibroid. The nerves present the features of a peripheral degenerative neuritis. The cord and the nerve-roots are, as a rule, uninvolved. In the primary atrophic form the ganglion cells of the anterior horns are probably implicated. In the acute fatal cases there may be the most intense entero-colitis.

Symptoms.—ACUTE FORM.—We do not refer here to the accidental or suicidal cases, which present vomiting, pain in the abdomen, and collapse symptoms. In workers in lead there are several manifestations which follow a short time after exposure and set in acutely. There may be, in the first place, a rapidly developing anæmia. Acute neuritis has been described, and convulsions, epilepsy, and a delirium, which may be not unlike that produced by alcohol. There are cases in which the gastro-intestinal symptoms are intense and rapidly prove fatal. These acute forms occur more frequently in persons recently exposed, and more often in winter than in summer. Da Costa reported the onset of hemiplegia after three days' exposure to lead.

CHRONIC POISONING.—(*a*) *Blood Changes.*—A moderate grade of *anæmia,* the so-called saturnine cachexia, is usually present. The corpuscles do not often fall below 50 per cent. Many of the red cells show a remarkable granular, *basophilic degeneration* when stained with Jenner's stain, or with polychrome methylene blue. Grawitz first demonstrated their presence in cases of pernicious anæmia, and Pepper (tertius) and White showed that they were constantly present in lead-poisoning. Observations by Vaughan and others have shown that such granulations are found in the blood in a great variety of conditions, even in normal blood, but that they are most numerous in lead-poisoning, in which their occurrence in large numbers is of value in diagnosis. Cadwalader has shown the constant presence of *nucleated red blood-corpuscles* even when the anæmia is of very slight grade.

(*b*) *The blue line* on the gums is a valuable indication, but is not invariably present. Two lines must be distinguished: one, at the margin between the gums and teeth, is on, not in the gums, and is readily removed by rinsing the mouth and cleansing the teeth. The other is the characteristic blue-black line at the margin of the gum. The color is not uniform, but being in the papillæ of the gums the line is, as seen with a magnifying-glass, interrupted. The lead is absorbed and converted in the tissues into a black sulphide by the action of sulphuretted hydrogen from the tartar of the teeth. The line may form in a few days after exposure (Oliver) and disappear within a few weeks, or may persist for many months. Philipson noted the occurrence of a black line in miners, due to the deposition of carbon.

The most important symptoms of chronic lead-poisoning are colic, lead-palsy, and the encephalopathy. Of these, the colic is the most frequent. Of Tanquerel's cases, there were 1,217 of colic, 101 of paralysis, and 72 of encephalopathy.

(*c*) Colic is the most common symptom of chronic lead-poisoning. It is often preceded by gastric or intestinal symptoms, particularly constipation. The pain is over the whole abdomen. The colic is usually paroxysmal and relieved by pressure. There is often between the paroxysms a dull, heavy pain. There may be vomiting. During the attack, as Riegel noted, the pulse is increased in tension and the heart's action is retarded. Attacks of pain with acute diarrhœa may recur for weeks or even for three or four years.

Certain of the cases with colic may present the features of an acute intra-abdominal inflammatory condition. A case may be admitted to the surgical wards with a diagnosis of appendicitis, or simulate intestinal obstruction. Localized pain, slight fever, and moderate leucocytosis may be present. The history, the presence of a blue line on the gums, and the blood changes are of importance in differential diagnosis.

(*d*) *Lead-palsy.*—This is rarely a primary manifestation. Among 54 cases of lead-poisoning treated in the J. H. H. and dispensary there were 30 cases of lead-paralysis (H. M. Thomas). The upper limbs are most frequently affected. In 26 cases the arms alone were affected, and 18 of these showed the typical double wrist-drop. In 7 the right arm alone was involved, and in one the left. In 4 cases both arms and legs were attacked. The onset may be acute, subacute, or chronic. It usually occurs without fever. In its distribution it may be partial, limited to a muscle or to certain muscle groups, or generalized, involving in a short time the muscles of the extremities and the trunk. The muscles most used are often attacked. Madame Dejerine-Klumpke described the following *localized forms:* (1) Antebrachial type, paralysis of the extensors of the fingers and of the wrist. In this the musculo-spiral nerve is involved, causing the characteristic wrist-drop. The supinator longus usually escapes. In the long-continued flexion of the carpus there may be slight displacement backward of the bones, with distention of the synovial sheaths, so that there is a prominent swelling over the wrist known as Gruebler's tumor. (2) Brachial type, which involves the deltoid, the biceps, the brachialis anticus, and the supinator longus, rarely the pectorals. The atrophy is of the scapulo-humeral form. It is bilateral, and sometimes follows the first form, but it may be primary. (3) The Aran-Duchenne type, in which the small muscles of the hand and of the thenar and hypothenar eminences are involved. The atrophy is marked, and may be the first manifestation. Möbius has shown that this form is particularly marked in tailors. (4) The peroneal type. According to Tanquerel, the lower limbs are involved in the proportion of 13 to 100 of the upper limbs. The lateral peroneal muscles, the extensor communis of the toes, and the extensor proprius of the big toe are involved, producing the *steppage* gait. (5) Laryngeal form. Adductor paralysis was noted by Morell Mackenzie and others in lead-palsy.

Generalized Palsies.—There may be a slow, chronic paralysis, gradually involving the extremities, beginning with the classical picture of wrist-drop. More frequently there is a rapid generalization, producing complete paralysis in all the muscles of the parts in a few days. It may pursue a course like an ascending paralysis, associated with rapid wasting of all four limbs. Such cases, however, are very rare. Death has occurred by involvement of the diaphragm. Oliver reports a case of Philipson's in which complete paralysis supervened. In one patient with generalized paralysis this began in the legs after but two weeks' work as an enameler. It spread rapidly, so that in a little over a week he was bedridden, and on admission to the hospital nearly every muscle below the neck was involved. The diaphragm was completely paralyzed. He was walking about when he left the hospital, though there was still some weakness. Dejerine-Klumpke also recognized a febrile form of general paralysis which may closely resemble the subacute spinal paralysis of Duchenne.

There is also a primary saturnine muscular atrophy in which the weakness and wasting come on together. It is this form, according to Gowers, which most frequently assumes the Aran-Duchenne type.

The electrical reactions are those of lesions of the lower motor segment. The reaction of degeneration in its different grades may be present, depending upon the severity. Usually with the onset of the paralysis there are pains in the legs and joints. Sensation may, however, be unaffected.

(*e*) The *cerebral symptoms* are numerous. Seven of our cases showed marked cerebral involvement. One had delusions and maniacal excitement and had to be removed to an asylum. In other cases there occurred transient delirium, attacks of unconsciousness, and in one case convulsions. Optic neuritis or neuro-retinitis may occur. Hysterical symptoms occasionally occur in girls. Convulsions are not uncommon, and in an adult the possibility of lead-poisoning should always be considered. True epilepsy may follow the convulsions. An acute delirium may occur with hallucinations. The patients may have trance-like attacks, which follow or alternate with convulsions. A few cases of lead encephalopathy finally drift into lunatic asylums. Tremor is one of the commonest manifestations of lead-poisoning.

(*f*) *Arterio-sclerosis.*—Lead-workers are notoriously subject to arterio-sclerosis with contracted kidneys and hypertrophy of the heart. The cases usually show distinct gouty deposits, particularly in the big-toe joint; but in the United States acute gout in lead-workers is rare. According to Sir William Roberts, the lead favors the precipitation of the crystalline urates.

Prognosis.—In the minor manifestations this is good. According to Gowers, the outlook is bad in the primary atrophic form of paralysis. Convulsions are, as a rule, serious, and the mental symptoms which succeed may be permanent. Occasionally the wrist-drop persists.

Treatment.—Prophylactic measures should be taken at all lead-works, but, unless employees are careful, poisoning is apt to occur even under the most favorable conditions. Cleanliness of the hands and of the finger-nails, frequent bathing, and the use of respirators when necessary should be insisted upon. When the lead is in the system the iodide of potassium should be given in from 5- to 10-grain (0.3-0.6 gm.) doses three times a day. For the colic local applications and, if severe, morphia may be used. A morning purge of magnesium sulphate may be given. For the anæmia iron should be used. In the very acute cases it is well not to give iodide, as, according to some writers, the liberation of the lead which has been deposited in the tissues may increase the severity of the symptoms. For the local palsies massage and the constant current should be used. Bulletin No. 95 (1911) of the Bureau of Labor, Washington, contains an elaborate study of industrial lead-poisoning in Europe by Oliver, and of the conditions in the United States by Alice Hamilton and John B. Andrews.

IV. BRASS POISONING

Workers in brass, a compound of copper and zinc, and in bronze, an alloy of copper and tin, are not nearly so subject to poisoning as workers in lead and arsenic. Brass polishers and those exposed to the dust have the hair stained somewhat green and there is often a slight greenish deposit in the teeth and gums. It is said that there may be a green tint to the perspiration, even after a thorough bath.

The dust may cause an itching of the skin, the so-called "brass itch." The fumes arising from molten brass give rise to very peculiar symptoms, the so-called "brass-workers' ague," with "smelters' shakes" and "zinc chills," not an uncommon malady among the outpatients at the Johns Hopkins Hospital. The symptoms are an acute chill, which comes on some hours after exposure to the molten metal, sweating and a feeling of nausea; there may be vomiting, great thirst, a rapid, feeble pulse, a rise of temperature, never high, and in the course of a couple of hours very profuse sweating. The entire attack may last for six or eight hours, or the patient may be ill for a day. Many of our patients used to say that they were more liable to it on Monday, after Sunday's rest. It occurs exclusively in the brass foundries and where zinc, either alone or with an alloy, is heated to boiling. A large percentage of the workers are susceptible. It does not seem to impair the health very much, yet it is notorious how short-lived are the brass-workers in Birmingham. Hayhurst has shown how widely spread the malady is among the workers in zinc in the United States.

In treatment an emetic and a brisk purge may give relief. The drinking of milk and taking of sodium bicarbonate are advised.

V. ARSENICAL POISONING

Acute poisoning by arsenic is common, particularly by Paris green and such mixtures as "Rough on Rats," which are used to destroy vermin and insects. The chief symptoms are intense pain in the stomach, vomiting, and, later, colic, with diarrhœa and tenesmus; occasionally the symptoms are those of collapse. If recovery takes place, paralysis may follow. The treatment should be similar to that of other irritant poisons—rapid removal with the stomach pump, the promotion of vomiting, and the use of milk and eggs. Moist ferric hydroxide (half an ounce of Tct. ferri chloridi in a glass of water and add magnesia to excess) should be given freely.

Chronic Arsenical Poisoning.—Arsenic is used extensively in the arts, particularly in the manufacture of colored papers, artificial flowers, and in many of the fabrics employed as clothing. The glazed green and red papers used in kindergartens also contain arsenic. It is present, too, in many wall-papers and carpets. Much attention has been paid to this question, as instances of poisoning have been thought to depend upon wall-papers and other household fabrics. The arsenic compounds may be either in the form of solid particles detached from the paper or as gaseous volatile bodies formed from arsenical organic matter by the action of several moulds, notably *Peni-*

cilium brevicaule, Mucor mucedo, etc. (Gosio). In moisture, and at a temperature of from 60° to 95° F., a volatile compound is set free, probably "an organic derivative of arsenic pentoxide" (Sanger). The chronic poisoning from fabrics and wall-papers may be due, according to this author, to the ingestion of minute continued doses of this derivative. Contaminated glucose, used in manufacturing beer, caused a widespread epidemic of poisoning at Manchester. The associated presence of selenium compounds may have played a part in the production of the poisoning (Tunnicliffe and Rosenheim). Arsenic is eliminated in all the secretions, and has been found in the milk. J. J. Putnam has shown that it is not uncommon to find traces of arsenic in the urine of many persons in apparent health. The effects of moderate quantities of arsenic are not infrequently seen in medical practice. In chorea and in pernicious anæmia steadily increasing doses are often given until the patient takes from 15 to 20 drops of Fowler's solution three times a day. Flushing and hyperæmia of the skin, puffiness of the eyelids or above the eyebrows, nausea, vomiting, and diarrhœa are the most common symptoms. Redness and sometimes bleeding of the gums and salivation occur. In the protracted administration of arsenic patients may complain of numbness and tingling in the fingers. Cutaneous pigmentation and keratosis are very characteristic, and, as a late rare sequence of the latter, epithelioma. In chorea neuritis has occurred, and a patient with Hodgkin's disease had multiple neuritis after taking ℥ iv ʒ j of Fowler's solution in seventy-five days, during which time there were fourteen days on which the drug was omitted.

In the Manchester epidemic nearly all cases presented signs of neuritis and lesions of the skin. In some the sensory disturbances predominated, in others the motor, the individuals being unable to walk or to use their hands. In a certain number there was muscular incoördination, resembling that of tabes dorsalis. Rapid muscular atrophy characterized some cases. In not a few a condition of erythromelalgia was present. Occasionally a catarrh of the respiratory and alimentary tracts was the chief feature. Pigmentation, keratosis, and herpes were the most characteristic cutaneous manifestations.

How far similar symptoms are to be attributed to the small quantities of arsenic absorbed from wall-papers and fabrics is by some considered doubtful. That children and adults may take with impunity large doses for months without unpleasant effects, and the fact of the gradual establishment of a toleration which enables Styrian peasants to take as much as 8 grains of arsenious acid in a day, speak strongly against it. On the other hand, as Sanger states, we do not know accurately the effects of many of the compounds in minute and long-continued doses, notably the arsenates.

Arsenical paralysis has the same characteristics as lead-palsy, but the legs are more affected than the arms, particularly the extensors and peroneal group, so that the patient has the characteristic *steppage* gait of peripheral neuritis. The electrical reaction in the muscles may be disturbed before there is any loss of power, and when the patient is asked to extend the wrist fully and to spread the fingers slight weakness may be detected early.

Treatment.—Active elimination by the bowels and kidneys is advisable and the treatment of special conditions as indicated.

VI. FOOD POISONING

There may be "death in the pot" from many causes. Food poisons mav be *endogenous* or *exogenous*. Those articles in which the poison is of endogenous origin can scarcely be designated as foods. The poisonous mushroom, for example, is often mistaken for the edible form. The former is injurious because it normally produces a highly poisonous alkaloid, muscarine. Certain fish also produce normal physiological but toxic products. When eaten by mistake, as frequently occurs in the West Indies and Japan, these fish may cause poisonous symptoms. The exogenous origin of food poisons is by far the commonest. Under this head come those foods which are rendered poisonous by accidental contamination from outside sources. Food may contain specific organisms, as of tuberculosis or trichinosis; milk and other foods may become infected with typhoid bacilli, and so convey the disease.

Animals (or insects, as bees) may feed on substances which cause their flesh or products to be poisonous to man. The grains used as food may be infected with fungi and cause the epidemics of ergotism, etc. Foods of all sorts may become contaminated with the bacteria of putrefaction, the products of which may be highly poisonous.

The term "ptomaine poisoning" has been popularized to such an extent that it is used synonymously with food poisoning but true ptomaine poisoning is very rare. The term *ptomaine* was introduced by the Italian chemist, Selmi, to designate basic alkaloidal products formed in putrefaction. Mytilotoxin, found in poisonous mussels, is of this class, and is by far the most poisonous of the known ptomaines.

Among the more common forms are the following:

Meat Poisoning.—Outbreaks of disease due to poisons of bacterial origin or due to chemical changes in meat are not uncommon. Several groups of cases have been recognized.

(*a*) From the colon bacillus or the typho-coli group of organisms, which occupy a position intermediate between the typhoid and colon bacillus. In severe forms symptoms come on a few hours after eating the meat; violent vomiting, purging, pains in the abdomen and collapse and death may occur within twenty-four hours. The temperature may be subnormal. Individuals react very differently, as shown in the remarkable outbreak investigated by McWeeney in Limerick. Among 73 cases every grade of severity was seen, from severe cholera nostras to headache with slight fever. Indeed, there were cases without symptoms, but with the typhoid blood reaction.

Some of these cases have a close resemblance to paratyphoid B infection, and, as Durham pointed out, the bacilli are divisible into two groups: The Gaertner type (*B. enteritidis*) and the Aertryck type. The organism may be isolated from the stools, rarely from the blood, and the specific serum reactions are found. Carriers have been the source of infection in some cases.

The important matter in connection with this type of poisoning is the unaltered appearance of the meat. The danger seems greatest from beef and veal, and in Germany has particularly followed the use of meat from cattle ill with some septic or diarrhœal condition. Pork is a not infrequent cause in England, and severe attacks have followed the eating of pork pies.

(*b*) Meat poisoning associated with putrefaction. Here alterations of appearance, of smell and taste are usually present. The products are those of protein hydrolysis, various aromatic compounds, but more particularly the bodies known as putrescine, cadaverine and sepsin. How far these bodies themselves are responsible for the symptoms, how far they are due to infection with associated organisms, particularly the proteus and the colon bacilli, has not been definitely settled. Many cases of food poisoning have been reported as due to proteus and its toxins. This organism was found to be the cause of a severe outbreak due to eating potato salad.

(*c*) *Botulism.*—Poisoning due to *Bacillus botulinus.* The organism was discovered by van Ermengem in a ham, the eating of which gave rise to 50 cases of botulism. Formerly regarded as exclusively a form of meat poisoning, it has been shown by Dickson and his co-workers that the toxin may be found in vegetable products, especially when "home-canned." The condition is a true intoxication, the toxin being formed in the food and absorbed by the gastro-intestinal tract. It is destroyed by heating to the boiling point. The toxin causes marked thrombus formation both in arteries and veins with hyperæmia and hæmorrhages in the meninges and central nervous system. It is doubtful if there is a specific action on the nerve ganglion cells. The symptoms, which appear in from four to thirty hours, are weakness, disturbance of vision, diplopia and loss of accommodation. Paralysis of the eye muscles is common and any of the motor cranial nerves may be involved. Vertigo and incoördination are common. Sensation remains undisturbed. Dryness of the mouth and pharynx, constriction of the throat with difficulty in speaking and swallowing follow. There is obstinate constipation. In fatal cases death occurs in from four to eight days from cardiac or respiratory failure. The *treatment* is symptomatic; the stomach should be washed and the bowels emptied. Water should be given freely.

Certain game birds, particularly the grouse, are poisonous in special districts and at certain seasons. It is interesting to note that mutton and lamb have thus far not been implicated as a cause of food poisoning.

Poisoning by Meat Products.—(*a*) The poisonous effects which follow the drinking of milk infected with saprophytic bacteria are considered in the section on the diarrhœa of infants.

(*b*) *Cheese Poisoning.*—Various milk products, ice cream, custard, and cheese, may prove highly poisonous. In one epidemic Vaughan and Novy isolated from cheese a substance belonging to the poisonous albumins, and in an extensive ice-cream epidemic Vaughan and Perkins found in the ice cream a highly pathogenic bacillus, but its toxin has not been separated. The symptoms are those of acute gastro-intestinal irritation.

Poisoning by Shell-fish and Fish.—(*a*) *Mussel Poisoning.*—Brieger separated a ptomaine—mytilotoxin—which exists chiefly in the liver of the mussel. The observations of Schmidtmann and Cameron have shown that the mussel from the open sea only becomes poisonous when placed in filthy waters.

Dangerous, even fatal, effects may follow the eating of either raw or cooked mussels. The symptoms are those of an acute poisoning with profound action on the nervous system, and without gastro-intestinal manifestations. There are numbness and coldness, no fever, dilated pupils, and rapid pulse; death occurs sometimes within two hours with collapse symptoms. In an epidemic at Wilhelmshafen, Germany, in 1885, nineteen persons were attacked, four of whom died. Salkowski and Brieger isolated the *mytilotoxin* from specimens of the mussels. Poisoning occasionally follows the eating of oysters which are stale or decomposed. The symptoms are usually gastro-intestinal.

(*b*) *Fish Poisoning.*—There are two distinct varieties: in one the poison is a physiological product of certain glands of the fish, in the other it is a product of bacterial growth. The salted sturgeon used in parts of Russia has sometimes proved fatal to large numbers of persons. In the middle parts of Europe the barb is stated to be sometimes poisonous, producing the so-called *"barben cholera."* In China and Japan various species of the *tetrodon* are also toxic, sometimes causing death within an hour, with symptoms of intense disturbance of the nervous system.

Grain and Vegetable Food Poisoning.—(*a*) *Ergotism.*—The prolonged use of meal made from grains contaminated with the ergot fungus (*claviceps purpurea*) causes a series of symptoms known as ergotism, epidemics of which have prevailed in different parts of Europe. Two forms of this chronic ergotism are described—the one, gangrenous, is believed to be due to the sphacelinic acid, the other, convulsive or spasmodic, is due to the cornutin. In the former gangrene affects the extremities—usually the toes and fingers, less commonly the ears and nose. Preceding the onset of the gangrene there are usually anæsthesia, tingling, pains, spasmodic movements of the muscles, and gradual blood stasis in certain vascular territories.

The *nervous* manifestations are very remarkable. After a prodromal stage of ten to fourteen days, in which the patient complains of weakness, headache, and tingling sensations in different parts of the body, perhaps accompanied with slight fever, symptoms of spasm develop, producing cramps in the muscles and contractures. The arms are flexed and the legs and toes extended. These spasms may last from a few hours to many days and relapses are frequent. In severer cases epilepsy develops and the patient may die in convulsions. Mental symptoms are common, manifested sometimes in a preliminary delirium, but more commonly, in the chronic poisoning, as melancholia or dementia. Posterior spinal sclerosis occurs in chronic ergotism. In the interesting group of 29 cases studied by Tuczek and Siemens 9 died at various periods after the infection, and four post mortems showed degeneration of the posterior columns. A condition similar to tabes dorsalis is gradually produced by this slow degeneration in the spinal cord.

(*b*) *Lathyrism* (Lupinosis).—An affection produced by the use of meal from varieties of vetches, chiefly the *Lathyrus sativus* and *L. cicera.* The grain is popularly known as the chick-pea. The grains are usually powdered and mixed with the meal from other cereals in the preparation of bread. As early as the seventeenth century it was noticed that the use of flour with which the seeds of the *Lathyrus* were mixed caused stiffness of the legs. The subject did not attract much attention before the studies of James Irving, in India, who, between 1859 and 1868 in several communications, described a form of spastic paraplegia affecting many of the inhabitants in certain regions of India and due to the use of meal made from the *Lathyrus* seeds. It also produces a spastic paraplegia in animals. The Italian observers describe a similar form of paraplegia, and it has been observed in Algiers. The condition is that of a spastic paralysis, involving chiefly the legs, which may proceed to complete paraplegia. The arms are rarely, if ever, affected. It is evidently a slow sclerosis due to the influence of this toxic agent.

(*c*) *Potato-poisoning.*—Potatoes contain normally a very small amount (about 0.06 per cent.) of the poisonous principle solanin, and, under certain circumstances, may contain the poison in amounts sufficient to cause grave disturbance. The increase is due to the action of at least two species of bacteria, *B. solaniferum non-colorabile* and *B. solaniferum colorabile,* and occurs in those tubers which, during growth, have lain partially exposed above ground, and in those which, during storage, have become well sprouted. An extensive outbreak of potato-poisoning occurred in 1899 in a German regiment, fifty-six members of which, after eating sprouted potatoes, were seized with chills, fever, headache, vomiting, diarrhœa, colic, and great prostration. Many were jaundiced and several collapsed, but all recovered. Samples of the remaining potatoes yielded 0.38 per cent. of solanin, and this would indicate that a full portion must have contained about 5 grains.

(*d*) The "Vomiting Sickness" of Jamaica is due to poisoning by spoiled ackees—the fruit of *Blighia sapida.* Children are especially susceptible; the main features are vomiting, convulsions and coma; the average duration is twelve hours; the death rate is 85 per cent. (Scott).

Anaphylaxis.—Some individuals have a hyper-susceptibility to certain proteins and this may result in very diverse phenomena. The sensitization may be natural or acquired and in the latter case may be due to absorption from the digestive tract. The features are very variable; in an infant susceptible to cow's milk there may be vomiting, diarrhœa, urticaria or erythema, dyspnœa and prostration with a weak and rapid pulse. Some chronic skin affections, such as eczema, perhaps psoriasis, certain forms of erythema and urticaria, and some cases of asthma are due to this cause. Milk, eggs, meat, shell fish, strawberries, etc., are among the foods concerned. The use of skin tests made with the isolated protein is an important diagnostic measure.

Treatment.—The source of the infection must be ascertained and the offending food destroyed. The stomach should be washed out and the bowels evacuated by a brisk saline purge. Saline infusions, hypodermic or intravenous, may promote the elimination of the toxins.

In the cases of *anaphylaxis* it may be possible to avoid the particular food to which the patient is sensitized. Otherwise an immunity may be obtained by giving very minute doses of the protein concerned, insufficient to produce a reaction, and gradually increasing the amount. Children often lose the hyper-susceptibility as they grow older.

SECTION IV

DEFICIENCY DISEASES

I. PELLAGRA

Definition.—A deficiency disease, with periodical manifestations characterized by gastro-intestinal disturbances, skin lesions, and a tendency to changes in the nervous system.

Historical.—The disease appears to have been endemic in Spain by 1735 and the first description is by Cazal (1762), who named it *mal de la rosa.* It existed in Italy in 1750 and was described in 1771 by Frapolli, who gave it the name of pellagra (rough skin). By the eighteenth century it had spread over northern Italy and had appeared in France and Roumania. It is quite probable that there have been sporadic cases in the United States for the last fifty years.

Distribution.—The disease is prevalent in parts of southern Europe, particularly in Italy and Roumania. It exists in Spain, Portugal, France, Egypt and the United States, in the southern part of which country the disease has spread with extraordinary rapidity. In 1917 there were 3,666 deaths in the registration area. Better diagnosis can hardly explain the frequency, as the disease is so striking in its manifestations that many cases could hardly be overlooked. There is evidence that the disease is to some extent one of particular localities, as beri-beri; it is also a disease of the country more than of the cities. This applies particularly to Europe, but in the United States many towns and villages show a number of cases. As regards the influence of place, the number of cases in the asylums of the United States is significant. A few cases have occurred in England.

Etiology.—There are two main views, one that it is due to a defect in the diet—a lack of vitamines, in other words, a deficiency disease, and the other that it is due to infection of some kind. If the latter be the case the infectious agent is apparently not conveyed directly from person to person. In the Italian institutions, where a large number of pellagrins are treated, no attendant has contracted the disease. If due to food deficiency, the accused article is corn (maize), comparable to the part thought to be played by rice in beri-beri. The experiments of Goldberger and Wheeler support the dietetic view. Eleven prisoners were kept on ordinary diet from February 4 to April 19, 1915, from which date until October 31, 1915, they received a restricted diet lacking meat, eggs, milk, beans, peas and other proteins. The food was chiefly maize, rice, sweet potatoes, brown gravy, syrup, sugar and coffee—all of the best quality. Within five months six of the eleven volunteers had dermatitis said by experts to be pellagra.

Age.—The disease occurs at any age, but the majority of cases are between twenty and forty years. As regards races, the negro is more susceptible than the white, and, in reference to sex, women are apparently slightly more susceptible than men.

Occupation.—In Europe the disease is almost confined to laborers of the poorer classes, but this is not true of the United States.

Season.—The disease occurs particularly in the spring and sometimes in the autumn, both in its onset and recurrences.

Pathology.—There is nothing characteristic in the morbid anatomy. In the acute cases there may be atrophy of the walls of the intestines, fatty degeneration of the internal organs and changes in the nervous system. The alterations in the cord are fairly constant. There is degeneration of the lateral columns in the dorsal region and of the posterior columns in the cervical and dorsal regions. In the brains of patients with mental deterioration atrophy of the cerebrum is found.

Symptoms.—These vary markedly in severity, usually appearing in the spring and sometimes in the autumn. There is always a tendency to recurrence, and with each succeeding attack more damage is done, particularly to the nervous system. The onset is usually in the spring with indefinite symptoms, such as weakness, headache, and depression.

Digestive Tract.—Disturbance of the alimentary tract is usually an early symptom. In the mouth there may be sensations of heat, with loss of taste. Stomatitis is common, the mucous membrane is very red, ulcers may appear and the epithelium is stripped off, leaving a raw surface so that chewing is painful. Anorexia, nausea and vomiting are common; there is also diarrhœa, sometimes dysentery, often severe and accompanied by pain, the stools being serous or bloody. It may alternate with constipation.

Skin.—The erythema usually begins on the backs of the hands and at first resembles an ordinary sunburn. There may be puffy swelling. The affected areas are symmetrical and sharply defined as a rule, extending above the wrist and down to the last finger joint. The face, neck and feet may be affected in the same way. The process may not advance any further, the skin becomes darker and desquamates, after which some pigmentation remains. In other cases vesicles and bullæ form, containing serum or pus. These dry gradually, with the production of fissures. After drying and desquamation the skin may have a dry appearance and a deep red color. With repeated attacks the skin may become indurated, thickened and dark in color; later atrophy and thinning may follow. Exposure to the sun may have an influence on the eruption, but is not the cause. The erythema occurs sometimes on protected parts.

Nervous System.—Headache and vertigo are common. Mental features are often marked, among which are confusion, dullness, lassitude, irritability, feelings of anxiety and depression, change in the disposition, and hallucinations of sight and hearing. These may progress to profound depression and ultimately to dementia. Mania occurs sometimes and suicidal tendencies are not uncommon. The symptoms due to changes in the *cord* vary with the lesion. A spastic condition, disturbances of sensation, paralysis of the sphincters, or loss of the reflexes of the legs may be found.

The blood shows no special features beyond those of a secondary anæmia. The temperature is usually normal except in some of the acute cases.

Clinical Forms.—The disease occurs in two main forms, an acute and a chronic recurrent form. In the acute form there are fever, marked prostration, severe diarrhœa, delirium or stupor and a rapid downward course. Death may occur in a few weeks from the onset. These cases seem to be more frequent in the United States than in Europe. In the chronic form the manifestations are not severe, but tend to recur each year, and each attack leaves the patient in a worse condition. There is always the tendency to mental deterioration which occurs in fully 10 per cent. of the cases. Death occurs from exhaustion and cachexia, or some intercurrent disease. Fortunately, succeeding attacks are not necessarily more severe than the preceding ones. There are instances of this form persisting for twenty-five years. Cases without the skin lesions—pellagra sine pellagra—have been described.

Diagnosis.—A typical case offers no difficulties, but in the absence of the skin lesions considerable difficulty may be experienced. Scurvy might give difficulty, but the absence of the other features of pellagra should be conclusive. Skin lesions of the nature of erythema might cause confusion, but the absence of the general features removes doubt. The study of the stools differentiates it from sprue. The psychical features might suggest general paresis, but the skin lesions and digestive disturbance should make the diagnosis clear. The acute cases might be mistaken for various infections, but the erythema and gastro-intestinal features should prevent this.

Prognosis.—In the United States the outlook is regarded as serious, if not as regards death, certainly as regards ultimate recovery. In Europe, where the disease has existed for a long time, the prognosis is more favorable, and in Italy in some years the mortality was only 4 per cent. In cases with acute features or fever the prognosis is grave and signs of severe toxæmia or of mental involvement are ominous. Erythema of a moist character is regarded as a grave sign. Any complications should be regarded seriously. The prognosis is best in the chronic cases without mental features. The outlook is serious in asylum cases.

Prophylaxis.—"Peasant life, poverty, and polenta (corn)" have been given as the causal factors. Improvement in the living conditions and good sanitation are important points in the prevention. Too much corn or maize should not be used, particularly in institutions. The experiments noted above suggest that it is a deficiency disease which may possibly be eradicated by a proper diet, as has been the case with beri-beri. A sufficient amount of milk, eggs, meat and vegetables, especially beans, is important.

Treatment.—The patient should be placed in the best general conditions and a change of diet and climate is advisable. Rest in bed is necessary while the symptoms are acute. The diet should be as nutritious as possible and the diarrhœa need not interfere with taking sufficient nourishment. Fresh milk, buttermilk, eggs, fresh meat and fresh or dried vegetables should be taken in full amounts. Salt should be given freely. There is no proof that we have any remedy with a specific influence. Arsenic has been given by the mouth or by injection. Atoxyl and arsphenamine have been used in ordinary dosage, but arsenic by mouth, as Fowler's solution, is apparently more useful. Transfusion of blood, both from healthy individuals and those who have recovered from the disease, has been done apparently with good results in some cases. Symptomatic treatment and a proper diet seem to have been as successful as any special measure and should be given as demanded by the conditions in each patient.

II. BERI-BERI

(*Kakke, Endemic Multiple Neuritis*)

Definition.—A deficiency disease due to the absence of certain elements of the food, the so-called vitamines, and characterized clinically by multiple neuritis, anasarca, and muscular atrophy.

It seems probable that several forms of multiple neuritis have been described under the term beri-beri. The form which is particularly common in China and Japan is due to a diet deficient in the special vitamine which occurs in the outer layer of rice.

History.—The disease is believed to be of great antiquity in China, and is possibly mentioned in the oldest known medical treatise. In the early years of the nineteenth century it attracted much attention among the Anglo-Indian surgeons, and we may date the modern scientific study of the disease from Malcolmson's monograph, published at Madras in 1835. The opening of Japan gave an opportunity to the European physicians holding university positions, particularly Anderson, Baelz, Scheube, and Grimm, to investigate the disease. The studies of Japanese physicians, particularly Miura and Takagi, and of Dutch physicians in the East, have contributed much to our knowledge. The studies of Schaumann, Fraser, Stanton, and others and the dietetic experiments in the Philippines have confirmed the older views that it is a disorder depending upon an imperfect dietary.

Distribution.—It is specially prevalent among the Malays, Chinese and Japanese, and during the Russian war more than 50,000 cases occurred in the Japanese army. It prevails excessively in the Philippines. In India it is less common. Localized outbreaks have occurred in Australia. It prevails in parts of South America, and in the West Indies. It is met with among the fishermen of Norway and of the Newfoundland Banks. It occurs also in asylums, in which there have been severe outbreaks in the United States, and in the Richmond Asylum, Dublin, in the years 1894, 1896 and 1897 under conditions of over-crowding.

Etiology.—Two main views have prevailed: That it is an acute infection and that it is a disorder of metabolism. Numerous bacteriological studies have not determined the presence of any definite organism. On the other hand, the work of the past few years has confirmed the food theory widely held in Japan. Studies in the Far East leave no doubt that the disease is there due to a diet of rice from which the pericarp has been removed, in what is called "polishing" or "milling." This is an old story, as the Dutch knew of the association of the disease with rice, and it was by modifying the rice diet of the sailors that Takagi eradicated beri-beri from the Japanese navy. Braddon showed the importance of the retention of the pericarp for the prevention of the disease. Schaumann's experiments, amply confirmed by Fraser and Stanton, leave no question that beri-beri is associated with a diet freed from the materials existing in the pericarp. Whether these are the phosphorus compounds, as Schaumann believes, or unknown substances, the so-called vitamines, as Fraser and Stanton hold, has not been settled.

That beri-beri occurs in ships and in institutions may be explained by the fact that in the dietary, though it may not be of rice, similar compounds are lacking. On the other hand, certain French workers in the East hold that white rice alone does not produce the disease, and that there must be some other factor, since the great majority of rice-eaters in the East are immune.

Other factors are overcrowding, as in ships, jails and asylums, hot and moist seasons, and exposure to wet. Males are more subject to the disease than females. Under good hygienic conditions Europeans rarely contract it.

Morbid Anatomy.—The most constant and striking features are changes in the peripheral nerves and degenerative inflammation involving the axis cylinder and medullary sheaths. In acute cases this is found not only in the peripheral nerves, but also in the vagus and phrenic. The fibres of the voluntary muscles, as well as of the myocardium, are much degenerated.

Symptoms.—The incubation period is unknown, but it probably extends over several months. The following forms are recognized by Scheube:

(*a*) The incomplete or rudimentary form which often sets in with catarrhal symptoms, followed by pains and weakness in the limbs and a lowering of the sensibility in the legs, with the occurrence of paræsthesia. Slight œdema sometimes appears. After a time paræsthesia is felt in other parts of the body, and the patient may complain of palpitation of the heart, uneasy sensations in the abdomen, and sometimes shortness of breath. There may be weakness and tenderness of the muscles. After lasting from a few days to many months, these symptoms all disappear, but with the return of the warm weather there may be a recurrence. One of Scheube's patients suffered in this way for twenty years.

(*b*) The atrophic form sets in with much the same symptoms, but the loss of power in the limbs progresses more rapidly, and very soon the patient is no longer able to walk or to move the arms. The atrophy, which is associated with a good deal of pain, may extend to the muscles of the face. The œdematous symptoms and heart troubles play a minor rôle in this form, which is known as the dry or paralytic variety.

(*c*) The Wet or Dropsical Form.—Setting in as in the rudimentary variety, the œdema soon becomes the most marked feature, extending over the whole subcutaneous tissue, and associated with effusions into the serous sacs. The atrophy of the muscles and disturbance of sensation are not such prominent symptoms, but palpitation and rapid action of the heart and dyspnœa are common. The wasting may not be apparent until the dropsy disappears.

(*d*) The acute, pernicious, or cardiac form is characterized by threatenings of an acute cardiac failure, coming on rapidly after the existence of slight symptoms, such as occur in the rudimentary form. Death may follow within twenty-four hours; more commonly the symptoms extend over several weeks. Widespread paralysis with anæsthesia may be present.

The mortality varies greatly, from 2 or 3 per cent. to 40 or 50 per cent. among the coolies in certain settlements of the Malay Archipelago.

Diagnosis.—In tropical countries there is rarely any difficulty. In cases of peripheral neuritis, associated with œdema, coming from tropical ports, the possibility of this disease should be remembered. The peculiar epidemic dropsy of Calcutta and Bengal is probably beri-beri. Greig has shown it to be a nutritional disorder associated with the use of polished rice.

Prophylaxis.—Much has been done to prevent the disease, particularly in Japan. There has been no more remarkable triumph of modern hygiene than Takagi's dietetic reforms in the Japanese navy. Everywhere in the East a change in the diet has been followed by the disappearance of the disease. In the Straits Settlements a group of men took No. 1 polished white Siam rice, and developed beri-beri within sixty days. A group that took unpolished rice remained free from the disease. By exchange of clothing, contact, living together, the disease was not conveyed from one group to the other. Then the group that had partaken of the unpolished rice was fed with polished rice, and within two months developed beri-beri.

The change of diet in the Philippine Scouts instituted on September 30th, 1909, has been followed by remarkable results. Instead of 20 ounces of highly milled rice, the amount was limited to 16 ounces of unpolished rice. The number of admissions for the disease in 1908 and 1909 in a strength of men of 5,000 was 619 and 558. In 1910 there were 50 cases, and in the first five months of 1911 only one case. Chamberlain states that the Philippine experiments bear out at every point the polished rice theory of the etiology. After having been continuously present for five years at the Culion Leper Colony in the Philippines, beri-beri disappeared entirely in the nine months after the use of unpolished rice was enforced (Heiser).

Treatment.—It is a very chronic and obstinate malady. A nutritious diet, without much rice, rest in bed, purgation for the dropsy, cardiac stimulants, and the usual measures for the neuritis are the important factors in the treatment. Salicylates and saline laxatives are used in Japan. If the cardiac features are marked the usual treatment with active stimulation should be employed. When the œdema has subsided massage, passive movements, and electricity may be used for the atrophic muscles.

III. SCURVY

(*Scorbutus*)

Definition.—A disorder of metabolism of unknown origin, characterized by great debility, with anæmia, a spongy condition of the gums, and a tendency to hæmorrhages.

Etiology.—The disease has been known from the earliest times, and has prevailed particularly in armies in the field and among sailors on long voyages. It has been well called "the calamity of sailors." Owing largely to the efforts of Lind and to a knowledge of the conditions upon which the disease depends, scurvy has gradually disappeared from the naval service. In the mercantile marine cases still occasionally occur, owing to the lack of proper and suitable food.

In parts of Russia scurvy is endemic. In the United States scurvy is not a very rare disease. To the hospitals in the seaport towns sailors are now and then admitted with it. In large almshouses outbreaks occasionally occur. A very great increase of foreign population of a low grade has in certain districts made the disease not at all uncommon. In the mining districts of Pennsylvania the Hungarian, Bohemian, and Italian settlers are not infrequently attacked. McGrew has reported 42 cases in Chicago, limited entirely to Poles. He ascertained that in a large proportion of the cases the diet was composed of bread, strong coffee, and meat. Occasionally one meets with scurvy among quite well-to-do people. Some years ago scurvy was not infrequent in the large lumbering camps in the Ottawa Valley. In Great Britain and Ireland it has become very rare; only 302 cases were admitted to the Seaman's Hospital in the twenty-two years ending 1896 (Johnson Smith). It is not uncommon in the South African natives.

The cause is unknown; there are three theories of the disease:

(*a*) That it is the result of an absence of those ingredients in the food which are supplied by fresh vegetables. What these constituents are has not yet been definitely determined, whether the potassium salts or the absence of the organic salts present in fruits and vegetables. It may be due to a diet lacking in physical rather than chemical constituents. Wright has brought forward evidence which suggests that it may be an acid intoxication. That it is not due to an absence of fresh vegetables or the salts of fruits and vegetables seems to have been settled by Nansen and his comrades, who, living for months under the most unfavorable hygienic surroundings, but eating fresh bear's meat and bear's blood, escaped scurvy.

(*b*) That it is due to toxic materials in the food—some unknown organic poison the product of decomposition.

(*c*) In opposition to these chemical views it is urged that the disease depends upon a specific (as yet unknown) micro-organism.

Other factors play an important part, particularly physical and moral influences—overcrowding, dwelling in cold, damp quarters, and prolonged fatigue under depressing influences, as during the retreat of an army. Among prisoners, mental depression plays an important rôle. It is stated that the disease has broken out in the French convict ships *en route* to New Caledonia even when the diet was amply sufficient. Nostalgia is sometimes an important element. It is an interesting fact that prolonged starvation in itself does not necessarily cause scurvy. Not one of the professional fasters displayed any scorbutic symptom. The disease attacks all ages, but the old are more susceptible to it. Sex has no special influence, but during the siege of Paris it was noted that the males attacked were greatly in excess of the females.

Morbid Anatomy.—The anatomical changes are marked, though by no means specific, and are chiefly those associated with hæmorrhage. The blood shows a severe anæmia, without leucocytosis. The skin shows the ecchymoses evident during life. There are hæmorrhages into the muscles, and occasionally about or even into the joints. Hæmorrhages occur in the internal organs, particularly on the serous membranes and in the kidneys and bladder. The gums are swollen and sometimes ulcerated. Ulcers are occasionally met with in the ileum and colon. Hæmorrhages into the mucous membranes are extremely common. The spleen is enlarged and soft. Parenchymatous changes are constant in the liver, kidneys, and heart.

Symptoms.—The disease is insidious in its onset. Early symptoms are loss in weight, progressive weakness, and pallor. Very soon the gums are noticed to be swollen and spongy, to bleed easily, and in extreme cases to present a fungous appearance. These changes, regarded as characteristic, are sometimes absent. The teeth may become loose and even fall out. Actual necrosis of the jaw is not common. The breath is excessively foul. The tongue is swollen, but may be red and not much furred. The salivary glands are occasionally enlarged. Hæmorrhages beneath the mucous membranes of the mouth, especially on the hard palate, are common. The skin becomes dry and rough, and ecchymoses soon appear, first on the legs and then on the arms and trunk, and particularly into and about the hair-follicles. They are petechial, but may become larger, and when subcutaneous may cause distinct swellings. In severe cases, particularly in the legs, there may be effusion between the periosteum and the bone, forming irregular nodes, which may break down and form foul-looking sores. The slightest bruise or injury causes hæmorrhages into the injured part. Œdema about the ankles is common. The "scurvy sclerosis," seen oftenest in the legs, is a remarkable infiltration of the subcutaneous tissues and muscles, forming a brawny induration, the skin over which may be blood-stained. Hæmorrhages from the mucous membranes are less constant; epistaxis is, however, frequent. Hæmoptysis and hæmatemesis are uncommon. Hæmaturia, often microscopic, is common and bleeding from the bowels may occur in severe cases.

Palpitation of the heart and feebleness and irregularity of the impulse are prominent symptoms. The heart may be enlarged, especially the right ventricle. The rate may be increased. A hæmic murmur can usually be heard at the base. Hæmorrhagic infarction of the lungs and spleen has been described. Respiratory symptoms are not common. The appetite is impaired, and owing to the soreness of the gums the patient is unable to chew the food. Constipation is more frequent than diarrhœa. The urine is often albuminous. The amount is usually reduced and the specific gravity is high. The statements with reference to the inorganic constituents are contradictory. Some authorities have found the phosphates and potassium salts to be deficient; others hold that they are increased.

There are mental depression, indifference, in some cases headache, and in the later stages delirium. Cases of convulsions, or hemiplegia, and of meningeal hæmorrhage have been described. Remarkable ocular symptoms are occasionally met with, such as night-blindness or day-blindness. Changes in the optic disk have been found.

In advanced cases necrosis of the bones may occur, and in young persons even separation of the epiphyses. There are instances in which the cartilages have separated from the sternum. The callus of a recently repaired fracture has been known to undergo destruction. Fever is not present, except in the later stages, or when secondary inflammations in the internal organs appear. The temperature may, indeed, be sometimes below normal. Acute arthritis is an occasional complication.

Diagnosis.—No difficulty is met in the recognition of scurvy when a number of persons are affected together. In isolated cases, however, the disease is distinguished with difficulty from certain forms of purpura. The association with manifest insufficiency in diet, and the rapid amelioration with suitable food, are points by which the diagnosis can be readily settled.

Prognosis.—The outlook is good, unless the disease is far advanced and the conditions persist which lead to its occurrence. The mortality now is rarely great. Death results from gradual heart-failure, occasionally from sudden syncope. Meningeal hæmorrhage, extravasation into the serous cavities, entero-colitis, and other intercurrent affections may prove fatal.

Prophylaxis.—The regulations of the Board of Trade require that a sufficient supply of antiscorbutic articles of diet be taken on each ship; so that now, except as the result of accident, scurvy is rare in sailors.

Treatment.—The juice of two or three lemons or oranges daily and a diet of plenty of meat and fresh vegetables suffice to cure all cases of scurvy, unless far advanced. When the stomach is much disordered, small quantities of scraped meat and milk should be given at short intervals, and orange juice in gradually increasing quantities. Mashed potato, mixed with milk, is useful. As the patient gains in strength the diet may be more liberal, and he may eat freely of potatoes, cabbage, water-cresses, and lettuce. The stomatitis causes the greatest distress and a permanganate of potash or dilute carbolic acid solution forms the best mouth-wash. A tolerably strong solution of nitrate of silver applied to the gums is very useful. The constipation is best treated with large enemata. For other conditions, such as hæmorrhages and ulcerations, suitable measures must be employed.

INFANTILE SCURVY

(Barlow's Disease)

A special form of scurvy occurs in children in consequence of imperfect food supply. W. B. Cheadle and Gee, in London, described in very young children a cachexia associated with hæmorrhage. Cheadle regarded the cases as scurvy ingrafted on a rickety stock. Gee called his cases periosteal cachexia. Cases had previously been regarded as acute rickets.

A few years later Barlow made an exhaustive study of the condition with careful anatomical observations. The affection is now recognized as infantile scurvy, and is called Barlow's disease. The American Pædiatric Society collected 379 cases in 1898 in the United States. Of these, the hygienic surroundings were good in 303. A majority of the patients were under twelve months. The proprietary foods, particularly malted milk and condensed milk, seem to be the most important factors in producing the disease. There are instances in which it has developed in breast-fed infants, and in others fed on the carefully prepared milk of the Walker-Gordon laboratories.

The following clinical summary is taken from Barlow's description:

"So long as it is left alone the child is tolerably quiet; the lower limbs are kept drawn up and still; but when placed in its bath or otherwise moved there is continuous crying, and it soon becomes clear that the pain is connected with the lower limbs. At this period the upper limbs may be touched with impunity, but any attempt to move the legs or thighs gives rise to screams. Next, some obscure swelling may be detected, first on one lower limb, then on the other, though it is not absolutely symmetrical. . . . The swelling is ill-defined, but is suggestive of thickening round the shafts of the bones, beginning above the epiphyseal junctions. Gradually the bulk of the limbs affected becomes visibly increased. . . . The position of the limbs becomes somewhat different from what it was at the outset. Instead of being flexed they lie everted and immobile, in a state of pseudo-paralysis. . . .

About this time, if not before, great weakness of the back becomes manifest. A little swelling of one or both scapulæ may appear, and the upper limbs may show changes. These are rarely so considerable as the alterations in the lower limbs. There may be swelling above the wrists, extending for a short distance up the forearm, and some swelling in the neighborhood of the epiphyses of the humerus. There is symmetry of lesions, but it is not absolute; and the limb affection is generally consecutive, though the involvement of one limb follows very close upon another. The joints are free. In severe cases another symptom may now be found—namely, crepitus in the regions adjacent to the junctions of the shafts with epiphyses. The upper and lower extremities of the femur, and the upper extremity of the tibia, are the common sites of such fractures; but the upper end of the humerus may also be so affected. . . . A very startling appearance may be observed at this period in the front of the chest. The sternum, with the adjacent costal cartilages and a small portion of the contiguous ribs, seems to have sunk bodily back, *en bloc,* as though it had been subjected to some violence which had fractured several ribs in the front and driven them back. Occasionally thickenings of varying extent may be found on the exterior of the vault of the skull, or even on some of the bones of the face. . . . Here also must be mentioned a remarkable eye phenomenon. There develops a rather sudden proptosis of one eyeball, with puffiness and very slight staining of the upper lid. Within a day or two the other eye presents similar appearances, though they may be of less severity. The ocular conjunctiva may show a little ecchymosis, or may be quite free. With respect to the constitutional symptoms accompanying the above series of events the most important feature is the profound anæmia which is developed. . . . The anæmia is proportional to the amount of limb involvement. As the case proceeds there is a certain earthy-colored or sallow tint, which is noteworthy in severe cases, and when once this is established bruise-like ecchymoses may appear, and more rarely small purpura. Emaciation is not a marked feature, but asthenia is extreme and suggestive of muscular failure. The temperature is very erratic; it is often raised for a day or two, when successive limbs are involved, especially during the tense stage, but is rarely above 101° or 102° F. At other times it may be normal or subnormal." If the teeth have appeared the gums may be spongy.

In young children with difficulty in moving the lower limbs, or in whom paralysis is suspected, the condition should always be looked for. What is known sometimes as Parrot's disease, or syphilitic pseudo-paralysis, may be confounded with it. In it the loss of motion is more or less sudden in the upper or lower limbs, or in both, due to a solution of continuity and separation of the cartilage at the end of the diaphysis. There are usually crepitation and much pain on movement.

The essential lesion is a subperiosteal blood extravasation, which causes the thickening and tenderness in the shafts of the bones. In some instances there is hæmorrhage in the intramuscular tissue.

The *prophylaxis* is most important. The proprietary forms of condensed milk and preserved foods for infants should not be used. The fresh cow's milk should be substituted, and a teaspoonful of meat-juice or gravy may be given with a little mashed potato. Orange-juice or lemon-juice should be given three or four times a day. Recovery is usually prompt and satisfactory.

SECTION V

DISEASES OF METABOLISM

I. GOUT

(Podagra)

Definition.—A disorder of metabolism associated with retention of uric acid and of other purin bodies in the body, characterized clinically by attacks of acute arthritis, the deposition of sodium-biurate in and about the joints, and by the occurrence of irregular constitutional symptoms.

Etiology.—The purin bodies, adenin, guanin, hypoxanthin, xanthin, and uric acid, result from the transformation of the nucleo-proteins of the food and of the tissues by ferments or enzymes, each one of which has its own specific action. Among the proteolytic enzymes nuclease has a universal distribution, and, no matter what the source of the nucleo-protein, it sets free adenin and guanin. Specific enzymes also liberate uric acid from the nucleo-proteins of the tissues and from the purins of the food. Once formed, the difficulty is to get rid of uric acid, and this appears to be one essential factor in the etiology of gout. Birds and serpents, unable to oxidize it, excrete large quantities. "All mammals, with the important exception of man, are able to destroy uric acid rapidly and in considerable quantities. This destruction is an oxidation accomplished by a specific enzyme called uricase, and the reaction seems to consist of the removal of one of the carbon atoms from the uric acid, thus converting it into the more readily soluble allantoin" (Wells). These transforming enzymes are very variously distributed in the body; nuclease is present in all cells, adenase and the xanthin enzyme are not so widely distributed. Uricase, on which the uricolytic power of the different tissues depends, is present chiefly in the liver and kidneys of mammals, and to a less degree in the muscles. Man alone seems to have a difficulty in oxidizing uric acid. Even on a purin-free diet he excretes daily a certain amount, and purin-rich food is at once followed by a rise. In other mammals it is readily oxidized into allantoin, of which human urine never contains more than a trace.

Gout, then, can not be regarded as loss of the power of a given individual to destroy uric acid; since this does not appear to be an active function in the human body. Loss of power to eliminate favors the deposition of uric acid, and individuals who can not get rid easily of their purins, endogenous or exogenous, may be said to be gouty.

There is a form of gout in swine, characterized by a deposit of guanin in the muscles—the chalky flakes which are so often seen in old Virginia and Westphalian hams—and it has been found that the pig's liver is deficient in the enzyme guanase, which in other animals oxidizes this purin body. We can not say yet how great is the part played by uric acid in human gout and how much by the other purin bodies, but recent work favors the view that *imperfect elimination* rather than imperfect oxidation of the purin bodies is the chief factor in the disease.

The normal daily output of uric acid is from 0.4 to 1.5 gm., and it is greater by day than by night. The amount from the intake of the exogenous oxy-purins varies from 40 to 60 per cent. of the total purin content. The more active the functions of the body the greater the discharge. Severe exertion, fever and exposure to cold increase the output. The amount is greatly influenced by food, particularly when rich in purin bases. For example, after a meal containing sweetbread the amount may be doubled. In gouty persons the output is low, and there are cases of tophaceous gout in which, in the intervals between the attacks, the excretion was nil (Futcher). With the onset of an attack the output rises, and the phosphoric acid is also greatly increased, as shown in Chart XIII.

Predisposing Factors.—*Heredity* is important. In from 50 per cent. to 60 per cent. of all cases the disease existed in the parents or grandparents, and the transmission is more marked on the male side. Males are more subject than females. It is rarely seen before the thirtieth year, though cases have occurred before puberty, and even in infants at the breast.

Alcohol is an important factor in the etiology. Fermented liquors are more apt to cause it than distilled spirits, and the disease is much more common in England and in Germany, the countries which consume the largest amount of beer *per capita*. The disease is common in the United States, and is perhaps on the increase. As Futcher pointed out, gout is only one-third less frequent at the Johns Hopkins Hospital than at St. Bartholomew's Hospital, London. Among 18,000 patients (J. H. H.) there were 59 cases of gout; all but three in whites, and all in males but two (Futcher).

Food pays a rôle of importance equal to alcohol. Overeating without exercise is a predisposing cause. But the disease is by no means confined to the well-to-do. A combination of poor food, defective hygiene and the excessive consumption of malt liquors makes "poor man's gout" not infrequent.

Occupation is of great importance, and the disease is much more common in workers in breweries, and in persons who deal in any way with alcohol.

It is not uncommon in persons of great mental and bodily vigor. Among distinguished members of our profession who have been terrible sufferers were the elder Scaliger, Jerome Cardan and Sydenham. This statement of the latter, however, that "more wise men than fools are victims" of the affection, does not hold good to-day. The celebrated Pirckheimer wrote a famous "Apology for Gout" (1521), and there is much truth in what Podagra says: "For I take no pleasure in those hard, rough, rusticke, agresticke kind of people, who never are at rest, but always exercise their bodies with hard labors, are ever moyling and toyling, do seldom or never give themselves to pleasure, do endure hunger, which are content with a slender diet." (English Edition, 1617.)

Among the directly exciting causes of an attack may be mentioned a meal with large quantities of rich food and too much to drink; worry, or a sudden mental shock, and in sensitive persons a slight injury or accident may be followed by acute arthritis.

Pathology.—The *blood* contains an excess of uric acid. The average amount in 156 non-gouty patients was 1.7 mgs. per 100 gm. of blood with variations from 0.7 to 4.5 mgs. (Adler and Ragle). Pratt's studies in 21 gouty patients showed an average of 3.7 mgs. per 100 gm. of blood. The high

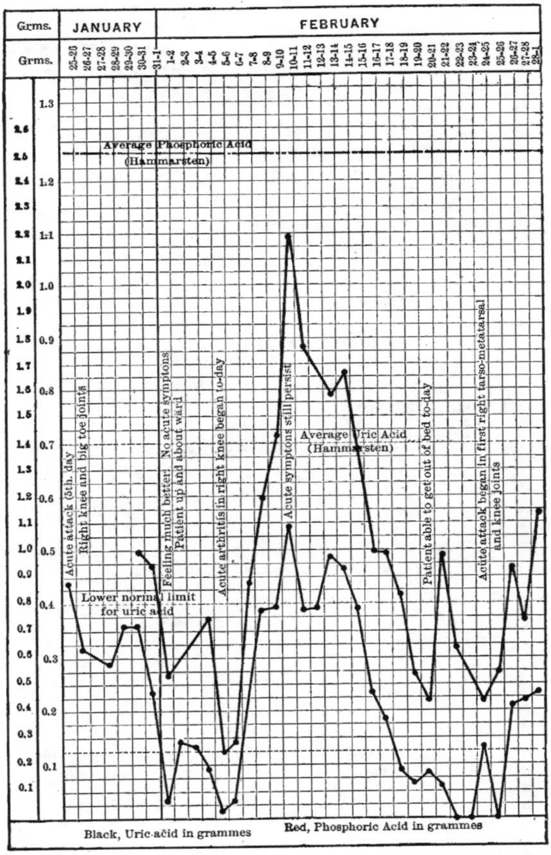

CHART XIII.—URIC ACID AND PHOSPHORIC ACID OUTPUT IN CASE OF ACUTE GOUT.

uric acid content is generally constant in gout and the amount is apparently greater during an attack than in the intervals. This excess, also, is not peculiar to gout, but occurs in leukæmia and chlorosis. The red cells in the "lead-gout" cases may show basophilic granular staining.

The important changes are in the articular tissues. The first joint of the great toe is most frequently involved; then the ankles, knees, and the small joints of the hands and wrists. The deposits may be in all the joints of the lower limbs and absent from those of the upper limbs (Norman Moore). If death takes place during an acute paroxysm, there are signs of inflammation, hyperæmia, swelling of the ligamentous tissues, and of effusion into the joint. The primary change, according to Ebstein, is a local necrosis, due to the presence of an excess of urates in the blood. This is seen in the cartilage and other articular tissues in which the nutritional currents are slow. In these areas of coagulation necrosis the reaction is always acid and the neutral urates are deposited in crystalline form, as insoluble acid urate. The articular cartilages are first involved. The gouty deposit may be uniform, or in small areas. Though it looks superficial, the deposit is invariably interstitial and covered by a thin lamina of cartilage. The deposit is thickest at the part most distant from the circulation. The ligaments and fibro-cartilage ultimately become involved and are infiltrated with biurate deposits, the so-called chalk-stones, or tophi. These are usually covered by skin; but in some cases, particularly in the metacarpo-phalangeal articulations, this ulcerates and the chalk-stones appear externally. The synovial fluid may also contain crystals. In very long-standing cases, owing to an excessive deposit, the joint becomes immobile. The marginal outgrowths in gouty arthritis are true exostoses (Wynne). The cartilage of the ear may contain tophi, which are seen as whitish nodules at the margin of the helix. The cartilages of the nose, eyelids, and larynx are less frequently affected.

Of changes in the internal organs those in the renal and vascular systems are the most important. The kidney changes believed to be characteristic of gout are: (*a*) A deposit of urates chiefly in the region of the papillæ. This, however, is less common than is usually supposed. Norman Moore found it in only 12 out of 80 cases. The apices of the pyramids show lines of whitish deposit. Ebstein described areas of necrosis in both cortex and medulla, in the interior of which were crystalline deposits of urate of soda. (*b*) An interstitial nephritis, either the ordinary "contracted kidney" or the arterio-sclerotic form, neither of which is in any way distinctive.

Arterio-sclerosis and cardiac hypertrophy are very constant lesions. Concretions of urate of soda may occur on the valves. Myocarditis is common.

Changes in the respiratory system are rare. Deposits have been found in the vocal cords, and uric-acid crystals have been found in the sputum of a gouty patient (J. W. Moore).

Symptoms.—Gout is usually divided into acute, chronic, and irregular forms.

Acute Gout.—Premonitory symptoms are common—twinges of pain in the small joints of the hands or feet, nocturnal restlessness, irritability of temper, and dyspepsia. The urine is acid, scanty, and high-colored. It deposits urates on cooling, and there may be transient albuminuria. There may be traces of sugar (gouty glycosuria). Before an attack the output of uric acid is low and is also diminished in the early part of the paroxysm. The relation of uric and phosphoric acids to the acute attacks is well represented in Chart XIII, prepared by Futcher. Both are extremely low in the intervals, but reach normal limits shortly after the onset of the acute symptoms. The phosphoric acid and uric acid show almost parallel curves. The patient was on a very light fixed diet at the time the determinations were made. In some instances the throat is sore, and there may be dyspnœa. The attack sets in usually in the early morning hours. The patient is aroused by a severe pain in the metatarso-phalangeal articulation of the big toe, and more commonly on the right than on the left side. The pain is agonizing, and, as Sydenham says, "insinuates itself with the most exquisite cruelty among the numerous small bones of the tarsus and metatarsus, in the ligaments of which it is lurking." The joint swells rapidly, and becomes hot, tense, and shiny. The sensitiveness is extreme, and the pain makes the patient feel as if the joint were being pressed in a vice. There is fever, and the temperature may rise to 102° to 103° F. Toward morning the severity of the symptoms subsides, and, although the joint remains swollen, the day may be passed in comparative comfort. The symptoms recur the next night, and the "fit," as it is called, usually lasts for from five to eight days, the severity of the symptoms gradually abating. There is usually a moderate leucocytosis during the acute manifestations. Other joints may be involved, particularly the tarsal joints. The inflammation, however intense, never goes on to suppuration. With the subsidence of the swelling the skin desquamates. The tarsus alone may be involved and so obstinate may be the inflammation that the question of surgical interference may be raised in the belief that it is tuberculous or suppurative. After the attack the general health may be much improved. As Aretæus remarks, a person in the interval has won the race at the Olympian games. Recurrences are frequent. Some patients have three or four attacks in a year; others suffer at longer intervals.

The term *retrocedent* or *suppressed* gout is applied to serious internal symptoms, coincident with a rapid disappearance or improvement of the local signs. Very remarkable manifestations may occur under these circumstances. The patient may have severe gastro-intestinal symptoms—pain, vomiting, diarrhœa, and great depression—and death may occur during such an attack. Or there may be cardiac manifestations—dyspnœa, pain, and irregular action of the heart. In some instances, in which the gout is said to attack the heart, an acute pericarditis proves fatal. So, too, there may be marked cerebral manifestations—delirium or coma, and even apoplexy—but in a majority of these instances the symptoms are, in all probability, uræmic.

Chronic Gout.—With increased frequency in the attacks, the articular symptoms persist for a longer time, and gradually many joints become affected. Deposits of urates take place, at first in the articular cartilages and then in the ligaments and capsular tissues; so that in the course of years the joints become swollen, irregular, and deformed. The feet are usually first affected, then the hands. In severe cases there may be extensive concretions about the elbows and knees and along the tendons and in the bursæ. The tophi appear in the ears. Finally, a unique clinical picture is produced which can not be mistaken for that of any other affection. The skin over the tophi may rupture or ulcerate, and about the knuckles the chalk-stones may be freely exposed. Patients with chronic gout are usually dyspeptic, often of a sallow complexion, and show signs of arterio-sclerosis. The pulse tension is increased, the vessels are stiff, and the left ventricle is hypertrophied. The urine is increased in amount, is of low specific gravity, and usually contains a slight amount of albumin, with a few hyaline casts. Severe cramps involving the calf, abdominal, and thoracic muscles are common. Intercurrent attacks of acute polyarthritis may occur, in which the joints become inflamed, and the temperature ranges from 101° to 103° F. There may be pain, redness, and swelling of several joints without fever. Uræmia, pleurisy, pericarditis, peritonitis, and meningitis are common terminal affections.

Irregular Gout.—This is a motley, ill-defined group of symptoms, manifestations of a condition of disordered nutrition, to which the terms *gouty diathesis* or *lithæmic state* have been given. Cases are seen in members of gouty families, who may never themselves have suffered from the acute disease, and in persons who have lived not wisely but too well, who have eaten and drunk largely, lived sedentary lives, and yet have been fortunate enough to escape an acute attack. It is interesting to note the various manifestations in a family with marked hereditary disposition. The daughters often escape, while one son may have gouty attacks of great severity, even though he lives a temperate life and tries in every way to avoid the conditions favoring the disorder. Another son has, perhaps, only the irregular manifestations and never the acute articular affection. While the irregular features are perhaps more often met with in the hereditary affection, they are by no means infrequent in persons who appear to have acquired the disease. The tendency in some families is to call every affection gouty. Even infantile complaints, such as eczema, naso-pharyngeal vegetations, and enuresis, are often regarded, without sufficient grounds, as evidences of the family ailment. Among the commonest manifestations of irregular gout are the following:

(*a*) *Cutaneous Eruptions.*—Garrod and others have called special attention to the frequent association of eczema with the gouty habit.

(*b*) *Gastro-intestinal Disorders.*—Attacks of what is termed "biliousness," in which the tongue is furred, the breath foul, and the bowels constipated, are not uncommon in gouty persons. A gouty parotitis is described.

(*c*) *Cardio-vascular Symptoms.*—With gout arterio-sclerosis is frequently associated. The blood tension is persistently high, the vessel walls become stiff, and cardiac and renal changes gradually occur. In this condition the symptoms may be renal, as when the albuminuria becomes more marked, or dropsical symptoms supervene. The manifestations may be cardiac, when the hypertrophy of the left ventricle fails and there are palpitation, irregular action, and ultimately a condition of asystole. Or, finally, the manifestations may be vascular, and thrombosis of the coronary arteries may cause sudden death, or, as most frequently happens, cerebral hæmorrhage occurs. It makes but little difference whether we regard this condition as primarily an arterio-sclerosis or as a gouty nephritis; the point to be remembered is that the nutritional disorder with which an excess of uric acid is associated induces in time increased tension, arterio-sclerosis, chronic interstitial nephritis, and changes in the myocardium. Pericarditis is not an infrequent terminal complication. Phlebitis is a troublesome and not very uncommon complication. It may arise in connection with varicose veins of the legs or occur in many venous districts in succession or simultaneously.

(*d*) *Nervous Manifestations.*—Headache, migraine attacks, neuralgias, sciatica, and paræsthesias are not uncommon. A common gouty manifestation, upon which Duckworth has laid stress, is the occurrence of hot or itching feet at night. Plutarch mentions that Strabo called this "the lisping of the gout." Cramps in the legs may be very troublesome. Hutchinson called attention to hot and itching eyeballs. Associated or alternating with this symptom there may be attacks of episcleral congestion. Apoplexy is a common termination and meningitis may occur, usually basilar.

(*e*) *Urinary Disorders.*—The urine is highly acid and high-colored, and may deposit crystals of uric acid on standing. Transient and temporary increase in this ingredient cannot be regarded as serious. In many cases of chronic gout the amount may be diminished, and increased only at certain periods, forming the so-called uric-acid showers. A sediment of uric acid in a urine does not necessarily mean an excess. It is often dependent on the inability of the urine to hold it in solution. Sugar is found intermittently in the urine of gouty persons—gouty glycosuria. It may pass into true diabetes, but is usually very amenable to treatment. Oxaluria may also be present. Gouty persons are specially prone to calculi, Jerome Cardan to the contrary, who reckoned freedom from stone among the chief of the *dona podagræ*. Minute quantities of albumin are very common in gouty persons, and, when the renal changes are well established, tube-casts. Urethritis, with a purulent discharge, may arise, so it is stated, usually at the end of an attack. It may occur spontaneously, or follow a pure connection.

(*f*) *Pulmonary Disorders.*—There are no characteristic changes, but chronic bronchitis occurs with great frequency in persons of a gouty habit.

(*g*) Of eye affections, iritis, glaucoma, hæmorrhagic retinitis, and suppurative panophthalmitis have been described.

X-rays.—The changes in the bones consist of small dark areas on the plates, circular in outline, with clear, sharp borders. They are usually found in the epiphysis of the affected joints, especially of the fingers, and are due to the absorption of bone areas in which sodium urate has been deposited.

Diagnosis.—Recurring attacks of arthritis, limited to the big toe or to the tarsus, occurring in a member of a gouty family, or in a man who has lived too well, leave no question as to the nature of the trouble. There are many cases of gout, however, in which the feet do not suffer most severely. After an attack or two in one toe, other joints may be affected, and it is just in such cases of polyarthritis that the difficulty in diagnosis is apt to arise. We have had cases admitted for the third or fourth time with involvement of three or more of the larger joints. The presence of tophi has settled the nature of a trouble which in the previous attacks had been regarded as rheumatic. The following are suggestive points in such cases: (1) The patient's habits and occupation. In the United States the brewery men and barkeepers are often affected. (2) The presence of tophi. The ears should always be inspected in a case of polyarthritis. The diagnosis may rest with a small tophus. The student should learn to recognize, on the ear margin, Woolner's tip, fibroid nodules, and small sebaceous tumors. The last are easily recognized microscopically. The needle-shaped sodium biurate crystals are distinctive of the tophi. (3) The condition of the urine. The uric-acid output is usually very low during the intervals of the paroxysm. At the height of the attack the elimination, as a rule, is greatly increased. (4) The gouty polyarthritis may be afebrile. A patient with three or four joints red, swollen, and painful in rheumatic fever has pyrexia, and, while it may be present and often is in gout, its absence is a valuable diagnostic sign. Many cases go a-begging for a diagnosis. A careful study of the patient's habits as to beer drinking, of the location of the initial arthritic attacks, and the examination for tophi in the ears will prevent many cases being mistaken for rheumatic fever or arthritis deformans. Lastly, in doubtful forms of arthritis a careful study of the purin metabolism is of value. The estimation of the amount of endogenous uric acid in the blood and the delayed excretion of exogenous purins are important.

Prognosis.—"Once gouty, always gouty" is usually true, but by care the frequency and intensity of attacks can be reduced. As regards the duration of life, the state of the circulation and kidneys is the important factor.

Treatment.—Hygienic.—Individuals who have inherited a tendency to gout, or who have shown any manifestations of it, should live temperately, abstain from alcohol, and eat moderately. An open-air life, with plenty of exercise and regular hours, does much to counteract an inborn tendency to the disease. The skin should be kept active and an occasional Turkish bath is advantageous. The patient should dress warmly, avoid rapid alterations in temperature, and be careful not to have the skin suddenly chilled.

Dietetic.—With few exceptions, persons over forty eat too much, and the first injunction to a gouty person is to keep his appetite within reasonable bounds, to eat at stated hours, and to take plenty of time at his meals. In the matter of food, quantity is a factor of more importance than quality with many gouty persons. As Sir William Roberts well says, "Nowhere perhaps is it more necessary than in gout to consider the man as well as the ailment, and very often more the man than the ailment."

The weight of opinion leans to the use of a modified nitrogenous diet, without excess in starchy and saccharine articles of food. Foods rich in purins, such as bouillon, beef extracts, sweetbreads, liver, kidneys, and brain, should be avoided. Milk and eggs are particularly useful, owing to their being purin free. Fresh vegetables and fruits may be used freely, but strawberries and bananas should be avoided.

Ebstein urged strongly the use of fat in the form of good fresh butter, from 2½ to 3½ ounces in the day. He held that stout gouty subjects not only do not increase in weight with plenty of fat in the food, but that they actually become thin and the general condition improves very much. Hot bread of all sorts and the various articles of food prepared from Indian corn should, as a rule, be avoided. Roberts advised gouty patients to restrict as far as practicable the use of common salt, since the sodium biurate very readily crystallizes out in tissues with a high percentage of sodium salts. In this matter of diet each individual case must receive separate consideration.

There are very few conditions in the gouty in which alcohol is required. Whenever indicated, whisky will be found perhaps the most serviceable. While all are injurious to these patients, some are much more so than others, particularly malted liquors, champagne, port, and a very large proportion of all the light wines.

Mineral Waters.—All forms may be said to be beneficial in gout, as the main element is the water, and the ingredients are usually indifferent. Much of the humbuggery in the profession still lingers about mineral waters, more particularly about the so-called lithia waters.

The question of the utility of alkalies in the treatment of gout is closely connected with this subject of mineral waters. This deep-rooted belief in the profession was shaken by Sir William Roberts, who claimed to have shown that alkalescence as such has no influence whatever on the sodium biurate. The sodium salts are believed by this author to be particularly harmful, but, in spite of all the theoretical denunciation of the use of the sodium salts, the gouty from all parts of the world flock to those very Continental springs in which these salts are most predominant. Of the mineral springs best suited for the gouty may be mentioned, in the United States, those of Saratoga, Bedford, and the White Sulphur; Buxton and Bath, in England; in France, Aix-les-Bains and Contrexeville; and in Germany, Carlsbad, Wildbad, Homburg, and Marienbad. Excellent results are claimed for mineral waters with special radio-active properties. The efficacy in reality is in the water, in the way it is taken, on an empty stomach, and in large quantities; and the important accessories in the modified diet, proper hours, regular exercises, with baths, douches, etc., play a very important rôle in the "cure."

Medical Treatment.—In an acute attack the limb should be elevated and the affected joint wrapped in cotton-wool. Warm fomentations, or Fuller's lotion, may be used. The local hot-air or passive hyperæmia treatment may be tried. A brisk mercurial purge is always advantageous at the outset. The wine or tincture of colchicum, in doses of 20 to 30 minims (1.2 to 2 c. c.) may be given every four hours in combination with the citrate of potash. The action of the colchicum should be carefully watched; its effect is most marked when free purgation follows. It has in a majority of the cases a powerful influence over the symptoms—relieving the pain, and reducing, sometimes with great rapidity, the swelling and redness. It should be stopped as soon as it has relieved the pain. Cinchophen (atophan) is often useful in doses of 15 grains, 1 gm., three or four times a day. It may also be helpful in the subacute and chronic forms. In cases in which the pain and sleeplessness are distressing and do not yield to treatment, morphia is necessary. The patient should be placed on a diet chiefly of milk and barley-water. During convalescence the diet should be increased slowly and gradually the patient may resume the diet previously laid down.

In some of the subacute intercurrent attacks sodium salicylate or acetyl-salicylic acid may be useful. The chronic and irregular forms are best treated by the dietetic and hygienic measures already noted. Potassium iodide is sometimes useful. Albu speaks favorably of lemon-juice as a remedy. The vegetable acids are converted in the system into alkaline carbonates, thus enabling the blood to keep the uric acid compounds in solution, and facilitating their elimination.

Where the arthritic attacks are confined to one joint, such as the great-toe joint, surgical interference may be considered. Riedel reports two successful cases in which he removed the entire joint capsule of the big-toe joint, with permanent relief.

II. DIABETES MELLITUS

Definition.—A disease of metabolism in general with especial disturbance of carbohydrate metabolism in which the normal utilization of carbohydrate is impaired with an increase in the sugar content of the blood and consequent glycosuria. There is a tendency to subsequent disturbance of the fat metabolism with resulting acidosis (Ketosis).

History.—The disease was known to Celsus. Aretæus first used the term diabetes, calling it a wonderful affection "melting down the flesh and limbs into urine." He suggested that the disease got its name from the Greek word signifying a syphon. Willis in the seventeenth century gave a good description and recognized the sweetness of the urine "as if there has been sugar and honey in it." Dobson in 1776 demonstrated the presence of sugar, and Rollo in 1797 wrote an admirable account and recommended the use of a meat diet. The modern study of the disease dates from Claude Bernard's demonstration of the glycogenic function of the liver in 1857.

Etiology.—The enzymes of the intestinal mucosa convert the starches and sugars of the food into monosaccharides—dextrose, galactose and levulose—which pass into the portal circulation, but the major portion remains in the liver, where it is converted into glycogen. The percentage of sugar in the systemic blood remains constant—0.06 to 0.11 per cent. Part of the sugar passes to the muscles, where it is stored as glycogen. The total storage capacity of the liver is estimated at about one-tenth of its weight, *i. e.*, about 150 gms. for an ordinary organ weighing 1,500 gms. Not all of the glycogen comes from the carbohydrates; a small part in health is derived from the proteins and fats. This treble process of transformation, storage and retransformation of the sugars is effected by special enzymes, which are furnished by internal secretions, chiefly of the pancreas and hypophysis, and are directly influenced by the nervous system. According to Claude Bernard the sugar is simply warehoused on demand in the liver, and given out to the muscles which need it in their work. In any case, the sugar, one of the chief fuels of the body, is burned up, supplying energy to the muscles, and is eliminated as CO_2 and water. The nature of the intermediate stages of the transformation is still under discussion.

The following are the conditions which influence the appearance of sugar in the urine:

(*a*) Excess of Carbohydrate Intake.—In a normal state the sugar in the blood is about 0.1 per cent. In diabetes the percentage is usually from 0.2 to 0.4 per cent. The hyperglycæmia is immediately manifested by the appearance of sugar in the urine. The healthy person has a definite limit of carbohydrate assimilation; the total storage capacity for glycogen is estimated at about 300 gms. Following the ingestion of enormous amounts of carbohydrates the liver and the muscles may not be equal to the task of storing it; the blood content of sugar passes beyond the normal limit and the renal cells immediately begin to get rid of the surplus. Like the balance at the Mint, which is sensitive to the correct weight of the gold coins passing over it, they only react at a certain point of saturation. Fortunately excessive quantities of pure sugar itself are not taken. The carbohydrates are chiefly in the form of starch, the digestion and absorption of which take place slowly, so that this so-called alimentary glycosuria very rarely occurs, though enormous quantities may be taken. The assimilation limit of a normal fasting individual for sugar itself is about 250 gms. of grape sugar, and considerably less of cane and milk sugar. Clinically one meets with many cases in which glycosuria is present as a result of excessive ingestion of carbohydrates, particularly in stout persons and heavy feeders—so-called lipogenic diabetes—a form very readily controlled.

(*b*) Disturbances in the Nervous System.—Bernard shows that there was a centre in the medulla—the diabetic centre—puncture of which is followed by hyperglycæmia due to an increased outflow of sugar from the liver warehouse. He demonstrated that the efferent path of this influence was through the splanchnic nerves and the afferent through the vagi. The exact location of this centre has never been determined, and its precise rôle in the carbohydrate metabolism is obscure. Clinically, however, it has long been known that many lesions of the nervous system cause glycosuria—tumors, particularly those in the neighborhood of the medulla, injuries both to the brain and to the upper part of the spinal cord, meningitis, and hæmorrhage. Some of these may disturb Bernard's centre in the medulla, but many of them disturb the internal secretion of the hypophysis. Clinically, glycosuria arising from disturbances in the nervous system is not an important variety.

(*c*) Disturbances of the Internal Secretions.—The part played in the carbohydrate metabolism by the ductless glands is of the first importance. Though not yet fully understood, the following are the chief points, so far as they bear on clinical work:

(1) *Pancreatic Secretion.*—Extirpation of the pancreas in a dog is followed by hyperglycæmia and prolonged glycosuria, which is not relieved by feeding pancreas to the animal, but which is checked if experimentally a portion of healthy organ from another dog is inserted into the portal circulation. The pancreas contains structures known as "the islands of Langerhans," which, from the work of Opie and others, are believed to furnish an internal secretion necessary to normal carbohydrate metabolism. A portion of the organ separated from the rest, and its duct ligated, atrophies, but a tissue remains composed of enlarged islands of Langerhans. If the remainder of the pancreas be removed, this atrophied portion is able to ward off glycosuria; but if this is removed glycosuria appears immediately (W. G. MacCallum). In some way the secretion furnished by this organ is essential to the proper preparation of the sugars. Cohnheim suggests a correlation of this internal secretion with a muscle enzyme, to which it acts as an amboceptor, and that it is by the combined action of these two glycolytic bodies that the sugars are normally burned up in the muscles. Many diseases of the pancreas are associated with glycosuria, some with permanent diabetes. Hæmorrhagic pancreatitis, cancer, calculus, chronic interstitial pancreatitis, catarrh of the ducts may all be associated with a profound disturbance in the metabolism of the sugars. In fact, there is no one organ the disease of which is more constantly associated with glycosuria, and the studies of Opie warrant the belief that the essential factor is a disturbance of the function of the internal secretion provided by the islands of Langerhans.

(2) *Hypophysis.*—It was long known that glycosuria occurred in tumors of the region of the hypophysis, particularly in acromegaly, and it follows fractures of the base of the skull. Experimentally, Cushing and his students have shown that the posterior lobe of the pituitary gland has an important influence in carbohydrate metabolism. The secretion of this portion of the gland is discharged into the third ventricle, and any operative disturbance of it, or of the infundibulum, is at once followed by glycosuria, and by a re-

markable lowering of the assimilation limit for sugars. On the other hand, a deficiency of this secretion, or the removal of this portion of the gland alone, is followed by a remarkable increased tolerance for carbohydrates.

Clinically, this sequence is not infrequently seen. A tumor which at first irritates the gland, as in the early stages of acromegaly, may cause glycosuria, but later, as the posterior lobe of the gland is destroyed, there is an extraordinarily high assimilation limit for sugars, and associated with it a great increase in the deposition of fat in the body, a syndrome to be referred to later. Intravenous or subcutaneous injection of the extract of the posterior lobe promptly lowers this high assimilation limit for carbohydrates.

(3) *Adrenals and Thyroids.*—We have less positive information about the relation of carbohydrate metabolism to the internal secretions of these glands. Glycosuria does not necessarily follow lesions of the adrenals, but epinephrin has a powerful influence on the carbohydrate metabolism, and glycosuria may be readily produced in animals by subcutaneous injection, and by the local application of epinephrin to the pancreas. Clinically, we know practically nothing of an adrenal glycosuria. It does not occur in Addison's disease. It has occasionally been noticed in the prolonged therapeutic use of epinephrin. In disturbances of the thyroid gland glycosuria is not uncommon. There is a lowered tolerance for sugar in Graves' disease which is sometimes associated with a true diabetes, and in the remarkable instances of acute myxœdema the amount of sugar in the urine may be large. The use of thyroid extract is occasionally followed by glycosuria. On the other hand, patients may take the extract continuously for many years without glycosuria.

Possibly the glycosuria associated with pregnancy is due to a disturbance in the internal secretions. It is a transient condition, usually disappearing with parturition, and rarely leads to diabetes. It may recur in successive pregnancies.

(*d*) Disturbances in the Function of the Liver.—One of the most remarkable features in carbohydrate metabolism is that the great warehouse of the sugars may be damaged to any degree without causing hyperglycæmia or glycosuria. Whether or not there is a type of disease to which the name of "liver diabetes" may be given is doubtful. There are cases of cirrhosis of the liver and of gallstones—particularly those associated with enlargement of the organ—in which glycosuria is present, but they are probably all associated with coincident affections of the pancreas. In the "bronze diabetes," which is accompanied by great hypertrophy of the liver, the glycosuria is probably pancreatic.

(*e*) Disturbances in the Kidney Functions.—Disease of the kidneys is rarely associated with glycosuria. Occasionally one finds it in chronic nephritis, but the existence of a true diabetes depending upon renal changes has not been proved. There is a remarkable experimental diabetes of great interest in connection with carbohydrate metabolism. If phloridzin, a glucoside prepared from the bark of the apple-tree, is given by mouth or subcutaneously to man or animals glycosuria results, and even continues on a nitrogenous diet, and in man when fasting. The amount of sugar excreted may be large, yet there is no hyperglycæmia. It seems that the sugar is directly manufactured by the kidney epithelium, and largely from the proteins.

(*f*) Miscellaneous Disturbances.—The carbohydrate metabolism may be upset in acute fevers, in many of which a transient glycosuria is present. It is not uncommon after the administration of ether, less so after chloroform. Metabolic disturbances in gout are not infrequently associated with glycosuria, and cachexias and profound anæmias may be accompanied by transient glycosuria. A mental shock, a severe nervous strain and worry precede many cases. Patients suffocated by smoke, or poisoned by coal gas, may have sugar in the urine.

Incidence.—According to statistics diabetes appears to be about as frequent in the United States as in European countries. In England and Wales the deaths increased from 2,767 in 1902 to 4,542 in 1916. The disease is on the increase in the United States. The statistics for 1870 gave 2.1; for 1890, 3.8; for 1900, 9.3; and for 1915, 17.5 deaths to the 100,000 population. This may be due to the great increase in the consumption of sugar. Among 27,618 patients admitted to the medical wards of the Johns Hopkins Hospital in twenty-two years there were 276 cases of diabetes, or one per cent.

Hereditary influences play an important rôle and cases are on record of its occurrence in many members of the same family. Morton, who calls the disease *hydrops ad matulam* (Phthisiologia, 1689), records a remarkable family in which four children were affected, one of which recovered on a milk diet and diascordium. An analysis of the cases in our series gave only 6 cases with a history of diabetes in relatives (Pleasants). Naunyn obtained a family history of diabetes in 35 out of 201 private cases, but in only 7 of 157 hospital cases. There are instances of the coexistence of the disease in man and wife. Among 516 married pairs collected by Senator, in which either husband or wife was diabetic, in 18 cases the second partner had become diabetic. Similarity in habits probably accounts for this.

Sex.—Men are more frequently affected than women, the ratio being about three to two. Of the 276 cases of diabetes referred to, 179 were in males and 97 in females (Futcher). It is a disease of adult life; a majority of the cases occur from the third to the sixth decade. Of the 276 cases, the largest number—70—occurred between fifty and sixty years of age.

Diabetes in Children.—This usually occurs among the better classes. Hereditary influences are marked. The course of the disease is, as a rule, much more rapid than in adults. While the disease is usually severe there are not infrequent cases of a mild type. One case is mentioned of a child apparently born with glycosuria, who recovered in eight months.

Persons of a neurotic *temperament* are often affected. It is a disease of the higher classes. Van Noorden states that the statistics for London and Berlin show that the number of cases in the upper ten thousand exceeds that in the lower hundred thousand inhabitants.

Race.—Hebrews seem especially prone to it; one-fourth of Frerichs' patients were of the Semitic race. Diabetes is comparatively rare in the colored race, but not so uncommon as was formerly supposed. Of the series of 276 cases, 29, or 10.6 per cent., were in negroes.

Metabolism in Diabetes.—Glycosuria, neurotic, dietetic or toxic, may be a matter of simple overflow, but the essence of true diabetes is a waste of the carbohydrates, which hurry through the body, in great part never warehoused as glycogen. Why this should be, whether the liver and muscles are at fault in refusing to transform the carbohydrate, or whether the defect is the enzymes of the ductless glands, are problems awaiting solution. Naunyn held that hyperglycæmia is due to a failure of the liver and muscles to store up glycogen as in health. On the other hand, Lépine, Opie, and others support the view that the glycolytic ferments are lacking—the former may depend on the latter. In either case the result is a failure of the normal oxidation of the carbohydrates. Hyperglycæmia is responsible for the thirst and the polyuria, and there is a very considerable daily loss of energy in warming the liquids taken to the temperature of the body, according to Benedict and Joslin nearly 6 per cent. of the total heat of the day; and it is this excess of sugar in the system that renders the body so favorable a culture medium for pus organisms. There is loss of energy with the steady waste of sugar fuel; practically every gram of sugar excreted in the urine results in a loss of 4.1 calories, consequently a diabetic patient excreting 100 grams of sugar and 20 grams of β-oxybutyric acid loses 500 calories in this way, so that the patients are apt to be underfed, unless this loss is made up by a full amount of other food (Benedict and Joslin). Studies upon the respiratory quotient—which is the ratio between the CO_2 given out and the O taken in by a healthy individual on a mixed diet (expressed by the fraction 0.9)—favor the view that there is failure in the proper combustion of the carbohydrates. Benedict and Joslin conclude that a respiratory quotient above 0.74 indicates a fairly liberal supply of glycogen stored in the body; while a respiratory quotient of 0.70, or below that, indicates that the patient has no available carbohydrates, and has lost in a measure the power of storing them. And here comes the special danger; as the carbohydrates pass through the body unburned, the energy must be provided from the proteins and fats. The metabolism of the former does not appear to be seriously disturbed, and the carbohydrate portion of the protein molecule is well tolerated and in part supplies the place of the lost sugars. The danger is in the metabolism of the fats. The carbohydrates are not used as fuel; the proteins are easily utilized, but apparently it takes so much draught to burn them that not enough is left to consume the fats completely; and the products of incomplete combustion accumulate in the system and suffocate the patient as effectually as does the CO of a charcoal stove. The chief product of this incomplete combustion of the fats is the β-oxybutyric acid, which itself is the source of the diacetic acid and acetone, and the special danger of the disease is now recognized to be the production of an acidosis in consequence of this imperfect fat metabolism. One of the most valuable advances in our knowledge of the metabolism of the disease has been the work of Beddard, Pembrey and Spriggs and more recently of Poulton, who have shown that the amount of CO_2 in the alveolar air may be taken as a measure of the acidosis. The acetone bodies in the urine indicate a large production in the body but this may have been completely compensated. The blood examination is more important to determine the degree of accumulation and with even slight degrees there are changes in the alveolar air.

The CO_2 tension of the alveolar air is reduced. In slight acidosis this is between 32 and 38 mm. Hg, in moderate acidosis 28 to 32 mm. Hg, and in severe acidosis less than 28 mm. Hg (normal 38-45 mm. Hg). The lowest figure noted by Joslin was 9 mm. Hg.

Renal Diabetes.—This term is applied to a condition in which there is glycosuria without increase of the sugar in the blood. In it the glycosuria is independent of the carbohydrate intake and the blood sugar is normal or decreased in amount. The kidney cells allow sugar to escape. As a rule it is discovered accidentally as there are rarely any symptoms. The condition is rare and the patients should be followed for a long time to exclude Diabetes Mellitus.

Morbid Anatomy.—The *nervous system* shows no constant lesions. In a few instances there have been tumors or sclerosis in the medulla, or a cysticercus has pressed on the floor. A secondary multiple neuritis is not rare, and to it the so-called diabetic tabes is probably due, and changes occur in the posterior columns of the cord similar to those which have been found in pernicious anæmia. In the sympathetic system the ganglia have been enlarged and in some instances sclerosed. The *heart* is hypertrophied in some cases. Endocarditis is very rare. Arterio-sclerosis is common. The *lungs* show important changes. Acute broncho-pneumonia or lobar pneumonia (either of which may terminate in gangrene) and tuberculosis are common. The so-called diabetic phthisis is always tuberculous and results from a caseating broncho-pneumonia. In rare cases there is a chronic interstitial pneumonia, non-tuberculous. Fat embolism of the pulmonary vessels may occur in connection with diabetic coma.

The *liver* is usually enlarged; fatty degeneration is common. In the so-called diabetic cirrhosis—the *cirrhosis pigmentaire*—the liver is enlarged and sclerotic, and cachexia develops with melanoderma. Dilatation of the stomach with enlargement of the duodenum and colonic stasis are common.

Pancreas.—Of 15 autopsies in 27 fatal cases, in 9 the pancreas was found atrophic. In one of these fat necroses were present, in another calculi. Hyaline degeneration of the islands of Langerhans is a special feature in certain cases. Chronic interstitial pancreatitis is common.

The *kidneys* show a diffuse nephritis with fatty degeneration. Hyaline change is often found in the tubal epithelium, particularly of the descending limb of the loop of Henle, and in the Malpighian tufts.

Symptoms.—*Acute* and *chronic* forms are recognized, but there is no essential difference between them, except that in the former the patients are younger, the course is more rapid, and the emaciation more marked.

The *onset* is gradual, and either frequent micturition or inordinate thirst first attracts attention. Very rarely it sets in rapidly, after a sudden emotion, an injury, or after a severe chill. When fully established the disease is characterized by great thirst, the passage of large quantities of saccharine urine, a voracious appetite, and, as a rule, progressive emaciation.

Among the GENERAL SYMPTOMS *thirst* is one of the most distressing. Large quantities of water are required to keep the sugar in solution and for its excretion in the urine. The amount of fluid consumed will be found to bear a definite ratio to the quantity excreted. Instances, however, are not uncommon of pronounced diabetes in which the thirst is not excessive; but in such cases the amount of urine passed is never large. The thirst is most intense an hour or two after meals. As a rule, the digestion is good and the appetite inordinate. The condition is sometimes termed *bulimia* or *polyphagia.* Lumbar pain is common.

The tongue is usually dry, red, and glazed, and the saliva scanty. The gums may become swollen, and in the later stages aphthous stomatitis is common. Constipation is the rule.

In spite of the enormous amount of food consumed a patient may become rapidly emaciated. This loss of flesh bears some ratio to the polyuria, and when, under suitable diet, the sugar is reduced, the patient may gain in flesh. The skin is dry and harsh, and sweating rarely occurs, except when tuberculosis coexists. Drenching sweats have been known to alternate with excessive polyuria. General pruritus or pruritus pudendi may be very distressing, and occasionally is one of the earliest symptoms. The temperature is often subnormal; the pulse is usually frequent, and the tension increased. Many diabetics do not show marked emaciation. Patients past the middle period of life may have the disease for years without much disturbance of the health, and may remain well nourished. These are the cases of the *diabète gras* in contradistinction to *diabète maigre*.

THE URINE.—The amount varies from 3 to 4 litres in mild cases to 15 to 20 litres in very severe cases. In rare instances the quantity of urine is not much increased. Under strict diet the amount is much lessened, and in intercurrent febrile affections it may be reduced to normal. The specific gravity is high, ranging from 1.025 to 1.045; but in exceptional cases it may be low, 1.013 to 1.020. The highest specific gravity recorded is by Trousseau—1.074. Very high specific gravities—1.070 + —suggest fraud. The urine is pale in color, almost like water, and has a sweetish odor and a distinctly sweetish taste. The reaction is acid. Sugar is present in varying amounts. In mild cases it does not exceed 1½ or 2 per cent., but it may reach from 5 to 10 per cent. The total amount excreted in the twenty-four hours may range from 10 to 20 ounces (320 to 640 grams) and in exceptional cases from 1 to 2 pounds.

Ketonuria.—The ketone bodies, acetone, diacetic acid and β-oxybutyric acid are present, sometimes in small amounts in mild cases but increasing with the severity of the disease; and are indications of acidosis. In coma the excretion of β-oxybutyric acid may be as much as 100 gm. or more a day.

Glycogen has also been found in the urine, and in rare instances sugars other than glucose occur, lactose, levulose, and pentose, and to these conditions the term *melituria* is sometimes applied. *Albumin* is not infrequent.

Pneumaturia, gas in the urine, due to fermentation in the bladder, is occasionally met with. Cammidge's reaction may be present. Fat may be passed in the urine in the form of a fine emulsion (lipuria).

BLOOD IN DIABETES.—The water content is lower than normal. Polycythæmia may be present to 6 or 8 millions of red cells per cmm. Towards the end and with complications there may be a leucocytosis and the leucocytes may contain glycogen. Hyperglycæmia is rarely above 0.4 per cent. The increase in the blood sugar may persist after glycosuria has disappeared.

The alkalinity is lessened and the specific gravity reduced. Lipæmia is present in many cases and may be readily recognized by the presence of dancing particles among the red cells in a slide of fresh blood. The blood lipoids are increased from the normal figure of about 0.6 per cent. to 0.83 per cent. in mild cases, to 0.9 in moderately severe and 1.4 per cent. in severe cases (Joslin). Lipæmia may be present without acidosis and is sometimes due to surcharging of the blood stream with the products of fatty digestion as in the normal lipæmia of sucklings.

Complications.—(*a*) COMA (*Acidosis*)—There are three groups of cases: (1) Typical dyspnœic coma, the air-hunger of Kussmaul, in which with loud and deep in- and expirations, the pulse grows weak, and the patient gradually fails and dies, sometimes within twenty-four hours. The breath very often has the fruity odor of acetone. It may come on without any premonition and the patient may waken out of sleep in dyspnœa. An acyanotic dyspnœa is one of the best indications of acidosis. (2) Cases in which, without any previous dyspnœa or distress, the patient is attacked with headache, a feeling of intoxication, thick speech and a staggering gait, and gradually falls into deep coma. (3) Cases in which, particularly after exertion, the patient is attacked suddenly with weakness, giddiness and fainting; the hands and feet are cold and livid, the pulse small, respiration rapid; the patient becomes drowsy, and death occurs within a few hours. Dyspepsia, constipation, abdominal pain, marked irritability and restlessness may precede the onset of coma and should suggest its possibility.

(*b*) CUTANEOUS.—Boils and carbuncles are extremely common. Painful onychia may occur. Eczema is also met with, and at times an intolerable itching. In women the irritation of the urine may cause the most intense pruritus pudendi, and in men a balanitis. Rarer affections are xanthoma and purpura. Gangrene is not uncommon, and is associated usually with arterio-sclerosis. Perforating ulcer of the foot occurred in 7 of 276 cases. Bronzing of the skin (*diabète bronzé*) occurs in certain cases in which the diabetes arises as a late event in the disease known as hæmochromatosis, which is further characterized by pigmentary cirrhosis of the liver and pancreas. With the onset of severe complications the tolerance of the carbohydrates is much increased. Profuse sweats may occur.

(*c*) PULMONARY.—The patients are not infrequently carried off by *acute pneumonia,* which may be lobar or lobular. *Gangrene* is very apt to supervene, but the breath does not necessarily have the foul odor of ordinary gangrene. Abscess following lobar pneumonia occurred in one of our cases. *Tuberculous broncho-pneumonia* is common and may run a rapid course.

(*d*) RENAL.—*Albuminuria* is a tolerably frequent complication. The amount varies greatly, and, when slight, does not seem to be of much moment. Œdema of the feet and ankles is not an infrequent symptom. General anasarca is rare, however, owing to the marked polyuria. It is sometimes associated with arterio-sclerosis. It occasionally precedes the occurrence of the diabetic coma. Occasionally cystitis is a troublesome symptom.

(*e*) NERVOUS SYSTEM.—*Peripheral Neuritis.*—Neuralgia, numbness and tingling, uncommon symptoms in diabetes, are probably minor neuritic manifestations. The involvement may be general of the upper and lower extremities. Sometimes it is unilateral, or the neuritis may be in a single nerve—the sciatic or the third nerve. Herpes zoster may occur.

Diabetic Tabes (so-called).—This is a peripheral neuritis, characterized by lightning pains in the legs, loss of knee-jerk—which may occur without the other symptoms—and a loss of power in the extensors of the feet. The gait is the characteristic *steppage,* as in alcoholic, and other forms of neuritic paralysis. Changes in the posterior columns of the cord have been found.

Diabetic Paraplegia.—This is also in all probability due to neuritis. There are cases in which power has been lost in both arms and legs.

Mental Symptoms.—The patients are often morose, and there is a strong tendency to become hypochondriacal. Some patients display an extraordinary degree of restlessness and anxiety.

(*f*) SPECIAL SENSES.—Cataract is liable to occur, and with rapidity in young persons. Diabetic retinitis closely resembles the albuminuric form. Hæmorrhages are common. Sudden amaurosis, similar to that which occurs in uræmia, may occur. Paralysis of the muscles of accommodation may be present; and, lastly, atrophy of the optic nerves. Aural symptoms may come on with great rapidity, either an otitis media, or in some instances inflammation of the mastoid cells. Ocular tension may be lowered in coma.

(*g*) SEXUAL FUNCTION.—Impotence is common, and may be an early symptom. Conception is rare; if it occurs, abortion is apt to follow. A diabetic mother may bear a healthy child; there is no known instance of a diabetic mother bearing a diabetic child. The course of the disease is usually aggravated after delivery.

Diagnosis.—There is no difficulty in determining the presence of sugar in the urine if the proper tests are applied. Alcapton may prove very deceptive, and in one reported case of ochronosis (Osler) a diagnosis of diabetes was made by four or five of the leading physicians in Europe, one of whom was an authority on diabetes. Deception may be practised. One patient had urine with a specific gravity of 1.065, but the reactions were for cane sugar; and there is a case in the literature in which, when the cane sugar fraud was detected, the woman bought grape sugar and put it into her bladder.

To determine whether the case is one of simple glycosuria or diabetes is not always easy, as the one readily merges into the other. The younger the individual the greater the probability that the case is true diabetes. It is well to test the assimilation limit; 100 grams of glucose given in solution two hours after a breakfast of a roll and butter with coffee should not give glycosuria. To do so indicates a deficiency in the capacity to store carbohydrates and a possibility that diabetes may follow. Transient glycosuria occurs in a great many conditions already mentioned. For practical purposes the common form is that met with in persons above 50 years of age, who eat and drink too much and tend to grow stout. The detection of a little sugar in the urine may have the great advantage of frightening the patient into a more rational mode of life. The forms following anæsthesia, accidents, business worries, fright and that which occurs in pregnancy are, as a rule, readily controlled.

Prognosis.—The younger the patient the less likely is recovery. In children the disease may run a very rapid course, and death may occur within a few weeks, or a child may die in coma before the condition has been recognized. On the other hand, in persons over fifty sugar may be present in the urine for years without any impairment of strength or health. The outlook is good in the fat, bad in the lean. It is particularly good in the stout, active, business man, whose glycosuria has come on as a result of worry, work, and excess in food and drink. An early diagnosis, obesity and a gain in tolerance are hopeful features.

The following steps should be taken to estimate the gravity of a case. The carbohydrate tolerance should be estimated and the presence of acetone and diacetic acid determined, as they usually indicate a serious disturbance in the fat metabolism. It is well to remember that the acetone bodies may be only temporarily present, and it is not necessary to sign the patient's death warrant so soon as they appear. A patient may live for many years with traces, and they may disappear after having been present for months.

Treatment.—In families with a marked predisposition to the disease the use of starchy and saccharine articles of diet should be restricted. The personal hygiene of a diabetic patient is of the first importance. Sources of worry should be avoided, and he should lead an even, quiet life, if possible in an equable climate. The heat waste should be prevented by wearing warm clothes and avoiding cold. A warm, or, if tolerably robust, a cold, bath should be taken every day. An occasional Turkish bath is useful. Systematic, moderate exercise should be taken. When this is not feasible, massage should be given.

Diet.—Each patient presents his own problem and must be studied individually. The endeavor should be made to keep the urine sugar free and acid free. In this the proper use of fasting, as advocated by Allen, is of great aid but it should not be employed carelessly. The object of treatment is to inincrease the carbohydrate tolerance; it is important not to overtax the patient's powers of using carbohydrates by giving more than he can utilize. In mild cases the carbohydrate intake may be gradually reduced, sugar as such being cut off first and the carbohydrate intake reduced by a certain proportion each day until the urine is sugar free. In the medium and severe cases fasting is useful. The purpose of it should be explained to the patient and his co-operation secured. The time of fasting required to render the urine sugar free varies from one to five days. The patient should be put to bed; water may be taken freely and tea or coffee allowed (without sugar or cream) if desired. If sugar persists after the second day of fasting 300 c. c. of meat broth or bouillon may be given. When the urine is sugar free it is necessary to determine the carbohydrate tolerance.

The profession, and much more the diabetic patient, owes much to E. P. Joslin of Boston for his studies on diabetes. We quote some of his directions:

"In severe, long-standing, complicated, obese and elderly cases, as well as in all cases with acidosis, or in any case if desired, without otherwise changing habits or diet, omit fat, after two days omit protein and then halve the carbohydrates daily until the patient is taking only 10 grams; then fast. In other cases begin fasting at once. Fast four days, unless earlier sugar-free. Allow water freely, tea, coffee and thin, clear meat broths as desired."

"If glycosuria persists at the end of four days, give 1 gram protein or 0.5 gram carbohydrate per kilogram body weight for two days and then fast again for three days unless earlier sugar-free. If glycosuria remains, repeat and then fast for one or two days as necessary. If there is still sugar, give protein as before for four days, then fast one, and then gradually increase the periods of feeding, one day each time, until fasting one day each week. I have seen no uncomplicated case fail to get sugar-free by this method."

"When the twenty-four-hour urine is free from sugar, give 5 to 10 grams carbohydrate (150 to 300 grams of 5 per cent. vegetables) and continue to add 5 to 10 grams carbohydrate daily up to 50 grams or more until sugar appears."

"When the urine has been sugar-free for three days, add about 20 grams protein and thereafter 15 grams protein daily in the form of egg-white, fish or lean meat (chicken) until the patient is receiving 1 gram protein per kilogram body weight or less if the carbohydrate tolerance is zero."

"Add no fat until the protein reaches 1 gram per kilogram body weight (unless the protein tolerance is below this figure) and the carbohydrate tolerance has been determined, but then add 5 to 25 grams daily, according to previous acidosis, until the patient ceases to lose weight or receives in the total diet about 30 calories per kilogram body weight."

"The return of sugar demands fasting for twenty-four hours or until sugar-free. Resume the former diet gradually, adding fat last in order to maintain as high a carbohydrate tolerance as possible, sacrificing body weight for this purpose. This rule should be inflexibly followed, especially with children."

"Whether sugar reappears in the urine or not it is desirable upon one day each week to rest that function of the body which controls the assimilation of sugar by either a complete fast day or a diet of low caloric value. My plan is patterned on the following rule: Whenever the tolerance is less than 20 grams carbohydrate, fasting should be practised one day in seven; when the tolerance is over 20 grams carbohydrate, cut the diet in half on one day each week (half-day)."

Days of Reduced Diet.—In every case it is wise to restrict the diet on one day a week. In mild cases the quantity of carbohydrate should be reduced to one-half or one-third of the usual amount. In moderate or severe cases a complete fast of one day is advisable. A day when only eggs and the 5 per cent. vegetables are taken is also an advantage. The exact amount allowed in any case must depend on the carbohydrate tolerance: the lower this is the greater importance of a fast day.

Saccharine may be used in place of sugar. It is an advantage in using vegetables which are boiled in cooking, to do the boiling in three different waters. All the water should be removed after each boiling. This reduces the amount of carbohydrate. It is well to do this with patients who demand bulk in the diet.

The patient should keep an accurate record of his diet and the amounts taken. It is well for him to have scales to determine the exact weights so that the intake is known accurately. Tables of food values are of assistance in determining the amount of protein, carbohydrate and fat in the diet. He should be taught to examine the urine for sugar, daily in severe cases, once or twice a week in milder cases. It is not necessary for the patient to gain weight or even to equal his former normal weight.

Medical Treatment.—This is not satisfactory and there is no drug which appears to have a direct curative influence. Opium and its derivatives are sometimes useful for irritable patients but are rarely required. Potassium bromide may be given for the same purpose. The use of arsenic has been recommended and is indicated, either alone or with iron in case of anæmia. The bowels should be kept freely open and for this such drugs as mineral oil, cascara, senna and phenolphthalein are most useful. Purging should be avoided.

Coma.—The urine should be watched carefully for acetone and diacetic acid. Their presence is a sign for reduction in the diet, especially the fats.

QUANTITY OF FOOD Required by a Severe Diabetic Patient Weighing 60 kilograms. (Joslin.)

Food	Quantity Grams	Calories per Gram	Total Calories
Carbohydrate	10	4	40
Protein	75	4	300
Fat	150	9	1,350
Alcohol	15	7	105
			1,795

STRICT DIET. (Foods without sugar.) Meats, Poultry, Game, Fish, Clear Soups, Gelatine, Eggs, Butter, Olive Oil, Coffee, Tea and Cracked Cocoa.

FOODS ARRANGED APPROXIMATELY ACCORDING TO CONTENT OF CARBOHYDRATES

	5% ±		10% ±	15% ±	20% ±
VEGETABLES	Lettuce Spinach Sauerkraut String Beans Celery Asparagus Cucumbers Brussels Sprouts Sorrel Endive Dandelion Greens Swiss Chard Vegetable Marrow	Cauliflower Tomatoes Rhubarb Egg Plant Leeks Beet Greens Water Cress Cabbage Radishes Pumpkin Kohl-Rabi Sea Kale	Onions Squash Turnip Carrots Okra Mushrooms Beets	Green Peas Artichokes Parsnips Canned Lima Beans	Potatoes Shell Beans Baked Beans Green Corn Boiled Rice Boiled Macaroni
FRUITS	Ripe Olives (20 per cent. fat) Grape Fruit		Lemons Oranges Cranberries Strawberries Blackberries Gooseberries Peaches Pineapples Watermelon	Apples Pears Apricots Blueberries Cherries Currants Raspberries Huckleberries	Plums Bananas
NUTS	Butternuts Pignolias		Brazil Nuts Black Walnuts Hickory Pecans Filberts	Almonds Walnuts (Eng.) Beechnuts Pistachios Pine Nuts	Peanuts **40%** Chestnuts
Miscel-laneous	Unsweetened and Unspiced Pickle Clams Scallops Fish Roe	Oysters Liver			

30 grams (1 oz.) CONTAIN APPROXIMATELY	Protein	Fat	Carbohydrates GRAMS	Calories
Oatmeal	5	2	20	110
Meat (uncooked)	6	2	0	40
" (cooked)	8	3	0	60
Potato	1	0	6	25
Bacon	5	15	0	155
Cream, 40%	1	12	1	120
" 20%	1	6	1	60
Milk	1	1	2	20
Bread	3	0	18	90
Rice	3	0	24	110
Butter	0	25	0	240
Egg (one)	6	5	0	75
Brazil Nuts	5	20	2	210
Orange (one)	0	0	10	40
Grape Fruit (one)	0	0	10	40
Vegetables from 5–6% groups	0.5	0	1	6

1 gram protein contains 4 calories.
1 " carbohydrate contains 4 calories.
1 " fat contains 9 calories.
1 " alcohol contains 7 calories.

1 kilogram—2.2 pounds.
6.25 grams protein contain 1 gram nitrogen.
A patient "at rest" requires 30 calories per kilogram body weight.

CHART XIV.—DIABETIC FOOD TABLES. (JOSLIN.)

If sugar is present fasting is usually indicated. If signs of coma appear the patient should be put to bed and kept as quiet as possible. The stomach should be washed out and the bowels moved by enema. Fluid should be given freely to an amount of 1,000 c. c. every six hours, as thin broth, tea, coffee or water by mouth. If necessary some may be given by rectum. If this is not possible the fluid should be given subcutaneously or intravenously. If the patient has been on full diet, cut out the fat, but continue the same amount of protein and carbohydrate, the latter being given in simple form, such as thin oatmeal gruel, orange juice, milk or bread. At least a gram of carbohydrate per kilo of body weight may be given. If the circulation is failing, digitalis should be given. Joslin advises against the use of alkalies and while the general practice has been to give sodium bicarbonate his opinion carries great weight. If alkali has been given he advises a reduction in the dose of 30 grams a day.

Of the complications, the *pruritus* and *eczema* are best treated by cooling lotions of boric acid or hyposulphite of soda (1 ounce; water, 1 quart), or the use of ichthyol and lanolin ointment. With co-existing pulmonary tuberculosis the usual diabetic treatment can be employed.

The decision as to the performance of an operation should be carefully made. The patient should be given a thorough study and put in the best possible condition so that he is sugar and acid free.

III. DIABETES INSIPIDUS

Definition.—A chronic affection characterized by the passage of large quantities of normal urine of low specific gravity.

The condition is to be distinguished from diuresis or polyuria, which is a frequent symptom in hysteria and some forms of nephritis. There may be excessive polyuria with abdominal tumors and aneurism, tuberculous peritonitis and carcinoma. Willis in 1674 first recognized the distinction between a saccharine and non-saccharine form of diabetes.

Etiology.—The disease is most common in young persons. Of the 85 cases collected by Strauss, 9 were under five years; 12 between five and ten years; 36 between ten and twenty-five years. Males are more frequently attacked than females. The affection may be congenital. A hereditary tendency has been noted in many instances, the most extraordinary of which has been reported by Weil. Of 91 members in four generations, 23 had persistent polyuria without any deterioration in health.

It may follow injury to the base of the skull. It is sometimes associated with adiposity and defective genital development (pituitary disease). Recent observations have shown a striking relationship between pituitary disease and diabetes insipidus. In some cases it is due to insufficiency of the pars intermedia of the pituitary body. In a case reported by Cushing there was polyuria for three months after a sellar decompression operation, regarded as due to an irritative lesion of the pituitary. Tumors, lesions of the medulla and pituitary, malignant metastases in the pituitary, injury and syphilis, usually basal and meningitic, are possible factors. Hemianopsia is present in a number of the cases. Disturbance of the function of the pituitary gland, more particularly the pars intermedia, may be regarded as the essential factor, certainly in a large percentage of cases. Cushing has advanced the suggestion that disturbance of the pituitary function through its autonomic nervous connections may be the explanation of the polyuria which occurs in functional nervous disturbance.

Clinical Classification.—There are two forms: primary or idiopathic, in which there is no evident organic basis, and secondary or symptomatic, in which there is evidence of disease in the brain or elsewhere. Of 9 cases reported by Futcher, 4 belonged to the former and 5 to the latter group. Trousseau stated that the parents of children with diabetes insipidus frequently have glycosuria or albuminuria. The disease has followed rapidly the copious drinking of cold water, or a drinking bout, or has set in during the convalescence from an acute disease. The secondary or symptomatic form is almost always associated with injury or disease of the nervous system, traumatism to the head or, in some cases, to the trunk. In some cases the functional capacity of the kidney to eliminate salt and urea is diminished.

Morbid Anatomy.—There are no constant anatomical lesions. The *kidneys* have been found enlarged and congested. The *bladder* has been found hypertrophied. Dilatation of the ureters and of the pelves of the kidneys has been present. Death has not infrequently resulted from chronic pulmonary disease. Very varied lesions have been met with in the nervous system.

Symptoms.—The disease may come on rapidly, as after a fright or an injury; more commonly it is gradual. A copious secretion of urine, with increased thirst, is the prominent feature. The amount of urine in the twenty-four hours may range from 20 to 40 pints, or even more. Trousseau speaks of a patient who consumed 50 pints of fluid daily and passed about 56 pints of urine in the twenty-four hours. In two of our cases the amount passed was greater than that ingested in liquids and solids. The specific gravity is low, 1.001 to 1.005; the color is extremely pale and watery. The total solid constituents may not be reduced. The amount of urea has sometimes been found in excess. Abnormal ingredients are rare. Muscle-sugar, inosite, has been occasionally found. Albumin is rare. Traces of sugar have been met with. Naturally, with the passage of such enormous quantities of urine, there is a proportionate thirst, and the only inconvenience of the disease is the necessity for frequent micturition and frequent drinking. The appetite is usually good, rarely excessive as in diabetes mellitus; but Trousseau tells of the terror inspired by one of his patients in the keepers of those eating-houses where bread was allowed without extra charge to the extent of each customer's wishes, and says that the man was paid to stay away. The patients may be well nourished and healthy-looking. The disease in many instances does not appear to interfere in any way with the general health. The perspiration is naturally slight and the skin is harsh. The amount of saliva is small and the mouth usually dry. The tolerance of alcohol is remarkable, and patients have been known to take a couple of pints of brandy, or a dozen or more bottles of wine, in the day.

Course.—This depends largely upon the nature of the primary trouble. Sometimes, with organic disease, either cerebral or abdominal, the general health is much impaired; the patient becomes thin, and rapidly loses strength. In the essential or idiopathic cases good health may be maintained for an indefinite period, and the affection has persisted for fifty years. Death usually results from some intercurrent affection. Spontaneous cure may take place.

Diagnosis.—A low specific gravity and the absence of sugar in the urine distinguish the disease from diabetes mellitus. Hysterical polyuria may sometimes simulate it very closely. The amount of urine may be enormous, and only the development of other hysterical manifestations may enable the diagnosis to be made. This condition is, however, always transitory. In certain cases of chronic nephritis a very large amount of urine of low specific gravity may be passed, but the presence of albumin and hyaline casts, high blood pressure, stiff vessels, and hypertrophied left ventricle make the diagnosis easy.

Treatment.—No attempt should be made to reduce the amount of liquid. In some cases gradual reduction of the protein and salt intake is useful. This should be done gradually. Administration of the posterior lobe of the pituitary has been useful. As a rule this has to be given by injection, but in some cases the giving of the gland extract by mouth has been effectual. Lumbar puncture has been followed by marked improvement and should be tried. Theocin is sometimes useful in doses of 5 grains (0.3 gm.) three times a day. Antisyphilitic treatment should be thoroughly tried in patients with a suspicious history or a positive Wassermann reaction.

IV. RICKETS (RACHITIS)

Definition.—A disease of infants, characterized by impaired nutrition of the entire body and alterations in the growing bones.

Glisson, the anatomist of the liver, accurately described the disease in 1650. The name is derived from the old English word *wrickken,* to twist. Glisson suggested to change the name of rachitis, from the Greek ῥάχις, the spine, as it was one of the first parts affected, and also from the similarity in the sound to rickets.

Etiology.—Rickets exists in all parts of the world, but is particularly marked among the poor of the larger cities, who are badly housed and ill fed. It is much more common in Europe than in America. In Vienna and London from 50 to 80 per cent. of all the children at the clinics present signs of rickets. It is a comparatively rare disease in Canada. In the cities of the United States it is very prevalent, particularly among the children of the negro and of the Italian races. Want of sunlight, impure air, confinement, and lack of exercise are important factors. Prolonged lactation and suckling the child during pregnancy are accessory influences in some cases.

There is no evidence that the disease is hereditary.

Rickets affects male and female children equally. It is a disease of the first and second years of life, rarely beginning before the sixth month. Jenner described a late rickets, in which form the disease may not appear until the ninth or even until the twelfth year, or later (the osteomalacia of puberty). A faulty diet is a factor in the production of the disease. A deficiency of fat assimilation is suggested. Like scurvy, rickets may be found in the families of the wealthy under perfect hygienic conditions. It is most common in children fed on condensed milk, the various proprietary foods, cow's milk, and food rich in starches. "An analysis of the foods on which rickets is most frequently and certainly produced shows invariably a deficiency in two of the chief elements so plentiful in the standard food of young animals—namely, animal fat and proteid" (Cheadle). Bland Sutton's interesting experiment with the lion's cubs at the "Zoo" illustrates this point. When milk, pounded bones, and cod-liver oil were added to the meat diet the rickets disappeared, and for the first time in the history of the society the cubs were reared. Associated with the defect in food is a lack of proper assimilation of the lime salts.

Morbid Anatomy.—Glisson's original description of the external appearances of a rickety child is remarkably complete; indeed, his monograph is an enduring monument to the skill and powers of observation of this great physician. "(1) An irregular or unusual proportion of its parts. The head is evidently larger than normal, and the face fatter in respect to the other parts. . . . (2) The external members and muscles of the whole body are seen to be delicate and emaciated, as though consumed by atrophy or tabes, and this (so far as we know) is always observed in those dead of this affection. (3) The whole skin, both the true and the fleshy and fatty layers, is flaccid and rather pendulous, like a loose glove, so that you think it could hold much more flesh. (4) About the joints, especially in the wrists and ankles, there are certain protuberances which, if opened, are seen to arise, not in the fleshy or membranous parts, but in the ends of the bones themselves, especially in their epiphyses. (5) The joints, limbs, and habitus of all these external parts are less firm and rigid, less inflexible than in other dead bodies, and the neck scarcely becomes rigid, *a frigore,* post mortem, or to a less extent than in other cadavers. (6) The chest externally is thin and much narrowed, especially beneath the scapulæ, as though compressed from the sides, and the sternum accuminated like the keel of a ship or the breast of a fowl. (7) The ends of the ribs which join with the cartilages of the sternum are nodular, like the ends of the wrists and ankles." He also described the prominent abdomen, the enlarged liver, and the changes in the mesenteric glands.

The *bones* show the most important changes, particularly the ends of the long bones and the ribs. Between the shaft and epiphyses a slight bulging is apparent, and on section the zone of proliferation, which normally is represented by two narrow bands, is greatly thickened, bluish in color, more irregular in outline, and very much softer. The width of this cushion of cartilage varies from 5 to 15 mm. The line of ossification is also irregular and more spongy and vascular than normal. The periosteum strips off very readily from the shaft, and beneath it there may be a spongy tissue not unlike decalcified bone. The practical outcome of these changes is an imperfect ossification, so that the bone has neither the natural rate of growth nor the normal firmness. In the cranium there may be large areas, particularly in the parieto-occipital region, in which the ossification is delayed, producing the so-called cranio-tabes, so that the bone yields readily to pressure with the finger. There are localized depressed spots of atrophy, which, on pressure, give the so-called "parchment crackling." Flat hyperostoses arise on the outer table, particularly on the frontal and parietal bones, producing the characteristic broad forehead with prominent frontal eminences, a condition sometimes mistaken for hydrocephalus. .

Kassowitz, the leading authority on the anatomy of rickets, regards the hyperæmia of the periosteum, the marrow, the cartilage, and of the bone itself as the primary lesion, out of which all the others arise. It is interesting to note that Glisson attributed rickets to disturbed nutrition by arterial blood, and believed the changes in the long bones to be due to excessive vascularity.

The chemical analysis of rickety bones shows a marked diminution in the calcareous salts, which may be as low as 25 or 35 per cent.

The liver and spleen are usually enlarged, and sometimes the mesenteric glands. As Gee suggested, these conditions probably result from the general state of the health associated with rickets. Beneke has described a relative increase in the size of the arteries in rickets.

Symptoms.—The disease comes on insidiously about the period of dentition, before the child begins to walk. Mild grades of it are often overlooked. In many cases digestive disturbances precede the appearance of the characteristic lesions, and the nutrition of the child is markedly impaired. There is usually slight fever, the child is irritable and restless, and sleeps badly. If he has already walked, he now shows a marked disinclination to do so, and seems feeble and unsteady in his gait. Sir William Jenner called attention to three general symptoms of great importance: First, a diffuse soreness of the body, so that the child cries when an attempt is made to move it, and prefers to keep perfectly still. Secondly, slight fever (100° to 101.5° F.), with nocturnal restlessness, and a tendency to throw off the bedclothes. This may be partly due to the fact that the general sensitiveness is such that even their weight may be distressing. Thirdly, profuse sweating, particularly about the head and neck, so that in the morning the pillow is soaked with perspiration.

The tissues become soft and flabby; the skin is pale; and from a healthy, plump condition the child becomes puny and feeble. The muscular weakness may be marked, particularly in the legs, and paralysis may be suspected. This so-called pseudo-paresis of rickets results in part from the flabby, weak condition of the legs and in part from the pain associated with the movements. Coincident with, or following closely upon, the general symptoms the characteristic skeletal lesions are observed. Among the first of these to appear are the changes in the ribs, at the junction of the bone with the cartilage, forming the so-called rickety rosary. When the child is thin these nodules may be distinctly seen, and in any case can be easily made out by touch. They very rarely appear before the third month. They may increase in size up to the second year, and are rarely seen after the fifth year. The thorax undergoes important changes. Just outside the junction of the cartilages with the ribs there is an oblique, shallow depression extending downward and outward. A transverse curve, sometimes called Harrison's groove, passes outward from the level of the ensiform cartilage toward the axilla, and may be deepened at each inspiration. It is rendered more prominent by the eversion and prominence of the costal border. The sternum projects, particularly in its lower half, forming the so-called pigeon or chicken breast. These changes in the thorax are not peculiar, however, to rickets, and are much more commonly associated with hypertrophy of the tonsils, or any trouble which interferes with the free entrance of air into the lungs. The spine is often curved posteriorly, the processes are prominent; lateral curvature is not so common.

The *head* of a rickety child usually looks large in proportion both to the body and the face, and the fontanelles remain open for a long time. There are areas, particularly in the parieto-occipital regions, in which ossification is imperfect; and the bone may yield to the pressure of the finger, a condition to which the term *cranio-tabes* has been given. Coincidently with this, hyperplasia proceeds in the frontal and parietal eminences, so that these portions of the skull increase in thickness, and may form irregular bosses. In one type the skull may be large and elongated, with the top considerably flattened. In another, and perhaps more common, case the shape of the skull, when seen from above, is rectangular—the *caput quadratum*. The skull looks large in proportion to the face. The forehead is broad and square, and the frontal eminences marked. The anterior fontanelle is late in closing, and may remain open until the third or fourth year. The skin is thin, the veins are full and prominent, and the hair is often rubbed from the back of the skull.

On placing the ear over the anterior fontanelle, or in the temporal region, a systolic murmur may frequently be heard. This condition, first described by John D. Fisher, of Boston, in 1833, is heard with the greatest frequency in rickets, but its presence and persistence in perfectly healthy infants have been amply demonstrated. The murmur is rarely present after the fifth year. A knowledge of the existence of this systolic brain murmur may prevent errors. A case has been reported as an instance of tumor of the brain.

Changes occur in the bones of the face, chiefly in the maxillæ, which are reduced in size. The normal process of dentition is much disturbed; indeed, late teething is one of the marked features in rickets. The teeth which appear may be small and badly formed.

In the upper limbs changes in the scapulæ are not common. The clavicle may be thickened at the sternal end, and there may be thickening near the attachment of the sterno-cleido muscle. The most noticeable changes are at the lower ends of the radius and ulna. The enlargement is at the junction-area of the shaft and epiphysis. Less evident enlargements may occur at the lower end of the humerus. In severe cases the natural shape of the bones of the arm may be much altered, since they have had to support the weight of the child in crawling on the floor. The changes in the pelvis are of special importance, particularly in female children, as in extreme cases they lead to great deformity, with narrowing. In the legs, the lower end of the tibia first becomes enlarged; and in slight cases it may alone be affected. In the severe forms the upper end of the bone, the corresponding parts of the fibula, and the lower end of the femur become greatly thickened. If the child walks, slight bowing of the tibiæ inevitably results. In more advanced cases the tibiæ, and even the femora, may be arched forward. In other instances the condition of knock-knee occurs. Unquestionably the chief cause of these deformities is the weight of the body, but muscular action takes part in it. The green-stick fracture is not uncommon in the soft bones of rickets.

These changes in the skeleton proceed slowly, and the general symptoms vary a good deal with their progress. The child becomes more or less emaciated, though "fat rickets" is by no means uncommon, and a child may be well nourished but "pasty" and flabby. Fever is not constant, but in actively progressing changes in the bone there is usually a slight pyrexia. The abdomen is large, "pot-bellied," due partly to flatulent distention, partly to enlargement of the liver, and in severe cases to diminution of the volume of the thorax. The spleen is often enlarged and readily palpable. The urine is stated to contain an excess of lime salts. There is usually slight anæmia, the hæmoglobin is absolutely and relatively decreased; a leucocytosis may or may not be present; it is more common with enlargement of the spleen (Morse). Many rickety children show marked nervous symptoms; irritability, peevishness, and sleeplessness are constantly present. Jenner called attention to the close relationship which existed between rickets and infantile convulsions, particularly to the fits which occur after the sixth month. Tetany is by no means uncommon. It involves most frequently the arms and hands; occasionally the legs as well. Laryngismus stridulus is a common complication, and though not, as some state, invariably associated, yet it is certainly much more frequent in rickety than in other children. Severe rickets interferes seriously with the growth of a child. Extreme examples of rickety dwarfs are not uncommon. Acute rickets, so-called, is in reality a manifestation of scurvy, and has been described with that disease.

Prognosis.—The disease is never in itself fatal, but the condition of the child is such that it is readily carried off by intercurrent affections, particularly those of the respiratory organs. Spasm of the larynx and convulsions occasionally cause death. In females the deformity of the pelvis is serious, as it may lead to difficulties in parturition.

Treatment.—The better the condition of the mother during pregnancy the less likelihood is there of the development of rickets in the child. Rapidly repeated pregnancies and suckling of a child during pregnancy seem important factors in the production of the disease. Of the general treatment, attention to the feeding of the child is the first consideration. If the mother is unhealthy, or cannot nurse the child, a suitable wet-nurse should be provided, or the child must be artificially fed, in which case cow's milk, diluted according to the age of the child, should constitute the chief food. Care should be taken to examine the stools, and if curds are present the child is taking too much, or it is not sufficiently diluted. Barley-water and carefully strained and well-boiled oatmeal gruel form excellent additions to the milk.

The child should be warmly clad and in the fresh air and sunshine the greater part of the day. The child should be bathed daily in warm water. Careful friction with sweet oil is very advantageous, and, if properly performed, allays rather than aggravates the sensitiveness. Special care should be taken to prevent deformity. The child should not be allowed to walk, and for this purpose splints applied so as to extend beyond the feet are very effective. Of medicines, phosphorus has been warmly recommended by Kassowitz, and also by Jacobi. The child may be given gr. 1/120 (0.0005 gm.) two or three times a day, dissolved in olive oil. The best preparation is the elixir phosphori, six to ten minims (0.36 to 0.6 c. c.) three times a day (Jacobi). Cod-liver oil, in doses of from a half to one teaspoonful, is very advantageous. The syrup of the iodide of iron may be given with the oil. The digestive disturbances, together with the complications, should receive appropriate treatment. Polyglandular therapy is said to have been useful, given on the possibility that the internal secretions are at fault.

V. OBESITY

Definition.—A disorder of metabolism characterized by excessive deposit of fat in the body.

Etiology.—Corpulence, an overgrowth of the bodily fat, an "oily dropsy," as Byron termed it, is a common condition which may be a source of great bodily and mental distress. Primarily it results from inadequate oxidation of the food stuffs, associated either with excessive absorption of the materials which produce fat, or with incomplete combustion. Both factors probably take part. It is not always due to excessive intake of food; many stout persons are light eaters. On the other hand, there are cases in which the increase in weight is directly due to an excessive consumption of food. There is a marked hereditary tendency. Certain races are prone to obesity, and women are more often affected than men.

Fat metabolism is as yet imperfectly understood; it is under the control of the internal secretions. We see the deposition of fat in connection with many processes with which the internal secretions are concerned. At puberty there is a great increase in the fat deposits, particularly of the skin. Following castration there is an increase in the amount of subcutaneous fat. Eunuchs as a rule are very stout. At the menopause increase in weight is common, and during both pregnancy and lactation the subcutaneous fat may be greatly increased.

In only one point have we positive knowledge as to the internal secretions controlling fat metabolism. It has been known that tumors of the pituitary gland or in its neighborhood may be associated with general adiposity and sexual infantilism (Fröhlich's syndrome). The studies of Cushing and his students have shown that the pituitary body influences carbohydrate metabolism, and that with the removal of the posterior lobe there is a great increase in the body weight. There seems to be a definite hypophysial syndrome of increased tolerance for carbohydrates with adiposity. Many of the cases of extreme obesity in young persons are due to hypopituitarism. The remarkable acute obesity, in which as much as 70 pounds may be gained in six months, probably depends upon perversions of some internal secretions.

Symptoms.—Inconvenience caused by the bulk, and loss of good looks in women, are the features for which we are usually consulted. While fat is no sign of health, the great bulk may be consistent with remarkable vigor and activity. Shortness of breath, embarrassed cardiac action, difficulty in walking are the most common complaints. In children obesity is very often associated with careless habits in eating and lack of proper control on the part of parents. The condition is increasing, particularly in the United States, where one sees an extraordinary number of very stout children. A remarkable phenomenon associated with excessive fat is an uncontrollable tendency to sleep—like the fat boy in Pickwick. It is probable that this narcolepsy is a manifestation of disturbed internal secretions.

Treatment.—In women obesity is a very distressing state, accompanied with all sorts of inconveniences and discomforts. With a marked hereditary tendency not much can be expected. The famous George Cheyne, who was a man of enormous bulk, reduced himself by dieting from thirty-two stones (448 pounds) to proper dimensions. One of his aphorisms says: "Every wise man after Fifty ought to begin and lessen at least the quantity of his Aliment, and if he would continue free from great and dangerous Distempers and preserve his Senses and Faculties clear to the last, he ought every seven years to go on abating gradually and sensibly, and at last descend out of life as he ascended into it, even into a Child's Diet." Put in other words, it reads —We eat too much after forty years of age.

In the case of children very much may be done by regulating the diet, reducing the starches and fats in the food, not allowing them to eat sweets, and encouraging systematic exercises. In the case of women who tend to grow stout after child-bearing or at the climacteric, in addition to systematic exercises, they should be told to avoid taking too much food, and particularly to reduce the starches and sugars. There are a number of methods or systems in vogue at present. In the celebrated one of Banting the carbohydrates and fats were excluded and the amount of food was greatly reduced.

Oertel's method is given under the treatment of fatty heart. He reduces the amount of liquid taken, and this is practically, too, the so-called Schweninger cure, in which liquids are allowed only two hours after the food.

Von Noorden's dietary is as follows: Eight o'clock, 80 grams of lean, cold meat, 25 grams of bread, one cup of tea, with a spoonful of milk, no sugar. Ten o'clock, one egg. Twelve o'clock, a cup of strong meat broth. One o'clock, a small plate of meat soup flavored with vegetables, 150 grams of lean meat of one or two sorts, partly fish, partly flesh, 100 grams of potatoes with salad, 100 grams of fresh fruit, or compote without sugar. Three o'clock, a cup of black coffee. Four o'clock, 200 grams of fresh fruit. Six o'clock, a quarter of a litre of milk, if desired, with tea. Eight o'clock, 125 grams of cold meat, or 180 grams of meat weighed raw and grilled, and eaten with pickles or radishes and salad, 30 grams of Graham bread, and two or three spoonfuls of cooked fruit without sugar. He believes it more satisfactory to give in addition to the three meals smaller quantities of food at shorter intervals, so as to obviate the tendency to weakness which these patients often experience. In addition he allows twice in the day a glass of wine. The use of mineral water, weak tea, or lemonade is not limited at the meal times or in the intervals. An occasional "hunger-day" is given.

In the *treatment* of extreme obesity it is very much better that the patient should be in hospital, or under the care of a nurse, who will undertake the proper weighing and administration of the food. The amount of fluid ingested should not be reduced below one litre a day. Many of these patients are anæmic, even with a florid appearance, and for them iron in full doses is advisable.

The thyroid extract should be used only in a systematic "cure." One grain three times a day is a sufficient dose at first. In conjunction with the diet and exercises it is useful, but it should not be ordered indiscriminately to fat persons. Pituitary gland extracts have also been used. The use of involuntary or passive exercise by means of electricity is useful, especially in the reduction of regional fat.

VI. THE LIPOMATOSES

Various forms of localized deposits of fat may be considered here, and we follow the division in Lyon's thorough study of these conditions (*Archives of Internal Medicine*, VI, 1).

I. Adiposis Dolorosa (*Dercum's Disease*).—In the words of the original description this is a disorder characterized by irregular symmetrical deposits of fatty masses in various portions of the body, preceded or attended by pain, and associated sometimes with asthenia and psychical changes.

The lipomatous masses are diffuse and symmetrical, involving the abdomen, chest, arms or legs; or localized on the limbs or trunk. The hands, face and feet are usually spared. The pain is sometimes spontaneous and is easily excited by pressure. Asthenia, not always present, may be a marked feature. The patients are often irritable and there are cases with mental changes. Sometimes the skin over the areas of infiltration is markedly hyperæsthetic. The affection is more common in females. Nine or ten autopsies have been made, none of which threw clear light on the pathology. Quite possibly it is a disturbance of the internal secretions.

II. Nodular Circumscribed Lipomatosis.—The cases are common. The lipomata are distributed in various localities and vary in size from small encapsulated nodules to large circumscribed tumors, solitary or multiple, sometimes symmetrically placed. They may be painful, and Lyon calls attention to the fact that the accessory features of asthenia and psychical changes may also be present.

III. Diffuse Symmetrical Lipomatosis of the Neck.—This remarkable affection, also called adeno-lipomatosis, is characterized by symmetrical fatty infiltrations, either simple or lobulated, of the subcutaneous tissues, forming a huge collar about the neck. It may occur in this part alone, or other limited lipomata are found elsewhere. Males are much more frequently attacked than females. The tumors interfere but little with health, but as they increase the condition becomes very disfiguring. There are sometimes constitutional symptoms. The name "*adeno*-lipomatosis" has been given because scattered throughout the diffuse fatty masses there are small firm nodules of lymphatic tissue—sometimes hæmo-lymph glands.

IV. Cerebral Adiposity (*Dystrophia Adiposo-Genitalis, Fröhlich*).—A condition of obesity may occur in connection with tumors of the hypophysis, or adjacent parts, associated with a hypoplasia of the genital organs and a condition of infantilism. The condition will be discussed in the section on internal secretions, as it appears from the researches of Cushing to be associated with the perversion of the function of the pituitary gland.

V. Pseudo-Lipoma.—Sydenham made the keen observation that in hysterical patients there were sometimes swellings, which neither yielded to the impress of the finger nor left a mark. Charcot described the condition as "hysterical œdema," of which there is both a blue and a white variety.

Many of these subcutaneous infiltrations, just as in the soft, supraclavicular pad, so common in stout women, are due to fat, and French writers describe all grades of transition from a pseudo-œdema to a true lipoma.

Treatment.—This is not satisfactory. A trial of thyroid extract in small doses is advisable, but it is well to suspend its use for a week in every month. Extracts of other glands may also be tried. In patients with signs of tumor of the hypophysis surgical measures should be considered.

VII. HÆMOCHROMATOSIS

Definition.—A disorder of metabolism characterized by a deposition of an iron-containing pigment in the glandular organs, and by an increase in the normal pigmentation with which is associated a progressive sclerosis of various organs, and, in a large proportion of the cases, diabetes. The disease was first described by von Recklinghausen.

Etiology.—Of the cases on record the great majority had diabetes. Only one occurred in a woman. In the majority of the patients, middle-aged men, there seemed to be no marked predisposing causes, though Blumer maintains that alcohol plays an important part.

Pathology.—On autopsy the ochre or bronze color of the organs is the striking feature. The liver is large and sclerotic; the spleen also enlarged, and the pancreas either small and atrophic or fatty and fibroid. The lymph nodes are also pigmented. The pigment is hæmosiderin or iron-reacting. It is chiefly in the cells of the glands, in the muscle cells of the heart, and in the lymph nodes. The amount in the various organs is enormous, a hundred times the normal in the liver, for example. The hæmofuscin, the non-iron-reacting pigment, varies in different amounts, and it has a yellow tint, and is found chiefly in the connective tissue cells. The blood shows no special changes.

The pathogenesis is obscure, and Sprunt, whose study (*Archives of Internal Medicine,* July, 1911) contains an admirable summary of our knowledge, concludes that there is no evidence of abnormal blood destruction, and that it is a primary disorder of metabolism, "implicating many of the body tissues, and manifested by a change in the chromogenic groups of the proteid molecule with the deposition of pigments."

Rous and Oliver produced an identical condition in rabbits by repeated transfusions of blood, so that large amounts were being constantly destroyed.

Clinical Features.—There are two groups of cases, the larger one in which diabetes is present, and the smaller in which there is no sugar in the urine. The former group is spoken of by the French as *diabète bronzé,* which has the features of a severe diabetes with weakness, progressive pigmentation of the skin, and an enlarged liver. The pigmentation of the skin which is the feature that attracts attention varies in color from a dark brown to a leaden or bluish black. Dr. Maude Abbott's case was known as *Blue Mary.* The liver shows cirrhosis with a smooth and uniform enlargement. The spleen may be enlarged secondarily. It was very large in two of our cases. The diabetes is usually severe, and runs a rapid course. Prior to the onset of diabetes the disease may last for years.

There is no special treatment beyond measures for the general health; in the patients with diabetes the usual treatment should be carried out.

VIII. OCHRONOSIS

Definition.—A rare disorder of metabolism associated with blackening of the cartilages and fibrous tissues and pigmentation of the skin, and the presence of dark urine due to alcapton or to derivatives of carbolic acid.

Etiology.—There are two groups of cases:

(*a*) There is a congenital life-long chemical malformation, sometimes a family affection, in which there is a failure to complete the catabolism of certain aromatic compounds, with the result that peculiar bodies, homogentisic acid and uroleucic acid are excreted in the urine, which blackens on exposure to air—alcaptonuria. The anomaly may be present in three generations.

(*b*) In the other group the dark urine and the blackening of the tissues are due to the prolonged use of carbolic acid, usually the application of strong solutions externally to ulcers. There may possibly be other causes.

Symptoms.—When well developed, ochronosis presents a very striking picture. The discoloration of the fibrous tissues is best seen about the knuckles, and in thin persons the tendons of the hands and feet show a bluish-gray appearance. The cartilage of the ear has a bluish tint, and there may be symmetrical black patches on the sclerotics. Widespread pigmentation of the skin has been observed. In one patient there was a coal-black discoloration of the skin over the nose and cheeks, and the same was beginning in the hands. This may occur also in the carboluria group, as well shown in the colored illustration of Dr. Pope's patient. Several of the reported cases had arthritis, and the two brothers in the Maryland family had a curious anterior inclination of the trunk, and a peculiar waddling gait. There are few symptoms directly due to the chemical malformation. The patients enjoy good health, but the disfigurement may be very great. Post mortem, the appearance is remarkable, as pictured in Virchow's original case; the cartilages, ligaments and fibrous structures are everywhere of a brown-black color.

IX. ACIDOSIS

Definition.—Acidosis may be defined as a decrease in the amount of fixed bases in the blood and other tissues of the body or in other words a relative increase in the acid ions. This involves a decrease in the alkali reserve of the body and hence a disturbance of the acid-base equilibrium. This might be described better as a decrease in the alkalinity; an actual acid condition is not present. The free carbon dioxide in the body converts the bases not bound by other acids to bicarbonate and hence the bicarbonate represents the excess of base remaining after non-volatile acids have been neutralized. Hence acidosis involves a depletion of the bicarbonate in the blood which has been termed the "first line of defence" against acidosis. A definite acid-base equilibrium is essential to life and any marked departure from it results in serious difficulty. This equilibrium is kept at a very constant level and any increase of acid or alkali is automatically guarded against. Under ordinary conditions of diet there is production of acid radicals. These are disposed of by oxidation, elimination, excretion and neutralization.

The means by which the normal ratio is maintained are as follows: (1) Elimination of carbon dioxide by the lungs, in which sodium bicarbonate plays a large part as a carrier; (2) elimination of acid by the kidneys; (3) neutralization of acid by ammonia, and (4) intake of fixed bases with the food. It is evident that oxidation plays a large part in the process. In disturbance of the usual acid-base relations the body endeavors to protect itself by an increase in the normal processes. One important means is increased neutralization of acid by ammonia. The ratio of this to the total N of the urine, which normally is 2 to 5 per cent., may rise to 25 or even 40 per cent. By an increased respiration rate the effort is made to excrete more carbon dioxide by the lungs. The kidneys may excrete more acid than in normal conditions. The reserve of alkali is used so far as it is available. These means, however, may not be sufficient and it is evident that a decrease in the amount of sodium bicarbonate will result in less CO_2 being carried from the tissues and hence an accumulation of it there. From this dyspnœa and air hunger result. So long as the reduction in the alkali reserve is not marked the condition is not serious, but if this does result many changes follow, disturbance in oxidation, disturbed renal function, altered N metabolism, dyspnœa, etc.

The mechanism of this decreased alkalinity is various. In diabetes mellitus there is excessive formation of acetone bodies. In certain of the diarrhœal diseases it may be that alkali is excreted by the bowel; this probably occurs in cholera. In conditions in which there is loss of fluids it may be that there is not sufficient fluid available. The kidneys may not excrete the normal amount of acid phosphates or may be unable to increase the excretion to meet an emergency.

Occurrence.—Acidosis may occur in many diseases, in some of which it is of slight significance only, in others of extreme gravity. The more important are as follows:

(1) Starvation.—This applies particularly to the absence of carbohydrates from the diet. It is probably a factor in the production of acidosis in acute infections in which there is difficulty in giving sufficient food, and may contribute to the acidosis after anæsthesia, especially in cases in which little or no food has been taken for sometime beforehand.

(2) Anæsthesia.—Slight grades of acidosis are common and in the majority unimportant, but in a critical case the incidence of acidosis may be enough to determine a fatal outcome. Hence the wisdom of taking measures to prevent it so far as possible.

(3) Pregnancy.—Here the acidosis is rarely of serious moment.

(4) In Children.—In certain of the diarrhœal diseases of children, acidosis may be marked and be sufficient to determine a fatal result. The cyclic vomiting of children is often associated with acidosis. An acid intoxication may be due to a disturbance in the metabolism of the fats and proteins. The condition may come on in a perfectly healthy child, with gastro-intestinal symptoms, vomiting, diarrhœa and slight fever. On the second or third day dyspnœa appears with abdominal distention, the child begins to get drowsy, and on the fourth or fifth day or even earlier there is coma. The urine usually contains acetone and diacetic acid.

(5) Infectious Diseases.—Rheumatic fever, pneumonia, asiatic cholera and typhoid fever are examples.

(6) Diabetes Mellitus.—In this acidosis is a serious factor. The term ketosis or ketone acidosis has been suggested as a designation.

(7) Renal and Cardio-Renal Disease.—In this group it appears that the decrease in the ability of the kidney to excrete acids is an important factor.

Diagnosis.—(1) Increase in the Respiration Rate.—In certain forms, as in diabetes mellitus, this suggests the diagnosis at once. In all cases of hyperpnœa for which no other cause is found, the possibility of acidosis should be considered. If the ketone bodies are responsible there is usually a fruity odor to the breath.

(2) Carbon Dioxide Tension in the Alveolar Air.—Marked lowering of this is evidence of acidosis except when due to the effect of high altitudes or conditions interfering with the exchange of gases between the alveolar air and the blood.

(3) Blood.—(*a*) Lowering of the CO_2 content. (*b*) Decreased alkalinity. (*c*) Determination of the oxygen-containing power of the hæmoglobin.

(4) Urine.—(*a*) Increase in the ammonia. (*b*) Excess of acid or the presence of abnormal acids. (*c*) Change in the fixed bases.

(5) Tolerance.—Tolerance to alkalies, especially bicarbonate, measured by the amount of sodium bicarbonate required to render the urine alkaline.

Prognosis.—As acidosis is not a disease in itself, it is difficult to speak of prognosis, but the outcome of the disease which it complicates may depend on the acidosis, as for example in the diarrhœal diseases of children. In diabetes mellitus, acidosis is often the terminal event. The response to treatment may be regarded as an important element in estimating the outcome.

Treatment.—Prevention should be used whenever possible. In diabetes mellitus this is essential and should always be considered in the treatment of that disease. Before anæsthesia and in the acute infections the useful measures are: (1) The giving of large amounts of water. (2) The administration of carbohydrate. This may be by mouth or by bowel as by the use of a 2 to 5 per cent. solution of glucose. (3) The giving of soda bicarbonate by mouth, bowel or intravenously until the urine is alkaline. This is important in the early stages, as for instance in children. In some cases the giving of sodium, calcium, potassium and magnesium salts may be of advantage. With established acidosis the treatment must depend on the underlying condition. In general the giving of sodium bicarbonate intravenously (2-5 per cent. solution) even up to 100 grams is advisable in severe cases. In milder ones the administration may be by mouth or by rectum. If possible large amounts of water should be given.

SECTION VI

DISEASES OF THE DIGESTIVE SYSTEM

A. DISEASES OF THE MOUTH

STOMATITIS

Acute Stomatitis.—Simple or erythematous stomatitis, the commonest form, results from the action of irritants of various sorts. Frequent at all ages, in children it is usually associated with dentition and with gastro-intestinal disturbance, particularly in ill-nourished, unhealthy subjects; in adults it may follow the abuse of tobacco, or the use of too hot or too highly seasoned food; it is a concomitant of indigestion, or of the specific fevers.

The affection may be limited to the gums and lips or may extend over the whole surface of the mouth and include the tongue. There are at first superficial redness and dryness of the membrane, followed by increased secretion and swelling of the tongue, which is furred and indented by the teeth. There is rarely any constitutional disturbance, but in children there may be slight fever. The condition causes discomfort, sometimes actual distress and pain, particularly in mastication.

In infants the mouth should be carefully sponged after each feeding. A mouth-wash of borax or glycerin and borax may be used, and in severe cases, which tend to become chronic, a one per cent. solution of nitrate of silver may be applied.

Aphthous Stomatitis.—This form, also known as *follicular* or *vesicular* stomatitis, is characterized by the presence of small, slightly raised spots, from 2 to 4 mm. in diameter, surrounded by reddened areolæ. The spots appear first as vesicles, which rupture, leaving small ulcers with grayish bases and bright-red margins. They are seen most frequently on the inner surfaces of the lips, the edges of the tongue, and the cheeks. They are seldom present on the mucous membrane of the pharynx. This form is met with most often in children under three years, either as an independent affection or in association with a febrile disease or with an attack of indigestion. The vesicles come out with great rapidity and the little ulcers may be fully formed within twenty-four hours. The child complains of soreness of the mouth and takes food with reluctance. The buccal secretions are increased and the breath is heavy, but not foul. The constitutional symptoms are usually those of the disease with which the aphthæ are associated. The disease must not be confounded with thrush. No special parasite has been found in connection with it. It is not a serious condition, and heals rapidly with the improvement of the constitutional state. In severe cases it may extend to the pillars of the fauces and to the pharynx, and produce ulcers which are irritating and difficult to heal.

Each ulcer should be touched with nitrate of silver and the mouth should be thoroughly cleansed after taking food. A wash of chlorate of potassium, or of borax and glycerin, may be used. The constitutional symptoms should receive careful attention.

A curious affection occurs in southern Italy sometimes in epidemic form, characterized by a pearly-colored membrane with induration, immediately beneath the tongue on the frænum (Riga's disease). There may be much induration and ultimately ulceration. It occurs in both healthy and cachectic children, usually about the time of the eruption of the first teeth.

Ulcerative Stomatitis.—This form, which is also known by the names of *fetid stomatitis,* or *putrid sore mouth,* occurs particularly in children after the first dentition. It may prevail as a widespread epidemic in institutions in which the sanitary conditions are defective. It has been met with in jails and camps. Insufficient and unwholesome food, improper ventilation, and prolonged damp, cold weather seem to be special predisposing causes. Lack of cleanliness of the mouth, the presence of carious teeth, and the collection of tartar around them favor the occurrence of the disease. The affection spreads like a specific disease, but the microbe has not been isolated. It has been held that the disease is the same as the foot-and-mouth disease and that it is conveyed by milk, but there is no positive evidence on these points.

The morbid process begins at the margin of the gums, which become swollen and red, and bleed readily. Ulcers form, the bases of which are covered with a grayish-white, firmly adherent membrane. In severe cases the teeth may become loosened and necrosis of the alveolar process may occur. The ulcers extend along the gum-line of the upper and lower jaws; the tongue, lips, and mucosa of the cheeks are usually swollen, but rarely ulcerated. There is salivation, the breath is foul, and mastication is painful. The submaxillary lymph-glands are enlarged. An exanthem may appear and be mistaken for measles. The constitutional symptoms are often severe, and in debilitated children death sometimes occurs.

In the *treatment* chlorate of potassium has been found to be almost specific. It should be given in doses of 5 grains (0.3 gm.), three times a day, to a child, and to an adult double that amount. Locally it may be used as a mouth-wash, or the powdered salt may be applied directly to the ulcerated surfaces. When there is much fetor, a solution of potassium permanganate may be used as a wash, and silver nitrate applied to the ulcers.

A *variety* of ulcerative sore mouth, which differs entirely from this form, is common in nursing women, and is usually seen on the mucous membrane of the lips and cheeks. The ulcers arise from the mucous follicles, and are from 3 to 5 mm. in diameter. They may cause little or no inconvenience; but in some instances they are very painful and interfere seriously with the taking of food and its mastication. As a rule they heal readily after the application of nitrate of silver, and the condition is an indication for tonics, fresh air, and a better diet.

Recurring outbreaks of an *herpetic,* even *pemphigoid,* stomatitis are seen in neurotic individuals (*stomatitis neurotica chronica,* Jacobi). It may precede or accompany the fatal form of *pemphigus vegetans.*

Parrot describes the occasional appearance in new-born, debilitated children of small ulcers symmetrically placed on the hard palate on either side of the middle line. They rarely heal, but tend to increase in size, and may involve the bone. Bednar's aphthæ consist of small patches and ulcers on the hard palate, caused as a rule in young infants by the artificial nipple or the nurse's finger.

Parasitic Stomatitis (*Thrush; Soor; Muguet*).—This affection, most commonly seen in children, is dependent upon a fungus, *Saccharomyces albicans,* called by Robin *Oïdium albicans.* It belongs to the order of yeast fungi, and consists of branching filaments, from the ends of which ovoid torula cells develop. The disease apparently does not arise in a normal mucosa. Improper diet, uncleanliness of the mouth, fermentation of remnants of food, or the occurrence, from any cause, of catarrhal stomatitis predispose to the growth. In institutions it is frequently transmitted by unclean feeding-bottles, spoons, etc. It is not confined to children, but is met with in adults in the final stages of fever, in chronic tuberculosis, diabetes, and in cachectic states. The parasite grows in the upper layers of the mucosa, and the filaments form a dense felt-work among the epithelial cells. The disease begins on the tongue and is seen in the form of slightly raised, pearly-white spots, which increase in size and gradually coalesce. The membrane thus formed can be readily scraped off, leaving an intact mucosa, or, if the process extends deeply, a bleeding, slightly ulcerated surface. The disease spreads to the cheeks, lips, and hard palate, and may involve the tonsils and pharynx. In very severe cases the entire buccal mucosa is covered by the grayish-white membrane. It may even extend into the œsophagus and to the stomach and cæcum. It is occasionally met with on the vocal cords. Robust, well-nourished children are sometimes affected, but it is usually met with in enfeebled, emaciated infants with digestive or intestinal troubles. In such cases the disease may persist for months.

The affection is readily recognized, and must not be confounded with aphthous stomatitis, in which the ulcers, preceded by the formation of vesicles, are perfectly distinctive. In thrush the microscopic examination shows the presence of the characteristic fungus throughout the membrane. In this condition, too, the mouth is usually dry—a striking contrast to the salivation accompanying aphthæ.

Thrush is more readily prevented than removed. The child's mouth should be kept scrupulously clean, and, if artificially fed, the bottles should be thoroughly sterilized. Lime-water or any other alkaline fluid, such as the bicarbonate of soda (a drachm to a tumbler of water), may be employed. When the patches are present these alkaline mouth-washes may be continued after each feeding. A spray of borax or of sulphite of soda (a drachm to the ounce) or the black wash with glycerine may be employed. The permanganate of potassium is also useful. The constitutional treatment is of equal importance, and it will often be found that the thrush persists, in spite of all local measures, until the general health of the infant is improved by change of air or the relief of the diarrhœa, or, in obstinate cases, the substitution of a natural for the artificial diet.

Gangrenous Stomatitis (*Cancrum Oris; Noma*).—An affection characterized by a rapidly progressing gangrene, starting on the gums or cheeks, and leading to extensive sloughing and destruction. This terrible, but fortunately rare, disease is seen only in children under very insanitary conditions or during convalescence from the acute fevers. It is more common in girls than in boys. It is met with between the ages of two and five years. In at least one-half of the cases the disease occurs during convalescence from measles. Cases have been seen also after scarlet fever and typhoid. The mucous membrane is first affected, usually of the gums or of one cheek. The process begins insidiously, and when first seen there is a sloughing ulcer of the mucous membrane, which spreads rapidly and leads to brawny induration of the skin and adjacent parts. The sloughing extends, and in severe cases the cheek is perforated. The disease may spread to the tongue and chin; it may invade the bones of the jaws and even involve the eyelids and ears. In mild cases an ulcer forms on the inner surface of the cheek, which heals or may perforate and leave a fistulous opening. Naturally in such a severe affection the constitutional disturbance is great, the pulse rapid, the prostration extreme, and death usually takes place within a week or ten days. The temperature may reach 103° or 104° F. Diarrhœa is usually present, and aspiration pneumonia is a common complication. No specific organism has been found. Destruction of the sore by the Paquelin cautery or fuming nitric acid is the most effectual treatment. Antiseptic applications should be used to destroy the fetor. The child should be carefully nourished and stimulants given freely.

Mercurial Stomatitis (*Ptyalism*).—It occurs in persons with a special susceptibility, rarely now as a result of the excessive use of the drug, and also in those whose occupation necessitates the constant handling of mercury. It may follow the administration of repeated small doses. Thus, a patient with heart-disease who was ordered an eighth of a grain of calomel every three hours for diuretic purposes had, after taking eight or ten doses, a severe stomatitis, which persisted for several weeks. It may follow the administration of small doses of gray powder. The patient complains first of a metallic taste in the mouth, the gums become swollen, red, and sore, mastication is difficult, the salivary glands become enlarged and painful, and there is a great increase in their secretion. The tongue is swollen, the breath is foul, and, if the affection progresses, there may be ulceration of the mucosa, and, in rare instances, necrosis of the jaw. Although troublesome and distressing, the disease is rarely serious, and recovery usually takes place in a couple of weeks. Instances in which the teeth become loosened or detached or in which the inflammation extends to the pharynx and Eustachian tubes are rarely seen.

The administration of mercury should be suspended so soon as the gums are "touched." Mild cases of the affection subside within a few days and require only a simple mouth-wash. In severer cases the chlorate of potassium may be given internally, and used to rinse the mouth. The bowels should be freely opened; the patient should take a hot bath every evening and should drink plentifully of alkaline mineral waters. Atropine is sometimes serviceable, and may be given in doses of 1/100 of a grain (0.00065 gm.) twice a day. Iodine is also recommended. When the salivation is severe and protracted the patient becomes much debilitated and anæmic, so that a supporting treatment is indicated. The diet is necessarily liquid, for the patient finds the chief difficulty in taking food. If the pain is severe Dover's powder may be given at night.

Here may be appropriately mentioned the influence of stomatitis, particularly the mercurial form, upon the developing teeth of children. The condition known as *erosion,* in which the teeth are honeycombed or pitted owing to defective formation of enamel, is indicative, as a rule, of infantile stomatitis. Such teeth must be distinguished carefully from those of congenital syphilis, which may coexist, but the two conditions are distinct. The honeycombing is frequently seen on the incisors; but, according to Jonathan Hutchinson, the test teeth of infantile stomatitis are the first permanent molars, then the incisors, "which are almost as constantly pitted, eroded, and of bad color, often showing the transverse furrow which crosses all the teeth at the same level." Magitot regards these transverse furrows as the result of infantile convulsions or of severe illness during early life, analogous to the furrows on the nails which may follow a serious disease.

Geographical Tongue (*Eczema of the Tongue*).—A remarkable desquamation of the superficial epithelium of the tongue in circinate patches, which spread while the central portions heal. Fusion of patches leads to areas with sinuous outlines. When extensive the tongue may be covered with these areas, like a geographical map. The affection causes a good deal of itching and heat, and it may be a source of much mental worry to the patients, who often dread lest it may be a commencing cancer.

The etiology is unknown. It occurs in infants and children, and it is not very infrequent in adults. It has been regarded as a gouty manifestation, and transient attacks may accompany indigestion. It is very liable to relapse. In adults it may prove very obstinate and in one instance the disease persisted in spite of all treatment for more than two years. Solutions of nitrate of silver give the most satisfactory results in relieving the intense burning.

There is a superficial glossitis, limited usually to the border and point of the tongue, which presents irregular reddish spots, looking as if the epithelium was removed, and the papillæ are reddened and swollen. The condition is sometimes known as Möller's glossitis. Local treatment with nitrate of silver as a rule gives relief.

Leukoplakia Buccalis.—Samuel Plumbe described the condition as *icthyosis lingualis.* It has also been called *buccal psoriasis* and *leuco-keratosis mucosæ oris.* The following forms occur: (*a*) Small white spots upon the tongue, slightly raised, even papillomatous—lingual corns. (*b*) Diffuse thickening of the epithelial coating of the tongue, either a thin, bluish-white color or opaque white, depending upon the thickness. It is patchy, and more often upon the dorsum and sides. (*c*) Diffuse oral leukoplakia, a remarkable condition in which the roof of the mouth, the gums, lips, and cheeks are covered with an opaque white, sometimes smooth, sometimes fissured, rugose layer. In this widespread form the tongue may be spared. The visible mucosa of the lips, occasionally the genital mucosa, and the pelves of the kidneys may be involved.

While appearing spontaneously, the condition is most common in heavy smokers, and has been called smoker's tongue. Epithelioma occasionally starts from the localized patches. A majority of the patients have had syphilis, but the condition does not yield, as a rule, to specific treatment.

Leukoplakia is a very obstinate affection. All irritants, such as smoke and very hot food, should be avoided. Local treatment with one-half-per-cent. corrosive sublimate or a one-per-cent. chromic-acid solution has been recommended. The propriety of active local treatment is doubtful. Papillomatous outgrowths should be cut off. The X-rays may be tried. The most extensive form may disappear spontaneously.

The *glossy flat atrophy* of the posterior part of the tongue, described by Virchow, is in a majority of instances of syphilitic origin. Scars may give an irregular appearance to the surface. Symmers found this smooth atrophy in 55 of 75 post mortems in syphilitic subjects.

Hyperæsthesia of the Tongue.—A very distressing affection, seen chiefly in women at or beyond the menopause, occurs as a sensation of burning felt at the top over the dorsum, along the edges or sometimes over the entire organ. On examination nothing is to be seen; there is no swelling, and there may be no irritation about the teeth. It is a very obstinate affection. Painting with iodine or in some cases the application of the X-rays may give relief.

Fetor Oris.—The practitioner is frequently consulted for foul breath, and is daily made aware of its prevalence. All unconscious, he is himself often a subject of the condition, to the disgust of his patients, with whom he has to come into such close contact. It is impossible to give even a list of all the causes. The following are a few of the more important: (*a*) In connection with indigestion and the associated catarrhal disturbances in the mouth, pharynx, and stomach. The breath is "heavy," as the mothers say. A simple mouth-wash and a mercurial purge suffice to remove it. In a more serious disease of the stomach the breath may be foul, and occasionally, in sloughing cancer, horribly stinking. (*b*) Local conditions in the mouth: (1) All the forms of stomatitis. Smokers should remember that, apart altogether from the smell of tobacco, their breath in the morning is usually, to say the least, "heavy." (2) Pyorrhœa alveolaris. This is the most common cause of foul breath in adults, and is almost constantly present after middle life, causing a perfectly distinctive odor. To test for the presence draw a bit of stout thread or the edge of a sheet of paper high up between the teeth and the gums and then smell it. Scrupulous treatment by a dentist is needed, and daily scouring, etc. (*c*) The tonsillar diseases. In the crypts of the tonsils the epithelial débris accumulates, and, invaded by micro-organisms, gradually forms the little round or triangular bodies, which can be squeezed out of the lacunæ, and when pressed between the fingers smell like Limburger cheese. The fetor oris from this cause is quite distinctive. To test the presence in child or adult, smell the finger after it has been rubbed firmly upon the tonsil. Local treatment is needed. (*d*) Decayed teeth, the foul odor of which is quite distinct from that of pyorrhœa or chronic tonsillitis. (*e*) Respiratory. Many diseases of the nose, larynx, bronchi, and lungs are associated with foul breath. (*f*) Hæmic. The halitus—the expired air from the lung—may be impregnated with odors from the blood. Of this there are many well-known instances. For practical purposes it is to be remembered that pyorrhœa alveolaris and chronic lacunar tonsillitis are the two most common causes of foul breath.

Oral Sepsis.—To William Hunter, of Charing Cross Hospital, is due the credit of insisting upon the importance of the mouth as the chief channel of entrance of the pyogenic organisms, and as itself the seat of septic processes. Necrosed teeth, pyorrhœa alveolaris, gingivitis, alveolar abscess, etc., are present in a great many people. A systemic infection may follow or the general health may be lowered by the continuous production of pus. In extensive pyorrhœa alveolaris the daily amount of pus must be considerable, and there can be no question that it has a debilitating influence on the general health and is sometimes associated with a moderate anæmia and with a pasty complexion. Hunter describes septic gastritis and septic enteritis as common sequences; indeed, he regards appendicular, pleuritic, gall-bladder and pyelitic inflammations as forms of "medical sepsis" due largely to infection from the mouth. One form of pernicious anæmia—infective hæmolytic anæmia—he believes to be due to oral sepsis, or an infective glossitis. Certain types of nephritis and forms of arthritis are believed to be due to oral infection.

There is no question of the importance of the subject, and we should insist upon scrupulous cleanliness of the mouth and teeth. An adult should have his teeth cleansed by a dentist once a month. We should, too, have less delicacy in telling our friends in whom the odor of the breath reveals the presence of pyorrhœa. It is a very difficult condition to cure. Locally much may be done to keep it under control. Vaccines have been used, sometimes, but not always, with success. If possible, the patient should be referred to a dentist who is specially competent to deal with it. The tartar should be removed and antiseptic mouth washes, such as carbolic acid (1 per cent.), used frequently. Hydrogen peroxide or equal parts of tincture of iodine and alcohol may be applied locally. A saturated solution of thymol is an effective mouth wash.

Affections of the mucous glands are not very common. In catarrhal troubles in children and in measles they may be swollen. They are enlarged and very prominent in Mikulicz's disease, with chronic symmetrical enlargement of the salivary and lachrymal glands. There is a singular affection of the mucous glands of the lips, chiefly of the lower, with much swelling and infiltration. It was described by Volkmann, and has been called Bälz's disease. The mucous glands are enlarged, the ducts much dilated, and on pressure a mucoid or muco-purulent secretion may exude. The skin over the lips may be reddened and swollen.

B. DISEASES OF THE SALIVARY GLANDS

Supersecretion (*Ptyalism*).—The normal amount of saliva varies from 2 to 3 pints in the twenty-four hours. The secretion is increased during the taking of food and in the physiological processes of dentition. A great increase, to which the term *ptyalism* is applied, is met with (1) occasionally in mental and nervous affections and in rabies; (2) occasionally in the acute fevers, particularly in small-pox; (3) sometimes with disease of the pancreas; (4) during gestation, usually early, though it may persist through the entire course; (5) occasionally at each menstrual period; and, lastly, it is a common effect of certain drugs—mercury, the iodine compounds, and (among vegetable remedies) jaborandi, muscarin, and tobacco excite the salivary secretion. Of these we most frequently see the effect of mercury in producing ptyalism. The salivation may be present without any inflammation of the mouth. For *treatment* atropine or the bromides may be given in small doses at first and the effect watched until the most efficient dosage is found.

Xerostomia (*Arrest of the Salivary and Buccal Secretions; Dry Mouth*).—In this condition, first described by Jonathan Hutchinson, the secretions of the mouth and salivary glands are suppressed. The tongue is red, sometimes cracked, and quite dry; the mucous membrane of the cheeks and of the palate is smooth, shining, and dry; and mastication, deglutition, and articulation are very difficult. A majority of the cases are in women, and in several instances have been associated with nervous phenomena. The general health, as a rule, is unimpaired. It may be due to involvement of some centre which controls the secretion of the glands. The free use of glycerin locally is sometimes of value and jaborandi or pilocarpine can be given cautiously.

Inflammation of the Salivary Glands.—(*a*) *Specific Parotitis.* (See Mumps.)

(*b*) *Symptomatic parotitis* or *parotid bubo* occurs:

(1) In the course of the infectious fevers—typhus, typhoid, pneumonia, pyæmia, etc. It was a common complication of the fevers during the recent war. In ordinary practice it occurs oftenest, perhaps, in typhoid fever. It is the result of infection through the blood or by the salivary duct. The process is usually intense and leads rapidly to suppuration. It is, as a rule, an unfavorable indication in the course of a fever. Parotitis may occur in secondary syphilis.

(2) In connection with injury or disease of the abdomen or pelvis, a condition to which Stephen Paget has called special attention. Of 101 cases of this kind, "10 followed injury or disease of the urinary tract, 18 were due to injury or disease of the alimentary canal, and 23 were due to injury or disease of the abdominal wall, the peritoneum, or the pelvic cellular tissue. The remaining 50 were due to injury, disease, or temporary derangement of the genital organs." By temporary derangement is meant slight injuries or natural processes—a slight blow on the testis, the introduction of a pessary, menstruation, or pregnancy. Bucknell has brought forward strong evidence to show that in all these cases infection takes place through the duct.

(3) In association with facial paralysis, as in a case of fatal peripheral neuritis described by Gowers; in diabetes and chronic metallic poisoning.

In the infectious diseases rigid cleanliness of the mouth is an important preventive measure. For the parotitis an ice bag often aids, or hot fomentations may be applied. A free incision should be made *early* if there are signs of suppuration.

(*c*) *Chronic parotitis,* a condition in which the glands are enlarged, rarely painful, may follow inflammation of the throat or mumps. Salivation may be present. It may be due to lead, mercury, or potassium iodide. It occurs also in chronic nephritis and in syphilis. Symmetrical enlargement of the parotids of moderate extent is not very uncommon among hospital patients. The cases at the Johns Hopkins clinic have been reported by C. P. Howard (*Internat. Clinics,* xix, 1). It may be associated with xerostomia. The parotid and submaxillary glands are affected with equal frequency. In one case the swelling recurred over a period of 20 years (Greig).

(*d*) *Mikulicz's Disease.*—In this remarkable affection, described in 1888, there is a chronic, indolent, painless, symmetrical enlargement of the salivary and lachrymal glands. The condition may last for several years. In some cases the process is tuberculous or luetic. The gland substance itself may not be disturbed, but there is a great infiltration of the interstitial connective tissue. In one case the lachrymal glands were replaced by fibrous tissue. In America the disease has been seen chiefly in negroes. The enlargement may subside after an acute fever. Good results have followed the use of arsenic, iodide and the X-rays. There is no tendency to recurrence after removal.

(*e*) *Gaseous Tumors of Steno's Duct and of the Parotid Gland.*—In glass-blowers and musicians Steno's duct may become inflated with air and form a tumor the size of a nut or of an egg. Some have contained a mixture of air, saliva, and pus. In rare cases there are gaseous tumors of the glands, which give a sensation of crepitation on palpation.

C. DISEASES OF THE PHARYNX

Circulatory Disturbances.—(*a*) *Huperæmia* is common in acute and chronic affections of the throat, and is frequently seen as a result of the irritation of tobacco smoke, and from the constant use of the voice. Venous stasis is seen in valvular disease of the heart, and in mechanical obstruction of the superior vena cava by tumor or aneurism. In aortic insufficiency the capillary pulse may sometimes be seen, and the intense throbbing of the internal carotid may be mistaken for aneurism.

(*b*) *Hæmorrhage* is found in association with bleeding from other mucous surfaces, or it is due to local causes—granulations, varicosities, or vegetations. It may be mistaken for hæmorrhage from the lungs or stomach. Sometimes the patient finds the pillow stained in the morning with bloody secretion. The condition is rarely serious, and requires only suitable local treatment. Occasionally a hæmorrhage takes place into the mucosa, producing a pharyngeal hæmatoma. A condition of the uvula resembling hæmorrhagic infarction may occur.

(*c*) *Œdema.*—An infiltrated œdematous condition of the uvula and adjacent parts is not very uncommon in conditions of debility, in profound anæmia, and in nephritis. The uvula is sometimes enormously enlarged from this cause, whence may arise difficulty in swallowing or in breathing.

Acute Pharyngitis (*Sore Throat; Angina Simplex*).—The entire pharyngeal structures, often with the tonsils, are involved. The condition may follow cold or exposure. In other instances it is associated with constitutional states, such as gout, or with digestive disorders. The patient complains of uneasiness and soreness in swallowing, of a feeling of tickling and dryness in the throat, together with a constant desire to hawk and cough. Frequently the inflammation extends into the larynx and produces hoarseness. Not uncommonly it is only part of a general naso-pharyngeal catarrh. The process may pass into the Eustachian tubes and cause slight deafness. There is stiffness of the neck, the lymph-glands of which may be enlarged and painful. The constitutional symptoms are rarely severe. The disease sets in with a chilly feeling and slight fever; the pulse is increased in frequency. Occasionally the febrile symptoms are more severe, particularly if the tonsils are specially involved. The examination of the throat shows general congestion of the mucous membrane, which is dry and glistening, and in places covered with sticky secretion. The uvula may be much swollen.

Acute pharyngitis lasts only a few days and requires mild measures. Cold compresses or an ice bag may be applied to the neck. If the tonsils are involved and the fever is high, aconite or sodium salicylate may be given. Guaiacum also is beneficial; but in a majority of the cases a calomel purge or a saline aperient and simple inhalations meet the indications.

Chronic Pharyngitis.—This may follow repeated acute attacks. It is very common in persons who smoke or drink to excess, and in those who use the voice very much, such as clergymen, hucksters, and others. It is frequently associated with chronic nasal catarrh. The naso-pharynx and the posterior wall are the parts most frequently affected. The mucous membrane is relaxed, the venules are dilated, and roundish bodies, from 2 to 4 mm. in diameter, reddish in color, project to a variable distance beyond the mucous membrane and represent proliferation of lymph tissue about the mucous glands. They may be very abundant, forming elongated rows in the lateral walls of the pharynx. There may be a dry glistening state of the pharyngeal mucosa, known as *pharyngitis sicca.* The pillars of the fauces and the uvula are often much relaxed. The secretion forms at the back of the pharynx and the patient may feel it drop down from the vault, or it is tenacious and adherent, and is removed only by repeated efforts at hawking.

In the *treatment* special attention must be paid to the general health. If possible, the cause should be ascertained. The condition is almost constant in smokers, and cannot be cured without stopping the use of tobacco. The use of food either too hot or too much spiced should be forbidden. When it depends upon excessive exercise of the voice, rest should be enjoined. In many of these cases change of air and tonics help very much. In the local treatment, gargles, washes, and pastilles of various sorts give temporary relief, but when the hypertrophic condition is marked the spots should be thoroughly destroyed by the galvano-cautery. In many instances this affords great and permanent relief, but in others the condition persists, and, as it is not unbearable, the patient gives up hope of permanent relief.

Ulceration of the Pharynx.—(*a*) *Follicular.*—The ulcers are usually small, superficial, and generally associated with chronic catarrh.

(*b*) *Syphilitic.*—Most frequently painless and situated on the posterior wall of the pharynx, they occur in the secondary stage as small, shallow excavations with the mucous patches. In the tertiary stage they are due to erosion of gummata, and in healing they leave whitish cicatrices.

(*c*) *Tuberculous.*—Not very uncommon in advanced cases of pulmonary tuberculosis, if extensive, they form one of the most distressing features of the disease. The ulcers are irregular, with ill-defined edges and grayish-yellow bases. The posterior wall of the pharynx may have an eroded, worm-eaten appearance. These ulcers are, as a rule, intensely painful. Occasionally the primary disease is about the tonsils and the pillars of the fauces.

(*d*) *Ulcers* occur in connection with pseudo-membranous inflammation, particularly the diphtheritic. In cancer and in lupus ulcers are also present.

(*e*) Ulcers are met with in certain of the fevers, particularly in typhoid.

In many instances the diagnosis of the nature of pharyngeal ulcers is very difficult. The tuberculous and cancerous varieties are readily recognized, but doubt frequently arises as to the syphilitic character of an ulcer. In many instances the local conditions may be uncertain. Other evidences of syphilis should be sought for, and the patient placed on mercury and iodide of potassium, under which remedies specific ulcers usually heal with great rapidity.

Acute Infectious Phlegmon of the Pharynx.—Under this term Senator has described cases in which, along with difficulty in swallowing, soreness of the throat, and sometimes hoarseness, the neck enlarges, the pharyngeal mucosa becomes swollen and injected, the fever is high, the constitutional symptoms are severe, and the inflammation passes on rapidly to suppuration. The symptoms are very intense. The swelling of the pharyngeal tissues early reaches such a grade as to impede respiration. Similar symptoms may be produced by foreign bodies in the pharynx.

Retro-pharyngeal abscess occurs: (*a*) In healthy children between six months and two years of age. The child becomes restless, the voice changes; it becomes nasal or metallic in tone, and there are pain and difficulty in swallowing. Inspection of the pharynx reveals a projecting tumor in the middle line, or, if not visible, it is felt, on palpation, projecting from the posterior wall. (*b*) As a not infrequent sequel of the fevers, particularly scarlet fever and diphtheria. (*c*) In caries of the bodies of the cervical vertebræ. The diagnosis is readily made, as the projecting tumor can be seen, or felt with the finger on the posterior wall of the pharynx.

Angina Ludovici (*Ludwig's Angina; Cellulitis of the Neck*).—In medical practice this is seen as a secondary inflammation in the specific fevers, particularly diphtheria and scarlet fever. It may occur idiopathically or result from trauma. It is probably always a streptococcus infection which spreads rapidly from the glands. The swelling at first is most marked in the submaxillary region of one side. The symptoms are, as a rule, intense, and, unless early and thorough surgical measures are employed, there is great risk of systemic infection. The various acute septic inflammations of the throat —acute œdema of the larynx, phlegmon of the pharynx and larynx, and angina Ludovici—"represent degrees varying in virulence of one and the same process" (Semon). The treatment is surgical and free incisions should be made.

D. DISEASES OF THE TONSILS

I. SUPPURATIVE TONSILLITIS

Etiology.—Acute suppuration of the tonsillar tissues is met with most frequently in young persons, with chronic enlargement of the glands, sometimes as a sequence of the acute follicular form, sometimes as a result of exposure to cold or wet.

Symptoms.—The constitutional disturbance is very great. The temperature rises to 104° or 105° F., and the pulse ranges from 110 to 130. Nocturnal delirium is not uncommon. The prostration may be extreme. There is no local disease of similar extent which so rapidly exhausts the strength of a patient. Soreness and dryness of the throat, with pain in swallowing, are the symptoms of which the patient first complains. One or both tonsils may be involved. They are enlarged, firm to the touch, dusky red and œdematous, and the contiguous parts are also much swollen. The swelling of the glands may be so great that they meet in the middle line, or one tonsil may even push the uvula aside and almost touch the other gland. The salivary and buccal secretions are increased. The glands of the neck enlarge, the lower jaw is fixed, and the patient is unable to open his mouth. In from two to four days the enlarged gland becomes softer, and fluctuation can be distinctly felt by placing one finger on the tonsil and the other at the angle of the jaw. The abscess points usually toward the mouth, but in some cases toward the pharynx. It may burst spontaneously, affording instant relief. Suffocation has followed the rupture of a large abscess and the entrance of the pus into the larynx. When the suppuration is peritonsillar and extensive, the internal carotid artery may be opened; but these are, fortunately, very rare accidents.

Occasionally a small focus of deep-seated suppuration is the cause of a fever lasting for weeks or months.

Treatment.—Hot applications in the form of poultices and fomentations are more comfortable than the ice-bag. The gland should be felt—it cannot always be seen—from time to time, and opened when fluctuation is distinct. The progress may be shortened and the patient spared several days of great suffering if an incision is made early. The curved bistoury, guarded nearly to the point with plaster or cotton, is the most satisfactory instrument. The incision should be made from above downward, parallel with the anterior pillar. There are cases in which, before suppuration takes place, the swelling is so great that the patient is threatened with suffocation. In such instances the tonsil must be excised or tracheotomy performed. Delavan refers to two cases in which he states that tracheotomy would have saved life. Patients with this affection require a nourishing liquid diet, and during convalescence iron in full doses.

Early removal of the tonsils should be practised when a child suffers with recurring attacks, and thorough local treatment should be given to the naso-pharynx. Particular care should be taken of the child's mouth and throat.

II. CHRONIC TONSILLITIS

(Chronic Naso-pharyngeal Obstruction; Adenoids; Mouth-breathing; Aprosexia)

Under this heading will be considered also hypertrophy of the adenoid tissue in the vault of the pharynx, sometimes known as the pharyngeal tonsil, as the affection usually involves both the tonsils proper and this tissue, and the symptoms are not to be differentiated.

Chronic enlargement of the tissues of the tonsillar ring is an affection of great importance, and may influence in an extraordinary way the mental and bodily development of children.

The lacunæ are really nothing but culture tubes in which an extraordinary number of organisms grow, the dominant one being the streptococcus. Other frequent organisms are the staphylococcus, pneumococcus, and *Micrococcus catarrhalis*. Normally these forms of organisms are kept at bay by the epithelium and by an army of leucocytes which constantly stream out from the lymphoid tissue. But in catarrhal conditions or by abrasion, the organisms may spread into the substance of the tonsil or even pass the capsule and enter the system through the lymphatics.

Etiology.—"Adenoids" have become recognized as one of the most common and important affections of childhood, occurring most frequently between the fifth and tenth years. The introduction of the systematic inspection of school children has done more than anything else to force upon the profession and the public the recognition of the condition as one influencing seriously the bodily and mental growth, disturbing hearing and furnishing a focus for the development of pathogenic organisms. Few children escape altogether. In many it is a trifling affair, easily remedied; in others it is a serious and obstinate trouble, taxing the skill and judgment of the specialist. It is not easy to say why the disease has become so prevalent. In the United States it is attributed to the dry, hot air of the houses, in England to the cold, damp climate. In winter nearly all the school children in England have the "snuffles," and a considerable proportion of them adenoids. American children may be especially prone, but the disease is even more prevalent in England.

Adenoids may be associated with slight enlargement of the lymph-glands, thymus and spleen in the condition of lymphatism.

Morbid Anatomy.—The tonsils are enlarged, due to multiplication of all the constituents of the glands. The lymphoid elements may be chiefly involved without much development of the stroma. In other instances the fibrous matrix is increased, and the organ is then harder, smaller, firmer, and is cut with much greater difficulty.

The adenoids, which spring from the vault of the pharynx, form masses varying in size from a small pea to an almond. They may be sessile, with broad bases, or pedunculated. They are reddish in color, of moderate firmness, and contain numerous blood-vessels. "Abundant, as a rule, over the vault, on a line with the fossa of the Eustachian tube, the growths may lie posterior to the fossa—namely, in the depression known as the fossa of Rosenmüller, or upon the parts which are parallel to the posterior wall of the pharynx. The growths appear to spring in the main from the mucous membrane covering the localities where the connective tissue fills in the inequalities of the base of the skull" (Harrison Allen). The growths are most frequently papillomatous with a lymphoid parenchyma. Hypertrophy of the pharyngeal adenoid tissue may be present without great enlargement of the tonsils proper. Chronic catarrh of the nose usually coexists.

Symptoms.—The direct effect of adenoids is the establishment of mouth-breathing. The indirect effects are deformation of the thorax, changes in the facial expression, sometimes marked alteration in the mental condition, in certain cases stunting of the growth, and in a great many subjects deafness. Woods Hutchinson has suggested that the embryological relation of these structures and the pituitary body may account for the interference with development. The establishment of *mouth-breathing* is the symptom which first attracts the attention. It is not so noticeable by day, although the child may present the vacant expression characteristic of this condition. At night the child's sleep is greatly disturbed; the respirations are loud and snorting, and there are sometimes prolonged pauses, followed by deep, noisy inspirations. The pulse may vary strangely during these attacks, and in the prolonged intervals may be slow, to increase greatly with the forced inspirations. The alæ nasi should be observed during the sleep of the child, as they are sometimes much retracted during inspiration, due to a laxity of the walls, a condition readily remedied by the use of a soft wire dilator. Night terrors are common. The child may wake up in a paroxysm of shortness of breath. Sometimes these attacks are of great severity and the dyspnœa may suggest pressure of enlarged glands on the trachea. Sometimes there is a nocturnal paroxysmal cough of a very troublesome character, usually excited by lying down. Children with adenoids are specially liable to bronchitis. The thin, ill-nourished mouth-breathing child with deformed chest, cough and scattered bronchial râles is a familiar figure in tuberculosis dispensaries.

When the mouth-breathing has persisted for a long time definite changes result in the face, mouth, and chest. The facies is so peculiar and distinctive that the condition may be evident at a glance. The expression is dull, heavy, and apathetic, due in part to the fact that the mouth is habitually open. In long-standing cases the child is stupid-looking, responds slowly to questions, and may be sullen and cross. The lips are thick, the nasal orifices small and pinched-in, the superior dental arch narrowed and the roof of the mouth considerably raised. Carious teeth are common.

The remarkable alterations in the shape of the chest in connection with enlarged tonsils were first carefully studied by Dupuytren (1828), who evidently fully appreciated the great importance of the condition. He noted "a lateral depression of the parietes of the chest consisting of a depression, more or less great, of the ribs on each side, and a proportionate protrusion of the sternum in front." J. Mason Warren (Medical Examiner, 1839) gave an admirable description of the constitutional symptoms and the thoracic deformities induced by enlarged tonsils. These, with the memoir of Lambron (1861), constitute the most important contributions to our knowledge on the subject. Three types of deformity may be recognized:

(*a*) The pigeon or chicken breast is the most common form, in which the sternum is prominent and there is a circular depression in the lateral zone (Harrison's groove), corresponding to the attachment of the diaphragm. The ribs are prominent anteriorly and the sternum is angulated forward at the manubrio-gladiolar junction. As a mouth-breather is watched during sleep one can see the lower and lateral thoracic regions retracted during inspiration by the action of the diaphragm.

(*b*) Barrel Chest.—Some children, the subject of chronic naso-pharyngeal obstruction, have recurring attacks of asthma, and the chest may be gradually deformed, becoming rounded and barrel-shaped, the neck short, and the shoulders and back bowed. A child of ten or eleven may have the thoracic conformation of an old man with emphysema.

(*c*) The Funnel Breast (*Trichterbrust*).—This remarkable deformity, in which there is a deep depression at the lower sternum, has excited much controversy as to its mode of origin. In some instances, at least, it is due to the obstructed breathing in connection with adenoid vegetations. In two cases in children seen while the condition was in process of formation during inspiration the lower sternum was forcibly retracted, so much so that at the height the depression corresponded to that of a well-marked "*Trichterbrust.*" While in repose, the lower sternal region was distinctly excavated.

The voice is altered and acquires a nasal quality. The pronunciation of certain letters is changed, and there is inability to pronounce the nasal consonants *n* and *m*. Bloch lays great stress upon the association of mouth-breathing with stuttering.

The *hearing* is impaired, usually owing to the extension of inflammation along the Eustachian tubes and the obstruction with mucus or the narrowing of their orifices by pressure of the adenoid vegetations. In some instances it may be due to retraction of the drums, as the upper pharynx is insufficiently supplied with air. Naturally the senses of taste and smell are much impaired. There may be little or no nasal catarrh or discharge, but the pharyngeal secretion of mucus is increased. Children do not notice this, as the mucus is usually swallowed, but older persons expectorate it with difficulty.

Among other symptoms are headache, which is by no means uncommon, general listlessness, and an indisposition for physical or mental exertion. Habit-spasm of the face has been described in connection with it and permanent relief has been afforded by the removal of the adenoid vegetations. Enuresis is occasionally an associated symptom. The influence upon the mental development is striking. Mouth-breathers are usually dull, stupid, and backward. It is impossible for them to fix the attention for long at a time, and to this impairment of the mental function Guye, of Amsterdam, gave the name *aprosexia*. Headaches, forgetfulness, inability to study without discomfort are frequent symptoms of this condition in students. There is more than a grain of truth in the aphorism *shut your mouth and save your life,* which is found on the title-page of Captain Catlin's celebrated pamphlet on mouth-breathing (1861), to which cause he attributed all the ills of civilization.

A symptom specially associated with enlarged tonsils is fetor of the breath. The inspissated secretion undergoes decomposition and the little cheesy masses may sometimes be squeezed from the crypts of the tonsils. In some cases of chronic enlargement the cheesy masses may be deep in the tonsillar crypts; and if they remain for a prolonged period lime salts are deposited and a tonsillar calculus is produced.

Children with adenoids are especially prone to take cold and to recurring attacks of follicular disease. They are also more liable to diphtheria, and in them the anginal features in scarlet fever are always more serious. The ultimate results of untreated adenoid hypertrophy are important. In some cases the vegetations disappear, leaving an atrophic condition of the vault of the pharynx. Neglect may also lead to the so-called Thornwaldt's disease, in which there is a cystic condition of the pharyngeal tonsil and constant secretion of muco-pus.

Diagnosis.—The facial aspect is usually distinctive. Enlarged tonsils are readily seen on inspection of the pharynx. There may be no great enlargement of the tonsils and nothing apparent at the back of the throat even when the naso-pharynx is completely blocked with adenoid vegetations. In children the rhinoscopic examination is rarely practicable. Digital examination is the most satisfactory. The growths can then be felt either as small, flat bodies or, if extensive, as velvety, grape-like papillomata.

Treatment.—If the tonsils are large and the general state is evidently influenced by them they should be removed. Important complications may follow the removal—hæmorrhage, hyperpyrexia, infarction and abscess of the lungs, general sepsis, cerebro-thrombosinusitis, subcutaneous emphysema, death from status lymphaticus. Applications of iodine and iron, or penciling the crypts with nitrate of silver, are of service in the milder grades, but it is waste of time to apply them to enlarged glands. There is a condition in which the tonsils are not much enlarged, but the crypts are constantly filled with cheesy secretions and give a foul odor to the breath. In such instances the removal of the secretion and thorough penciling of the crypts with chromic acid may be practised. The galvano-cautery is of service in many cases of enlarged tonsils when there is objection to removal.

The treatment of the adenoid growths should be thoroughly carried out. Parents should be frankly told that the affection is serious, one which impairs the mental not less than the bodily development of the child. In spite of the thorough ventilation of this subject by specialists, practitioners do not appear to have grasped the full importance of this disease. They are far too apt to temporize and unnecessarily postpone radical measures. The child must be anæsthetized. Severe hæmorrhage has followed in a few cases. Special examination should be made of the thymus and lymph glands, as if they are enlarged the operation should be postponed. In this state of lymphatism death during anæsthesia has occurred. The good effects of the operation are often apparent within a few days, and the child begins to breathe through the nose. In some instances the habit of mouth-breathing persists. As soon as the child goes to sleep the lower jaw drops and the air is drawn into the mouth. In these cases a chin strap can be readily adjusted, which the child may wear at night. In severe cases it may take months of careful training before the child can speak properly. An all-important point in the treatment of lesions of the naso-pharynx (and, indeed, in the prevention of this unfortunate condition) is to increase the breathing capacity of the chest by making the child perform systematic exercises, which cause the air to be driven freely and forcibly in and out through the naso-pharynx.

Throughout the entire treatment attention should be paid to hygiene and diet, and cod-liver oil and the iodide of iron may be administered with benefit.

E. DISEASES OF THE ŒSOPHAGUS

I. ACUTE ŒSOPHAGITIS

Etiology.—Acute inflammation occurs (*a*) in the catarrhal processes of the specific fevers; more rarely as an extension from catarrh of the pharynx. (*b*) As a result of intense mechanical or chemical irritation, produced by foreign bodies, very hot liquids, or strong corrosives. (*c*) In the form of pseudo-membranous inflammation in diphtheria, and occasionally in pneumonia, typhoid fever, and pyæmia. (*d*) As a pustular inflammation in smallpox, and, according to Laennec, as a result of a prolonged administration of tartar emetic. (*e*) In connection with local disease, particularly cancer either of the tube itself or extension to it from without. And, lastly, acute œsophagitis, occasionally with ulceration, may occur spontaneously in sucklings.

Morbid Anatomy.—It is extremely rare to see redness of the mucosa, except when chemical irritants have been swallowed. More commonly the epithelium is thickened and has desquamated, so that the surface is covered with a fine granular substance. The mucous follicles are swollen and occasionally there are small erosions. In the pseudo-membranous inflammation there is a grayish exudate, usually limited in extent, at the upper portion of the gullet. In the phlegmonous inflammation the mucous membrane is greatly swollen, and there is purulent infiltration in the submucosa. It may extend throughout a large part of the gullet. Gangrene occasionally supervenes. There is a remarkable fibrinous or membranous œsophagitis, most frequently met with in the fevers, sometimes also in hysteria, in which long casts of the tube may be vomited.

Symptoms.—Pain in deglutition is always present in severe inflammation of the œsophagus. A dull pain beneath the sternum is also present. In the milder forms of catarrhal inflammation there are usually no symptoms. The presence of a foreign body is indicated by dysphagia and spasm with the regurgitation of portions of the food. Later, blood and pus may be ejected. It is surprising how extensive the disease may be in the œsophagus without producing much pain or great discomfort, except in swallowing. The intense inflammation which follows the swallowing of corrosives, when not fatal, gradually subsides, and often leads to cicatricial contraction and stricture. In the cases in which there is danger of contraction œsophageal bougies should be passed before this is marked. The patient should swallow some oil before the passage of the bougie, the size of which should be gradually increased. Dilatation should be done every few days at first.

Treatment.—This is unsatisfactory, particularly in the severer forms. The slight catarrhal cases require no special treatment. When the dysphagia is intense it is best not to give food by the mouth, but to feed entirely by enemata. Fragments of ice may be given, and as the pain and distress subside, demulcent drinks. External applications of cold often give relief.

A *chronic* form of œsophagitis is described, but this results usually from the prolonged action of the causes which produce the acute form.

Catarrhal Ulceration.—Follicular ulcers are not uncommon. Tuberculous and syphilitic ulcers are rare. Very prominent varicose veins and small erosions are not uncommon. The other forms are the carcinomatous, the erosion due to aneurism, and the ulcerative action of corrosive substances. There are two other important varieties—the ulcers in acute infectious diseases, diphtheria, scarlet fever, and pneumonia; and the peptic ulcer, first described by Albers in 1839. Tileston has collected forty cases of peptic ulcer in the œsophagus. The pain, dysphagia, vomiting, and hæmorrhage have been the most important symptoms. Perforation occurred in six cases, in one instance into the aorta. Treatment is difficult; in severe cases gastrostomy should be done.

Œsophageal Varices.—Associated with chronic heart-disease and more frequently with the senile and the cirrhotic liver, the œsophageal veins may become distended and varicose. The mucous membrane is in a state of chronic catarrh, and the patient has frequent eructations of mucus. Rupture of these varices is one of the commonest causes of hæmatemesis in cirrhosis of the liver and in enlarged spleen. The blood may pass per rectum alone.

II. SPASM OF THE ŒSOPHAGUS

(*Œsophagismus*)

This is met with in nervous patients and hypochondriacs, also in chorea, epilepsy, and especially hydrophobia. It is sometimes associated also with the lodgment of foreign bodies, or with cases in which a patient has swallowed a foreign body and thinks it has stuck. For weeks there may be spasm, due perhaps to autosuggestion, though the bougie passes freely. The idiopathic form is found in females of a marked neurotic habit, but may also occur in elderly men. It may be present only during pregnancy. The patient complains of inability to swallow solid food, and in extreme instances even liquids are rejected. The attack may come on abruptly, and be associated with emotional disturbances and with substernal pain. The bougie, when passed, may be arrested temporarily at the seat of the spasm, which gradually yields, or it may slip through without the slightest effort. The condition is rarely serious, though it may persist for years. Spasm of the lower end of the gullet, associated with cardio-spasm, may be the cause of a remarkable fusiform dilatation of the œsophagus.

The *diagnosis* is not difficult, particularly in young persons with marked nervous manifestations. In elderly persons œsophagismus often occurs with hypochondriasis, but great care must be taken to exclude cancer.

In some cases a cure is at once effected by the passage of a bougie. The general neurotic condition also requires special attention. Atropine in full doses is sometimes helpful.

Paralysis of the œsophagus is a very rare condition, due most often to central disease, particularly bulbar paralysis. It may be peripheral in origin, as in diphtheritic paralysis. Occasionally it occurs in hysteria. The essential symptom is dysphagia.

III. STRICTURE OF THE ŒSOPHAGUS

This results from: (*a*) Congenital stenosis of the œsophagus.—There are two groups of cases, one in which there is complete occlusion, and the middle of the tube is converted into a fibrous cord; the other, the more common, in which the lower part opens into the trachea or one of the bronchi. There are some 19 cases on record (William Thomas). (*b*) The cicatricial contraction of healed ulcers, usually due to corrosive poisons, occasionally to syphilis, and in rare instances after the fevers. (*c*) The growth of tumors in the walls, as in the so-called cancerous stricture. Eighty-five per cent. of the cases are of this nature. (*d*) External pressure by aneurism, enlarged lymph-glands, enlarged thyroid, other tumors, and sometimes by pericardial effusion.

The cicatricial stricture may occur anywhere in the gullet, and in extreme cases may involve the whole tube, but in a majority of instances it is found either high up near the pharynx or low down toward the stomach. The narrowing may be extreme, so that only small quantities of food can trickle through, or the obstruction may be quite slight. When the stricture is low down the œsophagus is dilated and the walls are usually much hypertrophied. When the obstruction is high in the gullet, the food is usually rejected at once, whereas, if it is low, it may be retained and a considerable quantity collects before it is regurgitated. Any doubt as to its having reached the stomach is removed by the alkalinity of the material ejected and the absence of the characteristic gastric odor. Auscultation of the œsophagus may be practised and is sometimes of service. The patient takes a mouthful of water and the auscultator listens along the left of the spine. The normal œsophageal *bruit* may be heard later than seven seconds, the normal time, or there may be heard a loud splashing, gurgling sound. The secondary murmur, heard as the fluid enters the stomach, may be absent. The bismuth meal and the fluoroscope make the diagnosis very easy. The passage of the œsophageal bougie will determine accurately the locality. Conical bougies attached to a flexible whalebone stem are the most satisfactory, but the gum-elastic stomach tube may be used; a large one should be tried first. The patient should be placed on a low chair with the head well thrown back. The index finger of the left hand is passed far into the pharynx, and in some instances this procedure alone may determine the presence of a new growth. The bougie is passed beside the finger until it touches the posterior wall of the pharynx, then along it, more to one side than in the middle line, and so gradually pushed into the gullet. It is to be borne in mind that in passing the cricoid cartilage there is often a slight obstruction. Great gentleness should be used, as the bougie has been passed through a cancerous ulcer into the mediastinum or through a diverticulum. It is well always, as a precautionary measure, to examine carefully for aneurism, which may produce all the symptoms of organic stricture. In cases in which the narrowing is extreme there is always emaciation. For treatment, surgical works must be consulted.

IV. CANCER OF THE ŒSOPHAGUS

This is usually epithelioma. It is not a common disease; there were only 38 cases in the medical wards of the Johns Hopkins Hospital in twenty-three years. It may occur in quite young persons, and is more frequent in males than in females. The middle and lower thirds are most often affected. At first confined to the mucous membrane, the cancer gradually increases and soon ulcerates. The lumen of the tube is narrowed, but when ulceration is extensive in the later stages the stricture may be less marked. Dilatation of the tube and hypertrophy of the walls usually take place above the cancer. The ulcer may perforate the trachea or a bronchus, the lung, the pleura, the mediastinum, the aorta or one of its larger branches, the pericardium, or erode the vertebræ. The recurrent laryngeal nerves are not infrequently implicated. Perforation of the lung produces, as a rule, local gangrene.

Symptoms.—Dysphagia is usually an early symptom but may be absent throughout. If present it is progressive and becomes extreme, so that the patient emaciates rapidly. Regurgitation may take place at once; or, if the cancer is situated near the stomach, it may be deferred for ten or fifteen minutes, or even longer if the tube is much dilated. The rejected materials may be mixed with blood and may contain cancerous fragments. Tickling sensations in the throat, increased secretion and cough are not infrequent. In persons over fifty years of age persistent difficulty in swallowing accompanied by rapid emaciation usually indicates œsophageal cancer. Sudden transient attacks of difficulty in swallowing may occur. The cervical lymph-glands are frequently enlarged and may give early indication of the nature of the trouble. Pain may be persistent or be present only when food is taken. In certain instances the pain is very great. The latent cases are very rare. Bronchitis and broncho-pneumonia are common terminal events.

Diagnosis.—It is important, in the first place, to exclude pressure from without, as by aneurism or tumor. The history enables us to exclude cicatricial stricture and foreign bodies. The sound may be passed and the presence of the stricture determined but great care should be exercised. The œsophagoscope is of great aid. Fragments of carcinomatous tissue may be removed with the tube. The X-ray examination is of service both in showing the presence of a growth and its position.

Treatment.—In most cases milk and liquids can be swallowed, but supplementary nourishment should be given by the rectum. It may be advisable to pass a tube into the stomach and introduce food in this way. When there is difficulty in feeding the patient it is much better to have gastrostomy performed at once, as it gives comfort and prolongs the patient's life.

V. RUPTURE OF THE ŒSOPHAGUS

(*a*) Rupture may occur as a result of violent vomiting after a full meal, or when intoxicated. In 1914 Walker collected 22 cases, 20 of which were in males. In every case the rupture was at the lower end. Boerhaave described the first case in Baron Wassennar, who "broke asunder the tube of the œsophagus near the diaphragm, so that, after the most excruciating pain, the elements which he swallowed passed, together with the air, into the cavity of the thorax, and he expired in twenty-four hours." (*b*) In a few cases the rupture has occurred in a diseased and weakened tube, near the scar of an ulcer, for example. (*c*) Post mortem softening—œsophago-malacia—must not be mistaken for it. In spontaneous rupture the rent is clean-cut; in malacia it is rounded and the margins are softened. The contents of the stomach may be in the left pleura.

VI. DILATATIONS AND DIVERTICULA

Stenosis of the gullet is followed by secondary dilatation of the tube above the constriction and great hypertrophy of the walls. Primary dilatation, which is extremely rare, is associated with spasm of the lower end of the gullet and of the cardiac orifice or with contraction of the stomach as in scirrhous cancer. The tube may attain extraordinary dimensions, as in the specimen presented in 1904 to the Association of American Physicians by Kinnicutt. Regurgitation of food is the most common symptom. There may also be difficulty in breathing from pressure.

Diverticula are of two forms: (*a*) Pressure diverticula, which are most common at the junction of the pharynx and gullet, on the posterior wall. Owing to weakness of the muscles at this spot, local bulging occurs, which is gradually increased by the pressure of food, and finally forms a saccular pouch. (*b*) The traction diverticula situated on the anterior wall near the bifurcation of the trachea result, as a rule, from the extension of inflammation from the lymph-glands with adhesion and subsequent cicatricial contraction, by which the wall of the gullet is drawn out. The diagnosis of these forms is readily made by the X-rays. Diverticula have been successfully extirpated.

A rare and remarkable condition, of which a case has been recorded by MacLachlan, and of which a second was in attendance at the Hopkins clinic, is the œsophago-pleuro-cutaneous fistula. In this patient fluids were discharged at intervals through a fistula in the right infra-clavicular region, which communicated with a cavity in the upper part of the pleura or lung. The condition had persisted for more than twenty-five years.

F. DISEASES OF THE STOMACH

I. ACUTE GASTRITIS

(Simple Gastritis; Acute Gastric Catarrh; Acute Dyspepsia)

Etiology.—Acute gastritis occurs at all ages, and is usually traceable to errors in diet. It may follow the ingestion of more food than the stomach can digest, or it may result from taking unsuitable articles, which either themselves irritate the mucosa or, remaining undigested, decompose, and so excite an acute dyspepsia. A frequent cause is the taking of food which has begun to decompose, particularly in hot weather. In children these fermentative processes are very apt to excite acute catarrh of the bowels as well. Another very common cause is the abuse of alcohol, and the acute gastritis which follows a drinking-bout is one of the most typical forms. The tendency to gastric disturbance varies very much in different individuals, and, indeed, in families. We recognize this in using the expressions a "delicate stomach" and a "strong stomach."

Morbid Anatomy.—Beaumont's study of St. Martin's stomach showed that in acute catarrh the mucous membrane is reddened and swollen, less gastric juice is secreted, and mucus covers the surface. Slight hæmorrhages may occur or even small erosions. The submucosa may be somewhat œdematous. Microscopically the changes are chiefly noticeable in the mucous and peptic cells, which are swollen and more granular, and there is an infiltration of the intertubular tissue with leucocytes.

Symptoms.—In mild cases the symptoms are those of slight indigestion—an uncomfortable feeling in the abdomen, headache, depression, nausea, eructations, and vomiting, which usually gives relief. The tongue is heavily coated and the saliva is increased. In children there are intestinal symptoms—diarrhœa and colicky pains and often slight fever. The duration is rarely more than twenty-four hours. In the severer forms the attack may set in with a chill and febrile reaction, in which the temperature rises to 102° or 103° F. The tongue is furred, the breath heavy, and vomiting is frequent. The ejected substances, at first mixed with food, subsequently contain much mucus and bile-stained fluids. There may be constipation, but very often there is diarrhœa. The urine presents the usual febrile characteristics, and there is a heavy deposit of urates. The abdomen may be somewhat distended and slightly tender in the epigastric region. Herpes may appear on the lips. The attack may last from one to three days, and occasionally longer. The examination of the vomitus shows, as a rule, absence of hydrochloric acid, the presence of lactic and fatty acids, and marked increase in the mucus.

Diagnosis.—The ordinary æfebrile gastritis is readily recognized. The acute febrile form is so similar to the initial symptoms of many of the infectious diseases that it is impossible for a day or two to make a diagnosis, particularly in the cases which have come on, so to speak, spontaneously and independently of an error in diet. Some of these resemble closely an acute infection; the symptoms may be very intense, and if, as sometimes happens, the attack sets in with severe headache and delirium, the case may be mistaken for meningitis. When the abdominal pains are intense the attack may be confounded with gallstone colic. The gastric crises in tabes have been confounded with a simple acute gastritis, and it is always wise in adults to test the knee-jerks and pupillary reactions.

Treatment.—Mild cases recover spontaneously in twenty-four hours, and require no treatment other than a dose of castor oil in children or of blue mass in adults. In the severer forms, if there is much distress in the region of the stomach, the vomiting should be promoted by warm water, or the stomach tube may be employed for some patients. A dose of calomel, 2 to 3 grains (0.13 to 0.2 gm.), should be given, and followed, after some hours, by a saline cathartic. If there is eructation of acid fluid, bicarbonate of soda and bismuth may be given. The stomach should have, if possible, absolute rest, and it is a good plan in the case of strong persons, particularly in those addicted to alcohol, to cut off all food for a day or two. The patient may be allowed soda water and ice freely. It is well not to attempt to check the vomiting unless it is excessive and protracted. Recovery is usually complete, though repeated attacks may lead to subacute or chronic gastritis.

Phlegmonous Gastritis; Acute Suppurative Gastritis.—The disease is due to infection of the submucosa, probably through a minute abrasion. Males are more frequently affected than females, and most of the cases are in comparatively young people. In a majority of the instances in which the examination has been made streptococci have been present, but the pneumococcus has been found in a few cases. The disease is rare; Leith was able to collect only 85 cases. There is a widespread suppurative infiltration of the submucosa, with great thickening of the walls. Sometimes there is a localized abscess formation, with tumor, which may burst into the stomach or into the peritoneum.

The important symptoms are pain, high fever, vomiting, dry tongue, all the features of a severe infection, and sometimes jaundice. A diagnosis is rarely made; occasionally there is a large tumor mass to be felt. The outlook is very serious. In the case reported by Bovee, he cut down and opened an acute abscess, the size of a man's fist, in the anterior wall of the pyloric region.

Toxic Gastritis.—This most intense form of inflammation of the stomach is excited by the swallowing of concentrated mineral acids or strong alkalies, or by such poisons as phosphorus, corrosive sublimate, ammonia, arsenic, etc. In the non-corrosive poisons, such as phosphorus, arsenic, and antimony, the process consists of an acute degeneration of the glandular elements, and hæmorrhage. With the powerful concentrated poisons the mucous membrane is extensively destroyed, and may be converted into a brownish-black eschar. In the less severe grades there may be areas of necrosis surrounded by inflammatory reaction, while the submucosa is hæmorrhagic and infiltrated. The process is of course more intense at the fundus, but the active peristalsis may drive the poison through the pylorus into the intestine.

SYMPTOMS.—The symptoms are intense pain in the mouth, throat, and stomach, salivation, great difficulty in swallowing, and constant vomiting, the vomited materials being bloody and sometimes containing portions of the mucous membrane. The abdomen is tender, distended, and painful on pressure. In the most acute cases symptoms of collapse supervene; the pulse is weak, the skin pale and covered with sweat; there is restlessness, and sometimes convulsions. There may be albumin or blood in the urine, and petechiæ may occur on the skin. When the poison is less intense, the sloughs may separate, leaving ulcers, which too often lead, in the œsophagus to stricture, in the stomach to chronic atrophy, and finally to death from exhaustion.

DIAGNOSIS.—The diagnosis of toxic gastritis is usually easy, as inspection of the mouth and pharynx shows, in many instances, corrosive effects, while the examination of the vomit may indicate the nature of the poison.

In poisoning by acids, magnesia should be administered in milk or with egg albumen. When strong alkalies have been taken, the dilute acids should be administered. If the case is seen early, lavage should be used. For the severe inflammation which follows the swallowing of the stronger poisons palliative treatment is alone available, and morphia may be freely employed to allay the pain.

Diphtheritic or Membranous Gastritis.—This is met with occasionally in diphtheria, but more commonly as a secondary process in typhus or typhoid fever, pneumonia, pyæmia, small-pox, and occasionally in debilitated children. The exudation may be extensive and uniform or in patches. The condition is not recognizable during life, unless the membranes are vomited.

Mycotic and Parasitic Gastritis.—It occasionally happens that fungi grow in the stomach and excite inflammation. One of the most remarkable cases of the kind is that reported by Kundrat, in which the favus fungus occurred in the stomach and intestine.

In cancer and in dilatation of the stomach the sarcinæ and yeast fungi probably aid in maintaining the chronic gastritis. As a rule, the gastric juice is capable of killing the ordinary bacteria. Anthrax bacilli may produce swelling of the mucosa and ulceration. Acute emphysematous gastritis may be of mycotic origin. The larvæ of certain insects may excite gastritis.

II. CHRONIC GASTRITIS

(Chronic Catarrh of the Stomach; Chronic Dyspepsia)

Definition.—A condition of disturbed digestion associated with increased mucous formation, qualitative or quantitative changes in the gastric juice, enfeeblement of the muscular coats, so that the food is retained for an abnormal time in the stomach; and, finally, with alterations in the mucosa. The term chronic gastritis is used loosely to designate a variety of gastric disorders, in many of which there are no actual changes in the mucous membrane.

Etiology.—The causes may be classified as follows: (*a*) *Dietetic.* Unsuitable or improperly prepared food, and the persistent use of certain articles of diet, such as very fat substances or foods containing too much of the carbohydrates. The use in excessive quantity of hot bread, hot cakes, and pie is a fruitful cause, particularly in the United States. The use in excess of tea or coffee, and, above all, of alcohol in its various forms. Under this heading, too, may be mentioned the habits of eating at irregular hours or too rapidly, and imperfectly chewing the food. "The platter kills more than the sword." A common cause is drinking too freely of ice-water during meals, a practice which plays no small part in the prevalence of dyspepsia in America. Another frequent cause is the abuse of tobacco, particularly chewing. (*b*) *Constitutional causes.* Anæmia, chlorosis, chronic tuberculosis, gout, diabetes, and nephritis are often associated with chronic gastric catarrh. (*c*) *Local conditions:* (1) of the stomach, as in cancer, ulcer, and dilatation; (2) conditions of the portal circulation, causing chronic engorgement of the mucous membrane, as in cirrhosis, chronic heart-disease, and certain chronic lung affections. (*d*) *Oral sepsis,* particularly pyorrhœa, is regarded as a common cause of gastric disturbance. The evidence for this is chiefly of the *propter hoc* kind—the improvement in digestion after attention to the mouth. (*e*) The association of chronic *appendicitis* with gastric disturbance is well recognized. The frequency with which the stomach symptoms recur or persist after removal of the appendix suggests that both conditions are sometimes due to another common cause.

Morbid Anatomy.—In simple chronic gastritis the organ is usually enlarged, the mucous membrane pale gray in color, and covered with closely adherent, tenacious mucus. The veins are large, patches of ecchymosis are not infrequently seen, and in the chronic catarrh of portal obstruction and of chronic heart-disease small hæmorrhagic erosions. Toward the pylorus the mucosa is not infrequently irregularly pigmented, and presents a rough, wrinkled, mammilated surface, which may be so prominent that writers have described it as *gastritis polyposa.* The membrane may be thinner than normal, and much firmer. The minute anatomy shows the picture of a parenchymatous and an interstitial inflammation. The mucous membrane may undergo complete atrophy and be represented by a smooth cuticular membrane resembling that of the cardiac portion of the horse's stomach.

Symptoms.—The affection persists for an indefinite period, and, as is the case with most chronic diseases, changes from time to time. Many of the symptoms are due to functional disturbance. The disease itself probably does not cause many symptoms. The appetite is variable, sometimes greatly impaired, at others very good. Among early symptoms are feelings of distress or oppression after eating, which may become aggravated and amount to actual pain. When the stomach is empty there may also be a painful feeling. The pain differs in different cases, and may be trifling or of extreme severity. When localized and felt beneath the sternum or in the præcordial region it is known as heart-burn or sometimes cardialgia. There is pain on pressure over the stomach, usually diffuse and not severe. The tongue is coated, and the patient complains of a bad taste in the mouth. The tip and margin of the tongue are very often red. Associated with this catarrhal stomatitis there may be an increase in the salivary and pharyngeal secretions. Nausea is an early symptom, and is particularly apt to occur in the morning hours. It is not, however, nearly so constant a symptom as in cancer of the stomach, and in mild grades of the affection it may not occur at all. Eructation of gas, which may continue for some hours after taking food, is a very prominent feature in cases of so-called flatulent dyspepsia, and there may be marked distention of the intestines. With the gas, bitter fluids may be brought up. Vomiting, which is not very frequent, occurs either immediately after eating or an hour or two later. In the chronic catarrh of old topers a bout of morning vomiting is common, in which a slimy mucus is brought up. The vomitus consists of food in various stages of digestion and slimy mucus, and the chemical examination shows the presence of abnormal acids, such as butyric, or even acetic, in addition to lactic acid, while the hydrochloric acid, if present, is much reduced in quantity. The digestion may be delayed, but usually there is not much disturbance of motility.

Constipation is usually present, but in some instances there is diarrhœa, and undigested food passes rapidly through the bowels. The urine is often scanty, high-colored, and deposits a heavy sediment of urates.

Of other symptoms headache is common, and the patient feels constantly out of sorts, indisposed for exertion, and low-spirited. In aggravated cases melancholia may occur. Trousseau called attention to the occurrence of vertigo, a marked feature in certain cases. The pulse is small, sometimes slow, and there may be palpitation of the heart. Fever does not occur. Cough is sometimes present, but the so-called stomach cough of chronic dyspeptics is in all probability dependent upon pharyngeal irritation. J. T. Pilcher has called attention to the frequency with which absence of free hydrochloric acid is found with the presence of occult blood. In many of these the stomach condition appears to be secondary to local disease elsewhere in the abdomen, particularly the appendix, gall-bladder or the pancreas. The bleeding comes from small erosions, and is always of the so-called occult variety. Many varieties of pathogenic organisms are almost constantly found, of which the streptococci are the most important.

The Gastric Contents.—The fasting stomach usually contains much mucus.

The study of the gastric contents usually shows the appearance of the secretions to be much delayed but they gradually appear. The HCl is usually diminished, though it may be normal. In some cases the free HCl may be absent while in the advanced forms of atrophy of the mucosa there may be neither acids nor ferments. Mucus is not present in atrophic gastritis.

The symptoms of atrophy of the mucous membrane of the stomach, without contraction of the organ, are very complex, and cannot be said to present a uniform picture. The majority of the cases present the symptoms of an aggravated chronic dyspepsia, often of such severity that cancer is suspected. The persistent distress after eating, the vomiting, and the gradual loss of flesh and strength may lead to the diagnosis of cancer. The clinical picture may be that of a severe anæmia. As early as 1860 Flint called attention to this connection between atrophy of the gastric tubules and anæmia.

Diagnosis.—It is well in any patient complaining of gastric symptoms to decide first whether there is primary organic disease of the stomach or whether the condition is secondary to disease elsewhere. This involves a general study which should always be made thoroughly. It is easy to fix one's attention on the area of symptoms and fail to recognize the site of the cause. The organic causes of chronic stomach disturbance are usually readily recognized. Carcinoma may give the greatest difficulty, but a careful study of the gastric contents and the X-ray findings usually removes any doubt. With this excluded the problem is to decide whether there is any other organic change in the stomach or whether the symptoms are purely functional. If evidence of change is found the next problem is whether the condition is primary or secondary. In this the history and the general study of the patient are important. The causes mentioned before give an idea as to how varied the etiology may be.

Ewald distinguishes three forms of chronic gastritis: (1) Simple gastritis; (2) mucous gastritis; (3), atrophic gastritis. In (1) the fasting stomach contains only a small quantity of a slimy fluid, while after the test breakfast the HCl is diminished in quantity or may be absent. Lactic acid and the fatty acids may be present. The pepsin and rennin are always present. In (2) the acidity is always slight and the condition is distinguished from (1) chiefly by the large amount of mucus present. In (3) the fasting stomach is generally empty, while after the test breakfast HCl, pepsin, and rennin are wholly wanting.

The diagnosis of cancer of the stomach from chronic gastritis may be very difficult when a tumor is not present. The cases require most careful study, and it is important to decide whether the stomach is primarily at fault, or whether the symptoms are due to disease of other organs—liver, gall-bladder, appendix or pancreas.

Treatment.—When possible the cause in each case should be ascertained and an attempt made to determine the special form of indigestion. In the majority of cases the symptoms are secondary to disease elsewhere and in them the treatment is largely of the primary condition. Usually there is no difficulty in differentiating the ordinary catarrhal and the nervous varieties. A careful study of the phenomena of digestion should be made. Two important questions should be asked of every dyspeptic—first, as to the time taken at his meals; and, second, as to the quantity he eats. A number of all cases of disturbed digestion come from hasty and imperfect mastication and from overeating. Especial stress should be laid upon the former point. In some instances it will alone suffice to cure dyspepsia if the patient will count a certain number before swallowing each mouthful. The second point is of even greater importance. People habitually eat too much, and it is probably true that a greater number of maladies arise from excess in eating than from excess in drinking. Chittenden's researches have shown that we require much less nitrogenous food to maintain a standard of perfect health—a lesson that the Hindoos and Japanese have also taught us. George Cheyne's thirteenth aphorism, quoted under the section on Obesity, contains a volume of dietetic wisdom.

(*a*) General and Dietetic.—A careful and systematically arranged dietary is the first, sometimes the only, essential in the treatment of a case of chronic dyspepsia. It is impossible to lay down rules applicable to all cases but in general the diet should be low in protein and largely carbohydrate. Individuals differ extraordinarily in their capability of digesting different articles of food, and there is much truth in the old adage, "One man's food is another man's poison." The individual preferences for different articles of food should be permitted in the milder forms. Physicians have probably been too arbitrary in this direction, and have not yielded sufficiently to the intimations given by the appetite and desires of the patient.

A rigid milk diet may be tried. "Milk and sweet sound Blood differ in nothing but in Color: *Milk* is *Blood*" (George Cheyne). In the forms associated with nephritis and chronic portal congestion, as well as in many instances in which the dyspepsia is part of a neurasthenic or hysterical trouble, this plan in conjunction with rest is most efficacious. If milk is not digested well it may be diluted one-third with soda water or Vichy, or 5 to 10 grains of carbonate of soda, or a pinch of salt may be added to each tumblerful. In many cases the milk from which the cream has been taken is better borne. Buttermilk is particularly suitable, but can rarely be taken for so long a time alone, as patients tire of it much more quickly than they do of ordinary milk. Not only can the general nutrition be maintained on this diet, but patients sometimes increase in weight, and the gastric symptoms disappear entirely. It should be given at fixed hours and in definite quantities. A patient may take 6 or 8 ounces every three hours. The amount necessary varies a good deal, but at least 3 to 5 pints should be given in the twenty-four hours. This form of diet is not, as a rule, well borne when there is a tendency to dilatation of the stomach. The milk may be previously peptonized, but it is impossible to feed a chronic dyspeptic in this way. The stools should be carefully watched, and if more milk is taken than can be digested it is well to supplement the diet with eggs and dry toast or biscuits.

In a large proportion of the cases it is not necessary to annoy the patient with strict dietaries. It may be quite sufficient to cut off certain articles of food. Thus, if there are acid eructations or flatulency the farinaceous foods should be restricted, particularly potatoes and the coarser vegetables. A fruitful source of indigestion is the hot bread and this, as well as the various forms of pancakes, pies and tarts, with heavy pastry, and fried articles of all sorts, should be strictly forbidden. As a rule, white bread, toasted, is more readily digested than bread made from the whole meal. Persons, however, differ very much in this respect, and the Graham or brown bread is most digestible for many people. Sugar and very sweet articles of food should be taken in great moderation or avoided altogether. Many instances of aggravated indigestion are due to the prevalent practice of eating largely of ice-cream. One of the most powerful enemies of the American stomach is the soda-water fountain, which has usurped so important a place in the apothecary shop.

Fats, with the exception of a moderate amount of good butter, very fat meats, and thick, greasy soups should be avoided. Ripe fruit in moderation is often advantageous, particularly when cooked. Bananas are not, as a rule, well borne. Strawberries are to many persons a cause of an annual attack of indigestion and sore throat.

In the matter of special articles of food it is impossible to lay down rigid rules, and it is the common experience that one patient with indigestion will take with impunity the articles which cause distress to another.

Another detail of importance is the general hygienic management. These patients are often introspective, dwelling in a morbid manner on their symptoms, and much inclined to take a despondent view of their condition. Very little progress can be made unless the physician gains their confidence from the outset. Their fears and whims should not be made too light of or ridiculed. Systematic exercise, carefully regulated, particularly when, as at watering places, it is combined with a restricted diet, is of special service. Change of air and occupation, a prolonged sea voyage, or a summer in the mountains will sometimes cure the most obstinate dyspepsia.

(*b*) Medicinal.—The special measures may be divided into those which attempt to replace elements which are lacking in the digestive juices and those which stimulate the organ. In the first group come the hydrochloric acid and ferments, which are so freely employed. The former is the most important. It is the ingredient in the gastric juice most commonly deficient. It is not only necessary for its own important actions, but its presence is intimately associated with that of the pepsin, as it is only in the presence of a sufficient quantity that the pepsinogen is converted into the active digestive ferment. It is best given as the dilute acid taken in somewhat larger quantities than are usually advised. Ewald recommends large doses—of from 90 to 100 drops—at intervals of fifteen minutes after the meals. Leube and Riegel advise smaller doses. Probably from 15 to 20 drops is sufficient. The prolonged use of it does not appear to be hurtful. Its use should be restricted to cases of neurosis and atrophy of the mucous membrane. In actual gastritis its value is doubtful.

Nitrate of silver is a good remedy in some cases, used in solution in the lavage (1 to 1,500 or 1 to 2,000), or in pill form, one-eighth to one-fourth of a grain three times a day. Argyria has resulted after its protracted use.

The digestive ferments are extensively employed. The use of pepsin may be limited to the cases of advanced mucous catarrh and atrophy of the stomach, in which it should be given, in doses of from 10 to 15 grains, with dilute hydrochloric acid a quarter of an hour after meals. Pancreatin is of equal or even greater value and should be given in doses of from 15 to 20 grains, in combination with bicarbonate of soda. It is conveniently administered in tablets, each of which contains 5 grains of the pancreatin and the soda, and of these two or three may be taken fifteen or twenty minutes after each meal. Malt diastase is sometimes serviceable given with alkalies.

Of measures which stimulate the glandular activity *lavage* is the most important, particularly in the forms characterized by the secretion of a large quantity of mucus. Lukewarm water should be used, or, if there is much mucus, a 1-per-cent. salt solution, or a 3- to 5-per-cent. solution of bicarbonate of soda. If there is much fermentation the 3-per-cent. solution of boric acid may be used. It is best employed in the morning on an empty stomach, or in the evening some hours after the last meal in those cases in which there is much nocturnal distress and flatulency. Once a day is, as a rule, sufficient, or, in the case of delicate persons, every second day. The irrigation may be continued until the water which comes away is quite clear. It is not necessary to remove all the fluid after the irrigation. While in some hands this measure has been carried to extremes, it is one of value in certain cases. When there is an insuperable objection to lavage a substitute may be used in the form of warm alkaline drinks, taken slowly in the early morning or the last thing at night.

Of medicines which stimulate the gastric secretion the most important are the bitter tonics, such as nux vomica, gentian, and cardamom. These are probably of more value in chronic gastritis than the hydrochloric acid. Of these nux vomica is the most powerful, though none of them have probably any very great stimulating action on the secretion, and influence rather the appetite than the digestion. If a patient has been in the habit of taking beer or light wines or stimulants with his meals, the practice may be continued if moderate quantities are taken. Beer, as a rule, is not well borne. A dry sherry or a glass of claret is preferable.

(*c*) Treatment of Special Conditions.—*Flatulency.*—For this condition careful dieting may suffice, particularly forbidding such articles as tea, pastry, and the coarser vegetables. It is usually combined with pyrosis, in which the acid fluids are brought into the mouth. Bismuth and bicarbonate of soda sometimes suffice to relieve the condition. For acid dyspepsia Sir William Roberts recommended the bismuth lozenge of the British Pharmacopœia, the antacid properties of which depend on chalk and bicarbonate of soda. It should be taken an hour or two after meals, and only when the pain and uneasiness are present. The burnt magnesia is also a good remedy. Glycerin in from 20- to 60-minim doses, the essential oils, animal charcoal alone or in combination with compound cinnamon powder may be tried. If there is much pain, chloroform in 20-minim doses or a teaspoonful of Hoffman's anodyne may be used. In obstinate cases lavage is indicated and is sometimes striking in its effects. Alkaline solutions may be used.

Vomiting is not a feature which often calls for treatment in chronic dyspepsia; sometimes in children it is a persistent symptom. Creosote and carbolic acid in drop doses, a few drops of chloroform or of dilute hydrocyanic acid, cocaine, bismuth, and oxalate of cerium may be used. If obstinate, the stomach should be washed out daily.

Constipation is a frequent and troublesome feature of most forms of indigestion. Every effort should be made to remedy this without the use of purgatives. Regularity in going to stool, the taking of sufficient water especially before meals, proper exercise, and the use of agar-agar or mineral oil may be enough. If drugs are needed the simpler laxatives should be used, such as senna, cascara and phenolphthalein. In the cases secondary to other diseases, such as renal or cardiac, the use of salines is indicated. Glycerin suppositories and the injection of from half a teaspoonful to a teaspoonful of glycerin may be efficacious.

Many cases are greatly benefited by the use of mineral waters, particularly a residence at the springs with a careful supervision of the diet and systematic exercise.

III. CIRRHOSIS VENTRICULI

(*Plastic Linitis*)

Brinton described under the term *linitis plastica* a condition of diffuse sclerosis of the stomach with thickening of the walls and reduction of the lumen. It may be localized, but more commonly involves the whole organ, and a similar condition has been found in the colon, small bowel, and rectum. In one case, a patient of Dr. Drake's, Montreal, the stomach was no bigger than a cucumber, and the cæcum and part of the ascending colon showed the same thickening. The special lesion is an enormous hypertrophy of the submucosa, with atrophy of the gland elements and hypertrophy of the muscular layers, so that the wall is six to eight times the normal thickness; but, as Brinton remarks, the layers remain distinct. There are two forms, benign and malignant, which are not easy to separate without the most careful microscopic examination. Lyle collected 118 cases from the literature, more than half of which were the true plastic linitis of Brinton.

The *symptoms* are at first indefinite, but when well established vomiting becomes marked and there is inability to retain even small amounts of food. The presence of a sausage-shaped tumor in the epigastrium is important. Hæmorrhage may be present. The X-ray picture is of great help. The protracted history, the restriction in capacity of the stomach, and the tumor may give a characteristic clinical picture. Gastro-enterostomy is helpful if it can be done but in the majority it is impossible; total gastrectomy has been performed in some cases.

IV. DILATATION OF THE STOMACH

(*Gastrectasis*)

Etiology.—ACUTE DILATATION is a very serious condition, described by Hilton Fagge, characterized by sudden onset, vomiting of enormous quantities of fluid, and symptoms of collapse. Of 102 cases collected by Lewis A. Conner 42 followed operation with general anæsthesia. The next largest group occurs in the course of severe diseases, or during convalescence. Cases have followed injuries, particularly of the head and spine. In 9 cases the symptoms came on after a single large meal; 6 cases were associated with spinal disease, in 3 while the patients were in a plaster of Paris jacket, and in a few cases it has come on in persons in good health. There were 74 deaths. In 69 autopsies the duodenum was found dilated in 38 cases. In a majority of cases it is due to a constriction of the lower end of the duodenum by traction on the mesenteric root, which is particularly apt to occur when there is a long mesentery and when the coil of small bowel is empty and falls into the true pelvis. The diagnosis is usually easy—repeated vomiting of large quantities of bilious non-fæcal fluid, with subnormal temperature, pain, collapse symptoms, and distended abdomen are the common features. The treatment consists in repeated emptying of the stomach with the tube; change in posture from the dorsal to the belly position or the knee-elbow position has been followed by prompt relief. Operation has not proved very satisfactory.

Chronic dilatation results from: (*a*) *Pyloric obstruction* due to narrowing of the orifice or of the duodenum by the cicatrization of an ulcer, hypertrophic stenosis of the pylorus (whether cancerous or simple), congenital stricture, or occasionally by pressure from without of a tumor or of a floating kidney. The pylorus may be tilted up by adhesions to the liver or gall-bladder, or the stomach may be so dilated that the pylorus is dragged down and kinked. Adhesions about the gall-bladder may extend along the adjacent parts of the stomach and hitch up the pylorus into the hilus of the liver, forming a very acute kink. In some cases there is an *intermittent* retention lasting for some hours, often due to pyloric spasm. In such cases there are usually hyperacidity and the signs of vagotonia. It may be associated with disease of the duodenum, gall-bladder or appendix. In some cases it seems as if pyloric spasm leads to definite dilatation. (*b*) *Relative or absolute insufficiency of the muscular power* of the stomach, due on the one hand to repeated overfilling of the organ with food and drink, and on the other to atony of the coats induced by chronic inflammation or the degeneration of impaired nutrition, the result of constitutional affections.

The most extreme forms are met with as a sequence of the cicatricial contraction of an ulcer. There may be considerable stenosis without much dilatation, the obstruction being compensated by hypertrophy of the muscular coats. In the second group, due to atony of the muscular coats, we must distinguish between instances in which the stomach is simply enlarged and those with actual dilatation, conditions characterized by Ewald as *megalogastria* and *gastrectasis* respectively. The size of the stomach varies greatly and the maximum capacity of a normal organ Ewald places at about 1,600 c. c. Measurements above this point indicate absolute dilatation.

Atonic dilatation may result from weakness of the coats, due to repeated overdistention, to chronic catarrh of the mucous membrane, or to the general muscular debility associated with chronic wasting disorders of all sorts. The combination of chronic gastric catarrh with overfeeding and excessive drinking is a common cause of atonic dilatation. The condition is frequently seen in diabetics, in the insane, and in beer-drinkers. In Germany this form is common in men employed in breweries. Possibly muscular weakness of the coats may result in some cases from disturbed innervation. Dilatation of the stomach is most frequent in middle-aged or elderly persons, but the condition is not uncommon in children, especially in association with rickets.

Symptoms.—In *atonic dilatation* there may be no symptoms whatever, even with a very greatly enlarged organ; more frequently there are the associated features of neurasthenia, enteroptosis, and nervous dyspepsia; while in a third group there may be all the symptoms of pyloric obstruction—vomiting of enormous quantities, etc. There is no limit to the capacity of the organ in this condition. Gould and Pyle mention an instance in which the stomach held 70 pints!

The features of *pyloric obstruction,* from whatever cause, are usually very evident. Dyspepsia is present in nearly all cases, and there are feelings of distress and uneasiness in the region of the stomach. The patient may complain much of hunger and thirst and eat and drink freely. The most characteristic symptom is the vomiting at intervals of enormous quantities of liquid and of food, amounting sometimes to four or more litres. The material is often of a dark-grayish color, with a characteristic sour odor due to the organic acids present, and contains mucus and remnants of food. On standing it separates into three layers, the lowest consisting of food, the middle of a turbid, dark-gray fluid, and the uppermost of a brownish froth. The microscopic examination shows a large variety of bacteria, yeast fungi, and the sarcina ventriculi. There may also be cherry stones, plum stones, and grape seeds. The hydrochloric acid may be absent, diminished, normal, or in excess, depending upon the cause of the dilatation. The fermentation produces lactic, butyric, and, possibly, acetic acid and various gases. In the *intermittent* forms with pyloric spasm there is retention often for four to eight hours, usually with hyperacidity. Vagotonia is often present and disease of the gall-bladder, duodenum or appendix should be considered.

In consequence of the small amount of fluid which passes from the stomach or is absorbed there are constipation, scanty urine, and extreme dryness of the skin. The general nutrition of the patient suffers greatly; there is loss of flesh and strength, and in some cases the most extreme emaciation. The color may be retained and if there is much vomiting, there may be marked polycythæmia. The gastric tetany will be considered in the section on that disease.

PHYSICAL SIGNS.—*Inspection.*—The abdomen may be large and prominent, the greatest projection occurring below the navel in the standing posture. In some instances the outline of the distended stomach can be plainly seen, the small curvature a couple of inches below the ensiform cartilage, and the greater curvature passing obliquely from the tip of the tenth rib on the left side, toward the pubes, and then curving upward to the right costal margin. Too much stress can not be laid on the importance of inspection. Very often the diagnosis may be made *de visu.* Active peristalsis may be seen in the dilated organ, the waves passing from left to right. Occasionally anti-peristalsis may be seen. In cases of stricture, particularly of hypertrophic stenosis, as the peristaltic wave reaches the pylorus, the tumor-like thickening can sometimes be distinctly seen through the thin abdominal wall. To stimulate the peristalsis the abdomen may be flipped with a wet towel. Inflation may be practiced with carbonic-acid gas. A small teaspoonful of tartaric acid dissolved in an ounce of water is first given, then a rather larger quantity of bicarbonate of soda. In many cases the outline of the dilated stomach stands out with great distinctness, and waves of peristalsis are seen in it.

Palpation.—The peristalsis may be felt, and usually in stenosis a tumor is evident at the pylorus. The resistance of a dilated stomach is peculiar, and has been aptly compared to that of an air cushion. Bimanual palpation elicits a splashing sound—*clapotage*—which is, of course, not distinctive, as it can be obtained whenever there are much liquid and air in the organ. The splashing may be very loud, and the patient may produce it himself by suddenly depressing the diaphragm, or it may be readily obtained by shaking him. The gurgling of gas through the pylorus may be felt.

Percussion.—The note is tympanitic over the greater portion of a dilated stomach; in the dependent part the note is flat. In the upright position the percussion should be made from above downward, in the left parasternal line, until a change in resonance is reached. The line of this should be marked, and the patient examined in the recumbent position, when it will be found to have altered its level. When this is on a line with the navel or below it, dilatation of the stomach may generally be assumed to exist. The fluid may be withdrawn from the stomach with a tube, and the dulness so made to disappear, or it may be increased by pouring in more fluid. In cases of doubt the organ should be distended with carbonic-acid gas or inflated through a stomach-tube.

Auscultation.—The *clapotage* or succussion can be obtained readily. Frequently a curious sizzling sound is present, not unlike that heard when the ear is placed over a soda-water bottle when first opened. It can be heard naturally, and is usually evident when the artificial gas is being generated. The heart sounds may sometimes be transmitted with great clearness and with a metallic quality.

Diagnosis.—This can usually be made without much difficulty. Emphasis should be placed on the value of inspection, particularly in combination with inflation of the stomach. Curious errors are on record, one of the most remarkable of which was the confounding of dilated stomach with an ovarian cyst; even after tapping and the removal of portions of food and fruit seeds, abdominal section was performed and the dilated stomach opened. The diagnosis of ascites has been made and the abdomen opened. The *prognosis* depends upon the cause; it is good in simple atony, bad in cancerous stricture, fairly good in simple stricture, from whatever cause.

Treatment.—In the cases due to atony careful regulation of the diet and proper treatment of the associated catarrh will suffice to effect a cure. Strychnine, ergot, and iron are recommended. Washing out the stomach is of great service, though we do not see such striking and immediate results in this form. In cases of mechanical obstruction the stomach should be emptied and thoroughly washed, either with warm water or with an antiseptic solution. Three important things are accomplished: The weight which distends the organ is removed; the fermenting materials which irritate and inflame the stomach and impede digestion are washed out; and we cleanse the inner surface of the organ. The patient can usually be taught to wash out his own stomach, and in a case of dilatation from simple stricture the practice may be followed with great benefit. The rapid reduction in the size of the stomach is often remarkable, the vomiting ceases, food is taken readily, and in many cases the general nutrition improves rapidly. As a rule, once a day is sufficient, and it may be practised either the first thing in the morning or before going to bed. So soon as the fermentative processes have been checked lukewarm water alone should be used. In the *intermittent* form the use of atropine with small doses of bromide is often useful. Any lesion elsewhere in the abdomen should be properly treated.

The food should be taken in small quantities at frequent intervals, and as concentrated as possible. Fatty and starchy articles of diet are to be avoided. Liquids should be taken sparingly.

Surgery should be resorted to early in cases of organic stricture; in atonic dilatation after all other measures have been given a thorough trial, gastro-enterostomy may be practised but the results are not satisfactory.

V. THE PEPTIC ULCER, GASTRIC AND DUODENAL

The round, perforating, simple or peptic ulcer is usually single, and occurs in the stomach and in the duodenum as far as the papilla. Post mortem statistics show a great preponderance of the gastric ulcer, but the experience of surgeons has taught us that in more than fifty per cent. of cases which come to operation the ulcer is outside the pyloric ring.

Erosions.—Small abrasions of the mucosa—2 to 4 mm.—usually multiple, are common, extending half way or quite through the layer. They are often called hæmorrhagic erosions from their blood-stained appearance. They are met with in the new-born, in cachectic states in children, in chronic heart and arterial disease, in cirrhosis of the liver, etc. Of no clinical importance, as a rule, occasionally an acute hæmorrhagic erosion of quite small size opens a large artery, and the patient bleeds to death. There is no difference between this condition and the acute form of the gastric ulcer.

In certain acute infections with the pneumococcus (Dieulafoy) and septic organisms there may be hæmorrhagic erosions, which occasionally prove fatal by hæmatemesis. It is probable that the post-operative hæmatemesis, slight or grave, may be due to these erosions. The French have described them as if peculiar to operations for appendicitis but cases occur after all sorts of abdominal operations. It is probable that the slight gastric hæmorrhages which occur in connection with the throbbing aorta in neurotic women are due to these erosions.

Etiology of Peptic Ulcer.—Incidence.—The disease is much more common than medical and pathological statistics indicate. The surgical work of many men has taught us that the peptic ulcer exists in many cases which we had regarded as simple hyperchlorhydria. In two points surgical experience has completely changed our medical standpoint, viz.: the incidence of ulcer in the male is greater than in the female, and the duodenal is more common than the gastric ulcer. In a series of 1725 proved cases more than two-thirds were duodenal (Smithies). The surgical statistics have sent our medical figures to the scrap heap. The incidence appears to vary in different localities, and post mortem figures from the United States and Canada show a much lower percentage of cases (1.32) than on the continent of Europe (5 per cent.), and in London, 4.2 per cent. (C. P. Howard).

Sex.—Of 1,699 cases collected from hospital statistics by W. H. Welch and examined post mortem, 40 per cent. were in males and 60 per cent. were in females. Surgical statistics show an enormous preponderance of males.

Age.—In females the largest number of cases occurred between fifteen and twenty-five; in males between forty and fifty, in our series. It may occur in old people. E. G. Cutler studied a series of 29 cases in children. In 6 the symptoms came on immediately after birth. There were 8 cases under seven years of age, and 9 between eight and thirteen.

OCCUPATION.—It was impossible in our series to say that occupation had any influence. Among women, chlorotic, dyspeptic servant girls seem very prone. Shoemakers are thought to be specially liable. It appears relatively more common in the hospital classes.

TRAUMA.—Ulcers have been known to follow a blow in the region of the stomach. There was a history of injury in 7 cases in our series.

ASSOCIATED DISEASES.—Anæmia and chlorosis predispose strongly to gastric ulcer, particularly in women and in association with menstrual disorders. A very considerable number of all cases of gastric ulcer occur in chlorotic girls. It has been found also in connection with disease of the heart, arteriosclerosis, and disease of the liver. The tuberculous and syphilitic ulcers of the stomach have been considered.

BURNS.—The duodenal ulcer may follow large superficial burns. Perry and Shaw found it in 5 of 149 autopsies in cases of burns of the skin.

Infection.—This is the most important factor. Any focal infection may be responsible, as in the mouth. In cases of other associated abdominal infections, as in the appendix or gall-bladder, both may have come from a common source, or the ulcer may be secondary to the other.

Morbid Anatomy and Pathology.—Ninety per cent. of gastric ulcers are to be found at the pyloric end; nearly all duodenal ulcers are in the first or ascending portion, and more than one-half extend up to or within three-fourths of an inch of the pylorus, while twenty per cent. involve the margin of the pyloric ring (Mayo). In explanation of the greater frequency of the ulcer just outside the pyloric sphincter it is stated that this part of the duodenal mucosa is deficient in blood supply in comparison with the other. It is thought to be a bacteriological infection of the mucosa, the source being some focus in the territory of the portal vein, particularly the appendix. It may not be easy on the operating table to distinguish between an ulcer of the duodenum and that of the stomach, but Mayo says that the position of the pyloric vein gives the exact location. Multiple ulcers may occur, 8.2 per cent. in the Mayo series. From 5 to 34 have been found. In the stomach, post mortem statistics (Welch) give, in 793 cases, 288 on the lesser curvature, 235 on the posterior wall, 69 on the anterior wall, 95 at the pylorus, 50 at the cardia, 29 at the fundus, and 27 on the greater curvature.

The acute ulcer is usually small, punched out, the edges clean-cut, the floor smooth, and the peritoneal surface not thickened. The chronic ulcer is of larger size, the margins are no longer sharp, the edges are indurated, and the border is sinuous. It may reach an enormous size, as in the one reported by Peabody, which measured 19 by 10 cm. and involved all of the lesser curvature and spread over a large part of the anterior and posterior walls. The sides are often terraced. The floor is formed either by the submucosa, by the muscular layers, or, not infrequently, by the neighboring organs, to which the stomach has become attached. In the healing of the ulcer, if the mucosa is alone involved, the granulation tissue grows from the edges and the floor and the newly formed tissue gradually contracts and unites the margins, leaving a smooth scar. In larger ulcers which have involved the muscular coat the cicatricial contraction may cause serious changes, the most important of which is pyloric narrowing and consequent dilatation of the stomach. In the case of a girdle ulcer hour-glass contraction of the stomach may be produced. Large ulcers persist for years without any attempt at healing.

Among the more serious changes which may result are the following:

PERFORATION.—This occurred in 28.1 per cent. of 1,871 cases collected by Musser. In some series (Mayo's) duodenal perforation is the more common. Of 272 cases of duodenal ulcer in Mayo's series (to June 1, 1908), perforation was found sixty-six times, 16 acute, 13 subacute with abscess, and 37 chronic and protected. Perforation of the anterior wall of the stomach usually excites an acute peritonitis. On the posterior wall the ulcer penetrates directly into the lesser peritoneal cavity, in which case it may produce an air-containing abscess with the symptoms of the condition known as subphrenic pyopneumothorax. In rare instances adhesions and a gastrocutaneous fistula form, usually in the umbilical region. Fistulous communication with the colon may also occur, or a gastroduodenal fistula. The pericardium may be perforated, and even the left ventricle. Perforation into the pleura may also occur. It is to be noted that general emphysema of the subcutaneous tissues occasionally follows perforation of a gastric ulcer.

EROSION OF BLOOD-VESSELS.—In both forms of ulcer hæmorrhage occurs, in 8.1 per cent. of Musser's series of 1,871 cases. In Moynihan's 114 cases of duodenal ulcer, hæmorrhage occurred in 41. It is more common in the chronic form. Ulcers on the posterior wall may erode the splenic artery, but perhaps more frequently the bleeding proceeds from the artery of the lesser curvature. In the case of duodenal ulcer the pancreaticoduodenal artery may be eroded, or fatal hæmorrhage may result from the opening of the hepatic artery, or more rarely the portal vein. Embolism of the artery supplying the ulcerated region has been met with in several cases; in others diffuse endarteritis. Small aneurisms have been found in the floor of the ulcers. A rare event is emphysema of the sub-peritoneal tissue, which may be extensive and even pass on to the posterior mediastinum. Jurgensen ascribes it to entrance of air into the veins, but Welch thinks it represents an invasion with the gas bacillus.

CICATRIZATION.—Superficial ulcers often heal without leaving any serious damage. Stenosis of the pyloric orifice not infrequently follows the healing of an ulcer in its neighborhood. In other instances the large annular ulcer may cause in its cicatrization an hour-glass contraction of the stomach. The adhesion of the ulcer to neighboring parts may subsequently be the cause of much pain. The parts of the mucosa in the neighborhood of the ulcer frequently show signs of chronic gastritis.

PERIGASTRIC ADHESIONS.—The condition is common, as high as 5 per cent. of post mortem records. It follows ulcer, lesions of the gall-bladder, pancreatic disease, syphilitic disease of the liver, and chronic tuberculosis. In some instances the lesions are quite extensive, and the condition has been called *plastic perigastritis*. It may be associated, too, with hypertrophic thickening of the coats of the stomach and with chronic plastic peritonitis. In some instances the pylorus may be narrowed as a result of the adhesions, or a sort of hour-glass stomach may be produced, or the motility of the organ is interfered with. Pain is the most constant feature, and may simulate that of gastric ulcer or of hyperacidity, and may be present constantly or at intervals. It is much influenced by posture and usually relieved by pressure. Local tenderness is present in a majority of instances. The cases are chronic, the general health is but slightly interfered with, and there are not, as a rule, signs of gastric dilatation. A definite tumor may be present about the region of the pylorus. Chronic appendicitis and lesions of the gall-bladder are found in many cases.

Mode of Origin.—The mode of origin is unknown. The anatomical basis is an interference with the blood supply in a limited area of the mucosa, attributed to embolism, thrombosis, or spasm of the arteries. As they are not end vessels, simple obstruction can not account for it. Trophic influences, bacterial necrosis of the mucosa, spasm of the muscular coat in limited areas, etc., are among the hypotheses which have been advanced. The present tendency is to attach much importance to the part played by infection.

Jejunal Ulcer.—This may occur after gastrojejunostomy, but in many cases the ulcer involves both stomach and jejunum. The condition is rare, as after 1,141 gastrojejunostomies at the Mayo clinic not one developed an ulcer.

Carcinoma and Ulcer.—There has been much difference of opinion as to the number of cases in which carcinoma develops in an ulcer. There is no doubt of its occurrence but the percentage is probably small.

Symptoms.—The condition may be latent and only met with accidentally, post mortem. The first symptoms may be those of perforation. In other cases the patient has had gastric disturbance for years and the ulcer may not have been suspected until the occurrence of a sudden hæmorrhage. The *history* is almost always of an illness of long duration, usually of some years, in which there have been remissions often with complete relief from symptoms. The periodicity may be marked; the symptoms are rarely continuous. Many of the symptoms are due to associated conditions of which vagotonia is important. The ulcer alone may give few symptoms in some cases.

Dyspepsia may be slight and trifling or of a most aggravated character. Nausea and *vomiting* occur in a large proportion of the gastric cases, the latter not for two or more hours after eating. It is probably most common when the ulcer is near the pylorus. The vomitus usually contains a large amount of hydrochloric acid.

Hæmorrhage is present in at least one-third of all cases. A patient may feel faint and turn pale and sweat; the next day the stools may be tarry from the blood that has passed into the small bowel. The bleeding may be latent (occult). These concealed hæmorrhages are often small, and the blood is not readily seen in the vomitus or stools. These latent hæmorrhages may cause a slowly progressive anæmia. More commonly the bleeding is profuse, and the blood may be in such quantities and brought up so quickly that it is fluid, bright red in color, and quite unaltered. When it remains for some time in the stomach and is mixed with food it may be greatly changed, but the vomiting of a large quantity of unaltered blood is very characteristic of ulcer. As a rule, there are only one or two attacks; in our series 7 cases had one hæmorrhage, 7 two, 11 three, 1 four, and 15 many (Howard). Profuse bleedings may occur at intervals for many years. Death may follow directly. From 16 to 18 per cent. of the fatal cases are due to it (S. and W. Fenwick).

The immediate effect of the hæmorrhage is a severe anæmia, from which it may take months to rally; slight fever is common. Rare and untoward effects are convulsions, sometimes only the usual convulsions of extreme cerebral anæmia from which recovery takes place, or they may precede a hemiplegia, due probably to thrombosis. Amaurosis may follow the hæmorrhage and unfortunately may be permanent, due to degeneration of the retinal ganglion cells, or to a thrombosis of the cerebral arteries or veins.

Pain is perhaps the most constant and distinctive feature of ulcer. It varies greatly in character; it may be only a gnawing or burning sensation, which is particularly felt when the stomach is empty, and is relieved by taking food, but the more characteristic form comes on in paroxysms, in which the pain is not only felt in the epigastrium, but radiates to the back and to the sides. In many cases the two points of epigastric pain and dorsal pain, about the level of the tenth dorsal vertebra, are very well marked. These attacks are most frequently induced by taking food, and they may recur at a variable period after eating, sometimes within fifteen or twenty minutes, at others as late as two or three hours. The pain rarely comes on more than four hours after taking food. It is usually stated that when the ulcer is near the cardia the pain is apt to set in earlier, but there is no certainty on this point. In some cases it comes on in the early morning hours. The attacks may occur at intervals with great intensity for weeks or months at a time, so that the patient requires morphia, then again they may disappear entirely for a prolonged period. In the attack the patient is usually bent forward, and finds relief from pressure over the epigastric region; one patient during the attack would lean over the back of a chair; another would lie flat on the floor, with a hard pillow under the abdomen.

Tenderness on pressure is a common symptom and patients wear the waist-band very low. Pressure should be made with great care, as rupture of an ulcer is said to have been induced by careless manipulation.

In old ulcers with thickened bases an indurated mass may be felt in the neighborhood of the pylorus.

Gastric Contents.—There is often evidence of some retention. The findings as to acidity vary and too much importance should not be placed on them. Our ideas as to hyperacidity have had to be revised; high figures are not always present in ulcer. With marked retention there may be high acidity figures. If neoplasm has developed in an ulcer the HCl is reduced. Careful search should always be made for blood, either fresh or occult, both in the stomach contents and stools.

Of general symptoms, *loss of weight* results from the prolonged dyspepsia, but it rarely, except in association with cicatricial stenosis of the pylorus, reaches the high grade met with in cancer. The *anæmia* may be extreme, and in one case of duodenal ulcer, the blood-count was as low as 700,000 per c. mm. Of 44 cases in the wards of the Hopkins Hospital in which blood-counts were made, the lowest was 1,902,000 per c. mm. There are instances in which the anæmia can not be explained by the occurrence of hæmorrhage. In a few instances polycythæmia is present, even after a hæmorrhage, due to concentration of the blood in association with dilatation of the stomach. In a few cases *parotitis* occurs, with the perforation sometimes, or after a hæmorrhage.

PERFORATION.—The acute, perforating form is much more common in women than in men. The symptoms are those of perforative peritonitis. Particular attention must be given to this accident, since it has come so successfully within the sphere of the surgeon. Perforation may take place either into the lesser peritoneum or into the general peritoneal cavity, in both of which cases operation is indicated; in rare instances the ulcer may perforate the pericardium. This was the case in 10 of 28 cases in which the diaphragm was perforated (Pick). Localized, more frequently subphrenic, abscess may follow perforation.

URINE.—Albumin is occasionally present; in 14 of our series with dilatation of the stomach. Indican may be present. Acetone and diacetic acid (with syncopal attacks) have been described by Dreschfeld.

HOUR-GLASS STOMACH most frequently results from the cicatrization of an ulcer. It may follow perforation of an ulcer into the liver or pancreas. In a few cases it is congenital. The symptoms, fairly characteristic, are thus given by Moynihan:

(*a*) In washing out the stomach part of the fluid is lost. (*b*) If the stomach is washed clean, a sudden reappearance of stomach contents may take place. (*c*) "Paradoxical dilatation"; when the stomach has apparently been emptied, a splashing sound may be elicited by palpation of the pyloric segment. (*d*) After distending the stomach, a change in the position of the distention tumor may be seen in some cases. (*e*) Gushing, bubbling, or sizzling sounds are heard on dilatation with carbon dioxide at a point distinct from the pylorus. (*f*) In some cases, when both parts are dilated, two tumors with a notch or sulcus between are apparent to sight or touch. To these may be added (*g*) a most characteristic X-ray picture.

Prognosis.—In all statistics the acute and chronic ulcer have been considered together. The former is more amenable to medical treatment, but grave complications may occur even before the digestive symptoms have been very pronounced. The chronic ulcer may last for years—twelve, eighteen, or even twenty—with intervals of good health. Controversy as to the relative results of medical and surgical treatment is futile. Medical treatment is indicated in different conditions than surgical. In the early stages medical treatment is advisable and should have a thorough trial. With a chronic ulcer it may be a waste of time to attempt it. Many cases do well with medical treatment; others are not helped. Surgery is not always successful, for gastro-enterostomy, which is done so often, can not be regarded as a physiological operation. In private practice many series of cases have not a mortality above 6 per cent. The mortality of the chronic peptic ulcer in the hands of such experts as the Mayos and Moynihan is very low. In 670 operations for ulcer of the stomach the mortality was 3.5 per cent., and 47 cases required a secondary operation (Balfour). In Moynihan's cases of duodenal ulcer, 114 in number (exclusive of perforation), there were only two deaths.

Diagnosis.—The acute non-indurated ulcer may cause very few symptoms —nothing beyond gastric discomfort with pain. Hæmatemesis may be the first symptom of moment. This group of cases is seen chiefly in young girls, and appears to be more common in England than in the United States. A condition which may be confounded with it is *gastrostaxis,* described by Hale White. The stomach symptoms are marked, the bleeding may be profuse, but post mortem or at operation no ulcer is found. Careful inspection must be made, as fatal bleeding may come from a very small erosion.

In the chronic cases the nutrition at first may remain good, and the patient looks well. The whole complaint is of the stomach, of pain and distress, with belching and nausea or vomiting from two to four hours after meals. This special feature of the recurrence of the pain some hours after taking food, its extraordinary regularity, and the relief afforded by taking food clearly separate the dyspeptic features of ulcer from other types. In the early stages there is usually no alteration in secretion or motility, but sooner or later both are altered. The rhythm of gastric function is disturbed. With disturbance in motility, usually delay, the secretion is altered. The secretory findings depend partly on the extent and chronicity of the ulcer and the impairment of motility. The post-digestion secretion increases. The X-ray examination is of the greatest aid and may be the only means by which we can distinguish gastric from duodenal ulcer. In uncomplicated duodenal ulcer the stomach is usually hypertonic.

The presence of *adhesions,* especially between the gall-bladder and duodenum, may cause difficulty. The symptoms are long continued, present a great variety and may suggest gastric ulcer but in their irregularity are more like those of gall-stones. The taking of food may give relief which may suggest duodenal or gastric ulcer close to the pylorus. Blood is not found in the gastric contents or stools. The X-ray study may suggest duodenal ulcer. As operation is indicated in these cases, an error in diagnosis leading to operation is not serious.

Treatment.—The main principles are as follows: First, the control of foci of infection; second, the obtaining of gastric rest so far as possible, and, third, the neutralization of acidity. Unless there are definite indications for operation, it seems wise to try the effect of medical treatment, but this should be carried out systematically. The control of *infection* demands proper treatment of any foci, especially in the mouth. The control of *gastric acidity* means that there should not be free HCl in the stomach either while food is contained there or during the night.

The patient should be at rest in bed and kept there for several weeks. In the method advised by Sippy, food is given every hour from 7 A. M. to 7 P. M. during the day. At first three ounces of a mixture of equal parts of milk and cream are given. After a few days soft eggs and cooked cereals are gradually added. These may be given alternately with and in addition to the milk and cream. The total bulk at one feeding should not exceed six ounces. Later, cream soups, bread and butter, and soft foods may be added.

To control the *acidity,* alkali is given between each feeding. This is done by giving a powder of gr. x (0.6 gm.) each of heavy calcined magnesia and sodium bicarbonate alternating with a powder of gr. x (0.6 gm.) of bismuth carbonate and gr. xxx (2 gm.) of sodium bicarbonate. In addition, after the last feeding of the day, the powders should be given every half hour for four doses or until the stomach is empty. The powders are administered in about two ounces of water. It is well to aspirate the stomach about two hours after the last feeding to be sure that it is empty. If this amount of alkali is not sufficient, more sodium bicarbonate may be given. By examining the stomach contents occasionally it can be determined whether or not the free acidity is being controlled. After some weeks the patient may be given light meals, but the taking of equal parts of milk and cream each hour should be kept up. When the hourly feedings between meals are stopped, the alkaline powder should be taken every hour for three doses after each meal. It is usually well to continue this treatment longer than may seem necessary.

If the ulcer has caused pyloric obstruction, as a rule a larger amount of alkali is required and it is well to empty the stomach each night about half an hour after the last powder is taken. The important thing is to give sufficient alkali to control the acidity. A careful watch over the progress should be kept and the amount of retained material noted. The emptying of the stomach the last thing at night lessens the tendency to night secretion. Regular examinations of the stool for occult blood are an important guide as to the value of the treatment. In all cases it is important to obtain the co-operation of the patient so that after he passes from immediate observation he will be careful to follow instructions.

Medicinal measures, apart from the alkaline treatment, are of little value. Atropine may be useful in the dosage suitable for each patient. For the bowels the use of salines in the morning is usually best, or enemata may be given. The artificial Carlsbad salts (sulphate of sodium, 50 parts; bicarbonate of sodium, 6; chloride of sodium, 3) may be given.

The pain, if severe, requires opium. Unless it is intense morphia should not be given, as there is a very serious danger of establishing the morphia habit. Doses of an eighth of a grain (0.008 gm.), with bicarbonate of soda and bismuth, will allay the mild attacks, but the very severe ones require the hypodermic injection of a quarter (0.016 gm.) or often half (0.03 gm.) a grain. In the milder attacks Hoffman's anodyne, or 20 or 30 drops of spirit of chloroform, or the spirit of camphor, will give relief. Counter irritation over the stomach with mustard or cantharides is often useful.

When the stomach is irritable, the patient should be fed per rectum. He will sometimes retain food which is passed into the duodenum through a tube. Cracked ice, chloroform, oxalate of cerium, and bismuth may be tried. When *hæmorrhage* occurs the patient should be put under the influence of opium as rapidly as possible. No attempt should be made to check the hæmorrhage by administering medicines by the mouth; as the profuse bleeding is always from an eroded artery, frequently from one of considerable size, it is doubtful if acetate of lead, tannic and gallic acids, and the usual remedies have the slightest influence. The essential point is to give rest, which is best obtained by opium. Nothing should be given by the mouth except small quantities of ice. Not infrequently the loss of blood is so great that the patient faints. A fatal result is not, however, very common from hæmorrhage. Blood serum (15 to 30 c. c.) may be injected intramuscularly. Transfusion is advisable in severe conditions. The patients usually recover rapidly from the hæmorrhage and require iron in full doses, which may, if necessary, be given hypodermically.

Surgical interference is indicated: (1) For perforation; (2) in the chronic indurated ulcer. Experience has shown that after gastro-enterostomy the ulcer may heal rapidly, and in some cases the ulcer itself may be located; (3) in all cases when the ulcer has caused persistent, mechanical interference;

(4) in all cases associated with recurring hæmorrhages. In young girls the single severe attack of hæmatemesis may be a simple gastrorrhexis, or from a simple ulcer that heals readily, but in men severe hæmatemesis is almost always from the chronic ulcer; (5) in the perigastric adhesions after chronic ulcer operation is sometimes helpful; (6) in chronic cases in which medical treatment fails to give relief; and (7) when there is reason to suspect the development of carcinoma.

In the present state of our knowledge it is not easy to determine the limits of medical and surgical practice in the treatment of peptic ulcer. The old statistics are not of use, since it is quite clear that scores of cases have been masquerading under the names of hyperchlorhydria, acid dyspepsia, and so forth. The simple non-indurated ulcer is, in the majority of cases, a medical disease. A chronic indurated form is best treated surgically.

VI. CANCER OF THE STOMACH

Etiology.—Incidence.—In an analysis of 30,000 cases of cancer, W. H. Welch found the stomach involved in 21.4 per cent., this organ thus standing next to the uterus in order of frequency. Among 8,464 medical cases admitted to the Johns Hopkins Hospital, there were 150 cases of cancer of the stomach and 39 cases among the first 1,000 autopsies. The disease is more common in some countries. Figures indicate that cancer of the stomach is increasing in frequency.

Sex.—Of the 150 cases 126 were males and 24 females. Welch gives the ratio as 5 to 4.

Age.—Of our 150 cases the ages were as follows: Between twenty and thirty, 6; from thirty to forty, 17; forty to fifty, 38; fifty to sixty, 49; sixty to seventy, 36; seventy to eighty, 4. Fifty-eight per cent. occurred between the ages of forty and sixty. Of the 6 cases occurring under the thirtieth year, the youngest was twenty-two. Of the large number of cases analyzed by Welch, three-fourths occurred between the fortieth and seventieth years. Congenital cancer of the stomach has been described, and cases have been met with in children.

Race.—Among our 150 cases, 131 were white, 19 were negroes.

Previous Diseases, Habits, Etc.—A history of dyspepsia was present in only 33 cases; of these, 17 had had attacks at intervals, 11 had had chronic stomach trouble, and 5 had had dyspepsia for one or two years before the symptoms of cancer developed. Napoleon, discussing this point with his physician Antommarchi, said that he had always had a stomach of iron and felt no inconvenience until the onset of what proved to be his fatal illness.

Gastric Ulcer.—The relation to this condition is in dispute—the physicians are against, some surgeons are in favor. In only 4 cases in our series was there a history pointing to ulcer.

Morbid Anatomy.—The most common varieties of gastric cancer are the cylindrical-celled adeno-carcinoma and the encephaloid or medullary carcinoma; next in frequency is scirrhous, and then colloid cancer. With reference to the situation of the tumor, Welch analyzed 1,300 cases, in which the distribution was as follows: Pyloric region, 791; lesser curvature, 148; cardia,

104; posterior wall, 68; the whole or greater part of the stomach, 61; multiple tumors, 45; greater curvature, 34; anterior wall, 30; fundus, 19.

The medullary cancer occurs in soft masses, which involve all the coats of the stomach and usually ulcerate early. The tumor may form villous projections or cauliflower-like outgrowths. It is soft, grayish-white in color, and contains much blood. The cylindrical-celled epithelioma may also form large irregular masses, but the consistence is usually firmer, particularly at the edges of the cancerous ulcers. Cysts are not uncommon in this form. The scirrhous variety is characterized by great hardness, due to the abundance of the stroma and the limited amount of alveolar structures. It is seen most frequently at the pylorus, where it is a common cause of stenosis. It may be combined with the medullary form. It may be diffuse, involving all parts of the organ, and leading to a condition which can not be recognized macroscopically from cirrhosis. This form has also been seen in the stomach secondary to cancer of the ovaries. In connection with the diffuse carcinomatosis there may be simultaneous involvement of the small and large intestines. The colloid cancer is peculiar in its widespread invasion of all the coats. It also spreads with greater frequency to the neighboring parts, and it occasionally causes extensive secondary growths of the same nature in other organs. The appearance on section is very distinctive, and even with the naked eye large alveoli can be seen filled with the translucent colloid material. The term alveolar cancer is often applied to this form. Ulceration is not constantly present, and there are instances in which, with most extensive disease, digestion has been but slightly disturbed.

Secondary Cancer of the Stomach.—Of 37 cases collected by Welch, 17 were secondary to cancer of the breast. Among the first 1,000 autopsies at the Johns Hopkins Hospital there were 3 cases of secondary cancer.

Changes in the Stomach.—Cancer at the cardia is usually associated with wasting of the organ and reduction in its size. The œsophagus above the obstruction may be greatly dilated. On the other hand, annular cancer at the pylorus causes stenosis with great dilatation of the organ. In a few rare instances the pylorus has been extremely narrowed without any increase in the size of the stomach. In diffuse scirrhous cancer the stomach may be very greatly thickened and contracted. It may be displaced or altered in shape by the weight of the tumor, particularly in cancer of the pylorus; in such cases it has been found in every region of the abdomen, and even in the true pelvis. The mobility of the tumors is at times extraordinary and very deceptive, and they may be pushed into the right hypochondrium or into the splenic region, entirely beneath the ribs. Adhesions very frequently occur, particularly to the colon, the liver, and the anterior abdominal wall.

Secondary cancerous growths in other organs are very frequent, as shown by the following analysis by Welch of 1,574 cases: Metastasis occurred in the lymphatic glands in 551; in the liver in 475; in the peritoneum, omentum, and intestine in 357; in the pancreas in 122; in the pleura and lung in 98; in the spleen in 26; in the brain and meninges in 9; in other parts in 92. The lymph glands affected are usually those of the abdomen, but the cervical and inguinal glands are not infrequently attacked, and give an important clue in diagnosis. Secondary metastatic growths occur subcutaneously, either at the navel or beneath the skin in the vicinity, and are of value in diagnosis.

PERFORATION.—This occurred into the peritoneum in 17 of 507 cases of cancer of the stomach (Brinton). In our series perforation occurred in 4 cases. When adhesions form, the most extensive destruction of the walls may take place without perforation into the peritoneal cavity. In one instance a large portion of the left lobe of the liver lay within the stomach. Occasionally a gastro-cutaneous fistula is established. Perforation may occur into the colon, the small bowel, the pleura, the lung, or the pericardium.

Symptoms.—LATENT CARCINOMA.—There may be no symptoms pointing to the stomach, and the tumor may be discovered accidentally after death. In a second group the symptoms of carcinoma are present, not of the stomach, but of the liver or some other organ, or there are subcutaneous nodules, or, as in one of our cases, secondary masses on the ribs and vertebræ. In a third group, seen particularly in elderly persons in institutions, there is gradual asthenia, sometimes anasarca, without nausea, vomiting, or other local symptoms.

FEATURES OF ONSET.—Of the 150 cases in our series, 48 complained of pain, 44 of dyspepsia, 21 of vomiting, 13 of loss in weight, 3 of difficulty in swallowing, 1 of tumor. In 7 the features of onset suggested pernicious anæmia. In 37 cases there was a history of sudden onset.

GENERAL SYMPTOMS.—*Loss of Weight.*—Progressive emaciation is one of the most constant features. In 79 of our cases in which exact figures were taken: To 30 pounds, 32 cases; 30 to 50 pounds, 36 cases; 50 to 60 pounds, 5 cases; 60 to 70 pounds, 4; over 70 pounds, 1; 100 pounds, a case of cancer at the cardiac end with obstruction to swallowing. The loss in weight is not always progressive. We see increase in weight under three conditions: (*a*) Proper dieting, with treatment of the associated catarrh; (*b*) in cancer of the pylorus after relief of the dilatation of the organ by lavage, operation, etc.; (*c*) after a profound mental impression. The visit of an optimistic consultant may be followed by a gain in weight. In Keen and D. D. Stewart's case there was a gain of seventy pounds after an exploratory operation!

Loss in strength is usually proportionate to the loss in weight. One sees sometimes remarkable vigor almost to the close, but this is exceptional.

Anæmia is present in a large proportion of all cases, and with the emaciation gives the picture of cachexia. There is often a yellow or lemon tint of the skin. In 59 cases blood-counts were made; in 3 the red corpuscles were above 6,000,000 per c. mm. This occurs in the concentrated condition of the blood in certain cases of cancer of the pylorus with dilatation of the stomach. The average count in the 59 cases was 3,712,186 per c. mm. In only 8 cases was the count below 2,000,000, and in none below 1,000,000. The average of the hæmoglobin was 44.9 per cent. In only 9 was it below 30 per cent. In 62 cases in which the leucocytes were counted there were only 18 cases in which they were above 12,000 per c. mm.; in only 3 cases were they above 20,000. The features of onset may suggest a primary anæmia.

Among other general symptoms may be mentioned *fever,* which was present at some time in 74 of our 150 cases. In only 13 of these did the temperature rise above 101°. In 2 it was above 103°. Fifteen presented fairly constant elevation of temperature. Eight presented sudden rises. Two cases had *chills,* with elevation to 103° and 104°. Chills may be associated with suppuration at the base of the cancer.

Urine.—There may be no changes throughout or albumin and casts may be found. Glycosuria, peptonuria, and acetonuria have been described. Indican is common.

Œdema.—Swelling of the ankles is of frequent occurrence toward the close. With an early general anasarca in combination with extreme anæmia, the cancer is usually overlooked.

The *bowels* are often constipated. In only 12 cases in our series was diarrhœa present. In 2 cases blood was passed per rectum. There are no special *cardiac symptoms;* the pulse becomes progressively weaker. Thrombosis of one femoral vein may occur, or, as in one of our cases, widespread thrombosis in the superficial veins of the body.

Symptoms on the part of the nervous system are rare; consciousness is often retained to the end. *Coma* may occur similar to that seen in diabetes, and is believed to be due to an acid intoxication.

FUNCTIONAL DISTURBANCES.—*Anorexia,* loss of desire for food, is a frequent and valuable symptom, more constant perhaps than any other. *Nausea* is a striking feature in many cases; there is often a sudden repulsion at the sight of food. In exceptional cases the appetite is retained throughout.

Vomiting may come on early, or only after the dyspepsia has persisted for some time. It occurred in 128 cases in our series. At first it is at long intervals, but subsequently it is more frequent, and may recur several times in the day. There are cases in which it comes on in paroxysms and then subsides; in other cases it sets in early, persists with great violence, and may cause a fatal termination within a few weeks. Vomiting is more frequent when the cancer involves the orifices, particularly the pylorus, in which case it is usually delayed for an hour or more after taking the food. When the cardiac orifice is involved it may follow at a shorter interval. Extensive disease of the fundus or of the anterior or posterior wall may be present without the occurrence of vomiting. The food is sometimes very little changed, even after it has remained in the stomach for twenty-four hours.

Hæmorrhage occurred in 36 of our 150 cases; in 32 the blood was dark and altered, in 3 it was bright red. In 2 cases vomiting of blood was the first symptom. The bleeding is rarely profuse; more commonly there is slight oozing, and the blood is mixed with, or altered by, the secretions, and, when vomited, the material is dark brown or black, the so-called "coffee-ground" vomit. Occult blood is almost constantly present in carcinoma; in ulcer it is intermittent.

Pain, an early and important symptom, was present in 130 of our cases. It is very variable in situation and, while most common in the epigastrium, it may be referred to the shoulders, the back, or the loins. The pain is described as dragging, burning, or gnawing in character, and very rarely occurs in severe paroxysms, as in gastric ulcer. As a rule, it is aggravated by taking food. There is usually marked tenderness on pressure in the epigastric region. The areas of skin tenderness are referred, as Head has shown, to the region between the nipple and the umbilicus in front and behind from the fifth to the twelfth thoracic spine.

THE STOMACH CONTENTS.—The finding of pus and blood in the empty stomach and pus, blood and mucus two hours after the test meal is suggestive. Diminished motility may be an early finding in pyloric cancer. There is a tendency to a downward trend of gastric secretion, the opposite of the findings in gastric ulcer. The results of secondary infection and secondary gastric catarrh are added to the picture. The protein curve often shows a marked divergence from the acid curve which increases as digestion goes on and is most marked in cases of subacidity or achylia. The test for soluble albumin (Wolff-Junghans) is of value, especially two hours after the test meal. The tryptophan test and ereptic reaction are of doubtful value owing to frequent regurgitation of duodenal contents. Bacteria in large numbers occur, one, the Oppler-Boas bacillus—an unusually long non-motile form—is supposed to be of diagnostic value, and to be largely responsible for the formation of lactic acid. Blood is a most important ingredient; the persistent presence microscopically of red corpuscles in the early morning washings is always very suspicious. Later, when coffee-ground vomiting takes place, the macroscopic evidence is sufficient. Fragments of the new growth may be vomited or may appear in the washings.

Examination of the Gastric Contents.—As an outcome of the enormous number of observations, it may be said that free HCl is absent in a large proportion of all cases of cancer of the stomach. Of 94 cases in which the contents were examined in 84 free HCl was absent. In 5 undoubted cases the reaction was good; in 2 of these the history suggested previous ulcer. HCl may be absent in chronic gastritis and in atrophy of the gastric mucosa. The presence of lactic acid is regarded as a valuable sign.

PHYSICAL EXAMINATION.—*Inspection.*—After a preliminary survey, embracing the facies, state of nutrition, etc., particular attention is given to the abdomen. An all-important matter is to have the patient in a good light. Fullness in the epigastric region, inequality in the infracostal grooves, the existence of peristalsis, a wide area of aortic pulsation, the presence of subcutaneous nodules or small masses about the navel, and, lastly, a well-defined tumor mass—these, together or singly, may be seen on careful inspection. In 62 of the 150 cases a positive tumor could be seen. In 52 the tumor descended with inspiration; in 36 peristalsis was visible; in 3 cases movements were visible in the tumor itself. In 10 cases with visible peristalsis no tumor was seen, but could be felt on palpation. Inflation may be tried, except when hæmorrhage has been profuse or the cancer is very extensive. The dilatation often renders evident the peristalsis or may bring a tumor into view. The presence of subcutaneous and umbilical nodules may help. They were found in 5 of our series.

Palpation.—In 115 cases a tumor could be felt; in 48 in the epigastric region, in 25 in the umbilical, in 18 in the left hypochondriac, in 17 in the right hypochondriac region, while in 7 cases a mass descended in deep inspiration from beneath the left costal margin. These figures illustrate in how large a proportion of the cases the tumor is in evidence when the patient comes under observation. In rare cases examination in the knee-elbow position is of value. *Mobility* in gastric tumor is a point of much importance. First, the change with respiration, a mass may descend 3 or 4 inches in deep inspiration; secondly, the communicated pulsation from the aorta, which is often suggestive in its extent; thirdly, the intrinsic movements in the hypertrophied muscularis. This may give a remarkable character to the mass, causing it to appear and disappear, lifting the abdominal wall in the epigastric region; and, fourthly, mechanical movements, with inflation, with change of posture, or communicated with the hand. Tumors of the pylorus are the most movable, and in extreme cases can be displaced to either hypochondrium or pushed far down below the navel (see illustrative cases in Osler's Lectures on the Diagnosis of Abdominal Tumors). Pain on palpation is common; the mass is usually hard, sometimes nodular. Gas can at times be felt gurgling through the tumor at the pyloric region.

Percussion gives less important indications—the note over a tumor is rarely flat, more often a flat tympany. *Auscultation* may reveal the gurgling through the pylorus; sometimes a systolic bruit is transmitted from the aorta, and when a local peritonitis exists a friction may be heard.

Complications.—*Secondary growths* are common. In 44 autopsies in our series there were metastases in 38; in 29 the lymph-glands were involved; in 23 the liver, in 11 the peritoneum, in 8 the pancreas, in 8 the bowel, in 4 the lung, in 3 the pleura, in 4 the kidneys, and in 2 the spleen. In 8 no deposits were found.

Perforation may lead to peritonitis, but in 3 of our 4 cases there was no general involvement. Cancerous ascites is not very uncommon. Dock has called attention to the value of the examination of the fluid in such cases as a help to diagnosis. The cells show mitoses and are very characteristic. Secondary cancer of the *liver* is very common; the enlargement may be very great, and such cases are not infrequently mistaken for primary cancer of the organ. Involvement of the *lymph-glands* may give valuable indications. There may be early enlargement of a gland at the posterior border of the left sterno-cleido-mastoid muscle; later adjacent glands may become affected. This occurs also in uterine cancer.

A remarkable picture is presented when the cancer *sloughs* or becomes gangrenous; the vomitus has a foul odor, often of a penetrating nature, to be perceived throughout the room. In cases in which the ulcer perforates the colon the vomiting may be fæcal. The fæcal odor with incessant vomiting was present in a case in which there was no perforation of the colon at autopsy.

Course.—While usually *chronic* and lasting from a year to eighteen months, *acute* cancer of the stomach is by no means infrequent. Of the 69 cases in which we could determine accurately the duration, 15 lasted under three months, 16 from three to six months, 14 from six to twelve months—a total of 45 under one year. Four cases lasted for two years or over. One patient lived for at least two years and a half.

Diagnosis.—Every effort should be made to recognize carcinoma before a tumor is present. Persistent gastric symptoms in an individual over forty require that malignant disease be excluded. Repeated studies of the gastric contents with comparison of the findings and the X-ray examination are the greatest aids. The X-ray picture is modified, the peristaltic waves are interfered with, anti-peristalsis and shadows varying in intensity with the degree of induration of the carcinoma may be seen. In a doubtful case exploration should be advised without much delay if the findings are suspicious. There are cases in which a positive diagnosis can be reached in no other way.

In 115 of our 150 cases a tumor existed, and with this the recognition is rarely in doubt. The chief difficulty is in cases with gastric symptoms or anæmia, or both, without the presence of tumor. In the one a chronic gastritis is suspected; in the other a primary anæmia. In *chronic gastritis* the history of long-standing dyspepsia, the absence of cachexia, the absence of lactic acid in the test meal, and the less striking blood changes are the important points for consideration. The cases with grave *anæmia* without tumor offer the greatest difficulty. The blood-count is rarely so low as in pernicious anæmia. In only 8 of our 59 cases with careful blood examination was the number below 2,000,000 per c. mm. The lower color index, as in secondary anæmia, the absence of megaloblasts, and a leucocytosis speak for cancer. With metastases in the bone marrow the blood picture may be that of pernicious anæmia (Harrington and Teacher).

From *ulcer of the stomach* malignant disease is, as a rule, readily recognized. The *ulcus carcinomatosum* usually presents a well-marked history of ulcer for years. The greatest difficulty is offered when there is ulcer with tumor due to cicatricial contraction about the pylorus. In 3 such cases we mistook the mass for cancer, and even at operation it may (as in one of them) be impossible to say whether a neoplasm is present.

Treatment.—In early surgical treatment lies the only hope, but there is great difficulty in the diagnosis. Operated upon early, complete removal is sometimes possible. In a majority of cases the operation is only palliative. In suitable cases early exploration should be advised; the operation *per se* is sometimes beneficial and the patient is rarely the worse for it. W. J. Mayo reports 651 resections of the stomach in a period of twenty years. Of one series of 239 patients who recovered from the operation and were traced, 62 were alive five years or more afterwards.

The diet should consist of readily digested substances of all sorts. Many patients do best on milk alone. Washing out the stomach, which may be done, with a soft tube without any risk, is particularly advantageous when there is obstruction at the pylorus, and is by far the most satisfactory means of combating the vomiting. The excessive fermentation is also best treated by lavage. When the pain becomes severe, particularly if it disturbs the rest at night, morphia must be given. One-eighth of a grain (0.008 gm.), combined with bicarbonate of soda (gr. v, 0.3 gm.), bismuth (gr. v-x, 0.3-0.6 gm.), usually gives prompt relief, and the dose does not always require to be increased. Creosote (♏ j-ij, 0.06-0.12 c. c.) and carbolic acid are useful. The bleeding in gastric cancer is rarely amenable to treatment. In cases which are inoperable the use of radium or deep X-ray therapy with hard tubes is worthy of trial.

Other Forms of Tumor.—*Non-cancerous tumors* of the stomach rarely cause inconvenience. *Polypi* (polyadenomata) are common and they may be numerous; as many as 150 have been reported in one case. There is a form in which the adenoma exists as an extensive area slightly raised above the level of the mucosa—*polyadénome en nappe* of the French. An extraordinary multiple adenoma associated with multiple tumors throughout the intestines and subcutaneous hæmangio-endotheliomata was described by Winternitz. H. B. Anderson described a case of remarkable multiple *cysts* in the walls of the stomach and small intestine. *Sarcomata* are very rare. In an analysis of 61 cases Frazier found 23 spindle-cell, 16 small round cell, 3 large round cell forms, 6 lymphosarcoma, 7 myosarcoma, 5 myxosarcoma, and 1 cystic sarcoma. *Fibromata* and *lipomata* have been described. External polypoid tumors, myo- or fibro-sarcomata may grow from the peritoneal surface, usually the posterior, of which Sherran has collected 18 cases.

Foreign bodies, occasionally produce remarkable tumors of the stomach. The most extraordinary is the *hair tumor* which occurs in hysterical women who have been in the habit of eating their own hair. A specimen in the medical museum of McGill University is in two sections, which form an exact mold of the stomach. The tumors are large, very puzzling, and are usually mistaken for cancer. Of 7 cases operated upon, 6 recovered; in 9 cases the condition was found post mortem (Schulten).

VII. HYPERTROPHIC STENOSIS OF THE PYLORUS

In Adults.—Microscopically, the condition is found to be very largely hypertrophy of the muscularis and submucosa of the pylorus. It was well described by the older writers. The symptoms are those of dilatation of the stomach. Some of these cases may be congenital, as there have been instances reported in girls as early as the twelfth and sixteenth years.

Congenital.—This remarkable affection, first recognized by Beardsley of Connecticut, has been thoroughly studied by Hirschsprung, John Thomson, and others.

ETIOLOGY.—There are two conditions, congenital hypertrophy of the pylorus and spasm. The hypertrophy is frequent in first born children and in 80 per cent. is in boys. Symptoms are rare in the first week of life and usually appear from the second to the fourth week. Spasm is probably mainly responsible for the symptoms, as the tumor may persist after the symptoms have gone. The majority of the children are breast fed. How much hypertrophy of the pyloric ring may be caused by spasm is a question.

SYMPTOMS.—Vomiting of food and wasting are constantly present; the former begins, as a rule, during the second or third week, and in a few instances at birth; it occurs usually soon after nursing. It is often of the expulsive type; the wasting becomes extreme, there are marked constipation, great weakness, sometimes terminal diarrhœa, or a sudden fatal syncope.

PHYSICAL SIGNS.—These are distinctive—visible peristalsis and palpable tumor. The peristalsis is best seen after feeding, when the waves pass at intervals, in characteristic form, from left to right above the navel; two or three waves may be seen at once. The pyloric tumor may be felt as a firm, hard, freely movable body, to the right of the navel and a little above it, which varies in size and consistency, and through which gas may sometimes be felt to gurgle. The X-ray examination adds little.

TREATMENT.—Medical treatment consists in feeding with breast or modified milk, 1-3 ounces every 3 or 4 hours. Dextrose solution (200 c. c., 4 per cent.) can be given by the bowel. Lavage of the stomach should be done twice a day. The milder cases do well under this but there should not be delay in resorting to surgical measures if improvement does not occur. The division of the circular muscular layer (Rammstedt's operation) is a successful procedure (47 recoveries in 61 cases). The after care is important. The child should be kept warm, given fluid by bowel and subcutaneously, and fed carefully with a gradual increase in the amount.

VIII. HÆMORRHAGE FROM THE STOMACH

(*Hæmatemesis*)

Etiology.—Hæmatemesis may result from many conditions, local or general. (*a*) In local disease: (1) cancer; (2) ulcer; (3) disease of the blood-vessels, such as miliary aneurisms and occasionally varicose veins; (4) acute congestion, as in gastritis, and possibly in vicarious hæmorrhage; (5) following operations in the abdomen, particularly when the omentum is wounded, erosions of the gastric mucosa may occur, from which hæmorrhage takes place. It is a very fatal complication after appendicitis and is usually associated with peritonitis.

(*b*) Passive congestion due to obstruction in the portal system. This may be either (1) hepatic, as in cirrhosis of the liver, thrombosis of the portal vein, or pressure upon the portal vein by tumor, and secondarily in cases of chronic disease of the heart and lungs. (2) Splenic. Gastrorrhagia is by no means an uncommon symptom in enlarged spleen, and is explained by the intimate relations which exist between the vasa brevia and the splenic circulation.

(*c*) Toxic: (1) The poisons of the specific fevers, small-pox, measles, yellow fever; (2) poisons of unknown origin, as in acute yellow atrophy and in purpura; (3) phosphorus.

(*d*) Trauma: (1) Mechanical injuries, such as blows and wounds, and occasionally by the stomach-tube; (2) the result of severe corrosive poisons.

(*e*) Certain constitutional diseases: (1) Hæmophilia; (2) profound anæmias; (3) cholæmia.

(*f*) In certain nervous affections, particularly hysteria, and occasionally in general paresis and epilepsy.

(*g*) The blood may not always come primarily from the stomach but from the nose or pharynx. In hæmoptysis some of the blood may find its way into the stomach. Again, in bleeding from the œsophagus blood may trickle into the stomach, from which it is ejected. This occurs in the case of rupture of aneurism and of œsophageal varices. A child may draw blood with the milk from the mother's breast in considerable quantities and then vomit it.

(*h*) Gastrostaxis.—Under this name Hale White describes cases of hæmorrhage from the stomach in young girls without any lesion of the mucosa. They are often mistaken for ulcer. Surgeons have taught us that the condition is by no means uncommon. At operation the blood has been seen oozing from points in the mucosa. There may be no pain or any of the ordinary features of ulcer.

(*i*) Miscellaneous causes: Aneurism of the aorta or of its branches may rupture into the stomach. There are instances in which a patient has vomited blood once without any recurrence or without developing symptoms pointing to disease of the stomach. In new-born infants hæmatemesis may occur alone or in connection with bleeding from other mucous membranes.

In medical practice, hæmorrhage from the stomach occurs most frequently in connection with cirrhosis of the liver and ulcer of the stomach.

Morbid Anatomy.—When death has occurred from the hæmatemesis there are signs of intense anæmia. The lesion is evident in cancer and in ulcer of the stomach. Fatal hæmorrhage may come from a small miliary aneurism communicating with the surface by a pinhole perforation, or the bleeding may be due to the rupture of a submucous vein and the erosion in the mucosa may be small and readily overlooked. It may require a careful and prolonged search to avoid overlooking such lesions. In the large group associated with portal obstruction, whether due to hepatic or splenic disease, the mucosa is usually pale, smooth, and shows no trace of any lesion. In cirrhosis, fatal by hæmorrhage, one may sometimes search in vain for any local lesion and we must conclude that it is possible for even the most profuse bleeding to occur by diapedesis. The stomach may be distended with blood and yet the source of the hæmorrhage be not apparent. In such cases the œsophagus should be examined, as the bleeding may come from that source. In toxic cases there are invariably hæmorrhages in the mucous membrane itself.

Symptoms.—In rare instances fatal syncope may occur without any vomiting. In a case of the kind, in which the woman had fallen over and died in a few minutes, the stomach contained between three and four pounds of blood. The sudden profuse bleedings rapidly lead to profound anæmia. When due to ulcer or cirrhosis the bleeding usually recurs for several days. Fatal hæmorrhage from the stomach is met with in ulcer, cirrhosis, enlargement of the spleen, and in instances in which an aneurism ruptures into the stomach or œsophagus. Gastrorrhagia may occur in splenic anæmia or in leukæmia before the condition has aroused attention.

The vomited blood may be fluid or clotted; it is usually dark in color, but in the basin the outer part becomes red from the action of the air. The longer blood remains in the stomach the more altered it is when ejected.

The amount of blood lost is very variable, and in the course of a day the patient may bring up three or four pounds, or even more. In a case under the care of George Ross, in the Montreal General Hospital, the patient lost during seven days ten pounds, by weight, of blood. The usual symptoms of anæmia develop rapidly, and there may be slight fever, and subsequently œdema may occur. Syncope, convulsions, and occasionally hemiplegia occur after very profuse hæmorrhage. Blindness may follow, the result either of thrombosis of the retinal arteries or veins, or an acute degeneration of the ganglion cells of the retina.

Diagnosis.—In a majority of instances there is no question as to the origin of the blood. Occasionally it is difficult, particularly if the case has not been seen during the attack. Examination of the vomit readily determines whether blood is present or not. The materials vomited may be stained by wine, the juice of strawberries, raspberries, or cranberries, which give a color very closely resembling that of fresh blood, while iron and bismuth and bile may produce the blackish color of altered blood. In such cases the microscope will show the shadowy outlines of the red blood-corpuscles, and, if necessary, spectroscopic and chemical tests may be applied.

Deception is sometimes practised by hysterical patients, who swallow and then vomit blood or colored liquids. With a little care such cases can usually be detected. The cases must be excluded in which the blood passes from the nose or pharynx, or in which infants swallow it with the milk.

There is not often difficulty in distinguishing between hæmoptysis and hæmatemesis, though the coughing and the vomiting are not infrequently combined. The following are points to be borne in mind in the diagnosis:

HÆMATEMESIS	HÆMOPTYSIS
1. Previous history points to gastric, hepatic, or splenic disease.	1. Cough or signs of some pulmonary or cardiac disease precedes, in many cases, the hæmorrhage.
2. The blood is brought up by vomiting, prior to which the patient may experience a feeling of giddiness or faintness.	2. The blood is coughed up, and is usually preceded by a sensation of tickling in the throat. If vomiting occurs, it follows the coughing.
3. The blood is usually clotted, mixed with particles of food, and has an acid reaction. It may be dark, grumous, and fluid.	3. The blood is frothy, bright red in color, alkaline in reaction. If clotted, rarely in such large coagula, and muco-pus may be mixed with it.
4. Subsequent to the attack the patient passes tarry stools, and signs of disease of the abdominal viscera may be detected.	4. The cough persists, physical signs of local disease in the chest may usually be detected, and the sputum may be blood-stained for many days

Prognosis.—Except in the case of rupture of an aneurism or of large veins, hæmatemesis rarely proves fatal. In our experience death has followed more frequently in cases of cirrhosis and splenic enlargement than in ulcer or cancer. In ulcer it is to be remembered that in the chronic hæmorrhagic form the bleeding may recur for years. The treatment of hæmatemesis is considered under gastric ulcer.

IX. NEUROSES OF THE STOMACH

(Nervous Dyspepsia)

Serious functional disturbances of the stomach may occur without any discoverable anatomical basis. The cases are most frequent in those who have either inherited a nervous constitution or who have gradually, through indiscretions, brought about a condition of nervous prostration. Not infrequently, the gastric symptoms stand so far in the foreground that the general neuropathic character of the patient quite escapes notice. Sometimes the gastric manifestations have a reflex origin depending on organic disturbances in other parts, such as the gall-bladder, appendix or colon.

In all disturbance of the digestive tract, attention must be given to the whole and not to one part only. The digestive tube is a complicated mechanism which requires perfect coördination for proper function. Disease of one part may disturb the working elsewhere as, for example, disease of the appendix may cause gastric symptoms. Great importance attaches to proper motor function and many disturbances are due to this being disturbed. Motility may be increased, slowed, reversed or stopped, and any of these may result in symptoms. Contraction of a segment causes inhibition of the segment distal to it and this is particularly important in special zones, e. g., the pylorus and duodenum. Irregularities and blocks may occur as in the heart, especially where one zone passes into another, e. g., at the pylorus and ileo-cæcal valve. The nervous control plays a large part and the importance of vagotonia must always be kept in mind. Keith divides the digestive tract into neuro-muscular sections, each separated from the adjoining one by a sphincter which blocks the passage of waves of contraction. He compares these to the blocks on a railroad, in which if one is blocked, the others are also.

Alvarez has drawn attention to the part played by *reversed peristalsis* in causing symptoms. For example, regurgitation may be due to a distended and over-active colon or irritation from a diseased appendix. Vomiting may be due to increased tone and activity in the jejunum for which an irritable colon may be responsible. Belching of gas may represent reversed peristalsis set up by some organic lesion. Nausea is due more often to intestinal lesions, e. g., in the colon with reversed peristalsis, than to disease of the œsophagus and stomach. As to the cause of a coated tongue there is no proof that it is always due to gastric disease. It may be due to regurgitation, as particles of material from the colon may easily reach the tongue. The condition termed "biliousness" is often a result of reversed intestinal activity originating in the colon and when this is emptied relief is obtained.

The sufferer from nervous dyspepsia presents a varying picture. All grades occur, from the emaciated skeleton-like patient with anorexia nervosa to the well-nourished, healthy-looking, fresh-complexioned individual whose only complaint is distress and uneasiness after eating.

Motor Neuroses.—(*a*) HYPERMOTILITY.—An increase in the normal motor activity of the stomach results in disturbance if there is pyloric spasm. It is more commonly a secondary neurosis but it may occur primarily, possibly from reflex causes. The diagnosis is made by the stomach-tube or X-ray examination. It gives rise to no characteristic clinical symptoms.

(*b*) PERISTALTIC UNREST.—This is a common and distressing symptom. Shortly after eating, the peristaltic movements of the stomach are increased, and borborygmi and gurgling may be heard, even at a distance. The subjective sensations are most annoying, and it appears as if in the hyperæsthetic condition of the nervous system the patient felt normal peristalsis, just as in these states the usual beating of the heart may be perceptible to him. A further analogy is afforded by the fact that emotion increases this peristalsis. It may extend to the intestines, particularly to the duodenum, and on palpation over this region the gurgling is marked. The cause is usually reversed peristalsis due sometimes to disease elsewhere.

(*c*) ERUCTATIONS.—*Aerophagia.*—In this condition severe attacks of noisy eructations, following one another often in rapid succession, occur. When violent they last for hours or days. At other times they occur in paroxysms, depending often upon mental excitement. They are more commonly observed in hysterical women and neurasthenics, but also, not infrequently, in children. The hysterical nature of the affection is sometimes testified to by the occurrence, especially in children, of several instances in one household. The expelled gas in these cases is atmospheric air, which is swallowed or aspirated from without. Sometimes the whole process may be clearly observed, but in other instances the act of swallowing may be almost or quite imperceptible.

(*d*) Nervous Vomiting.—In some cases this is not associated with anatomical changes in the stomach or with any state of the contents, but is due to nervous influences acting either directly or indirectly upon the vomiting centres. The patients are, as a rule, women and the subject of more or less marked nervous manifestations. A special feature of this form is the absence of preliminary nausea and of the straining efforts of the ordinary act of vomiting. It is rather a regurgitation, and without visible effort and without gagging the mouth is filled with the contents of the stomach, which are then spat out. It comes on, as a rule, after eating, but may occur at irregular intervals. In some cases the nutrition is not impaired, a feature which may give a clue to the true nature of the disease, as there may be no other hysterical manifestation present. It may occur in children but in many cases this recurring vomiting is associated with acidosis. Nervous vomiting may be a very serious condition. We have had at least two fatal cases. In some instances, after persisting for weeks or months at home, the patient gets well in a few days in hospital. In other instances the course is protracted, and the cases are among the most trying we are called upon to treat.

One type of vomiting is associated with certain diseases of the nervous system—particularly tabes—forming part of the gastric crises. Leyden reported cases of primary periodic vomiting, which he regarded as a neurosis.

(*e*) Rumination; Merycismus.—In this remarkable condition the patients regurgitate and chew the cud like ruminants. It occurs in neurasthenic or hysterical persons, epileptics, and idiots. In some patients it is hereditary. In one instance a governess taught it to two children. The habit may persist for years, and does not necessarily impair the health.

(*f*) Cardiospasm.—Spasmodic, usually painful, contraction of the circular muscle fibres at the cardiac orifice may follow the introduction of a sound, hasty eating, or the taking of too hot or too cold food. It may occur in tetanus and also in hysterical and neurasthenic individuals, especially in air swallowers, in whom, if it be combined with pyloric spasm, it may result in painful gastric distention—"pneumatosis." Here the spasm may be of considerable duration. Vagotonia is often responsible. Some cases represent failure of the sphincter to relax, rather than actual spasm.

(*g*) Pyloric Spasm.—This is usually a secondary occurrence, following superacidity, supersecretion, ulcer, or the introduction of irritating substances. The spasm often causes pain in the region of the pylorus and increased gastric peristalsis. In cases in which the spasm is combined with superacidity and supersecretion marked dilatation with atony may follow. Sometimes the pylorus may be felt as an oval, hard tumor, which relaxes under the fingers as gas passes through it. It is not easy to distinguish organic stricture and pylorospasm, but the duodenal tube will pass the latter. Atropine usually has a relaxing effect on pylorospasm, especially if vagotonia is present.

(*h*) Atony.—Motor insufficiency is generally due to injudicious feeding, to organic disease of the stomach itself, or to general wasting processes. In some otherwise normal individuals of neurotic temperaments an atony may, however, occur which possibly deserves to be classed among the neuroses. The symptoms are usually those of a moderate dilatation, and are often associated with marked sensory disturbances—feelings of weight and pressure, distention, eructations, and so forth. Great care must be taken in the diagnosis to rule out all other possible causes.

(*i*) INSUFFICIENCY OR INCONTINENCE OF THE PYLORUS.—This condition was described first by de Séré and later by Ebstein. It may be recognized by the rapid passing of gas from the stomach into the bowel on attempts at inflation of the former, as well as by the presence of intestinal contents in the stomach. There are no distinctive clinical symptoms.

(*j*) INSUFFICIENCY OF THE CARDIA.—This condition is only recognized by the occurrence of eructations or in rumination.

Secretory Neuroses.—(*a*) HYPERACIDITY; HYPERCHLORHYDRIA. — The work of Hawk and Rehfuss and their co-workers has altered materially our views as to hyperacidity. They have shown that grades of acidity which we thought abnormal are normal in certain healthy individuals. Each of us has his own figure of gastric acidity and no general standard can be given. It is a question what symptoms are due to hyperacidity. Other disturbances, as in the motor function and pyloric spasm, have to be taken into account. Organic disease, especially ulcer and reflex causes lower in the digestive tract, should always be considered. Yet there are some symptoms apparently associated with hyperacidity especially in nervous individuals. They do not, as a rule, immediately follow the ingestion of food, but occur one to three hours later, at the height of digestion. There is a sense of weight and pressure, sometimes of burning in the epigastrium, commonly associated with acid eructations. If vomiting occurs, the pain is relieved. The patient is usually relatively well nourished, and the appetite is often good, though the sufferer may be afraid to eat on account of the anticipated pain. There is commonly constipation.

(*b*) SUPERSECRETION, INTERMITTENT AND CONTINUOUS.—This is a form long recognized, but specially studied by Reichmann and others. The increased flow of the gastric juice may be intermittent or continuous. The secretion under such circumstances is usually superacid, though this is not always the case. The periodical form—the *gastroxynsis* of Rossbach—may be quite independent of the time of digestion. Great quantities of highly acid gastric juice may be secreted in a very small space of time. Such cases are rare, and are especially associated either with profound neurasthenia or with tabes. The attack may last for several days. It usually sets in with a gnawing, unpleasant sensation in the stomach, severe headache, and shortly after the patient vomits a clear, watery secretion of such acidity that the throat is irritated and made raw and sore. The attacks may be quite independent of food. *Continuous supersecretion* is more common. The constant presence of fluid in the stomach, together with the pyloric spasm, which commonly results from the irritation of the overacid gastric juice, is followed by more or less dilatation. Digestion of the starches is retarded, and there are eructations of acid fluid and gastric distress. This secretion of highly acid gastric juice may continue when the stomach is free from food. In these cases pain, burning acid eructations, and even vomiting, occur during the night and early in the morning.

(*c*) SUBACIDITY OR ANACIDITY; ACHYLIA GASTRICA NERVOSA.—Lack of the normal amount of acid is found in chronic catarrh, and particularly in cancer. A reduction in the normal amount of acid may exist with the most pronounced symptoms of nervous dyspepsia and yet the stomach will be free from food within the regular time. A condition in which free acid is absent in the gastric juice may occur in cancer, in extreme sclerosis of the mucous membrane, as a nervous manifestation, and occasionally in tabes. In most of these cases, though there be no free acid, yet the digestive ferments are present. There may be a complete absence of the gastric secretion. To these cases Einhorn has given the name of *achylia gastrica*. In the true form the enzymes are absent. This condition was at first thought to occur only in cases of total atrophy of the gastric mucosa, but recent observations have shown that it may occur as a neurosis. In a case of Einhorn's the gastric secretions returned after five years of total *achylia gastrica*.

The symptoms of subacidity, or even of *achylia gastrica*, vary greatly in intensity; they may be almost or quite absent in cases of advanced atrophy of the mucosa, and, as a rule, are not marked so long as the motor activity of the stomach remains good. If atony, however, occurs and abnormal fermentative processes arise, severe gastric and intestinal symptoms may follow. In the cases associated with hysteria and neurasthenia, even though the food may be well taken care of by the intestines, there are very commonly grave sensory disturbances in the region of the stomach, in addition to the general nervous symptoms.

Sensory Neuroses.—(*a*) HYPERÆSTHESIA.—In this condition the patients complain of fullness, pressure, weight, burning, and so forth, during digestion, just such symptoms as accompany a variety of organic diseases of the stomach, and yet in all other respects the gastric functions appear quite normal. Sometimes these distressing sensations are present even when the stomach is empty. These symptoms are usually associated with other manifestations of hysteria and neurasthenia. The pain often follows particular articles of food. An hysterical patient may apparently suffer excruciating pain after taking the smallest amount of food of any sort, while anything prescribed as a medicine may be well borne. In severe cases the patient may be reduced to an extreme degree by starvation.

(*b*) GASTRALGIA.—Severe pains in the epigastrium, paroxysmal in character, occur (1) as a manifestation of a functional neurosis, independent of organic disease, and usually associated with other nervous symptoms (it is this form which will here be described); (2) in chronic disease of the nervous system, forming the so-called gastric crises; and (3) in organic disease of the stomach, such as ulcer or cancer.

The functional neurosis occurs chiefly in women, very commonly in connection with disturbed menstrual function or with pronounced nervous symptoms. The affection may set in as early as puberty, but it is more common at the menopause. Anæmic, constipated women who have worries and anxieties at home are most prone to the affection. Attacks of it sometimes occur in robust, healthy men. More often it is only one feature in a condition of general neurasthenia or a manifestation of that form of nervous dyspepsia in which the gastric juice or hydrochloric acid is secreted in excess.

The *symptoms* are very characteristic; the patient is suddenly seized with severe pains in the epigastrium, which pass toward the back and around the lower ribs. The attack is usually independent of the taking of food, and may recur at definite intervals, a periodicity which has given rise to the supposition in some cases that the affection is due to malaria. The most marked periodicity, however, may be in the gastralgic attacks of ulcer. They frequently come on at night. Vomiting is rare; more commonly the taking of food relieves the pain. To this, however, there are striking exceptions. Pressure upon the epigastrium commonly gives relief, but deep pressure may be painful. Stress has been laid upon the occurrence of painful points, but they are so common in neurasthenia that little importance can be attributed to them.

The *diagnosis* offers many difficulties. Organic disease either of the stomach or of the nervous system, particularly the gastric crises of tabes, must be excluded. In the case of ulcer or cancer this is not always easy. Disease elsewhere, such as in the gall-bladder or appendix, may be the etiological factor and search should be made for such lesions. The prolonged intervals between the attacks and their independence of diet are important features in simple gastralgia; but in many instances it is less the local than the general symptoms of the case which enable us to make the diagnosis. In gall-stone colic jaundice is frequently absent, and in any long-standing case of gastralgia the question of cholelithiasis should be considered. There may be hyperacidity associated with gastric atony. Such a case may be treated for months as one of nervous dyspepsia until a more severe attack than usual is followed by jaundice.

(*c*) Anomalies of the Sense of Hunger and Repletion; Bulimia.—Abnormally excessive hunger coming on often in paroxysmal attacks, which cause the patient to commit extraordinary excesses in eating. This condition may occur in diabetes mellitus and sometimes in gastric disorders, particularly those associated with supersecretion. It is, however, more commonly seen in hysteria and in psychoses. It may occur in cerebral tumors, in Graves' disease, and in epilepsy.

The attacks often begin suddenly at night, the patient waking with a feeling of faintness and pain, and an uncontrollable desire for food. Sometimes such attacks occur immediately after a large meal. The attack may be relieved by a small amount of food, while at other times enormous quantities may be taken. In obstinate cases gastritis, atony, and dilatation frequently result from the abuse of the stomach.

Akoria.—An absence of the sense of satiety. This condition is commonly associated with bulimia and polyphagia, but not always. The patient always feels "empty." There are usually other well-marked manifestations of hysteria or neurasthenia.

Anorexia Nervosa.—This condition, which is a manifestation of a neurotic temperament, is discussed under the general heading of Hysteria.

Treatment of Neuroses of the Stomach.—The most important part of the treatment of nervous dyspepsia is often that directed toward the improvement of the general physical and mental condition of the patient. The possibility that the symptoms may be of reflex origin should be borne in mind. The possibility of eye-strain, cholelithiasis, or chronic appendicitis should be considered. A large proportion of cases of nervous dyspepsia are dependent upon mental and physical exhaustion or worry, and a vacation or a change of scene will often accomplish what treatment at home has failed to do. The manner of life should be investigated and a proper amount of physical exercise in the open air and systematic hydrotherapy insisted upon. This alone will in some cases be sufficient to cause the disappearance of the symptoms.

Many cases of nervous dyspepsia with marked neurasthenic or hysterical symptoms do well on the Weir Mitchell treatment, and in obstinate forms it should be given a thorough trial. The most striking results are perhaps seen in the case of anorexia nervosa. It is also of value in nervous vomiting.

In *cardiospasm* care should be taken to eat slowly, to avoid swallowing too large morsels or irritating substances. The methodical introduction of thick sounds may be of value.

The treatment in *atony* of the stomach should be similar to that adopted in moderate dilatation—the administration of small quantities of food at frequent intervals; the limitation of fluids, which should be taken in small amounts at a time; lavage. Strychnine in full doses may be of value.

In the distressing cases of *hyperacidity,* in addition to the treatment of the general neurotic condition, alkalies must be employed either in the form of magnesia or bicarbonate of soda. These should be given in large doses and at the *height of digestion.* The burning acid eructations may be relieved in this way. In hyperacidity and hypersecretion the use of atropine frequently gives relief. It should be given before food and in small doses at first, beginning with 1/150 grain (0.0004 gm.) and gradually increasing. The combination of bromide and belladonna is sometimes useful. The diet should be mainly albuminous. Stimulating condiments and alcohol should be avoided. Starches should be sparingly allowed, and only in most digestible forms. Fats are fairly well borne.

Limiting the patient to a strictly meat diet is a valuable procedure in many cases of dyspepsia associated with hyperacidity. The meat should be taken either raw or, if an insuperable objection exists to this, very slightly cooked. It is best given finely minced or grated on stale bread. An ample dietary is 3¼ ounces (100 grams) of meat, two medium slices of stale bread, and an ounce (30 grams) of butter. This may be taken three times a day with a glass of water or soda water. The fluid should not be taken too cold. The use of fats, as cream, butter, and olive oil, is often of value. Special care should be taken in the examination of the meat to guard against tapeworm infection. Many obstinate cases yield satisfactorily to a month or six weeks of this treatment, after which time the less readily digested articles of food may be gradually added to the dietary.

In *supersecretion* the use of the stomach-tube is of the greatest value. In the periodical form it should be used as soon as the attack begins. The stomach may be washed with alkaline solutions or solutions of nitrate of silver, 1 to 1,000, may be used. Where this is impracticable the taking of albuminous food may give relief. Alkalies in large doses are indicated. In cases of *continued supersecretion* there are usually atony and dilatation. The diet here should be much as in superacidity, but should be administered in smaller quantities at frequent intervals. Lavage with alkaline solutions or with nitrate of silver is of great value. To relieve pain large quantities of bicarbonate of soda or magnesia should be given at the height of digestion.

In *subacidity* a carefully regulated, easily digestible mixed diet, not too rich in protein, is advisable. Bitter tonics before meals are sometimes of value. In *achylia gastrica* the use of predigested foods and of hydrochloric acid in full doses may be of assistance.

In marked *hyperæsthesia,* besides the treatment of the general condition, nitrate of silver in doses of gr. ¼-½ (0.016 to 0.032 gm.), taken in three or four ounces of water on an empty stomach, is advised by Rosenheim. In some instances rectal feeding may have to be used.

For pain large doses of alkalies should be given, of which the light magnesia and bicarbonate of soda are the best. A teaspoonful of either or of a mixture of equal parts may be given after food and when required. A combination of potassium bromide (gr. xv, 1 gm.) with codein (gr. 1/3, 0.02 gm.) or atropine (gr. 1/100, 0.00065 gm.) is sometimes useful. Chloroform in small doses or Hoffman's anodyne will sometimes allay the severe pains. The general condition should receive careful attention, and in many cases the attacks recur until the health is restored by change of air with the prolonged use of arsenic. If there is anæmia iron may be given freely.

There are forms of nervous dyspepsia occurring in women who are often well nourished and with a good color, yet who suffer—particularly at night—with flatulency and abdominal distress. The sleep may be quiet and undisturbed for two or three hours, after which they are aroused with painful sensations in the abdomen and eructations. The appetite and digestion may appear to be normal. Constipation is, however, usually present. In many of these patients the condition seems rather intestinal and the distress is due to the accumulation of gases and reversed peristalsis. The fats, starches, and sugars should be restricted. Some of these cases obtain relief from thorough irrigation of the colon at bedtime. The state of the nervous system should be carefully studied.

In all forms of gastric neurosis special care should be taken to prevent constipation.

G. DISEASES OF THE INTESTINES

I. DISEASES OF THE INTESTINES ASSOCIATED WITH DIARRHŒA

CATARRHAL ENTERITIS; DIARRHŒA

In the classification of catarrhal enteritis the anatomical divisions of the bowel have been too closely followed, and a duodenitis, jejunitis, ileitis, typhlitis, colitis, and proctitis have been recognized; whereas in a majority of cases the entire intestinal tract, to a greater or lesser extent, is involved, sometimes the small most intensely, sometimes the large bowel; but during life it may be quite impossible to say which portion is specially affected.

Etiology.—The causes may be either *primary* or *secondary.* Among the causes of *primary* catarrhal enteritis are: (*a*) Improper food, one of the most frequent, especially in children, in whom it follows overeating, or the ingestion of unripe fruit. In some individuals special articles of diet will always produce a slight diarrhœa, which may not be due to a catarrh of the mucosa, but to increased peristalsis induced by the offending material. (*b*)

Various toxic substances. Many of the organic poisons, such as those produced in the decomposition of milk and articles of food, excite the most intense intestinal catarrh. Certain inorganic substances, as arsenic and mercury, act in the same way. (*c*) Gastrogenous diarrhœa. This is secondary to the absence of free hydrochloric acid in the stomach. (*d*) Changes in the weather. A fall in the temperature of from twenty to thirty degrees, particularly in the spring or autumn, may induce—how, it is difficult to say—an acute diarrhœa. We speak of this as a catarrhal process, the result of cold or of chill. On the other hand, the diarrhœal diseases of children are associated in a very special way with the excessive heat of summer months. (*e*) Changes in the constitution of the intestinal secretions. We know too little about the *succus entericus* to be able to speak of influences induced by change in its quantity or quality. It has long been held that an increase in the amount of bile poured into the bowel might excite a diarrhœa; hence the term bilious diarrhœa, so frequently used by the older writers. Possibly there are conditions in which an excessive amount of bile is poured into the intestine, increasing the peristalsis, and hurrying on the contents; but the opposite state, a scanty secretion, by favoring the natural fermentative processes, much more commonly causes an intestinal catarrh. Absence of the pancreatic secretion from the intestine is associated in certain cases with a fatty diarrhœa. (*f*) Nervous influences. Mental states may profoundly affect the intestinal canal. These probably act through the autonomic system. As a result of stimulation of the vagus, peristalsis is increased. These influences should not properly be considered under catarrhal processes, as they result from disturbed peristalsis and are usually described under the heading *nervous diarrhœa.* In children it frequently follows fright. It is common, too, in adults as a result of emotional disturbances. Canstatt mentions a surgeon who always, before an important operation, had watery diarrhœa. In hysterical women it is an occasional occurrence, due to excitement, or a chronic, protracted diarrhœa, which may last for months or years.

Among the *secondary* causes of intestinal catarrh may be mentioned: (*a*) Infectious diseases. Dysentery, cholera, typhoid fever, pyæmia, septicæmia, tuberculosis, and pneumonia are occasionally associated with intestinal catarrh. In dysentery and typhoid fever the ulceration is in part responsible but in cholera it is probably a direct influence of the bacilli or of the toxic materials produced by them. (*b*) The extension of inflammatory processes from adjacent parts. Thus, in peritonitis, catarrhal swelling and increased secretion are always present in the mucosa. In cases of invagination, hernia, tuberculosis, or cancerous ulceration catarrhal processes are common. (*c*) Circulatory disturbances cause a catarrhal enteritis, usually of a very chronic character. This is common in diseases of the liver, such as cirrhosis, and in chronic affections of the heart and lungs—all conditions, in fact, which produce engorgement of the terminal branches of the portal vessels. (*d*) In the cachectic conditions in cancer, profound anæmia, Addison's disease, and nephritis intestinal catarrh may occur as a terminal event.

Morbid Anatomy.—It is rare to see the mucous membrane injected; more commonly it is pale and covered with mucus. In the upper part of the small intestine the tips of the valvulæ conniventes may be deeply injected. Even in extreme grades of portal obstruction intense hyperæmia is not often seen.

The entire mucosa may be softened and infiltrated, the lining epithelium swollen, or even shed, and appearing as large flakes among the intestinal contents. This is, no doubt, a post mortem change. The lymph follicles are almost always swollen, particularly in children. The Peyer's patches may be prominent and the solitary follicles may stand out with distinctness and present erosions, the so-called follicular ulcers. This may be a striking feature in the intestine in all forms of catarrhal enteritis in children, irrespective of the intensity of the diarrhœa. When the process is more chronic the mucosa is firmer, in some instances thickened, in others distinctly thinned, and the villi and follicles present a slaty pigmentation.

Symptoms.—Acute and chronic forms may be recognized. The important symptom of both is *diarrhœa,* which, in the majority of instances, is the sole indication of this condition. It is not to be supposed that diarrhœa is invariably caused by, or associated with, catarrhal enteritis, as it may be produced by nervous and other influences. It is probable that catarrh of the jejunum may exist without any diarrhœa; indeed, it is common to find post mortem a catarrhal state of the small bowel in persons who have not had diarrhœa during life. The stools vary extremely in character. The color depends upon the amount of bile with which they are mixed, and they may be of a dark or blackish brown, or of a light yellow, or even of a grayish-white tint. The consistence is usually very thin and watery, but in some instances the stools are pultaceous like thin gruel. Portions of undigested food can often be seen (lienteric diarrhœa), and flakes of yellowish-brown mucus. Microscopically there are innumerable micro-organisms, epithelium and mucous cells, crystals of phosphate of lime, oxalate of lime, and occasionally cholesterin and Charcot's crystals. In *enteritis* there is unchanged bile, the stools may be green, cellulose is not digested and the mucus is intimately mixed with the stool. In *colitis* the stool is usually browner, cellulose is largely digested and the mucus is on the outside of the fæces and may be in large masses.

Pain in the abdomen is usually present in acute enteritis, particularly when due to food. It is of a colicky character, and when the colon is involved there may be tenesmus. More or less tympanites exists, and there are gurgling noises due to the rapid passage of fluid and gas from one part to another. In the very acute attacks there may be vomiting. Fever is not, as a rule, present, but there may be a slight elevation of one or two degrees. The appetite is lost, there is intense thirst, and the tongue is dry and coated. In very acute cases, when the quantity of fluid lost is great and the pain excessive, there may be collapse symptoms. The number of evacuations varies from four or five to twenty or more in the course of the day. The attack lasts for two or three days, or may be prolonged for a week or ten days.

Chronic catarrh may follow the acute form, or may come on gradually as an independent affection or as a sequence of obstruction in the portal circulation. It is characterized by diarrhœa, with or without colic. The dejections vary; when the small bowel is chiefly involved the diarrhœa is of a lienteric character, and when the colon is affected the stools are thin and mixed with much mucus. A special form of mucous diarrhœa will be subsequently described. The general nutrition in these chronic cases is greatly disturbed;

there may be much loss of flesh and great pallor. The patients are inclined to suffer from depression or hypochondriasis.

Carbohydrate Indigestion.—This may involve both the stomach and bowels. The main symptom is distention from gas. The stools are acid and contain much undigested starch. If there is much fermentation the stools in addition are mushy and contain bubbles of gas. The result of a protein-fat diet is an important point in the diagnosis.

Diagnosis.—It is important, in the first place, to determine, if possible, whether the large or small bowel is chiefly affected. In catarrh of the small bowel the diarrhœa is less marked, the pains are of a colicky character, borborygmi are not so frequent, the fæces usually contain portions of food, and are more yellowish-green or grayish-yellow and flocculent and do not contain much mucus. When the large intestine is at fault there may be no pain whatever, as in the catarrh of the large intestine associated with tuberculosis and nephritis. When present, the pains are most intense, and, if the lower portion of the bowel is involved, there may be marked tenesmus. The stools have a uniform soupy consistence; they are grayish in color and granular throughout, with here and there flakes of mucus, or they may contain very large quantities of mucus.

Duodenitis is usually associated with acute gastritis and, if the process extends into the bile-duct, with jaundice. The study of the duodenal contents aids in the diagnosis. Neither jejunitis nor ileitis can be separated from general intestinal catarrh.

The Cœliac Affection.—Under this heading Gee described an intestinal disorder, most common in children between the ages of one and five, characterized by the occurrence of pale, loose stools, not unlike gruel or oatmeal porridge. They are bulky, not watery, yeasty, frothy, and extremely offensive. The affection has received variоus names, such as *diarrhœa alba* or *diarrhœa chylosa*. It is not associated with tuberculosis or other hereditary disease. It begins insidiously and there are progressive wasting, weakness, and pallor. The belly becomes doughy and inelastic. There is often flatulency. Fever is usually absent. The disease is lingering and a fatal termination is common. So far nothing is known of the pathology of the disease. Ulceration of the intestines has been met with, but it is not constant.

Sprue or Psilosis.—It is difficult to decide where this disease should be placed. Various theories of etiology are held—disease of the pancreas, bacterial, infection by a mould (*Monilia*), or a fat deficiency disease. It occurs especially in the tropics (India, China and Java) but is not infrequent in the United States, a point which Wood has emphasized.

The chief features are: (1) *Diarrhœa.* The stools are very large, acid, light in color and contain a large amount of fat. It is a fatty diarrhœa, without pain or tenesmus, and the stools are like those of pancreatic insufficiency. The stools are usually passed between midnight and 10 A. M. The loss of fat may vary from 30 to 50 per cent. There is also marked nitrogen loss in the stools. (2) *Tongue.* This may be inflamed and show eroded patches or superficial cracks. (3) *Anæmia.* The color index may be high and the picture resemble that of pernicious anæmia. (4) The disease is chronic and remissions are common. There is often marked emaciation. The diagnosis from pellagra has given difficulty but the study of the stools should prevent this.

In *treatment,* absolute rest in bed, a diet of finely chopped beef, cooked lightly and given four times a day, and at least four pints of hot water, have been found useful. The giving of pancreatic ferments and the use of autogenous streptococcus vaccine should be tried.

DIPHTHEROID OR CROUPOUS ENTERITIS

A croupous or diphtheroid inflammation of the mucosa of the small and large intestines occurs (*a*) most frequently as a secondary process in the infectious diseases—pneumonia, pyæmia in its various forms, and typhoid fever; (*b*) as a terminal process in many chronic affections, such as nephritis, cirrhosis of the liver, or cancer; and (*c*) as an effect of certain poisons—mercury, lead, and arsenic. The ulcerative colitis of chronic disease may be only a terminal event in these diphtheroid processes.

There are three different anatomical pictures. In one group of cases the mucosa presents on the top of the folds a thin grayish-yellow diphtheroid exudate situated upon a deeply congested base. In some cases all grades may be seen between the thinnest film of superficial necrosis and involvement of the entire thickness of the mucosa. In the colon similar transversely arranged areas of necrosis are seen situated upon hyperæmic patches, and it may be here much more extensive and involve a large portion of the membrane. There may be most extensive inflammation without any involvement of the solitary follicles of the large or small bowel.

In a second group the membrane has rather a croupous character. It is grayish-white in color, more flake-like and extensive, limited, perhaps, to the cæcum or to a portion of the colon; thus, in pneumonia this flaky adherent false membrane may be found sometimes forming patches 1 to 2 cm. in diameter, in form not unlike rupia crusts.

In a third group the affection is really a follicular enteritis, involving the solitary glands, which are swollen and capped with an area of diphtheroid necrosis or are in a state of suppuration. Follicular ulcers are common in this form. The disease may run its course without any symptoms, and the condition is unexpectedly met with post mortem. In other instances there are diarrhœa, pain, but not often tenesmus or the passage of blood-stained mucus. In the toxic cases the intestinal symptoms may be very marked, but in the terminal colitis of the fevers and of constitutional affections the symptoms are often trifling.

PHLEGMONOUS ENTERITIS

As an independent affection this is excessively rare, even less frequent than its counterpart in the stomach. It is seen occasionally in connection with intussusception, strangulated hernia, and chronic obstruction. Apart from these conditions it occurs most frequently in the duodenum, and leads to suppuration in the submucosa and abscess formation. Except when associated with hernia or intussusception the affection can not be diagnosed. The symptoms usually resemble those of peritonitis.

ULCERATIVE ENTERITIS

In addition to the specific ulcers of tuberculosis, syphilis, and typhoid fever, the following forms of ulceration occur in the bowels:

Follicular Ulceration.—As mentioned, this is very common in the diarrhœal diseases of children, and also in the secondary or terminal inflammations in many fevers and constitutional disorders. The ulcers are small, punched out, with sharply cut edges, and are usually limited to the follicles. With this form may be placed the catarrhal ulcers of some writers.

Stercoral ulcers, which occur in long-standing cases of constipation. Very remarkable indeed are the cases in which the sacculi of the colon become filled with rounded small scybala, some of which produce distinct ulcers in the mucous membrane. The fæcal masses may have lime salts deposited in them, and thus form little enteroliths.

Simple Ulcerative Colitis.—Apart from dysentery of the Shiga type, the amœbic and terminal forms, there is a variety of ulcerative colitis, sometimes of great severity, not uncommon in England and the United States. It is a disease of adults, of unknown origin. The sexes are equally affected; of 177 cases collected by Eric Smith, 89 were in males. Some patients have had previous bowel trouble; sometimes there have been intermittent attacks of diarrhœa and constipation. Post mortem, the colon is dilated, often without hypertrophied walls; the ulceration, as a rule, limited to it and very extensive, the ulcers ranging in size from a pin's head to large areas, with infiltrated, rarely undermined, edges. The Shiga bacillus is not present; colon bacilli are found but no one organism has apparently any definite relation to the disease.

When established, the main features are:

(*a*) Diarrhœa: the motions very frequent in the day, up to 20 or 30, usually small, bile-stained, with mucus, pus, and blood, sometimes mixed with the motion or separate. There may be clotted lumps of blood, or the blood is uniformly mixed, and the motions look like anchovy sauce. The pain, while severe, is usually diffuse, abdominal, and colicky, and, not so frequently, in the rectum. Many of the motions pass without pain.

(*b*) Fever, which occurs in the majority of the cases, though severe forms may be free throughout.

(*c*) Wasting, debility, and progressive anæmia.

(*d*) With the proctoscope the mucous membrane is seen to be red and œdematous. Later the œdema subsides and ulceration appears.

The disease may run a very acute course, but most frequently it is chronic, lasting from eight weeks to three or four months. Transient improvement may follow, and a relapse. Death is most commonly from exhaustion, occasionally from hæmorrhage, and in a few instances from perforation.

Ulceration from External Perforation.—This may result from the erosion of new growths or, more commonly, from localized peritonitis with abscess formation and perforation of the bowel. This is met with most frequently in tuberculous peritonitis, but it may occur in the abscess which follows perforation of the appendix or suppurative or gangrenous pancreatitis. Fatal hæmorrhage may result from the perforation.

Cancerous Ulcers.—In very rare instances of multiple cancer or sarcoma the submucous nodules break down and ulcerate. In one case the ileum contained eight or ten sarcomatous ulcers secondary to an extensive sarcoma in the neighborhood of the shoulder-joint.

Solitary Ulcer.—Occasionally a solitary ulcer is met with in the cæcum or colon, which may lead to perforation. Two instances of ulcer of the cæcum, both with perforation, have come under our observation, and in one instance a simple ulcer of the colon perforated and led to fatal peritonitis.

Diagnosis of Intestinal Ulcers.—As a rule, diarrhœa is present in all cases, but exceptionally there may be extensive ulceration, particularly in the small bowel, without diarrhœa. Very limited ulceration in the colon may be associated with frequent stools. The character of the dejections is of great importance. Pus, shreds of tissue, and blood are the most valuable indications. *Pus* occurs most frequently in connection with ulcers in the large intestine, but when the bowel alone is involved the amount is rarely great, and the passage of any quantity of pure pus is an indication that it has come from without, most commonly from the rupture of a pericæcal abscess, or in women of an abscess of the broad ligament. Pus may also be present in cancer of the bowel or it may be due to local disease in the rectum. A purulent mucus may be present in the stools in cases of ulcer, but it has not the same diagnostic value. The swollen, sago-like masses of mucus which are believed by some to indicate follicular ulceration are met with also in mucous colitis. *Hæmorrhage* is an important and valuable symptom of ulcer in the bowel, particularly if profuse. It occurs under so many conditions that taken alone it may not be specially significant, but with other coexisting circumstances it may be the most important indication of all.

Fragments of tissue are occasionally found in the stools in ulcer, particularly in the extensive and rapid sloughing in dysenteric processes. Definite portions of mucosa, shreds of connective tissue, and even bits of the muscular coat may be found. Pain occurs in many cases, either of a diffuse, colicky character, or sometimes, in the ulcer of the colon, very limited and well defined. Examination by means of tubes should always be done, as by them ulcers in the lower bowel may be viewed directly.

Perforation is an accident liable to happen when the ulcer extends deeply. In the small bowel it leads to a localized or general peritonitis. In the large intestine, too, a fatal peritonitis may result, or, if perforation takes place in the posterior wall of the ascending or descending colon, the production of a large abscess cavity in the retro-peritoneum.

Treatment of the Previous Conditions

Acute Dyspeptic Diarrhœa.—The patient should be in bed and in acute cases no food should be allowed for twenty-four hours. If there is vomiting the stomach should be washed with an alkaline solution. If the attack has followed the eating of large quantities of indigestible material, castor oil or calomel is advisable, but is not necessary if the patient has been freely purged. If the pain is severe, 20 drops (1.3 c. c.) of laudanum and a drachm (4 c. c.) of spirit of chloroform may be given, or, if the colic is very intense, a hypodermic of a quarter of a grain (0.016 gm.) of morphia. It is not well to check the diarrhœa unless it is profuse, as it usually stops spontaneously within forty-eight hours. If persistent, the aromatic chalk powder or large doses of bismuth (30 to 40 grains, 2 gm.) may be given. A small enema of starch (2 ounces, 60 c. c.), with 20 drops (1.3 c. c.) of laudanum, every six hours, is a most valuable remedy. The diet should be increased very gradually during convalescence.

Chronic diarrhœa, including chronic catarrh and ulcerative enteritis. It is important, in the first place, to ascertain, if possible, the cause and whether ulceration is present or not. So much in treatment depends upon the careful examination of the stools—as to the amount of mucus, the presence of pus, the occurrence of parasites, and, above all, the state of digestion of the food—that the practitioner should pay special attention to them. Many patients simply require rest in bed and a restricted diet. Chronic diarrhœa of many months' or even of several years' duration may be sometimes cured by strict confinement to bed and a diet of boiled milk and albumen water.

The *gastrogenous diarrhœa* may be promptly relieved by giving dilute hydrochloric acid in full doses. Calcium lactate (gr. xv, 1 gm.) and pancreatin are also useful.

In that form in which immediately after eating there is a tendency to loose evacuations it may be that some one article of diet is at fault. The patient should rest for an hour or more after meals. Sometimes this alone is sufficient to prevent the occurrence of the diarrhœa. Arsenic in moderate doses taken at the end of the meal is sometimes helpful. In those forms which depend upon abnormal conditions in the small intestine, bismuth is indicated. It must be given in large doses—from half a dram to a dram (2 to 4 gm.) three times a day. The smaller doses are of little use. Salol and the salicylate of bismuth may be tried.

In the form due to *carbohydrate indigestion,* the carbohydrate should be greatly reduced or a protein-fat diet given. If the diarrhœa lessens, vegetables with a low carbohydrate content (see page 433) should be added gradually.

An extremely obstinate and intractable form is the diarrhœa of hysterical and nervous women. A systematic rest cure will be found most advantageous, and if a milk diet is not well borne the patient may be fed on egg albumen. The condition seems to be associated in some cases with increased peristalsis, and in such the bromides may do good, or preparations of opium may be necessary. There are instances which prove most obstinate and resist all forms of treatment, and the patient may be greatly reduced. A change of air and surroundings may do more than medicines.

In a large group of the chronic diarrhœas the mischief is seated in the *colon* and is due to ulceration. Medicines by the mouth are here of little value. The stools should be carefully watched and a diet arranged which shall leave the smallest possible residue. Boiled or peptonized milk may be given, but the stools should be examined to see whether there is an excess of food or of curds. Meat is, as a rule, badly borne in these cases. The diarrhœa is best treated by enemata. The starch and laudanum should be tried, but when ulceration is present it is better to use astringent injections. From 2 to 4 pints of warm water, containing from half a dram to a dram (2 to 4 gm.) of nitrate of silver, may be used. In the chronic diarrhœa which follows dysentery this is particularly advantageous. In giving large injections the patient should be in the dorsal position, with the hips elevated, and it is best to allow the injection to flow in gradually from a siphon bag. In this way the entire colon can be irrigated and the patient can retain the injection for some time. The silver injections may be very painful, but they are invaluable in all forms of ulcerative colitis. Acetate of lead, boracic acid, sulphate of copper, suphate of zinc, and salicylic acid may be used in 1 per cent. solutions. Any ulcers which can be reached should be treated by local applications, of which the silver salts are particularly useful. In obstinate cases appendicostomy or cæcostomy should be done and the bowel irrigated through the opening.

In the intense forms of choleraic diarrhœa in adults associated with constant vomiting and frequent watery discharges the patient should be given at once a hypodermic of a quarter of a grain (0.016 gm.) of morphia, which should be repeated in an hour if the pains return or the purging persists. This gives prompt relief, and is often the only medicine needed in the attack. The patient should be given stimulants, and, when the vomiting is allayed by suitable remedies, small quantities of milk and lime water.

II. DIARRHŒAL DISEASES IN CHILDREN

Children are particularly susceptible to disorders of the alimentary tract. Although several forms are recognized, they so often merge the one into the other that a sharp differentiation is impossible.

General Etiology.—Certain factors predispose to diarrhœa. Age.—The largest number of cases occur just after the nursing period; the highest mortality is in the second half of the first year, when this period falls in the hot weather; hence the dread of the "second summer."

Diet.—Diarrhœa is most frequent in artificially fed babies. Of 1,943 fatal cases collected by Holt, only 3 per cent. were breast-fed. The agitation for pure milk in the large cities has decreased materially the number of diarrhœa cases among bottle-fed infants.

Among the poor the bowel complaint comes with artificial feeding, and is due either to milk ill-suited in quantity or poor in quality, or to indigestible articles of diet. Many of the fatal cases have been fed upon condensed milk. In some cases the absorption of partially digested food protein may be responsible, or protein from bacteria in the milk.

Temperature.—The relation of the atmospheric temperature to the prevalence of the disease in children has long been recognized. The mortality curve begins to rise in May, increases in June, reaching the maximum in July, and gradually sinks through August and September. The maximum corresponds closely with the highest mean temperature, yet we can not regard the heat itself as the direct agent, but only as one of several factors. Thus the mean temperature of June is only four or five degrees lower than that of July, and yet the mortality is not more than one-third. Seibert, who analyzed the mortality and the temperature month by month in New York for ten years, fails to find a constant relation between the degrees of heat and the number of cases of diarrhœa. Neither barometric pressure nor humidity appears to have any influence.

BACTERIOLOGY.—The discovery by Duvall and Bassett of a bacillus apparently identical with the Shiga bacillus in the dejecta of children suffering from summer diarrhœa awakened renewed interest in the relation of bacteria to these disorders in children. The Rockefeller Institute research showed that this organism was present in a large number of cases of so-called "summer diarrhœa." The studies of Martini and Lentz, Flexner, Hiss, Parke, and others indicate that there is a group of closely allied forms of bacilli differing slightly from the original Shiga bacillus in their action on certain sugars and in agglutinating properties. The type of organisms most frequently associated with the diarrhœas of children belongs to the so-called "acid type," and, unlike the Shiga cultures, ferments mannite with acid production.

The causal connection of this group of bacteria with all the diarrhœal diseases of children has not been proved. In the hands of some workers they have been found in the fæces of a large proportion of all cases examined, and also less frequently in the sporadic diarrhœas occurring throughout the year. These organisms are often found in comparatively small numbers, and are more easily isolated from mucus or blood-stained stools. They occur in the acute primary intestinal infection in children, in subacute infection without previous symptoms coincident with or following other acute diseases such as measles, pneumonia, etc., and in the terminal intestinal infection following malnutrition or marasmus. They have been found in breast-fed infants as well as bottle-babies.

The mode of entrance of the organism has not been determined. Simultaneous outbreaks of many cases in remote parts of a community where there can be no common milk supply, and occurrence of the disease in breast- and condensed-milk-fed babies, indicate that cow's milk is not the only conveyor of the infection, and point to some common cause, possibly to the water, as a means of contamination.

The importance of other organisms must not be overlooked. The observations of Escherich showed the remarkable simplicity of bacterial flora in the intestines of healthy milk-fed children, *Bacterium lactis aërogenes* being present in the upper portion of the bowel and *Bacterium coli commune* in the lower bowel, each almost in pure culture.

When diarrhœa is set up the number and varieties of bacteria are greatly increased, although heretofore no forms had been found to bear a constant or specific relationship to the diarrhœal fæces. Certain diarrhœas in children are apparently induced by the lactic acid organisms in milk, others by *colon* or *proteus bacilli,* and others, again, by the *pyogenic cocci* and other forms; all these bacteria may be associated with the dysentery bacilli. There is considerable evidence to support the view that the destructive lesions of the intestines may be produced by the *Streptococcus pyogenes* after an initial infection with a member of the dysentery group.

Morbid Anatomy.—In mild cases there may be only a slight catarrhal swelling of the mucosa of both small and large bowel, with enlargement of the lymph follicles. The mucous membrane may be irregularly congested; often this is most marked at the summit of the folds. The submucosa is usually infiltrated with serum and small round cells. In more severe cases ulceration may take place. The loss of substance begins, usually, in the mucosa, over swollen lymph follicles. About the ulcer there is a more or less distinctly marked inflammatory zone. The destruction of the tissue is limited to the region of the follicles and becomes progressive by the union of several adjoining ulcers. This process is usually confined to the lower bowel, and may be so extensive as to leave only ribbons of intact mucosa. The ulcers never perforate. Rarely there is a croupous or pseudo-membranous enteritis affecting the lower ileum, colon, and rectum. The constant features are the increased secretion of mucus and the lymphoid hyperplasia. The mesenteric glands are enlarged.

The changes in the other organs are neither numerous nor characteristic. Broncho-pneumonia occurs in many cases. The liver is often fatty, the spleen may be swollen. Brain lesions are rare; the membranes and substance are often anæmic, but meningitis or thrombosis is very uncommon.

Clinical Forms.—ACUTE INTESTINAL INDIGESTION.—This form occurs in children of all ages, and is associated with improper food. The symptoms often begin abruptly with nausea and vomiting, or, especially in stronger children, several hours or a day or two after the disturbing diet. The local symptoms are colicky pains, moderate tympanites, and diarrhœa. The stools are four to ten in twenty-four hours; at first fæcal, then fluid, with more or less mucus and particles from undigested material. There is no blood. The usual intestinal bacteria are found. Occasionally, when there is mucus, dysentery bacilli are present. There is always fever. It is rarely very high, and never continues. The pulse may be rapid and the prostration marked in very young or weak children. These symptoms usually subside shortly after the emptying of the bowel.

In weakened infants, or when the treatment has been delayed or the diet remains unchanged, this disturbance may lead to more serious conditions. Attacks of intestinal indigestion tend to recur.

FERMENTATIVE DIARRHŒA.—This form is characterized by more severe constitutional symptoms. It may begin after an intestinal indigestion of several days in which the stools are fluid and offensive, and contain undigested food and curds. In other cases the disease sets in abruptly with vomiting, griping pains, and fever, which may rapidly reach 104°-105° F.

Nervous symptoms are usually prominent. The child is irritable and sleeps poorly. Convulsions may usher in the acute symptoms or occur later. An increasing drowsiness, ending in coma, has been noted in many cases. The stools, which vary from four to twenty in twenty-four hours, soon lose their fæcal character and become fluid. Later they consist largely of green or translucent mucus. An occasional fleck of blood is noticed in the mucus, but this is never present in large amounts. Microscopically, besides the food residue and mucous strands are a moderate number of leucocytes and red blood-corpuscles. Epithelial cells are found with numerous bacteria.

The acute symptoms generally pass away in a few days with judicious treatment. Relapses are frequent, following any indiscretion. The attack may be the beginning of severe ileo-colitis. These gastro-intestinal intoxications are largely confined to the summer months and form an important group of the summer diarrhœas of children.

CHOLERA INFANTUM.—This term should be reserved for the fulminating form of gastro-intestinal intoxication. The typical cases are rare and form only a very small proportion of the diarrhœal diseases of infants. The disease sets in with vomiting, which is incessant and is excited by an attempt to take food or drink. The stools are profuse and frequent; at first fæcal in character, brown or yellow in color, and finally thin, serous, and watery. The stools first passed are very offensive; subsequently they are odorless. The thin, serous stools are alkaline. There is fever, but the axillary temperature may register three or more degrees below that of the rectum. From the outset there is marked prostration; the eyes are sunken, the features pinched, the fontanelles depressed, and the skin has a peculiar ashy pallor. At first restless and excited, the child subsequently becomes heavy, dull, and listless. The tongue is coated at the onset, but subsequently becomes red and dry. As in all choleraic conditions, the thirst is insatiable; the pulse is rapid and feeble, and toward the end becomes irregular and imperceptible. Death may occur within twenty-four hours, with symptoms of collapse and great elevation of the internal temperature. Before the end the diarrhœa and vomiting may cease. In other instances the intense symptoms subside, but the child remains torpid and semi-comatose, with fingers clutched, and there may be convulsions. The head may be retracted and the respirations interrupted, irregular, and of the Cheyne-Stokes type. The child may remain in this condition for some days without any signs of improvement. It was to this group of symptoms in infantile diarrhœa that Marshall Hall gave the term "hydrencephaloid," or spurious hydrocephalus. As a rule, no changes in the brain or other organs are found. The condition of sclerema is described as a sequel of cholera infantum. The skin and subcutaneous tissue becomes hard and firm, and the appearance has been compared to that of a half-frozen cadaver.

No constant organism has been found in these cases. Baginsky considers the disease the result of the action on the system of the poisonous products of decomposition encouraged by the various bacteria present—a *Fäulniss* disease. The clinical picture is that produced by an acute bacterial infection, as in Asiatic cholera.

Diagnosis.—The diagnosis is readily made. There is no other intestinal affection in children for which it can be mistaken. The constant vomiting, the frequent watery discharges, the collapse symptoms, and the elevated temperature make an unmistakable clinical picture. The outlook in the majority of cases is bad, particularly in children artificially fed. Hyperpyrexia, extreme collapse, and incessant vomiting are the most serious symptoms.

Ileo-colitis (*Entero-colitis, Inflammatory Diarrhœa*).—In this form there is evidence of an inflammatory alteration of the intestinal wall, usually of the lower ileum and large intestine. Several sub-varieties are recognized according to the nature and site of the lesions. Many of the cases are grafted on the simple forms above described. The mucous discharges continue, mingled with food residue and often streaked with blood. Pus cells are numerous under the microscope. The temperature remains elevated or may be remittent. After two or three weeks the symptoms gradually subside, the stools become fewer in number, and the fæcal character returns.

In other instances the severe involvement of the intestines seems evident within a few hours of the onset, with abdominal pain, vomiting, and fever. Blood and pus may be present in nearly every stool. Tenesmus is frequent and prolapsus ani is not uncommon. In severe attacks the prostration is marked, the tongue is dry, the mouth covered with sordes, and death may ensue in a few days from profound sepsis, or the patient may continue desperately ill for weeks and gradually recover or die from asthenia.

Hæmorrhage of large amount is extremely rare. The appearance of bright red stains on the napkin indicates, usually, ulceration of the lower bowel or rectum. When the blood is dark brown the lesion is in the ileum or near the valve. The extent of the ulceration can not be accurately determined by the quantity of the blood passed.

Membranous-colitis is usually only to be distinguished by the discovery of the membrane in the rectum through a speculum or in prolapsus, or by the passage of a fragment of the membrane in the stools.

Inflammation of the colon often occurs in marantic infants. It may consist of a catarrhal or follicular inflammation of the lower bowel without destructive lesion, and is frequently a terminal infection.

Ileo-colitis may become chronic and persist for months. The signs of active inflammation subside; there is little pain or fever, but more or less mucus remains in the stools. The general condition suffers. There is a continuous loss in weight; the skin is dry and hangs in folds; nervous symptoms are always present. There may be stiffness and contraction of the extremities, with opisthotonos. The progress is irregular, marked by short periods of improvement. Death is often due to a relapse, to asthenia, or to broncho-pneumonia. In many of these cases, both acute and chronic, the dysentery bacilli have been found in association with other organisms. In all these forms *acidosis* may occur and should always be kept in mind. Increase in the respiration rate, for which no other explanation is found, should excite suspicion of acidosis.

Prevention.—Unquestionably, most of the intestinal disorders of children can be prevented. In many large cities the mortality from the summer diarrhœas has been greatly reduced by prophylactic measures. The infant should have abundance of air-space in the home, with plenty of sunlight and fresh air. In hot weather it may be well for him to sleep out of doors, day and night. The clothing must not be too heavy in midsummer; often only a binder and thin dress. This clothing should be altered with every change of the temperature. The greatest cleanliness should surround the life of the baby, and the nursing-bottles and nipples are to be boiled each day and kept scrupulously clean. Breast-feeding is continued whenever possible.

With bottle-babies, in warm weather, the diet should be reduced in strength —i. e., weaker milk mixtures used and more water given. In all crowded communities the milk should be sterilized or pasteurized during the summer months, and all the water given the baby, either with or between the nourishment, boiled. It is better that a child should be in the country during the hot weather, but when this is impossible the parks in the large cities afford much relief.

Treatment.—Hygienic Management.—Even after the illness has begun, much can be done by hygienic measures to diminish the severity. Change of air to seashore or mountain is often followed by a marked improvement in the child's condition. The patient must not be too warmly clad. The temperature may be lowered and nervous symptoms allayed by hydrotherapy.

Baths, warm and cool, are helpful. Colon irrigations serve the double purpose of flushing the bowel and stimulating the nervous system. They should be given cool when there is much fever.

DIET.—The dietetic management is of the utmost importance. In acute cases with fever the milk, whether breast or cow's milk, and all its modifications, must be stopped at once. It is best to give the infant nothing but water for several hours, it may be for two or three days, or until the acute symptoms subside; a cereal water may then be substituted, to which may be added egg albumen, broth, or beef juice. The time at which it is safe to return to a milk diet varies with each case, and no definite rules can be laid down. It is usually better to defer milk until the temperature is nearly normal.

If the stools are alkaline from protein decomposition, a diet consisting largely of carbohydrates—i. e., barley water—is indicated; whereas protein diet, such as beef juice and egg albumen, is more helpful when the stools are strongly acid.

Experience has shown that the ingredient in the milk that is not well borne is the fat; hence skimmed milk, diluted or partially digested, can often be safely given before diluted whole milk. Whey is often helpful. In Germany buttermilk has been widely used in convalescence from intestinal disturbances. The various proprietary foods, or condensed milk mixed with water, although not to be given over long periods, may be found serviceable in the gradual return of the child to a normal diet.

In children from three to seven years of age these acute derangements are rarely serious, and usually respond promptly after purgation and restricted diet, consisting largely of boiled milk.

It must be borne in mind that injudicious treatment, either in diet or medication, may interrupt what otherwise would be a prompt recovery and bring on the most serious intestinal lesions. The chronic cases, both in infants and old children, especially those with ileo-colitis and ulceration, present unusual difficulties. Each case must be studied by itself. Food which is digested in the upper portion of the intestinal tract is preferable. Milk, properly modified with cereal water or predigested, if intelligently prescribed, offers the best chance of success. The percentage system of milk modification, which enables the physician to alter the proportion of fat or carbohydrate in the milk mixture, is of great service in feeding these long-standing cases.

Care must be taken not to over-feed, although occasionally, when there is persistent anorexia, gavage may be necessary. This is best accomplished through a nasal tube. Some infants will retain food given through a catheter when they will vomit the same mixture taken from a bottle. Beef juice is frequently useful. It should always be given with considerable fluid.

MEDICINAL.—In all cases of diarrhœa there are more or less congestion of the intestinal mucosa, hypersecretion of mucus, and increased peristalsis due in part to the irritant action of improper food. In certain forms toxic symptoms are noticed early. In other instances inflammatory lesions in the wall of the bowel are present. The keynote, then, of the treatment is promptness. Nature's effort to remove the disturbing cause should be assisted, not checked.

Castor oil and calomel are to be preferred as purgatives, especially for infants. A dram (4 c. c.) of the former, repeated, if necessary, will usually sweep the intestinal tract and relieve the irritation. Where there is much nausea or intestinal fermentation, calomel is indicated. It may be given in divided doses at short intervals until one or two grains (0.065 or 0.13 gm.) have been taken, or until the characteristic green stools appear. Very early in the attack, if nausea is marked, nothing relieves so quickly as gastric lavage with warm water or a weak soda solution. In older children a large draught of boiled water may be substituted. In many cases irrigation of the lower bowel with large quantities of salt solution flushes the colon, removing the irritating material, and diminishes the absorption of toxins. It also reduces the temperature and allays nervous symptoms. The irrigating fluid should be cool when there is much fever. The infant is placed in the dorsal position or turned a little to the left, with hips elevated, and the fluid from a fountain syringe, about three feet above the patient, is allowed to flow into the rectum through a large soft rubber catheter. Usually about a pint can be retained before expulsion. If desired, the catheter can be gently pushed into the bowel as it becomes distended with fluid. Two or three quarts should be used at one irrigation, which may be repeated several times in twenty-four hours if it is beneficial.

Where there is ulceration of the lower bowel various astringents, such as alum, witch hazel (one or two teaspoonfuls to one quart), silver nitrate, 1-4,000, or a weak solution of permanganate of potassium, may be used as the irrigating fluid. In great local irritation and tenesmus, enemata (2 ounces, 60 c. c.) of flaxseed or starch, with 2 to 5 drops (0.12 to 0.3 c. c.) of laudanum, are soothing and beneficial.

Water should be given freely by whichever method is indicated. With signs of *acidosis*, as much water as possible should be given and sodium bicarbonate in full doses, gr. xv-lx (1-4 gm.) by mouth or by the bowel every two hours, until the urine is alkaline. When there is much loss of fluid from the body or when toxic symptoms are marked infusion of normal salt solution under the skin may be tried. One to three hundred c. c. can be readily introduced. This procedure is not so permanently helpful as it was thought to be some years ago. There is rarely any necessity to transfuse unless in severe acidosis.

Of the many drugs vaunted as intestinal astringents and antiseptics, bismuth, either as subgallate or subnitrate, has proved most serviceable. It should not be given until the disturbing material has been removed and the temperature is falling; then it should be administered in large doses, 5 to 10 grains (0.3 to 0.6 gm.) every hour, until there is discoloration of the stools. In some cases this may be hastened by lac sulphur in grain doses. Opium should be very sparingly used, and then only for a specific purpose, to check excessive peristalsis, violent colic, or very numerous passages. It may be given to an infant as Dover's powder, ¼-1 grain (0.016 to 0.065 gm.); or paregoric, 5-10 minims (0.3 to 0.6 c. c.) every four hours; or morphia, hypodermically, 1/200-1/50 grain (0.00032 to 0.0013 gm.), when prompt action is desired. Occasionally it is well to combine it with atropine, 1/1,000-1/250 grain (0.000065-0.00026 gm.) The bowels should not be locked when the stools are foul or the temperature is high. When there is prostration stimulants, such as camphor or strychnine (gr. 1/200-1/100, 0.0003-0.0006 gm.), are indicated.

Serum Therapy.—Thus far the results of serum therapy have been disappointing. It is only in the very early cases that any improvement results. The marked reduction in the mortality in adult dysentery in Japan, reported by Shiga, should encourage the further trial of this treatment in the epidemic diarrhœa, as no ill effects have been ascribed to its use. It is given in 10-40 c. c. doses, hypodermically.

Treatment of Cholera Infantum.—In cholera infantum serious symptoms may occur with great rapidity, and here the incessant vomiting and frequent purging render the administration of remedies extremely difficult. Irrigation of the stomach and large bowel is of great service, and when the fever is high ice-water injections may be used, or a graduated bath. As in the acute choleraic diarrhœa of adults, morphia hypodermically is the remedy which gives greatest relief, and in the conditions of extreme vomiting and purging, with restlessness and collapse symptoms, this drug alone commands the situation. A child of one year may be given from 1/100 to 1/80 of a grain (0.00065 to 0.0008 gm.) to be repeated in an hour, and again if not better.

In all cases of diarrhœa convalescence requires very careful management. An infant which has suffered from a severe attack should be especially watched throughout the remainder of the hot weather. During this time it is rarely safe to return to a full diet.

III. APPENDICITIS

Inflammation of the vermiform appendix is the most important of acute intestinal disorders. Formerly the "iliac phlegmon" was thought to be due to disease of the cæcum—typhlitis—or of the peritoneum covering it—perityphlitis; but we now know that with rare exceptions the cæcum itself is not affected, and even the condition formerly described as stercoral typhlitis is in reality appendicitis. The contribution of Fitz in 1886 served to put the whole question on a rational basis. For historical and special details the reader is referred to the monograph of Kelly and Hurdon.

Etiology.—The exciting causes of appendicitis are not always evident. An infection is the essential factor. The lumen of the appendix forms a sort of test-tube, in which the fæces lodge and are with difficulty discharged, so that the mucosa is liable to injury from retention of the secretions or from the presence of inspissated fæces or occasionally foreign bodies. The anatomical features of the appendix render it liable to ulceration, strangulation and perforation. In some instances the appendicitis is a local expression of a general infection. The causes of the undoubted increase of the disease are not known; some have attributed it to the prevalence of influenza. The acute catarrhal form may be associated with pneumonia or typhoid fever or any of the acute infections. Direct injury, as in straining and heavy lifting, is an occasional exciting cause. Other conditions, tuberculosis and actinomycosis, may present the features of acute appendicitis. Cancer was found in 22 of 5,000 appendices removed at the Mayo Clinic and in 4 among 7,000 cases reported by Adams.

The bacteriology is most varied. The *Bacillus coli* is present in a large number of cases, and the pyogenic organisms, particularly the *Streptococcus pyogenes.* A fresh conception of the etiology is suggested by the work of Rosenow. As is well known, the dominant parasite in appendicitis is the colon bacillus, either in pure culture or with streptococci and staphylococci; the former chiefly in the lumen, the latter in the walls of the tube. Rosenow claims that in most cases appendicitis is a blood infection secondary to a distant focus such as the tonsil: and it would appear that streptococci circulating in the blood have an elective affinity for the appendix. In 19 of 29 animals appendicitis was produced by injection of human tonsillar strains of organisms.

AGE.—Appendicitis is a disease of young persons, 50 per cent. of the cases occurring before the twentieth year. It has been met with as early as the seventh week, but it is rarely seen prior to the fifth year. Of 1,223 cases at the Johns Hopkins Hospital only 9 cases were under 5 years, 59 in children under 10, 140 between 11 and 15, 199 between 16 and 20, and 255 between 21 and 25 (Churchman).

SEX.—It is about equally common in males and in females.

In England since 1901 the mortality has increased from 38 per million to 75 in 1911, and 68 in 1913. There is an increase in the years of high diarrhœal mortality. The figures do not bear out any belief that the increased frequency is a result of changes in diet. There were 9,374 deaths in the registration area of the United States in 1917.

Indiscretions in diet are very prone to bring on an attack, particularly in the recurring form of the disease, in which pain in the appendix region not infrequently follows the eating of indigestible articles of food.

Varieties.—McCarty from a study of 5,000 appendices removed at the Mayo clinic makes the following classification:

(*a*) APPENDICITIS CATARRHALIS ACUTA, a condition in which the mucosa is infiltrated with leucocytes and congested with inflammatory reaction in the lymph follicles and lymphatic tissues of the submucosa.

(*b*) APPENDICITIS CATARRHALIS CHRONICA, following repeated mild or severe acute catarrh, marked by increase of scar tissue, and distortion of the normal regularity of the structure. Blood pigment is often present.

(*c*) APPENDICITIS PURULENTA NECROTICA, an advanced stage of the acute catarrhal condition, plus the formation of intramural abscesses, necrosis, and perforation.

(*d*) PERI-APPENDICITIS ACUTA, an extension to the peritoneum of the conditions just described.

(*e*) OBLITERATION, a condition of the lumen, the result of destruction of the mucosa and the formation of scar tissue, occurring in about 24 per cent. of all cases, and an inflammatory, not an involutionary, process.

There are cases, too, in which the appendix becomes sphacelated *en masse,* and may slough off.

Fæcal Concretions.—The lumen of the appendix may contain a mould of fæces, which can readily be squeezed out. Even while soft the contents of the tube may be moulded in two or three sections with rounded ends. Concretions —enteroliths, coproliths—are also common. Of 700 cases of foreign bodies there were 45 per cent. of fæcal concretions (J. F. Mitchell). The enteroliths often resemble date stones in shape. The importance of these concretions is shown by the great frequency with which they are found in all acute inflammations of the appendix.

Foreign Bodies.—Of 1,400 cases of appendicitis collected by J. F. Mitchell these were present in 7 per cent.; in 28 cases pins were found. It is well to bear in mind that some of the concretions bear a very striking resemblance to cherry and date stones.

Symptoms.—In a large proportion of all cases of acute appendicitis the following symptoms are present: (*a*) Sudden pain in the abdomen, usually referred to the right iliac fossa; (*b*) fever, often of moderate grade; (*c*) gastro-intestinal disturbance—nausea, vomiting, and frequently constipation; (*d*) tenderness or pain on pressure in the appendix region.

Pain.—A sudden, violent pain in the abdomen is the most constant, first, decided symptom of perforating inflammation of the appendix, and occurred in 84 per cent. of the cases analyzed by Fitz. In fully half of the cases it is localized in the right iliac fossa, but it may be central, diffuse, but usually in the right half of the abdomen. Even in the cases in which the pain is at first not in the appendix region it is usually felt here within thirty-six or forty-eight hours. It may extend toward the perineum or testicle. It is sometimes very sharp and colic-like, and cases have been mistaken for nephritic or for biliary colic. Some patients speak of it as a sharp, intense pain—serous-membrane pain; others as a dull ache—connective-tissue pain. While a very valuable symptom, pain is at the same time one of the most misleading. Some of the forms of recurring pain in the appendix region Talamon called appendicular colic. The condition is believed to be due to partial occlusion of the lumen, leading to violent and irregular peristaltic action of the circular and longitudinal muscles.

Fever.—Fever is always present in the early stage, even in the mildest forms, and is a most important feature. J. B. Murphy stated that he would not operate on a case in which he was confident that no fever had been present in the first thirty-six hours of the disease. An initial chill is very rare. The fever may be moderate, from 100° to 102°; sometimes in children at the very outset the thermometer may register above 103.5°. The thermometer is one of the most trustworthy guides in the diagnosis of acute appendicitis. Appendicular colic of great severity may occur without fever. When a localized abscess has formed, and in some very virulent cases of general peritonitis, the temperature may be normal, but at this stage there are other symptoms which indicate the gravity of the situation. The pulse is quickened in proportion to the fever.

Gastro-intestinal Disturbance.—The tongue is usually furred and moist, seldom dry. Nausea and vomiting may be absent, but are commonly present in the acute perforative cases. The vomiting rarely persists beyond the second day in favorable cases. Constipation is the rule, but the attack may set in with diarrhœa, particularly in children.

Lymphoid hyperplasia. This occurs in children or young adults, subjects of status lymphaticus, and is marked by repeated attacks of colic without any marked change in temperature or pulse rate, or leucocytosis (Symmers).

Local Signs.—Inspection of the abdomen is at first negative; there is no distention, and the iliac fossæ look alike. On palpation there are usually from the outset rigidity or muscle spasm of the right rectus muscle, and tenderness or actual pain on deep pressure. The muscular rigidity may be so great that a satisfactory examination can not be made without an anæsthetic. McBurney called attention to a localized point of tenderness on deep pressure, situated at the intersection of a line drawn from the navel to the anterior-superior spine of the ilium, with a second, vertically placed, corresponding to the outer edge of the right rectus muscle. Firm, deep, continuous pressure with one finger at this spot causes pain, often of the most exquisite character. In addition to the tenderness, rigidity, and actual pain on deep pressure, there is to be felt, in some cases, an induration or swelling. This may be a boggy, ill-defined mass in the situation of the cæcum; more commonly the swelling is circumscribed and definite, situated in the iliac fossa, two or three fingers' breadth above Poupart's ligament. Some have been able to feel and roll beneath the fingers the thickened appendix. The later the case comes under observation the greater the probability of the existence of a well-marked tumor mass. It is not to be forgotten that there may be neither tumor mass nor induration to be felt in some of the most intensely virulent cases of perforative appendicitis. The pain may be mistaken for that of hip joint disease.

In addition may be mentioned marked frequency of micturition, especially in children, which may be an early symptom. The urine is scanty and often contains albumin and indican. The attitude is somewhat suggestive, the decubitus is dorsal, and the right leg is semi-flexed. Pulling on the right spermatic cord may cause pain. Examination *per rectum* in the early stages rarely gives any information of value. The symptoms may be entirely pelvic when the appendix dips over the brim and the inflamed area is in direct contact with the uterine adnexa.

LEUCOCYTOSIS.—The blood picture is of value equal to the pulse and temperature. As a rule, in acute attacks there is a leucocytosis of 12,000 to 15,000, chiefly of the polynuclears. In mild catarrhal cases there may be no increase. Usually the degree is an expression of the peritoneal irritation. A low leucocytosis or a leucopenia is an indication of a virulent infection.

Albuminuria is common. Sometimes there is an acute nephritis, and Dieulafoy described an acute toxic form. He thinks that the kidneys are not infrequently damaged in the disease.

There are three possibilities in any case: (1) Gradual recovery, (2) the formation of a local abscess, and (3) general peritonitis.

RECOVERY is the rule in the mild catarrhal cases. The pain lessens at the end of the second or third day, the temperature falls, the tongue becomes cleaner, the vomiting ceases, the local tenderness is less marked, and the bowels are moved. By the end of a week the acute symptoms have subsided. So liable is the attack to recur that relapsing appendicitis is spoken of.

LOCAL ABSCESS FORMATION.—As a result of ulceration and perforation, sometimes following the necrosis, by the end of the fourth or fifth day there is an extensive area of induration in the right iliac fossa, with great tenderness, and operations have shown that even at this very early date an abscess cavity may have formed. Though as a rule the fever becomes aggravated with the onset of suppuration, this is not always the case. The two most important elements in the diagnosis of abscess formation are the gradual increase of the local tumor and the aggravation of the general symptoms. Nowadays, when operation is so frequent, we have opportunities of seeing the abscess in various stages of development. Quite early the pus may lie between the cæcum and the coils of the ileum, with the general peritoneum shut off by fibrin, or there is a sero-fibrinous exudate with a slight amount of pus between the lower coils of the ileum. The abscess cavity may be small and lie on the psoas muscle, or at the edge of the promontory of the sacrum, and never reach a palpable size. The sac, when larger, may be roofed in by the small bowel and present irregular processes and pockets leading in different directions. In larger collections in the iliac fossa the roof is generally formed by the abdominal wall. Some of the most important of the localized abscesses are those which are situated entirely within the pelvis. The various directions and positions into which the abscess may pass or perforate are many and left alone, it may discharge externally, burrow in various directions, or be emptied through the rectum, vagina, or bladder. Death may be caused by septicæmia, by perforation into an artery or vein, or by pylephlebitis.

General Peritonitis.—This may be caused by direct perforation of the appendix and general infection of the peritoneum before any delimiting inflammation is excited. In a second group of cases there has been an attempt at localizing the infective process, but it fails, and the general peritoneum becomes involved. In a third group of cases a localized focus of suppuration exists about an inflamed appendix, and from this perforation takes place.

Death in appendicitis is due usually to general peritonitis.

The gravity of appendix disease lies in the fact that from the very onset the peritoneum may be infected; the initial symptoms of pain, with nausea and vomiting, fever, and local tenderness, present in all cases, may indicate a wide-spread infection of this membrane. The onset is usually sudden, the pain diffuse, not always localized in the right iliac fossa, but it is not so much the character as the greater intensity of the symptoms from the outset that makes one suspicious of a general peritonitis. Abdominal distention, diffuse tenderness, and absence of abdominal movements are the most trustworthy local signs, but they are not really so trustworthy as the general symptoms. The initial nausea and vomiting persist, the pulse becomes more rapid, the tongue is dry, the urine scanty. In very acute cases, by the end of twenty-four hours the abdomen may be distended. By the third and fourth days the classical picture of a general peritonitis is well established—a distended and motionless abdomen, a rapid pulse, a dry tongue, dorsal decubitus with the knees drawn up, and an anxious, pinched, Hippocratic facies. The picture may be that of septicopyæmia or sapræmia; high fever, chills, sweats, without local reaction. These are generally acute, gangrenous cases with anomalous position of the appendix, behind the colon, or deep in the pelvis. Even when looked for carefully there may be no local indications. Sometimes there have been gastro-intestinal symptoms for a few days before, to which no attention has been paid. In one case, seen by the family physician at 2 p. m. for the first time, by the senior author at 4.30 p. m., at 7 p. m. by a surgeon who refused to operate, death occurred within 12 hours after the physician was first called.

Remote Effects.—The remote effects of perforative appendicitis are interesting. Hæmorrhage may occur. In one of our cases the appendix was adherent to the promontory of the sacrum, and the abscess cavity had perforated in two places into the ileum. Death resulted from profuse hæmorrhage. Cases are on record in which the internal iliac artery or the deep circumflex iliac artery has been opened. Suppurative pylephlebitis may result from inflammation of the mesenteric veins near the perforated appendix. The appendix may perforate in a hernial sac. Distant disorders attributed to disease of the appendix are various types of gastric dyspepsia, ulcer, spasm of the pylorus, pancreatitis, bile tract infection and cirrhosis of the liver.

After operation, thrombosis of the iliac or femoral veins is not uncommon, and sudden death from pulmonary embolism has followed. The leg may be permanently enlarged. Hernia may occur in the wound. Strangulation of the bowel is an occasional sequence. Recurrence of the symptoms after operation has been noted, due in some cases to incomplete removal.

Diagnosis.—Appendicitis is by far the most common inflammatory condition, not only in the cæcal region, but in the abdomen generally in persons under thirty. The surgeons have taught us that, almost without exception, sudden pain in the right iliac fossa, with fever and localized tenderness, with or without tumor, means appendix disease. There are certain diseases of the abdominal organs characterized by pain which are apt to be confounded with appendicitis. Biliary colic, kidney colic, and the colicky pains at the menstrual period in women have to be carefully considered.

Diseases of the tubes and pelvic peritonitis may simulate appendicitis very closely, but the history and the local examination under ether should in most cases enable the practitioner to reach a diagnosis. Some cases supposed to be recurring appendicitis prove to be tubo-ovarian disease.

The Dietl's crises in floating kidney have been mistaken for appendicitis.

Acute hæmorrhagic pancreatitis may produce symptoms very like those of appendicitis with general peritonitis. The relation of typhoid fever and appendicitis is interesting. The gastro-intestinal symptoms, particularly the pain and the fever, may at the onset suggest appendicitis. Operations have been comparatively frequent. In the second and third weeks of typhoid fever perforation of the appendix may occur, and occasionally late in the convalescence perforation of an unhealed ulcer of the appendix.

In a great many patients with *chronic appendicitis* stomach symptoms predominate, and an appendicular dyspepsia has been recognized particularly by the French writers and by surgeons. Many of the patients are neurotic. The dyspeptic symptoms are irregular, and food rarely gives relief, as in ulcer. Pain is the prevailing symptom, often caused by food, and more abdominal than epigastric, without radiation, and there are frequently pain and tenderness at McBurney's point. Vomiting is rare, but there is usually much flatulency. Without being seriously ill, the patient's condition is constantly below par, and he may go the rounds of physicians for years. In an analysis of 100 cases of this type at the Mayo clinic by Graham and Guthrie, reported on a year after operation, 77 per cent. were cured by the removal of the appendix. As a majority of these patients are neurotic, it is not easy to say how far the good results have been due directly to the removal of the appendix, the pathological condition of which, as reported upon by Graham and Guthrie, did not seem to differ much from that which is met with, according to Aschoff, in a majority of individuals in the fourth decade. In a certain number of these patients the relief after removal of the appendix is not permanent.

There is a well-marked appendicular hypochondriasis. Through the pernicious influence of the daily press, appendicitis has become a sort of fad, and the physician has often to deal with patients who have almost a fixed idea that they have the disease. Hysteria may simulate appendicitis very closely, and it may require a very keen judgment to make a diagnosis. Mucous colitis with enteralgia in nervous women is sometimes mistaken for appendicitis.

Perinephritic and pericæcal abscess from perforation of ulcer, either simple or cancerous, and circumscribed peritonitis in this region from other causes, can rarely be differentiated until an exploratory incision is made.

Chronic obliterative appendicitis can not always be differentiated from the perforative form, and in intensity of pain, severity of symptoms, and, in rare instances, even in the production of peritonitis, the two may be identical.

Briefly stated, localized pain in the right iliac fossa, with or without induration or tumor, the existence of McBurney's tender point, fever, furred tongue, vomiting, with constipation or diarrhœa, indicate appendicitis. The occurrence of general peritonitis is suggested by increase and diffusion of the abdominal pain, tympanites (as a rule), marked aggravation of the constitutional symptoms, particularly elevation of fever and increased rapidity of the pulse. Obliteration of hepatic dulness is rarely present, as the peritoneum in these cases does not often contain gas.

Appendicitis and Pregnancy.—The association is not uncommon. Of 103 perforative or gangrenous cases 89 were operated upon, with 36 deaths. Of 14 cases not operated upon all died. Of the 103 cases 80 aborted before or after operation. Of 104 non-perforative cases 50 were operated upon with 1 death; of the remaining 54, 4 died; 13 of these non-perforative cases aborted (Babler). Mild cases recover; in the severer forms it is safer to operate at once.

Prognosis.—*There would be no percentage of deaths from appendicitis if every case commencing with acute pain and developing tenderness and rigidity of the abdomen and quickening of the pulse were operated upon within twelve hours* (Rutherford Morison).

The mortality from the operative cases is steadily diminishing. At the London Hospital, the mortality in the 1,000 cases operated upon between January, 1900, and August, 1904, was 17.2 per cent., whilst in the 1,000 consecutive cases operated upon between 1912 and the first six weeks of 1913 the mortality was 3.2 per cent., and only 4 per cent for the 698 cases operated upon during the attack (Lett). The earlier the operation the lower the mortality. It would be interesting to know how many of the 9,374 fatal cases in 1917 in the United States had been operated upon and at what period.

Treatment.—Gradually the profession has learned to recognize that appendicitis is a surgical disease. In hospital practice the cases should be admitted directly to the surgical wards. Many lives are lost by temporizing. The general practitioner does well to remember—whether his leanings be toward conservative or radical methods of treatment—that the surgeon is often called too late, never too early.

There is no medicinal treatment of appendicitis. There are remedies which will allay the pain, but there are none capable in any way of controlling the course of the disease. Rest in bed, no food, no purgation, the use of an enema if necessary, gastric lavage if there is vomiting, are the wisest measures till a decision as to operation is reached. The practice of giving opium in some form in appendicitis and peritonitis is decreasing, but is still too common. The persistent use of ice locally may be employed to relieve the pain. General opinion is opposed to the use of purges.

Operation is indicated in all cases of acute inflammatory trouble in the cæcal region, whether tumor is present or not, when the general symptoms are severe, and *when at the end of twelve hours, or even earlier, the features of the case point to a progressive lesion.* The mortality from early operation under these circumstances is very slight.

In recurring appendicitis, when the attacks are of such severity and frequency as seriously to interrupt the patient's occupation, the mortality in the hands of capable operators is very small.

IV. INTESTINAL OBSTRUCTION

Intestinal obstruction may be caused by strangulation, intussusception, twists and knots, strictures and tumors, by abnormal contents, and by paralysis of the muscular coat of the bowel.

Etiology and Pathology.—(*a*) STRANGULATION.—This is the most frequent cause of acute obstruction, and occurred in 34 per cent. of the 295 cases analyzed by Fitz, and in 35 per cent. of the 1,134 cases of Leichtenstern. Of the 101 cases of strangulation in Fitz's table, which has the special value of having been carefully selected from the literature since 1880, the following were the causes: Adhesions, 63; vitelline remains, 21; adherent appendix, 6; mesenteric and omental slits, 6; peritoneal pouches and openings, 3; adherent tube, 1; peduncular tumor, 1. The bands and adhesions result, in a majority of cases, from former peritonitis. A number of instances have been reported following operations upon the pelvic organs in women. The strangulation may be recent and due to adhesion of the bowel to the abdominal wound or a coil may be caught between the pedicle of a tumor and the pelvic wall. Such cases are only too common. Late occlusion after recovery from the operation is due to bands and adhesions.

The vitelline remains are represented by Meckel's diverticulum, which forms a finger-like projection from the ileum, usually within eighteen inches of the ileo-cæcal valve. The coils of the intestine may be strangulated about the diverticulum when its end is attached to the abdominal wall, to the mesentery, or to another portion of the intestine, or a long diverticulum unattached may be twisted, or there may be inversion of the diverticulum into the lumen of the bowel causing obstruction or leading to intussusception.

Seventy per cent. of the cases of obstruction from strangulation occur in males; 40 per cent. of all the cases occur between the ages of fifteen and thirty years. In 90 per cent. of the cases of obstruction from these causes the site of the trouble is in the small bowel; the position of the strangulated portion was in the right iliac fossa in 67 per cent. of the cases, and in the lower abdomen in 83 per cent.

(*b*) INTUSSUSCEPTION.—In this condition one portion of the intestine slips into an adjacent portion, forming an invagination or intussusception. The two portions make a cylindrical tumor, which varies in length from a half inch to a foot or more. The condition is always a descending intussusception, and, as the process proceeds, the middle and inner layers increase at the expense of the outer layer. An intussusception consists of three layers of bowel: the outermost, known as the intussuscipiens, or receiving layer; a middle or returning layer; and the innermost or entering layer. The student can obtain a clear idea of the arrangement by making the end of a glove-finger pass into the lower portion. The actual condition can be very clearly studied in the post mortem invaginations which are so common in the small bowel of children. In the statistics of Fitz, 93 of 295 cases of acute intestinal obstruction were due to this cause. Of these, 52 were in males and 27 in females. The cases are most common in early life, 34 per cent. under one year and 56 per cent. under the tenth year. Of 103 cases in children, nearly 50 per cent. occurred in the fourth, fifth, and sixth months (Wiggin). No definite causes could be assigned in 42 of the cases; in the others diarrhœa or habitual constipation had existed.

The site of the invagination varies. We may recognize (1) an *ileo-cæcal,* when the ileo-cæcal valve descends into the colon. There are cases in which this is so extensive that the valve has been felt *per rectum.* This form occurred in 75 per cent. of the cases; in 89 per cent. of Wiggin's collected cases. In the *ileo-colic* the lower part of the ileum passes through the ileo-cæcal valve. (2) The *ileal,* in which the ileum is alone involved. (3) The *colic,* in which it is confined to the large intestine. (4) *Colico-rectal,* in which the colon and rectum are involved. (5) Intussusception of the appendix is rare, but there are cases on record, most of them in children.

Irregular peristalsis is the essential cause of intussusception. Nothnagel found in the localized peristalsis caused by the faradic current that it was not the descent of one portion into the other, but the drawing up of the receiving layer by contraction of the longitudinal coat. Invagination may follow any limited, sudden, and severe peristalsis.

In the post mortem examination, in a case of death from intussusception, the condition is very characteristic. Peritonitis may be present or an acute injection of the serous membrane. When death occurs early, as it may do from shock, there is little to be seen. The portion of bowel affected is large and thick, and forms an elongated tumor with a curved outline. The parts are swollen and congested, owing to the constriction of the mesentery between the layers. The entire mass may be of a deep livid-red color. In very recent processes there is only congestion, and perhaps a thin layer of lymph, and the intussusception can be reduced, but when it has lasted for a few days, lymph is thrown out, the layers are glued together, and the entering portion of the gut can not be withdrawn.

The anatomical condition accounts for the presence of the tumor, which exists in two-thirds of all cases; and the engorgement, which results from the compression of the mesenteric vessels, explains the frequent occurrence of blood in the discharges, which has so important a diagnostic value. If the patient survives, necrosis and sloughing of the invaginated portion may occur, and, if union has taken place between the inner and outer layers, the calibre of the gut may be restored and a cure in this way effected. Many cases of the kind are on record. In the Museum of McGill University are 17 inches of small intestine, which were passed by a lad who had symptoms of internal strangulation, and who made a complete recovery.

(*c*) Twists, Knots, and Traction Kinks.—Volvulus or twist occurred in 42 of the 295 cases (Fitz). Sixty-eight per cent. were in males. It is most frequent between the ages of thirty and forty. In the great majority of all cases the twist is axial and associated with an unusually long mesentery. In 50 per cent. of the cases it was in the sigmoid flexure. The next most common situation is about the cæcum, which may be twisted upon its axis or bent upon itself. As a rule, in volvulus the loop of bowel is simply twisted upon its long axis, and the portions at the end of the loop cross each other and so cause the strangulation. It occasionally happens that one portion of the bowel is twisted about another.

Traction kinks occur at three regions—the third portion of the duodenum, the last part of the ileum, and the sigmoid flexure. What is known as gastromesenteric ileus is caused by compression of the lower portion of the duodenum by the root of the mesentery with its contained blood-vessels. The condition has been described under acute dilatation of the stomach.

The *ileum kink* occurs within a few inches of the cæcum. This portion has a short tight mesentery and a large loose cæcum sags over the brim of the pelvis and may cause a definite kink of the ileum with constipation, pain in the right iliac fossa, and symptoms which simulate appendicitis.

Traction of a very full sigmoid flexure may, without any special twist, compress and obstruct a neighboring coil of the colon.

(*d*) Strictures and Tumors.—These are very much less important causes of acute obstruction, as may be judged by the fact that there are only 15 instances out of the 295 cases, in 14 of which the obstruction occurred in the large intestine (Fitz). On the other hand, they are common causes of chronic obstruction. Lipoma may occur, growing from the submucosa, and cause intussusception. In a number of cases the tumor has been passed *per rectum.* S. B. Ward collected 9 cases.

The obstruction may result from: (1) *Congenital stricture.* These are exceedingly rare. Much more commonly the condition is that of complete occlusion, either forming the imperforate anus or the congenital defect by which the duodenum is not united to the pylorus. (2) *Simple cicatricial stenosis,* which results from ulceration, tuberculous or syphilitic, more rarely from dysentery, and most rarely of all from typhoid ulceration. (3) *New growths.* The malignant strictures are due chiefly to cylindrical epithelioma, which forms an annular tumor, most commonly met with in the large bowel, about the sigmoid flexure, or the descending colon. Of benign growths, papillomata, adenomata, lipomata, and fibromata occasionally induce obstruction. (4) *Compression and traction.* Tumors of neighboring organs, particularly of the pelvic viscera, may cause obstruction by adhesion and traction. In the healing of tuberculous peritonitis the contraction of the thick exudate may cause compression and narrowing of the coils.

(*e*) Abnormal Contents.—Foreign bodies, such as fruit stones, coins, pins, needles, or false teeth, are occasionally swallowed. Round worms may become rolled into a tangled mass and cause obstruction. In reality, however, the majority of foreign bodies, such as coins, buttons, and pins, swallowed by children, cause no inconvenience whatever, but in a day or two are found in the stools. Occasionally such a foreign body as a pin will pass through the œsophagus and will be found lodged in some adjacent organ, as in the heart (Peabody), or a barley ear may reach the liver (Dock).

Medicines, such as magnesia or bismuth, have been known to accumulate in the bowels and produce obstruction, but in the great majority of the cases the condition is caused by fæces, gall-stones, or enteroliths. Of 44 cases, in 23 the obstruction was by gall-stones, in 19 by fæces, and in 2 by enteroliths. Obstruction by fæces may happen at any period of life. As mentioned when speaking of the dilatation of the colon, it may occur in young children and persist for weeks. In fæcal accumulation the large bowel may reach an enormous size and the contents become very hard. The retained masses may be channeled, and small quantities of fæcal matter are passed until a mass too large enters the lumen and causes obstruction. There may be very few symptoms, as the condition may be borne for weeks or even for months.

Obstruction by *gall-stones* is not very infrequent, as may be gathered from the fact that 23 cases were reported in the literature in eight years. Eighteen of these were in women and 5 in men. In six-sevenths of the cases it occurred about the fiftieth year. The obstruction is usually in the ileo-cæcal region, but it may be in the duodenum. These large solitary gall-stones ulcerate through the gall-bladder, usually into the small intestine, occasionally into the colon. In the latter case they rarely cause obstruction. Courvoisier has collected 131 cases in the literature.

Enteroliths may be formed of masses of hair, more commonly of the phosphates of lime and magnesia, with a nucleus formed of a foreign body or of hardened fæces. Nearly every museum possesses specimens of this kind. They are not so common in men as in ruminants, and, as indicated in Fitz's statistics, are very rare causes of obstruction.

(*f*) Paralytic Ileus.—Without any obstruction in the lumen, in a localized area or in a wide section of the bowel, the muscular walls may be so paralyzed that no movement of the contents occurs, causing a condition which virtually amounts to obstruction. The best illustrations of local paralytic ileus are seen in the embolic and thrombotic processes in the mesenteric arteries, when the corresponding portions of the intestinal wall are in a state of infarct. This occurs in the verminous aneurism in a horse, and is associated with the common intestinal colic. It is more common in the small than in the large bowel, but in one instance of paralytic ileus due to localized involvement of about eight inches of the wall of the transverse colon there was not, so far as one could discover, any affection of the blood-vessels; the symptoms were those of acute obstruction.

Following operations, particularly on the abdomen, after injuries, following paracentesis in ascites, in pneumonia, pleurisy, and occasionally in heart disease, a paralytic state of the bowel may occur, with cessation of peristalsis, distention of the abdomen, vomiting, and other signs of obstruction. There are remarkable cases of hysteria with symptoms of chronic obstruction of the bowels and fæcal vomiting—the so-called ileus hystericus.

Symptoms.—(*a*) Acute Obstruction.—Constipation, pain in the abdomen and vomiting are the three important symptoms. Pain sets in early and may come on abruptly while the patient is walking, or, more commonly, during the performance of some action. It is at first colicky in character, but subsequently it becomes continuous and very intense. Vomiting follows quickly and is a constant and most distressing symptom. At first the contents of the stomach are voided, and then greenish, bile-stained material, and soon, in cases of acute and permanent obstruction, the material vomited is a brownish-black liquid, with a distinctly fæcal odor. This sequence of gastric, bilious, and, finally, stercoraceous vomiting is perhaps the most important diagnostic feature of acute obstruction. The constipation may be absolute, without the discharge of either fæces or gas. Very often the contents of the bowel below the stricture are discharged. Distention of the abdomen usually occurs, and, when the large bowel is involved, it is extreme. On the other hand, if the obstruction is high up in the small intestine, there may be very slight tympany. At first the abdomen is not painful, but subsequently it may become acutely tender.

The constitutional symptoms from the outset are severe. The face is pallid and anxious, and finally collapse symptoms supervene. The eyes become sunken, the features pinched, and the skin is covered with a cold, clammy sweat. The pulse becomes rapid and feeble. There may be no fever; the axillary temperature is often subnormal. The tongue is dry and parched and the thirst is incessant. The urine is high-colored, scanty, and there may be suppression, particularly when the obstruction is high up in the bowel. This is probably due to the constant vomiting and the small amount of liquid which is absorbed. The case terminates, as a rule, in from three to six days. In some instances the patient dies from shock or sinks into coma. A leucocytosis of 75,000 or 80,000 may be present.

(*b*) Symptoms of Chronic Obstruction.—When due to fæcal impaction, there is a history of long-standing constipation. There may have been discharge of mucus, or, in some instances, the fæcal masses have been channeled, and so have allowed the contents of the upper portion of the bowel to pass through. In elderly persons this is not infrequent; but examination, either *per rectum* or externally, in the course of the colon, will reveal the presence of hard scybalous masses. There may be retention of fæces for weeks without exciting serious symptoms. In other instances there are vomiting, pain in the abdomen, gradual distention, and finally the ejecta become fæcal. The hardened masses may excite an intense colitis or even peritonitis.

In stricture, whether cicatricial or cancerous, the symptoms of obstruction are very diverse. Constipation gradually comes on, is extremely variable, and it may be months or even years before there is complete obstruction. There are transient attacks, in which from some cause the fæces accumulate above the stricture, the intestine becomes greatly distended, and in the swollen abdomen the coils can be seen in active peristalsis. In such attacks there may be vomiting, but it is very rarely of a fæcal character. In the majority of these cases the general health is seriously impaired; the patient gradually becomes anæmic and emaciated, and, finally, in an attack in which the obstruction is complete, death occurs with all the features of acute occlusion, or the case may be prolonged for ten or twelve days.

Diagnosis.—(*a*) The Situation of the Obstruction.—Hernia must be excluded, which is by no means always easy, as fatal obstruction may occur from the involvement of a very limited portion of the gut in the external ring or in the obturator foramen. A thorough rectal and, in women, a vaginal examination should be made, which will give important information as to the condition of the pelvic and rectal contents, particularly in cases of intussusception, in which the descending bowel can sometimes be felt. In cases of obstruction high up the empty coils sink into the pelvis and can there be detected. In the inspection of the abdomen there are important indications, as the special prominence in certain regions, the occurrence of well-defined masses, and the presence of hypertrophied coils in active peristalsis. John Wyllie called attention to the great value in diagnosis of the "patterns of abdominal tumidity." In obstruction of the lower end of the large intestine not only may the horseshoe of the colon stand out plainly, when the bowel is in rigid spasm, but even the pouches of the gut may be seen. When the cæcum or lower end of the ileum is obstructed the tumidity is in the lower central region, and during spasm the coils of the small bowel may stand out prominently, one above the other, either obliquely or transversely placed—the so-called "ladder pattern." In obstruction of the duodenum or jejunum there may only be slight distention of the upper part of the abdomen, associated usually with rapid collapse and anuria. The acute toxæmia may be due to proteose intoxication.

In the ileum and cæcum the distention is more in the central portion of the abdomen; the vomiting is distinctly fæcal and occurs early. In obstruction of the colon tympanites is much more extensive and general. Tenesmus is more common, with the passage of mucus and blood. The course is not so quick, the collapse does not supervene so rapidly, and the urinary secretion is not so much reduced.

In obstruction from stricture or tumor the situation can in some cases be accurately localized, but in others it is very uncertain. Digital examination of the rectum should first be made. The rectal tube may then be passed, but it is impossible to get beyond the sigmoid flexure. In the use of the rigid tube there is danger of perforation of the bowel in the neighborhood of a stricture. The quantity of fluid which can be passed into the large intestine should be estimated. The capacity of the large bowel is about six quarts. Wiggin advises about a pint and a half from a height of three feet for an infant. For diagnostic purposes the rectum may be inflated with air. In certain cases these measures give important indications as to the situation of the obstruction in the large bowel. Whenever possible an X-ray examination should be made.

(*b*) NATURE OF THE OBSTRUCTION.—This is often difficult, not infrequently impossible, to determine. *Strangulation* is not common in very early life. In many instances there have been previous attacks of abdominal pain, or there are etiological factors which give a clue, such as old peritonitis or operation on the pelvic viscera. Neither the onset nor the character of the pain gives us any information. In rare instances nausea and vomiting may be absent. The vomiting usually becomes fæcal from the third to the fifth day. A tumor is not common in strangulation, and was present in only one-fifth of the cases. Fever is not of diagnostic value.

Intussusception is an affection of childhood, and is of all forms of internal obstruction the one most readily diagnosed. The onset is acute with pain and signs of shock after which the symptoms may decrease for a time. Vomiting is not constant. The presence of tumor, bloody stools, and tenesmus are the important factors. The tumor is usually sausage-shaped and felt in the region of the transverse colon. It existed in 66 of 93 cases. It became evident the first day in more than one-third of the cases, on the second day in more than one-fourth, and on the third day in more than one-fifth. Blood in the stools occurs in at least three-fifths of the cases, either spontaneously or following the use of an enema. The blood may be mixed with mucus. Tenesmus is present in one-third of the cases. Fæcal vomiting is not very common and was present in only 12 of the 93 instances. Abdominal tympany is a symptom of slight importance, occurring in only one-third of the cases.

Volvulus can rarely be diagnosed. The frequency with which it involves the sigmoid flexure is to be borne in mind. The passage of a flexible tube or injecting fluids might in these cases give valuable indications.

In fæcal obstruction the condition is usually clear, as the fæces can be felt *per rectum* and also in the distended colon. Fæcal vomiting, tympany, abdominal pain, nausea, and vomiting are late and are not so constant. In obstruction by gall-stone a few of the patients gave a previous history of gall-stone colic. Jaundice was present in only 2 of the 23 cases. Pain and vomiting, as a rule, occur early and are severe, and fæcal vomiting is present in two-thirds of the cases. A tumor is rarely evident.

(*c*) Diagnosis from Other Conditions.—Acute enteritis with great relaxation of the intestinal coils, vomiting, and pain may be mistaken for obstruction. Instances have been reported in which peritonitis following disease of the appendix has been mistaken for acute obstruction. The intense vomiting, the general tympany and abdominal tenderness, and, in some instances, the suddenness of the onset are very deceptive. In appendix disease the temperature is more frequently elevated, the vomiting is never fæcal, and in many cases there is a history of previous attacks in the cæcal region. Acute hæmorrhagic pancreatitis may produce symptoms which simulate closely intestinal obstruction.

Treatment.—Purgatives should not be given. For the pain hypodermic injections of morphia are indicated. To allay the distressing vomiting, the stomach should be washed out. Not only is this directly beneficial, but Kussmaul claimed that abdominal distention is relieved, pressure in the bowel above the seat of obstruction lessened, and the violent peristalsis diminished. It may be practised three or four times a day, and in some instances has proved beneficial; in others curative. Thorough irrigation of the large bowel with injections should be done, the warm fluid being allowed to flow in slowly and the amount carefully estimated.

Inflation may also be tried, by forcing the air into the rectum, but this is not without risk, as instances of rupture of the bowel have been reported. Of 39 cases in children treated by inflation or enemata 16 recovered (Wiggin). In cases of acute obstruction surgical measures should be resorted to early.

For the tympanites turpentine stupes and hot applications may be applied. In cases of chronic obstruction the diet must be carefully regulated, and opium and belladonna are useful for the paroxysmal pains. Enemata should be employed, and, if the obstruction becomes complete, resort must be had to surgical measures.

V. CONSTIPATION

(*Costiveness*)

Definition.—Retention of fæces from any cause.

Constipation in Adults.—The causes are varied and may be classed as general and local.

General Causes.—(*a*) Constitutional peculiarities: Torpidity of the bowels is often a family complaint and is found more often in dark than in fair persons. (*b*) Sedentary habits, particularly in persons who eat too much and neglect the calls of nature. (*c*) Certain diseases, such as anæmia, neurasthenia, and hysteria, chronic affections of the liver, stomach, and intestines, and the acute fevers. Under this heading may appropriately be placed that most injurious of all habits, *drug-taking*. (*d*) Either a coarse diet, which leaves too much residue, or a diet which leaves too little.

Local Causes.—Weakness of the abdominal muscles in obesity or from overdistention in repeated pregnancies. Atony of the large bowel from chronic disease of the mucosa; the presence of tumors, physiological or pathological, pressing upon the bowel; enteritis; foreign bodies, large masses of scybala, and strictures of all kinds. An important local cause is atony of the colon, particularly of the muscles of the sigmoid flexure by which the fæces are propelled into the rectum. An obstinate form is that associated with a contracted state of the bowel, sometimes spoken of as *spasmodic* constipation. This is met with—first, as a sequence of chronic dysentery or ulcerative colitis; secondly, in cases of hysteria and neurasthenia, usually with vagotonia; and, thirdly, in very old persons often without any definite cause. It may be that the sigmoid flexure and lower colon are in a condition of contraction and spasm, while the transverse and ascending parts are in a state of atony and dilatation. The most characteristic sign of this variety is the presence of hard, globular masses, or, more rarely, small and sausage-like fæces.

Radiography has taught us much of the conditions favoring intestinal stasis. The upward position in man favors visceroptosis, with which we find associated many of the most obstinate cases of constipation. Arbuthnot Lane has emphasized the fact of this dropping or dragging of the intestines, particularly at certain points—e. g., the third part of the duodenum, at the end of which there may be an abrupt kink associated with a considerable dilatation of the duodenum itself. This is of course relieved immediately when the patient lies down. The second is the ileal kink, caused by a dropping of the cæcum, and the lower coil of the ileum itself. The obstruction may result in considerable dilatation of the end of the ileum, with delay in the passage of the fluid fæces. A third point is the fixed splenic flexure of the colon, and the X-ray may show an ascending colon as low as the level of the iliac crest, and the transverse in the pelvis, necessarily causing delay in the passage of the fæces past this angle. The sigmoid loop seems specially designed to promote stasis; the rectum may also present an elongated S-shaped loop, and, finally, there is the sharp pelvi-rectal flexure, above which the fæces accumulate.

The rate of the passage of the fæces through the large bowel may be estimated accurately with the X-rays. After a bismuth meal the cæcum is reached in about four hours, the hepatic flexure two hours later, the splenic flexure three hours after that, and the beginning of the pelvic colon twelve hours after the commencement of the meal. The fæces do not pass beyond the pelvi-rectal flexure until just before defæcation.

Hurst divides all cases of constipation into two main groups. In one the delay occurs in the passage through the colon, particularly in the distal half; in the other the passage as far as the pelvic colon is normal, but defæcation is not properly performed. Every case of chronic constipation ought to be carefully studied with the X-rays.

Symptoms.—The most persistent constipation for weeks or even months may exist with fair health. Debility, lassitude, and a mental depression are frequent symptoms in constipation, particularly in persons of a nervous temperament. Headache, loss of appetite, a furred tongue, and foul breath may also occur. In girls the skin is "muddy," acne is common, chlorosis may follow, and there is a flabby state of the system generally.

When persistent, the accumulation of fæces leads to unpleasant, sometimes serious, local symptoms, such as piles, ulceration of the colon, distention of the sacculi, perforation, enteritis, and occlusion. In women pressure may cause pain at the time of menstruation and a sensation of fullness and distention in the pelvic organs. Neuralgia of the sacral nerves may be caused by an overloaded sigmoid flexure. The fæces collect chiefly in the colon. Even in extreme grades of constipation it is rare to find dry fæces in the cæcum. The fæces may form large tumors at the hepatic or splenic flexures, or a sausage-like, doughy mass above the navel, or an irregular lumpy tumor in the left inguinal region. In old persons the sacculi of the colon become distended and the scybala may remain in them and undergo calcification, forming enteroliths.

In cases with prolonged retention the fæcal masses become channeled and diarrhœa may occur for days before the true condition is discovered by rectal or external examination. In women who have been habitually constipated attacks of diarrhœa with nausea and vomiting should excite suspicion and lead to a thorough examination of the large bowel. Fever may occur and Meigs reported an instance in which the condition simulated typhoid fever.

Captivated by the theories of Metchnikoff we have been for some years on the crest of a colonic wave, and "intestinal toxæmia" has been held responsible for many of the worst of the ills that flesh is heir to, more particularly arterio-sclerosis and old age. The seniles and preseniles of two continents have been taking sour milk and lacto-bacillary compounds, to the great benefit of the manufacturing chemists! Much of what is regarded as intestinal toxæmia is really intestinal infection.

Constipation in infants is a common and troublesome disorder. The causes are congenital, dietetic, and local. There are instances in which the child is constipated from birth and may not have a natural movement for years, and yet thrive and develop. There are cases of enormous dilatation of the large bowel with persistent constipation. The condition appears sometimes to be a congenital defect. In some of these patients there may be constricting bands, or, as in a case of Cheever's, a congenital stricture.

Dietetic causes are more common. In sucklings it often arises from an unnatural dryness of the small residue which passes into the colon, and it may be very difficult to decide whether the fault is in the mother's milk or in the digestion of the child. Most probably it is in the latter, as some babies may be persistently costive on natural or artificial foods. Deficiency of fat in the milk is believed by some writers to be the cause. In older children it is of the greatest importance that regular habits should be enjoined. Carelessness on the part of the mother in this matter often lays the foundation of troublesome constipation in after life. Impairment of the contractility of the intestinal wall in consequence of inflammation, disturbance in the normal intestinal secretions, and mechanical obstruction by tumors, twists, and intussusception are the chief local causes.

Treatment.—Much may be done by systematic habits, particularly in the young. The patient should go to stool at a fixed hour every day, whether there is desire or not, and the desire should always be granted. Exercise in moderation is helpful. In stout persons and in women with pendulous abdomens the muscles should have the support of a bandage. Friction or regularly applied massage is useful in the more chronic cases. A good substitute is a metal ball weighing from four to six pounds, which may be rolled over the abdomen every morning for five or ten minutes. The function of the stomach should be thoroughly studied and any disturbance properly treated. The diet should be low in protein, with plenty of fruit and vegetables, particularly salads and tomatoes. It is often advisable to cut meat from the diet and substitute cereals, milk and milk foods. Oatmeal is usually laxative, though not to all; brown or bran bread is better than that made from fine white flour. Of liquids, water and aërated mineral waters may be taken freely. A tumblerful of hot or cold water on rising, taken slowly, is efficacious in many cases. A glass of hot water at night may also be tried alone. A pipe or a cigar after breakfast is with many men an infallible remedy.

When the condition is not very obstinate it is well to try to relieve it by hygienic and dietetic measures. If drugs must be used they should be the milder saline laxatives or the compound liquorice powder. Enemata are often necessary, and it is much preferable to employ them early than to constantly use purgative pills. Glycerine either in the form of suppository or as a small injection is very valuable. Injections of tepid water, with or without soap, may be used for a prolonged period with good effect and without damage. The patient should be in the dorsal position with the hips elevated, and it is best to let the fluid flow in slowly from a fountain syringe.

The usual remedies employed are often useless in spastic constipation. A very satisfactory measure is the olive or cotton seed oil injection. The patient lies on the back with the hips elevated, and from 15 to 20 ounces of oil are allowed to flow slowly (or are injected) into the bowel. The operation should take at least fifteen minutes. This may be repeated every day until the intestine is cleared, and subsequently a smaller injection every few days will suffice. In the cases with a spastic colon the injection of oil at bedtime, which is retained during the night, is often effectual.

There are various drugs which are of special service, particularly the combination of ipecacuanha, nux vomica, or belladonna, with aloes, or podophyllin. Cascara sagrada, phenolphthalein, and agar agar are useful. Persistent effort should be made to reduce the dosage by attention to hygienic measures. At present petroleum oil in some form is much in vogue. It was introduced in 1885 by Randolph. It is given in doses from half an ounce to one ounce one to three times a day. It is harmless, sometimes effective, very often without any influence whatever. In anæmia and chlorosis, a sulphur confection taken in the morning, and a pill of iron, rhubarb, and aloes throughout the day, are very serviceable. Certain very severe cases are benefited by "short-circuiting," the lower end of the ileum being joined to the lower end of the colon.

In children the indications should be met, as far as possible, by hygienic and dietetic measures. In the constipation of sucklings a change in the diet of the mother may be tried, or from one to three teaspoonfuls of cream may be given before each nursing. In artificially fed children the top milk with the cream should be used. Drinking of water, barley water, or oatmeal water will sometimes obviate the difficulty. If laxatives are required, simple syrup, manna, or olive oil may be sufficient. The conical piece of soap, so often seen in nurseries, is sometimes efficacious. Massage along the colon may be tried. Small injections of cold water may be used. Large injections should be avoided, if possible. If it is necessary to give a laxative by the mouth, castor oil or fluid magnesia is the best. The saline purgatives appear to act by increasing the muscular and glandular activity of the bowel. If there are signs of gastro-intestinal irritation, rhubarb and soda or gray powder may be given. In older children the diet should be carefully regulated.

VI. ENTEROPTOSIS

(Glénard's Disease)

Definition.—"Dropping of the viscera," visceroptosis, is not a disease, but a sympton group characterized by looseness of the mesenteric and peritoneal attachments, so that the stomach, the intestines, particularly the transverse colon, the liver, the kidneys, and the spleen occupy an abnormally low position in the abdominal cavity.

Symptoms and Physical Signs.—There are two varieties: in one, which may be called constitutional or *congenital,* it is an expression of an anomaly of development, a narrow upper abdominal opening, low diaphragm and elongated visceral ligaments, all of which combined lead to a greater or less degree of prolapse of the abdominal viscera. The second group, or the *acquired* enteroptosis, is largely due to relaxation of the abdominal wall. The support of the viscera is due to the integrity of the reflex arc and abdominal muscles, the tonic action of which, as shown by the studies of Keith and of Sherrington, is brought into play by a reflex, the afferent end organs of which are the peritoneal nerves and Pacinian bodies.

In the first group is embraced a somewhat motley series of cases, in which, with a pronounced nervous or, as we call it now, neurasthenic basis, there are displacements of the viscera *with symptoms.* The patients are usually young, more frequently women than men, and of spare habit. The condition may follow an acute illness with wasting. They complain, as a rule, of dyspepsia, throbbing in the abdomen, and dragging pains or weakness in the back, and inability to perform the usual duties of life. A very considerable proportion of all the cases of neurasthenia present the local features of enteroptosis. When preparing for the examination one notices usually an erythematous flushing of the skin; the scratch of the nail is followed instantly by a line of hyperæmia, less often of marked pallor. The pulsation of the abdominal aorta is readily seen.

In the second group inspection of the abdomen shows a very relaxed abdominal wall, and, as a rule, the lineæ albicantes of recurring pregnancies. Peristalsis of the intestines may be seen, and in extreme cases the outlines of the stomach itself with its waves of peristalsis. On inflating the stomach the organ stands out with great prominence, and the lesser and greater curvatures are seen, the latter extending perhaps a hand's breadth below the level of the navel. The waves of peristalsis are feeble and without the vigor and force of those seen in the stomach dilated from stricture of the pylorus. The condition of descensus ventriculi with atony is best studied in this group of cases. An important point to remember is that it may exist in an extreme grade without symptoms.

Radiography has given much information of the position of the viscera. The stomach is vertically placed and reaches far below the navel; its motility may be normal, but there may be stasis from associated pyloric spasm or from kinking of the duodenum. Clapotâge or splashing is usually distinct.

Nephroptosis, or displacement of the *kidney,* is one of the most constant phenomena in enteroptosis. It is well, perhaps, to distinguish between the kidney which one can just touch on deep inspiration—palpable kidney—one which is freely movable, and which on deep inspiration descends so that one can put the fingers of the palpating hand above it and hold it down, and, thirdly, a floating kidney, which is entirely outside the costal arch, is easily grasped in the hand, readily moved to the middle line, and low down toward the right iliac fossa. It is held by some that the designation floating kidney should be restricted to the cases in which there is a meso-nephron, but this is excessively rare, while extreme grades of renal mobility are common. Some of the more serious sequences of movable kidney, namely, Dietl's crises and intermittent hydronephrosis, will be considered with diseases of the kidney.

Displacement of the *liver* is very much less common. In thin women who have laced, the organ is often tilted forward, so that a very large surface of the lobes comes in contact with the abdominal wall; it is a very common mistake under these circumstances to think that the organ is enlarged. Dislocation of the liver itself will be considered later.

Mobility of the *spleen* is sometimes very marked in enteroptosis. In an extreme grade it may be found in almost any region of the abdomen. It is very frequently mistaken for a fibroid or ovarian tumor. A considerable proportion of the cases come first under the care of the gynæcologist.

There is usually much relaxation of the mesentery and of the peritoneal folds which support the intestines. The colon is displaced downward (coloptosis), with consequent kinking at the flexures. The descent may be so low that the transverse colon is at the brim of or even in the pelvis. It may indeed be fixed or bent in the form of a V. It is frequently to be felt, as Glénard states, as a firm cord crossing the abdomen at or below the level of the navel. This kinking may take place not only in the colon, but at the pylorus, where the duodenum passes into the jejunum, and where the ileum enters the cæcum.

The *cæcum* may be very movable and with this there may be pain, attacks of colic and constipation. There may be fullness in the cæcal region and on palpation the distended cæcum is easily felt. The mass may be very movable.

The explanation of the phenomena accompanying enteroptosis is by no means easy. It has been suggested by Glénard and others that overfilling of the splanchnic vessels in consequence of displacements and kinking accounts for the feelings of exhaustion and general nervousness. In a large proportion of the cases, however, no symptoms occur until after an illness or some protracted nervous strain.

Treatment.—In a majority of all cases four indications are present: To treat the existing neurasthenia, to relieve the nervous dyspepsia, to overcome the constipation, and to afford mechanical support to the organs. Three of these are considered under their appropriate sections. In cases in which the enteroptosis has followed loss in weight after an acute illness or worries and cares an important indication is to fatten the patient.

A well-adapted abdominal bandage is one of the most important measures in enteroptosis. In many of the milder grades it alone suffices. There is no single simple measure which affords relief to distressing symptoms in so many cases as the abdominal bandage. It is best made of linen, should fit snugly, and should be arranged with straps so that it can not ride up over the hips. A special form must be used for movable kidney. In some cases support may be given by the use of adhesive strapping. Exercises to strengthen the abdominal muscles and proper abdominal breathing are aids. General "setting-up" exercises are often helpful. Some of the more aggravated types of enteroptosis are combined with such features of neurasthenia that a rigid Weir Mitchell treatment is indicated. In a few very refractory cases surgical interference may be called for.

And, lastly, the physician must be careful in dealing with the subjects of enteroptosis not to lay too much stress on the disorder. It is well never to tell the patient that a kidney is movable; the symptoms may date from a knowledge of the existence of the condition.

VII. MISCELLANEOUS AFFECTIONS

I. MUCOUS COLITIS

Known by various names, such as *membranous enteritis, tubular diarrhœa, mucous colic,* and *myxoneurosis intestinalis,* this remarkable disease has been recognized for several centuries. An exhaustive description of it is given by Woodward in vol. ii of the Medical and Surgical Reports of the Civil War. The passage of mucus in large quantities from the bowel is met with, *first,* in catarrh of the intestine, due to various causes. It is not uncommon in children, and may be associated with disturbances of digestion and slight colic. *Secondly,* in local disease or irritation of the bowel, in cancer of the colon and of the rectum. In tubo-ovarian disease much mucus and slime may be passed. *Thirdly,* true mucous colitis, a secretion neurosis of the large intestine met with particularly in nervous and hysterical patients. It is more common in women than in men. It has increased greatly of late years, and has become the fashionable complaint, displacing neuritis to a great extent. There is an abnormal secretion of a tenacious mucus, which may be slimy and gelatinous, like frog-spawn, or it is passed in strings or strips, more rarely as a continuous tubular membrane. The membrane *in situ* adheres closely to the mucosa, but is capable of separation without any lesion of the surface. Microscopically the casts are mucoid, of a uniform granular ground substance through which there are remnants of cells, some of which have undergone a definite hyaline transformation. Triple phosphate, cholesterin, and fatty crystals are present, and occasionally fine, sand-like concretions. The epithelium of the mucosa seems to be intact.

Symptoms.—In a large proportion of all the cases the subjects are nervous in greater or less degree. Some cases have had hysterical outbreaks, and there may be hypochondriasis or melancholia. The patients are self-centred and often much worried about the mucous stools. Some of the cases are among the most distressing with which we have to deal, invalids of many years' standing, neurasthenic to an extreme degree, with recurring attacks of pain and the passage of large quantities of mucus or even intestinal casts.

In many cases the attacks may come on in paroxysms, associated with colicky pains, or occasionally crises of the greatest severity, so that appendicitis may be suspected. Emotional disturbances, worry of all sorts, or an error in diet may bring on an attack. Constipation is a special feature in many cases. Sometimes there are attacks of nervous diarrhœa. Some patients have a movement after each meal. This is due to an active gastro-colic reflex, so that fæces reach the rectum after each meal.

While the disease is obstinate and distressing, it is rarely serious, though Herringham states that he knew of three cases of mucous colitis in which death occurred suddenly, in all with great pain in the left side of the abdomen. The abdomen itself is rarely distended. There is often a painful spot between the navel and the left costal border, tender on pressure, and sometimes the paroxysms of pain seem centred in this region. A spastic condition of the colon frequently exists and is easily recognized by palpation.

Diagnosis.—This is rarely doubtful, but it is important not to mistake the membranes for other substances; thus, the external cuticle of asparagus and undigested portions of meat or sausage-skins sometimes assume forms not unlike mucous casts, but microscopic examination will quickly differentiate them. The presence of ulcers and polypi should be excluded. Mucous colitis with severe pain may be mistaken for appendicitis.

Treatment.—Drugs are of little value. It is quite useless to give bismuth and so-called intestinal remedies. First the basic neurasthenic state is to be dealt with, and this may suffice for a cure. Secondly, daily irrigations of the colon through a long tube—one to two pints of warm alkaline fluid. At Plombières, Harrogate, and other spas this treatment is most successfully carried out. The injection of olive oil at bedtime is sometimes helpful. It should be retained during the night. Thirdly, the coarser sorts of food which leave a large residue should be eaten, and, should these measures fail, the question of irrigating through the appendix or cæcum may be considered.

II. DILATATION OF THE COLON

There are four groups of cases. In the first the distention is entirely gaseous, and occurs not infrequently as a transient condition. In many cases it has an important influence, inasmuch as it may be extreme, pushing up the diaphragm and seriously impairing the action of the heart and lungs. It is an occasional cause of sudden heart-failure. In pneumonia and other acute diseases this inflation of the colon may be extreme.

In the second group are the cases in which the distention of the colon is caused by solid substances, as fæcal matter, occasionally by foreign bodies introduced from without, and more rarely by gall-stones. In institutions, particularly in insane asylums, it is not infrequent to find the aged with great distention of the colon.

When, thirdly, the dilatation is due to an organic obstruction in front of the dilated gut, the colon may reach a very large size. These cases are common enough in malignant tumors and sometimes in volvulus. Dilatation of the sigmoid flexure occurs particularly when this portion of the bowel is congenitally very long. In such cases the bowel may be so distended that it occupies the greater part of the abdomen, pushing up the liver and the diaphragm. An acute condition is sometimes caused by a twist in the meso-colon. And, fourthly—

Idiopathic Dilatation.—Hirschsprung's disease. The cases are not uncommon, occurring in children and in young adults. The sigmoid flexure alone or the entire colon is involved, and the size may be colossal. In Formad's case the circumference of the colon was from fifteen to thirty inches, and the weight of the contents forty-seven pounds. The origin is obscure. In some the condition is congenital, and the dilatation and hypertrophy increase progressively; in others there is an unusually long sigmoid flexure; in others again narrowing of the terminal portion of the descending colon or a valve-like structure has been found. The *symptoms* are very definite—constipation, an enlarged abdomen, attacks of pain with increasing distention, and then diarrhœa, either natural or induced, with relief. Such attacks may occur from birth and continue to the twentieth or thirtieth year. The abdominal picture is distinctive—the great enlargement of the upper half of the abdomen, the spreading of the costal arch, the remarkable length from the ensiform cartilage to the navel, and in the attacks the coils of the colon stand out prominently, and even the longitudinal bands may be seen.

The outlook is uncertain. Medical treatment is of little avail. Scrupulous care of the bowels may check the progress; but, as a rule, it is a progressive malady for which surgery alone offers complete relief. Resection of the enlarged colon has been done in a good many cases. Colotomy gives relief; colostomy has also been successful. Of 44 cases treated surgically, 15 were completely cured and 7 were improved (Finney).

III. INTESTINAL SAND

"Sable Intestinal."—There are two groups of cases in which sand-like material is passed with the stools. The *false,* in which it is made up of the remains of vegetable food and fruits which have resisted digestion or which have become encrusted with earthy salts. *True* intestinal sand of animal origin, gritty fine particles, usually gray, black or brown, is formed in the bowel and is made up largely of lime salts. In mucous colitis this material may be passed at intervals for months.

IV. DIVERTICULITIS—PERISIGMOIDITIS

Congenital diverticula, of which Meckel's is the type, may cause strangulation or obstruction.

Acquired diverticula, commonly hernial protrusion of the mucous and serous coats, occur anywhere in the intestinal tract. In the small bowel they rarely cause symptoms, though in a case reported by one of us with scores of herniæ ranging in size from a marble to an orange, there were distressing audible borborygmi, and Gardinier and Sampson met with an instance of obstruction. The site of election of the common form is the sigmoid flexure near the junction with the rectum and the clinical interest in the frequency with which they are the seat of inflammation—diverticulitis, perisigmoiditis. Teller and Gruner analyzed 324 cases. The evaginations of the mucosa are usually the result of high intra-colic pressure with gas or fæces in the aged. Sixty-eight per cent. of the cases were males.

The secondary pathological processes are *mechanical,* as torsion, formation of concretions and lodgment of foreign bodies; and *inflammatory,* acute diverticulitis, which may rapidly become gangrenous; chronic inflammation leading to thickening, and tumor formation and narrowing; perforation, causing local abscess, general peritonitis or fistula. Other changes are chronic local peritonitis with adhesions, metastatic suppuration, and in late stages cancer may develop.

The *symptoms* rarely permit of more than a tentative diagnosis. Pain in the left lower quadrant with tenderness, rigidity and a mass in a person over sixty, who has been constipated, should suggest diverticulitis as well as cancer. The absence of blood in the stools, the long history of pain, negative sigmoidoscopy, slight fever and good nutrition or even obesity are in favor of the former. Unless specially contra-indicated, the condition calls for operation. W. J. Mayo reports (1917) resection in 42 cases. An important point is that carcinoma coexisted in 13. The mortality was high in the series, 14 per cent.

V. AFFECTIONS OF THE MESENTERY

Hæmorrhage (*Hæmatoma*).—Instances in which the bleeding is confined to the mesenteric tissues are rare; more commonly the condition is associated with hæmorrhagic infiltration of the pancreas and with retroperitoneal hæmorrhage. It occurs in rupture of aneurisms, either of the abdominal aorta or of the superior mesenteric artery, in malignant forms of the infectious fevers, small-pox, and in individuals in whom no predisposing conditions exist.

Affections of the Mesenteric Vessels.—(*a*) ANEURISM (see page 853).

(*b*) EMBOLISM AND THROMBOSIS.—*Infarction of the Bowel.*—When the mesenteric vessels are blocked by emboli or thrombi the condition of infarction follows in the territory supplied, which may pass on to gangrene or to perforation and peritonitis. If the superior mesenteric artery is blocked the result is fatal. In the veins the thrombosis may be primary, following infective processes in the intestines, particularly about the appendix, or it occurs in cachectic states. Secondary thrombosis is met with in cirrhosis of the liver, syphilis, and pylephlebitis, or may result from the stasis caused by arterial emboli. Jackson, Porter, and Quimby made an exhaustive study of 30 Boston cases, and collected 214 cases. They recognize two groups—acute and chronic. In the former the onset is sudden, with colic, nausea, vomiting, and a bloody diarrhœa, so that the picture is one of acute obstruction. The abdomen becomes distended and death occurs in collapse within a few days. In the chronic cases the onset is insidious, and there may be no symptoms referable to the abdomen. Of the 214 cases, 64 per cent. were in men. The diagnosis is extremely difficult, and the acute cases are usually regarded as obstruction. Exploratory operation has been made in 47 cases, 4 of which have recovered. In J. W. Elliot's successful case 48 inches of the bowel were resected. In the horse, infarction of the intestine, commonly in connection with the verminous aneurisms of the mesenteric arteries, is the usual cause of colic.

Diseases of the Mesenteric Veins.—Dilatation and sclerosis occur in cirrhosis of the liver. In instances of prolonged obstruction there may be large saccular dilatations with calcification of the intima, as in a case of obliteration of the venæ portæ described by the senior author. Suppuration of the mesenteric veins is not rare, and occurs usually in connection with pylephlebitis. The mesentery may be much swollen and is like a bag of pus, and it is only on careful dissection that one sees that the pus is really within channels representing extremely dilated mesenteric veins.

Disorders of the Chyle Vessels.—Varicose, cavernous, and cystic chylangiomata are met with in the mucosa and submucosa of the small intestine, occasionally of the stomach. Extravasation of chyle into the mesenteric tissue is sometimes seen. Chylous cysts may occur at the root of the mesentery. Bramann records a case in a man aged sixty-three, in which a cyst of this kind the size of a child's head was healed by operation. There is an instance on record of a congenital malformation of the thoracic duct, in which the receptaculum formed a flattened cyst which discharged into the peritoneum, and a chylous ascitic fluid was withdrawn on several occasions. Homans reported the case of a girl who, from the third to the thirteenth year, had an enlarged abdomen. Laparotomy showed a series of cysts containing clear fluid. They were supposed to be dilated lymph vessels connected with the intestines.

Cysts of the Mesentery.—They may be either dermoid, hydatid, serous, sanguineous, or chylous. They occur at any portion of the mesentery, and range from a few inches in diameter to large masses occupying the entire abdomen. They are frequently adherent to the neighboring organs, to the liver, spleen, uterus, and sigmoid flexure.

The *symptoms* usually are those of a progressively enlarging tumor in the abdomen. Sometimes a mass develops rapidly, particularly in the hæmorrhagic forms. Colic and constipation or acute obstruction are present in some cases. The general health, as a rule, is well maintained in spite of the progressive enlargement of the abdomen, which is most prominent in the umbilical region. Mesenteric cysts may persist for many years, even ten or twenty.

The *diagnosis* is extremely uncertain, and no single feature is in any way distinctive. The important signs are: the great mobility, the situation in the middle line, and the zone of tympany in front of the tumor. Of these, the second is the only one which is at all constant, as when the tumors are large the mobility disappears, and at this stage the intestines, too, are pushed to one side. It is most frequently mistaken for ovarian tumor. Movable kidney, hydronephrosis, and cysts of the omentum have also been confused with it. The only treatment is surgical.

VI. DILATATION OF THE DUODENUM

This is often associated with visceroptosis and compression of the terminal portion of the duodenum by the root of the mesentery. Adhesions from local peritonitis are responsible in some cases. The symptoms are (1) *pain* in the upper abdomen, sometimes described as a pulling or dragging sensation, sometimes more severe, and suggesting ulcer or gall-bladder disease; (2) *vomiting* which is frequent and sometimes persistent; (3) constipation; and (4) marked vagotonic features. The X-ray study is an important aid in the diagnosis. In treatment, position may be useful, the patient lying on the face with the feet elevated, or on the left side, or taking the knee-chest position. Correction of the visceroptosis by an abdominal support or by gaining weight may give relief. In severe cases surgical intervention is advisable.

H. DISEASES OF THE LIVER

I. JAUNDICE

(*Icterus*)

Definition.—Jaundice or icterus is a condition characterized by coloration of the skin, mucous membranes, and fluids of the body by bile-pigment.

Like albuminuria, jaundice is a symptom and not a disease, and is met with in a variety of conditions. Bile pigment and bile salts may be in the blood and not appear in the urine or be in the tissues. In *dissociated jaundice* the bile pigments and salts reach the plasma independently; the kidneys may excrete one and not the other.

I. OBSTRUCTIVE JAUNDICE

The chief causes of obstructive jaundice are: (1) Obstruction by foreign bodies within the ducts, as gall-stones and parasites; (2) by inflammatory tumefaction of the duodenum or of the lining membrane of the duct; (3) by stricture or obliteration of the duct; (4) by tumors closing the orifice of the duct or growing in its interior; (5) by pressure on the duct from without, as by tumors of the liver itself, of the stomach, pancreas, kidney, or omentum; by pressure of enlarged glands in the fissures of the liver, and, more rarely, of abdominal aneurism, fæcal accumulation, or the pregnant uterus.

In these cases of extra-hepatic or obstructive jaundice the pressure within the biliary capillaries, usually low, becomes increased and the bile is absorbed by the lymphatics of the liver and not by the blood capillaries. To these causes some add lowering of the blood pressure in the portal system so that the tension in the smaller bile-ducts is greater than in the blood-vessels. For this view there is no positive evidence. In this class may perhaps be placed the cases of jaundice from mental shock or depressed emotions, which "may conceivably cause spasm and reversed peristalsis of the bile-duct" (W. Hunter).

General Symptoms of Obstructive Jaundice.—(*a*) *Icterus, or tinting of the skin and conjunctivæ.* The color ranges from a lemon-yellow in catarrhal jaundice to a deep olive-green or bronzed hue in permanent obstruction. In some instances the color of the skin is greenish black, the so-called "black jaundice." Except the central nervous system, all of the tissues are stained.

(*b*) In the more chronic forms *pruritus* is a most distressing symptom. There is a curious pre-icteric itching, which Riesman thinks is suggestive of cancer, but it is often marked in gall-stone cases. Sweating is common, and may be curiously localized to the abdomen or to the palms of the hands. Lichen, urticaria, and boils may occur. *Xanthoma multiplex* is rare. Usually in the flat form, rarely nodular, they are most common in the eyelids and on the hands and feet. They may be very numerous over the whole body. Occasionally the tumors are found in the bile duct. After persisting for years they may disappear. In very chronic cases telangiectases develop in the skin, sometimes in large numbers over the body and face, occasionally on the mucous membrane of the tongue and lips, forming patches of a bright red color from 1 to 2 cm. in breadth.

(*c*) The blood serum is tinged with bilirubin. By this an early diagnosis may be made.

(*d*) The *secretions* are colored with bile-pigment. The sweat tinges the linen; the tears and saliva and milk are rarely stained. The expectoration is not often tinted unless there is inflammation, as when pneumonia coexists with jaundice. The urine may contain the pigment before it is apparent in the skin or conjunctiva. The color varies from light greenish yellow to a deep black-green. In cases of jaundice of long standing or great intensity the urine usually contains albumin and always bile-stained tubecasts.

(*e*) *No bile passes into the intestine.* The stools therefore are of a pale drab or slate-gray color, and usually very fetid and pasty. The "clay-color" of the stools is also in part due to the presence of undigested fat which, according to Müller, may be increased from 7 to 10 per cent., which is normal, to 55 or 78.5 per cent. There may be constipation; in many instances, owing to decomposition, there is diarrhœa.

(*f*) *Slow pulse.* The heart's action may fall to 40, 30, or even to 20 per minute. It is particularly noticeable in the cases of catarrhal and recent jaundice, and is not as a rule an unfavorable symptom. Whether this is due to interrupted conductivity or to direct poisoning of the auriculo-ventricular bundle has not been determined. It occurs only in the early stages of jaundice. At this time bile acids pass into the blood, but are produced in very small quantities when jaundice is established. The respirations may fall to 10 or even to 7 per minute. Xanthopsia, or yellow vision, may occur.

(*g*) *Hæmorrhage.* The tendency to bleeding in chronic icterus is a serious feature and in some cases the blood coagulation time is much retarded. This is an important point as incontrollable hæmorrhage is a well-recognized accident in operating upon patients with chronic jaundice. Purpura, large subcutaneous extravasations, more rarely hæmorrhages from the mucous membranes, occur in protracted jaundice, and in the more severe forms.

(*h*) *Cerebral symptoms.* Irritability, great depression of spirits, or even melancholia may be present. In any case of persistent jaundice special nervous phenomena may develop and rapidly prove fatal—such as sudden coma, acute delirium, or convulsions. Usually the patient has a rapid pulse, slight fever, and a dry tongue, and he passes into the so-called "typhoid state." These features are not nearly so common in obstructive as in febrile jaundice, but they not infrequently terminate a chronic icterus in whatever way produced. The group of symptoms has been termed *cholæmia,* or, on the supposition that cholesterin is the poison, *cholesteræmia;* but its true nature has not been determined. In some cases the symptoms may be due to uræmia.

II. TOXIC AND HÆMOLYTIC JAUNDICE

The term hæmatogenous jaundice was formerly applied to this group in contradistinction to the hepatogenous jaundice, associated with manifest obstructive changes in the bile-passages. The toxic jaundice cases are essentially obstructive in origin, and it is doubtful whether there are any true non-obstructive cases. For this type the name "hæmohepatogenous" jaundice has been suggested. Rolleston refers to them as cases of "intrahepatic" jaundice. Toxic substances, bacterial or chemical, circulate in the blood and cause destruction of red blood cells. The toxin and its products cause a degeneration of the liver cells and an inflammatory condition of the bile capillaries. The bile becomes viscid and the fine ducts are narrowed (intrahepatic obstruction). The bile pigments are absorbed by the lymphatics and blood capillaries. "The absorbed bile in toxæmic jaundice is usually rich in bile pigments which arise from the increased destruction of hæmoglobin; it is deficient in bile salts owing to the impaired function of the liver cells" (Willcox). The mucous membrane of the duodenum may be swollen and show hæmorrhages. Hunter groups the causes as follows: 1. Jaundice produced by the action of poisons, such as toluylendiamin, phosphorus, arsenic, snake-venom. 2. Jaundice met with in various infections, such as yellow fever, malaria, pyæmia, relapsing fever, typhus, typhoid fever, scarlatina. 3. Jaundice in various conditions of more or less infective nature, and variously designated as epidemic, infectious, febrile, malignant jaundice, icterus gravis, Weil's disease, acute yellow atrophy and the form due to *Spirochæta ictero-hæmorrhagica.*

The *symptoms* are not nearly so striking as in the obstructive variety. The bile is present in the stools. The skin has in many cases only a slight lemon tint. The urine may contain no bile-pigment, but the urinary pigments are considerably increased. In the severer forms, as in acute yellow atrophy, the color may be more intense, but in malaria and pernicious anæmia the tint is usually light. The constitutional disturbance may be very profound, with high fever, delirium, convulsions, suppression of urine, black vomit, and cutaneous hæmorrhages. In certain cases of hæmolytic jaundice the fragility of the red corpuscles is greatly increased and they may be smaller than normal (Widal, Chauffard) and show granular degeneration. This is particularly the case in the group of congenital icterus with enlarged spleen.

The study of digestive lipæmia may be of value in the diagnosis of the cause of jaundice. A light supper without fat is taken and the blood examined next morning before breakfast and again two to five hours after breakfast at which fat is eaten freely. Normally the blood contains many fat particles. In total obstruction of the bile passages there is no absorption of fat into the blood. If jaundice is due to retention of the bile pigment alone, absorption is not altered, but if there is retention of the bile salts fat does not appear in the blood. For dissociation of bile and retention of part of its elements, the liver must be responsible.

Certain special forms deserve notice.

Tetrachloride of Ethane.—The vapor inhaled in the coating of aeroplane wings is a not uncommon cause of illness. Headache, nausea, and abdominal discomfort may be present for a week or more before the jaundice appears. If quickly removed from the influence of the vapor, recovery is prompt, but *icterus gravis* may occur with purpura, convulsions, suppression of urine and coma. Fever is absent and there is no anæmia, and the jaundice is unusually deep. There is extensive degeneration of the liver cells, and if the disease lasts many weeks, a "replacement cirrhosis." Contraction of the liver with ascites may follow.

Trinitrotoluene.—Many munition workers suffered severely, some from the local effects, dermatitis or erythema, many more from the inhalation of the dust or the swallowing of the powder. The toxic symptoms come on after a variable period of exposure from a few days to months. Nausea, weakness and pallor, with signs of irritation of the throat are early symptoms. Then jaundice begins, and if severe, there are the usual toxic features. The anæmia resembles the pernicious type, with a high color index and leucopenia. At first enlarged, the liver may subsequently shrink, and some of the cases have the clinical and anatomical picture of acute yellow atrophy with purpura and hæmorrhages. In both these forms when jaundice is severe, full alkaline treatment is helpful—sodium citrate and sodium bicarbonate, 30 grain (2 gm.) doses of each every two or three hours and intravenous injection of normal saline with two drams (8 gm.) of bicarbonate of soda to the pint (Willcox). Other substances used in munition factories such as dinitrophenol, dinitrobenzene and picric acid may cause toxic jaundice.

Salvarsan and its *substitutes.*—Occasional fever with nausea, irritation of the skin and scattered purpura may follow a full dose. The severer symptoms usually come on in two or three days with fever, delirium, jaundice and death in coma or with convulsions. The purpura may be very extensive with hæmorrhage from the mucous membranes. Death has followed within two days. The liver presents widespread necroses with fatty degeneration.

III. HEREDITARY ICTERUS

A family form of icterus has long been known. We must recognize, indeed, several groups. First, icterus neonatorum, as in the remarkable instance described by Glaister (Lancet, March, 1879), in which a woman had eight children, six of whom died of jaundice shortly after birth; one of the cases had stenosis of the common duct, which, as John Thomson has shown, is, with angiocholitis, a common lesion in this affection. Still more remarkable is it that the mother of this woman had twelve children, all of whom were icteric after birth, but the jaundice gradually disappeared. A brother of the woman had several children who also were jaundiced at birth. Glaister states that all of the children of Morgagni, fifteen in number, had icterus neonatorum. Secondly, the congenital *acholuric icterus*. Minkowski reported eight cases in three generations. Cases without hereditary basis are not uncommon. The jaundice is slight, the stools are not clay colored, the urine has no bile pigment but contains urobilin, the general health is little if at all disturbed. Splenic enlargement is a marked feature. There is a tendency to hæmolysis of the red blood cells. The blood serum contains bile pigment. No special changes have been found in the liver or bile passages. Thirdly, a group of cases with enlargement of the spleen and liver and marked constitutional disturbances, anæmia, dwarfing of stature, infantilism, and slight jaundice. Cases which have been described as Hanot's cirrhosis have occurred in two or three members of a family, and the jaundice has dated from early childhood. Two special affections may here receive consideration, the icterus of the new-born and acute yellow atrophy.

II. ICTERUS NEONATORUM

New-born infants are liable to jaundice, which in some instances rapidly proves fatal. A mild and a severe form may be recognized.

The *mild or physiological icterus* of the new-born is a common disease in foundling hospitals, and is not very infrequent in private practice. In 900 consecutive births at the Sloane Maternity icterus was noted in 300 cases (Holt). The discoloration appears early, usually on the first or second day, and is of moderate intensity. The urine may be bile-stained and the fæces colorless. The nutrition of the child is not usually disturbed, and in the majority of cases the jaundice disappears within two weeks. This form is never fatal. The cause of this jaundice is not at all clear. Some have attributed it to stasis in the smaller bile-ducts, which are compressed by the distended radicals of the portal vein. Others hold that the jaundice is due to the destruction of a large number of red blood-corpuscles during the first few days after birth.

The *severe form* of icterus in the new-born may depend upon (*a*) congenital absence of the common or hepatic duct, of which many instances are on record; (*b*) congenital syphilitic hepatitis; and (*c*) septic infection, associated with phlebitis of the umbilical vein. This is a severe and fatal form, in which hæmorrhage from the cord may also occur.

Curiously enough, in contradistinction to other forms, the brain and cord may be stained yellow in icterus neonatorum, sometimes diffusely, more rarely in definite foci corresponding to the ganglion cells which have become deeply stained (Schmorl).

III. ACUTE YELLOW ATROPHY

(*Malignant Jaundice; Icterus Gravis*)

Definition.—An acute widespread autolytic necrosis of the liver cells of unknown origin, characterized by jaundice, toxæmia and a reduction in the volume of the liver.

Etiology.—The first authentic account was given by the famous old Paris doctor Ballonius—sometimes called the French Hippocrates (1538-1616). Bright gave a good description in 1836. It is a rare disease, as among 28,000 medical cases admitted to the Johns Hopkins Hospital in nearly twenty-three years there were only 3 cases. It varies in frequency in different countries, and seems to be rarer in the United States than in Germany and England. The majority of cases occur between the tenth and the fortieth year. Rolleston collected 22 cases occurring within the first ten years of life.

Acute necrosis of the liver occurs under many conditions: (*a*) In the infections, syphilis, typhoid fever, diphtheria, septicæmia, these necroses may be widespread. (*b*) Non-bacterial poisons. The remarkable delayed chloroform poisoning is a hepatic necrosis resembling very closely acute yellow atrophy. Phosphorus produces a similar condition, and possibly mercury. (*c*) Autogenous poisons, produced in connection with pregnancy and parturition. The ordinary necrotic foci of the liver in pregnancy are the same kind but less in degree than those of acute yellow atrophy.

An exaggeration of any of these types may lead to a clinical condition which we call acute yellow atrophy. Its association with pregnancy is remarkable. More than one-half of the cases occur in women, and in a large proportion of these during the middle or latter half of pregnancy. The disease has followed a profound shock, or mental emotion. It occurs occasionally in syphilis and other acute infections, and there are cases of cirrhosis of the liver, particularly of the hypertrophic form, associated with diffuse necrosis, intense jaundice and toxæmia. We are as yet ignorant of the conditions under which the poisons, bacterial or metabolic, cause this widespread necrosis.

Morbid Anatomy.—The liver is greatly reduced in size, looks thin and flattened, and sometimes does not reach more than one-half or even one-third of its normal weight. It is flabby and the capsule is wrinkled. Externally the organ has a greenish-yellow color. On section the color may be yellowish-brown, yellowish-red, or mottled, and the outlines of the lobules are indistinct. The yellow and dark-red portions represent different stages of the same process—the yellow an earlier, the red a more advanced stage. The organ may cut with considerable firmness. The liver-cells are seen in all stages of necrosis, and in spots appear to have undergone complete destruction, leaving a fatty, granular *débris* with pigment grains and crystals of leucin and tyrosin. Hæmorrhages occur between the liver-cells. There is a cholangitis of the smaller bile-ducts. Marchand, MacCallum, and others have described regenerative changes in the cases which do not run an acute course.

The other organs show extensive bile-staining, and there are numerous hæmorrhages. The kidneys may show marked granular degeneration of the epithelium, and usually there is fatty degeneration of the heart. In a majority of the cases the spleen is enlarged.

Symptoms.—In the initial stage there is gastro-duodenal catarrh, and at first the jaundice is thought to be of a simple nature. In some instances this lasts only a few days, in others two or three weeks. Then severe symptoms set in—headache, delirium, trembling of the muscles, and, in some instances, convulsions. Vomiting is a constant symptom, and blood may be brought up. Hæmorrhages occur into the skin or from the mucous surfaces; in pregnant women abortion may occur. The jaundice usually increases, coma sets in and gradually deepens until death. The body temperature is variable; in a majority of the cases the disease runs an afebrile course, though sometimes just before death there is an elevation. In some instances, however, there has been marked pyrexia. The pulse is usually rapid, the tongue coated and dry, and the patient is in a "typhoid state." There may be complete obliteration of the liver dulness. This is due to the flabby organ falling away from the abdominal walls and allowing the intestinal coils to take its place.

The urine is bile-stained and often contains tube-casts. Frequently albuminuria and occasionally albumosuria occur. Urea is markedly diminished. There is a corresponding increase in the percentage of nitrogen present as ammonia. Herter finds it may be increased from the normal 2 to 5 per cent. up to 17 per cent. The diminution in urea is probably partly due to the liver-cells failing to manufacture urea from ammonia, but it may also be in part due to organic acids seizing on the ammonia, and thus preventing the formation of urea out of the basic ammonia. Leucin and tyrosin are not constantly present; of 23 cases collected by Hunter, in 9 neither was found; in 10 both were present; in 3 tyrosin only; in 1 leucin only. The present view is that the leucin and tyrosin are derived from the liver-cells themselves as a result of their extensive destruction. In the majority of cases no bile enters the intestines, and the stools are clay-colored. The disease is almost invariably fatal. In a few instances recovery has been noted. The senior author saw in Leube's clinic, at Würzburg, a patient who was convalescent.

The duration and the type of the disease depend upon the extent and the rapidity of progress of the necrosis. Cases have lasted as long as forty days, while death has occurred as early as the second day. A sub-acute form has been described by Milne, a slow necrosis lasting many months, associated with jaundice—a protracted stage from which recovery is possible by regeneration of liver tissue, but consecutive cirrhosis is the rule.

Diagnosis.—Jaundice with vomiting, diminution of the liver volume, delirium, and the presence of leucin and tyrosin in the urine, form a characteristic and unmistakable group of symptoms. Leucin and tyrosin are not, however, distinctive. They may be present in cases of afebrile jaundice with slight enlargement of the liver.

It is not to be forgotten that any severe jaundice may be associated with intense cerebral symptoms. The clinical features in certain cases of hypertrophic cirrhosis are almost identical, but the enlargement of the liver, the more constant occurrence of fever, and the absence of leucin and tyrosin are distinguishing signs. Phosphorus poisoning may closely simulate acute yellow atrophy, particularly in the hæmorrhages, jaundice, and the diminution in the liver volume, but the gastric symptoms are usually more marked, and leucin and tyrosin are stated not to occur in the urine.

Treatment.—No known remedies have any influence on the course of the disease. Theoretically, efforts should be made to eliminate the toxins before they produce their degenerative effects by free elimination, the giving of alkalies and the use of subcutaneous and intravenous saline injections. Gastric sedatives may be used to allay the distressing vomiting.

IV. AFFECTIONS OF THE BLOOD-VESSELS OF THE LIVER

Anæmia.—When the liver looks anæmic, as in the fatty or amyloid organ, the blood-vessels, which during life were probably well filled, can be readily injected. There are no symptoms indicative of this condition.

Hyperæmia.—(*a*) Active Hyperæmia.—After each meal the rapid absorption by the portal vessels induces transient congestion of the organ, which, however, is entirely physiological: but it is quite possible that in persons who persistently eat and drink too much this active hyperæmia may lead to functional disturbance, or, in the case of drinking too freely of alcohol, to organic change. In the fevers an acute hyperæmia may be present.

The *symptoms* are indefinite. Possibly the sense of distress or fullness in the right hypochondrium, so often mentioned by dyspeptics and by those who eat and drink freely, may be due to this cause. There are probably diurnal variations in the volume of the liver. In cirrhosis with enlargement the rapid reduction in volume after a copious hæmorrhage indicates the important part which hyperæmia plays even in organic troubles. Andrew H. Smith described a case of periodical enlargement of the liver.

(*b*) Passive Congestion.—This is much more common and results from an increase of pressure in the efferent vessels or sub-lobular branches of the hepatic veins. Every condition leading to venous stasis in the right heart at once affects these veins.

In chronic valvular disease, myocardial insufficiency, cirrhosis of the lung, and in intrathoracic tumors mechanical congestion occurs and finally leads to very definite changes. The liver is enlarged, firm, and of a deep-red color; the hepatic vessels are greatly engorged, particularly the central vein in each lobule and its adjacent capillaries. On section the organ presents a peculiar mottled appearance, owing to the deeply congested hepatic and the anæmic portal territories; hence the term *nutmeg* given to this condition. Gradually the distention of the central capillaries reaches such a grade that atrophy of the intervening liver-cells is induced. Brown pigment is deposited about the centre of the lobules and the connective tissue is greatly increased. In this cyanotic induration or cardiac liver the organ is large in the early stage, but later it may become contracted. Occasionally in this form the connective tissue is increased about the lobules as well, but the process usually extends from the sub-lobular and central veins.

The *symptoms* of this form are not always to be separated from those of the associated conditions. Gastro-intestinal catarrh is usually present and hæmatemesis may occur. The portal obstruction in advanced cases leads to ascites, which may precede the development of general dropsy. There is often slight jaundice, the stools may be clay-colored, and the urine contains bile-pigment. The liver is increased in size, may be a full hand's breadth below the costal margin and tender on pressure. It is in this condition particularly that we meet with pulsation of the liver. We must distinguish the communicated throbbing of the heart, which is very common, from the heaving, diffuse impulse due to regurgitation into the hepatic veins, in which the whole liver can be felt to dilate with each impulse.

The indications for *treatment* in hyperæmia are to restore the balance of the circulation and to unload the engorged portal vessels. In cases of intense hyperæmia 18 or 20 ounces of blood may be directly aspirated from the liver, as advised by George Harley and practised by many Anglo-Indian physicians. Good results sometimes follow this hepato-phlebotomy. The prompt relief and marked reduction in the volume of the organ which follow an attack of hæmatemesis or bleeding from piles suggest this practice. Salts administered by Matthew Hay's method deplete the portal system freely and thoroughly. As a rule, the treatment must be that of the condition with which it is associated.

Diseases of the Portal Vein.—(*a*) THROMBOSIS; ADHESIVE PYLEPHLEBITIS.—Coagulation of blood in the portal vein is met with in cirrhosis, in syphilis of the liver, invasion of the vein by cancer, proliferative peritonitis involving the gastro-hepatic omentum, perforation of the vein by gall-stones, and occasionally follows sclerosis of the walls of the portal vein or of its branches. In rare instances a complete collateral circulation is established, the thrombus undergoes the usual change, and ultimately the vein is represented by a fibrous cord, a condition which has been called *pylephlebitis adhesiva.* In a case of this kind the portal vein was represented by a narrow fibrous cord; the collateral circulation, which must have been completely established for years, ultimately failed, ascites and hæmatemesis supervened and rapidly proved fatal. The diagnosis of obstruction of the portal vein can rarely be made. A suggestive symptom, however, is a *sudden* onset of the most intense engorgement of the branches of the portal system, leading to hæmatemesis, melæma, ascites, and swelling of the spleen.

Infarcts are not common in the liver and may be anæmic or hæmorrhagic. They are met with in obstruction of the portal vessels, or of the portal and hepatic veins at the same time, occasionally in disease of the hepatic artery.

(*b*) SUPPURATIVE PYLEPHLEBITIS is considered in the section on abscess.

Affections of the hepatic vein are extremely rare. Dilatation occurs in cases of chronic enlargement of the right heart, from whatever cause. Emboli occasionally pass from the right auricle into the hepatic veins.

Stenosis of the orifices of the hepatic veins may occur as a primary lesion with a special syndrome described by Craven Moore—a progressive enlargement of the liver, signs of involvement of the inferior vena cava, and ascites.

Hepatic Artery.—Enlargement of this vessel is seen in cases of cirrhosis of the liver. It may be the seat of extensive sclerosis. Aneurism of the hepatic artery is rare and will be referred to in the section on arteries.

V. DISEASES OF THE BILE-PASSAGES AND GALL-BLADDER

I. ACUTE CATARRH OF THE BILE-DUCTS

(*Catarrhal Jaundice*)

Definition.—Jaundice due to swelling and obstruction of the terminal portion of the common duct.

Etiology.—General catarrhal inflammation of the bile-ducts is usually associated with gall-stones. The process now under consideration is usually an extension of a gastro-duodenal catarrh, and the process is most intense in the *pars intestinalis* of the duct, which projects into the duodenum. The mucous membrane is swollen, and a plug of inspissated mucus fills the diverticulum of Vater, and the narrower portion just at the orifice, completely obstructing the outflow of bile. It is not known how widespread this catarrh is in the bile-passages, and whether it really passes up the ducts. It is possible that an infection of the finer ducts within the liver may initiate the attack, but the evidence for this is not strong, and it seems more likely that the terminal portion of the duct is first involved. In one case at post mortem the orifice was found plugged with inspissated mucus, the common and hepatic ducts were slightly distended and contained a bile-tinged, not a clear, mucus, and there were no observable changes in the mucosa of the ducts.

This catarrhal or simple jaundice results from the following causes: (*a*) Duodenal catarrh, in whatever way produced, most commonly following an attack of indigestion. It is most frequently met with in young persons, but may occur at any age, and may follow not only errors in diet, but also cold, exposure, and malaria, as well as the conditions associated with portal obstruction, chronic heart-disease, and nephritis. (*b*) Emotional disturbances may be followed by jaundice, which is believed to be due to catarrhal swelling. Cases of this kind are rare and the anatomical condition is unknown. (*c*) Simple or catarrhal jaundice may occur in epidemic form. (*d*) Catarrhal jaundice is occasionally seen in the infectious fevers, such as pneumonia and typhoid fever. The nature of acute catarrhal jaundice is still unknown, but it is probably an acute infection. In favor of this view are the occurrence in epidemic form and the presence of slight fever. The spleen, however, is not often enlarged. In only 4 out of 23 cases was it palpable.

Symptoms.—There may be neither pain nor distress, and the patient's friends may first notice the yellow tint, or the patient himself may observe it in the looking-glass. In other instances there are dyspeptic symptoms and uneasy sensations in the hepatic region or pains in the back and limbs. In the epidemic form the onset may be more severe, with headache, chill, and vomiting. Fever is rarely present, though the temperature may reach 101°, sometimes 102°. All the signs of obstructive jaundice are present, the stools are clay-colored, and the urine contains bile-pigment. The skin has a bright-yellow tint; the greenish, bronzed color is never seen in the simple form. Spider angiomata may occur on the face in catarrhal jaundice. They disappear in a few months. The pulse may be normal, but occasionally it is remarkably slow, and may fall to 40 or 30 beats in the minute, and the respirations to as low as 8 per minute. Sleepiness may be present and rarely a comatose state. The liver may be normal in size, but is usually slightly enlarged, and the edge can be felt below the costal margin. Occasionally the enlargement is more marked. As a rule the gall-bladder can not be felt. The spleen may be increased in size. The duration is from four to eight weeks. There are mild cases in which the jaundice disappears within two weeks; on the other hand, it may persist for three months or even longer. The stools should be carefully watched, for they give the first intimation of removal of the obstruction.

Diagnosis.—This is rarely difficult. The onset in young, comparatively healthy persons, the moderate grade of icterus, the absence of emaciation or of evidences of cirrhosis or cancer usually make the diagnosis easy. Cases which persist for two or three months cause uneasiness, as the suspicion is aroused that it may be more than simple catarrh. The absence of pain, the negative character of the physical examination, and the maintenance of the general nutrition are the points in favor of simple jaundice. There are instances in which time alone can determine the true nature of the case. The possibility of other forms must be borne in mind in anomalous types.

Treatment.—The diet should be simple and the fats restricted. Measures should be used to allay gastric catarrh, if it is present. A dose of calomel may be given, and the bowels kept open subsequently by salines. The patient should not be violently purged. Daily lavage of the stomach with water at 95° is useful. Bismuth and bicarbonate of soda may be given, and the patient should drink freely of the alkaline mineral waters, of which Vichy is the best. The method devised by Lyon, in which a 25 per cent. solution of magnesium sulphate is introduced into the duodenum, relaxing the sphincter of the common duct, by which large amounts of bile can be drained from the bile passages is of great value. By the use of this method the duration is usually greatly shortened.

II. CHRONIC CATARRHAL ANGIOCHOLITIS

This may possibly occur also as a sequel of the acute catarrh but it is unusual to see a chronic, persistent jaundice attributed to this cause. A chronic catarrh always accompanies obstruction in the common duct, whether by gall-stones, malignant disease, stricture, or external pressure. There are two groups of cases:

With Complete Obstruction of the Common Duct.—In this form the bile-passages are greatly dilated, the common duct may reach the size of the thumb or larger, there is usually dilatation of the gall-bladder and of the ducts within the liver. The contents of the ducts and of the gall-bladder are a clear, colorless mucus. The mucosa may be everywhere smooth and not swollen. The clear mucus is usually sterile. The patients are the subjects of chronic jaundice, usually without fever.

With Incomplete Obstruction of the Duct.—There is pressure on the duct or there are gall-stones, single or multiple, in the common duct or in the diverticulum of Vater. The bile-passages are not so much dilated, and the contents are a bile-stained, turbid mucus. The gall-bladder is rarely much dilated. In a majority of all cases stones are found in it.

The symptoms of this type of angiocholitis are sometimes very distinctive. With it is associated most frequently the so-called hepatic intermittent fever, recurring attacks of chills, fever, and sweats. It is important to bear in mind that the chills, fever, and sweats do not necessarily mean suppuration.

III. SUPPURATIVE AND ULCERATIVE ANGIOCHOLITIS

The condition is a diffuse, purulent angiocholitis involving the larger and smaller ducts. In a large proportion of all cases there is associated suppurative disease of the gall-bladder. In all forms of infection of the bile passages cultures of the duodenal contents may give information as to the infecting organism.

Etiology.—It is the most serious of the sequels of gall-stones. Occasionally a diffuse suppurative angiocholitis follows the acute infectious cholecystitis; this, however, is rare, since fortunately in the latter condition the cystic duct is usually occluded. Cancer of the duct, or foreign bodies, such as lumbricoids or fish bones, are occasional causes. There may be extension from a suppurative pylephlebitis. In rare instances suppurative cholangitis occurs in the acute infections, as pneumonia and influenza.

The common duct is greatly dilated and may reach the size of the index finger or the thumb; the walls are thickened, and there may be fistulous communications with the stomach, colon, or duodenum. The hepatic ducts and their extensions in the liver are dilated and contain pus mixed with bile. On section of the liver small abscesses are seen, which correspond to the dilated suppurating ducts. The gall-bladder is usually distended, full of pus, and with adhesions to the neighboring parts, or it may have perforated.

Symptoms.—The symptoms of suppurative cholangitis are usually very severe. A previous history of gall-stones, the development of a septic fever, the swelling and tenderness of the liver, the enlargement of the gall-bladder, and the leucocytosis are suggestive features. Jaundice is always present, but is variable. In some cases it is very intense, in others it is slight. There may be very little pain. There are progressive emaciation and loss of strength. In one case parotitis developed which subsided without suppuration.

Treatment.—With infection of the bile passage, the diet should be simple and water taken freely. Hexamine may be given in full dosage. In some cases drainage of the gall-bladder has been of use. Vaccines prepared from duodenal cultures may be tried. The procedure used by Lyon to aid drainage of the bile-passages is often very useful.

IV. ACUTE INFECTIOUS CHOLECYSTITIS

Etiology.—Acute inflammation of the gall-bladder is usually due to bacterial invasion, with or without the presence of gall-stones. Three varieties or grades may be recognized: the catarrhal, the suppurative, and the phlegmonous. The condition is very serious, may be fatal, and may require prompt surgical intervention for its relief.

Acute non-calculous cholecystitis is a result of bacterial invasion. The colon bacillus, the typhoid bacillus, the pneumococcus and staphylococci and streptococci have been the organisms most often found. The frequency of gall-bladder infection in the fevers is a point already referred to, particularly in typhoid fever. In many cases the organisms are found in the wall of the gall-bladder when the contents are sterile.

The association of appendix lesions with cholecystitis is interesting, fully 69 per cent. at the Mayo clinic; but this is not surprising in view of studies which show a normal appendix to be a rarity. There are indications, however, that chronic changes in this organ may reflexly disturb the mechanism of the secretion, storage, and outflow of bile.

Condition of the Gall-bladder.—The organ is usually distended and the walls tense. Adhesions may have formed with the colon or the omentum. In the acute stage the mucous membrane is swollen and the amount of mucin increased. As the process continues the mucosa becomes thickened, the epithelium desquamates, there are areas of necrosis, and the villi may be much hypertrophied and stand out, giving a strawberry appearance. With the obstruction of the duct and pyogenic infection there may be acute necrotic cholecystitis, with rapid perforation, or a more chronic purulent cholecystitis—empyema of the gall-bladder.

Symptoms.—Severe paroxysmal pain is, as a rule, the first indication, most commonly in the right side of the abdomen in the region of the liver. It may be in the epigastrium or low down in the region of the appendix. "Nausea, vomiting, rise of pulse and temperature, prostration, distention of the abdomen, rigidity, general tenderness becoming localized" usually follow (Richardson). In this form, without gall-stones, jaundice is not often present. Leucocytosis is common. The local tenderness is extreme, but it may be deceptive in its situation. Associated probably with the adhesion and inflammatory processes between the gall-bladder and the bowel are the intestinal symptoms, and there may be complete stoppage of gas and fæces; indeed, the operation for acute obstruction has been performed in several cases. The distended gall-bladder may sometimes be felt. As a sequel there may be purulent distention or empyema.

Diagnosis.—This is by no means easy, as the symptoms may not indicate the section of the abdomen involved. Appendicitis or acute intestinal obstruction may be diagnosed. The history is often a valuable guide. Occurring during convalescence from typhoid fever, after pneumonia, or in a patient with previous cholecystitis, such a group of symptoms as mentioned would be highly suggestive. The differentiation of the variety of the cholecystitis can not be made. In the acute suppurative and phlegmonous forms the symptoms are usually more severe, perforation is very apt to occur, with local or general peritonitis, and unless operative measures are undertaken death ensues.

There is an acute cholecystitis, probably an infective form, in which the patient has recurring attacks of pain in the region of the gall-bladder. The diagnosis of gall-stones is made, but an operation shows simply an enlarged gall-bladder filled with mucus and bile, and the mucous membrane perhaps swollen and inflamed. In some of these cases gall-stones may have been present and have passed before the operation.

Treatment.—In the milder catarrhal forms the inflammation subsides spontaneously; in severer form operation is indicated and the results are excellent. Increase in the local signs, an enlarged palpable gall-bladder, increasing leucocytosis and fever, are usually indications for operation. In 675 cholecystectomies at the Mayo clinic there were only 17 deaths.

V. CHRONIC CHOLECYSTITIS

This occurs in a number of different forms, as, for example, an atrophic sclerotic and an ulcerative form.

Etiology.—It often results from a previous attack of acute cholecystitis or may be associated with gall-stones. In some cases it is undoubtedly chronic from the onset, resulting from a persistent infection which is never acute enough to set up an active attack. It may be associated with chronic infection of the ducts.

Pathology.—The gall-bladder is usually distended and contains thick bile and mucus. The walls may be thickened. The mucosa may be atrophic and sometimes the gall-bladder is small and sclerotic; it may be surrounded by a mass of dense adhesions. The relationship between the lymphatics of the gall-bladder and pancreas is important in explaining the association of infection in these organs.

Symptoms.—These are much the same as those from gall-stones and a differential diagnosis may be impossible. There may be attacks of acute pain. In the intervals there may be an entire absence of any tenderness in the gall-bladder region. Sometimes the gall-bladder is palpable. Of special importance is the frequency of gastric symptoms. W. J. Mayo has called attention to a form of chronic cholecystitis without gall-stones and accompanied with chronic interlobular pancreatitis. The mucous membrane shows a strawberry-like appearance covered with yellow specks representing the tufts of exposed villi stripped of their covering of epithelium. The process is confined to the gall-bladder; the glands along the ligament may be enlarged. The chief symptom is pain in the region of the gall-bladder, but there is no distention and the chronic pancreatitis is not always expressed clinically.

Treatment.—The medical management is much the same as in gall-stones; a simple diet, large amounts of water, keeping the bowels freely open and taking regular exercise. The administration of salicylate of sodium and hexamine seems sometimes to be of use. The taking of salines before breakfast is often helpful. The decision as to surgical interference must depend on the severity of the symptoms and the interference with health due to the condition. In some cases adhesions are present between the gall-bladder and the colon, pylorus and duodenum, which are usually best recognized by the X-ray examination. Operation may be justified to correct them. If there is distinct evidence of a chronic suppurative process in the gall-bladder, surgical measures are indicated and should not be delayed.

VI. CANCER OF THE BILE-PASSAGES

Incidence.—Of 3,908 operations on the gall-bladder and biliary passages, in 85 or 2.1 per cent. cancer was found (Mayo). It is more common in women, 3 to 1 (Musser), and in three-fourths of the cases gall-stones are or have been present. The fundus of the bladder is usually attacked first.

Symptoms.—When the disease involves the *gall-bladder,* a tumor can be detected extending diagonally downward and inward toward the navel, variable in size, occasionally very large, due either to great distention of the gall-bladder or to involvement of contiguous parts. It is usually very firm and hard. Jaundice is usually due to involvement of the liver; it was present in 69 per cent. of Musser's cases; pain is often of great severity and paroxysmal in character. The pain and tenderness on pressure persist in the intervals between the paroxysmal attacks. There is loss of weight, sometimes fever and sweats. When the liver becomes involved the picture is that of carcinoma of the organ.

Primary malignant disease in the *bile-ducts* is less common, and rarely forms tumors that can be felt externally. The tumor is usually in the common duct, 57 of 80 cases collected by Rolleston. There is usually an early, intense, and persistent jaundice. The gall-bladder is usually enlarged in obstruction of the common duct by malignant disease. The dilated gall-bladder may rupture. At best the diagnosis is very doubtful, unless cleared up by an exploratory operation. A very interesting form of malignant disease of the ducts is that which involves the diverticulum of Vater. Rolleston has collected 16 cases.

VII. STENOSIS AND OBSTRUCTION OF THE BILE-DUCTS

Stenosis.—Stenosis or complete occlusion may follow ulceration, most commonly after the passage of a gall-stone. In these instances the obstruction is usually situated low down in the common duct. Instances are extremely rare. Foreign bodies, such as the seeds of various fruits, may enter the duct, and occasionally round worms crawl into it. Liver-flukes and echinococci are rare causes of obstruction in man.

Obstruction.—Obstruction by *pressure* from without is more frequent. Cancer of the head of the pancreas, less often a chronic interstitial inflammation, may compress the terminal portion of the duct; rarely, cancer of the pylorus. Secondary involvement of the lymph-glands of the liver is a common cause of occlusion of the duct, and is met with in many cases of cancer of the stomach and other abdominal organs. Rare causes of obstruction are aneurism of a branch of the cœliac axis of the aorta, and pressure of very large abdominal tumors.

Symptoms.—The symptoms produced are those of chronic obstructive jaundice. At first, the liver is enlarged, but in chronic cases it may be reduced in size, and be found of a deeply bronzed color. The hepatic intermittent fever is not often associated with complete occlusion of the duct from any cause, but it is most frequently met with in chronic obstruction by gall-stones. Permanent occlusion of the duct terminates in death. In a majority of the cases the conditions which lead to the obstruction are in themselves fatal. The liver, which is not necessarily enlarged, presents a moderate grade of cirrhosis. Cases of cicatricial occlusion may last for years.

Diagnosis.—A history of colic, jaundice of varying intensity, paroxysms of pain, and intermittent fever point to gall-stones. In cancerous obstruction the tumor mass can sometimes be felt in the epigastric region. In cases in which the lymph-glands in the transverse fissure are cancerous the primary disease may be in the pelvic organs or the rectum, or there may be a limited cancer of the stomach, which has not given any symptoms. In these cases the examination of the other lymphatic glands may be of value. Involvement of the clavicular groups of lymph-glands may also be serviceable in diagnosis. The gall-bladder is usually enlarged in obstruction of the common duct, except in the cases of gall-stones (Courvoisier's law). Great and progressive enlargement of the liver with jaundice and moderate continued fever is more commonly met with in cancer.

Congenital Obliteration of the Ducts.—John Thomson, in 1892, collected 49 cases and studied the condition thoroughly. C. P. Howard and Wolbach, reviewing the literature, bring the cases up to 76, exclusive of those associated with syphilis. Jaundice sets in early, but may be delayed for ten or twelve days, and is progressive and deep. Hæmorrhages in the skin, from the gastro-intestinal tract, and from the umbilical cord have occurred in fully 50 per cent. Nearly one-half of the cases die within the first month, a few live on for five or six months, but rarely as long as the tenth or twelfth.

Thomson regards congenital malformation as the chief cause, others are due to cholangitis and a few to congenital cirrhosis of the liver.

VI. CHOLELITHIASIS

No chapter in medicine is more interesting than that which deals with the question of gall-stones. Few affections present so many points for study—chemical, bacteriological, pathological, and clinical. There has been a great advance in our knowledge in two directions: First, as to the mode of formation of the stones, and, secondly, as to the surgical treatment of the cases.

Origin of Gall-stones.—There are three mechanisms specially concerned: (1) infection, (2) stasis, and (3) the cholesterol content of the blood.

(1) *Infection.*—The route may be (1) hæmatogenous, probably the most common, (2) by elimination through the liver, and (3) retrograde. Hæmatogenous infection may be from a focus of infection in any part of the body; disease of the appendix is sometimes responsible. The gall-bladder is a peculiarly favorable habitat for organisms. Streptococci, staphylococci, pneumococci, colon bacilli and typhoid bacilli have all been found with varying conditions of the bile. The typhoid bacillus may live indefinitely in the gall-bladder and has been grown in pure culture from the interior of gall-stones. The experimental production of gall-stones has been accomplished by injecting organisms into the gall-bladders of animals. The calculus associated with infection is composed largely of calcium salts, a point emphasized by Rosenbloom.

(2) *Stasis.*—An inspissated condition of the bile occurs with this and precipitation is likely to occur. A nucleus is thus formed and other elements are deposited on it. The work of Boysen showed that the gall-bladder was not affected when the gall-stones were of the primary bile-pigment calcium type. Inspissation of the bile is favored by pregnancy and the acute infectious diseases. The views of Meltzer on disturbed contrary innervation of the gall-bladder with retention of bile are of interest in this connection.

(3) *Cholesterol.*—In probably 75 per cent. of cases of cholelithiasis there is an increase in the cholesterol content of the blood. In some cases this may be temporary and not present when the existence of gall-stones is recognized. Cholesterol may be of exogenous or endogenous origin. There is often an increase in the blood cholesterol during typhoid fever. In favor of the importance of the cholesterol is the number of cases in which the gall-bladder is sterile. It is evident that with a foreign body present there may be subsequent infection. A study of the cases in which cholesterol stones are found shows that a history of infection is generally lacking. The formation of a cholesterol stone may be favored by an increase in the cholesterol in the blood, by its increased excretion by the liver, or by deposit of material from inspissated bile.

Country.—Gall-stones are less frequent in the United States than in Germany, 6.94 to 12 per cent. (Mosher). They are less common in England than on the Continent.

Age.—Nearly 50 per cent. of all the cases occur in persons above forty years of age. They are rare under twenty-five. They have been met with in the new-born, and in infants (John Thomson).

Sex.—Three-fourths of the cases occur in women. Pregnancy has an important influence. Naunyn states that 90 per cent. of women with gall-stones have borne children.

All conditions which favor *stagnation of bile* in the gall-bladder predispose to the formation of stones. Among these may be mentioned corset-wearing, enteroptosis, nephroptosis, and occupations requiring a "leaning forward" position. Lack of exercise, sedentary occupations, particularly when combined with over-indulgence in food, constipation, and depressing mental emotions are also to be regarded as favoring circumstances.

Physical Characters of Gall-stones.—They may be single, in which case the stone is usually ovoid and may attain a very large size. Instances are on record of gall-stones measuring more than 5 inches in length. They may be extremely numerous, ranging from a score to several hundreds or even several thousands, in which case the stones are very small. When moderately numerous, they show signs of mutual pressure and have a polygonal form, with smooth facets; occasionally, however, five or six gall-stones of medium size are met with in the bladder which are round or ovoid and without facets. They are sometimes mulberry-shaped and very dark, consisting largely of bile-pigments. Again there are small, black calculi, rough and irregular in shape, and varying in size from grains of sand to small shot. These are sometimes known as gall-sand. On section, a calculus contains a nucleus, which consists of bile-pigment, rarely a foreign body. The greater portion of the stone is made up of cholesterin, which may form the entire calculus and is arranged in concentric laminæ showing also radiating lines. Salts of lime and magnesia, bile acids, fatty acids, and traces of iron and copper are also found in them. Most gall-stones consist of from 70 to 80 per cent. of cholesterin, in either the amorphous or the crystalline form. As above stated, it is sometimes pure, but more commonly it is mixed with the bile-pigment. The outer layer of the stone is usually harder and brownish in color.

Seat of Formation.—Within the liver itself calculi are occasionally found, but are here usually small and not abundant, and in the form of ovoid, greenish-black grains. A large majority of all calculi are formed within the gall-bladder. The stones in the larger ducts have usually had their origin in the gall-bladder.

Symptoms.—In some cases gall-stones cause no symptoms directly referable to the gall-bladder. The gall-bladder will tolerate the presence of large numbers for an indefinite period of time, and post mortem examinations show that they are present in 25 per cent. of all women over sixty years of age (Naunyn). Moynihan claims that in most cases there are early symptoms—a sense of fullness, weight, and oppression in the epigastrium; a catch in the breath, a feeling of faintness or nausea, and a chilliness after eating. Attacks of indigestion are common, and it is important to remember that persistent gastric symptoms are often due to gall-stones. The gastric secretion may be increased or decreased, more often the latter. Obstinate attacks of urticaria may occur.

The main symptoms of cholelithiasis may be divided into (1) the aseptic, mechanical accidents in consequence of migration of the stone or of obstruction, either in the ducts or in the intestines; (2) the septic, infectious accidents, either local (the angiocholitis and cholecystitis with empyema of the gall-bladder, and the fistulæ and abscess of the liver and infection of the neighboring parts) or general, fever and secondary visceral lesions.

BILIARY COLIC.—Gall-stones may become engaged in the cystic or the common duct without producing pain or severe symptoms. More commonly the passage of a stone excites the violent symptoms known as biliary colic. The attack sets in abruptly with agonizing pain in the right hypochondriac region, which radiates to the shoulder, or is very intense in the epigastric and in the lower thoracic regions. It is often associated with a rigor and a rise in temperature from 102° to 103°. The pain is usually so intense that the patient rolls about in agony. There are vomiting, profuse sweating, and great depression of the circulation. There may be marked tenderness in the region of the liver, which may be enlarged, and the gall-bladder may become palpable and very tender. In other cases the fever is more marked. The spleen is enlarged (Naunyn) and the urine contains albumin with red blood-corpuscles. Ortner holds that *cholecystitis acuta*, occurring in connection with gall-stones, is a septic (bacterial) infection of the bile-passages. The symptoms of acute infectious cholecystitis and those of what we call gall-stone colic are very similar, and surgeons have frequently performed cholecystotomy for the former condition, believing calculi were present. In a large number of the cases jaundice occurs, but it is not a necessary symptom. It does not happen during the passage of the stone through the cystic duct but only when it becomes lodged in the common duct. The pain is due (*a*) to the slow progress in the cystic duct, in which the stone takes a rotary course owing to the arrangement of the Heisterian valve; the cystic duct is poor in muscle fibres but rich in nerves and ganglia; (*b*) to the acute inflammation which usually accompanies an attack; (*c*) to the stretching and distention of the gall-bladder by retained secretions.

The attack varies in duration. It may last for a few hours, several days, or even a week or more. If the stone becomes impacted in the orifice of the common duct, the jaundice becomes intense; much more commonly it is a slight transient icterus. The attack of colic may be repeated at intervals for some time, but finally the stone passes and the symptoms disappear.

Occasionally accidents occur, such as rupture of the duct with fatal peritonitis. Fatal syncope during an attack and the occurrence of repeated convulsive seizures have come under observation but these are rare events. Palpitation and distress about the heart may be present, and occasionally a mitral murmur occurs during the paroxysm, but the cardiac conditions described by some writers as coming on acutely in biliary colic are possibly preëxistent in these patients.

The *diagnosis* of acute hepatic colic is generally easy. The pain is in the upper abdominal and thoracic regions, whereas the pain in nephritic colic is in the lower abdomen. A chill, with fever, is much more frequent in biliary colic than in gastralgia, with which it is liable, at times, to be confounded. A history of previous attacks is an important guide, and the occurrence of jaundice, however slight, determines the diagnosis. To look for the gall-stones, the stools should be thoroughly mixed with water and carefully filtered through a narrow-meshed sieve. Pseudo-biliary colic is not infrequently met with in nervous women, and the diagnosis of gall-stones made. This nervous hepatic colic may be periodical; the pain may be in the right side and radiating; sometimes associated with other nervous phenomena, often excited by emotion, fatigue or excesses. The liver may be tender, but there are neither icterus nor inflammatory conditions. The combination of colic and jaundice, so distinctive of gall-stones, is not always present. The pains may not be colicky, but more constant and dragging in character. A remarkable xanthoma of the bile-passages has been found in association with hepatic colic. Many patients with gall-stones have stomach symptoms—flatulency, regurgitation, and distress after eating. Sometimes the pain may be much increased by food or on exertion. In chronic gall-bladder cases, with adhesions and perforation, the clinical picture may resemble closely that of ulcer. The presence of gall-stones may be proved by X-ray examination in a considerable proportion of cases.

Obstruction of the Cystic Duct.—The effects may be thus enumerated: (*a*) *Dilatation* of the gall-bladder. In acute obstruction the contents are bile mixed with much mucus or muco-purulent material. In chronic obstruction the bile is replaced by a clear fluid mucus. This is an important point in diagnosis, particularly as a dropsical gall-bladder may form a very large tumor. The reaction is not always constant. It is either alkaline or neutral; the consistence is thin and mucoid. Albumin is usually present. A dilated gall-bladder may reach an enormous size, and in one instance Tait found it occupying the greater part of the abdomen. In such cases, as is not unnatural, it has been mistaken for an ovarian tumor. In one case it was attached to the right broad ligament. The dilated gall-bladder can usually be felt below the edge of the liver, and in many instances it has a characteristic outline like a gourd. An enlarged and relaxed organ may not be palpable, and in acute cases the distention may be upward toward the hilus of the liver. The dilated gall-bladder usually projects directly downward, rarely to one side or the other, though occasionally toward the middle line. It may reach below the navel, and in persons with thin walls the outline can be accurately defined. Riedel called attention to a tongue-like projection of the anterior margin of the right lobe in connection with enlarged gall-bladder. It is to be remembered that distention of the gall-bladder may occur without jaundice; indeed, the greatest enlargement has been met with in such cases.

Palpation.—There are two conditions in which gall-stones may be felt; the large, loose, flaccid pouch with numerous stones in a person with a very relaxed abdominal wall—a well-known surgeon described the palpation of gall-stones in himself—and the hard top of the single large ovoid stone about which the walls of the gall bladder have contracted.

(*b*) *Acute cholecystitis.* The simple form is common, and to it are due probably very many of the symptoms of the gall-stone attack. Phlegmonous cholecystitis is rare. Perforation may occur with fatal peritonitis.

(*c*) *Suppurative cholecystitis,* empyema of the gall-bladder, is much more common, and in the great majority of cases is associated with gall-stones. There may be enormous dilatation, and over a litre of pus has been found. Perforation and the formation of abscesses in the neighborhood are not uncommon.

(*d*) *Calcification* of the gall-bladder may be a termination of the previous condition. There are two forms: incrustation of the mucosa with lime salts and the true infiltration of the wall with lime, the so-called ossification.

(*e*) *Atrophy* of the gall-bladder. This is by no means uncommon. The organ shrinks into a small fibroid mass, not larger, perhaps, than a good-sized pea or walnut, or even has the form of a narrow fibrous string; more commonly the gall-bladder tightly embraces a stone. This condition is usually preceded by hydrops of the bladder.

Occasionally the gall-bladder presents *diverticula,* which may be cut off from the main portion, and usually contain calculi.

Obstruction of the Common Duct.—There may be a single stone tightly wedged in the duct in any part of its course, or a series of stones, sometimes extending into both hepatic and cystic ducts, or a stone lies in the diverticulum of Vater. There are three groups of cases: (*a*) In rare instances a stone tightly corks the common duct, causing *permanent occlusion;* or it may partly rest in the cystic duct, and may have caused thickening of the junction of the ducts; or a big stone may compress the hepatic or upper part of the common duct. The jaundice is deep and enduring, and there are no septic features. The pains, the previous attacks of colic, and the absence of enlarged gall-bladder help to separate the condition from obstruction by new growths, although it cannot be differentiated with certainty. The ducts are usually much dilated and everywhere contain a clear mucoid fluid.

(*b*) *Incomplete obstruction, with infective cholangitis.* There may be a series of stones in the common duct, a single stone which is freely movable, or a stone (ball-valve stone) in the diverticulum of Vater. These conditions may be met with at autopsy, without the subjects having had symptoms pointing to gall-stones; but in a majority there are characteristic features.

The common duct may be as large as the thumb; the hepatic duct and its branches through the liver may be greatly dilated, and the distention may be even apparent beneath the liver capsule. Great enlargement of the gall-bladder is rarer. The mucous membrane of the ducts is usually smooth and clear, and the contents consist of a thin, slightly turbid bile-stained mucus.

Naunyn gave as the distinguishing signs of stone in the common duct: "(1) The continuous or occasional presence of bile in the fæces; (2) distinct variations in the intensity of the jaundice; (3) normal size or only slight enlargement of the liver; (4) absence of distention of the gall-bladder; (5) enlargement of the spleen; (6) absence of ascites; (7) presence of febrile disturbance; and (8) duration of the jaundice for more than a year."

In connection with the ball-valve stone, which is most commonly found in the diverticulum of Vater, though it may be in the common duct itself, there is a special symptom group: (*a*) Ague-like paroxysms, chills, fever, and sweating; the *hepatic intermittent fever* of Charcot; (*b*) jaundice of varying intensity, which persists for months or even years, and deepens after each paroxysm; (*c*) at the time of the paroxysm, pains in the region of the liver with gastric disturbance. These symptoms may continue on and off for three or four years, without the development of suppurative cholangitis. The condition has lasted from eight months to three years. The rigors are of intense severity, and the temperature rises to 103° or 105° F. The chills may recur daily for weeks, and present a tertian or quartan type, so that they are often attributed to malaria, with which, however, they have no connection. The jaundice is variable, and deepens after each paroxysm. The itching may be most intense. Pain, which is sometimes severe and colicky, does not always occur. There may be marked vomiting and nausea. As a rule there is no progressive deterioration of health. In the intervals between the attacks the temperature is normal.

The clinical history and post mortem examinations show conclusively that this condition may persist for years without a trace of suppuration within the ducts. It is probable that the toxic symptoms develop only when a certain grade of tension is reached. An interesting and valuable diagnostic point is the absence of dilatation of the gall-bladder in cases of obstruction from stone —Courvoisier's rule.

(*c*) *Incomplete obstruction, with suppurative cholangitis.*—When suppurative cholangitis exists the mucosa is thickened, often eroded or ulcerated; there may be extensive suppuration in the ducts throughout the liver, and even empyema of the gall-bladder. Occasionally the suppuration extends beyond the ducts, and there is localized liver abscess, or there is perforation of the gall-bladder with the formation of abscess between the liver and stomach.

Clinically it is characterized by a fever which may be intermittent, but more commonly is remittent and without prolonged intervals of apyrexia. The jaundice is rarely so intense, nor do we see the deepening of the color after the paroxysms. There is usually greater enlargement of the liver, and tenderness and more definite signs of septicæmia. The cases run a shorter course, and recovery never takes place.

The More Remote Effects of Gall-stones.—(*a*) *Biliary Fistulæ.*—(1) *Cutaneous.*—The external fistula is the most common, 184 out of 384 cases (Naunyn). A majority occur in the region of the navel, to which part the falciform ligament directs the suppuration. The number of stones discharged varies from one or two to many hundreds. Of the 184 cases in Courvoisier's statistics recovery took place in 78. In rare instances the fistula is in the right iliac fossa, or even in the thigh.

(2) *Gastro-intestinal Fistulæ.*—The duodenal is the most frequent, 108 of 384 cases (Naunyn). Usually the opening is between the fundus of the gall-bladder and the first part of the duodenum. A big stone may ulcerate through, leaving little or no damage. In other instances the cicatrization leads to obstruction. Communication with the ileum and jejunum is rare.

Fistulæ between the common duct and the duodenum occurred in 15 cases in Naunyn's series. Biliary gastric fistulæ are rare. The vomiting of gall-stones is not necessarily proof of the perforation, but in the majority of such cases the stones probably pass up through the pylorus.

(3) *Broncho-biliary Fistulæ.*—Of J. E. Graham's collected series of 35 cases, 19 were due to gall-stones; 11 to hydatids; 2 to round-worms; and in 2 the cause was doubtful. In many cases the amœbic liver abscess perforating into the lung is followed by a permanent biliary fistula.

(4) Perforation may occur into the *portal vein,* of which there are a few cases on record, one of which, according to tradition, was the famous Ignatius Loyola.

(5) Perforation into the *hepatic artery* or one of its branches is exceed-

ingly rare. Either an erosion from the common duct or an hepatic aneurism may rupture into the gall-bladder.

(6) Fistula into the *urinary passages* may be with the pelvis of the kidney in which the gall-stone has been found, or into the urinary bladder, of which there are few cases on record.

(7) Lastly, the communication between the *pericardium* and the biliary tract is referred to by Naunyn in a single case.

(*b*) *Perforation into the Peritoneum.*—Of 119 cases (Courvoisier) in 70 the rupture occurred directly into the peritoneal cavity; in 49 an encapsulated abscess formed. As a rule, the condition is due to an acute cholecystitis.

(*c*) *Obstruction of the Bowel by Gall-stones.*—Reference has been made to this; its frequency appears from the fact that of 295 cases of obstruction, occurring during eight years, analyzed by Fitz, 23 were by gall-stones. Courvoisier's statistics give a total number of 131 cases, in 6 of which the calculi had a peculiar situation, as in a diverticulum or in the appendix. Of the remaining 125 cases, in 70 the stone was spontaneously passed, usually with severe symptoms. The post mortem reports show that in some of these cases even very large stones have passed, as the gall-duct has been enormously distended, its orifice admitting the finger freely. This, however, is extremely rare. The stones have been found most commonly in the ileum.

Treatment of Gall-stones and Their Effects.—General Treatment.—In an attack of biliary colic the patient should be kept under morphia, given hypodermically, in quarter-grain (0.016 gm.) doses. In an agonizing paroxysm it is well to give a whiff or two of chloroform until the morphia has had time to act. Great relief is experienced from the hot bath and from fomentations in the region of the liver. The patient should be given laxatives and drink copiously of alkaline mineral waters. Olive oil has proved useless in our hands. When taken in large quantities, fatty concretions are passed with the stools, which have been regarded as calculi; and concretions due to eating pears have been also mistaken, particularly when associated with colic attacks. Since the days of Durande, whose mixture of ether with turpentine is still largely used in France, various remedies have been advised to dissolve the stones within the gall-bladder, none of which are efficacious.

Foci of infection should be treated and special attention given to the mouth. The patient should take regular exercise. The diet should be simple and in some cases a cholesterol free diet seems useful. Water should be taken freely. The soda salts are believed to prevent the concentration of the bile and the formation of gall-stones. Either the sulphate or the phosphate may be taken in doses of from 1 to 2 drams daily. For the itching McCall Anderson's dusting powder may be used: starch, an ounce (30 gm.); camphor, a drachm and a half (6 gm.); and oxide of zinc, half an ounce (15 gm.). Some of this should be finely dusted over the skin. Powdering with starch, strong alkaline baths (hot), pilocarpin hypodermically (gr. 1/8-1/6, 0.008-0.01 gm.), and antipyrin (gr. v, 0.3 gm.), may be tried. Ichthyol and lanolin ointment or menthol ointment sometimes gives relief.

Surgical Treatment.—The indications for operation are: (*a*) Repeated attacks of gall-stone colic. The patient is much safer in the hands of a surgeon than when left to Nature, with the feeble assistance of drugs and mineral waters. (*b*) The presence of a distended gall-bladder, associated with attacks of pain or with fever. (*c*) When a gall-stone is permanently lodged in the common duct the question of advising operation depends largely upon the personal methods and success of the surgeon who is available. (*d*) Persistent ill health or gastric disturbance due to infection of the biliary tract or gall-stones.

Of 4,000 operations performed by the Mayo brothers to February 20th, 1911, the mortality was 2.57 per cent. Of 2,920 cases in which the gall-bladder alone was involved the mortality was 1.8 per cent. Of 492 cases in which the common duct was involved the mortality was 8 per cent. In 2.25 per cent. there was the complication of malignant disease.

The question comes up as to the re-formation of stones, but the possibility of this is very slight. In the Mayo series there were but 3 cases and it is probable that in the majority of instances the stones had not re-formed, but were incompletely removed. Deaver reports an instance in which 200 stones were removed two years after the extraction of 120. After removal of the gall-bladder stones may be formed in the hepatic ducts.

VII. THE CIRRHOSES OF THE LIVER

General Considerations.—The many forms of cirrhoses of the liver have one feature in common—an increase in the connective tissue. We use the term cirrhosis (by which Laennec characterized the tawny, yellow color of the common atrophic form) to indicate similar changes in other organs.

Etiology.—There are five types of primary lesion, any one of which may lead to cirrhosis.

1. *Toxic Cirrhosis.*—This is the only acute type and it is seen post partum, in chloroform narcosis and sometimes as a terminal lesion in any form of disease. There is a central necrosis about the hepatic vein which may be slight in amount, or in some cases an acute yellow atrophy, very extensive so that the liver is rapidly reduced in size. Into the necrotic areas leucocytes migrate, the dead liver cells are quickly removed and there is an apparent increase of the connective tissue. Great regeneration of the liver cells is possible. Clinically this type can scarcely be spoken of as cirrhosis.

2. *Infectious Cirrhosis.*—Adami and his school hold that in many cases the colon bacilli from the bowel pass to the liver and there gradually excite a slow proliferation of connective tissue, regarding it as a kind of subinfection. Mallory, whose classification is followed, thinks that the only type of true infectious cirrhosis is through the bile ducts, usually when there is bile stasis or gall-stones or other obstructions are present. Cases are described in which invasion occurs along apparently normal bile ducts and the organisms cause necrosis of the liver cells, proliferation of the fibroblasts, and thickening of the walls of the smaller bile ducts which may be dilated and tortuous. Clinically this type is rare, and characterized by a chronic jaundice and enlargement of the liver.

3. *Pigment Cirrhosis.*—This may be an external pigment as in antharcosis in which the irritation of the coal particles reaching the liver through the lymphatics may excite a moderate grade of cirrhosis. The endogenous pig-

ment is a transformation of hæmoglobin either as in malaria or as in the remarkable affection known as hæmochromatosis.

4. *Syphilitic Cirrhosis.*—Whether congenital or acquired, the essential lesion is produced by the *Treponema pallidum,* either a diffuse proliferation of fibroblasts, or a more localized lesion, the gumma.

5. *Alcoholic Cirrhosis.*—As a result of the toxic action of the alcohol, the liver cells, singly or in groups, undergo a slow necrosis, following which there is a multiplication of the fibroblasts with a hyalin degeneration of some cells and multiplication of others and an increase in the smaller bile ducts. Fatty infiltration is common, so that the organ may be enlarged.

Of these types the toxic and one form of the alcoholic are associated with shrinkage, the infectious, the pigmentary and the fatty cirrhosis with enlargement of the organ. Clinically we may consider four forms, the portal, the hypertrophic (of Hanot), the syphilitic, and the capsular.

I. PORTAL CIRRHOSIS

Etiology.—The disease occurs most frequently in middle-aged males who have been addicted to drink. Whisky, gin, and brandy are more potent to cause cirrhosis than beer. It is more common in countries in which strong spirits are used than in those in which malt liquors are taken. It is not always due to alcohol. Symmers believes that syphilis is an important factor in the etiology in the Laennec cirrhosis. Among 1,000 autopsies in the Johns Hopkins Hospital there were 63 cases of small atrophic liver, and 8 cases of the fatty cirrhotic organ. Lancereaux claims that the *vin ordinaire* of France is a common cause. Of 210 cases, excess in wine alone was present in 68 cases. He thinks it is the sulphate of potash in the plaster of Paris used to give the "dry" flavor which damages the liver.

Cirrhosis of the liver in young children is not very rare. In a certain number of the cases there is an alcoholic history, in others syphilis has been present, while a third group, due to the poisons of the infectious diseases, embraces a certain number of the cases of Hanot's hypertrophic cirrhosis.

Morbid Anatomy.—Portal cirrhosis occurs in two well-characterized forms:

THE ATROPHIC CIRRHOSIS OF LAENNEC.—The organ is greatly reduced in size and may be deformed. The weight is sometimes not more than a pound or a pound and a half. It presents numerous granulations on the surface; is firm, hard, and cuts with great resistance. The substance is seen to be made up of greenish-yellow islands surrounded by grayish-white connective tissue. W. G. MacCallum has shown that regenerative changes in the cells are almost constantly present. This yellow appearance of the liver induced Laennec to give to the condition the name of cirrhosis.

THE FATTY CIRRHOTIC LIVER.—Even in the contracted form the fat is increased, but in typical examples of this variety the organ is not reduced in size, but is enlarged, smooth or very slightly granular, anæmic, yellowish-white in color, and resembles an ordinary fatty liver. It is, however, firm, cuts with resistance, and microscopically shows a great increase in the connective tissue. This form occurs most frequently in beer-drinkers.

The two essential elements in cirrhosis are destruction of liver-cells and obstruction to the portal circulation.

In an autopsy on a case of cirrhosis with contraction the peritoneum is usually found to contain a large quantity of fluid, the membrane is opaque, and there is chronic catarrh of the stomach and of the small intestines. The spleen is enlarged, in part, at least, from the chronic congestion, possibly due in part to a toxic influence. The pancreas frequently shows interstitial changes. The kidneys are sometimes cirrhotic, the bases of the lungs may be much compressed by the ascitic fluid, the heart often shows marked degeneration, and arterio-sclerosis is usually present. A remarkable feature is the association of acute tuberculosis with cirrhosis. In seven cases of our series the patients died with either acute tuberculous peritonitis or acute tuberculous pleurisy. Rolleston has found that tuberculosis was present in 28 per cent. of 706 fatal cases of cirrhosis. Peritoneal tuberculosis was found in 9 per cent. of a series of 584 cases.

The compensatory circulation is usually readily demonstrated. It is carried out by the following set of vessels: (1) The accessory portal system of Sappey, of which important branches pass in the round and suspensory ligaments and unite with the epigastric and mammary systems. These vessels are numerous and small. Occasionally a large single vein, which may attain the size of the little finger, passes from the hilus of the liver, follows the round ligament, and joins the epigastric veins at the navel. Although this has the position of the umbilical vein, it is usually, as Sappey showed, a para-umbilical vein—that is, an enlarged vein by the side of the obliterated umbilical vessel. There may be produced about the navel a large bunch of varices, the so-called caput Medusæ. Other branches of this system occur in the gastro-epiploic omentum, about the gall-bladder, and, most important of all, in the suspensory ligament. These latter form large branches, which anastomose freely with the diaphragmatic veins, and so unite with the vena azygos. (2) By the anastomosis between the œsophageal and gastric veins. The veins at the lower end of the œsophagus may be enormously enlarged, producing varices which project on the mucous membrane. (3) The communications between the hæmorrhoidal and the inferior mesenteric veins. The freedom of communication in this direction is very variable, and in some instances the hæmorrhoidal veins are not much enlarged. (4) The veins of Retzius, which unite the radicles of the portal branches in the intestines and mesentery with the inferior vena cava and its branches. To this system belong the whole group of retroperitoneal veins, which are in most instances enormously enlarged, particularly about the kidneys, and which serve to carry off a considerable proportion of the portal blood.

Symptoms.—The most extreme grade of portal cirrhosis may exist without symptoms. *So long as the compensatory circulation is maintained* the patient may suffer little or no inconvenience. The remarkable efficiency of this collateral circulation is well seen in those rare instances of permanent obliteration of the portal vein. The symptoms may be divided into two groups —obstructive and toxic.

Obstructive.—The overfilling of the blood-vessels of the stomach and intestine leads to chronic catarrh, and the patients suffer with nausea and vomiting, particularly in the morning; the tongue is furred and the bowels are irregular. Hæmorrhage from the stomach may be an early symptom; it is often profuse and liable to recur. It seldom proves fatal. The amount vomited may be remarkable as in a case in which ten pounds were ejected in seven days. Following the hæmatemesis melæna is common; but hæmorrhages from the bowels may occur for several years without hæmatemesis. The bleeding very often comes from œsophageal varices. Very frequently epistaxis occurs. Enlargement of the spleen may be due to a toxæmia. The organ can usually be felt. Evidences of the establishment of the collateral circulation are seen in the enlarged epigastric and mammary veins, more rarely in the presence of the caput Medusæ and the development of hæmorrhoids. The distended venules in the lower thoracic zone along the line of attachment of the diaphragm are not specially marked in cirrhosis. The most striking feature of failure in the compensatory circulation is *ascites,* the effusion of serous fluid into the peritoneal cavity, which may appear suddenly. The conditions under which this occurs are still obscure. In some cases it is due more to chronic peritonitis than to the cirrhosis. The abdomen gradually distends, may reach a large size, and contain as much as 15 to 20 litres. Œdema of the feet may precede or develop with the ascites. The dropsy is rarely general.

Jaundice is usually slight, and was present in 107 of 293 cases of cirrhosis collected by Rolleston. The skin has frequently a sallow, slightly icteroid tint. The urine is often reduced in amount, contains urates in abundance, often a slight amount of albumin, and, if jaundice is intense, tube-casts. The disease may be afebrile throughout, but in many cases, as shown by Carrington, there is slight fever, from 100° to 102.5° F.

Examination at an early stage of the disease may show an enlarged and painful liver. In many of the cases of portal cirrhosis the organ is "enlarged at all stages of the disease, and, whether enlarged or contracted, the clinical symptoms and course are much the same" (Foxwell). The patient may first come under observation for dyspepsia, hæmatemesis, slight jaundice, or nervous symptoms. Later in the disease the patient has an unmistakable hepatic facies; he is thin, the eyes are sunken, the conjunctivæ watery, the nose and cheeks show distended venules, and the complexion is muddy or icteroid. On the enlarged abdomen the vessels are distended, and a bunch of dilated veins may surround the navel. A venous hum, sometimes accompanied by a thrill, may be present in the epigastrium or over varicosities. Nævi of a remarkable character may appear on the skin, either localized stellate varices—spider angiomata—usually on the face, neck, and back, and also "mat" nævi—areas of skin of a reddish or purplish color due to the uniform distention of small venules. When much fluid is in the peritoneum it is impossible to make a satisfactory examination, but after withdrawal the area of liver dulness is found to be diminished, particularly in the middle line, and on deep pressure the edge of the liver can be detected, and occasionally the hard, firm, and even granular surface. The spleen can be felt in the left hypochondriac region. Examination of the anus may reveal the presence of hæmorrhoids.

Toxic Symptoms.—At any stage of cirrhosis the patient may have cerebral symptoms, either a noisy, joyous delirium, or stupor, coma, or even convulsions. The condition is not infrequently mistaken for uræmia. The nature of the toxic agent is not yet settled. Without jaundice, and not attributable to cholæmia, the symptoms may come on in hospital when the patient has not had alcohol for weeks.

The fatty cirrhotic liver may produce symptoms similar to those of the contracted form, but more frequently it is latent and is found accidentally in topers who have died from various diseases. The greater number of the cases clinically diagnosed as cirrhosis with enlargement come in this division.

Diagnosis.—With ascites, a well-marked history of alcoholism, the hepatic facies, and hæmorrhage from the stomach or bowels, the diagnosis is rarely doubtful. If, after withdrawal of the fluid, the spleen is found to be enlarged and the liver either not palpable or, if it is enlarged, hard and regular, the probabilities in favor of cirrhosis are very great. In the early stages of the disease, when the liver is increased in size, it may be impossible to say whether it is a cirrhotic or a fatty liver. The differential diagnosis between common and syphilitic cirrhosis can usually be made. A marked history of syphilis or the existence of other syphilitic lesions, with great irregularity on the surface or at the edge of the liver, are in favor of the latter. Thrombosis or obliteration of the portal vein can rarely be differentiated. In a case of fibroid transformation of the portal vein which came under observation, the collateral circulation had been established for years, and the symptoms were simply those of extreme portal obstruction, such as occur in cirrhosis. Thrombosis of the portal vein may occur in cirrhosis and be characterized by a rapidly developing ascites.

Prognosis.—The outlook is bad. When the collateral circulation is fully established the patient may have no symptoms whatever. There are instances of enlargement of the liver, slight jaundice, cerebral symptoms, and even hæmatemesis, in which the liver becomes reduced in size, the symptoms disappear, and the patient may live in comparative comfort for many years. There are cases, too, possibly syphilitic, in which, after one or two tappings, the symptoms have disappeared and the patients have apparently recovered. Ascites is a very serious event, especially if due to the cirrhosis and not to an associated peritonitis. Of 34 cases with ascites 10 died before tapping was necessary; 14 were tapped, and the average duration of life after the swelling was first noticed was only eight weeks; of 10 cases the diagnosis was wrong in 4, and in the remaining 6, who were tapped oftener than once, chronic peritonitis and perihepatitis were present (Hale White).

II. HYPERTROPHIC BILIARY CIRRHOSIS (*Hanot*)

This well-characterized form was first described by Requin in 1846, but our accurate knowledge of the condition dates from the work of Hanot (1875), whose name in France it bears—*maladie de Hanot.*

Cirrhosis with enlargement occurs in the portal cirrhosis; there is an enlarged fatty and cirrhotic liver of alcoholics, a pigmentary form occurs in hæmochromatosis, and in association with syphilis the organ is often very large. The hypertrophic cirrhosis of Hanot is easily distinguished from these forms.

Etiology.—Males are more often affected than females—in 22 of Schachmann's 26 cases. The subjects are young; some of the cases in children probably belong to this form. Alcohol plays a minor part, and not one of our patients had been a heavy drinker. The absence of all known etiological factors is a remarkable feature.

Morbid Anatomy.—The organ is enlarged, weighing from 2,000 to 4,000 grams. The form is maintained, the surface is smooth, or presents small granulations; the color in advanced cases is of a dark olive green; the consistence is greatly increased. The section is uniform, greenish yellow in color, and the liver nodules may be seen separated by connective tissue. The bile-passages present nothing abnormal. The cirrhosis is mono- or multilobular, with a connective tissue rich in round cells. The bile-vessels are the seat of an angiocholitis, catarrhal and productive, and there is an extraordinary development of new biliary canaliculi. The liver-cells are neither fatty nor pigmented, and may be increased in size and show karyokinetic figures. From the supposed origin about the bile-vessels it has been called biliary cirrhosis, but the histological details have not been worked out fully, and the separation of this as a distinct form rests upon clinical rather than anatomical grounds. The spleen is greatly enlarged and may weigh 600 or more grams.

Symptoms.—The cases occur in young persons; there is not, as a rule, an alcoholic history, and males are usually affected. The features are: (*a*) A remarkably chronic course of from four to six, or even ten years. (*b*) Jaundice, usually slight, often not more than a lemon tint, or a tinging of the conjunctivæ. At any time during the course an *icterus gravis,* with high fever and delirium, may develop. There is bile in the urine; the stools are not clay-colored as in obstructive jaundice, but may be very dark and "bilious." (*c*) Attacks of pain in the region of the liver, which may be severe and associated with nausea and vomiting. The pain may be slight and dragging, and in some cases is not at all a prominent symptom. The jaundice may deepen after attacks of pain. (*d*) Enlarged liver. A fullness in the upper abdominal zone may be the first complaint. On inspection the enlargement may be very marked. In one of our cases the left lobe was unusually prominent and stood out almost like a tumor. An exploratory operation showed only an enlarged, smooth organ without adhesions. On palpation the hypertrophy is uniform, the consistence is increased, and the edge distinct and hard. The gall-bladder is not enlarged. The vertical flatness is much increased and may extend from the sixth rib to the level of the navel. (*e*) The spleen is enlarged, easily palpable, and very hard. (*f*) Certain negative features are of moment—the usual absence of ascites and of dilatation of the subcutaneous veins of the abdomen. Among other symptoms may be mentioned hæmorrhages. One patient had bleeding at the gums for a year; another had had for years most remarkable attacks of purpura with urticaria. Pruritus, xanthoma, lichen, and telangiectasis may be present in the skin. The skin may become very bronzed, almost as deeply as in Addison's disease. Slight fever may be present, which increases during the crises of pain. There may be a marked leucocytosis. A curious attitude of the body has been seen, in which the right shoulder and right side appear dragged down. The patients die with the symptoms of icterus gravis, from hæmorrhage, from an intercurrent infection, or in a profound cachexia. Certain of the cases of cirrhosis of the liver in children are of this type; the enlargement of the spleen may be very pronounced.

III. SYPHILITIC CIRRHOSIS

This is considered in the section on syphilis (p. 279). It is referred to again to emphasize (1) its frequency; (2) the great importance of its differentiation from the alcoholic form; (3) its curability in many cases; and (4) the tumor formations in connection with it.

IV. CAPSULAR CIRRHOSIS—PERIHEPATITIS

Local capsulitis is common in many conditions of the liver. The form of disease here described is characterized by an enormous thickening of the entire capsule, with great contraction of the liver, but not necessarily with special increase in the connective tissue of the organ itself. Our chief knowledge of the disease we owe to the Guy's Hospital physicians, particularly to Hilton Fagge and to Hale White, who collected 22 cases from the records. The liver substance itself was "never markedly cirrhotic; its tissue was nearly always soft." Chronic capsulitis of the spleen and a chronic proliferative peritonitis are almost invariably present. In 19 of the 22 cases the kidneys were granular. Hale White regards it as a sequel of interstitial nephritis. The youngest case in his series was twenty-nine. The symptoms are those of portal cirrhosis —ascites, often recurring and requiring many tappings. Jaundice is not often present. There are two groups of cases—the one in adults usually with ascites is regarded as ordinary cirrhosis and the diagnosis is rarely made. Signs of interstitial nephritis, recurring ascites, and absence of jaundice are regarded by Hale White as important diagnostic points. In the second group the perihepatitis, perisplenitis, and proliferative peritonitis are associated with adherent pericardium and chronic mediastinitis. In one such case the diagnosis of capsular hepatitis was very clear, as the liver could be grasped in the hand and formed a rounded, smooth organ resembling the spleen. The child was tapped 121 times (Archives of Pædiatrics, 1896).

Treatment.—The portal function of the liver may be put out of action without much damage to the body. There may be an extreme grade of cirrhotic atrophy without symptoms; the portal vein may be obliterated, or, experimentally, the portal vein may be anastomosed with the cava. So long as there is an active compensatory circulation a patient with portal cirrhosis may remain well. In the hypertrophic form toxæmia is the special danger and we have no means of arresting the progress of the disease. In the alcoholic form it is too late, as a rule, to do much after symptoms have occurred. In a few cases an attack of jaundice or hæmatemesis may prove the salvation of the patient, who may afterward take to a temperate life. The diet should be very simple and large amounts of water taken to aid elimination. The bowels should be kept open, for which the use of the salines is generally best. An occasional course of potassium iodide may be given. With the advent of ascites the critical stage is reached. Restriction of fluid intake and free purgation may relieve a small exudate, rarely a large one, and it is best to tap early. In the syphilitic cirrhosis much more can be done, and a majority of the cases of cure after ascites are of this variety. Iodide of potassium in moderate doses, 15 to 30 drops of the saturated solution, and mercury save a number of cases even after repeated tapping. The diagnosis may be reached only after removal of the fluid, but in every case with a history of syphilis, a positive Wassermann reaction, or with irregularity of the liver this treatment should be tried.

Surgical Treatment.—(*a*) *Tapping.*—When the ascites increases it is better to tap early. As Hale White remarks, a case of cirrhosis of the liver which is tapped rarely recovers, but there are instances in which early and repeated paracentesis is followed by cure. Accidents are rare; hæmorrhage, acute peritonitis, or erysipelas at the point of puncture occasionally follow; collapse may occur during the operation, to guard against which Mead advised the use of the abdominal binder. Continuous drainage with Southey's tubes is not often practicable and has no special advantages. (*b*) *Laparotomy,* with complete removal of the fluid, and freshening or rubbing the peritoneal surfaces, to stimulate the formation of adhesions. (*c*) *Omentopexy,* the stitching of the omentum to the abdominal wall, and the establishment of collateral circulation in this way between the portal and the systemic vessels. This operation is sometimes successful. In 224 cases there were 84 deaths and 129 recoveries; 11 cases doubtful. Among the 129 successful cases, in 25 the ascites recurred; 70 appeared to have completely recovered. (*d*) *Fistula of Eck.* The porto-caval anastomosis has been performed once in man in cirrhosis of the liver (Widal, *La Semaine Médicale,* 1903). The patient lived for three months. (*e*) *Auto-drainage,* in which the fluid is drained into the subcutaneous tissues.

VIII. ABSCESS OF THE LIVER

Etiology.—Suppuration within the liver, either in the parenchyma or in the blood or bile-passages, occurs under the following conditions:

(*a*) The *tropical abscess,* also called the *solitary,* commonly follows amœbic dysentery. It frequently occurs among Europeans in India, particularly those who drink alcohol freely and are exposed to great heat. Cases may occur without a history of previous dysentery, and there have been fatal cases without any affection of the large bowel. In the United States the large solitary abscess is not very infrequent. The relation of this form of abscess to amœbic dysentery has been considered. The number of cases has been much reduced since the introduction of the emetine treatment.

(*b*) *Traumatism* is an occasional cause. The injury is generally in the hepatic region. Instances occur in trainmen injured while coupling cars. Injury to the head is not infrequently followed by liver abscess.

(*c*) *Embolic or pyæmic abscesses* are the most numerous, occurring in a general pyæmia or following foci of suppuration in the territory of the portal vessels. The infective agents may reach the liver through the hepatic artery, as in those cases in which the original focus of infection is in the area of the systemic circulation; though it may happen occasionally that the infective agent, instead of passing through the lungs, reaches the liver through the inferior vena cava and the hepatic veins. A remarkable instance of multiple abscesses of arterial origin was shown by the case of aneurism of the hepatic artery reported by Ross and Osler. Infection through the portal vein is more common. It results from dysentery and other ulcerative affections of the bowels, appendicitis, occasionally after typhoid fever, in rectal affections, and in abscesses in the pelvis. In these cases the abscesses are multiple and, as a rule, within the branches of the portal vein—suppurative pylephlebitis.

(*d*) A not uncommon cause is *inflammation of the bile-passages* caused by gall-stones, more rarely by parasites—suppurative cholangitis. In some instances of tuberculosis of the liver the affection is chiefly of the bile-ducts, with the formation of multiple tuberculous abscesses containing a bile-stained pus.

(*e*) *Foreign bodies and parasites.* In rare instances foreign bodies, such as a needle, may pass from the stomach or gullet, lodge in the liver, and excite an abscess, or a foreign body, such as a needle or a fish-bone, has perforated a branch or the portal vein itself and induced pylephlebitis. Echinococcus cysts frequently cause suppuration, the penetration of round worms into the liver less commonly, and most rarely of all the liver-fluke.

Morbid Anatomy.—(*a*) Of the Solitary or Tropical Abscess.—This has been described under amœbic dysentery.

(*b*) Of Septic and Pyæmic Abscesses.—These are usually multiple, though occasionally, following injury, there may be a large solitary abscess. In suppurative pylephlebitis the liver is uniformly enlarged. The capsule may be smooth and the external surface of normal appearance. On section there are isolated pockets of pus, either having a round outline or in some places distinctly dendritic, and from these the pus may be squeezed. The entire portal system within the liver may be involved; sometimes territories are cut off by thrombi. The suppuration may extend into the main branch or even into the mesenteric and gastric veins. In suppurative cholangitis there is usually obstruction by gall-stones, the ducts are greatly distended, the gall-bladder enlarged and full of pus, and the branches within the liver are extremely distended, having an appearance not unlike that described in pylephlebitis. An abscess may have a sponge-like appearance due to the fusion of numerous points of suppuration. Suppuration about the echinococcus cysts may be very extensive, forming enormous abscesses, the characters of which are at once recognized by the remnants of the cysts.

Symptoms.—(*a*) Of the Large Solitary Abscess.—The abscess may be latent and run a course without definite symptoms; death may occur suddenly from rupture.

Fever, pain, enlargement of the liver, and a septic condition are the important symptoms of hepatic abscess. The temperature is elevated at the outset and is of an intermittent or septic type. It is irregular, and may remain normal or even subnormal for a few days; then the patient has a rigor and the temperature rises to 103° F. or higher. Owing to this intermittent character of the fever the disease is often mistaken for malaria. The fever may rise every afternoon without a rigor. Profuse sweating is common, particularly when the patient falls asleep. In chronic cases there may be little or no fever. Patients with a liver abscess perforating the lung, may cough up pus after the temperature has been normal for weeks. The pain is variable and usually referred to the back or shoulder; or there is a dull aching sensation in the right hypochondrium. When turned on the left side, the patient often complains of a heavy, dragging sensation, so that he usually prefers to lie on the right side. Pain on pressure over the liver is usually present, particularly on deep pressure at the costal margin in the nipple line.

The *enlargement* of the liver is most marked in the right lobe, and, as the abscess cavity is usually situated more toward the upper than the under surface, the increase in volume is upward and to the right, not downward, as in cancer and the other affections producing enlargement. Percussion in the mid-sternal and parasternal lines may show a normal limit. At the nipple-line the curve of liver dulness begins to rise, and in the mid-axillary it may reach the fifth rib, while behind, near the spine, the area of dulness may be almost on a level with the angle of the scapula. There are instances in which this characteristic feature is not present, as when the abscess occupies the left lobe. The enlargement of the liver may be so great as to cause bulging of the right side, and the edge may project a hand's-breadth or more below the costal margin. In such instances the surface is smooth. Palpation is painful, and there may be fremitus on deep inspiration. In some instances fluctuation may be detected. Adhesions may form to the abdominal wall and the abscess may point below the margin of the ribs, or even in the epigastric region. In many cases the appearance of the patient is suggestive. The skin has a sallow, slightly icteroid tint, the face is pale, the complexion muddy, the conjunctivæ are infiltrated, and often slightly bile-tinged. There is in the facies and in the general appearance of the patient a strong suggestion of the existence of abscess. There is no internal affection associated with suppuration which gives just the same hue as certain instances of abscess of the liver. Marked jaundice is rare. Diarrhœa may be present and give an important clue to the nature of the case, particularly if amœbæ are found in the stools. Constipation may occur.

Perforation of the lung occurred in 9 of the 27 cases in our series. The symptoms are most characteristic. The extension may occur through the diaphragm, without actual rupture, and with the production of a purulent pleurisy and invasion of the lung. With cough of an aggravated and convulsive character, there are signs of involvement at the base of the right lung, defective resonance, feeble tubular breathing, and increase in the tactile fremitus; but the most characteristic feature is the presence of a reddish-brown expectoration of a brick-dust color, resembling anchovy sauce. Amœbæ are present in variable numbers and display active amœboid movements. The brownish tint of the expectoration is due to blood-pigment and blood-corpuscles, and there may be orange-red crystals of hæmatoidin.

The abscess may perforate externally, as mentioned already, or into the stomach or bowel; occasionally into the pericardium. The duration of this form is very variable. It may run its course and prove fatal in six or eight weeks or may persist for several years.

The prognosis is serious, as the mortality is more than 50 per cent. The death-rate has been lowered of late years, owing to the great fearlessness with which the surgeons now attack these cases.

(*b*) Of the Pyæmic Abscess and Suppurative Pylephlebitis.—Clinically these conditions cannot be separated. Occurring in a general pyæmia, no special features may be added to the case. When there is suppuration within the portal vein the liver is uniformly enlarged and tender, though pain may not be a marked feature. There is an irregular, septic fever, and the complexion is muddy, sometimes distinctly icteroid. The features are indeed those of pyæmia, plus a slight icteroid tinge, and an enlarged and painful liver. The latter features alone are peculiar. The sweats, chills, prostration, and fever have nothing distinctive.

Diagnosis.—Abscess of the liver may be confounded with intermittent fever, a common mistake in malarial regions. Practically an *intermittent* *fever* which resists quinine is not malarial. Laveran's organisms are also absent from the blood. When the abscess bursts into the pleura a right-sided empyema is produced and perforation of the lung usually follows. When the liver abscess has been latent and dysenteric symptoms have not been marked, the condition may be considered empyema or abscess of the lung. In such cases the anchovy-sauce-like color of the pus and the presence of the amœbæ will enable one to make a definite diagnosis. Perforation externally is readily recognized, and yet in an abscess cavity in the epigastric region it may be difficult to say whether it has proceeded from the liver or is in the abdominal wall. When the abscess is large, and the adhesions are so firm that the liver does not descend during inspiration, the exploratory needle does not make an up-and-down movement during aspiration. The diagnosis of suppurating echinococcus cyst is rarely possible, except in Australia and Iceland, where hydatids are so common.

Perhaps the most important affection from which suppuration within the liver is to be separated is the *intermittent hepatic fever* associated with gall-stones. Of the cases reported a majority have been considered due to suppuration, and in two cases the liver had been repeatedly aspirated. Post mortem examinations have shown conclusively that the high fever and chills may recur at intervals for years without suppuration in the ducts. The distinctive features of this condition are paroxysms of fever with rigors and sweats—which may occur with great regularity, but which more often are separated by long intervals—the deepening of the jaundice after the paroxysms, the entire apyrexia in the intervals, and the maintenance of the general nutrition. The time element also is important, as in some of these cases the disease has lasted for several years. Finally, it is to be remembered that abscess of the liver, in temperate climates at least, is invariably secondary, and the primary source must be carefully sought for, either in dysentery, slight ulceration of the rectum, suppurating hæmorrhoids, ulcer of the stomach, or in suppurative disease of other parts of the body, particularly within the skull or in the bones. Leucocytosis may be absent in the amœbic abscess of the liver; in septic cases it may be very high.

In suspected cases, whether the liver is enlarged or not, exploratory aspiration may be performed. The needle may be entered in the anterior axillary line in the lowest interspace, or in the seventh interspace in the mid-axillary line, or over the centre of the area of dulness behind. The patient should be placed under ether, for it may be necessary to make several deep punctures. It is not well to use too small an aspirator. Operation should be done at once if pus is found. Extensive suppuration may exist, and yet be missed in the aspiration, particularly when the branches of the portal vein are distended with pus.

Treatment.—Pyæmic abcess and suppurative pylephlebitis are invariably fatal. Treves, however, reports a case of pyæmic abscess following appendicitis in which the patient recovered after an exploratory operation. Surgical measures are not justified in these cases, unless an abscess shows signs of pointing. As the abscesses associated with dysentery are often single, they afford a reasonable hope of benefit from operation. If, however, the patient is expectorating the pus, if the general condition is good and the hectic fever not marked, it is best to defer operation, as many of these instances recover spontaneously. The large single abscesses are the most favorable for operation. The general medical treatment of the cases is that of ordinary septicæmia.

IX. NEW GROWTHS IN THE LIVER

These may be cancer, either primary or secondary, adenoma, sarcoma, or angioma.

Etiology.—Cancer of the liver is third in order of frequency of internal cancer. It is rarely primary, usually secondary to cancer in other organs. It is a disease of late adult life. According to Leichtenstern, over 50 per cent. of the cases occur between the fortieth and the sixtieth years. It occasionally occurs in children. Women are attacked less frequently than men but some authors state that secondary cancer is more common in women, owing to the frequency of cancer of the uterus. In many cases trauma is an antecedent, and cancer of the bile-passages is associated in many instances with gall-stones. Cancer is stated to be less common in the tropics.

Morbid Anatomy.—The following forms of new growths occur in the liver and have a clinical importance:

CANCER.—*Primary Cancer.*—This is rare. Of 163 cases collected by Eggel, 63.3 per cent. were in males. There are several varieties. Nodular forms, in which there are scattered growths throughout the organ; the massive form in which the solitary tumor occupies a large area, either a lobe or the greater part of it; and small metastatic nodules. A very important form is that in which the liver is diffusely infiltrated with small growths, with much hyperplasia of the connective tissue—the so-called cancer with cirrhosis. The course of the disease is rapid, jaundice often occurs, splenic enlargement is not infrequent, ascites and œdema are common and toxic features are frequent toward the close.

Secondary Cancer.—The organ may reach an enormous size, 30½ pounds (Osler), 33 pounds (Christian). The cancerous nodules project beneath the capsule, and can be felt during life or even seen through the thin abdominal walls. They are usually disseminated equally, though in rare instances they may be confined to one lobe. The consistence of the nodules varies; in some cases they are firm and hard and those on the surface show a distinct umbilication, due to the shrinking of the fibrous tissue in the centre. These superficial masses are sometimes spoken of as "Farre's tubercles." More frequently the masses are on section grayish-white in color, or hæmorrhagic. Rupture of blood-vessels is not uncommon; in one specimen there was an enormous clot beneath the capsule of the liver, together with hæmorrhage into the gall-bladder and into the peritoneum. The secondary cancer shows the same structure as the initial lesion, and is usually an alveolar or cylindrical carcinoma. Degeneration is common in these secondary growths; thus the hyaline transformation may convert large areas into a dense, dry, grayish-yellow mass. Extensive areas of fatty degeneration may occur, sclerosis is not uncommon, and hæmorrhages are frequent. Suppuration sometimes follows.

Cancer of the bile-passages which has been already considered.

PRIMARY ADENOMA.—Gordinier and Sawyer collected 44 cases, 28 of which were multiple, and of these 21 were associated with the cirrhosis of Laennec.

In a majority of the cases the process appears to be secondary to a cirrhosis, a compensatory cell hypertrophy to offset the destruction of the liver cells. In some cases, however, it may be a primary affair. The clinical picture is that of cirrhosis, often of the Hanot type.

Sarcoma.—Of primary sarcoma of the liver very few cases have been reported. Secondary sarcoma is more frequent, and many examples of lympho-sarcoma and myxo-sarcoma are on record, less frequently glio-sarcoma or the smooth or striped myoma. The most important form is the *melano-sarcoma,* secondary to sarcoma of the eye or of the skin. Very rarely melano-sarcoma occurs primarily in the liver. In this form the liver is greatly enlarged, is either uniformly infiltrated with the growth, which gives the cut surface the appearance of dark granite, or there are large nodular masses of a deep black or marbled color. There are usually extensive metastases, and in some instances every organ of the body is involved. Nodules of melano-sarcoma of the skin may give a clue to the diagnosis.

Other Forms of Liver Tumor.—Angioma occurs as a small, reddish body the size of a walnut, and consists simply of a series of dilated vessels. Occasionally in children angiomata grow and produce large tumors.

Cysts are occasionally found, either single, which is not very uncommon, or multiple, when they usually coexist with congenital cystic kidneys.

Symptoms.—It is often impossible to differentiate primary and secondary cancer of the liver unless the primary seat of the disease is evident, as in the case of scirrhus of the breast, cancer of the rectum, or of a tumor in the stomach. As a rule, cancer of the liver is associated with progressive enlargement; but in some cases of primary nodular cancer and in the cancer with cirrhosis the organ may not be enlarged. Gastric disturbance, loss of appetite, nausea, and vomiting are frequent. Progressive loss of flesh and strength may be the first symptoms. Pain or a sensation of uneasiness in the right hypochondriac region may be present, but enormous enlargement of the liver may occur without the slightest pain. Jaundice, which is present in at least half of the cases, is usually of moderate extent, unless the common duct is occluded. Ascites is rare, except in the form of cancer with cirrhosis, in which the picture is that of the atrophic form. Pressure by nodules on the portal vein or extension of the cancer to the peritoneum may induce ascites.

Inspection shows the abdomen to be distended, particularly in the upper zone. In late stages, when emaciation is marked, the cancerous nodules can be plainly seen beneath the skin, and in rare instances even the umbilications. The superficial veins are enlarged. On palpation the liver is felt, a hand's-breadth or more below the costal margin, descending with each inspiration. The surface is usually irregular, and may present large masses or smaller nodular bodies, either rounded or with central depressions. In instances of diffuse infiltration the liver may be greatly enlarged and present a perfectly smooth surface. The growth is progressive, and the edge of the liver may ultimately extend below the level of the navel. Although generally uniform and producing enlargement of the whole organ, occasionally the tumor in the left lobe forms a solid mass occupying the epigastric region. By percussion the outline can be accurately limited and the progressive growth of the tumor estimated. The spleen is rarely enlarged. Pyrexia is present in many cases, usually a continuous fever, ranging from 100° to 102° F.; it may be intermittent, with rigors. This may be associated with the cancer alone, or, as in one of our cases, with suppuration. Œdema of the feet, from anæmia, usually supervenes. Cancer of the liver kills in from three to fifteen months. One of our patients lived for more than two years.

Diagnosis.—The diagnosis is easy when the liver is greatly enlarged and the surface nodular. The smoother forms of diffuse carcinoma may at first be mistaken for fatty or amyloid liver, but the presence of jaundice, the rapid enlargement, and the more marked cachexia will usually suffice to differentiate it. Perhaps the most puzzling conditions occur in the cases of enlarged syphilitic liver with irregular gummata. The large echinococcus liver may present a striking similarity to carcinoma, but the nodules are usually softer, the disease lasts much longer, and the cachexia is not marked.

Hypertrophic cirrhosis may at first be mistaken for carcinoma, as the jaundice is usually deep and the liver very large; but the absence of a marked cachexia and wasting and the painless, smooth character of the enlargement are points against cancer. In large, rapidly growing secondary cancers the superficial rounded masses may almost fluctuate and these soft tumor-like projections may contain blood. The form of cancer with cirrhosis can scarcely be separated from atrophic cirrhosis itself. Perhaps the wasting is more extreme and more rapid, but the jaundice and the ascites are identical. *Melano-sarcoma* causes great enlargement of the organ. There are frequently symptoms of involvement of other viscera, as the lungs, kidneys, or spleen. Secondary tumors may occur in the skin. A very important symptom, not present in all cases, is melanuria, the passage of a very dark-colored urine, which may, however, when first voided, be quite normal in color. The existence of a melanosarcoma of the eye, or the history of blindness in one eye, with subsequent extirpation, may indicate at once the true nature of the hepatic enlargement.

There are several conditions in which the liver itself, or portions of it, may be mistaken for tumor. (*a*) In a progressive cirrhosis with enlargement the left lobe may increase out of all proportion to the right, and form a prominent mass in the epigastrium. (*b*) Riedel's tongue-like lobe projecting from the edge in the neighborhood of the gall-bladder, and often associated with distention of this organ. (*c*) The extreme left portion of the organ may be almost separated by a broad, flat band, containing little or no liver tissue. In a very thin person this section may feel like a separate tumor mass. A small portion of the liver may rest directly upon the cœliac axis, connected with the left lobe by a mesentery. Lastly, the contracted, deformed organ in perihepatitis may form a visible, freely movable tumor in the upper portion of the abdomen, without a semblance of the normal liver. Such an instance is figured in Osler's lectures on *Abdominal Tumors*.

Treatment.—Resection of tumors of the liver has been performed in many cases. Otherwise the treatment is symptomatic.

X. FATTY LIVER

Two different forms of this condition are recognized—the fatty infiltration and fatty degeneration. Fatty *infiltration* occurs, to a certain extent, in normal livers, since the cells always contain minute globules of oil. In fatty *degenera-*

tion, which is much less common, the protoplasm of the liver-cells is destroyed and the fat takes its place, as seen in cases of malignant jaundice and in phosphorus poisoning.

Fatty liver occurs under the following conditions: (*a*) In association with general obesity, in which case the liver appears to be one of the storehouses of the excessive fat. (*b*) In conditions in which the oxidation processes are interfered with, as in cachexia, profound anæmia, and in pulmonary tuberculosis. The fatty infiltration of the liver in heavy drinkers is to be attributed to the excessive demand made by the alcohol upon the oxygen. (*c*) Certain poisons, of which phosphorus is the most characteristic, produce an intense fatty degeneration with necrosis of the liver-cells. The poison of acute yellow atrophy, whatever its nature, acts in the same way.

The liver is uniformly increased in size. The edge may reach below the level of the navel. It is smooth, looks pale and bloodless; on section it is dry, and renders the surface of the knife greasy. The liver may weigh many pounds, but the specific gravity is so low that the entire organ floats in water.

The *symptoms* of fatty liver are not definite. Jaundice is never present; the stools may be light colored, but even in the most advanced grades the bile is still formed. Signs of portal obstruction are rare. Hæmorrhoids are not very infrequent. Altogether, the symptoms are chiefly those of the disease with which the degeneration is associated. In cases of great obesity the physical examination is uncertain; but in cachectic conditions the organ can be felt to be greatly enlarged, though smooth and painless. Fatty livers are among the largest met with at the bedside.

XI. AMYLOID LIVER

The waxy, lardaceous, or amyloid liver occurs as part of a general degeneration, associated with cachexias, particularly when the result of long-standing suppuration. It is rare in the United States.

In practice, it is found oftenest in the prolonged suppuration of tuberculous disease, either of the lungs or of the bones. Next in order of frequency are the cases associated with syphilis. Here there may be ulceration of the rectum, with which it is often connected, or chronic disease of the bone, or it may be present when there are no suppurative changes. It is found occasionally in rickets, in prolonged convalescence from the infectious fevers, and in the cachexia of cancer.

The amyloid liver is large, and may attain dimensions equalled only by those of the cancerous organ. Wilks speaks of a liver weighing fourteen pounds. It is solid, firm, resistant, on section anæmic, and has a semitranslucent, infiltrated appearance. Stained with a dilute solution of iodine, the areas infiltrated with the amyloid matter assume a rich mahogany-brown color.

There are no characteristic *symptoms*. Jaundice does not occur; the stools may be light-colored, but the secretion of bile persists. The physical examination shows the organ to be uniformly enlarged and painless, the surface smooth, the edge rounded, and the consistence greatly increased. Sometimes the edge, even in great enlargement, is sharp and hard. The spleen may be involved, but there are no evidences of portal obstruction.

The *diagnosis* is, as a rule, easy. Progressive and great enlargement in connection with suppuration of long standing or with syphilis is almost always of this nature. In rare instances, however, the amyloid liver is reduced in size. In *leukæmia* the liver may attain considerable size and be smooth and uniform, resembling, on physical examination, the fatty organ. The blood condition at once indicates the true nature of the case.

XII. ANOMALIES IN FORM AND POSITION OF THE LIVER

In transposition of the viscera the right lobe of the organ may occupy the left side. A common and important anomaly is the tilting forward of the organ, so that the antero-posterior axis becomes vertical, not horizontal. Instead of the edge of the right lobe presenting just below the costal margin, a considerable portion of the surface of the lobe is in contact with the abdominal parietes, and the edge may be felt as low, perhaps, as the navel. This anteversion is apt to be mistaken for enlargement of the organ.

The "lacing" liver is met with in two chief types. In one the anterior portion, chiefly of the right lobe, is greatly prolonged, and may reach the transverse navel line, or even lower. A shallow transverse groove separates the thin extension from the main portion of the organ. The peritoneal coating of this groove may be fibroid, and in rare instances the deformed portion is connected with the organ by an almost tendinous membrane. The liver may be compressed laterally and have a pyramidal shape, and the extreme left border and the hinder margin of the left lobe may be much folded and incurved. The projecting portion of the liver, extending low in the right flank, may be mistaken for a tumor, or more frequently for a movable right kidney. Its continuity with the liver itself may not be evident on palpation or on percussion, as coils of intestine may lie in front. It descends, however, with inspiration, and usually the margin can be traced continuously with that of the left lobe of the liver. The greatest difficulty arises when this anomalous lappet is naturally very thick and united to the liver by a very thin membrane, or when it is swollen in conditions of great congestion of the organ.

The other principal type of lacing liver is quite different in shape. It is thick, broader above than below, and lies almost entirely above the transverse line of the cartilages. There is a narrow groove just above the anterior border, which is placed more transversely than normal.

Movable Liver.—This rare condition has received much attention, and J. E. Graham collected 70 cases from the literature. In a very considerable number of these there had been a mistaken diagnosis. A slight grade of mobility of the organ is found in the pendulous abdomen of enteroptosis, and after repeated ascites.

The organ is so connected at its posterior margin with the inferior vena cava and diaphragm that any great mobility from this point is impossible, except on the theory of a meso-hepar or congenital ligamentous union between these structures. The ligaments, however, may show an extreme grade of relaxation (the suspensory 7.5 cm., and the triangular ligament 4 cm., in one of Leube's cases); and when the patient is in the erect posture the organ may drop down so far that its upper surface is entirely below the costal margin. The condition is rarely met with in men; 56 of the cases were in women.

I. DISEASES OF THE PANCREAS

I. PANCREATIC INSUFFICIENCY

Failure of the internal secretion is followed by disturbance in the carbohydrate metabolism, of the external secretion by disturbances of digestion, or by the injurious effects of the retained secretion. The low sugar tolerance, the chief sign of impairment of the internal secretion, has been considered under diabetes. Insufficiency of the external secretion is indicated by:

Changes in the Character of the Stools.—(*a*) STEATORRHŒA.—The proportion of fat in the fæces varies; above 30 per cent. of the dried weight suggests pancreatic insufficiency. The stools are either oily like butter, or gray like asbestos. The ability to digest fat differs greatly and there are healthy persons who constantly have a high percentage of fat in the stools. Steatorrhœa may last for years without impairment of health. There is also a disturbance in the ratio between the neutral fats and the fatty acids. Cammidge gives the following average figures: Normal per cent., total fats 21, neutral fats 11, fatty acids 10; malignant disease, total fats 77, neutral fats 50, fatty acids 27; chronic pancreatitis, total fats 50, neutral fats 32, fatty acids 18.

(*b*) AZOTORRHŒA, the presence of undigested protein materials in the stools, has long been known as an association of pancreatic disease. Normally only 5 or 6 per cent. of the undigested proteins appears in the fæces, but in pancreatic disease as much as 30 or 40 per cent. may be recovered. Schmidt claims that the nuclear material of meat is digested by the pancreatic juice alone and that persistence of the nuclei of the meat fibres in the stools indicates defective tryptic digestion.

In jaundice due to malignant disease of the head of the pancreas stercobilin is absent; in that due to chronic pancreatitis or gall-stones it is either absent or present only in traces.

Cammidge's Pancreatic Reaction.—For details of the reaction the student must consult special manuals. It is claimed that the reaction is positive in all cases of active inflammatory changes in the pancreas, and that by it acute forms of pancreatitis can be differentiated from intestinal obstruction, and that by it chronic pancreatitis causing blocking of the common duct can be diagnosed from gall-stones. In malignant disease the reaction is negative in about three-fourths of the cases. The studies at the Mayo clinic under Wilson's direction lead to the conclusion that "if knowledge of the clinical histories and other factors of the personal equation be eliminated, the end results, judged by Cammidge's own criteria, must be considered, as a means of diagnosing disease of the pancreas, as both valueless and misleading." From observations of Whipple and others it seems that rapid disintegration of any of the body cells, particularly the polynuclear leucocytes, may give rise to the reaction.

II. PANCREATIC NECROSIS

The entire series of pancreatic lesions, from hæmorrhage to gangrene, and from fat necrosis to pancreatic cyst, may result from tryptic auto-digestion (Chiari). This is met with under four conditions: (*a*) Trauma, as in gunshot wounds, blows, or perforation of a peptic ulcer. (*b*) Primary thrombosis in the venous radicles of the glands. (*c*) Obstruction of the free flow of secretion in the duct. (*d*) Entrance of bile into the ducts.

In the mildest forms there are only a few small hæmorrhages or circumscribed areas of necrosis of the gland tissue with fat necrosis in the neighborhood; in severer forms groups of acini or the whole gland may be involved.

Fat necrosis occurs whenever the pancreatic juice, obstructed from any cause and dammed back on the gland, infiltrates its tissues, or escaping by the lymph spaces finds its way to structures at some distance from the gland. The necrosis is due to the fat-splitting ferment in the secretion (Opie).

Balser first called attention to this remarkable change which is found in the interlobular pancreatic tissue, in the mesentery, in the omentum, in the abdominal fatty tissue generally, and occasionally in the pericardial and subcutaneous fat. The necroses are most frequent in the acute and necrotic forms of pancreatitis, less common in the suppurative. In the pancreas the lobules are seen to be separated by a dead white necrotic tissue, which gives a remarkable appearance to the section. In the abdominal fat the areas are usually not larger than a pin's head; they at once attract attention, and may be mistaken, on superficial examination, for miliary tubercles or neoplasms. They may be larger; instances have been reported in which they were the size of a hen's egg. On section they have a soft tallowy consistence, and the substance is a combination of lime with certain fatty acids. The necroses may be crusted with lime.

III. HÆMORRHAGE

Both Spiess (1866) and Zenker (1874) were acquainted with hæmorrhage into the pancreas as a cause of sudden death, but the great medico-legal importance of the subject was first fully recognized by F. W. Draper, of Boston, whose townsmen, Harris, Fitz, Whitney, and others, have contributed additional studies. In 4,000 autopsies Draper met with 19 cases of pancreatic hæmorrhage, in 9 or 10 of which no other cause of death was found. When the bleeding is extensive the entire tissue of the gland is destroyed and the blood invades the retro-peritoneal tissue. In other instances the peritoneal covering is broken and the blood fills the lesser peritoneum (see hæmoperitoneum). The hæmorrhage may be in connection with an acute pancreatitis or with necrotic inflammation of the gland.

The *symptoms* are thus briefly summarized by Prince: "The patient, who has previously been perfectly well, is suddenly taken with the illness which terminates his life. . . . When the hæmorrhage occurs the patient may be quietly resting or pursuing his usual occupation. The pain which ushers in the attack is usually very severe and located in the upper part of the abdomen. It steadily increases in severity, is sharp or perhaps colicky in character. It is almost from the first accompanied by nausea and vomiting; the latter becomes frequent and obstinate, but gives no relief. The patient soon becomes anxious, restless, and depressed; he tosses about, and only with difficulty can he be restrained in bed. The surface is cold and the forehead is covered with a cold sweat. The pulse is weak, rapid, and sooner or later imperceptible. The abdomen becomes tender, the tenderness being located in the upper part of the abdomen or epigastrium. Tympanites is sometimes marked. The temperature is usually normal or subnormal. The bowels are constipated." A well marked tumor may sometimes be felt in the epigastrium. There may be tenderness and swelling in the course of the descending colon, with frequent stools, containing blood and mucus, and suggesting intussusception.

IV. ACUTE PANCREATITIS

Acute Pancreatitis.—While for convenience a distinction is made between hæmorrhagic, suppurative, and gangrenous pancreatitis, yet they are practically different manifestations of the same process. The principal *etiological* factors are stasis and infection. The latter is probably metastatic from some abdominal focus. This may be in the gall-bladder, an ulcer, or in the bowel, more often the colon. The appendix does not seem to be responsible in many cases. Infection from the biliary duct occurs, but probably is not the common cause. It seems likely that the infection may be carried to the pancreas by the lymphatics in the retroperitoneal tissues. Association with cholelithiasis is common, but the calculi are usually in the gall-bladder and rarely in the ampulla, which suggests that direct regurgitation of bile into the pancreatic duct occurs rarely. Injection of bile into the pancreatic duct of dogs reproduces the lesion.

Pathology.—The fat necrosis is probably due to the action of the fat splitting ferment. It has been suggested that the hæmorrhages may be due to trypsin digesting the walls of the vessels. The pancreatic juice is activated by calcium salts, by the action of bacteria or by the products of aseptic necrosis. It has been suggested that the toxic features may be much the same as those found in acute intestinal obstruction, of which the symptoms are due to proteose, one of the earliest productions of the action of trypsin on protein.

The pancreas is found enlarged, and the interlobular tissue infiltrated with blood, and perhaps with clots. The anatomical appearances are very characteristic. The tissues about the gland are infiltrated with blood and there may be fluid in the lesser peritoneum. Areas of fat necrosis are seen in the retroperitoneal fat, the mesocolon and mesentery. The gland itself is swollen and in section the stroma has a mottled dark brown appearance and the outlines of the acini may be lost.

Symptoms.—In some cases there have been premonitory attacks of pain which may be general or in the upper part of the abdomen, which may suggest gastric ulcer or gall-stones. The onset is very sudden with severe pain usually referred to the epigastrium. In the most acute cases there is a condition of shock. The symptoms of the attack are those of a very acute abdominal condition suggesting the perforation of an ulcer or sudden intestinal obstruction. There may be persistent vomiting and constipation is common. Examination shows fullness and tenderness in the upper abdomen and usually increasing distention. The tenderness may be specially marked across the epigastrium and there may be a distinct sense of resistance over the region of the pancreas. There is not likely to be any tumor mass felt until at least the third day. There may be marked leucocytosis. The temperature is usually low or subnormal, and the pulse rapid. The most acute cases, often termed fulminating, show a very severe onset with marked shock and collapse. This has been explained as probably due to pressure on the cœliac axis. In these cases there is profuse hæmorrhage into the pancreas and death usually follows in two or three days.

In the acute cases of average severity, the onset is sudden, but less severe than in the preceding. Only part of the pancreas may be damaged by the hæmorrhagic process and the most greatly damaged part may go on to necrosis and gangrene. Suppuration may follow, giving the picture of an *acute suppurative pancreatitis.* There may be either a single abscess or numerous small ones. In one series of 38 cases, in 24 there was a single abscess. In some cases there is a diffuse purulent infiltration. Among the results are peripancreatic abscess with perforation into the stomach, duodenum or peritoneum and thrombosis of the portal vein. The course of the suppurative form is likely to be chronic. Jaundice, diarrhœa, and glycosuria have occurred, but these are rare. A tumor mass in the epigastrium may result. In the less acute forms the process may be limited to only a part of the pancreas, usually the head, and the hæmorrhage is slight. The main symptoms are pain in the abdomen with nausea and vomiting, but the pulse and temperature may show no change and the condition may be overlooked, especially as it is often associated with cholecystitis.

In *gangrenous pancreatitis,* complete necrosis of the gland, or part of it, may follow either hæmorrhage or hæmorrhagic inflammation, and in exceptional cases may occur after suppurative infiltration or after injury or perforation of an ulcer of the stomach. Symptoms of hæmorrhagic pancreatitis may precede or be associated with it. Death usually follows in from ten to twenty days, with symptoms of collapse. The pancreas may present a dry necrotic appearance, but as a rule the organ is converted into a dark slaty-colored mass lying nearly free in the omental cavity or attached by a few shreds. In other instances the totally or partially sequestrated organ may lie in a large abscess cavity, forming a palpable tumor in the epigastric region. The necrotic pancreas may be discharged per rectum, with recovery.

Diagnosis.—The sudden dramatic onset in the severe forms should always suggest the possibility of acute pancreatitis. Perforation of the stomach or bowel and intestinal obstruction give features very similar, also the rupture of an aneurism. "Acute pancreatitis is to be suspected when a previously healthy person or a sufferer from occasional attacks of indigestion is suddenly seized with a violent pain in the epigastrium followed by vomiting and collapse, and in the course of twenty-four hours by a circumscribed epigastric swelling, tympanitic or resistant, with slight elevation of temperature. Circumscribed tenderness in the course of the pancreas and tender spots throughout the abdomen are valuable diagnostic signs" (Fitz). The mild forms are more difficult to recognize and are usually mistaken for cholecystitis. The presence of a tumor mass is of the greatest moment. Consideration of the possibility of acute pancreatitis is the best safeguard against error.

Treatment.—It is well to stop all intake by mouth and give fluid by rectum. Morphia should be given in full doses to control the pain. The decision as to exploration must depend on the condition; in the fulminant cases it may not be possible, in the less severe cases it is usually wise, in the mild cases it is not necessary. With signs of suppuration and abscess formation drainage is indicated. Otherwise symptomatic measures are indicated.

V. CHRONIC PANCREATITIS

Forms.—There is still a great deal of uncertainty about this condition. The truth is if operators regard an indurated or even nodular head of the pancreas as indicating a chronic pancreatitis they will find it in 80 per cent. of all adults. Those who follow Virchow's technique in post mortem work and open the stomach and duodenum and press on the course of the bile duct know how almost invariable is this sensation over the head of the organ, which may be sliced with the conviction that there must be some special morbid change. W. J. Mayo remarks how frequently he has found the pancreas enlarged, indurated and nodulated in cases in which no symptomatic evidence whatever existed of pancreatic inflammation. Anatomically there are two forms:

(*a*) Interlobular pancreatitis which follows occlusion of the duct, or an infection, such as occurs in the presence of calculi, biliary or pancreatic, with which organisms of the colon group, streptococci, or occasionally the typhoid bacillus are associated. Even in advanced sclerosis of this type the islands of Langerhans are spared. It may occur as an independent affection. It is not at all uncommon in the bodies of adults to find the head of the pancreas extraordinarily hard and so dense that it feels like scirrhus; surgeons have long noted this. The condition is often present without symptoms of pancreatic disease during life. A very special form is the chronic interstitial pancreatitis which accompanies hæmochromatosis, described elsewhere. Mayo Robson, Moynihan and other surgeons have called attention to the fact that sclerosis of the head of the pancreas may cause obstruction of the duct.

(*b*) Chronic interacinar pancreatitis is characterized by a diffuse fibrosis penetrating between the acini, with little or no involvement of the interlobular tissues. It may follow infection through the duct, but is more common in association with cirrhosis of the liver and arterio-sclerosis.

The possibility of *syphilis* as an etiological factor should be kept in mind. Warthin has shown that syphilis of the pancreas is not uncommon.

So much influenced is our present picture of chronic pancreatitis by personal equation on the part of surgical and laboratory workers that we are not in a position to speak very definitely on several important points.

Symptoms.—It must be confessed that the clinical picture is very obscure, in spite of the good work done by our surgical colleagues. Cammidge, who has had the advantage of seeing Mayo Robson's cases, describes four types: (*a*) The dyspeptic, in which the disease is due to morbid conditions of the bowels, and the symptoms are mainly referred to the digestive organs. (*b*)

The cholelithic, associated with the presence of gall-stones in the common duct; there is usually chronic jaundice and the dominant symptoms are hepatic. (*c*) A miscellaneous group in which the pancreatitis is secondary to malignant disease, etc. (*d*) The diabetic group with glycosuria, into which the members of the preceding groups may merge in course of time.

Symptoms of pancreatic insufficiency of the internal or external secretion are generally present; there is pain after food, very often jaundice, and on deep pressure the head of the pancreas may sometimes be felt. Bulky stools are suggestive. With Schmidt's test diet the average weight of the dried stools is from 45 to 65 grams. With pancreatic disease weights of 125 to 400 grams may be found. The stools are fatty and light and greasy in appearance. There is marked loss of fat and nitrogen in the stools. There is a large amount of unsplit fat present. The extent of digestion of cell nuclei is of some value. The estimation of diastase in the fæces and urine is of assistance in some cases. The stools may show both steatorrhœa and azotorrhœa.

Treatment.—Owing to the difficulty of diagnosis in the early stages it is impossible to speak positively in a great many cases, but in the forms which are associated with pain, jaundice, the presence of calculi, and infection of the ducts excellent results have followed free drainage of the bile passages. Removal of the gall-bladder is sometimes more effectual than drainage alone.

VI. PANCREATIC CYSTS

Of 121 cases operated upon 60 were in males and 56 in females, in 5 the sex was not given (Körte). Sixty-six of the cases occurred in the fourth decade. Railton's case (not in Körte's series), an infant aged six months, and Shattuck's case in a child of thirteen and a half months are the youngest in the literature. According to the origin Körte recognizes three varieties.

Varieties.—Traumatic Cases.—In this list of 33 cases 30 were in men and only 3 in women. Blows on the abdomen or constantly repeated pressure are the most common forms of trauma. One case followed severe massage. Usually with the onset there are inflammatory symptoms, pain, and vomiting, sometimes suggestive of peritonitis. The contents of the cyst are usually bloody, though in 13 of the traumatic cases it was clear or yellowish.

Cysts Following Inflammatory Conditions.—In 51 cases the trouble began gradually after attacks of dyspepsia with colic, simulating somewhat that of gall-stones. Occasionally the attack set in with very severe symptoms, suggestive of obstruction of the bowel. In this group the tumor appeared in 19 cases soon after the onset of the pain; in others it was delayed for a period of from a few weeks to two or three years. McPhedran reported a remarkable instance in which the tumor appeared in the epigastrium with signs of severe inflammation. It was opened and drained and believed to be a hydrops of the lesser peritoneal cavity. Three months later a second cyst developed, which appeared to spring directly from the pancreas.

Cysts without Any Inflammatory or Traumatic Etiology.—Of 33 cases in this group 26 were in women. A remarkable feature is the prolonged period of their existence—in one case for forty-seven years, in one for between sixteen and twenty years, in others for sixteen, nine, and eight years, in the majority for from two to four years.

Morbid Anatomy.—Anatomically Körte recognizes (1) *retention cysts* due to plugging of the main duct; (2) *proliferation cysts* of the pancreatic tissue —and cysto-adenoma; (3) *retention cysts* arising from the alveoli of the gland and of the smaller ducts, which become cut off and dilate in consequence of chronic interstitial pancreatitis; (4) *pseudo-cysts* following inflammatory or traumatic affections of the pancreas, usually the result of injury, causing hæmorrhage and hydrops of the lesser peritoneum.

Situation.—In its growth the cyst may (1) be in the lesser peritoneum, push the stomach upward, and reach the abdominal wall between the stomach and the transverse colon; (2) more rarely the cyst appears above the lesser curvature and pushes the stomach downward; in both of these cases the situation of the tumor is high in the abdomen; but (3) it may develop between the leaves of the transverse meso-colon and lie below both the colon and the stomach. The relation of these two organs to the tumor is variable, but in the majority of cases the stomach lies above and the transverse colon below the cyst. Occasionally, too, as in T. C. Railton's case, the cyst may arise in the tail of the pancreas and project far over in the left hypochondrium in the position of the spleen or of a renal tumor.

General Symptoms.—Apart from the features of onset already referred to, the patient may complain of no trouble unless the cyst reaches a very large size. Painful colicky attacks, with nausea and vomiting and progressive enlargement of the abdomen, have frequently been noted. Fatty diarrhœa from disturbance of the function of the pancreas is rare. Sugar in the urine has been present in a number of cases. Increased secretion of the saliva, the so-called pancreatic salivation, is also rare. Pressure of the cyst may sometimes cause jaundice, and in rare instances dyspnœa. Very marked loss of flesh has been present in a number of cases. A remarkable feature often noticed has been the transitory disappearance of the cyst. In one of Halsted's cases the girth of the abdomen decreased from 43 to 31 inches in ten days with profuse diarrhœa. Sometimes the disappearance has followed blows.

Diagnosis.—The cyst occupies the upper abdomen, usually forming a semicircular bulging in the median line, rarely to either side. In 16 cases Körte states that the chief projection was below the navel. In one case operated upon by Halsted the tumor occupied the greater part of the abdomen. The cyst is immobile, respiration having little or no influence on it. As already mentioned, the stomach, as a rule, lies above it and the colon below.

In a majority of the cases the fluid is of a reddish or dark-brown color, and contains blood or blood coloring matter, cell detritus, fat granules, and sometimes cholesterin. The consistence of the fluid is usually mucoid, rarely thin. The reaction is alkaline, the specific gravity from 1.010 to 1.020. In 22 cases Körte states that the fluid was not hæmorrhagic.

The existence of ferments is important. In 54 cases they were present in the fluid or in the material from the fistula. In 20 cases only one ferment was present, in 20 cases two, and in 14 cases all three of the pancreatic ferments were found. In view of the wide occurrence of disastatic and fat-emulsifying ferments in various exudates, the only positive sign in the diagnosis of the pancreatic secretion is the digestion of fibrin and albumin.

Operation.—Of 160 cases of operation there were 150 recoveries. Incision and drainage were done in 138 cases and in 15 excision.

VII. TUMORS OF THE PANCREAS

Of new growths in the organ carcinoma is the most frequent. Sarcoma, adenoma, and lymphoma are rare.

Frequency.—At the General Hospital in Vienna in 18,069 autopsies there were 22 cases of cancer of the pancreas (Biach). In 11,472 post mortems at Milan Segré found 132 tumors of the pancreas, 127 of which were carcinomata, 2 sarcomata, 2 cysts, and 1 syphiloma. In 6,000 autopsies at Guy's Hospital there were only 20 cases of primary malignant disease of the organ (Hale White). In the first 1,500 autopsies at the Johns Hopkins Hospital there were 6 cases of adeno-carcinoma, and 1 doubtful case in which the exact origin could not be stated. There were 8 cases of secondary malignant disease of the pancreas. The head of the gland is most commonly involved, but the disease may be limited to the body or to the tail. The majority of the patients are in the middle period of life.

Symptoms.—The diagnosis is not often possible. The following are the most important and suggestive features: (*a*) Epigastric pains, often occurring in paroxysms. (*b*) Jaundice, due to pressure of the tumor in the head of the pancreas on the bile-duct. The jaundice is intense and permanent, and associated with dilatation of the gall-bladder, which may reach a very large size. (*c*) The presence of a tumor in the epigastrium. This is very variable. In 137 cases Da Costa found the tumor present in only 13. Palpation under anæsthesia with the stomach empty would probably give a very much larger percentage. As the tumor rests directly upon the aorta there is usually a marked degree of pulsation, sometimes with a bruit. There may be pressure on the portal vein, causing thrombosis and its usual sequels. (*d*) Symptoms due to loss of function of the pancreas are less important. Fatty diarrhœa is not very often present. In consequence of the absence of bile the stools are usually very clay-colored and greasy. Diabetes also is not common. (*e*) A very rapid wasting and cachexia. Of other symptoms nausea and vomiting are common. In some instances the pylorus is compressed and there is great dilatation of the stomach. In a few cases there has been profuse salivation.

The points of greatest importance in the diagnosis are the intense and permanent jaundice, with dilatation of the gall-bladder, rapid emaciation, and the presence of a tumor in the epigastric region. Of less importance are features pointing to disturbance of the functions of the gland.

Of other new growths sarcoma and lymphoma have been occasionally found. Miliary tubercle is not very uncommon in the gland. Syphilis, which the work of Warthin shows to be common, may occur as a chronic interstitial inflammation, or in the form of gummata.

The outlook in tumors of the pancreas is, as a rule, hopeless; but of late years a number of successful cases of operation have been reported.

VIII. PANCREATIC CALCULI

Pancreatic lithiasis is comparatively rare. Lazarus in 1904 collected 57 cases of which 47 were males. The majority were between 30 and 50 years of age. In 1,500 autopsies at the Johns Hopkins Hospital there were 2 cases.

The stones are usually numerous, either round in shape or rough, spinous and coral-like. The color is opaque white. They are composed chiefly of carbonate of lime. The effects of the stones are: (1) A chronic interstitial inflammation of the gland substance with dilatation of the duct; sometimes there is cystic dilatation of the gland; (2) acute inflammation with suppuration; (3) the irritation of the stones may lead to carcinoma.

Symptoms.—The cases are not often diagnosed. Pains in the epigastrium, often very severe, but not characteristic and the signs of pancreatic insufficiency already described, are suggestive features. The X-rays may be of aid in diagnosis. An analysis of the calculi passed with the stools may alone serve to distinguish a case from one of gall-stones. Operation has been performed successfully.

J. DISEASES OF THE PERITONEUM

I. ACUTE GENERAL PERITONITIS

Definition.—Acute inflammation of the peritoneum.

Etiology.—The condition may be primary or secondary.

(*a*) Primary Peritonitis.—In this the organisms, usually the penumococcus or streptococcus, reach the peritoneum by the blood or lymphatics. It is often a terminal infection, as seen in nephritis, gout, and arterio-sclerosis. Of 102 cases of peritonitis which came to autopsy at the Johns Hopkins Hospital, 12 were of this form.

(*b*) Secondary peritonitis is due to extension of inflammation from, or perforation of, one of the organs covered by the peritoneum. Peritonitis from extension may follow inflammation of the stomach or intestines, ulceration in these parts, cancer, acute suppurative inflammations of the spleen, liver, pancreas, retroperitoneal tissues, and the pelvic viscera.

Perforative peritonitis is the most common, following external wounds, perforation of an ulcer of the stomach or bowels, perforation of the gall-bladder, abscess of the liver, spleen, or kidneys. Two important causes are appendicitis and suppurating inflammation about the Fallopian tubes and ovaries. There are instances in which peritonitis has followed rupture of an apparently normal Graafian follicle.

Of the above 102 cases, 56 originated in an extension from some diseased abdominal viscus. The remaining 34 followed surgical operations upon the peritoneum or the contained organs.

The peritonitis of septicæmia and pyæmia is almost invariably the result of a local process. An exceedingly acute form of peritonitis may be caused by the development of tubercles on the membrane.

Morbid Anatomy.—In recent cases, on opening the abdomen the intestinal coils are distended and glued together with lymph, and the peritoneum presents a patchy, sometimes a uniform injection. The exudation may be: (*a*) Fibrinous, with little or no fluid, except a few pockets of clear serum between the coils. (*b*) Sero-fibrinous. The coils are covered with lymph, and there is in addition a large amount of a yellowish, sero-fibrinous fluid. In instances in which the stomach or intestine is perforated this may be mixed with food or fæces. (*c*) Purulent, in which the exudate is either thin and greenish yellow in color, or opaque white and creamy. (*d*) Putrid. Occasionally in puerperal and perforative peritonitis, particularly when the latter has been caused by cancer, the exudate is thin, grayish green in color, and has a gangrenous odor. (*e*) Hæmorrhagic. This is sometimes found as an admixture in cases of acute peritonitis following wounds, and occurs in the cancerous and tuberculous forms. (*f*) A rare form occurs in which the injection is present, but almost all signs of exudation are wanting. Close inspection may be necessary to detect a slight dulling of the serous surfaces.

The amount of the effusion varies from half a litre to 20 or 30 litres. There are essential differences between the various kinds of peritonitis.

Bacteriology.—A large number of organisms have been found. In the cases following operation the staphylococcus was present alone in 12 out of 33, the streptococcus in 5, and the colon bacillus in 5. Other organisms were the pneumococcus, bacillus pyocyaneus, and bacillus aërogenes. Of 56 cases of peritonitis following intestinal infections, the colon bacillus occurred in 43, usually in connection with streptococci. The bacillus lactis aërogenes has also been found as the sole organism. The gonococcus is present in the form which arises from salpingitis and may occur in the gonorrhœal infections of children.

Much attention has been paid to the *pneumococcus* as an agent in the causation of peritonitis, and many cases are of the primary form without recognizable portal of entry; but there are many latent pneumococcic lesions, particularly those of the middle ear, and of the accessory sinuses of the nose. Cameron makes two groups of cases; a diffuse form setting in with abdominal pain, high fever, vomiting, and diarrhœa, in which death may occur within 36 hours. In the other group the peritonitis is local, and the symptoms may suggest appendicitis. Gradually a localized abscess develops, which may rupture internally. The creamy greenish yellow odorless pus is very characteristic.

Symptoms.—In the perforative and septic cases the onset is marked by chilly feelings or an actual rigor with intense pain in the abdomen. In typhoid fever, when the sensorium is benumbed, the onset may not be noticed. The pain is general, and is usually intense and aggravated by movements and pressure. A position is taken which relieves the tension of the abdominal muscles, so that the patient lies on the back with the thighs drawn up and the shoulders elevated. The greatest pain is usually below the umbilicus, but in peritonitis from perforation of the stomach pain may be referred to the back, the chest, or the shoulder. The respiration is superficial—costal in type—as it is painful to use the diaphragm. For the same reason the action of coughing is restrained, and even the movements necessary for talking are limited. In this early stage the sensitiveness may be great and the abdominal muscles are often rigidly contracted. If the patient is at perfect rest the pain may be very slight, and there are instances in which it is not at all marked, and may, indeed, be absent.

The abdomen gradually becomes distended and tense and is tympanitic on percussion. The pulse is rapid, small, and hard, and often has a peculiar wiry quality. It ranges from 110 to 150. The temperature may rise rapidly after the chill and reach 104° or 105° F., but the subsequent elevation is moderate. In some very severe cases there may be no fever throughout. The leucocyte count varies with the grade of infection. In the severe cases it may not be increased. The tongue at first is white and moist, but subsequently becomes dry and often red and fissured. Vomiting is an early and prominent feature and causes great pain. The contents of the stomach are first ejected, then a yellowish and bile stained fluid, and finally a greenish and, in rare instances, a brownish black liquid with slight fæcal odor. The bowels may be loose at the onset and then constipation may follow. Frequent micturition may be present, less often retention. The urine is usually scanty and high-colored, and contains a large quantity of indican.

The appearance of the patient when these symptoms have fully developed is very characteristic. The face is pinched, the eyes are sunken, and the expression is very anxious. The constant vomiting of fluids causes a wasted appearance, and the hands sometimes present the washer-woman's skin. Except in cholera, we see the Hippocratic facies more frequently in this than in any other disease—*"a sharp nose, hollow eyes, collapsed temples; the ears cold, contracted, and their lobes turned out; the skin about the forehead being rough, distended, and parched; the color of the whole face being brown, black, livid, or lead-colored."* There are one or two additional points about the abdomen. The tympany is usually excessive, owing to the great relaxation of the walls of the intestines by inflammation and exudation. There is absence of the sounds of peristalsis and the breath and heart sounds may be heard loudly. The splenic dulness may be obliterated, the diaphragm pushed up, and the apex beat of the heart dislocated to the fourth interspace. The liver dulness may be greatly reduced, or may, in the mammary line, be obliterated. It has been claimed that this is a distinctive feature of perforative peritonitis, but the liver dulness in the mammary line may be obliterated by tympanites alone. In the axillary line, on the other hand, the liver dulness, though diminished, may persist. Pneumo-peritoneum following perforation more certainly obliterates the hepatic dulness. In such cases the fluid effused produces a dulness in the lateral region; but with gas in the peritoneum, if the patient is turned on the left side, a clear note is heard beneath the seventh and eighth rib. Acute peritonitis may present a flat, rigid abdomen throughout its course.

Effusion of fluid—ascites—is usually present except in some acute, rapidly fatal cases. The flanks are dull on percussion. The dulness may be movable, though this depends altogether upon the degree of adhesions. There may be considerable effusion without either movable dulness or fluctuation. A friction rub may be present, as first pointed out by Bright, but it is not nearly so common in acute as in chronic peritonitis.

Prognosis.—In the cases due to injury or perforation of an abdominal organ much depends on the interval between this and operation. Every hour of delay increases the risk. In the group due to extension from the pelvic organs the outlook is more favorable. The acute diffuse peritonitis usually terminates in death. The most intense forms may kill within thirty-six to forty-eight hours; more commonly death results in four or five days, or the attack may be prolonged to eight or ten days. The pulse becomes irregular, the heart-sounds weak, the breathing shallow; there are lividity with pallor, a cold skin with high rectal temperature—a group of symptoms indicating profound failure of the vital functions. Occasionally death occurs with great suddenness. A low temperature, rapid pulse, marked distention, absence of leucocytosis and severe toxæmia point to a fatal ending. The causal organism influences the outlook; cases due to the gonococcus and some forms of staphylococci are more favorable than those due to the streptococcus. There are different views as to the gravity of the colon bacillus infections.

Diagnosis.—In typical cases the severe pain at onset, the distention of the abdomen, the tenderness, the fever, the gradual onset of effusion, collapse, and the vomiting give a characteristic picture. Careful inquiries should at once be made concerning the previous condition, from which a clue can often be had as to the starting-point of the trouble. In young adults a considerable proportion of all cases depends upon perforating appendicitis, and there may be an account of previous attacks of pain in the iliac region, or of constipation alternating with diarrhœa. In women the most frequent causes are suppurative processes in the pelvic viscera, associated with salpingitis, abscesses in the broad ligaments, or acute puerperal infection. It is not always easy to determine the cause. Many cases come under observation for the first time with the abdomen distended and tender, and it is impossible to make a satisfactory examination. In such instances the pelvic organs should be examined with the greatest care. Suggestive points in the pneumococcus form in children are the sudden onset, the severe toxæmia, high fever, marked leucocytosis, vomiting, and diarrhœa with markedly less abdominal pain and tenderness as compared with other acute forms. The following conditions are most apt to be mistaken for acute peritonitis:

(*a*) *Acute Entero-colitis.*—Here the pain and distention and the sensitiveness on pressure may be marked. The pain is more colicky in character, the diarrhœa is more frequent, and the collapse is more extreme.

(*b*) *The So-called Hysterical Peritonitis.*—This has deceived the very elect, as almost every feature of genuine peritonitis, even the collapse, may be simulated. The onset may be sudden, with severe pain in the abdomen, tenderness, vomiting, diarrhœa, difficulty in micturition, and the characteristic decubitus. Even the temperature may be elevated. There may be recurrence of the attack. A case has been reported by Bristowe in which four attacks occurred within a year, and it was not until special hysterical symptoms developed that the true nature of the trouble was suspected.

(*c*) *Obstruction of the bowel* may simulate peritonitis, both having pain, vomiting, tympanites, and constipation. It may be impossible to make a diagnosis before exploration in the absence of a satisfactory history.

(*d*) *Rupture of an abdominal aneurism or embolism of the superior mesenteric artery* may cause symptoms which simulate peritonitis. In the latter, a sudden onset with severe pain, the collapse symptoms, frequent vomiting, and great distention of the abdomen may be present.

(*e*) Acute hæmorrhagic pancreatitis or a ruptured tubal pregnancy may be mistaken for peritonitis.

Treatment.—Something can be done in prevention by recognition and prompt treatment of conditions which may lead to general peritonitis, such as gastric ulcer, appendicitis, cholecystitis, etc. An early surgical consultation is important. With signs or suspicion of peritonitis, the patient should be at absolute rest and propped up in bed in a sitting position; nothing should be given by mouth; a solution of glucose (5 per cent.) and sodium bicarbonate (2 per cent.) should be given per rectum by the drop method. Purgatives should not be given. If there is shock from perforation, fluid may be given subcutaneously, and epinephrin (♏ xv, 1 c. c.) and camphorated oil (gr. iii, 2 gm.) as indicated. If there is much vomiting gastric lavage is indicated. If there is constant secretion into the stomach a small tube may be kept in position so that frequent lavage is possible without disturbing the patient. The rectal tube may be used to relieve tympanites. Turpentine stupes, an ice bag or hot applications may be applied to the abdomen if they give comfort. It is usually well to withhold morphia until a definite course of action is decided upon. In general, operation is indicated and as soon as possible, especially after perforation. In some cases delay may be advisable, for example until shock has passed, but this should be left to the judgment of the surgeon. In pneumococcus peritonitis delay is advisable unless an abscess forms.

II. PERITONITIS IN INFANTS

Peritonitis may occur in the fetus as a consequence of syphilis, and may lead to constriction of the bowel by fibrous adhesions.

In the new-born a septic peritonitis may extend from an inflamed cord. Distention of the abdomen, slight swelling and redness about the cord, and not infrequently jaundice are present. It is uncommon and existed in only 4 of 51 infants dying with inflammation of the cord and septicæmia (Runge).

During childhood peritonitis arises from causes similar to those affecting the adult. Perforative appendicitis is common. Peritonitis following blows or kicks on the abdomen occurs more frequently at this period. In boys injury while playing football may be followed by diffuse peritonitis. A rare cause in children is extension through the diaphragm from an empyema. There are on record instances of peritonitis occurring in several children at the same school. It was in investigating an epidemic of this kind at the Wandsworth school, in London, that Anstie received the post mortem wound of which he died. It is to be remembered that peritonitis in children may follow the gonorrhœal vulvitis so common in infant homes and hospitals.

III. LOCALIZED PERITONITIS

Subphrenic Peritonitis.—The general peritoneum covering the right and left lobes of the liver may be involved in an extension from the pleura of suppurative, tuberculous, or cancerous processes. In various affections of the liver—cancer, abscess, hydatid disease, and in affections of the gall-bladder—the inflammation may be localized to the peritoneum covering the upper surface of the organ. These forms of localized subphrenic peritonitis in the greater sac are not so important in reality as those which occur in the lesser peritoneum. The anatomical relations of this structure are as follows: It lies behind and below the stomach, the gastro-hepatic omentum, and the anterior layer of the great omentum. Its lower limit forms the upper layer of the transverse meso-colon. On either side it reaches from the hepatic to the splenic flexure of the colon, and from the foramen of Winslow to the hilus of the spleen. Behind it covers and is tightly adherent to the front of the pancreas. Its upper limit is formed by the transverse fissure of the liver, and by that portion of the diaphragm which is covered by the lower layer of the right lateral ligament of the liver; the lobus Spigelii lies bare in the cavity. The foramen of Winslow, through which the lesser communicates with the greater peritoneum, is readily closed by inflammation.

Inflammatory processes, exudates, and hæmorrhages may be confined entirely to the lesser peritoneum. The exudate of tuberculous peritonitis may be confined to it. Perforations of certain parts of the stomach, of the duodenum, and of the colon may excite inflammation in it alone; and in various affections of the pancreas, particularly trauma and hæmorrhage, the effusion into the sac has often been confounded with cyst of this organ.

Special mention must be made of the remarkable form of subphrenic abscess containing air, which may simulate closely pneumothorax, and hence was called by Leyden *pyo-pneumothorax subphrenicus*. The affection has been thoroughly studied by Scheurlen, Mason, Meltzer, and Lee Dickinson. In 142 out of 170 recorded cases the cause was known. In a few instances, as in one reported by Meltzer, the subphrenic abscess seemed to have followed pneumonia. Pyothorax is an occasional cause. By far the most frequent condition is gastric ulcer, which occurred in 80 of the cases. Duodenal ulcer was the cause in 6 per cent. In about 10 per cent. of the cases the appendix was the starting-point of the abscess. Cancer of the stomach is an occasional cause. Other rare causes are trauma, perforation of an hepatic or a renal abscess, lesions of the spleen, abscess, and cysts of the pancreas. In a majority of all the cases in which the stomach or duodenum is perforated—sometimes, indeed, in the cases following trauma—the abscess contains air.

The *symptoms* of subphrenic abscess vary very considerably, depending a good deal upon the primary cause. The onset, as a rule, is abrupt, particularly when due to perforation of a gastric ulcer. There are severe pain, vomiting, often of bilious or of bloody material; respiration is embarrassed, owing to the involvement of the diaphragm; then the constitutional symptoms occur associated with suppuration, chills, irregular fever, and emaciation. Subsequently perforation may take place into the pleura or into the lung, with severe cough and abundant purulent expectoration.

The perihepatic abscess beneath the arch of the diaphragm, whether to the right or left of the suspensory ligament, when it does not contain air, is almost invariably mistaken for empyema. Remarkable features are superadded when the abscess cavity contains air. On the right side, when the abscess is in the greater peritoneum, above the right lobe of the liver, the diaphragm may be pushed up to the level of the second or third rib, and the physical signs on percussion and auscultation are those of pneumothorax, particularly the tympanitic resonance and the movable dulness. The liver is usually greatly depressed and there is bulging on the right side. Still more obscure are the cases of air-containing abscesses due to perforation of the stomach or duodenum, in which the gas is contained in the lesser peritoneum. Here the diaphragm is pushed up and there are signs of pneumothorax on the left side. In a large majority of all the cases which follow perforation of a gastric ulcer the effusion lies between the diaphragm above, and the spleen, stomach, and the left lobe of the liver below. The X-ray is of value and on the left side the sign described by Fussell and Pancoast in perinephritic abscess may be helpful. This consists in a wave in the fluid seen with the fluoroscope when the patient's body is moved quickly from side to side.

The prognosis in subphrenic abscess is not very hopeful. Of the cases on record about 20 per cent. only have recovered.

Appendicular.—The most frequent cause of localized peritonitis in the male is appendicitis. The situation varies with the position of this extremely variable organ. The adhesion, perforation, and intraperitoneal abscess cavity may be within the pelvis, or to the left of the median line in the iliac region, in the lower right quadrant of the umbilical region—a not uncommon situation—or, of course, most frequently in the right iliac fossa. In the most common situation the localized abscess lies upon the psoas muscle, bounded by the cæcum on the right and the terminal portion of the ileum and its mesentery in front and to the left. In many of these cases the limitation is perfect, and post mortem records show that complete healing may take place with the obliteration of the appendix in a mass of firm scar tissue.

Pelvic Peritonitis.—The most frequent cause is inflammation about the uterus and Fallopian tubes. Puerperal septicæmia, gonorrhœa, and tuberculosis are the usual causes. The tubes are the starting-point in a majority of the cases. The fimbriæ become adherent and closely matted to the ovary, and a thickening of the parts, in which the individual organs are scarcely recognizable, is gradually produced. The tubes are dilated and filled with cheesy matter or pus, and there may be small abscess cavities in the broad ligaments. Rupture of one of these may cause general peritonitis, or the membrane may be involved by extension, as in tuberculosis of these parts.

The *treatment* of these forms is surgical.

IV. CHRONIC PERITONITIS

The following varieties may be recognized:

Local adhesive peritonitis, a very common condition, which occurs particularly about the spleen, forming adhesions between the capsule and the diaphragm, about the liver, less frequently about the intestines and mesentery. Points of thickening or puckering on the peritoneum occur sometimes with union of the coils or with fibrous bands. In a majority of such cases the condition is met accidentally post mortem. Two sets of symptoms may, however, be caused by these adhesions. When a fibrous band is attached in such a way as to form a loop or snare, a coil of intestine may pass through it. Thus, of the 295 cases of intestinal obstruction analyzed by Fitz, 63 were due to this cause. The second group is less serious and comprises cases with persistent abdominal pain of a colicky character, sometimes rendering life miserable. A careful X-ray study is the greatest aid in determining the situation of and results from the adhesions.

Diffuse Adhesive Peritonitis.—This is a consequence of an acute inflammation, either simple or tuberculous. The peritoneum is obliterated. On cutting through the abdominal wall, the coils of intestines are uniformly matted together and can neither be separated from each other nor can the visceral and parietal layers be distinguished. There may be thickening of the layers, and the liver and spleen are usually involved in the adhesions.

Proliferative Peritonitis.—Apart from cancer and tubercle, which produce typical lesions of chronic peritonitis, the most characteristic form is that which may be described under this heading. The essential anatomical feature is great thickening of the peritoneal layers, usually without much adhesion. The cases are sometimes seen with sclerosis of the stomach. It may occur in connection with a sclerotic condition of the cæcum and the first part of the colon. It is not uncommon with cirrhosis of the liver. In a case of this kind there is usually moderate effusion, more rarely extensive ascites. The peritoneum is opaque white in color, and everywhere thickened, often in patches. The omentum is usually rolled and forms a thickened mass transversely placed between the stomach and the colon. The peritoneum over the stomach, intestines, and mesentery is sometimes greatly thickened. The liver and spleen may simply be adherent, or there is a condition of chronic perihepatitis or perisplenitis, so that a layer of firm, almost gristly connective tissue of from one-fourth to half an inch in thickness encircles these organs. Usually the volume of the liver is in consequence greatly reduced. The gastro-hepatic omentum may be constricted by this new growth and the calibre of the portal vein much narrowed. A serous effusion may be present. On account of the adhesions which form, the peritoneum may be divided into three or four different sacs, as is described under tuberculous peritonitis. In these cases the intestines are usually free, though the mesentery is greatly shortened. There are instances of chronic peritonitis in which the mesentery is so shortened by this proliferative change that the intestines form a ball not larger than a cocoanut situated in the middle line, and after the removal of the exudation can be felt as a solid tumor. The intestinal wall is greatly thickened and the mucous membrane of the ileum is thrown into folds like the valvulæ conniventes. This proliferative peritonitis is found frequently in the subjects of chronic alcoholism. In cases of long-continued ascites the serous surfaces generally become thickened and present an opaque, dead white color. This condition is observed especially in hepatic cirrhosis, but attends tumors, chronic passive congestion, etc.

In all forms of chronic peritonitis a friction may be felt usually in the upper zone of the abdomen. Polyorrhomenitis, *polyserositis,* general chronic inflammation of the serous membranes, Concato's disease (as the Italians call it) may occur with this form as well as in the tuberculous variety. The pericardium and both pleuræ may be involved. The pericardial pseudocirrhosis described by Pick is an allied condition.

In some instances of chronic peritonitis the membrane presents numerous nodular thickenings, which may be mistaken for tubercles. J. F. Payne described a case of this sort associated with disseminated growths throughout the liver which were not cancerous. It has been suggested that some of the cases of tuberculous peritonitis cured by operation have been of this nature, but histological examination should determine between the conditions. Miura, in Japan, reported a case in which these nodules contained the ova of a parasite. One case has been reported in which the exciting cause was regarded as cholesterin plates, which were contained within the granulomatous nodules.

Chronic Hæmorrhagic Peritonitis.—Blood-stained effusions in the peritoneum occur particularly in cancerous and tuberculous disease. A chronic inflammation analogous to the hæmorrhagic pachymeningitis of the brain was described first by Virchow, and is localized most commonly in the pelvis. Layers of new connective tissue form on the surface of the peritoneum with large wide vessels from which hæmorrhage occurs. This is repeated from time to time with the formation of regular layers of hæmorrhagic effusion. It is rarely diffuse, more commonly circumscribed. Probably the spontaneous peritoneal hæmorrhage with the features of an "acute abdomen" (Churchman) may represent the primary form of this rare condition.

Treatment.—In cases with *adhesions* which are causing symptoms, great caution should be exercised in advising operation and a thorough X-ray study made to determine, if possible, the exact condition. For local adhesions of the pylorus, duodenum, and colon, causing obstruction, surgery may be beneficial. In the cases with extensive adhesions about the cæcum and ascending colon, the chances are less favorable. Every effort should be made to help the action of the bowels by medical measures. For the cases of *chronic proliferative peritonitis* very little can be done. If a primary cause is present, such as renal and cardiac disease or syphilis of the liver, treatment should be directed to that. The treatment in general is practically that of ascites and tapping should be done whenever necessary. The injection of epinephrin (♏ xv, 1 c. c.) into the peritoneal cavity after tapping has been of benefit in some cases. As a rule operation is not advisable and no benefit results from an attempt to produce additional adhesions.

V. NEW GROWTHS IN THE PERITONEUM

Tuberculous Peritonitis.—This has already been considered.

Cancer of the Peritoneum.—Although, as a rule, secondary to disease of the stomach, liver, or pelvic organs, cases of primary cancer have been described. It is probable that the so-called primary cancers of the serous membranes are endotheliomata and not carcinomata. Secondary malignant peritonitis occurs in connection with all forms of cancer. It is usually characterized by a number of round tumors scattered over the entire peritoneum, sometimes small and miliary, at other times large and nodular, with puckered centres. The disease most commonly starts from the stomach or the ovaries. The omentum is indurated and, as in tuberculous peritonitis, forms a mass which lies transversely across the upper portion of the abdomen. Primary malignant disease of the peritoneum is extremely rare. Colloid sometimes occurs, forming enormous masses, which in one case weighed over 100 pounds. Cancer of this membrane spreads, either by the detachment of small particles which are carried in the lymph currents and by the movements to distant parts, or by contact of opposing surfaces. It occurs more frequently in women than in men, and more commonly at the later period of life than in the young.

The *diagnosis* of cancer of the peritoneum is easy with a history of a local malignant disease; as when it occurs with ovarian tumor or with cancer of the pylorus. In cases in which there is no evidence of a primary lesion the diagnosis may be doubtful. The clinical picture is usually that of chronic ascites with progressive emaciation. There may be no fever. If there is much effusion nothing definite can be felt on examination. After tapping, irregular nodules or the curled omentum may be felt lying transversely across the upper portion of the abdomen. Multiple nodules, if large, indicate cancer, particularly in persons above middle life. Nodular tuberculous peritonitis is most frequent in children. The presence about the navel of secondary nodules and indurated masses is more common in cancer. Inflammation, suppuration, and the discharge of pus from the navel rarely occur except in tuberculous disease. Considerable enlargement of the inguinal glands may be present in cancer. The nature of the fluid in cancer and in tubercle may be much alike. It may be hæmorrhagic in both; more often in the latter. The histological examination in cancer may show large multinuclear cells or groups of cells—the sprouting cell-groups of Foulis—which are extremely suggestive. The colloid cancer may give a different picture; instead of ascitic fluid, the abdomen is occupied by semi-solid gelatinous substance, and is firm, not fluctuating. Echinococci in the peritoneum may simulate cancer very closely.

Free solid tumors are sometimes met with, usually fibroid or calcareous, as in the case reported by Campbell and Ower, in which a man had had a movable tumor in his abdomen for more than twenty years. It had increased in size, and at his death was a rounded mass 8 by 9 cm.

VI. ASCITES

(Hydro-peritoneum)

Definition.—The accumulation of serous fluid in the peritoneal cavity.

Etiology.—Local Causes.—(*a*) Chronic inflammation of the peritoneum, either simple, cancerous, or tuberculous. (*b*) Portal obstruction in the terminal branches within the liver, as in cirrhosis, syphilis and chronic passive congestion, or by compression of the vein in the gastro-hepatic omentum, by proliferative peritonitis, gumma, new growths, or aneurism. (*c*) Thrombosis of the portal vein. (*d*) Tumors of the abdomen. The solid growths of the ovaries may cause considerable ascites, which may completely mask the true condition. It is important to bear in mind this possibility in the obscure ascites of women. The enlarged spleen in leukæmia, less commonly in malaria, may be associated with recurring ascites.

General Causes.—The ascites is part of a general dropsy, the result of mechanical effects, as in heart-disease. In cardiac lesions the effusion is sometimes confined to the peritoneum, in which case it is due to secondary changes in the liver, or it has been suggested to be connected with a failure of the suction action of this organ by which the peritoneum is kept dry. Ascites occurs also in the dropsy of nephritis and in hydræmic states of the blood.

Symptoms.—A gradual uniform enlargement of the abdomen is the characteristic sign of ascites. (*a*) *Inspection.*—According to the amount of fluid the abdomen is protuberant and flattened at the sides. With large effusions, the skin is tense and may present the lineæ albicantes. Frequently the navel itself and the parts about it are very prominent. In many cases the superficial veins are enlarged and a plexus joining the mammary vessels can be seen. Often it can be determined that the current is from below upward. In some instances, as in thrombosis or obliteration of the portal vein, these superficial abdominal vessels may be extensively varicose. About the navel in cases of cirrhosis there is occasionally a large bunch of distended veins, the so-called caput Medusæ. The heart may be displaced upward.

(*b*) *Palpation.*—Fluctuation is obtained by placing one hand upon one side of the abdomen and giving a sharp tap on the opposite side with the other hand, when a wave is felt to strike as a definite shock against the applied hand. Even comparatively small quantities of fluid may give this fluctuation shock. When the abdominal walls are thick or very fat, an assistant may place the edge of the hand in front of the abdomen. A different precedure is adopted in palpating for the solid organs in case of ascites. Instead of placing the hand flat upon the abdomen, as in the ordinary method, the pads of the fingers only are placed lightly upon the skin, and then by a sudden depression of the fingers the fluid is displaced and the solid organ or tumor may be felt. By this method of "dipping" or displacement, the liver may be felt below the costal margin, or the spleen, or sometimes solid tumors of the omentum or intestine.

(*c*) *Percussion.*—In the dorsal position with a moderate quantity of fluid in the peritoneum the flanks are dull, while the umbilical and epigastric regions, in which the intestines float, are tympanitic. This area of clear resonance may have an oval outline. Having obtained the lateral limit of the dulness on one side, if the patient turns on the opposite side, the fluid gravitates to the dependent part and the uppermost flank is now tympanitic. In moderate effusions this movable dulness changes greatly in the different postures. Small amounts of fluid, probably under a litre, would scarcely give movable dulness, as the pelvis and the renal regions hold a considerable quantity. In such cases it is best to place the patient in the knee-elbow position, when a dull note will be determined at the most dependent portion. By careful attention to these details mistakes are usually avoided.

Differential Diagnosis.—The following are among the conditions which may be mistaken for dropsy: *Ovarian tumor,* in which the sac develops, as a rule, unilaterally, though when large it is centrally placed. The dulness is anterior and the resonance is in the flanks, into which the intestines are pushed by the cyst. Examination *per vaginam* may give important indications. In those rare instances in which gas develops in the cyst the diagnosis may be very difficult. Succussion has been obtained in such cases. A *distended bladder* may reach above the umbilicus. In such instances some urine dribbles away, and suspicion of ascites or a cyst is occasionally entertained. A trocar may be thrust into a distended bladder, supposed to be an ovarian cyst, and it is stated that John Hunter tapped a bladder, thinking it to be ascites. Such a mistake should be avoided by careful catheterization prior to any operative procedures. And lastly, there are large pancreatic or hydatid cysts in the abdomen which may simulate ascites.

Nature of the Ascitic Fluid.—Usually this is a clear serum, light yellow in the ascites of anæmia and nephritis, often darker in color in cirrhosis of the liver. The specific gravity is low, seldom more than 1.010 or 1.015, whereas in the fluid of ovarian cysts or chronic peritonitis the specific gravity is over 1.015. It is albuminous and sometimes coagulates spontaneously. Dock has called attention to the importance of the study of the cells in the exudate. In cancer very characteristic forms, with nuclear figures, may be found. Hæmorrhagic effusion usually occurs in cancer and tuberculosis, occasionally in cirrhosis and with ruptured tubal pregnancy.

CHYLOUS ASCITES.—Of the cases tabulated by MacKenzie, Wallis, and Scholberg, 81 were in association with tumors, 46 with the infections, chiefly tuberculosis, 37 in association with affections of the thoracic duct and lymphatic system, and 78 in connection with general diseases such as cirrhosis of the liver, cardiac disease, nephritis, amyloid disease, and thrombosis of the blood-vessels. In a certain number of cases the cause of the condition is unknown. Quincke recognized that there were two types, one in which there was a true milky or fatty fluid, the other in which the turbidity is due to fatty degeneration of cells or to chemical substances of a non-fatty nature. The fluid of the true chylous ascites is yellowish-white in color, contains fine fat globules, a creamy layer collects on standing, the specific gravity generally exceeds 1.012, and the fat content is high. As a rule, it tends to accumulate rapidly and large amounts may be removed. The fluid of pseudo-chylous ascites is milky white, the opacity often may vary at different tappings. Microscopically there are many fine refractile granules, but they do not give reactions for fat, the cellular elements may be numerous, and a creamy layer rarely forms. The specific gravity is less than 1.012, and the total solids rarely exceed 2 per cent. The fat content is low. Lecithin combined with globulin appears to be the cause of the opalescence. These authors conclude that milky ascites is characteristic of no specific morbid lesion. The prognosis is usually grave.

Treatment.—This depends somewhat on the nature of the case. Treatment should be directed to the underlying cause if this is possible. In cirrhosis early and repeated tapping may give time for the establishment of the collateral circulation, and temporary cures have followed this procedure. The injection of epinephrin (ʒ ss, 2 c. c. of a 1-1000 solution) into the peritoneal cavity after tapping has been useful in some cases. Permanent drainage with Southey's tube, incision, and washing out the peritoneum have also been practised. In the ascites of cardiac and renal disease the cathartics are most satisfactory, particularly the bitartrate of potash, given alone or with jalap, and the large doses of salts given an hour before breakfast with as little water as possible. These sometimes cause rapid disappearance of the effusion, but are not so successful in ascites as in pleurisy with effusion. The stronger cathartics may sometimes be necessary. The ascites forming part of the general anasarca of nephritis will receive consideration under another section.

K. DISEASES OF THE OMENTUM

Torsion.—Though the first case was reported by Oberst in 1882, Bookman collected 131 cases in 1915. It is one of the recognized causes of the "acute abdomen." The torsion may occur with or without the presence of a hernial sac, with which fully 90 per cent. of the cases have occurred. The twist is usually associated with adhesion of the free extremity to some structure. As the cases are usually in connection with hernia, the diagnosis of strangulation is made. Pain, muscular rigidity and vomiting are the usual symptoms and the condition is mistaken for hernia, acute appendicitis, or intestinal obstruction. The existence of a hernia and the sudden appearance of an abdominal mass are suggestive. Early operation with removal of the strangulated portion is the only treatment.

SECTION VII

DISEASES OF THE RESPIRATORY SYSTEM

A. DISEASES OF THE NOSE

EPISTAXIS

Etiology.—Among local causes may be mentioned traumatism, small ulcers, picking or scratching the nose, new growths, and the presence of foreign bodies. In chronic nasal catarrh bleeding is not infrequent. The blood may come from one or both nostrils. The flow may be profuse after an injury.

Among general conditions the following are the most important: It occurs in growing children, particularly about the age of puberty; more frequently in the delicate than in the strong and vigorous. There is a family form in which many members in several generations are affected, a *hereditary multiple telangiectasis,* a special feature of which is recurring epistaxis. The disease has nothing to do with hæmophilia, with which it has been confounded. The bleeding occurs from the telangiectasis in the nasal mucosa, and from those in the lips, tongue, and skin. In 1915, Gjessing found reports of nineteen families in which it occurred.

Epistaxis is common in persons of so-called plethoric habit. It is stated sometimes to precede, or to indicate a liability to, apoplexy. There may be a most extreme grade of cyanosis without its occurrence. It is frequent in hepatic cirrhosis. In balloon and mountain ascensions epistaxis is common. In hæmophilia the nose ranks first of the mucous membranes from which bleeding arises. It occurs in all forms of chronic anæmias and in chronic interstitial nephritis. It precedes the onset of certain fevers and is associated in some special way with typhoid fever. Vicarious epistaxis has been described in suppression of the menses. Lastly, it is said to be brought on by certain psychical impressions; but the observations on this point are not trustworthy. The blood comes from capillary oozing or diapedesis but may come from a small vessel or from capillary angiomata situated in the respiratory portion of the nostril and upon the cartilaginous septum.

Symptoms.—Slight hæmorrhage is not associated with any special features. When the bleeding is protracted the patients have the more serious manifestations of loss of blood. In the slow dripping which takes place in some instances of hæmophilia, a remarkable blood tumor projecting from one nostril and extending even below the mouth may be formed.

Death from ordinary epistaxis is very rare. The more blood is lost the greater is the tendency to clotting with spontaneous cessation of the bleeding.

Diagnosis.—This is usually easy. One point only need be mentioned; namely, that bleeding from the posterior nares occasionally occurs during sleep and the blood trickles into the pharynx and may be swallowed. If vomited, it may be confounded with hæmatemesis; or, if coughed up, with hæmoptysis.

Treatment.—In a majority of the cases the bleeding ceases of itself. Various simple measures may be employed, such as holding the arms above the head, the application of ice to the nose, or the injection of cold or hot water into the nostrils. Astringents, such as zinc, alum, or tannin, may be used; and the tincture of the perchloride of iron, diluted with ice-water, may be introduced into the nostrils. If the bleeding comes from an ulcerated surface, an attempt should be made to apply chromic acid or the cautery. If the bleeding is at all severe and obstinate, the posterior nares should be plugged. A patient with epistaxis and spider angiomata of the skin and mucous membranes used a finger of a rubber glove with a small rubber tube and stopcock by which he could dilate the glove finger, inserted into the nostril, and so effectually control the bleeding. A solution of gelatine, epinephrine or thromboplastine may be injected into the nostril. The injection of blood serum may be tried or transfusion done in severe cases.

B. DISEASES OF THE LARYNX

I. ACUTE CATARRHAL LARYNGITIS

This may come on as an independent affection or in association with general catarrh of the upper respiratory passages.

Etiology.—Many cases are due to catching cold or to overuse of the voice; others come on in consequence of the inhalation of irritating gases especially in the recent war. Very severe laryngitis is excited by traumatism, either injuries from without or the lodgment of foreign bodies. It may be caused by the action of very hot liquids or corrosive poisons. It may occur in the general catarrh associated with influenza and measles. The pneumococcus, influenza bacillus and *Micrococcus catarrhalis* are the organisms most commonly found.

Symptoms.—There is a sense of tickling referred to the larynx; the cold air irritates and, owing to the increased sensibility of the mucous membrane, the act of inspiration may be painful. There is a dry cough, and the voice is altered. At first it is simply husky, but soon phonation becomes painful, and finally the voice may be completely lost. In adults the respirations are not increased in frequency, but in children dyspnœa is not uncommon and may occur in spasmodic attacks and become urgent if there is much œdema with the inflammatory swelling.

The laryngoscope shows a swollen mucous membrane of the larynx, particularly the ary-epiglottidean folds. The vocal cords have lost their smooth and shining appearance and are reddened and swollen. Their mobility also is greatly impaired, owing to the infiltration of the adjoining mucous membrane and of the muscles. A slight mucoid exudation covers the parts. The constitutional symptoms are not severe. There is rarely much fever, and in many cases the patient is not seriously ill. Occasionally cases come on with greater intensity, the cough is very distressing, deglutition is painful, and there may be urgent dyspnœa.

Diagnosis.—There is rarely any difficulty in determining the nature of a case if a satisfactory laryngoscopic examination can be made. The severer forms may simulate œdema of the glottis. When the loss of voice is marked, the case may be mistaken for one of nervous aphonia, but the laryngoscope decides the question at once. Much more difficult is the diagnosis of acute laryngitis in children, particularly in the very young, in whom it is so hard to make a proper examination. From ordinary laryngismus it is to be distinguished by the presence of fever, the mode of onset, and particularly the coryza and the previous symptoms of hoarseness or loss of voice. Membranous laryngitis may at first be quite impossible to differentiate, but in a majority of cases of this affection there are patches on the pharynx and early swelling of the cervical glands. The symptoms, too, are much more severe.

Treatment.—Rest of the larynx should be enjoined, so far as phonation is concerned; smoking should be forbidden. In cases of any severity the patient should be kept in bed. The room should be at an even temperature and the air saturated with moisture. Inhalations of menthol and eucalyptus are helpful. Early in the disease, if there is much fever, aconite and citrate of potash may be given, and for the irritating painful cough a full dose of Dover's powder or heroin at night. An ice-bag externally often gives great relief.

II. CHRONIC LARYNGITIS

Etiology.—The disease usually follows repeated acute attacks. The most common cause is overuse of the voice, particularly in persons whose occupation necessitates shouting in the open air. The constant inhalation of irritating substances, as tobacco-smoke, may also cause it.

Symptoms.—The voice is usually hoarse and rough and in severe cases may be almost lost. There is usually very little pain; only the unpleasant sense of tickling in the larynx, which causes a frequent desire to cough. With the laryngoscope the mucous membrane looks swollen, but much less red than in the acute condition. In association with the granular pharyngitis, the mucous glands of the epiglottis and of the ventricles may be involved.

Treatment.—The nostrils should be carefully examined, since in some instances chronic laryngitis is associated with and even dependent upon obstruction to the free passage of air through the nose. Local application must be made directly to the larynx, either with a brush or by means of a spray. Among the remedies most recommended are the solutions of nitrate of silver, chlorate of potash, perchloride of zinc, and tannic acid. Insufflations of bismuth are sometimes useful. Among directions to be given are the avoidance of heated rooms and loud speaking, and abstinence from tobacco and alcohol. The throat should not be too much muffled, and morning and evening the neck should be sponged with cold water.

III. ŒDEMATOUS LARYNGITIS

It was described by Matthew Baillie (1812) and Pitcairn (one of the owners of the famous Gold-headed Cane) was one of the first cases.

Etiology.—Œdema of the structures which form the glottis is met with (*a*) as a rare sequence of ordinary acute laryngitis; (*b*) in chronic diseases of the larynx, as syphilis or tubercle; (*c*) in severe inflammatory diseases like diphtheria, in erysipelas of the neck, and in various forms of cellulitis; (*d*) occasionally in the acute infections—scarlet fever, typhus, or typhoid; in nephritis, either acute or chronic, there may be a rapidly developing œdema; (*e*) in angio-neurotic œdema.

Symptoms.—There is dyspnœa, increasing in intensity, so that within an hour or two the condition becomes very critical. There is sometimes marked stridor in respiration. The voice becomes husky and disappears. The laryngoscope shows enormous swelling of the epiglottis, which can sometimes be felt with the finger or even seen when the tongue is strongly depressed with a spatula. The ary-epiglottidean folds are the seat of the chief swelling and may almost meet in the middle line. Occasionally the œdema is below the true cords. The *diagnosis* is rarely difficult, inasmuch as even without the laryngoscope the swollen epiglottis can be seen or felt with the finger. The condition is very often fatal.

Treatment.—An ice-bag should be placed on the larynx, and the patient given ice to suck. The air of the room should be moist. If the symptoms are urgent, the throat should be sprayed with a strong solution of cocaine or epinephrin and the swollen epiglottis scarified. If relief does not follow, tracheotomy should immediately be performed. The high rate of mortality is due to the fact that this operation is, as a rule, too long delayed.

IV. SPASMODIC LARYNGITIS

(*Laryngismus stridulus*)

Definition.—Spasmodic contraction of the intrinsic muscles of the larynx, usually in children, leading to closure of the glottis and dyspnœa.

Etiology.—In children it may be a purely nervous affection, without any inflammatory condition of the larynx, and is most commonly seen in connection with rickets. The disease has close relations with tetany and may display many of the accessory phenomena of this disease. Often the attack comes on when the child has been crossed or scolded. Mothers sometimes call the attacks "passion fits" or attacks of "holding the breath." It was supposed at one time that they were associated with enlargement of the thymus, and the condition therefore received the name of *thymic asthma*.

In adults it may follow irritation of the pneumogastric nerves, as in aneurism or mediastinal tumor. The crises in tabes dorsalis are due to sudden spasm of the intrinsic muscles. It is occasionally seen in hysteria. There are attacks of spasmodic cough in adults with distressing spasm of the glottis, lasting two or three months and arousing the suspicion of aneurism or tumor.

The actual state of the larynx during a paroxysm is a spasm of the adductors, but the precise nature of the influences causing it is not yet known, whether centric or reflex from peripheral irritation. The disease is not so common in America as in England.

Symptoms.—The attacks may come on either in the night or in the day; often just as the child awakes. There is no cough, no hoarseness, but the respiration is arrested and the child struggles for breath, the face gets congested, and then, with a sudden relaxation of the spasm, the air is drawn into the lungs with a high-pitched crowing sound, which has given to the affection the name of "child-crowing." Convulsions may occur during an attack or there may be carpo-pedal spasms. Death may, but rarely does, occur during the attack. With the cyanosis the spasm relaxes and respiration begins. The attacks may recur with great frequency throughout the day.

Treatment.—The gums should be carefully examined and, if swollen and hot, freely lanced. The bowels should be carefully regulated and, as these children are usually delicate or rickety, nourishing diet and cod-liver oil should be given. By far the most satisfactory method of treatment is the cold sponging. In severe cases, two or three times a day the child should be placed in a warm bath, and the back and chest thoroughly sponged for a minute or two with cold water. It may be employed when the child is in a paroxysm, though if the attack is severe and the lividity is great it is much better to dash cold water into the face. Sometimes the introduction of the finger far back into the throat relieves the spasm. Small doses of sodium bromide, chloral hydrate or antipyrine are sometimes useful.

Spasmodic croup, believed to be a functional spasm of the muscles of the larynx, is an affection seen most commonly between the ages of two and five years. According to Trousseau's description, the child goes to bed well, and about midnight or in the early morning hours awakes with oppressed breathing, harsh, croupy cough, and perhaps some huskiness of voice. The oppression and distress for a time are very serious, the face is congested, and there are signs of approaching cyanosis. The attack passes off abruptly, the child falls asleep and awakes the next morning feeling perfectly well. These attacks may be repeated for several nights in succession, and usually cause great alarm to the parents. There are instances in which the child is somewhat hoarse throughout the day, and has slight catarrhal symptoms and a brazen, croupy cough. There is probably slight catarrhal laryngitis with it. These cases are not infrequently mistaken for laryngeal diphtheria. To allay the spasm a whiff of chloroform may be administered, which will in a few moments give relief, or the child may be placed in a hot bath. A prompt emetic, such as wine of ipecac, will usually relieve the spasm, and is specially indicated if the child has overloaded the stomach through the day.

V. TUBERCULOUS LARYNGITIS

Etiology.—Tubercles may arise primarily in the laryngeal mucosa, but in the great majority of cases the affection is secondary to pulmonary tuberculosis, in which it is met with in a variable proportion of from 18 to 30 per cent. Laryngitis may occur very early in pulmonary tuberculosis. There may be well-marked involvement of the larynx with signs of very limited trouble at one apex.

Morbid Anatomy.—The mucosa is at first swollen and presents scattered tubercles, which seem to begin in the neighborhood of the blood-vessels. By their fusion small tuberculous masses arise, which caseate and finally ulcerate, leaving shallow irregular losses of substance. The ulcers are usually covered with a grayish exudation, and there is a general thickening of the mucosa about them, which is particularly marked upon the arytenoids. The ulcers may erode the true cords and finally destroy them, and passing deeply may cause perichondritis with necrosis and occasionally exfoliation of the cartilages. The disease may involve the pharynx and fauces and the mucous membrane, covering the cricoid cartilage toward the œsophagus. The epiglottis may be entirely destroyed. There are rare instances in which cicatricial changes go on to such a degree that stenosis of the larynx is induced.

Symptoms.—The first indication is slight huskiness of the voice, which finally deepens to hoarseness, and in advanced stages there may be complete loss of voice. There is something very suggestive in the early hoarseness of tuberculous laryngitis. The attention may be directed to the lungs simply by the quality of the voice.

The cough is in part due to involvement of the larynx. Early in the disease it is not very troublesome, but when the ulceration is extensive it becomes husky and ineffectual. Of the symptoms, none is more aggravating than the dysphagia, which is met with particularly when the epiglottis is involved, and when the ulceration has extended to the pharynx. In instances in which the epiglottis is in great part destroyed, with each attempt to take food there are distressing paroxysms of cough, and even of suffocation.

With the laryngoscope there is seen early in the disease a pallor of the mucous membrane, which also looks thickened and infiltrated, particularly that covering the arytenoid cartilages. The ulcers are very characteristic. They are broad and shallow, with gray bases and ill-defined outlines. The vocal cords are infiltrated and thickened, and ulceration is very common.

The diagnosis is rarely difficult, as it is usually associated with well-marked pulmonary disease. In case of doubt the secretion from the base of an ulcer should be examined for bacilli.

Treatment.—The voice should not be used. In the early stages no method of treatment is more effectual. Applications of lactic acid in glycerine and the electro-cautery are the best local measures. The insufflation, three times a day, of a powder of iodoform with morphia, after cleansing the ulcers with a spray, relieves the pain in a majority of the cases. Cocaine (4-per-cent. solution) applied with the atomizer will often enable the patient to swallow his food comfortably. There are, however, distressing cases of extensive laryngeal and pharyngeal ulceration in which even cocaine loses its good effects. With loss of the glottis the difficulty in swallowing is less when the patient hangs the head over and sucks food through a tube. Heliotherapy has given good results.

VI. SYPHILITIC LARYNGITIS

Syphilis attacks the larynx with great frequency. It may be congenital or a secondary or tertiary manifestation of the acquired form.

Symptoms.—In secondary syphilis there is occasionally erythema of the larynx, which may go on to definite catarrh, but has nothing characteristic. The process may proceed to the formation of superficial whitish ulcers, usually symmetrically placed on the cords or ventricular bands. Mucous patches and condylomata are rarely seen. The symptoms are practically those of slight loss of voice with laryngeal irritation, as in the simple catarrhal form.

The tertiary laryngeal lesions are numerous and serious. True gummata, varying in size from the head of a pin to a small nut, arise in the submucous tissue, most commonly at the base of the epiglottis. They go through the characteristic changes and may break down, producing extensive and deep ulceration, or—and this is more characteristic of syphilitic laryngitis—in their healing form a fibrous tissue which shrinks and produces stenosis. The ulceration may involve the cartilage, inducing necrosis and exfoliation, and even hæmorrhage from erosion of the arteries. Œdema may suddenly prove fatal. The cicatrices which follow the sclerosis of the gummata or the healing of the ulcers produce great deformity. The epiglottis may be tied down to the pharyngeal wall or to the epiglottic folds, or even to the tongue; and eventually a stenosis results, which may necessitate tracheotomy.

The laryngeal symptoms of congenital syphilis have the usual course of these lesions and appear either early, within the first five or six months, or after puberty; most commonly in the former period. The gummatous infiltration leads to ulceration, most commonly of the epiglottis and in the ventricles, and the process may extend deeply and involve the cartilage. Cicatricial contraction may also occur.

The diagnosis of syphilis of the larynx is rarely difficult, since it occurs most commonly in connection with other symptoms of the disease.

Treatment.—The administration of anti-syphilitic remedies is the most important, and under these the secondary lesions usually subside promptly. The tertiary laryngeal manifestations are always serious and difficult to treat. The deep ulceration is specially hard to combat, and the cicatrization may necessitate tracheotomy or gradual dilatation.

C. DISEASES OF THE BRONCHI

I. ACUTE TRACHEO-BRONCHITIS

Acute catarrhal inflammation of the trachea and larger bronchi is a very common disease, rarely serious in healthy adults, but very fatal in the old and in the young, owing to associated pulmonary complications. It is bilateral and affects either the larger and medium sized tubes or the smaller bronchi, in which case it is known as capillary bronchitis. We shall speak only of the former, as the latter is part and parcel of broncho-pneumonia.

Etiology.—In a majority of cases it is an acute infection beginning as a simple coryza and extending to the air passages. It is very contagious, as noted by Benjamin Franklin, and prevails at times in epidemic form; even apart from influenza with which it is usually associated. It prevails in the cold changeable months of the year. The association with cold is indicated in the popular expression "cold on the chest." It attacks person of all ages, but more particularly the young and the old. Some individuals have a special disposition and the slightest exposure may bring on an attack.

Acute bronchitis is associated with many infections, notably measles and typhoid fever. It is present also in asthma and whooping-cough. The subjects of spinal curvature are specially liable to the disease. The bronchitis of nephritis, gout, and heart-disease is usually a chronic form. Inhalation of dust is a contributing factor in many cases. Irritating gases of all sorts may cause bronchitis. Some of the worst types ever seen have followed the various gases used in the recent war. Ether inhalation is only too often followed by bronchitis. There is a spirochætal form which may be acute or chronic. The spirochætes are found in the sputum.

Bacteriology.—The pneumococcus is responsible for many cases both in young and old. The infection may follow pneumonia, and bronchitis may recur winter after winter, with the sputum showing an almost pure culture of the pneumococcus. These germs may persist in the sputum for many years, with an almost daily cough, aggravated in the winter. The influenza bacillus is very common and may be found alone or with streptococci. The *Micrococcus catarrhalis* is present in a number of the ordinary cases, very often in combination with other organisms. Less frequently the staphylococci, colon bacillus, and typhoid bacilli have been found. It is not possible to separate clinical groups of bronchitis to correspond with the chief infective agent found in the sputum. The pneumococcus carrier appears to be very liable to recurring attacks. The influenza bacillus may cause more prostration and there is a greater tendency to chronicity and bronchiectasis.

Morbid Anatomy.—The mucous membrane of the trachea and bronchi is reddened, congested, and covered with mucus and muco-pus, which may be seen oozing from the smaller bronchi, some of which are dilated. The finer changes in the mucosa consist in desquamation of the ciliated epithelium, swelling and œdema of the submucosa, and infiltration of the tissue with leucocytes. The mucous glands are much swollen.

Symptoms.—General.—The symptoms of an ordinary "cold" accompany the onset; the coryza extends to the larynx, producing hoarseness, and then to the trachea and bronchi, causing cough. A chill is rare, but there is a sense of oppression, with heaviness and languor and pains in the bones and back. In mild cases there is scarcely any fever, but in severer forms the range is from 101° to 103° F. The bronchial symptoms set in with a feeling of tightness and rawness beneath the sternum and a sensation of oppression in the chest. The cough is rough at first, and often of a ringing character. It comes on in paroxysms which rack and distress the patient extremely. The pain may be very intense beneath the sternum and along the attachments of the diaphragm. At first the cough is dry and the expectoration scanty and viscid, but in a few days the secretion becomes muco-purulent and abundant, and finally purulent. With the loosening of the cough great relief is experienced. The sputum is made up largely of pus-cells, with a variable number of the large round alveolar cells, many of which contain carbon grains, while others have undergone the myelin degeneration.

Physical Signs.—The respiratory movements are not greatly increased in frequency unless the fever is high. There are instances, however, in which the breathing is rapid and when the smaller tubes are involved there is dyspnœa. On palpation the bronchial fremitus may often be felt. On auscultation in the early stage, piping sibilant râles are everywhere to be heard. They are very changeable, and appear and disappear with coughing. With the relaxation of the bronchial membranes and the greater abundance of the secretion, the râles change and become mucous and bubbling in quality. The bronchi of the posterior and lower parts of the lungs are most involved. The bases of the lungs should be examined each day, particularly in children and the aged.

Course.—This depends on the conditions under which the disease arises. In healthy adults, by the end of a week the fever subsides and the cough loosens. In another week or ten days convalescence is fully established. In young children the chief risk is in the extension of the process downward. In measles and whooping-cough the ordinary bronchial catarrh is very apt to descend to the finer tubes, which become dilated and plugged with muco-pus, inducing areas of collapse, and finally broncho-pneumonia. This extension is indicated by changes in the physical signs. Usually at the base the râles are subcrepitant and numerous and there may be areas of defective resonance and of feeble or distant tubular breathing. In the aged and debilitated there are similar dangers if the process extends from the larger to the smaller tubes. In old age the bronchial mucosa is less capable of expelling the mucus, which is more apt to sag to the dependent parts and induce dilatation of the tubes with extension of the inflammation to the contiguous air-cells.

Diagnosis.—This is rarely difficult. Although the mode of onset may be brusque and perhaps simulate pneumonia, yet the absence of dulness and blowing breathing, and the general character of the bronchial inflammation, render the diagnosis easy. The complication of broncho-pneumonia is indicated by the greater severity of the symptoms, particularly the dyspnœa, the more paroxysmal and insistent cough, the changed color, and the physical signs.

Treatment.—We should do all in our power to lessen the risks of contagion. The patient should sleep alone, the sputum should be carefully collected and disinfected, and, when possible, there should be an abundance of sunlight and fresh air. In mild cases household measures suffice. The hot foot-bath, or the warm bath, a drink of hot lemonade, and a mustard plaster on the chest will often give relief. In severe cases the patient should be in bed: liquids should be taken freely. For the dry, racking cough, the symptom most complained of by the patient, Dover's powder is a useful remedy. It is a popular belief that quinine, in full doses, will check an oncoming cold on the chest, but this is doubtful. It is a common custom when persons feel the approach of a cold to take a Turkish bath, and though the tightness and oppression may be relieved by it, there is in a majority of the cases great risk. Hydrotherapy is most useful in the form of compresses to the thorax or a wet pack. Relief is obtained from the unpleasant sense of rawness by keeping the air of the room saturated with moisture, and in this dry stage the old-fashioned mixture of the wines of antimony and ipecacuanha with liquor ammonii acetatis and nitrous ether is useful. If the pulse is very rapid, tincture of aconite may be given, particularly in the case of children. The use of inhalations, such as the compound tincture of benzoin, often gives relief. For the cough, when dry and irritating, opium should be freely used in the form of Dover's powder or paregoric. In the very young and the aged care must be exercised in the use of opium, particularly if the secretions are free; but for the distressing, irritative cough, which keeps the patient awake, opium in some form gives the only relief. Heroin is often helpful. As the cough loosens and the expectoration is more abundant, the patient becomes more comfortable. In this stage it is customary to ply him with expectorants of various sorts. Though useful occasionally, they should not be given as a routine. *Vaccine treatment* is very uncertain, even when a single organism has been recovered, but occasionally prompt and satisfactory results are seen, both in prophylaxis and treatment.

In the acute bronchitis of children, if the amount of secretion is large and difficult to expectorate, or if there is dyspnœa and the color begins to get dusky, an emetic (a tablespoonful of ipecac wine) should be given at once and repeated if necessary.

II. CHRONIC BRONCHITIS

Etiology.—This affection may follow repeated attacks of acute bronchitis, but it is most commonly met with in chronic lung affections, heart-disease, aneurism of the aorta, gout, and renal disease. It is most frequent in the aged and in males. Climate and season have an important influence. It is the cause of the winter cough of the aged, which recurs with regularity as the weather gets cold and changeable. Owing to the more uniform heating of the houses, it is much less common in Canada and in the United States than in England.

Morbid Anatomy.—The bronchial mucosa presents a variety of changes, depending somewhat upon the disease with which chronic bronchitis is associated. In some cases the mucous membrane is very thin, so that the longitudinal bands of elastic tissue stand out prominently. The tubes are dilated, the muscular and glandular tissues atrophied, and the epithelium is in great part shed. In other instances the mucosa is thickened and infiltrated. There may be ulceration, particularly of the mucous follicles. Bronchial dilatations are not uncommon and emphysema is a constant accompaniment.

Symptoms.—In the form met with in old men, associated with emphysema, gout, or heart-disease, the chief symptoms are as follows: Shortness of breath, which may not be noticeable except on exertion. The patients "puff and blow" on going up hill or up a flight of stairs. This is due not so much to the chronic bronchitis itself as to associated emphysema or even to cardiac weakness. They complain of no pain. The cough is variable, changing with the weather and with the season. During the summer they may remain free, but each succeeding winter the cough comes on with severity and persists. There may be only a spell in the morning, or the chief distress is at night. The sputum in chronic bronchitis is very variable. In cases of the so-called dry catarrh there is no expectoration. Usually, however, it is abundant, mucopurulent, or distinctly purulent in character. There are instances in which the patient for years coughs up a thin fluid sputum. There is rarely fever. The general health may be good and the disease may present no serious features apart from the liability to induce emphysema and bronchiectasis. In many cases it is an incurable affection. Patients improve and the cough disappears in the summer time only to return during the winter months.

Physical Signs.—The chest is usually distended, the movements are limited, and the condition is often that which we see in emphysema. The percussion note is clear or hyperresonant. On auscultation, expiration is prolonged and wheezy, and rhonchi of various sorts are heard—some high-pitched and piping, others deep-toned and snoring. Crepitant râles are common at the bases.

In children apart from chronic disease of the lungs, chronic bronchitis with cough, chiefly nocturnal, is a common accompaniment of enlarged tonsils and adenoids. The child, a mouth breather, with the characteristic facies and chest, is often thin and underdeveloped, with an evening temperature of 99.5°. Diffuse râles are present at the apices, or, more commonly, the bases. The cough, the fever and the chest condition may lead to the diagnosis of tuberculosis.

Clinical Varieties.—The description just given is of the ordinary chronic bronchitis which occurs in connection with emphysema and heart-disease and in many elderly men. There are certain forms which merit special description: (*a*) There is a form in women which comes on between the ages of twenty and thirty and may continue indefinitely without serious impairment of the health. In some cases it follows influenza, and there may be slight bronchiectasis.

(*b*) BRONCHORRHŒA.—Excessive bronchial secretion is met with under several conditions. It must not be mistaken for the profuse expectoration of bronchiectasis. The secretion may be very liquid and watery—*bronchorrhœa serosa*—and in extraordinary amount. More commonly, it is purulent though thin, and with greenish or yellow-green masses. It may be thick and uniform. This profuse bronchial secretion is usually a manifestation of chronic bronchitis, and may lead to dilatation of the tubes and ultimately to fetid bronchitis. In the young the condition may persist for years without impairment of health and without apparently damaging the lungs.

(*c*) PUTRID BRONCHITIS.—Fetid expectoration is met with in connection with bronchiectasis, gangrene, abscess, or with decomposition of secretions within tuberculous cavities and in an empyema which has perforated the lung. There are instances in which, apart from any of these states, the expectoration has a fetid character. The sputum is abundant, usually thin, grayish-white in color, and separates into an upper fluid layer capped with frothy mucus and a thick sediment in which may sometimes be found dirty yellow masses the size of peas or beans—the so-called *Dittrich's* plugs. The affection is very rare apart from the above-mentioned conditions. In severe cases it leads to changes in the bronchial walls, pneumonia, and often to abscess or gangrene. Metastatic brain abscess has followed in a number of cases.

(*d*) DRY CATARRH.—The *catarrhe sec* of Laennec, a not uncommon form, is characterized by paroxysms of coughing of great intensity, with little or no expectoration. It is usually met with in elderly persons with emphysema, and is one of the most obstinate of all varieties of bronchitis.

The bronchitis with an unusual number of eosinophiles in the sputum is really a form of asthma.

Treatment.—Removal to a southern latitude may prevent the onset. In England the milder climate of Falmouth, Torquay, and Bournemouth is suitable for those who cannot go elsewhere. Egypt, southern France, southern California, and Florida furnish winter climates in which the subjects of chronic bronchitis live with the greatest comfort. With care chronic bronchitis may prove to be the slight ailment that, as Oliver Wendell Holmes remarked, promotes longevity.

The first endeavor is to ascertain, if possible, whether there are constitutional or local affections with which it is associated. In many instances the urine is found to be highly acid, perhaps slightly albuminous, and the arteries are stiff. In the form associated with this condition, sometimes called gouty bronchitis, the attacks seem related to the defective renal elimination, and to this condition the treatment should be first directed. In other instances there are heart-disease and emphysema. In the form occurring in the old prophylaxis is most important. There is no doubt that with prudence even in the most changeable winter weather much may be done to prevent the onset of chronic bronchitis. Woollen undergarments should be used and especial care should be taken in the spring months not to change them for lighter ones before the warm weather is established. The use of autogenous vaccines as a preventive is sometimes successful and is worthy of trial. A careful bacteriological study of the sputum should be made and the causal organism or organisms identified.

Cure is seldom effected by medicinal remedies. There are instances in which iodide of potassium acts with remarkable benefit, and it should always be given a trial in cases of paroxysmal bronchitis of obscure origin. For the morning cough, bicarbonate of sodium (gr. xv, 1 gm.), chloride of sodium (gr. v, 0.3 gm.), spirit of chloroform (♏ v, 0.3 c. c.) in anise water and taken with an equal amount of warm water will be found useful (Fowler). When there is much sense of tightness and fullness of the chest, the portable Turkish bath may be tried. When the secretion is excessive atropine is sometimes useful. When the heart is feeble, the combination of digitalis and strychnia is very beneficial. Turpentine, the old-fashioned remedy so warmly recommended by the Dublin physicians, has in many quarters fallen undeservedly into disuse. Preparations of tar, creosote, and terebene are sometimes useful. Of other balsamic remedies, the compound tincture of benzoin and the balsam of Peru or tolu may be used. Inhalations of eucalyptus and of the spray of ipecacuanha wine are often useful. If fetor be present, carbolic acid in the form of spray (1 per cent. solution) will lessen the odor, or thymol (1 to 1,000), but the intratracheal medication is the most efficient. After the larynx is anæsthetized with a 4 per cent. cocaine solution, inject with a suitable syringe about two drams (8 c. c.) of olive oil, with gr. ½ (0.032 gm.) of iodoform, and gr. ⅛ (0.008 gm.) of morphia if there is irritating cough. For urgent dyspnœa with cyanosis, venesection gives most relief. In the form in children associated with adenoids, complete removal, followed by respiratory exercises, is indicated.

III. BRONCHIECTASIS

Etiology.—Dilatation follows various affections of the bronchi themselves, of the lungs, and of the pleura. The condition may be unsuspected clinically and is much more common than indicated in the literature. Either the cases are now more often recognized or the disease has become more frequent. It occurs in from 2 to 4 per cent. of the post mortems in general hospitals. A majority of the cases occur between the ages of 20 and 40 years. Males are more often affected. Following Fowler's classification, the causes are:

A. Intrinsic, *acting directly through the bronchi.*

1. *Bronchitis.*—Chronic cough is a common antecedent, and the dilatation

is a mechanical effect of constant forced expiration acting on bronchial walls weakened by disease. There are three groups: (*a*) the remarkable form of generalized dilatation of the smaller bronchi seen in children after the infections, particularly measles, described by Sharkey, Carr and others. (*b*) Following an infective bronchitis, pneumococcal or influenzal, the cough persists and gradually the signs of diffuse bronchiectasis appear with fetid sputum. Such cases are not easy to differentiate from, some indeed are, fetid bronchitis. (*c*) The bronchitis following prolonged exposure to dust, as in miners and potters, is very often associated with bronchiectasis.

2. *Stenosis* of a bronchus, either by compression from without by a tumor or aneurism, a growth in the wall as in syphilis, or a foreign body within. The last is an important cause. As a result of the narrowing the secretions accumulate, the walls are weakened and dilatation follows.

B. Extrinsic Causes associated with changes in the lung tissue or pleura. (*a*) Fibrosis of the lung from whatever cause, syphilis, chronic pneumonia, anthracosis, and chronic fibroid pleurisy. (*b*) Acute broncho-pneumonia. It is rare after delayed resolution in lobar pneumonia but it may occur with broncho-pneumonia. In a patient dead six weeks from the onset there were areas of broncho-pneumonia, dilatation of the bronchi of both lower lobes, several spots of gangrene, and secondary abscess of the brain. (*c*) Compression of the lung. The tubes are rarely found dilated in the extreme compressed form of chronic empyema. Local compression by tumor or aneurism may be a cause without stenosis of the bronchus. The atelectatic bronchiectasis occurs in an area of lung which has not developed or not expanded after birth. The bronchial walls show an overgrowth of cartilage. (*d*) Tuberculosis. It is rare to dissect a lung in the chronic ulcerative form without finding somewhere a dilated bronchus. The more chronic the disease and the greater the fibrosis the more widespread the dilatation, and most often in the upper lobes.

C. Congenital.—This rare form, described by Grawitz, occurs as a universal saccular distention of the bronchi, usually of one lung; or it may be confined to the bronchi of the third and fourth order in local areas of atelectasis.

Morbid Anatomy.—Two chief forms are recognized—the *cylindrical* and the *saccular*—which may exist together in the same lung. The condition may be general or partial. Universal bronchiectasis is usually unilateral, occurs in rare congenital cases and is occasionally seen as a sequence of interstitial pneumonia. The entire bronchial tree is represented by a series of sacculi opening one into the other. The walls are smooth and possibly without ulceration or erosion except in the dependent parts. The lining membrane of the sacculi is usually smooth and glistening. The dilatations may form large cysts immediately beneath the pleura. Intervening between the sacculi is a dense cirrhotic lung tissue. The partial dilatations—the saccular and cylindrical—are common in chronic tuberculosis, particularly at the apex, in chronic pleurisy at the base, and in emphysema. Here the dilatation is more commonly cylindrical, sometimes fusiform. The bronchial mucous membrane is much involved and sometimes there is a narrowing of the lumen. Occasionally one meets with a single saccular bronchiectasis in connection with chronic bronchitis or emphysema. Some of these look like simple cysts, with smooth walls, without fluid contents. Bronchiolectasis as an acute condition may follow the infectious diseases.

Symptoms.—There are *acute* cases, usually the bronchiolectasis of children; but a case of the broncho-pneumonic form died in six weeks from the onset. In the limited dilatations of tuberculosis, emphysema, and chronic bronchitis the symptoms are in great part those of the original disease, and often the condition is not suspected during life.

In extensive *saccular bronchiectasis* the characters of the cough and expectoration are distinctive. The patient will pass the greater part of the day without any cough and then in a severe paroxysm will bring up a large quantity of sputum. Of 23 cases the amount for twenty-four hours was in 2 less than 100 c. c., in 11 from 100-300 c. c., in 2 almost 500 c. c., in 7 over 600 c. c. In one case with over one litre per day the cavities found were very small. Sometimes change of position will bring on a violent attack, probably due to the fact that some of the secretion flows from the dilatation to a normal tube. The daily spell of coughing is usually in the morning. The expectoration is in many instances very characteristic, grayish or grayish brown in color, fluid, purulent, with a peculiar acid, sometimes fetid, odor. Placed in a conical glass, it separates into a thick granular layer below and a thin mucoid intervening layer above, which is capped by a brownish froth. Microscopically it consists of pus-corpuscles, often large crystals of fatty acids, which are sometimes in enormous numbers over the field and arranged in bunches. Hæmatoidin crystals are sometimes present. Elastic fibres are seldom found except when there is ulceration of the bronchial walls. Tubercle bacilli are not present. In some cases the expectoration is very fetid. Nummular expectoration, such as comes from tuberculous cavities, is not common. Hæmorrhage occurred in 14 out of 35 cases analyzed by Fowler, in 17 of our 24 cases, slight in 8, and extreme in 3. Arthritis may occur, and it is one of the conditions with which the pulmonary osteo-arthropathy is commonly associated. Clubbing of the fingers and toes is common. There is a remarkable association of bronchiectasis with abscess of the brain. Among 13,700 autopsies at the London Hospital and the Brompton Hospital there were 19 instances of cerebral abscess with pulmonary disease, usually bronchiectasis (Schörstein).

Physical Signs.—The associated conditions are so various that the signs vary greatly. In deep-seated cases there may be no signs. The co-existence of tuberculosis, chronic bronchitis, emphysema or fibrosis gives a complicated picture. The signs on inspection, palpation and percussion are influenced by these factors. Dilatations near the surface yield a tympanitic note. In saccular bronchiectasis the signs vary as the cavity is empty or filled with secretion. On auscultation the breath sounds depend on associated changes unless the bronchiectasis is superficial, when cavernous breathing may be heard. Many varieties of râles are heard. In diffuse early cases they may have a very intense crackling quality which is sometimes suggestive of dilatation.

Diagnosis.—In the extensive sacculated forms, unilateral and associated with interstitial pneumonia or chronic pleurisy, the diagnosis is easy. There is contraction of the side, which in some instances is not at all extreme. The cavernous signs may be chiefly at the base and may vary according to the condition of the cavity, whether full or empty. There may be the most exquisite amphoric phenomena and loud resonant râles. The condition persists for years and is not inconsistent with a tolerably active life. The patients frequently show signs of marked embarrassment of the circulation with dyspnœa and cyanosis on exertion. A condition very difficult to distinguish from bronchiectasis is a limited pleural cavity communicating with a bronchus. The X-ray examination is of value in localizing the area of the lung in which the tubes are chiefly involved. The intensity of the shadow in plates taken before and after evacuation may be very suggestive.

The disease is often regarded as *tuberculosis,* which may co-exist, but proper sputum examination should prevent this. The acuteness of abscess of the lung and the character of the sputum are usually distinctive. From chronic bronchitis the diagnosis is difficult but the sputum and clubbing of the fingers are aids.

Treatment.—Medical treatment is not satisfactory, since it is impossible to heal the cavities. Postural treatment is important, and the most favorable position should be studied for each patient. Sleeping with the head low favors "drainage." The reduction of the fluid intake to a minimum is sometimes useful. Intratracheal injections have been recommended; with a suitable syringe a dram may be injected twice a day of the following solution: Menthol 10 parts, guaiacol 2 parts, olive oil 88 parts. Or better still when the odor is very offensive iodoform in olive oil. The creosote vapor bath may be given in a small room. The patient's eyes must be protected with well-fitting goggles, and the nostrils stuffed with cotton-wool. Twenty to thirty drops of creosote are poured upon water in a saucer and vaporized by placing the saucer over a spirit lamp. At first the vapor is very irritating and disagreeable, but the patient gets used to it. This should be done at first every other day for fifteen minutes, then gradually increased to an hour daily. This should be continued for three months and is a most satisfactory method.

Surgical treatment.—Collapse of the affected lung by nitrogen displacement has been tried. Drainage of the cavities in the lower lobe and subperiosteal resection of three or four ribs with the application of a compression pad have given good results. The bronchiectatic lobe has been resected. Sauerbruch in seven cases ligated the branch of the pulmonary artery going to the affected lobe, which is followed by cicatrization. Morriston Davies advises section of the phrenic nerves in the neck, causing paralysis of the diaphragm, when bronchiectasis begins to develop in interstitial pneumonia.

IV. HAY FEVER AND BRONCHIAL ASTHMA

Definition.—A reaction of an anaphylactic nature in sensitized persons, in others possibly a reflex neurosis, characterized by swelling of the nasal or respiratory mucous membrane, increased secretion, and, in asthma, spasm of the bronchial muscles with dyspnœa, chiefly expiratory. There are no essential differences between hay fever and asthma; in the one the nasal portion of the respiratory tract is affected, in the other the bronchial, in many instances both.

Etiology.—The word "Asthma," which means a panting, was used by the older writers as we use the term dyspnœa. We still speak of "cardiac and renal asthma," but the term should be restricted to the independent disease, first separated in the 17th century by Van Helmont and by Willis. The latter speaks of the "tyranny and cruelty" of the disease, and suspected the cause to lurk in the "Muscular coats of the pneumonic vessels," meaning the bronchi. Floyer (1698), who gives a good account of his own case in his "*Treatise of the Asthma,*" held the same views. With the introduction of accurate methods of diagnosis by Laennec the independent disease was separated from a host of maladies with dyspnœa as a prominent symptom.

Our modern conception of *hay fever* dates from the description by Bostock in 1819 and 1828 of the summar catarrh—Catarrhus estivus. He recognized the periodicity, the disturbance of respiration as sometimes the only feature, and the association with the "effluvium from new hay." Elliotson (1831) first suggested that it was caused by the "effluvia of the grass and probably the pollen." Morrill Wyman (1854) separated the spring and autumn forms of hay fever. Blackley (1873) demonstrated that "pollen possesses the power of producing hay fever both in its asthmatic and catarrhal forms," and, as early as 1865, showed that skin reactions were present in sensitive persons. Then came many observations on the relation of nasal conditions to asthma and hay fever. Dunbar applied modern methods to the study of the pollen problem, separated the toxins, studied their reactions, cutaneous and serological, and introduced a specific therapy.

Finally Meltzer and his pupils Auer and Lewis (1910) brought the disease into the category of anaphylactic phenomena. Following an injection of normal horse serum a guinea-pig has no reaction, but ten days later if a second dose be given the animal will be found to have been "sensitized" by the first dose, and, in consequence, has alarming symptoms—sneezing, dyspnœa at first, and the more laboured breathing and choreic convulsions. Anatomically the lungs are voluminous, do not collapse, and the bronchi show marked congestion of the mucosa. An asthmatic subject, sensitive, say, to eggs, if injected with a small amount of egg albumen will have an attack with difficulty in expiring, not inspiring. The lungs become distended and, as seen with the fluoroscope, the diaphragm does not move. The alveolar air has a low carbon dioxide content. An injection of epinephrin relieves the condition; just as, if given in time, it will remove the anaphylactic symptoms in the guinea-pig. The only possible explanation of the pulmonary features is that the air is imprisoned in the alveoli by the spasmodic contraction of the bronchial muscles; there is marked over-distention of the lungs, great difficulty in inspiration and still greater difficulty in expiration. The prompt relief by atropine and epinephrin supports this view of bronchial spasm. With it there is in both forms marked swelling with increased secretion from the mucous membrane. The subjects of hay fever and of asthma are sensitized to various "asthmogenic" agents, usually proteins, which may be inhaled, injected, or autogenous, the result of bacterial or other activity. The effect of pollen on the mucous membrane is direct by irritation and indirect by absorption of the protein. Sensitive individuals give skin reactions to the agents causing the asthma. In children sensitive to eggs, even the rubbing of egg albumen on the thoroughly cleansed skin may cause an urticaria (Talbot). Longcope and Rackemann demonstrated the presence of antibodies after artificial sensitization.

Walker's study of 400 cases of asthma gives the following results:—191 patients were sensitive to some protein by skin tests, animal hair protein in 78, food proteins in 68, pollen protein in 92, and bacterial proteins in 33. Many of the patients were sensitive to more than one protein (multiple sensitization). The same patient may be sensitive to plant, animal and bacterial proteins. Practically the majority of patients with bronchial asthma are sensitive to pollens, horse dandruff, staphylococci, cat hair and a few common foods as wheat, eggs and meat. In the nonsensitive group the disease appears later, after the fortieth year, and many of them have chronic bronchitis and cardiorenal changes. "As the age of onset increases the frequency of sensitization decreases."

We may group the exciting agents into:—

1. INSPIRATORY.—Vegetable, the pollens of various grasses and flowers. *Animal,* the emanations from horses, cats, birds and other substance contained in dust.

2. INGESTED.—A host of vegetable and animal proteins, various grasses, wheat, oats; leguminous foods, peas, beans and lentils; fruits and nuts. Many animal substances, meat, milk and eggs, oysters, lobsters and crabs.

3. METABOLIC.—Abnormal products of primary digestion in stomach or bowels; faulty transmutation in the liver; lack of quantity or quality in the internal secretions; imperfect assimilation in the tissues is probably responsible for many of the obscure cases which do not react to the ordinary animal and vegetable products.

4. BACTERIAL.—The studies of Goodale and others have shown that many asthmatic and hay fever patients are sensitized to the staphylococcus and various organisms, reacting to one or another. The exciting cause may exist in the air passages themselves. It is difficult in any other way to explain severe asthma following whooping cough in a woman who never had attacks previously.

The causes under 3 and 4 demand careful study, as in Walker's list 45 per cent. of 150 patients did not react to the ordinary animal and vegetable proteins.

The disease may "run" in families. Transmission of hypersensitiveness to certain substances has long been recognized, and the females of animals sensitized to a foreign protein, such as horse serum, transmit the susceptibility to this protein to their offspring. An extraordinary variety of circumstances may induce the paroxysms, among which local conditions of atmosphere are most important. A person may be free in the city and invariably suffer from an attack in the country or in one place. In many of these cases the individual becomes exposed to the special agent to which he is sensitized. Sleeping on a horsehair mattress or on a feather pillow may cause attacks in persons susceptible to these substances. There are children naturally sensitized to extraordinarily minute quantities of egg or meat.

The subjects of asthma, particularly of horse asthma, are liable to serious attacks of serum sickness after the administration of antitoxin. The symptoms are identical with anaphylactic shock in animals. The site of the injection becomes red and swollen, there is irritation of the skin, often with urticaria, sudden dyspnœa, cyanosis, great cardiac weakness, and death may follow within a few minutes. Of 28 cases collected by Gillette (quoted by Lord) death followed in fifteen. Inquiry should always be made as to previous asthma before giving either prophylactic or curative doses of antitoxin.

Asthma as a Reflex Neurosis.—Prior to the recent studies the disease was regarded as following irritation in various localities, nose, stomach and bowels, etc., and the subjects were regarded as neurotic. Emotional disturbances as fright, apprehension, the smelling of an artificial rose in a person the subject of "rose" cold, may cause attacks, and it is difficult to bring such cases into the anaphylactic category. The prompt and permanent relief which sometimes follows removal of irritation, e. g. a polypus of the nose, supports the view that this factor may prevail in the group of asthmatics not sensitive to animal or vegetable proteins. There is a morbid sensitiveness of the nasal mucous membrane in many patients with hay fever.

Pathology.—We have no knowledge of the *morbid anatomy* of true asthma. In long-standing cases the lesions are those of chronic bronchitis and emphysema.

Symptoms.—Bostock's account of his attacks of *hay fever* (1819) may be abstracted. "A sensation of heat and fulness is experienced in the eyes with redness and a discharge of tears. There is much smarting and itching, the eyes become inflamed and discharge copiously. This state of the eyes recurs in paroxysms in June and July. There follow fulness in the head, particularly the fore part, irritation of the nose causing sneezing which may occur in fits of extreme violence. There is tightness in the chest, with difficulty in breathing and a feeling of want of air. The voice may be husky and to these symptoms may be added languor, loss of appetite, incapacity for exertion, restless nights often with profuse perspiration." In his second paper (1828) Bostock recognized that the eyes, the nose, the fauces and the lungs may be involved in varying degrees.

The *asthma* fit is thus described by Floyer (1698). "At first waking about one or two o'clock in the night the fit begins, the breath is very slow, but after a little time more strait, the diaphragm seems stiff and tied and is with difficulty moved downwards, but for enlarging the breast in inspiration the intercostal muscles, which serve for the raising of the ribs and the scapular muscles all join their force, and strain themselves for the enlarging of the cavity of the breast. He has to rise out of his bed and sit erect that the weight of the viscera may pull down the diaphragm. The muscles which serve for expiration cannot easily perform the contraction of the thorax, being hindered by the stiffness and inflation of the membranes. The expiration is slow, leisurely and wheezing, and the muscular fibres of the bronchi and the vesiculæ of the lungs are contracted, and that produces the wheezing noise which is best heard in expiration." There is not much to add to this description.

The attack may last from a few minutes to several hours. When severe there are signs of defective aëration, cyanosis, with sweating, feeble pulse and cold extremities. Coughing is difficult, very tight and dry at first, and then more violent, with the expectoration of the distinctive sputum.

Physical Signs.—The chest looks full and fixed, and in spite of the active muscular efforts there is very little expansion. The breathing is costal, the diaphragm is low and the movement much restricted. Inspiration is short, expiration much prolonged, labored and accompanied by wheezing râles. Percussion may be hyperresonant—Biermer's "box tone"—the cardiac flatness is obliterated, and the liver dulness low. On auscultation inspiration is feeble, expiration prolonged and in both the normal characters are obscured by sibilant and sonorous râles. Towards the end the râles become moister. It is remarkable with what rapidity they may disappear. The sputum is distinctive. Early in the attack it is brought up with difficulty and consists of small round masses, gelatinous, like sago balls in a thin mucus, the so-called "perles" of Laennec. Spread on glass with a black background, they can be unfolded and are seen to be moulds of the smaller tubes, many of which have a twisted appearance. A smaller number show the spirals described by Curschmann, of which there are two forms, one a simple loose twist in which are entangled leucocytes and larger cells with coarse granulations—eosinophiles. The other, a form of spiral probably never met with except in true asthma, is a tightly coiled skein of mucus in which cells are entangled and through the centre of which runs a thread of clear translucent mucin. Curschmann's spirals are found in nearly all cases when looked for early and in the right way. In addition to the spirals and the eosinophiles, a third element is often present, the Charcot-Leyden crystals, hexagonal, elongated pointed structures. They are found more often when the sputum changes to muco-purulent or if it is let stand for twenty-four hours. The remarkable character of the sputum in bronchial asthma points to a process which differs from the ordinary forms of bronchitis. The small size of many of the casts indicates involvement of the smaller tubes and Curschmann suggested the name *bronchiolitis exudativa.* There is no satisfactory explanation of the spiral form, or the central thread, unless it be that the former is due to a rotary action of the ciliated epithelium, and the latter to a compression of mucous filaments by the spasm of the bronchial muscles in the smaller tubes.

The eosinophiles in the blood are much increased, up to 53 per cent. in one of our cases, and the increase may persist in moderate grade in the intervals between attacks.

The *course* is variable. Hay fever usually recurs year by year, in spring or autumn, varying with the pollen to which the individual is sensitive. Forms of asthma depending on protein intoxication are more variable. A child may recover completely after years of severe attacks. The milder forms may persist through long life, and be, as Oliver Wendell Holmes said of his asthma, "the slight ailment that promotes longevity." In long standing cases emphysema and chronic bronchitis complicate the disease, and later is added hypertrophy of the heart. Even with these complications, in a suitable climate or with great care, the patients may survive well into the seventh decade.

Diagnosis.—There is not any difficulty in recognizing hay fever but it is necessary to determine the particular pollen which is responsible if specific treatment is to be given. This is done by trying the skin reaction with extracts of various pollens. A positive result is shown by a local reaction. The picture of asthma is distinctive but to determine the particular protein (if any) responsible requires careful tests.

Treatment.—For *hay fever* change of locality during the pollen season may give freedom. Local treatment of the nose, if required, sometimes gives relief. The use of a cocaine spray is helpful, but is a dangerous remedy. Epinephrin (1-1000 solution) may be applied. Remedies which sometimes are of benefit are sodium bicarbonate internally in full dosage and locally as a spray, and calcium lactate which should be taken for a considerable period in doses of gr. xv (1 gm.) three times a day. Active immunization by pollen extracts is sometimes effective as a prophylactic. The particular pollen to which the patient is sensitive having been determined, an alcoholic solution of it is used, the first dose having a dilution insufficient to produce a skin reaction. The strength of the injections is increased very gradually; they are repeated every four or five days until ten to twenty have been given. This should be done if possible before the usual time for the attacks. It is wise to repeat the treatment at least for two successive years. The prevention of recurrence offers many difficulties, and each case should be studied in the light of recent investigations. Change of climate relieves many hay fever patients and, when the offending protein is found, immunization is practicable though unfortunately the duration is short. In the non-sensitive forms a study of the bronchial flora may show some dominant organism from which a vaccine may be prepared.

Careful study of each case of *asthma* by modern methods is an essential preliminary. The tests are not very difficult, but the intelligent coöperation of the patient or of the parents of a child is essential. The reactions should first be studied. The nonsensitive group comprise as a rule older patients in whom the disease has come on late and who are subject to bronchitis or show cardio-renal changes. The treatment of these conditions may give relief and it is in these patients that the iodide of potassium is helpful. To be of any service it should be used freely, increasing the dose until symptoms are caused. Vaccines may be prepared from the dominant organism in the sputum. The teeth and tonsils should be eliminated as factors of infection, and the condition of the intestines and bowels carefully studied. Nasal and sinus disease should be excluded and it is in the elderly patients that one sees striking relief from cauterization or from the removal of polypi.

In the *sensitive* groups—ingestion, inhalation, and bacterial—separation from the exciting factor is important; this may be in occupation, environment, contact with animals or in diet. Desensitization for the responsible food protein occurs if it is totally abstained from for a long period. The best results are obtained from dieting in this group. Walker could not increase the tolerance for the wheat proteins by subcutaneous injections, and, as in the case of eggs and meat and milk, it is better to cut out the articles from the diet. Special care has to be taken in the case of eggs as very minute quantities of the protein may cause attacks. Such articles as cakes, custards and puddings containing eggs must be excluded. The proteins of the cereals, wheat, barley, rice, rye, oat, buckwheat, may be the cause, and, as Goodale points out, the hay fever patient sensitive to the pollen of the grasses will react also to the proteins of wheat or rye. Protection may be obtained by giving small doses of the protein over long periods.

The horse asthmatics may be treated by beginning with the injection of a dilution of the hair protein of 1:100,000 and this must be slowly and gradually increased. Injections of horse serum is of little or no value in the treatment of horse asthma (Walker). Treatment with horse hair protein does not desensitize against cat hair protein. The prophylactic treatment is not without risks as in the case of an asthmatic of fifteen years' standing who received an injection on successive days of 0.01 and 0.02 mg. of an extract of horse hair, on the fourth day she had another of 0.03 mg. Within two minutes she complained of feeling hot, in three minutes the face was flushed, the eyes and nose "running" and the skin prickling. In five minutes asthma began with a choking sensation in the throat. Twelve minims of a 1:1000 epinephrin solution was injected which relieved the attack. Urticaria appeared and the attack was over in an hour and a half. In another patient a severe attack of serum disease followed a desensitizing dose of horse hair extract. In the bacterial cases the best results have been obtained by the use of vaccines of *Staphylococcus pyogenes aureus, Streptococcus hæmolyticus,* and diphtheroid organisms, when these have been the predominating organisms in the sputum.

Nose and throat operations appear to be of very little value in the sensitive group. The liability to colds and bronchitis disappears with the successful treatment with proteins, but when of the bacterial, not the anaphylactic, type vaccines may be more helpful.

Treatment of the Attack.—Hypodermics of epinephrin (♏ xv, 1 c. c., of a 1-1000 solution) or of atropine (gr. 1/100, 0.00065 gm.) may give prompt relief, but individual cases vary greatly. Smaller doses of epinephrin are sometimes efficient. Some patients are helped by injections of epinephrin given once a week over a long period. Caution should be exerted in patients with sclerosis or high blood pressure. Morphia (gr. 1/6-1/4, 0.01-0.016 gm.) hypodermically is one of the best remedies. The inhalation of amyl nitrite may give prompt relief or a whiff of chloroform may relieve the spasm. Pilocarpin (gr. 1/8, 0.008 gm.) hypodermically may be tried.

Usually a chronic asthmatic has some favorite substance to inhale or to smoke. Most of the cigarettes used for the purpose contain leaves of the Solanaceæ, to which nitrate of potash is added. Stramonium leaves and potassium nitrate burnt together on a plate may be used. A majority of patients use the patent cures, the virtues of which are largely, in many entirely, due to the solanaceous leaves or potassium nitrate, in a few to iodide or opium. Ordinary tobacco cigarettes are sometimes helpful.

V. FIBRINOUS BRONCHITIS

(*Plastic or Croupous Bronchitis*)

Definition.—An acute or chronic affection, characterized by the formation in certain of the bronchial tubes of fibrinous casts, which are expelled in paroxysms of dyspnœa and cough.

Fibrinous moulds of the bronchi are formed in diphtheria (with extension into the trachea and bronchi) in pneumonia, and occasionally in pulmonary tuberculosis, conditions which, however, have nothing to do with true fibrinous bronchitis. As to tuberculosis Landis states that no instance has occurred during thirteen years at the Phipps Institute, nor was it found in any of the 662 autopsies on tuberculous subjects. Fibrinous casts are expectorated in connection with chronic heart-disease and in the albuminous expectoration following tapping of a pleural exudate. In hæmoptysis blood-casts may be expectorated, and they are not to be confounded with the casts of true fibrinous bronchitis which may be coughed up with profuse hæmorrhage. In pneumonia small fibrinous plugs are not uncommon in the sputum, and in a few rare instances quite large moulds of the tubes may be coughed up. The mycelium of *Aspergillus fumigatus* may form membranous casts in the bronchi.

Pathology.—This is obscure. The membrane is identical with that to which the term croupous is applied, and the obscurity relates not so much to the mechanism of the production, which is probably the same as in other mucous surfaces, as to the curious limitation of the affection to certain bronchial territories and in the chronic form to the remarkable recurrence at stated or irregular intervals throughout a period of many years. In the fatal cases the bronchial mucous membrane may be found injected or pale. In Biermer's case the epithelial lining was intact beneath the cast, but in that of Kretschy the bronchi were denuded of their epithelium. Emphysema is almost invariably present. Evidences of recent or antecedent pleurisy are sometimes found.

Clinical Description.—Bettman (1901) analyzed the cases from the literature since 1869, grouping them into different classes. The most important is *chronic idiopathic fibrinous bronchitis.* It is a rare affection and most common at the middle period of life. Of 27 cases, 15 were in males. The attacks may occur at definite intervals for months or years. The form and size of the casts may be identical at each attack as though each time precisely the same bronchial area was involved. The expectoration of the casts is associated with paroxysms of dyspnœa and coughing, which occur at longer or shorter intervals. Fever and hæmoptysis may be present during the attack. Physical signs usually indicate the portion of the lung affected, as there are suppressed breath sounds and numerous râles on coughing. A very dry râle, called the *"bruit de drapeau,"* has been described, caused by the vibration of a loosened portion of the cast.

In five cases there were skin lesions. Tuberculosis is rarely present. The casts are usually rolled up and mixed with mucus and blood. When unrolled they are large white branching structures. The main stem may be as thick as the little finger. From the consistency and appearance they have been described as fibrinous, but they consist mainly of mucin. On cross-section they show a concentrically stratified structure, with leucocytes and alveolar epithelium. Leyden's crystals and Curschmann's spirals are sometimes found, and in Bettman's case there were protozoan-like bodies. Death occurred in only one case of the series.

The *acute form,* of which Bettman collected 15 cases, comes on most frequently during some fever, as typhoid, pneumonia, or the eruptive fevers. After a preliminary bronchitis the dyspnœa increases, and then the casts are coughed up. Chills and fever have been present. Four of the 15 cases proved fatal, and the casts were found *in situ.* It is much more serious than the chronic form into which it may pass. Night after night distressing attacks of coughing may occur, with dyspnœa and cyanosis, only relieved by the expectoration of large quantities of sputum with casts of all sizes, sometimes very small ones which "tail off" into true spirals. In a case of this type there were attacks of fever with toxæmia and delirium. The casts may have an arborescent structure or come from a single tube or its bifurcation.

Treatment.—In the acute cases the treatment should be that of ordinary acute bronchitis. We know of nothing which can prevent the recurrence of the attacks in the chronic form. In the uncomplicated cases there is rarely any danger during the paroxysm, even though the symptoms may be most distressing and the dyspnœa and cough very severe. Inhalations of ether, steam, or atomized lime-water aid in the separation of the membranes. Intratracheal injections of olive oil with iodoform may be tried. Pilocarpine might be useful, as in some instances it increases the bronchial secretion. The employment of emetics may be necessary, and in some cases they are effective in promoting the removal of the casts.

VI. FOREIGN BODIES IN THE BRONCHI

Largely as a result of the splendid work of Chevalier Jackson of Philadelphia, we have learned that foreign bodies in the bronchi are not infrequent. A great variety of objects may gain entrance to the trachea, the majority of which (75 per cent.) pass into the right bronchus. There is not necessarily any occurrence of severe symptoms with this and the history may be quite negative. No age is exempt but the accident is particularly apt to occur in children.

Symptoms.—These are very varied, depending principally on the character of foreign body. A very acute general process may result which ends fatally in a few days, as seen after the inhalation of a peanut, or there may be an acute process which gradually subsides into a chronic condition. Cough is common and resulting conditions such as abscess or bronchiectasis give their usual symptoms.

Physical Signs.—These are very varied and no set picture can be described. The most acute signs result from the inhalation of a nut, the peanut being most common in the United States. To this the name *Arachidic Bronchitis* has been given. The condition is an œdematous, purulent tracheo-bronchitis which often results in lung abscess. The cases are in children; the symptoms come on rapidly with high irregular fever, severe toxæmia and the signs of an intense general bronchitis, with a great variety of râles mostly coarse and bubbling. The "asthmatoid wheeze" is often present. The dyspnœa is extreme, cyanosis is marked and there is tenacious purulent sputum. If a bronchus is plugged there is dulness with absence of breath and voice sounds. The lung supplied by the plugged bronchus contains much secretion and is described as "drowned" lung.

The signs in the more chronic cases vary greatly depending on the character of the substance, the reaction set up, whether the bronchus is plugged and the changes in the supplied lung. In all cases there may be auscultation signs on the unaffected side due to extension of inflammation. Decreased expansion is the rule on the affected side. Two special signs are important. One is the occurrence of very fine râles over a small area in the case of metallic bodies which do not plug the bronchus and the other the *"asthmatoid wheeze"* described by Jackson. This is a wheezing sound heard with the ear or stethoscope close to the patient's mouth. It varies in pitch and loudness and may be with in- and expiration.

Diagnosis.—The acute features may lead to the diagnosis of pneumonia which a careful examination should prevent. In the chronic cases tuberculosis is often diagnosed but the frequency of the lesions in the lower lobes should prevent this. The X-rays are of great aid in many cases but not all foreign bodies show in the plates. The thought of the possibility of foreign body is the surest aid against error.

Treatment.—This is removal by *bronchoscopy* done by skilled hands. No one should attempt it without special training.

D. DISEASES OF THE LUNGS

I. CIRCULATORY DISTURBANCES IN THE LUNGS

Congestion.—There are two forms—active and passive.

1. ACTIVE CONGESTION.—About this much doubt and confusion still exist. French writers regard it as an independent primary affection (*maladie de Woillez*), and allot much space to it. English and American authors more correctly regard it as a symptomatic affection. Active fluxion to the lungs occurs with increased action of the heart, and when very hot air or irritating substances are inhaled. In diseases which interfere locally with the circulation the capillaries in the adjacent unaffected portions may be greatly distended. The importance of this collateral fluxion, as it is called, is probably exaggerated. In a whole series of pulmonary affections there is this associated congestion—in pneumonia, bronchitis, pleurisy, and tuberculosis.

The symptoms of active congestion of the lungs as given by French writers are of an affection difficult to distinguish from anomalous or larval forms of pneumonia. The chief features are initial chill, pain in the side, dyspnœa, moderate cough, and temperature from 101° to 103° F. The physical signs are defective resonance, feeble breathing, sometimes bronchial in character, and fine râles. A majority of physicians would undoubtedly class such cases under pneumonia. In many epidemics the abnormal and larval forms are specially prevalent.

The occurrence of an intense and rapidly fatal congestion of the lung, following extreme heat or cold or sometimes violent exertion, is recognized by some authors. Renforth, the oarsman, is said to have died from this cause during a race near St. John, N. B. Leuf has described cases in which, in association with drunkenness, exposure, and cold, death occurred suddenly, or within twenty-four hours, the only lesion found being an extreme, almost hæmorrhagic, congestion of the lungs. It is by no means certain that in these cases death really occurs from pulmonary congestion in the absence of specific statements with reference to the coronary arteries and the heart.

2. PASSIVE CONGESTION.—Two forms of this may be recognized, the mechanical and the hypostatic.

(*a*) *Mechanical congestion* occurs whenever there is an obstacle to the return of the blood to the heart. It is a common event in many affections of the left heart, particularly mitral stenosis. The lungs are voluminous, russet brown in color, cutting and tearing with great resistance. On section they show at first a brownish red tinge, and then the cut surface, exposed to the air, becomes rapidly of a vivid red color from oxidation of the abundant hæmoglobin. This is the condition known as *brown induration* of the lung. Occasionally this mechanical hyperæmia of the lung follows pressure by tumors. So long as compensation is maintained the mechanical congestion of the lung in heart disease does not produce any symptoms, but with enfeebled heart action the engorgement becomes marked and there are dyspnœa, cough, and expectoration with the characteristic alveolar cells.

(*b*) *Hypostatic Congestion.*—In fevers and adynamic states generally it is very common to find the bases of the lungs deeply congested, a condition induced partly by the effect of gravity, the patient lying recumbent in one posture for a long time, but chiefly by weakened heart action. That it is not an effect of gravity alone is shown by the fact that a healthy person may remain in bed an indefinite time without its occurrence. The posterior parts of the lung are dark in color and engorged with blood and serum; in some instances to such a degree that the alveoli no longer contain air and portions of the lung sink in water. The terms *splenization* and hypostatic pneumonia have been given to these advanced grades. It is a common affection in protracted cases of typhoid fever and in long debilitating illness. In ascites, meteorism, and abdominal tumors the bases of the lungs may be compressed and congested. In this connection must be mentioned the form of passive congestion met with in injury to, and organic disease of, the brain. In cerebral apoplexy the bases of the lungs are deeply engorged, not quite airless, but heavy, and on section drip with blood and serum. This condition may occur in an extreme grade throughout the lungs in death from morphia poisoning. In some instances the lung tissue has a blackish, gelatinous, infiltrated appearance, almost like diffuse pulmonary apoplexy. Occasionally this congestion is most marked in, and even confined to, the hemiplegic side. In prolonged coma the hypostatic congestion may be associated with patches of consolidation, due to the aspiration of portions of food into the air-passages.

The symptoms of hypostatic congestion are not at all characteristic. There are shortness of breath and cough with abundant sputum containing alveolar epithelium filled with yellow and black pigment—the so-called "heart-failure cells." On examination slight dulness, feeble, sometimes blowing, breathing and liquid râles can be detected.

Treatment.—The treatment is usually that of the condition with which the congestion is associated. In the intense pulmonary engorgement, which may possibly occur primarily, and which is met with in heart disease and emphysema, free bleeding should be practised. From 20 to 30 ounces of blood should be taken and if the blood does not flow freely and the condition is desperate aspiration of the right auricle may be performed.

Œdema.—In all forms of intense congestion of the lungs there is a transudation of serum from the engorged capillaries chiefly into the air-cells, but also into the alveolar walls. Not only is it very frequent in congestion, but also with inflammation, with new growths, infarcts, and tubercles. When limited to the neighborhood of an affected part, the name collateral œdema is sometimes applied to it.

Acute œdema is met with: (1) in the infections; (2) in nephritis; (3) in heart disease, particularly angina pectoris, myocarditis, and valve lesions; (4) in arterio-sclerosis with high tension; (5) pregnancy; (6) angio-neurotic œdema; (7) as a complication of the epileptic fit, and (8) after thoracentesis. The theory most generally accepted is that of W. H. Welch, whose experiments indicate that pulmonary œdema is due to a disproportionate weakness of the left ventricle, so that the blood accumulates in the lung capillaries until transudation occurs. Cardiac failure is the most important cause. Others regard it is an effect of disturbance in the vasomotor mechanism of the lungs with increased permeability of the capillaries. In some cases there are recurring attacks of acute œdema without obvious cause.

Anatomically the lung is anæmic, heavy, sodden, pits on pressure, and on section a large quantity of clear or blood-tinged serum flows out. It may have in places a gelatinous aspect.

Symptoms.—The onset is sudden with a feeling of oppression and pain in the chest and rapid breathing which soon becomes dyspnœic or orthopnœic. There may be an incessant short cough and a copious frothy, sometimes blood-tinged, expectoration, which may be expelled in a gush from the mouth and nose. The face is pale and covered with a cold sweat; the pulse is feeble and the heart's action weak. Over the entire chest may be heard piping and bubbling râles. The attack may be fatal in a few hours or may persist for twelve or twenty-four hours and then pass off. Steven, of Glasgow, reported a case with 72 attacks in two and a half years. This recurrent form may be associated with angina pectoris.

Treatment.—Venesection should be done at once and is often most helpful. Morphia (gr. 1/4, 0.016 gm.) with atropine (gr. 1/100, 0.0006 gm.) should be given hypodermically and the atropine repeated in fifteen minutes if there is no change. Aromatic spirit of ammonia (ʒ i, 4 c. c.) may be given by mouth. One of the digitalis preparations should be given intramuscularly and repeated every three hours if indicated. If hypertension is present nitroglycerine (gr. 1/100, 0.0006 gm.) is to be given under the tongue and repeated until an effect is produced. Inhalation of chloroform, artificial respiration, dry cupping and the use of oxygen may be helpful. Patients who have repeated attacks should be warned against over-exertion and with the first symptoms of an attack should be given ammonia, and morphia and atropine hypodermically.

Pulmonary Hæmorrhage.—This occurs in two forms—*broncho-pulmonary hæmorrhage,* sometimes called bronchorrhagia, in which the blood is poured into the bronchi and expectorated, and *pulmonary apoplexy* or pneumorrhagia, in which the hæmorrhage takes place into the air-cells and lung tissue.

1. Broncho-pulmonary Hæmorrhage; Hæmoptysis.—Spitting of blood, to which the term hæmoptysis should be restricted, results from a variety of conditions, among which the following are the most important: (*a*) In young healthy persons hæmoptysis may occur without warning, and after continuing for a few days disappear and leave no ill traces. There may be at the time of the attack no physical signs indicating pulmonary disease. In such cases good health may be preserved for years and no further trouble occur. These cases are not very uncommon, but in spite of the good health tuberculosis should be suspected. In Ware's important contribution, of 386 cases of hæmoptysis noted in private practice 62 recovered and pulmonary disease did not subsequently develop. (*b*) *Hæmoptysis in pulmonary tuberculosis,* which is considered on page 194. (*c*) In connection with certain diseases of the lung, as pneumonia (in the initial stage) and cancer, occasionally in gangrene, abscess, and bronchiectasis. (*d*) In many heart affections, particularly mitral lesions. It may be profuse and recur at intervals for years. (*e*) *In ulcerative affections of the larynx, trachea, or bronchi.* Sometimes the hæmorrhage is profuse and rapidly fatal, as when the ulcer erodes a large branch of the pulmonary artery. (*f*) *Aneurism.* It may be sudden and rapidly fatal when the sac bursts into

the air-passages. Slight bleeding may continue for weeks or months, due to pressure on the mucous membrane or erosion of the lung; or in some cases the sac "weeps" through the exposed laminæ of fibrin. (*g*) *Vicarious hæmorrhage,* which occurs in rare instances in cases of interrupted menstruation. The instances are well authenticated. Flint mentions a case which he had had under observation for four years, and Hippocrates refers to it in the aphorism. "Hæmoptysis in a woman is removed by an eruption of the menses." Periodical hæmoptysis has been met with after the removal of both ovaries. Fatal hæmorrhage has occurred from the lung during menstruation when no lesion was found to account for it. (*h*) *Permanent high arterial tension.* Hæmoptysis, sometimes profuse and lasting for days, may occur at intervals. In this group probably come the cases described by Sir Andrew Clark in arthritic subjects. (*i*) Hæmoptysis occurs sometimes *in malignant fevers* and *in purpura hæmorrhagica.* (*j*) With gun-shot injuries and foreign bodies in the lung. Lastly, there is endemic hæmoptysis, due to the bronchial fluke, an affection confined to parts of China and Japan.

Symptoms.—Hæmoptysis sets in, as a rule, suddenly. Often without warning the patient experiences a warm, saltish taste as the mouth fills with blood. Coughing is usually induced. There may be only an ounce or so brought up before the hæmorrhage stops, or the bleeding may continue for days, the patient bringing up small quantities. In other instances, particularly when a large vessel is eroded or an aneurism bursts, the amount is large, and the patient, after a few attempts at coughing, shows signs of suffocation and death is produced by inundation of the bronchial system. Fatal hæmorrhage may occur into a large cavity in a patient debilitated by tuberculosis without the production of hæmoptysis. The blood from the lungs generally has characters which render it readily destinguishable from vomited blood. It is alkaline in reaction, frothy, mixed with mucus, and air-bubbles are present in the clot. Blood-moulds of the smaller bronchi are sometimes seen. Patients can usually tell whether the blood has been brought up by coughing or by vomiting, and in a majority of cases the history gives important indications. In paroxysmal hæmoptysis connected with menstrual disturbances the practitioner should see that the blood is actually coughed up, since deception may be practised. The spurious hæmoptysis of hysteria is considered with that disease. Naturally, the patient is alarmed at the occurrence of bleeding, but, unless very profuse, as when due to rupture of an aneurism in a pulmonary cavity, the danger is rarely immediate. The attacks, however, are apt to recur for a few days and the sputum may remain blood-tinged for a longer period. In the great majority of cases the hæmorrhage ceases spontaneously. Blood may be swallowed and produce vomiting, and, after a day or two, the stools may be dark in color. It is not advisable to examine the chest during an attack of hæmoptysis.

2. PULMONARY "APOPLEXY"; HÆMORRHAGIC INFARCT.—The blood is effused into the air-cells and interstitial tissue. It is usually diffuse, the parenchyma not being broken, as is the brain tissue in cerebral apoplexy. Sometimes, in disease of the brain, in septic conditions, and in the malignant forms of fevers, the lung tissue is uniformly infiltrated with blood and has, on section, a black, gelatinous appearance.

As a rule, the hæmorrhage is limited and results from the blocking of a branch of the pulmonary artery either by a thrombus or an embolus. The condition is most common in chronic heart-disease. Although the pulmonary arteries are terminal ones, blocking is not always followed by infarction; partly because the wide capillaries furnish sufficient anastomosis, and partly because the bronchial vessels may keep up the circulation. The infarctions are chiefly at the periphery of the lung, usually wedge-shaped, with the base of the wedge toward the surface. When recent, they are dark in color, hard and firm, and look on section like an ordinary blood-clot. Gradual changes go on, and the color becomes a reddish brown. The pleura over an infarct is usually inflamed. A microscopic section shows the air-cells to be distended with red blood corpuscles, which may also be in the alveolar walls. The infarcts are usually multiple and vary in size from a walnut to an orange. Very large ones may involve the greater part of a lobe. In the artery passing to the affected territory a thrombus or an embolus is found. The globular thrombi, formed in the right auricular appendix, play an important part in the production of hæmorrhagic infarction. In many cases the source of the embolus can not be discovered, and the infarct may have resulted from thrombosis in the pulmonary artery, but it is not infrequent to find total obstruction of a large branch of a pulmonary artery without hæmorrhage into the corresponding lung area. The further history of an infarction is variable. It is possible that in some instances the circulation is re-established and the blood removed. More commonly, if the patient lives, the usual changes go on in the extravasated blood and ultimately a pigmented, puckered, fibroid patch results. Sloughing may occur with the formation of a cavity. Occasionally gangrene results. A gangrenous infarct may rupture and produce fatal pneumothorax.

The *symptoms* of pulmonary infarction are by no means definite. The condition may be suspected in chronic heart-disease when hæmoptysis occurs, particularly in mitral stenosis, but the bleeding may be due to the extreme engorgement. When the infarcts are very large, and particularly in the lower lobe, in which they most commonly occur, there may be signs of consolidation with blowing breathing and a pleuritic friction.

Treatment of Pulmonary Hæmorrhage.—The pressure within the pulmonary artery is considerably less than that in the aortic system. The system is under vaso-motor control, but our knowledge of the mutual relations of pressure in the aorta and in the pulmonary artery, under varying conditions, is imperfect (Bradford). There may be an influence on the systemic blood-pressure without any on the pulmonary, and the pressure in the one may rise while it falls in the other, or it may rise and fall in both together. The researches of Brodie and Dixon indicate that drugs which raise the peripheral blood pressure by vaso-constriction increase the total blood in the lung. Thus ergot, a remedy commonly used, causes a distinct rise in the pulmonary blood-pressure, while aconite produces a definite fall.

The question is beset with difficulties, and experimental work is by no means in accord. Wiggers concludes that in the early stages of hæmoptysis, when the breathing is not altered, lowering of the blood pressure within the pulmonary circuit can not be accomplished by the nitrites, but only by the cardiac depressants, and in the later stages of an attack, when the heart is very rapid, pituitary extract is the only drug that raises systemic pressure while simultaneously lowering that in the pulmonary circuit.

The anatomical condition in hæmoptysis is either hyperæmia of the bronchial mucosa (or of the lung tissue) or a perforated vessel. In the latter case the patient often passes rapidly beyond treatment, though there are instances of the most profuse hæmorrhage, which must have come from a perforated artery or a ruptured aneurism, in which recovery has occurred. Practically, for treatment, we should separate these cases, as the remedies which would be applicable in the case of congested and bleeding mucosa would be as much out of place in a case of hæmorrhage from ruptured aneurism as in a cut radial artery. When the blood is brought up in large quantities, it is almost certain either that an aneurism has ruptured or a vessel has been eroded. In the instances in which the sputum is blood tinged or when the blood is in smaller quantities, bleeding comes by diapedesis from hyperæmic vessels. In such cases the hæmorrhage may be beneficial in relieving congestion.

The indications are to reduce the frequency of the heart-beats and to lower the blood-pressure. The truth, *Das Blut ist ein ganz besonderer Saft,* is strikingly emphasized by the frightened state of the patient. Rest of the body and peace of the mind—*"quies, securitas, silentium"* of Celsus—should be secured. If there is marked restlessness, morphia hypodermically (gr. 1/6, 0.011 gm.) is advisable. Turn the patient on the affected side, if known, as regurgitation is less apt to occur into the bronchi of the sound lung. As Aretæus remarks, in hæmoptysis the patient despairs from the first, and needs to be strongly reassured. Death is rarely due directly to hæmoptysis; patients die after, not of it (S. West). In the majority of cases of mild hæmoptysis this is sufficient. Even when the patient insists upon going about, the bleeding may stop spontaneously. The diet should be light and unstimulating. Alcohol should not be used. The patient may, if he wishes, have ice to suck. Small doses of aromatic sulphuric acid may be given, but unless the bleeding is protracted styptic and astringent medicines are not indicated. For cough, which is always present and disturbing, opium should be freely given, and is of all medicines most serviceable in hæmoptysis. Digitalis should not be used, as it raises the blood-pressure in the pulmonary artery. Aconite may be used when there is much vascular excitement. Ergot, tannic acid, and lead have little or no influence in hæmoptysis; ergot probably does harm. One of the most satisfactory means of lowering the blood-pressure is purgation, and when the bleeding is protracted salts may be freely given. In profuse hæmoptysis, as from erosion of an artery or rupture of an aneurism, a fatal result is common, and yet post mortem evidence shows that thrombosis may occur with healing in a rupture of considerable size. The fainting induced by the loss of blood is probably the most efficient means of promoting thrombosis, and it was on this principle that formerly patients were bled from the arm, or from both arms, as in the case of Laurence Sterne. Ligatures, or Esmarch's bandages, placed around the legs may serve temporarily to check the bleeding. The ice-bag is of doubtful utility. In protracted cases pneumothorax has been induced, sometimes with success.

Briefly, then, we may say that hæmorrhage from rupture of aneurism or erosion of a blood-vessel usually proves fatal. The fainting induced by the loss of blood is beneficial, and, if the patient can be kept alive for twenty-four hours, a thrombus of sufficient strength to prevent further bleeding may form. The chief danger is the inundation of the bronchial system with the blood, so that while the hæmorrhage is profuse the cough should be encouraged. Opium should not then be used, and stimulants should be given with caution.

In the other group, in which the hæmorrhage comes from a congested area and is limited, the patient gets well if kept absolutely quiet, and fatal hæmorrhage probably never occurs from this source. Rest, reduction of the blood-pressure by minimum diet, purging, if necessary, and the administration of some preparation of opium to allay the cough are the main indications.

II. CHRONIC INTERSTITIAL PNEUMONIA

A fibroid change may have its starting point in the tissue about the bronchi and blood-vessels, the interlobular septa, the alveolar walls, or in the pleura. So diverse are the forms and so varied the conditions under which this change occurs that a proper classification is difficult. We may recognize two chief forms—the *local,* involving only a limited area of the lung substance, and the *diffuse,* invading either both lungs or an entire organ.

Etiology.—(*a*) LOCAL fibroid change in the lungs is common. It is a constant accompaniment of tubercle, in the evolution of which interstitial changes play a very important rôle. In tumors, abscess, gummata, hydatids, and emphysema it also occurs. Fibroid processes are frequently met with at the apices of the lung and may be due either to a limited healed tuberculosis, to fibroid induration in consequence of pigment, or, in a few instances, may result from thickening of the pleura.

(*b*) DIFFUSE INTERSTITIAL PNEUMONIA is met with: (1) As a sequence of *acute fibrinous pneumonia.* Although extremely rare, this is recognized as a possible termination. From unknown causes resolution fails to take place. Organization goes on in the fibrinous plugs within the air-cells and the alveolar walls become greatly thickened by a new growth, first of nuclear and subsequently of fibrillated connective tissue. Macroscopically there is produced a smooth, grayish, homogeneous tissue which has the peculiar translucency of all new-formed connective tissue. This has been called gray induration. A majority of the cases terminate within a few months, but instances which have been followed from the outset are very rare.

(2) *Chronic Broncho-pneumonia.*—The relation of broncho-pneumonia to cirrhosis of the lung was specially studied by Charcot, who stated that it may follow the acute or subacute form of this disease, particularly in children. The fibrosis extends from the bronchi, which are usually dilated. Bronchiectasis may be followed by fibrosis of the lung. The alveolar walls are thickened and the lobules converted into firm grayish masses, in which there is no trace of normal lung tissue. This may go on and involve an entire lobe or even the whole lung. Many of these cases are tuberculous from the outset.

(3) *Pleurogenous Interstitial Pneumonia.*—Charcot applied this term to that form of cirrhosis of the lung which follows invasion from the pleura. Doubt has been expressed by some writers whether this really occurs. While Wilson Fox was probably correct in questioning whether an entire lung can become cirrhosed by the gradual invasion from the pleura, there can be no doubt that there are instances of primitive dry pleurisy, which, as Sir Andrew Clark pointed out, gradually compress the lung and lead to interstitial cirrho-

sis. This may be due in part to the fibroid change which follows prolonged compression. In some cases there seems to be a distinct connection between the greatly thickened pleura and the dense strands of fibrous tissue passing from it into the lung substance. Instances occur in which one lobe or the greater part of it presents, on section, a mottled appearance, owing to the increased thickness of the interlobar septa—a condition which may exist without a trace of involvement of the pleura. In many other cases, however, the extension seems to be so definitely associated with pleurisy that there is no doubt as to the causal connection between the two processes. In these instances the lung is removed with great difficulty, owing to the thickness and close adhesion of the pleura to the chest wall.

(4) *Chronic interstitial pneumonia,* due to inhalation of dust, which is considered in a separate section.

(5) *Syphilis* of the lung may present the features of a chronic fibrosis.

(6) Indurative changes in the lung may follow the compression by aneurism or new growth or the irritation of a foreign body in a bronchus.

Morbid Anatomy.—There are two chief forms, the massive or lobar and the insular or broncho-pneumonic form. In the massive type the disease is unilateral; the chest of the affected side is sunken, deformed, and the shoulder much depressed. On opening the thorax the heart is seen drawn far over to the affected side. The unaffected lung is emphysematous and covers the greater portion of the mediastinum. It is scarcely credible in how small a space, close to the spine, the cirrhosed lung may lie. The adhesions between the pleural membranes may be extremely dense and thick, particularly in the pleurogenous cases; but when the disease has originated in the lung there may be little thickening of the pleura. The organ is airless, firm, and hard. It strongly resists cutting, and on section shows a grayish fibroid tissue of variable amount, through which pass the blood-vessels and bronchi. The latter may be either slightly or enormously dilated. There are instances in which the entire lung is converted into a series of bronchiectatic cavities and the cirrhosis is apparent only in certain areas or at the root. The tuberculous cases can usually be differentiated by the presence of an apical cavity, not bronchiectatic, often large, and the other lung almost invariably shows tuberculous lesions. Aneurisms of the pulmonary artery are not infrequent in the cavities. The other lung is always enlarged and emphysematous. The heart is hypertrophied, particularly the right ventricle, and there may be marked atheromatous changes in the vessels. An amyloid condition of the viscera is found in some cases.

In the broncho-pneumonic form the areas are smaller, often centrally placed, and most frequently in the lower lobes. They are deeply pigmented, show dilated bronchi, and when multiple are separated by emphysematous lung tissue.

A *reticular form* of fibrosis of the lung has been described by Percy Kidd and W. McCollum, in which the lungs are intersected by grayish fibroid strands following the lines of the interlobular septa.

Symptoms and Course.—The disease is essentially chronic, extending over a period of many years, and when once the condition is established the health may be fairly good. In a well marked case the patient complains only of his chronic cough, perhaps a slight shortness of breath. In other respects he is quite well, and is usually able to do light work. The cases are commonly regarded as tuberculous, though there may be scarcely a symptom of that affection except the cough. There are instances, however, of fibroid tuberculosis which can not be distinguished from cirrhosis of the lung except by the presence of tubercle bacilli in the expectoration. As the bronchi are usually dilated, the symptoms and physical signs may be those of bronchiectasis. The cough is paroxysmal and the expectoration is generally copious and of a muco-purulent or sero-purulent nature. It is sometimes fetid. Hæmorrhage is by no means infrequent, and occurred in more than one-half of the cases analyzed by Bastian. Walking on the level and in the ordinary affairs of life, the patient may show no shortness of breath, but in the ascent of stairs and on exertion there may be dyspnœa.

Physical Signs.—*Inspection.*—The affected side of the chest is immobile, retracted, and shrunken, and contrasts in a striking way with the voluminous healthy one. The intercostal spaces are obliterated and the ribs may even overlap. The shoulder is drawn down and from behind it is seen that the spine is bowed. The muscles of the shoulder-girdle are wasted. The heart is greatly displaced, being drawn over by the shrinkage of the lung to the affected side. When the left lung is affected there may be a large area of visible impulse in the second, third, and fourth interspaces. Mensuration shows a great diminution in the affected side, and with the saddle-tape the expansion may be seen to be negative. The *percussion* note varies with the condition of the bronchi. It may be absolutely flat, particularly at the base or at the apex. In the axilla there may be a flat tympany or even an amphoric note over a large sacculated bronchus. On the opposite side the percussion note is usually hyperresonant. On auscultation the breath-sounds have either a cavernous or amphoric quality at the apex, and at the base are feeble, with mucous, bubbling râles. The voice-sounds are usually exaggerated. Cardiac murmurs are not uncommon, particularly late in the disease, when the right heart fails. These are, of course, the physical signs of the disease when it is well established. They naturally vary considerably, according to the stage of the process. The disease is essentially chronic, and may persist for fifteen or twenty years. Death occurs sometimes from hæmorrhage, more commonly from gradual failure of the right heart with dropsy, and occasionally from amyloid degeneration of the organs.

Diagnosis.—This is never difficult but it may be impossible to say, without a clear history, whether the origin is pleuritic or pneumonic. Between cases of this kind and fibroid tuberculosis it is not always easy to discriminate, as the conditions may be almost identical. When tuberculosis is present, however, even in long-standing cases, bacilli are present in the sputum, and there may be signs of disease in the other lung.

Treatment.—It is only for an intercurrent affection or for an aggravation of the cough that the patient seeks relief. Nothing can be done for the condition itself. When possible the patient should live in a mild climate, and avoid exposure to cold and damp. A distressing feature in some cases is the putrefaction of the contents of the dilated tubes, for which the same measures may be used as in fetid bronchitis.

III. PNEUMOCONIOSIS

Definition.—Under this term, introduced by Zenker, are embraced those forms of fibrosis of the lung due to the inhalation of dusts in various occupations. They have received various names, according to the nature of the inhaled particles—*anthracosis*, or coal-miner's disease, *siderosis, chalicosis* and *silicosis.*

Etiology.—The dust is inorganic or organic; the former is the more common and more dangerous. The following are the chief forms:—(1) *Anthracosis.* Dwellers in cities inhale coal dust and soot, and the lungs gradually become carbonized. Klotz has shown that the lungs of the inhabitants of Pittsburgh have an excessive amount of carbon, which leads to varying degrees of fibrosis. (2) *Silicosis,* from the dust of flint in small angular particles, occurs in the South African gold mines and the zinc mines in Missouri. (3) *Chalicosis,* from the dust of quarries and potteries, and occupations of grinding steel, etc. (4) *Siderosis,* from iron dust, in workers with red oxide of iron, and in brass and bronze. (5) Dust from crushed slag which may cause an acute inflammation of a lower lobe.

Organic dust is not nearly so serious, and it is doubtful if pneumoconiosis is ever produced by it alone. The workers in cotton and woolen mills have a high death rate from tuberculosis, but the dust is probably not a serious factor. In the grinding of rags, new workers may have attacks of catarrh and fever with shivering ("Shoddy fever," Oliver). The dust of grain in threshing may cause irritation of the bronchi, headache and sometimes fever. The dust particles inhaled into the lungs are dealt with by the ciliated epithelium and by the phagocytes. The ordinary mucous corpuscles take in a large number of the particles, which fall upon the trachea and main bronchi. The cilia sweep the mucus out to a point from which it can be expelled by coughing. It is mucosa, reaching the lymph spaces, where they are attacked at once by the cells (in which they are in numbers) probably pick them up on the way. The mucous and the alveolar cells are the normal respiratory scavengers. In dwellers in the country, where the air is pure, they are able to prevent the access of dust particles to the lung tissue, so that even in adults these organs present a rosy tint, very different from the dark, carbonized appearance of the lungs of dwellers in cities. When the impurities in the air are very abundant, a certain proportion of the dust particles escapes these cells and penetrates the mucosa, reaching the lymph spaces, where they are attacked at once by the cells of the connective-tissue stroma, which are capable of ingesting and retaining a large quantity. In coal-miners, coal-heavers, and others whose occupations necessitate the constant breathing of a very dusty atmosphere even these forces are insufficient. Pulmonary anthracosis may be induced by passing an emulsion of china ink into the stomach of an animal through a catheter so that anthracosis may be due to the intestinal absorption of carbon particles arrested in the nose and pharynx, and then swallowed. The experimental work shows that both the tracheal and intestinal routes are used—through the former the particles reach the bronchi and external portions of the alveoli, through the latter the parenchyma of the lung. Occasionally in anthracosis the carbon grains reach the general circulation, and the coal dust is found in the liver and spleen. This occurs when the densely pigmented bronchial glands closely adhere to the pulmonary veins, through the walls of which the carbon particles pass to the general circulation. The lung tissue has a remarkable tolerance for these particles; but by constant exposure a limit is reached, and a definite pathological condition, an interstitial sclerosis, results. In coal-miners this may occur in patches, even before the lung tissue is uniformly infiltrated. In others it appears only after the entire organs have become so laden that they are dark in color, and an ink-like juice flows from the cut surface. The lungs of a miner may be black throughout and yet show no local lesions and be everywhere crepitant.

Morbid Anatomy.—In anthracosis the particles of carbon are found deposited in large numbers in the follicular cords of the tracheal and bronchial glands and of the peri-bronchial and peri-arterial lymph nodules, and in these they finally excite proliferation of the connective tissue elements. It is by no means uncommon to find in persons whose lungs are only moderately carbonized the bronchial glands sclerosed and hard. In anthracosis the fibroid changes usually begin in the peri-bronchial lymph tissue, and in the early stage of the process the sclerosis may be largely confined to these regions. A Nova Scotian miner, aged thirty-six, died at the Montreal General Hospital, of black smallpox, after an illness of a few days. In his lungs (externally coal-black) there were round and linear patches ranging in size from a pea to a hazel-nut, of an intensely black color, airless and firm, and surrounded by a crepitant tissue, slate gray in color. In the centre of each of these areas was a small bronchus. Many were situated just beneath the pleura, and formed typical examples of limited fibroid broncho-pneumonia. In addition there is usually thickening of the alveolar walls, particularly in certain areas. By the gradual coalescence of these fibroid patches large portions of the lung may be converted into firm areas of cirrhosis, grayish black in the coal-miner, steel gray in the stone-worker. In the case of a Cornish miner, aged sixty-three, one of these fibroid areas measured 18 by 6 cm. and 4.5 cm. in depth.

A second important factor is *chronic bronchitis*, which is present in a large proportion and really causes the chief syptoms. A third is the occurrence of *emphysema,* which is almost invariably associated with long-standing cases of pneumoconiosis. With the changes so far described, unless the cirrhotic area is unusually extensive, the case may present the features of chronic bronchitis with emphysema, but finally another element comes into play. In the fibroid areas softening occurs, probably a process of necrosis similar to that by which softening is produced in fibro-myomata of the uterus. At first these are small and contain a dark liquid. Charcot calls them *ulcères du poumon.* They rarely attain a large size unless a communication is formed with the bronchus, in which case they may become converted into suppurating cavities.

Anthracosis and Tuberculosis.—In the Pennsylvania anthracite district tuberculosis is relatively less common among the miners, the figures for ten years at Scranton for male adults being 3.37 per cent. in mine workers, 9.97 per cent. in those of other occupations (Wainwright). Goldman in Germany, Oliver and Trotter in England, all agree upon the comparative rarity of tuberculosis among coal miners. Dust does not favor tuberculosis because it excites fibrosis which is opposed to tuberculosis.

Haldane points out that the death rate among old miners from bronchitis is exceptionally high.

Symptoms.—The symptoms do not come on until the patient has worked for a variable number of years, usually twelve, in the dusty atmosphere. As a rule there are cough and failing health for a prolonged period of time before complete disability. The coincident emphysema is responsible in great part for the shortness of breath and wheezy condition of these patients. The expectoration is usually muco-purulent, often profuse, and in anthracosis very dark in color—the so-called "black spit," while in chalicosis there may be seen under the microscope the bright angular particles of silica.

Even with the physical signs of cavity, tubercle bacilli are not usually present. It is remarkable for how long a coal-miner may bring up sputum laden with coal particles even when there are signs only of a chronic bronchitis. Many of the particles are contained in the cells of the alveolar epithelium. In these instances it appears that an attempt is made by the leucocytes to rid the lungs of the carbon grains. In the late stages the condition is that of cirrhosis of the lungs.

Diagnosis.—This is rarely difficult; the expectoration is usually characteristic. It must always be borne in mind that chronic bronchitis and emphysema form essential parts of the process and that in late stages there may be tuberculous infection. The X-ray picture in the early stages shows a broadening of the normal shadows and as the disease advances there are circumscribed dense areas throughout both lungs.

Prophylaxis.—Much has been done to reduce the prevalence of the disease by proper ventilation of works and the protection of the men. The conversion of dry into wet mining prevents the distribution of injurious dust. On the whole the health of British miners is good. Silicosis is a dangerous condition and in the Rand and Missouri mines the average age at death of 198 cases was 36.7 years (Lanza).

Treatment.—This is practically that of chronic bronchitis and emphysema.

IV. EMPHYSEMA

Definition.—The condition in which the infundibular passages and the alveoli are dilated and the alveolar walls atrophied.

Floyer of Litchfield first described the anatomical condition and spoke of the disease as "flatulent asthma" (1698), meaning a disorder in which the lungs were blown up with air.

A practical division may be made into compensatory, hypertrophic, and atrophic forms, the acute vesicular emphysema, and the interstitial forms. The last two do not in reality come under the above definition, but for convenience they may be considered here.

I. COMPENSATORY EMPHYSEMA

Whenever a region of the lung does not expand fully in inspiration, either another portion of the lung must expand or the chest wall sink in order to occupy the space. The former almost invariably occurs. We have already mentioned that in broncho-pneumonia there is a vicarious distention of the air-vesicles in the adjacent healthy lobules, and the same happens in the neighborhood of tuberculous areas and cicatrices. In general pleural adhesions there is often compensatory emphysema, particularly at the anterior margins of the lung. The most advanced example of this form is seen in cirrhosis, when the unaffected lung increases greatly in size, owing to distention of the air-vesicles. A similar though less marked condition is seen in extensive pleurisy with effusion and in pneumothorax.

At first, this distention is a simple physiological process and the alveolar walls are stretched but not atrophied. Ultimately, however, in many cases they waste and the contiguous air-cells fuse, producing true emphysema.

II. HYPERTROPIC EMPHYSEMA

The large-lunged emphysema of Jenner, also known as substantive or idiopathic emphysema, is a well-marked clinical affection, characterized by enlargement of the lungs, due to distention of the air-cells and atrophy of their walls, and clinically by imperfect aëration of the blood and more or less marked dyspnœa.

Etiology.—Emphysema is the result of persistently high intra-alveolar tension acting upon a congenitally weak lung tissue. Strongly in favor of the view that the nutritive change in the air-cells is the primary factor are the markedly *hereditary* character of the disease and the frequency with which it starts early in life. To James Jackson, Jr., of Boston, we owe the first observations on the hereditary character of emphysema. Working under Louis' direction, he found that in 18 out of 28 cases one or both parents were affected.

In childhood it may follow recurring asthmatic attacks due to adenoid vegetations. It may occur, too, in several members of the same family. We are still ignorant as to the nature of this congenital pulmonary weakness. Cohnheim thinks it probably due to a defect in the development of the elastic-tissue fibres—a statement which is borne out by Eppinger's observations.

Heightened pressure within the air-cells may be due to forcible inspiration or expiration. Much discussion has taken place as to the part played by these two acts in the production of the disease. The inspiratory theory was advanced by Laennec and subsequently modified by Gairdner, who held that in chronic bronchitis areas of collapse were induced, and compensatory distention took place in the adjacent lobules. This unquestionably does occur in the vicarious or compensatory emphysema, but it probably is not a factor of much moment in the form now under consideration. The expiratory theory, supported by Mendelssohn and Jenner, accounts for the condition in a more satisfactory way. In all straining efforts and violent attacks of coughing the glottis is closed and the chest walls strongly compressed by muscular efforts, so that the strain is thrown upon those parts of the lung least protected, as the apices and the anterior margins, where we always find the emphysema most advanced. The sternum and costal cartilages gradually yield to the heightened intrathoracic pressure and are, in advanced cases, pushed forward, giving the characteristic rotundity to the thorax.

Freund's Theory.—A primary disease of the costal cartilages—a chronic hyperplasia with premature ossification brings about gradually a state of rigid dilatation of the chest, to which the emphysema is secondary. It is probable that there is a group of cases in which such changes occur in young persons, particularly in the cartilages of the first three ribs. Niemeyer met with a few such cases, and instances have been reported in which the cartilages increased in size and stood out prominently. For such a condition what is called Freund's operation (of resection) would be indicated.

Of other etiological factors *occupation* is the most important. The disease is met with in players on wind instruments, in glass-blowers, and in occupations necessitating heavy lifting or straining. Whooping-cough and bronchitis play an important rôle, not so much in the changes which they induce in the bronchi as in consequence of the prolonged attacks of coughing.

Morbid Anatomy.—The thorax is capacious, usually barrel-shaped, and the cartilages are calcified. On removal of the sternum, the anterior mediastinum is found completely occupied by the margins of the lungs, and the pericardial sac may not be visible. The organs are very large and have lost their elasticity, so that they do not collapse either in the thorax or when placed on the table. The pleura is pale and there is often an absence of pigment, sometimes in patches, termed by Virchow *albinism* of the lung. To the touch they have a peculiar, downy, feathery feel, and pit readily on pressure. This is one of the most marked features. Beneath the pleura greatly enlarged air-vesicles may be readily seen. They vary in size from .5 to 3 mm., and irregular bullæ, the size of a walnut or larger, may project from the free margins. The best idea of the extreme rarefaction of the tissue is obtained from sections of a lung distended and dried. At the anterior margins the structure may form an irregular series of air-chambers, resembling the frog's lung. On careful inspection, remnants of the interlobular septa or even of the alveoli may be seen on these large emphysematous vesicles. Though general, the distention is more marked, as a rule, at the anterior margins, and is often specially marked at the inner surface of the lobe near the root, where in extreme cases air-spaces as large as a hen's egg may sometimes be found. Microscopically there is atrophy of the alveolar walls, by which is produced a coalescence of neighboring air-cells. In this process the capillary network disappears before the walls are completely atrophied. The loss of the elastic tissue is a special feature. In certain cases there may be a congenital defect in the development of this tissue. The epithelium of the air-cells undergoes a fatty change, but the large distended air-spaces retain a pavement layer.

The *bronchi* show important changes. In the larger tubes the mucous membrane may be rough and thickened from chronic bronchitis; often the longitudinal lines of submucous elastic tissue stand out prominently. In the advanced cases many of the smaller tubes are dilated, particularly when, in addition to emphysema, there are peri-bronchial fibroid changes. Bronchiectasis is not an invariable accompaniment of emphysema, but, as Laennec remarks, it is difficult to understand why it is not more common. Of associated morbid changes the most important are found in the heart. The right chambers are dilated and hypertrophied, the tricuspid orifice is large, and the valve segments are often thickened at the edges. In advanced cases the cardiac hypertrophy is general. The pulmonary artery and its branches may be wide and show marked atheromatous changes.

The changes in the other organs are those commonly associated with prolonged venous congestion. Pneumothorax may follow the rupture of an emphysematous bleb.

Symptoms.—The disease may be tolerably advanced before any special symptoms occur. A child, for instance, may be somewhat short of breath on going upstairs or may be unable to run and play as other children without great discomfort; or, perhaps, has attacks of slight lividity. Doubtless much depends upon the completeness of cardiac compensation. When this is perfect, there may be no special interruption of the pulmonary circulation and, except with violent exertion, there is no interference with the aëration of the blood. In well-marked cases the following are the most important symptoms: *Dyspnœa,* which may be felt only on slight exertion, or may be persistent, and aggravated by intercurrent attacks of bronchitis. The respirations are often harsh and wheezy, and expiration is distinctly prolonged.

Cyanosis of an extreme grade is more common in emphysema than in other affections with the exception of congenital heart-disease. It is one of the few diseases in which a patient may be able to go about and walk into the hospital or consulting-room with a lividity of startling intensity. The contrast between the extreme cyanosis and the comparative comfort of the patient is very striking. In other affections of the heart and lungs associated with a similar degree of cyanosis the patient is invariably in bed and usually in a state of orthopnœa. One condition must be referred to, viz., the extraordinary cyanosis in cases of poisoning by aniline products, which is in most part due to the conversion of the hæmoglobin into methæmoglobin.

Bronchitis with associated cough is frequent and often the direct cause of the pulmonary distress. The contrast between emphysematous patients in the winter and summer is marked in this respect. In the latter they may be comfortable and able to attend to their work, but with the cold and changeable weather they are laid up with attacks of bronchitis. Finally the two conditions become inseparable and the patient has persistently more or less cough. The acute bronchitis may produce attacks not unlike asthma. In some instances this is true spasmodic asthma, with which emphysema is frequently associated.

As age advances, and with successive attacks of bronchitis, the condition grows slowly worse. In hospital practice it is common to admit patients over sixty with well marked signs of advanced emphysema. The affection can generally be told at a glance—the rounded shoulders, barrel chest, the thin yet oftentimes muscular form, and sometimes a characteristic facial expression. There is another group of patients from twenty-five to forty years of age who, winter after winter, have attacks of intense cyanosis in consequence of an aggravated bronchial catarrh. On inquiry we find that these patients have been short-breathed from infancy, and they belong to a category in which there has been a primary defect of structure in the lung tissue.

PHYSICAL SIGNS.—*Inspection.*—The thorax is markedly altered in shape; the antero-posterior diameter is increased and may be even greater than the lateral, so that the chest is barrel-shaped. The appearance is somewhat as if the chest was in a permanent inspiratory position. The sternum and costal cartilages are prominent. The lower zone of the thorax looks large and the intercostal spaces are much widened, particularly in the hypochondriac regions. The sternal fossa is deep, the clavicles stand out with great prominence, and the neck looks shortened from the elevation of the thorax and the sternum. A zone of dilated venules may be seen along the line of attachment of the diaphragm. Though this is common in emphysema, it is by no means peculiar to it or indeed to any special affection.

The curve of the spine is increased and the back is remarkably rounded, so that the scapulæ seem to be almost horizontal. Mensuration shows the rounded form of the chest and the very slight expansion on deep inspiration. The respiratory movements, which may look energetic and forcible, exercise little or no influence. The chest does not expand, but there is a general elevation. The inspiratory effort is short and quick; the expiratory movement is prolonged. There may be retraction instead of distention in the upper abdominal region during inspiration, and a transverse curve crossing the abdomen at the level of the twelfth rib is sometimes seen. The apex beat of the heart is not visible, and there is usually marked pulsation in the epigastric region. The cervical veins stand out prominently and may pulsate.

Palpation.—The vocal fremitus is somewhat enfeebled but not lost. The apex beat can rarely be felt. There is a marked shock in the lower sternal region and very distinct pulsation in the epigastrium. *Percussion* gives greatly increased resonance, full and drum-like—hyperresonance. The note is not often distinctly tympanitic. There may be marked variations in the note in local areas. The area of resonance is greatly extended, the heart dulness may be obliterated, the upper limit of liver dulness is greatly lowered, and the resonance may extend to the costal margin. Behind, a clear percussion note extends to a much lower level than normal. The level of splenic dulness, too, may be lowered.

On *auscultation* the breath-sounds are usually enfeebled and may be masked by bronchitic râles. The most characteristic feature is the prolongation of the expiration, and the normal ratio may be reversed—4 to 1 instead of 1 to 4. It is often wheezy and harsh and associated with coarse râles and sibilant rhonchi. It is said that in interstitial emphysema there may be a friction sound heard, not unlike that of pleurisy. The heart-sounds are usually feeble but clear; in advanced cases, when there is marked cyanosis, a tricuspid regurgitant murmur may be heard. Accentuation of the pulmonary second sound may be present.

Course.—This is slow but progressive, the recurring attacks of bronchitis aggravating the condition. Death may occur from intercurrent pneumonia, either lobar or lobular, and dropsy may supervene from cardiac failure. Occasionally death results from overdistention of the heart, with extreme cyanosis. Duckworth has called attention to the occasional occurrence of fatal hæmorrhage in emphysema. In an old emphysematous patient at the Montreal General Hospital death followed the erosion of a main branch of the pulmonary artery by an ulcer near the bifurcation of the trachea.

Treatment.—Practically, the measures mentioned in connection with bronchitis should be employed. In children with asthma and emphysema the nose should be carefully examined. No remedy is known which has any influence over the progress of the condition itself. Bronchitis is the great danger of these patients, and therefore when possible they should live in an equable climate. They do well in southern California and in Egypt. In consequence of the venous engorgement they are liable to gastric and intestinal disturbance, and it is particularly important to keep the bowels regulated and to avoid flatulency, which often seriously aggravates the dyspnœa. Patients who come into the hospital in a state of urgent dyspnœa and lividity, with great engorgement of the veins, particularly if they are young and vigorous, should be bled freely. Inhalation of oxygen may be used. Epinephrin hypodermically (♏ xv, 1 c. c.) often gives relief. Strychnine will be found useful. In children, with insufficiency of expiration and the lower edge of the lungs below the usual level, pressure on the lower ribs may correct this. Breathing exercises to aid expiration are helpful. Breathing of compressed air in a pneumatic cabinet gives temporary relief. Resection of the first costal cartilage or of the first three cartilages on either side has been practised (Freund's operation). It is not likely to be of any benefit in the aged in whom the condition is established, but in a special group in the young in which the primary trouble appears to be in the cartilages good results may follow.

III. ATROPHIC EMPHYSEMA

A senile change, called by Sir William Jenner small-lunged emphysema, is really a primary atrophy of the lung, coming on in advanced life, and scarcely constitutes a special affection. It occurs in "withered-looking old persons" who may perhaps have had a winter cough and shortness of breath for years. In striking contrast to the essential hypertrophic emphysema, the chest is small and the ribs obliquely placed. The thoracic muscles are usually atrophied. The lung is converted into a series of large vesicles, on the walls of which the remnants of air-cells may be seen.

IV. ACUTE VESICULAR EMPHYSEMA.

When death occurs from bronchitis of the smaller tubes or diffuse bronchopneumonia, when strong inspiratory efforts have been made, the lungs are large in volume and the air-cells much distended. Clinically, this condition may occur rapidly in cardiac dyspnœa and angina pectoris. The area of pulmonary resonance is much increased, and piping râles and prolonged expiration are heard everywhere. A similar condition may follow pressure on the vagi.

V. INTERSTITIAL EMPHYSEMA

Beads of air are seen in the interlobular and subpleural tissue, sometimes forming large bullæ beneath the pleura. A rare event is rupture close to the root of the lung, and the passage of air along the trachea into the subcutaneous tissues of the neck. After tracheotomy just the reverse may occur and the air may pass from the tracheotomy wound along the windpipe and bronchi and appear beneath the surface of the pleura. From this interstitial emphysema spontaneous pneumothorax may arise in healthy persons.

V. GANGRENE OF THE LUNG

Etiology.—Gangrene of the lung is not an affection *per se,* but occurs in a variety of conditions when necrotic areas undergo putrefaction. It is not easy to say why gangrene should occur in one case and not in another, as the germs of putrefaction are always in the air-passages, and yet necrotic territories rarely become gangrenous. Total obstruction of a pulmonary artery, as a rule, causes infarction, and the area shut off does not often, though it may, slough. Another factor would seem to be necessary—probably a lowered tissue resistance, the result of general or local causes. It is met with (1) as a sequence of lobar pneumonia. This rarely occurs in a previously healthy person—more commonly in the debilitated or in the diabetic subject. (2) Gangrene is very prone to follow aspiration pneumonia, since the foreign particles rapidly undergo putrefactive changes. Of a similar nature are the cases of gangrene due to perforation of cancer of the œsophagus into the lung or into the bronchus. (3) The putrid contents of a bronchiectatic, more commonly of a tuberculous, cavity may excite gangrene in the neighboring tissues. The pressure bronchiectasis following aneurism or tumor may lead to extensive sloughing. (4) Gangrene may follow simple embolism of the pulmonary artery. More commonly, however, the embolus is derived from a part which is mortified or comes from a focus of bone disease. In typhus and in typhoid fever gangrene of the lung may follow thrombosis of one of the larger branches of the pulmonary artery. Lastly, gangrene of the lung may occur in conditions of debility during convalescence from protracted fever—occasionally, indeed, without our being able to assign any reasonable cause.

Morbid Anatomy.—Laennec, who first accurately described pulmonary gangrene, recognized a diffuse and a circumscribed form. The former, though rare, is sometimes seen in connection with pneumonia, more rarely after obliteration of a large branch of the pulmonary artery. It may involve the greater part of a lobe, and the lung tissue is converted into a horribly offensive greenish-black mass, torn and ragged in the centre. In the circumscribed form there is well-marked limitation between the gangrenous area and the surrounding tissue. The focus may be single or there may be two or more. The lower lobe is more commonly affected than the upper, and the peripheral more than the central portion of the lung. A gangrenous area is at first uniformly greenish brown in color; but softening rapidly takes place with the formation of a cavity with shreddy, irregular walls and a greenish, offensive fluid. The lung tissue in the immediate neighborhood shows a zone of deep congestion, often consolidation, and outside this an intense œdema. In the embolic cases the plugged artery can sometimes be found. When rapidly extending, vessels may be opened and a copious hæmorrhage ensue. Perforation of the pleura is not uncommon. The irritating decomposing material usually excites the most intense bronchitis. Embolic processes are not infrequent. There is a remarkable association in some cases between circumscribed gangrene of the lung and abscess of the brain.

Symptoms and Course.—Usually definite symptoms of local pulmonary disease precede the characteristic features of gangrene. These, of course, are very varied, depending on the primary disease. The sputum is very characteristic. It is intensely fetid—usually profuse—and, if expectorated into a conical glass, separates into three layers—a greenish brown, heavy sediment; an intervening thin liquid, which sometimes has a greenish or a brownish tint; and, on top, a thick, frothy layer. Spread on a glass plate, the shreddy *débris* of lung tissue can readily be picked out. Even large fragments of lung may be coughed up. Robertson, of Onancock, Va., sent one several centimetres in length, which had been expectorated by a lad of eighteen, who had severe gangrene and recovered. Microscopically, elastic fibres are found in abundance, with granular matter, pigment grains, fatty crystals, bacteria, and leptothrix. It is stated that elastic tissue is sometimes absent. The peculiar plugs of sputum which occur in bronchiectasis are not found. Blood is often present, and, as a rule, is much altered. The sputum has, in a majority of the cases, an intensely fetid odor, which is communicated to the breath and may permeate the entire room. It is much more offensive than in fetid bronchitis or in abscess of the lung. The fetor is particularly marked when there is free communication between the gangrenous cavities and the bronchi. Localized gangrene, unsuspected during life and in which there had been no fetor of the breath, may be found post mortem.

The physical signs, when extensive destruction has occurred, are those of cavity, but the limited circumscribed areas may be difficult to detect. Bronchitis is always present. The X-ray examination aids in diagnosis.

Among the general symptoms may be mentioned fever, usually of moderate grade; the pulse is rapid, and very often the constitutional depression is severe. But the only special features indicative of gangrene are the sputum and the fetor of the breath. The patient generally sinks from exhaustion. Fatal hæmorrhage may ensue.

Treatment.—This is very unsatisfactory. The indication is to disinfect the gangrenous area, but this is often impossible. An antiseptic spray of carbolic acid may be employed. A good plan is for the patient to use over the mouth and nose an inhaler, which may be charged with a solution of carbolic acid or guaiacol; the latter drug has also been used hypodermically, with, it is said, happy results in removing the odor. If the signs of cavity are distinct an attempt should be made to cleanse it by direct injections of an antiseptic solution. If the patient's condition is good and the gangrenous region can be localized, surgical interference is indicated. The general condition of the patient is always such as to demand the greatest care in the matter of diet and nursing.

VI. ABSCESS OF THE LUNG

Etiology.—Suppuration occurs in the lung under the following conditions: (1) As a sequence of inflammation, either lobar or lobular. Apart from the purulent infiltration this is rare, and even in lobar pneumonia the abscesses are of small size and usually involve, as Addison remarked, several points at the same time. On the other hand, abscess formation is frequent in the deglutition and aspiration forms of broncho-pneumonia. After wounds of the neck or operations upon the throat, particularly the tonsils, in suppurative disease of the nose or larynx, occasionally even of the ear (Volkmann), infective particles reach the bronchi by aspiration and excite an intense inflammation which often ends in abscess. Cancer of the œsophagus, perforating the root of the lung or into the bronchi, may produce extensive suppuration. The abscesses vary in size from a walnut to an orange, have ragged and irregular walls, and purulent, sometimes necrotic, contents.

(2) Embolic, so-called metastatic, abscesses, the result of infective emboli, are extremely common in pyæmia. They may be numerous and present very

definite characters. As a rule they are superficial, beneath the pleura, and often wedge-shaped. At first firm, grayish red in color, and surrounded by a zone of intense hyperæmia, suppuration soon follows with the formation of a definite abscess. The pleura is usually covered with greenish lymph, and perforation sometimes takes place with the production of pneumothorax.

(3) Perforation of the lung from without, lodgment of foreign bodies, and, in the right lung, perforation from abscess of the liver or a suppurating echinococcus cyst are occasionally causes of pulmonary abscess.

(4) Suppurative processes play an important part in chronic pulmonary tuberculosis, many of the symptoms of which are due to them.

Symptoms.—Abscess following pneumonia is easily recognized by an aggravation of the general symptoms and by the physical signs of cavity and the character of the expectoration. Embolic abscesses can not often be recognized, and the local symptoms are generally masked in the general pyæmic manifestations. The character of the sputum is of great importance in determining the presence of abscess. The odor is offensive, yet it rarely has the horrible fetor of gangrene or of putrid bronchitis. Fragments of lung tissue and elastic tissue with alveolar arrangement may be found. The presence of this with the physical signs and the X-ray examination rarely leave any question as to the diagnosis. Embolic cases usually run a fatal course. Recovery occasionally occurs after pneumonia. In a case following typhoid fever Kerr removed two ribs and found free in the pus of a localized empyema a sequestered piece of lung, the size of the palm of the hand, which had sloughed off from the lower lobe. The patient made a good recovery.

Treatment.—The patient should lie with the affected side uppermost as much as possible. The X-ray picture is sometimes a guide as to the best position to favor drainage. The foot of the bed should be elevated and the patient lie without a pillow. The head should be lowered over the side of the bed during paroxysms of coughing. When the abscess is well defined and superficial, an attempt may be made to open and drain it. Artificial pneumothorax has been suggested when the abscess is connected with a bronchus. The patient should be kept in the open air if possible and given a liberal diet.

VII. NEW GROWTHS IN THE LUNGS

Etiology and Morbid Anatomy.—While primary tumors are rare, secondary growths are not uncommon. Carcinoma is the most common primary form. Endothelium and sarcoma are less frequent. Hypernephroma often has metastases in the lungs.

Varieties.—The following groups may be recognized:

(*a*) Acute pleuro-pneumonic form, with a very rapid course—dyspnœa, cough, asphyxia, rapid emaciation and death in from six to twelve weeks. Most of these cases are secondary, sometimes to unrecognized disease elsewhere, but there are instances of primary disease of this type. It is a remarkable fact that cobalt miners of Schneeberg are very liable to a primary carcinoma of the lung which may run this acute course.

(*b*) Chronic pleuro-pulmonary carcinoma, of which there are several types: (1) *Broncho-pulmonary Form.*—This, the most typical variety, begins with bronchial symptoms, bloody sputum, loss of weight and strength, and anæmia. The physical signs may be suggestive of tuberculosis, but the earliest indications are usually at the root of the lung. Later there may be cavity formation, with a bronchiectatic type of sputum. Tubercle bacilli are absent and there may be very large round cells with many fatty granules, representing degenerate cancer cells. The X-ray picture is not distinctive and the cases are usually taken for tuberculosis.

(2) *Mediastinal Type.*—Quite early in this form the glands become involved, increase rapidly, compress the adjoining structures and the type of the disease is that of a mediastinal tumor with its dominant pressure symptoms.

(3) *Pleuritic Type.*—Many of the cases are primary endothelioma of the pleura of which Keilty found 9 in 5,000 autopsies. The earliest and dominant symptoms are at the back with pleuritic pain, cough, friction, progressive effusion, and shortness of breath. On tapping, the effusion is usually bloody, though at first it may be clear. In other instances the pleura is early involved with rapid extension, but no effusion. There may be little or no cough, and very slight dyspnœa, with progressive weakness, emaciation, and anæmia as the chief features. Subcutaneous nodules may occur along the ribs, with widespread metastases in the lymph glands and internal organs.

From the standpoint of *treatment* not much is to be expected. The new surgical technique has made the thoracic cavity accessible, and it is possible that early explorations may become common in doubtful cases. In a few instances operation has been done; in Lenhartz' case the patient remained well for a year, and died two and a half years after operation.

E. DISEASES OF THE PLEURA

I. ACUTE PLEURISY

Anatomically, the cases may be divided into dry or adhesive pleurisy and pleurisy with effusion. Another classification is into primary or secondary forms. According to the course, a division may be made into *acute* and *chronic pleurisy,* and as it is impossible, at present, to group the various forms etiologically, this is perhaps the most satisfactory division.

I. FIBRINOUS OR PLASTIC PLEURISY

In this the pleural membrane is covered by a sheeting of lymph of variable thickness, which gives it a turbid, granular appearance, or the fibrin may exist in distinct layers. It occurs (1) as an independent affection, following cold or exposure. This form of acute plastic pleurisy without fluid exudate is not common in perfectly healthy individuals. Cases are met with, however, in which the disease sets in with the usual symptoms of pain in the side and slight fever, and there are the physical signs of fibrinous pleurisy. After persisting for a few days, the friction murmur disappears and no exudation occurs. Union takes place between the membranes, and possibly the pleuritic adhesions which are found in such a large percentage of all bodies examined after death originate in these slight fibrinous pleurisies.

Fibrinous pleurisy occurs (2) as a secondary process in acute diseases of the lung, such as pneumonia, which is always accompanied by a certain amount of pleurisy, usually of this form. Cancer, abscess, and gangrene also cause plastic pleurisy when the surface of the lung becomes involved. This condition is specially associated in a large number of cases with tuberculosis. Pleural pain, stitch in the side, and a dry cough, with marked friction sounds on auscultation, are the initial phenomena in many instances of pulmonary tuberculosis. The pleural signs are usually basic.

II. SERO-FIBRINOUS PLEURISY

In a majority of cases there is, with the fibrin, a variable amount of fluid exudate, which produces the condition known as pleurisy with effusion.

Etiology.—Of 194 cases in fifteen years in the Hopkins Hospital, there were 161 males and 33 females. Under twenty years of age there were 20 patients; 18 were over sixty years of age. The greatest number was in the fifth decade, 59. Cold acts as a predisposing agent, which permits the action of various micro-organisms. A majority of the cases are tuberculous. This view is based upon: (1) Post mortem evidence. Tubercles have been found in acute cases, thought to have been "rheumatic" or due to cold. (2) The not infrequent presence of tuberculous lesions, often latent, in the lung or elsewhere. (3) The character of the exudate. If coagulated and the coagulum digested and centrifugalized, tubercle bacilli are frequently found. Injected into a guinea pig, in amounts of 15 c. c. or more, tuberculosis followed in 62 per cent. (Eichhorst). The cytodiagnosis shows that as in other tuberculous exudates the mono-nuclear leucocytes predominate. (4) The tuberculin reaction is given in a considerable percentage of the cases. (5) The subsequent history. Of 90 cases of acute pleurisy which had been under the observation of H. I. Bowditch between 1849 and 1879, 32 died of or had pulmonary tuberculosis. Among 130 patients with primary pleurisy with effusion, followed for a period of seven years by Hedges, 40 per cent. became tuberculous.

Of 300 uncomplicated cases of pleural effusion in the Massachusetts General Hospital, followed by R. C. Cabot, the subsequent history was ascertained in 221; followed five years until death or pulmonary tuberculosis, 117; well after five years, 96. In 172 of the cases of pleurisy with effusion in the Johns Hopkins Hospital Hamman got reports from 88; of these 48 were living and well, 30 later became tuberculous, in 2 the result was questionable, and 8 died of other diseases. Twelve of the 88 had tubercle bacilli in the sputum while in the hospital without discoverable pulmonary lesion; 3 of the 12 were living and well; in 8 the signs became well marked; one died of unknown cause. Hamman collected 562 cases (including the above) in which the subsequent history was sought; of these 167, 29.7 per cent. became tuberculous.

Bacteriology of Acute Pleurisy.—From a bacteriological standpoint we may recognize three groups of cases, caused by the tubercle bacillus, the pneumococcus, and the streptococcus, respectively.

Bacillus tuberculosis is present in a very large proportion of all cases of primary or so-called idiopathic pleurisy. The exudate is usually sterile on cover slips or in the culture and inoculation tests made in the ordinary way, as the bacilli are very scanty. It has been demonstrated clearly that a large amount of the exudate must be taken to make the test complete, either in cultures or in the inoculation of animals. Eichhorst found that more than 62 per cent. were demonstrated as tuberculous when as much as 15 c. c. of the exudate was inoculated into test animals, while less than 10 per cent. of the cases showed tuberculosis when only 1 c. c. of the exudate was used. This is a point to which observers should pay very special attention. Le Damany has demonstrated the tuberculous character of all but 4 in 55 primary pleurisies. He used large quantities of the fluid for his inoculation experiments.

The *pneumococcus* pleurisy is almost always secondary to a focus of inflammation in the lung. It may, however, be primary. The exudate is usually purulent and the outlook is favorable.

The *streptococcus* pleurisy is the typical septic form which may occur either from direct infection of the pleura through the lung in broncho-pneumonia, or in cases of streptococcus pneumonia; in other instances it follows infection of more distant parts. The acute streptococcus pleurisy is the most serious and fatal of all forms.

Among other bacteria which have been found are the staphylococcus, Friedländer's bacillus, the typhoid bacillus, and the diphtheria bacillus.

Morbid Anatomy.—In sero-fibrinous pleurisy the serous exudate is abundant and the fibrin is found on the pleural surfaces and scattered through the fluid in the form of flocculi. The proportions of these constituents vary a great deal. In some instances there is very little membranous fibrin; in others it forms thick, creamy layers and exists in the dependent part of the fluid as whitish, curd-like masses. The fluid is of a lemon color, either clear or slightly turbid, depending on the number of formed elements. In some instances it has a dark brown color. The microscopic examination shows leucocytes, occasional swollen cells, which may be derived from the pleural endothelium, shreds of fibrillated fibrin, and a variable number of red blood-corpuscles. A large number of cells undergoing mitotic division is diagnostic of malignant disease. The fluid is rich in albumin and sometimes coagulates spontaneously. Its composition closely resembles that of blood serum. Cholesterin, uric acid, and sugar are occasionally found. The amount of the effusion varies from ½ to 4 litres. Enormous amounts are sometimes removed, 188 ounces in one case (E. C. Carter). The lung in serofibrinous pleurisy is more or less compressed. If the exudation is limited the lower lobe alone is atelectatic; but in an extensive effusion which reaches to the clavicle the entire lung will be found lying close to the spine, dark and airless, or even bloodless—*i. e.,* carnified.

In large exudations the adjacent organs are displaced; the liver is depressed and the heart dislocated. With reference to the position of the heart, the following statements may be made: (1) Even in the most extensive left sided exudation there is no rotation of the apex of the heart, which in no case was to the right of the mid-sternal line; (2) the relative position of the apex and base is usually maintained; in some instances the apex is lifted, in others the whole heart lies more transversely; (3) the right chambers of the heart occupy the greater portion of the front, so that the displacement is rather a definite dislocation of the mediastinum, with the pericardium, to the right, than any special twisting of the heart itself; (4) the kink or twist in the inferior vena cava described by Bartels may be present.

Symptoms.—Prodromes are not uncommon, but the disease may set in abruptly with a chill, followed by fever and a severe pain in the side. In very many cases, however, the onset is insidious, particularly in children and in elderly persons. A little dyspnœa on exertion and an increasing pallor may be the only features. Washbourn has called attention to the frequency with which the pneumococcus pleurisy sets in with the features of pneumonia. The pain in the side is the most distressing symptom, and is usually referred to the nipple or axillary regions. It must be remembered, however, that pleuritic pain may be felt in the abdomen or low down in the back, particularly when the diaphragmatic surface of the pleura is involved. It is lancinating, sharp, and severe, and is aggravated by cough. At this early stage, on auscultation, sometimes indeed on palpation, a dry friction rub can be detected. The fever rarely rises so rapidly as in pneumonia, and does not reach the same grade. A temperature of from 102° to 103° F. is an average pyrexia. It may drop to normal at the end of a week or ten days without any definite change in the physical signs, or may persist for several weeks. The temperature of the affected is higher than that of the sound side. Cough is an early symptom in acute pleurisy, but is rarely so distressing or frequent as in pneumonia. There are instances in which it is absent. The expectoration is usually slight in amount, mucoid, and occasionally streaked with blood.

At the outset there may be dyspnœa, due partly to the fever and partly to the pain in the side. Later it results from the compression of the lung, particularly if the exudation has taken place rapidly. In the cases with very rapid effusion the dyspnœa may be marked. When, however, the fluid is effused slowly, one lung may be entirely compressed without inducing shortness of breath, except on exertion, and the patient will lie quietly in bed without evincing the slightest respiratory distress. When the effusion is large the patient usually prefers to lie upon the affected side.

Physical Signs.—Inspection shows some degree of immobility on the affected side, depending upon the amount of exudation; and in large effusions an increase in volume, which may appear to be much more than it really is as determined by mensuration. The intercostal depressions are obliterated. In right sided effusions the apex beat may be lifted to the fourth interspace, be pushed beyond the left nipple, or even be seen in the axilla. When the exudation is on the left side, the heart impulse may not be visible; but if the effusion is large it is seen in the third and fourth spaces on the right side, and sometimes as far out as the nipple, or even beyond it. In massive effusion on the left side there may be a prominence below the left costal margin.

Palpation enables us to determine the deficient movements on the affected side, the obliteration of the intercostal spaces, and more accurately to define the position of the heart's impulse. In simple serofibrinous effusion there is rarely any œdema of the chest walls. It is scarcely ever possible to obtain fluctuation. Tactile fremitus is greatly diminished or abolished. If the effusion is slight there may be only enfeeblement. The absence of the voice vibrations in effusions of any size is the most valuable physical sign. In children and occasionally in adults there may be much effusion with retention of fremitus.

In rare cases the vibrations may be communicated to the chest walls through localized pleural adhesions.

Mensuration.—With the cyrtometer, if the effusion is excessive, a difference of from half an inch to an inch, or even, in large effusions, an inch and a half, may be found between the two sides. Allowance must be made for the fact that the right side is naturally larger than the left.

Percussion.—Early in the disease there may be no alteration, but with the gradual accumulation of the fluid the resonance becomes defective, and finally gives place to flatness. From day to day the gradual increase in height of the fluid may be studied. In a pleuritic effusion rising to the fourth rib in front the percussion signs are usually very suggestive. In the subclavicular region the attention is often aroused at once by a tympanitic note, the so-called Skoda's resonance, which is heard perhaps more commonly in this situation with pleural effusion than in any other condition. It shades into a flat note in the lower mammary and axillary regions. Tympany may be obtained also behind, just above the limit of effusion. The dulness has a peculiarly resistant, wooden quality, differing from that of pneumonia and readily recognized by skilled fingers. When the patient is in the erect posture the upper line of dulness is not horizontal, but is higher behind than in front, forming a parabola. The curve marking the intersection of the plane of contact of lung and fluid with the chest wall is known as "Ellis's line" which Garland verified clinically and by animal experiments. With medium-sized effusions this line begins lowest behind, advances upward and forward in a letter-S curve to the axillary region, whence it proceeds in a straight decline to the sternum. This curve is demonstrable only when the patient is in the erect position. Grocco, in 1902, called attention to the existence in pleural effusion of a triangular area of relative dulness, along the spine, on the side opposite to the pleurisy, in width from 2 to 5 cm., and with the apex upward. It can be demonstrated in a large majority of all cases, particularly in young and thin persons. It is possibly due to the bulging of the mediastinum, by the fluid, across the middle line, the anatomical possibility of which has been pointed out by Calvert.

On the right side the dulness passes without change into that of the liver. On the left side in the nipple line it extends to and may obliterate Traube's semilunar space. If the effusion is moderate, the phenomenon of movable dulness may be obtained by marking carefully, in the sitting posture, the upper limit in the mammary region, and then in the recumbent posture, noting the change in the height of dulness. This sign of fluid can not always be obtained. In very copious exudation the dulness may reach the clavicle and even extend beyond the sternal margin of the opposite side.

Auscultation.—Early in the disease a friction rub may be heard, which disappears as the fluid accumulates. It is a to-and-fro dry rub, close to the ear, and has a leathery, creaking character. There is another pleural friction sound which closely resembles, and is scarcely to be distinguished from, the fine crackling crepitus of pneumonia. This may be heard at the commencement of the disease, and also, as pointed out in 1844 by MacDonnell, Sr., of Montreal, when the effusion has receded and the pleural layers come together again.

With even a slight exudation there is weakened or distant breathing. Often inspiration and expiration are distinctly audible, though distant, and have a tubular quality. Sometimes only a puffing tubular expiration is heard, which may have a metallic or amphoric quality. Loud resonant râles accompanying this may forcibly suggest a cavity. These pseudo-cavernous signs are met with more frequently in children, and often lead to error in diagnosis. Above the line of dulness the breath sounds are usually harsh and exaggerated, and may have a tubular quality.

The vocal resonance is usually diminished or absent. The whispered voice is said to be transmitted through a serous and not through a purulent exudate (Baccelli's sign), but this is not always true. This author advises direct auscultation in the antero-lateral region of the chest. There may, however, be intensification—bronchophony. The voice sometimes has a curious nasal, squeaking character, which was termed by Laennec *ægophony,* from its supposed resemblance to the bleating of a goat. In typical form this is not common, but it is by no means rare to hear a curious twang-like quality in the voice, particularly at the outer angle of the scapula.

In the examination of the heart it is well to bear in mind that when the apex of the heart lies beneath the sternum there may be no impulse. The determination of the situation of the organ may rest with the position of maximum loudness of the sounds. Over the displaced organ a systolic murmur may be heard. When the lappet of lung over the pericardium is involved on either side there may be a pleuro-pericardial friction.

Blood Count.—Emerson studied the histories of 89 cases of acute pleurisy with effusion in which blood counts were made before the temperature reached normal. Only 26 had a leucocytosis between 10,000 and 15,000; one only above 15,000. In 12 of the cases the count was below 5,000.

The X-ray pictures are of great interest and of much value in diagnosis. They show that the effusion is not always in the lower portion of the chest with the patient in the upright position, but that it may represent a vertical column in the lateral aspect of the chest, compressing the lung toward the spine. The effusion is not always mobile, but may be fixed by adhesions in one position.

Course.—The course of acute sero-fibrinous pleurisy is very variable. After persisting for a week or ten days the fever subsides, the cough and pain disappear, and a slight effusion may be quickly absorbed. In cases in which the effusion reaches as high as the fourth rib recovery is usually slower. Many instances come under observation for the first time, after two or three weeks' indisposition, with the fluid at a level with the clavicle. The fever may last from ten to twenty days without exciting anxiety, though, as a rule, in ordinary pleurisy, the temperature in cases of moderate severity is normal within eight or ten days. Left to itself, the natural tendency is to resorption; but this may take place very slowly. With the absorption of the fluid there is a redux-friction crepitus, either leathery and creaking or crackling and râle-like, and for months, or even longer, the defective resonance and feeble breathing are heard at the base. Rare modes of termination are perforation and discharge through the lung, and externally through the chest wall, examples of which have been recorded by Sahli.

The immediate *prognosis* in pleurisy with effusion is good. Of 320 cases at St. Bartholomew's Hospital, only 6.1 per cent. died before leaving the hospital (Hedges). A sero-fibrinous exudate may persist for months without change, particularly in tuberculous cases, and will sometimes reaccumulate after aspiration and resist all treatment. After persistence for more than twelve months, in spite of repeated tapping, a serous effusion was cured by incision without deformity of the chest (S. West). When one pleura is full and the heart is greatly dislocated, the condition, although in a majority of cases producing remarkably little disturbance, is not without risk.

III. PURULENT PLEURISY

(*Empyema*)

Etiology.—Pus in the pleura is due to (*a*) infection from within, as a rule directly from a patch of pneumonia or a septic focus in the lung, or in some cases a tuberculous broncho-pneumonia; (*b*) involvement from without, as in fracture of a rib, penetrating wound, disease of œsophagus, etc. It frequently follows the infectious diseases, particularly scarlet fever. It is very often latent, and due to undiscovered pneumonia. It is common in children, more in boys than in girls, and between the ages of one and five and eight and nine.

The pneumococcus is the most common organism, then the ordinary pus organisms and tubercle bacilli; in rare cases the influenza bacillus, and even psorosperms, have been found.

Morbid Anatomy.—On opening an empyema post mortem we usually find that the effusion has separated into a clear, greenish yellow serum above and the thick, cream-like pus below. The fluid may be scarcely more than turbid, with flocculi of fibrin through it. In the pneumococcus empyema the pus is usually thick and creamy. It usually has a heavy, sweetish odor, but in some instances—particularly those following wounds—it is fetid. In cases of gangrene of the lung or pleura the pus has a horribly stinking odor. Microscopically it has the characters of ordinary pus. The pleural membranes are greatly thickened, and present a grayish white layer from 1 to 2 mm. in thickness. On the costal pleura there may be erosions, and in old cases fistulous communications are common. The lung may be compressed to a very small limit, and the visceral pleura also may show perforations.

Symptoms.—Purulent pleurisy may begin abruptly, with the symptoms already described. More frequently it comes on insidiously in the course of other diseases or follows an ordinary sero-fibrinous pleurisy. There may be no pain in the chest, very little cough, and no dyspnœa, unless the side is very full. Symptoms of septic infection are rarely wanting. If in a child, there is a gradually developing pallor and weakness; sweats occur, and there is irregular fever. A cough is by no means constant. The leucocytes are usually much increased; in one fatal case they numbered 115,000 per c. mm.

Physical Signs.—Practically they are those already considered in pleurisy with effusion but there are one or two additional points to be mentioned. In empyema, particularly in children, the disproportion between the sides may be extreme. The intercostal spaces may not only be obliterated, but may bulge. Not infrequently there is œdema of the chest walls. The network of subcutaneous veins may be very distinct. It must not be forgotten that in children the breath-sounds may be *loud and tubular* over a purulent effusion of considerable size. The dislocation of the heart and displacement of the liver are more marked in empyema than in serous effusion—probably, as Senator suggests, owing to the greater weight of the fluid.

A curious phenomenon associated generally with empyema, but sometimes occurring in the sero-fibrinous exudate, is *pulsating pleurisy,* first described by MacDonnell, Sr., of Montreal. In 95 cases collected by Sailer it was much more frequent in males than in females. In 38 there was a tumor; that is, empyema necessitatis. In all but one case the fluid was purulent. Pneumothorax may be present. There are two groups of cases, the intrapleural pulsating pleurisy and the pulsating *empyema necessitatis,* in which there is an external pulsating tumor. No satisfactory explanation has been offered how the heart impulse is thus forcibly communicated through the effusion.

Empyema is a chronic affection, which in a few instances terminates naturally in recovery, but a majority of cases, if left alone, end in death. The following are some modes of natural cure: (*a*) By absorption of the fluid. In small effusions this may take place gradually. The chest wall sinks. The pleural layers become greatly thickened and enclose between them the inspissated pus, in which lime salts are gradually deposited. Such a condition may be seen once or twice a year in the post mortem room of any large hospital. (*b*) By perforation of the lung. Although in this event death may take place rapidly, by suffocation, as Aretæus says, yet in cases in which it occurs gradually recovery may follow. Empyema may discharge either by opening into the bronchus and forming a fistula, or, as Traube pointed out, by producing necrosis of the pulmonary pleura, sufficient to allow the soaking of the pus through the spongy lung tissue into the bronchi. In the first way pneumothorax usually, though not always, develops. In the second way the pus is discharged, without formation of pneumothorax. Even with a bronchial fistula recovery is possible. (*c*) By perforation of the chest wall—*empyema necessitatis.* This is by no means an unfavorable method, as many cases recover. The perforation may occur anywhere in the chest wall, but is, as Cruveilhier remarked, more common in front. It may be anywhere from the third to the sixth interspace, usually, according to Marshall, in the fifth. It may perforate in more than one place, and there may be a fistulous communication which opens into the pleura at some distance from the external orifice. The tumor, when near the heart, may pulsate. The discharge may persist for years. In Copeland's Dictionary is mentioned an instance of a Bavarian physician who had a pleural fistula for thirteen years and enjoyed fairly good health.

An empyema may perforate the neighboring organs, the œsophagus, peritoneum, pericardium, or the stomach. A remarkable sequel is a pleuro-œsophageal fistula, of which cases have been reported by Voelcker, Thursfield, and Osler. In one case there was a fistulous communication through the chest wall. Very remarkable cases are those which pass down the spine and along the psoas into the iliac fossa, and simulate a psoas or lumbar abscess.

Encapsulated Empyema.—In lobar or broncho-pneumonia, pockets of pus from the size of an egg to an orange may form. A good many cases were met with in the streptococcus empyema during the War, and H. M. Thomas, Jr., calls attention to the frequency of abdominal pain and meteorism, the early prostration, the high leukocytosis, and the danger of rupture into the pleura. The condition may be revealed only by the X-ray picture.

IV. TUBERCULOSIS PLEURISY

This has already been considered (p. 178), and the symptoms and physical signs do not require any description other than that already given in connection with the sero-fibrinous and purulent forms.

V. OTHER VARIETIES OF PLEURISY

Hæmorrhagic Pleurisy.—A bloody effusion is met with under the following conditions: (*a*) In the pleurisy of *asthenic states,* such as cancer, nephritis, and occasionally in the malignant fevers. It is interesting to note the frequency with which hæmorrhagic pleurisy is found in cirrhosis of the liver. It occurred in the very patient in whom Laennec first accurately described this disease. While this may be a simple hæmorrhagic pleurisy, in a majority of the cases it has been tuberculous. (*b*) *Tuberculous pleurisy,* in which the bloody effusion may result from the rupture of newly formed vessels in the soft exudate accompanying the eruption of miliary tubercles, or it may come from more slowly formed tubercles in a pleurisy secondary to extensive pulmonary disease. (*c*) *Cancerous pleurisy,* whether primary or secondary, is frequently hæmorrhagic. (*d*) Occasionally hæmorrhagic exudation is met with in perfectly healthy individuals, in whom there is not the slightest suspicion of tuberculosis or cancer. In one such case, a large, able-bodied man, the patient was healthy and strong eight years afterward. And, lastly, it must be remembered that during aspiration the lung may be wounded and blood in this way be mixed with the sero-fibrinous exudate. The condition of hæmorrhagic pleurisy is to be distinguished from hæmothorax.

Diaphragmatic Pleurisy.—The inflammation may be limited partly or chiefly to the diaphragmatic surface. This is often a dry pleurisy, but there may be effusion, either sero-fibrinous or purulent, which is circumscribed on the diaphragmatic surface. In these cases the pain is low in the zone of the diaphragm and may simulate that of acute abdominal disease. It may be intensified by pressure at the point of insertion of the diaphragm at the tenth rib. The diaphragm is fixed and the respiration is thoracic and short. Andral noted severe dyspnœa and attacks simulating angina in some cases. The effusion is usually plastic, not serous. Serous or purulent effusions of any size limited to the diaphragmatic surface are extremely rare. Intense subjective with trifling objective features are suggestive of diaphragmatic pleurisy.

Encysted Pleurisy.—The effusion may be circumscribed by adhesions or separated into two or more pockets or loculi, which communicate with each other. This is most common in empyema. In these cases there have usually been, at different parts of the pleura, multiple adhesions by which the fluid is limited. In other instances the recent false membranes may encapsulate the exudation on the diaphragmatic surface, for example, or the part of the pleura posterior to the mid-axillary line. In some cases the tactile fremitus is retained along certain lines of adhesion. The condition may be very puzzling and present special difficulties in diagnosis. The exploratory needle should be freely used and the X-rays employed.

Interlobar pleurisy forms an interesting and not uncommon variety. In nearly every instance of acute pleurisy the interlobar serous surfaces are also involved and closely agglutinated together, and sometimes the fluid is encysted between them. In this position tubercles are to be carefully looked for. In a case of this kind following pneumonia there was an enormous purulent collection between the lower and upper and middle lobes of the right side which looked at first like a large abscess of the lung. These collections may perforate the bronchi, and the cases present special difficulties in diagnosis.

Chylothorax.—This is a rare condition first described by Bartolet in 1633. E. H. Funk found only 54 cases of chylous effusion reported (1918). Three forms of milk-like effusion occur; (1) chylous, (2) chyliform, and (3) pseudo-chylous. The cause of the *chylous* effusion is trauma, in which the thoracic duct is ruptured, or pressure causing a backward flow along the pulmonary and pleural lymphatics. The fluid accumulates rapidly. The signs are those of a serous effusion and the diagnosis is made only by aspiration. The fluid is milky in appearance and contains fat in minute globules. The fat may be as high as 4 per cent. The specific gravity exceeds 1.012. The *chyliform* effusion is usually associated with tuberculosis or neoplasm and accumulates slowly. The milky appearance is regarded as due to fat liberated by the breaking down of leucocytes and endothelial cells which have undergone fatty degeneration. The *pseudo-chylous* fluid has a specific gravity below 1.012 and is poor in solids. It occurs in heart disease, amyloid disease, and nephritis (syphilitic?).

Treatment.—Injury to the thoracic duct during operation may require ligation. For the effusion tapping is indicated if pressure symptoms are present but a large amount should not be removed at one time. Any underlying condition should receive proper treatment.

Diagnosis of Pleurisy

Acute plastic pleurisy is readily recognized. In the diagnosis of pleuritic effusion the first question is, Does a fluid exudate exist? the second, What is its nature? In large effusions the increase in the size of the affected side, the immobility, the absence of tactile fremitus, together with the displacement of organs, give infallible indications of the presence of fluid. The chief difficulty arises in effusions of moderate extent, when the dulness, the presence of bronchophony, and, perhaps, tubular breathing may simulate *pneumonia.* The chief points to be borne in mind are: (*a*) Differences in the onset and in the general characters of the two affections, more particularly the initial chill, the higher fever, more urgent dyspnœa, and the rusty expectoration, which characterize pneumonia. As already mentioned, some of the cases of pneumococcus pleurisy set in like pneumonia. (*b*) Certain physical signs—the more wooden character of the dulness, the greater resistance, and the marked diminution or the absence of tactile fremitus in pleurisy. The auscultatory signs may be deceptive. It is usually, indeed, the persistence of tubular breathing, particularly the high-pitched, even amphoric expiration, heard in some cases of pleurisy, which has raised the doubt. The intercostal spaces are more commonly obliterated in pleuritic effusion than in pneumonia.

The displacement of organs is a very valuable sign. Nowadays with an exploring needle the question is easily settled. In cases of doubt the exploratory puncture should be made without hesitation. Pus is sometimes not obtained if too small a needle is used. Pneumothorax is an occasional sequence. The needle is especially useful in those cases in which there are pseudo-cavernous signs at the base. In cases, too, of massive pneumonia, in which the bronchi are plugged with fibrin, if the patient has not been seen from the outset, the diagnosis may be impossible without it.

On the left side it may be difficult to differentiate a very large *pericardial* from a pleural effusion. The retention of resonance at the base, the presence of tympany toward the axilla, the absence of dislocation of the heart-beat to the right of the sternum, the feebleness of the pulse and of the heart-sounds, and the urgency of the dyspnœa, out of all proportion to the extent of the effusion, are the chief points to be considered. Hydrothorax, which is not uncommon in heart-disease, presents signs identical with those of sero-fibrinous effusion. Certain *tumors* within the chest may simulate pleural effusion. It should be remembered that many intrathoracic growths are accompanied by exudation. Malignant disease of the lung and of the pleura and hydatids of the pleura produce extensive dulness, with suppression of the breath-sounds, simulating closely effusion.

On the right side, abscess of the liver, subdiaphragmatic abscess, and hydatid cysts may rise high into the pleura and produce dulness and enfeebled breathing. Often in these cases there is a friction sound, which should excite suspicion, and the upper outline of the dulness is sometimes plainly convex. In a case of cancer of the kidney the growth involved the diaphragm very early, and for months there were signs of pleurisy before our attention was directed to the kidney. In all cases of doubt the X-ray examination is a great aid; exploratory puncture should be done without hesitation.

The second question, as to the nature of the fluid, is quickly decided by the use of the needle. The persistent fever, the occurrence of sweats, a leucocytosis, and the increase in the pallor suggest the presence of pus. In children the complexion is often sallow and earthy. In protracted cases, even in children, when the general symptoms and the appearance of the patient have been most strongly suggestive of pus, the syringe has withdrawn clear fluid. On the other hand, effusions of short duration may be purulent, even when the general symptoms do not suggest it. In pneumonia the practitioner should be on the alert if the crisis is delayed or the temperature rises after the crisis, if chills and sweats follow, or if the cough changes to one of paroxysmal type of great intensity. There are three groups: (*a*) The presence of the empyema is readily detected. (*b*) It is suspected, but it is not possible to locate the pus by the ordinary physical means. The exploratory needle should be freely used. (*c*) In a few instances small interlobar collections, small mural abscesses, and the diaphragmatic form may escape detection until an exploratory operation is performed. The prognostic import of the bacteriological examination of the aspirated fluid is as follows: The pneumococcus is of favorable significance, as such cases usually get well rapidly, even with a single aspiration. The streptococcus empyema is the most serious form, and even after a free drainage the patient may succumb to a general septicæmia. A sterile fluid indicates in a majority of instances a tuberculous origin. In the distinction between an exudate (pleurisy) and a transudate (hydrothorax) from the fluid, the points are: Specific gravity above 1.020 in exudate, below 1.015 in transudate; albumin 30 to 65 gms. per litre and fibrinogen 1 in exudate, and in transudate 10 to 30 gms. albumin and fibrinogen 0.1 gm. per litre.

Treatment

Acute Fibrinous Pleurisy.—The patient should be in bed. At the onset the severe pain may be relieved by hot or cold applications, but a hypodermic of morphia is more effective. The Paquelin cautery may be lightly applied. It is well to administer a mercurial or saline purge. Fixing the side by strapping with adhesive plaster, which should pass well over the middle line, applied tightly and evenly at full expiration, gives great relief. Dry cupping may be employed. Blisters are of no special service in the acute stages, although they relieve the pain. The ice-bag may be used as in pneumonia. The open-air treatment should be begun early, as a majority of the cases are tuberculous. Medicines are rarely required and mercurials are not indicated. Dover's powder or codein may be given at night.

When *effusion* has taken place, mustard plasters or iodine, producing slight counter-irritation, appear useful, particularly in the later stages. Iodide of potassium is of doubtful benefit. By some the salicylates are believed to be of special efficacy; but drug treatment of the disease is unsatisfactory. A dry diet and frequent saline purges (in concentrated form before breakfast) may be tried and it has been advised to use a salt-free diet, but these measures are disappointing.

Early and if necessary repeated *aspiration* is the most satisfactory treatment. The results obtained by Delafield in 200 cases treated by early aspiration have never been equalled by any other method. The credit of introducing aspiration in pleuritic effusions is due to Morrill Wyman, of Cambridge, Mass., and Henry I. Bowditch, of Boston. Years prior to Dieulafoy's work, aspiration was in constant use at the Massachusetts General Hospital and advocated repeatedly by Bowditch. As the question is one of some historical interest, we give Bowditch's conclusions concerning aspiration, expressed more than sixty years ago, and which practically represent the opinion of to-day: "(1) The operation is perfectly simple, but slightly painful, and can be done with ease upon any patient in however advanced a stage of the disease. (2) It should be performed forthwith in *all* cases in which there is complete filling up of one side of the chest. (3) He had determined to use it in *any* case of even *moderate* effusion lasting more than a few weeks and in which there should seem to be a disposition to resist ordinary modes of treatment. (4) He urged this practice upon the profession as a very important measure in practical medicine; believing that by this method death may frequently be prevented from ensuing either by sudden attack of dyspnœa or subsequent phthisis, and, finally, from the gradual wearing out of the powers of life or inability to absorb the fluid." When the fluid reaches to the clavicle the indication for aspiration is imperative. Fever is not a contra-indication; indeed, sometimes with serous exudates the temperature falls after aspiration.

The operation is simple and practically without risk. The spot selected for puncture should be either in the sixth intercostal space in the mid-axilla or at the outer angle of the scapula in the eighth space. The arm of the patient should be brought forward with the hand on the opposite shoulder, so as to widen the spaces. The needle should be thrust in close to the upper margin of the rib, so as to avoid the intercostal artery, the wounding of which, however, is exceedingly rare. The fluid should be withdrawn slowly. The amount will depend on the size of the exudate. If the fluid reaches to the clavicle a litre or more may be withdrawn with safety. As the fluid is withdrawn it may be replaced by oxygen, run in under a pressure of 4 mm. Hg. In chronic cases of serous pleurisy after the failure of repeated tappings S. West showed the value of free incision and drainage. He reported cases of recovery after effusions of fifteen and eighteen months' standing.

Repeated tapping may be required in some cases. In the chronic cases the injection of epinephrin (20 to 30 drops of a 1 to 1,000 solution) into the pleural cavity after aspiration has proved of value.

Symptoms and Accidents during Paracentesis.—Pain is usually complained of after a certain amount of fluid has been withdrawn; it is sharp and cutting in character. *Coughing* occurs toward the close, and may be severe and paroxysmal. *Pneumothorax* may follow an exploratory puncture or aspiration. *Subcutaneous emphysema* may develop from the point of puncture, without the production of pneumothorax. *Cerebral symptoms.*—Faintness is not uncommon. Convulsions may occur during the withdrawal or while irrigating the pleura. These symptoms are regarded by most authors as of reflex origin. Hemiplegia may follow. And lastly *sudden death* may occur either from syncope or during the convulsions.

As A. E. Russell has pointed out, these serious and even fatal events may follow exploratory puncture of the lung. Such accidents of paracentesis and of washing out the pleura are explained by the studies of Capps and Lewis, who have shown that a sudden and sometimes fatal fall in blood pressure may follow the experimental irrigation of the pleura in dogs. Occasionally toxic symptoms arise resembling those of the "serum illness"—pains in the joints, albumin in the urine, and œdema—suggestive of the absorption of toxins that act like a heterogeneous serum. Expectoration of a large quantity of *albuminous fluid* may occur suddenly after the tapping, associated with dyspnœa. Some cases have proved rapidly fatal, with the features of an acute œdema of the lungs. It occurs usually after large amounts are removed.

The after-treatment of pleurisy is important and the patients should be handled exactly as if they had an early tuberculous lung lesion.

Empyema.—A majority of the cases get well, provided that free drainage is obtained, and it makes no difference practically what measures are followed so long as this indication is met. In a few cases with turbid fluid, between sero-fibrinous and purulent, recovery follows aspiration. The good results in any method depend upon the thoroughness with which the cavity is drained. Irrigation of the cavity is rarely necessary unless the contents are fetid. In the subsequent treatment a point of great importance in facilitating the closure of the cavity is the distention of the lung on the affected side. This may be accomplished by the method advised by Ralston James, which has been practised with great success, especially in children. The patient daily, for a certain length of time, increasing gradually with the increase of his strength, transfers by air-pressure water from one bottle to another. The bottles should be large, holding at least a gallon each, and by the arrangement of tubes, as in the Wolff's bottle, an expiratory effort of the patient forces the water from one bottle into the other. Equally efficacious is the plan advised by Naunyn. The patient sits in an arm-chair grasping strongly one of the rungs with the hand and forcibly compressing the sound side against the arm of the chair; then forcible inspiratory efforts are made which act chiefly on the compressed lung, as the sound side is fixed. The abscess cavity is gradually closed, partly by the falling in of the chest wall and partly by the expansion of the lung. In some instances it is necessary to resect portions of one or more ribs.

Until recently efficient drainage has been regarded as the most important consideration, and both operative and drainage proceedings have been directed toward making the chest wall conform to the lung. While thoracotomy and free drainage have done a great deal, it must be confessed that in a not inconsiderable number of cases the obliteration of the pus cavity has been a long and sometimes hopeless matter. In its place continuous drainage and intermittent siphonage have been used.

The physician is often asked, in cases of empyema with emaciation, fever and feeble, rapid pulse, whether the patient can stand the operation. Even in the most desperate cases one should never hesitate to make a free incision.

II. CHRONIC PLEURISY

This affection occurs in two forms:

Chronic pleurisy with effusion in which the disease may set in insidiously or may follow an acute sero-fibrinous pleurisy. There are cases in which the fluid persists for months or even years without undergoing any special alteration and without becoming purulent. Such cases have the characters which we have described under pleurisy with effusion.

Chronic Dry Pleurisy.—The cases are met with (*a*) *as a sequence of ordinary pleural effusion.* When the exudate is absorbed and the layers of the pleura come together there is left between them a variable amount of fibrinous material which gradually undergoes organization, and is converted into a layer of firm connective tissue. This process goes on at the base, and is represented clinically by a slight grade of flattening, deficient expansion, defective resonance on percussion, and enfeebled breathing. After recovery from empyema the flattening and retraction may be still more marked. In both cases it is a condition which can be greatly benefited by pulmonary gymnastics. In these firm, fibrous membranes calcification may occur, particularly after empyema. It is not very uncommon to find between the false membranes a small pocket of fluid forming a sort of pleural cyst. In the great majority of these cases the condition need not cause anxiety. There may be an occasional dragging pain at the base of the lung or a stitch in the side, but patients may remain in perfectly good health for years. The most advanced grade of this secondary dry pleurisy is seen in those cases of empyema which have been left to themselves and have perforated and ultimately healed by a gradual absorption or discharge of the pus, with retraction of the side of the chest and permanent carnification of the lung. Traumatic lesions, such as gunshot wounds, may be followed by an identical condition. Post mortem, it is quite impossible to separate the layers of the pleura, which are greatly thickened, particularly at the base, and surround a compressed, airless, fibroid lung. Bronchiectasis may gradually ensue, sometimes not only on the affected side, but also in the lower lobe of the other lung.

(*b*) *Primitive dry pleurisy.*—This condition may directly follow the acute plastic pleurisy already described; but it may set in without any acute symptoms whatever, and the patient's attention may be called to it by feeling the pleural friction. A constant effect of this primitive dry pleurisy is the adhesion of the layers. This is probably an invariable result, whether the pleurisy is primary or secondary. The organization of the thin layer of exudation in a pneumonia will unite the two surfaces by delicate bands. Pleural adhesions are extremely common, and it is rare to examine a body entirely free from them. They may be limited in extent or universal. Thin fibrous adhesions do not produce any alteration in the percussion characters, and, if limited, there is no special change heard on auscultation. When, however, there is general synechia on both sides the expansile movement of the lung is considerably impaired. We should naturally think that universal adhesions would interfere materially with the function of the lungs, but practically we see many instances in which there has not been the slightest disturbance. The physical signs of total adhesion are by no means constant. It has been stated that there is a marked disproportion between the degree of expansion of the chest walls and the intensity of the vesicular murmur, but the latter is a very variable factor, and under perfectly normal conditions the breath-sounds, with very full chest expansion, may be extremely feeble. The diaphragm phenomenon—Litten's sign—is absent.

It is probable that a primitive dry pleurisy may lead to great thickening of the membranes, and ultimate invasion of the lung, causing a cirrhosis.

Lastly, there is a primitive dry pleurisy of tuberculous origin. In it both parietal and costal layers are greatly thickened—perhaps from 2 to 3 mm. each—and present firm fibroid, caseous masses and small tubercles, while uniting these two greatly thickened layers is a reddish-gray fibroid tissue, sometimes infiltrated with serum. This may be a local process confined to one pleura, or it may be in both. These cases are sometimes associated with a similar condition in the pericardium and peritoneum.

Occasionally remarkable vaso-motor phenomena occur in chronic pleurisy, whether simple or in connection with tuberculosis of an apex. Flushing or sweating of one cheek or dilatation of the pupil are the common manifestations. They appear to be due to involvement of the first thoracic ganglion at the top of the pleural cavity.

Treatment.—It is well to carry out the general treatment for tuberculosis. In some cases the use of exercises may be of value, but the chances of helping the local condition materially by any treatment are not good.

III. HYDROTHORAX

Hydrothorax is a transudation of simple non-inflammatory fluid into the pleural cavities, and occurs as a secondary process in many affections. The fluid is clear, without any flocculi of fibrin, and the membranes are smooth. It is met with more particularly in connection with general dropsy, either renal, cardiac, or hæmic. It may, however, occur alone, or with only slight œdema of the feet. A child was admitted to the Montreal General Hospital with urgent dyspnœa and cyanosis, and died the night after admission. She had extensive bilateral hydrothorax, which had come on early in the nephritis of scarlet fever. In renal disease hydrothorax is almost always bilateral, but in heart affections one pleura is more commonly involved. The physical signs are those of pleural effusion, but the exudation is rarely excessive. In kidney and heart-disease, even when there is no general dropsy, the occurrence of dyspnœa should at once direct attention to the pleura, since many patients are carried off by a rapid effusion. In chronic valvular disease the effusion is usually on the right side, and may recur for months. The greater frequency of the dextral effusion has been attributed to compression of the azygos vein, but compression of the pulmonary veins by the dilated right auricle seems more probable. Post mortem records show the frequency with which this condition is overlooked. The saline purges will in many cases rapidly reduce the effusion, but, if necessary, aspiration should be practised repeatedly.

IV. HÆMOTHORAX

This is a common sequence of wounds of the chest by bullets, shrapnel or bayonet; thousands of cases occurred in the recent war. A high velocity bullet may pass through the chest and lung without causing serious damage and the man may be walking about within a week. The blood usually comes from the lung. The amount varies from a few ounces to four or five pints. When withdrawn the blood forms a scanty clot. The fluid is not all blood, but mixed with serous exudate with many leucocytes, endothelial and eosinophile cells. Even when large amounts are present there may be no signs of anæmia. The pleural surfaces are covered with a thin film of fibrin. Pneumothorax and pneumo-hæmothorax are rare, 8 cases of the latter and 4 of the former in 328 cases of gunshot wounds of the chest (Bradford and Elliott).

Symptoms.—Shock, cough, dyspnœa, and spitting of blood are present in a majority of the cases. Slight fever is frequent and the pulse is quickened. If not infected the progress is uneventful. The cough lessens, slight fever persists, but with moderate exudates the absorption is rapid. A slight icteric tinge of the skin may be present.

The *physical signs* vary with the amount of fluid. With a massive exudate there is a flat or Skodaic note on percussion, absence of fremitus, and distant or feeble tubular breathing. The signs are often less distinctive than with simple effusion. With the fluoroscope the diaphragm is seen to be high. A remarkable phenomenon, not seen in ordinary effusion, is the early flattening and immobility of the side, which with the high level of the diaphragm speaks for massive collapse of the lung, with displacement of the heart towards the affected side. This may take place with moderate effusion and may disappear rapidly. Contralateral collapse of the unaffected lung is met with not infrequently, indicated by flatness at the opposite base with tubular breathing and increased fremitus.

Complications.—Septic infection is indicated by increasing fever and pulse rate, persistence of cough, increase of the exudate, sweats, etc. Secondary hæmorrhage is rare. Pneumonia, pericarditis, purulent bronchitis, abscess and gangrene, and general streptococcus infection may occur.

Treatment.—Without infection a majority of the cases get well with rest in bed, but increase of the dyspnœa may demand aspiration. Oxygen replacement is useful in large effusions. Infection calls for free drainage.

V. PNEUMOTHORAX

(*Hydro-Pneumothorax and Pyo-Pneumothorax*)

Air alone in the pleural cavity, to which the term pneumothorax is strictly applicable, is an extremely rare condition. It is almost invariably associated with a serous fluid—hydro-pneumothorax, or with pus—pyo-pneumothorax.

Etiology.—There exists normally within the pleural cavity of an adult a negative pressure of several (3 to 5) millimetres of mercury, due to the recoil of the distended, perfectly elastic lung. Hence, through any opening connecting the pleural cavity with the external air we should expect air to rush in until this negative pressure is relieved. To explain the absence of pneumothorax in a few cases of injury laying the pleura bare, in which it would be expected, S. West assumed the existence of a cohesion between the pleuræ, but this force has not as yet been satisfactorily demonstrated.

If the opening causing the pneumothorax remains patent, which occurs in some external wounds and in perforations through consolidated areas of the lung, the intrathoracic pressure will be that of the atmosphere. The lung will be found to have collapsed as much as possible by virtue of its own elastic tension, the intercostal grooves are obliterated, the heart is displaced, and the diaphragm depressed, because the negative pressure by which these organs are partly retained in their ordinary position has been relieved. If the opening becomes closed the intrathoracic pressure may rise above the atmospheric and the displacements be much increased. But most perforations through the lung are valvular, a property of lung tissue, and the intrapleural pressure is soon about 7 mm. of mercury. If there be a fluid exudate the pressure may be higher, but the high pressures supposed are more apparent than real, and that measured at the autopsy table is quite surely not that during life. It is more a question of the amount of distention than the actual pressure which determines the discomfort of the patient.

Pneumothorax arises: (1) In perforating wounds of the chest, in which case it is sometimes associated with extensive cutaneous emphysema. It may follow exploratory puncture either with a small needle or an aspirator. Pneumothorax rarely follows fracture of the rib, even though the lung may be torn. (2) In perforation of the pleura through the diaphragm, usually by malignant disease of the stomach or colon, or abscess of the liver. The pleura may also be perforated in cases of cancer of the œsophagus. (3) When the lung is perforated, by far the most common cause: (*a*) In the normal lung from rupture of the air-vesicles during straining or even when at rest. The air may be absorbed and no ill effect follow. It does not necessarily excite pleurisy, as pointed out many years ago by Gairdner, but inflammation and effusion are the usual result. (*b*) From perforation due to local disease of the lung, either the softening of a caseous focus or the breaking of a tuberculous cavity. According to S. West, 90 per cent. of all the cases are due to this cause. Less common are the cases due to septic broncho-pneumonia and to gangrene. A rare cause is the breaking of a hæmorrhagic infarct in chronic heart-disease. (*c*) Perforation of the lung from the pleura, which arises in certain cases of empyema and produces a pleuro-bronchial fistula. (4) Spontaneously, by the development in pleural exudates of the gas bacillus (*B. aërogenes capsulatus* Welch). Of 48 cases, the basis of Emerson's monograph (J. H. H. Reports, vol. xi), 22 were tuberculous, 6 were the result of trauma, 10 of aspiration, 2 were spontaneous, 2 followed bronchiectasis, 2 abscess of the lung, 1 gangrene, 2 an empyema, and 1 abscess of the liver perforating through the lung.

Pneumothorax occurs chiefly in adults, is rare in young children and more frequent in males than in females.

A remarkable recurrent variety has been described by S. West, Goodhart, and Furney. In Goodhart's case the pneumothorax developed first in one side and then in the other.

Morbid Anatomy.—If the trocar or blow-pipe is inserted between the ribs, there may be a jet of air of sufficient strength to blow out a lighted match. On opening the thorax the mediastinum and pericardium are seen to be displaced to the opposite side; but the heart is not rotated, and the relation of its parts is maintained much as in the normal condition. A serous or purulent fluid is usually present, and the membranes are inflamed. The cause of the pneumothorax can usually be found without difficulty. In the great majority of instances it is the perforation of a tuberculous cavity or a breaking of a superficial caseous focus. The orifice of rupture may be extremely small. In chronic cases there may be a fistula of considerable size communicating with the bronchi. The lung is usually compressed and carnified.

Symptoms.—Pain on the affected side and dyspnœa are the usual symptoms of onset. The rupture may be felt or even heard by the patient. The cough may be aggravated with an increase in the amount of sputum. In severe cases the color becomes livid, the pulse feeble and rapid, there is sweating with signs of great respiratory distress—the pneumothorax acutissimus of Unverricht. The patient may become unconscious and die within twenty-four hours. In 23 per cent. of 385 cases the onset was insidious (O. H. P. Pepper). The "splash" may be the first indication to the patient of any change.

Physical Signs.—*Inspection* shows marked enlargement of the affected side with immobility. The patient usually lies on the affected side. The heart impulse is usually much displaced. On *palpation* the fremitus is greatly diminished or more commonly abolished. It may be increased in front due possibly to bands of adhesions or a lung pressed up against the chest wall. On *percussion* the resonance has a tympanitic or an amphoric quality. This, however, is not always the case. It may be a dull tympany, resembling Skoda's resonance. In some instances it may be a full, hyperresonant note, like emphysema; while in others there is dulness. These extreme variations depend doubtless upon the degree of intrapleural tension. Error in diagnosis may result from ignorance of the fact that the percussion note may be "muffled, toneless, almost dull" (Walshe). There is usually dulness at the base from effused fluid, which can readily be made to change by altering the position of the patient. When recumbent the tympanitic note on the right side may reach the costal border, when erect the dulness may be at the third rib. The liver flatness may be obliterated. On *auscultation* the breath-sounds are suppressed. Sometimes there is only a distant feeble inspiratory murmur of marked amphoric quality. The contrast between the loud exaggerated breath-sounds on the normal side and the absence of the breath-sounds on the other is very suggestive. The râles have a peculiar metallic quality, and on coughing or deep inspiration there may be what Laennec termed the metallic tinkle. This sound, like striking a glass vessel with a pin, may even be heard some distance from the patient or in all parts of the room (Allbutt). A gurgling sound may be heard during inspiration, the so-called "water whistle noise." The voice has a curious metallic echo. The coin-sound, termed by Trousseau the *bruit d'airain,* is very characteristic. To obtain it the auscultator should place one ear on the back of the chest wall while the assistant taps one coin on another on the front of the chest. The metallic echoing sound which is produced in this way is one of the most constant and characteristic signs of pneumothorax. The Hippocratic succussion splash may be obtained when the auscultator's head is placed upon the chest while the patient's body is shaken. A splashing sound is produced, which may be audible at a distance. A patient may himself notice it in making abrupt changes in posture. The metallic phenomena are best heard in cases with a consolidated lung and thickened pleura, as in tuberculosis. The movable dulness and splash depend on fluid. Of other physical signs displacement of organs is most constant. The heart may be "drawn over" to the opposite side, and the liver greatly displaced, so that its upper surface is below the level of the costal margin, a degree of dislocation rarely seen in simple effusion.

Gas analysis.—Emerson determined experimentally that of the air introduced, the oxygen rapidly diminishes, but the nitrogen remains very constant. An increasing amount of oxygen suggests an open fistula. Air is absorbed rapidly from the normal pleura and in spontaneous cases the signs may disappear within a week; in other instances weeks or months may elapse.

Diagnosis.—In cases in which the percussion note is dull the condition may be mistaken for effusion. Diaphragmatic or congenital hernia following a crush or other accident may closely simulate it. Pneumothorax in a patient with emphysema may cause difficulty. Percussion of the lower border of the lung on the affected side shows that the resonance in pneumothorax extends to the lowest part of the pleural cavity and is fixed, not changing with in- and expiration.

Very large cavities with tympanitic percussion resonance and râles of an amphoric, metallic quality, may simulate pneumothorax. In total excavation of one lung the amphoric and metallic phenomena may be intense, but the absence of dislocation of the organs, of the succussion splash, and of the coin-sound suffices to differentiate this condition. While this is true in the great majority of cases, the coin sound may be heard over a large cavity in the right upper lobe. The condition of pyo-pneumothorax subphrenicus may simulate closely true pneumothorax.

X-ray Examination.—The characteristic features are an abnormally clear zone without the normal lung markings, the shadow of the collapsed lung not always easy to see, and the visceral displacements. The fluid shows as an opaque shadow and with the fluoroscope a wavy outline of the fluid may be seen in shaking the patient. An aneurism pressing on one bronchus may cause great inflation of the lung and a condition which gives clinical and X-ray features suggestive of pneumothorax.

Prognosis.—This depends largely upon the cause. S. West gives a mortality of 70 per cent. The tuberculous cases usually die within a few weeks. Of 22 tuberculous cases 20 died, and 5 of the 10 cases following aspiration (J. H. H. Series). There are tuberculous cases in which the pneumothorax, if occurring early, seems to arrest the progress of the tuberculosis. There is a chronic pneumothorax which may last between three and four years. The outlook in spontaneous pneumothorax is good. It may recur or it may appear later in the other side. Though usually not tuberculous and due to a ruptured bleb or a tear, it may be followed years later by tuberculosis of the lung (Hamman).

Treatment.—The patient should be kept as quiet as possible and morphia given to secure this if necessary. He should be encouraged to suppress cough and avoid deep respirations. Strapping the affected side and the giving of sedatives, such as codein and heroin, may lessen cough. With fluid present it may be necessary to remove some if there are pressure symptoms, but it is better left alone if possible for two weeks or until the fistula is closed. There are three groups of cases: First, in the pneumothorax acutissimus, with urgent dyspnœa, great displacement of the heart, cyanosis, and low blood pressure, an opening should be made in the pleura and kept open, converting a valvular into an open variety. Immediate aspiration with a trocar has saved life. Secondly, the spontaneous cases which usually do well, as the air is quickly absorbed; so also with the traumatic variety. Very many of the tuberculous cases are best let alone, if the patient is doing well, or if the disease in the other lung is advanced. Thirdly, when there is pus, and the patient is not doing well, or in the tuberculous variety if the other lung is not involved, pleurotomy, or resection of one or two ribs, may be done. Of nine cases in our series two recovered. Repeated aspiration may result in marked improvement.

VI. AFFECTIONS OF THE MEDIASTINUM

Lymphadenitis.—The greater number of glands are on the right side, and the right bronchus passes off at a higher level (fifth dorsal vertebra) than the left. The glands are constantly enlarged in all inflammatory affections of the lungs. In all the acute affections of childhood they are found swollen. They are almost constantly involved in tuberculosis of the lungs and they are not infrequently the only organs found tuberculous. Often in children the glands on the lung root become enlarged and caseous and penetrate deeply into the hilus and into the lung itself.

The *symptoms* of enlarged mediastinal glands are very uncertain in the simple and tuberculous forms. On the other hand in Hodgkin's disease and in sarcoma pressure symptoms are the rule.

Much attention has been paid to the diagnosis of this condition and authors speak lightly of the possibility of recognizing by percussion various grades of enlargement. It is claimed that the pressure of the glands on the right bronchus may cause a dulness in the right lung apex due to slight collapse. Examined by the X-rays, the percentage of children with enlarged mediastinal glands is very high, 50 to 60 in some series. D'Espine says there is a change in the whispered voice which has a bronchial ring at the level of the seventh cervical and last dorsal, and the respiratory murmur may be rougher and harsher.

Suppurative Lymphadenitis.—Occasionally abscess in the bronchial or tracheal lymph-glands is found. It may follow the simple adenitis, but is most frequently associated with tubercle. The liquid portion may gradually be absorbed and the inspissated contents undergo calcification. Serious accidents occasionally occur, as perforation into the œsophagus or into a bronchus, or in rare instances, as in the case reported by Sidney Phillips, perforation of the aorta, as well as a bronchus, which did not prove fatal rapidly, but caused repeated attacks of hæmoptysis during a period of sixteen months.

Tumors.—Sarcoma is by far the most frequent tumor. Ross, in a study of 60 cases, found 44 cases of sarcoma and 10 of carcinoma. The lung was usually involved. In nearly 70 per cent. the anterior glands were affected. There are three chief points of origin, the thymus, the lymph-glands, and the pleura and lung. Males are more frequently affected than females. The age is most commonly between thirty and fifty.

Symptoms.—The signs of mediastinal tumor are those of intrathoracic pressure. In some cases almost the entire chest is filled with the masses. The heart and lungs are pushed back and it is marvelous how life can be maintained with such dislocation and compression of the organs. *Dyspnœa* is one of the earliest and most constant symptoms, and may be due either to pressure on the trachea or on the recurrent laryngeal nerves. It may, indeed, be cardiac, due to pressure upon the heart or its vessels. In a few cases it results from the pleural effusion which so frequently accompanies intrathoracic growths. Associated with the dyspnœa is a *cough,* often severe and paroxysmal in character, with the brazen quality of the so-called aneurismal cough when a recurrent nerve is involved. The voice may also be affected from a similar cause. Hæmoptysis may occur and the picture suggest pulmonary tuberculosis. Pressure on the vessels is common. The superior vena cava may be compressed and obliterated, and when the process goes on slowly the collateral circulation may be completely established. Less commonly the inferior vena cava or one or other of the subclavian veins is compressed. The arteries are much more rarely obstructed. There may be dysphagia, due to compression of the œsophagus. There may be pupillary changes, usually contraction. Expectoration of blood, pus, and hair is characteristic of the dermoid cyst, of which Christian noted 64 cases in 1914.

Physical Signs.—On inspection there may be orthopnœa and marked cyanosis of the upper part of the body. In such instances, if of long duration, there are signs of collateral circulation and the superficial mammary and epigastric veins are enlarged. In these cases of chronic obstruction the finger-tips may be clubbed. There may be bulging of the sternum or the tumor may erode the bone and form a prominent subcutaneous growth. The rapidly growing lymphoid tumors more commonly than others perforate the chest wall. In 4 of 13 cases of Hodgkin's disease there was mediastinal growth, and in 3 instances the sternum was eroded and perforated. The perforation may be on one side of the breast-bone. The projecting tumor may pulsate; the heart may be dislocated and its impulse much out of place. Contraction of one side of the thorax has been noted in a few instances. On palpation the fremitus is absent wherever the tumor reaches the chest wall. If pulsating, it rarely has the forcible, heaving impulse of an aneurismal sac. On auscultation there is usually silence over the dull region. The heart-sounds are not transmitted and the respiratory murmur is feeble or inaudible, rarely bronchial. Vocal resonance is, as a rule, absent. Signs of pleural effusion occur in a great many instances of mediastinal growth, and in doubtful cases the aspirator needle should be used.

Tumors of the *anterior mediastinum* originate usually in the thymus, or its remnants, or in the connective tissue; the sternum is pushed forward and often eroded. The growth may be felt in the suprasternal fossa; the cervical glands are usually involved. The pressure symptoms are chiefly upon the venous trunks. Dyspnœa is a prominent feature.

Intrathoracic tumors in the *middle* and *posterior mediastinum* originate most commonly in the lymph-glands. The symptoms are out of all proportion to the signs; there is urgent dyspnœa and cough, which is sometimes loud and ringing. The pressure symptoms are chiefly upon the gullet, the recurrent laryngeal, and sometimes upon the azygos vein.

In a third group, tumors originating in the *pleura* and the *lung,* the pressure symptoms are not so marked. Pleural exudate is very much more common; the patient becomes anæmic and emaciation is rapid. There may be secondary involvement of the lymph-glands in the neck.

DIAGNOSIS.—The diagnosis of mediastinal tumor from aneurism is sometimes extremely difficult. An interesting case reported and figured by Sokolosski, in Bd. 19 of the Deutsches Archiv für klinische Medicin, in which Oppolzer diagnosed aneurism and Skoda mediastinal tumor, illustrates how in some instances the most skillful of observers may be unable to agree. Scarcely a sign is found in aneurism which may not be duplicated in mediastinal tumor. This is not strange, since the symptoms in both are largely due to pressure. The cyanosis, the venous engorgement, the signs of collateral circulation are, as a rule, much more marked in tumor. The time element is important. If a case has persisted for more than eighteen months the disease is probably aneurism. There are, however, exceptions to this. By far the most valuable sign of aneurism is the diastolic shock so often to be felt, and in a majority of cases to be heard, over the sac. This is rarely, if ever, present in mediastinal growths, even when they perforate the sternum and have communicated pulsation. Tracheal tugging is rarely present in tumor. Another point of importance is that a tumor, advancing from the mediastinum, eroding the sternum, and appearing externally, if aneurismal, has forcible, heaving, and distinctly expansile pulsations. The radiating pain in the back and arms and neck is rather in favor of aneurism, as is also a beneficial influence on it of iodide of potassium. The remarkable traumatic cyanosis of the upper half of the body which follows compression injuries of the thorax could scarcely be mistaken for the effect of tumor. The X-ray picture is rarely at fault in differentiating aneurism and tumor.

The frequency of *pleural effusion* in connection with mediastinal tumor is to be constantly borne in mind. It may give curiously complex characters to the physical signs—characters which are profoundly modified after aspiration of the liquid. Occasionally a tumor of the mediastinum is operable.

Abscess of the Mediastinum.—Hare collected 115 cases of mediastinal abscess, in 77 of which there were details sufficient to permit the analysis. Of these cases the great majority occurred in males. Forty-four were instances of acute abscess. The anterior mediastinum is most commonly the seat of the suppuration. The cases are most frequently associated with trauma. Some have followed erysipelas or occurred in association with eruptive fevers. Many cases, particularly the chronic abscesses, are of tuberculous origin. Of *symptoms,* pain behind the sternum is the most common. It may be of a throbbing character, and in the acute cases is associated with fever, sometimes with chills and sweats. If the abscess is large there may be dyspnœa. The pus may burrow into the abdomen, perforate through an intercostal space, or erode the sternum. Instances are on record in which the abscess has discharged into the trachea or œsophagus. In chronic abscess the pus becomes inspissated and produces no ill effect. The *physical signs* are indefinite. A pulsating and fluctuating tumor may appear at the border of the sternum or at the sternal notch. The absence of *bruit,* of the diastolic shock, and of the expansile pulsation usually enables a correct diagnosis to be made. When in doubt a needle may be inserted.

Mediastinitis, Acute and Indurative.—The *acute* form occurs in pericarditis and pleurisy, sometimes as a primary disease in the infections, particularly pneumonia and syphilis. The symptoms are indefinite and it is rarely recognized clinically. Pain behind the sternum and pressure signs may be present and a well marked creaking friction with dulling of the percussion note on the sternum (C. P. Howard). It may pass on to abscess formation or more commonly to the *indurative form,* in which there is great increase in the fibrous tissues in the mediastinum, usually with adherent pericarditis. The process may extend and seriously compress or even obliterate the vessels. Certain of the cases of fibroid obliteration of the superior vena cava originate in this way. It is sometimes associated with chronic fibroid polyserositis. The process may begin about the aorta and is then usually syphilitic. Cyanosis, dyspnœa and cough are the prominent symptoms. The superficial veins are enlarged, the sternal note is flat, the X-ray picture shows a broad mediastinal shadow, there may be visible pulsation of the larynx and trachea and sometimes a loud creaking friction is heard. Swelling of the feet and ascites may be present, and when the thoracic duct is involved the ascitic fluid may be chylous. The heart may be enlarged with an associated adherent pericardium and the clinical picture at the end may be that of cardiac dropsy.

Miscellaneous Affections.—In Hare's study of 520 cases there were 7 instances of fibroma, 11 cases of dermoid cyst, 8 cases of hydatid cyst, and cases of lipoma and gumma.

Emphysema of the Mediastinum.—Air in the cellular tissues of the mediastinum is met with in cases of trauma, and occasionally in fatal cases of diphtheria and in whooping-cough. It may extend to the subcutaneous tissues. Champneys called attention to its frequency after tracheotomy, in which, he says, the conditions favoring the production are division of the deep fascia, obstruction in the air-passages, and inspiratory efforts. The deep fascia, he says, should not be raised from the trachea. It is often associated with pneumothorax, and more often in rupture of the lung without pneumothorax, the pleura remaining intact and the air dissecting its way along the bronchi into the mediastinum and into the neck. The condition seems by no means uncommon. Angel Money found it in 16 of 28 cases of tracheotomy, and in 2 of these pneumothorax also was present.

F. DISEASES OF THE DIAPHRAGM

From its importance in respiration any disturbance of the function of the diaphragm may result in marked symptoms, especially in respiration. With inflammation of either surface the proper contraction is affected. *Paralysis* may occur with central lesions or injury or disease of the phrenic nerves. It is seen with diphtheria and acute polio-myelitis. The arch of the diaphragm is high and there may be massive collapse of the lower lobe on the affected side. Bilateral paralysis is always serious. There is severe dyspnœa, the movements of the epigastrium and hypochondria are reversed, the lower thorax expands horizontally to a marked extent and with the fluoroscope the high position of the arches and absence of movement can be seen. Clonic *spasm* is present with hiccough, which, in acute illness, is a sign of gravity. Tonic spasm is sometimes seen in patients with emphysema and severe bronchitis. Diaphragmatic hernia has to be distinguished from pneumothorax. In case of doubt the X-ray study renders the diagnosis clear. *Inflammation* is common and usually secondary to some process in the thorax or abdomen. The lymphatic supply favors infection. The best example of an acute process is seen in diaphragmatic pleurisy. The most important causes of more chronic inflammation are pleuritis and tuberculosis. As a result of an acute process changes in the muscle and adhesions are common with resulting restriction of motion. This causes dyspnœa and possibly the pain and soreness in the lower thorax so common after pleurisy. Diminished expansion of the lower thorax, absence of Litten's sign, dulness and feeble breath sounds are found, due in part to thickened pleura. The X-ray study confirms the diagnosis and by it the exact condition can be determined. The extent of deformity of the diaphragm and restriction of motion are often striking. In pulmonary tuberculosis there may be decreased movement of the diaphragm even when the lung lesion is apical. In pneumoconiosis, in some cases of emphysema and of fibroid change, the deformity of the diaphragm and its restricted function are marked. In advanced stages of all these diseases this plays a considerable part in causing the symptoms, especially dyspnœa.

SECTION VIII

DISEASES OF THE KIDNEYS

I. MALFORMATIONS

Newman classifies them as follows: A. Displacements without mobility—(1) congenital displacement without deformity; (2) congenital displacement with deformity; (3) acquired displacements. B. Malformations of the kidney. I. Variations in number—(*a*) supernumerary kidney; (*b*) single kidney, congenital absence of one kidney, atrophy of one kidney; (*c*) absence of both kidneys. II. Variations in form and size—(*a*) general variations in form, lobulation, etc.; (*b*) hypertrophy of one kidney; (*c*) fusion of two kidneys—horseshoe kidney, sigmoid kidney, disk-shaped kidney. In the *horseshoe* kidney, the commonest form of fusion, the lower poles are usually joined. The condition sometimes may be recognized during life by palpation. C. Variations in pelvis, ureters, and blood-vessels.

The *fused* kidneys may form a large mass, which is often displaced, being either in an iliac fossa, in the mid line of the abdomen, or even in the pelvis. Under these circumstances it may be mistaken for a new growth. The organ has been removed under the belief that it was a floating kidney. One patient lived eleven days with complete anuria.

Congenital Hydro-Ureter and Hydronephrosis.—In this rare condition one kidney may be involved or one kidney with the ureters. A man aged 21 under the care of Halsted had from his second year severe attacks of abdominal pain in which a swelling would appear between the hip and costal margin and subside with the passage of a large amount of urine; a huge hydronephrotic sac was opened and drained. Of the bilateral congenital form there are two varieties. (1) A remarkable hypertrophy and dilatation of the bladder and ureters, associated with congenital defect of the abdominal muscles. The bladder may form a large abdominal tumor, and the ureters may be visible through the thin abdominal walls as coils resembling the small intestine. (2) There is a form of dilatation of the bladder, enlargement of the ureters and pelvis, with a clinical picture of chronic pyelonephritis and retention of the urine, resembling obstruction, but in which, post mortem, there is no demonstrable organic obstruction. There appears to be a congenital maldevelopment of the musculature of the pelves, ureters and bladder wall, or "an acquired vesical paresis, so that efforts of micturition become weaker and weaker as time goes on." The bladder distends, the ureteral meatuses become insufficient, secondary infection follows, and the child from three to six years of age comes under observation with all the signs of an extensive pyelonephritis.

II. MOVABLE KIDNEY

(*Floating Kidney; Palpable Kidney; Ren mobilis; Nephroptosis*)

Known to Riolan in the 17th century and to Matthew Baillie and to Rayer in the first half of the 19th century, it is only in the past forty years that the condition has attracted widespread attention.

The kidney is held in position by its fatty capsule, by the peritoneum which passes in front of it, and by the blood-vessels. Usually fixed, under certain circumstances one or the other organ, more rarely both, becomes movable. In very rare cases the kidney is surrounded, to some extent, by the peritoneum, and is anchored at the hilus by a mesonephron. Some would limit the term floating kidney to this condition.

Movable kidney is almost always acquired. It is more common in women. Of the 667 cases collected by Kuttner, 584 were in women and only 83 in men. It is more common on the right than on the left side. Of 727 cases analyzed by this author, it occurred on the right in 553 cases, on the left in 81, and on both sides in 93. The greater frequency in women may be attributed to compression of the lower thoracic zone by tight lacing, and, more important still, to the relaxation of the abdominal walls which follows repeated pregnancies. Movable kidney, however, is by no means uncommon in nulliparæ. There may be a congenitally relaxed condition of the peritoneal attachments as the condition has been met with in infants and children. Wasting of the fat about the kidney, trauma and the lifting of heavy weights are occasionally factors. The kidney is sometimes dragged down by tumors. The greater frequency on the right side is probably associated with the position of the kidney just beneath the liver, and the depression to which the organ is subjected with each descent of the diaphragm in inspiration.

Many cases present that combination of neurasthenia with gastro-intestinal disturbance which has been described by Glénard as *enteroptosis* (see p. 538).

To determine the presence of a movable kidney the patient should be in the dorsal position, with the head moderately low and the abdominal walls relaxed. The left hand is placed in the lumbar region behind the eleventh and twelfth ribs; the right hand in the hypochondriac region, in the nipple line, just under the edge of the liver. Bimanual palpation may detect the presence of a firm, rounded body just below the edge of the ribs. If nothing is felt, the patient should be asked to draw a deep breath, when, if the organ is palpable, it is touched by the fingers of the right hand. Various grades of mobility may be recognized. It may be possible barely to feel the lower edge on deep palpation—*palpable kidney*—or the organ may be so far displaced that on drawing the deepest breath the fingers of the right hand may be, in a thin person, slipped above the upper end of the organ, which can be readily held down, but can not be pushed below the level of the navel—*movable kidney*. In a third group the organ is freely movable, and may even be felt just above Poupart's ligament, or in the mid line of the abdomen, or can even be pushed over beyond this point. To this the term *floating kidney* is appropriate.

The movable kidney may be tender on pressure, especially when it is grasped very firmly, when there is a dull pain, or sometimes a sickening sensation. Examination of the patient from behind may show a distinct flattening in the lumbar region on the side in which the kidney is mobile.

Symptoms.—In a large majority of cases there are no symptoms, and if detected accidentally it is well not to let the patient know of its presence. Too much stress may be laid upon the condition. Pain in the lumbar region or a sense of dragging and discomfort may be present or there may be intercostal neuralgia. In a large group the symptoms are those of neurasthenia with dyspepsia. In women the hysterical symptoms may be marked, and in men various grades of hypochondriasis; and various forms of insanity have been attributed to it! Dilatation of the stomach has been observed, due to pressure of the dislocated kidney upon the duodenum. The association with a *depressed* stomach is common in women. Constipation is not infrequent. Some writers have described pressure upon the gall-ducts, with jaundice, but this is very rare. Fæcal accumulation and even obstruction may be associated with the displaced organ.

DIETL'S CRISES.—In connection with movable kidney, nearly always in women, and on the right side, there are remarkable attacks characterized by pain, chill, nausea, vomiting, fever, and collapse. They were described first by Dietl, in 1864, and attributed to twist or kink of the renal vessels or of the ureter. In the subject of movable kidney they may recur at intervals for months or years. A sudden exertion, an error in diet, or standing for a long time may bring on an attack. The pain is in the renal region, of great intensity, simulating colic, and radiates down to the ureter and through to the back. The patient feels nauseated and cold, or there may be a severe chill; vomiting is common. The urine is scanty and contains an excess of urate and oxalates; sometimes it is bloody. The affected side is tender, the muscular tension increases, and the kidney may be felt enlarged, sensitive to pressure and less movable; but there is no positive tumor. In other cases a tumor rapidly forms from dilatation of the pelvis of the kidney. Appearing, first anteriorly, at the edge of the epigastric region, it may gradually reach the size of a large orange or a cocoanut and fills the entire renal region. This may happen within thirty-six or forty-eight hours. The nausea persists, there is fever, the patient looks ill, and the urine may be scanty or bloody. The general symptoms abate, the local tenderness lessens, the amount of urine may increase rapidly, and in ten or twelve hours the tumor may disappear. In a month or two with a return of the symptoms the tumor reappears, and again subsides. This is the condition of *intermittent hydronephrosis,* one of the most serious and distressing of the sequels of movable kidney.

Diagnosis.—The diagnosis of movable kidney is rarely doubtful. Tumors of the gall-bladder, ovarian growths, and tumors of the bowels may in rare instances be confounded with it.

Treatment.—In many instances the greatest relief is experienced from a bandage and pad. It should be applied in the morning, with the patient in the dorsal or knee-breast position, and she should be taught how to push up the kidney. An air pad may be used if the organ is sensitive. In other cases a support in the lower abdominal zone has the same effect. In the attacks of severe colic morphia may be required. The intermittent hydronephrosis may be relieved by the pad and bandage. It rarely demands immediate operation. The kidney may have to be fixed in position. This is a suitable procedure for severe cases, and relief is afforded in many instances by the operation, though not in all. Treatment designed to increase fat-formation often helps to hold the kidney in place. Attention should always be given to the state of the nervous system and in some cases a prolonged rest treatment is indicated.

III. CIRCULATORY DISTURBANCES

The secretion of urine is accomplished by the maintenance of a certain blood pressure within the glomeruli and by the activity of the renal epithelium. The watery elements are filtered from the glomeruli, the amount depending on the rapidity and the pressure of the blood current; the quality, whether normal or abnormal, depending upon the condition of the capillary and glomerular epithelium; while the greater portion of the solid ingredients are excreted by the epithelium of the convoluted tubules. The integrity of the epithelium covering the capillary tufts within Bowman's capsule is essential to the production of a normal urine. If under any circumstances their nutrition fails, as when, for example, the rapidity of the blood current is lowered, so that they are deprived of the necessary amount of oxygen, the material which filters through is no longer normal, but contains serum albumin. The renal epithelium is extremely sensitive to circulatory changes, and compression of the renal artery for only a few minutes causes serious disturbance.

The circulation of the kidney is influenced by reflex stimuli coming from the skin. Exposure to cold causes heightened blood pressure within the kidneys and increased secretion of urine. Bradford has shown that after excision of portions of the kidney, to as much as one-third of the total weight, there is a remarkable increase in the flow of urine.

Congestion of the Kidneys.—(1) Active Congestion; Hyperæmia.—Acute congestion of the kidney is met with in the early stage of nephritis, whether due to cold or to the action of poisons and severe irritants. Turpentine, cubebs, cantharides, and copaiba cause extreme hyperæmia of the organ. The most typical congestion of the kidney which we see post mortem is that in the early stage of acute nephritis, when the organ may be large, soft, of a dark color, and on section blood drips from it freely.

It has been held that in all the acute fevers the kidneys are congested, and that this explained the scanty, high colored, and often albuminous urine. On the other hand, the kidney in acute fever may be small, pale, and bloodless; this anæmia, increasing with the pyrexia and interfering with the nutrition of the glomerular epithelium, may account for the scanty, dark-colored urine and the presence of albumin. In the prolonged fevers, however, it is probable that relaxation of the arteries again takes place. Certainly it is rare to find post mortem marked anæmia; on the contrary, the kidney of fever is commonly swollen, the blood-vessels are congested, and the cortex frequently shows traces of cloudy swelling. The circulatory disturbances in acute fevers are probably less important than the irritative effects of the specific agents of the disease or the products produced in their growth or by the altered metabolism. The urine is diminished in amount, and may contain albumin and tube-casts, sometimes much of the former and few of the latter.

(2) Passive Congestion; Mechanical Hyperæmia.—This is found in

cases of chronic disease of the heart or lung, with impeded circulation, and as a result of pressure upon the renal veins by tumors, the pregnant uterus, or ascitic fluid. In the cardiac kidney, as it is called, the cyanotic induration associated with chronic heart disease, the organs are enlarged and firm, the capsule strips off, as a rule, readily, the cortex is of a deep red color, and the pyramids of a purple red. The section is coarse looking, the substance is very firm, and resists cutting and tearing. The interstitial tissue is increased, and there is a small-celled infiltration between the tubules. Here and there the Malpighian tufts have become sclerosed. The blood-vessels are usually thickened, and there may be more or less granular, fatty, or hyaline changes in the epithelium of the tubules. The condition is indeed a diffuse nephritis. The urine is usually reduced, is of high specific gravity, and contains more or less albumin. Hyaline tube casts and blood corpuscles are not uncommon. In some cases (over half) with macroscopically no signs of chronic or acute nephritis the urinary features lead to the diagnosis of acute nephritis (Emerson). In uncomplicated cases of the cyanotic induration uræmia is rare. In the cardiac cases with extensive arterio-sclerosis, the kidneys are more involved and the renal function is likely to be disturbed.

IV. ANOMALIES OF THE URINARY SECRETION

I. ANURIA

Total suppression of urine occurs under the following conditions:

(*a*) As an event in the intense congestion of acute nephritis. For a time no urine may be formed; more often the amount is greatly reduced.

(*b*) More commonly complete *anuria* is seen in subjects of renal stone, fragments of which block both ureters; or the calculus blocks the only kidney, the other being represented by a shell of tissue. In this "obstructive suppression," as it is called, there is a condition which has been called latent uræmia. There may be very little discomfort, and the symptoms are very unlike those of ordinary uræmia. Convulsions occurred in only 5 of 41 cases (Herter); headache in only 6; vomiting in only 12. Consciousness is retained; the pupils are usually contracted; the temperature may be low; there are twitchings and perhaps occasional vomiting. Of 41 cases, 35 occurred in males. Of 36 cases in which there was absolute anuria, in 11 the condition lasted more than four days, in 18 cases from seven to fourteen days, and in 7 cases longer than fourteen days (Herter). Obstructive suppression is met with also when cancer compresses both ureters and involves their orifices in the bladder.

(*c*) Cases occur occasionally in which the cause is prerenal. The following are among the more important conditions with which this form of anuria may be associated: Fevers and inflammations; acute poisoning by phosphorus, mercury, lead, and turpentine; aortic thrombosis involving the renal arteries; in the collapse after severe injuries or after operations, or, indeed, after the passing of a catheter; in the collapse stage of cholera and yellow fever; and, lastly, there is an hysterical anuria, of which Charcot reported a case in which the suppression lasted for eleven days. Bailey reports the case of a young girl, aged eleven, inmate of an orphan asylum, who passed no urine from October 10th to December 12th (when 8 ounces were withdrawn), and again from this date to March 1st! The question of hysterical deception was considered in the case.

A patient may live for from ten days to two weeks with complete suppression. In Polk's case, in which the only kidney was removed, the patient lived eleven days. It is remarkable that in many instances there are no toxic features. Adams reports a case of recovery after nineteen days of suppression.

Treatment.—In the obstructive cases surgical interference should be resorted to. In the non-obstructive cases, particularly when due to extreme congestion of the kidney, cupping over the loins, hot applications, free purging, and sweating with pilocarpine and hot air are indicated. When the secretion is once started diuretin often acts well. Large hot irrigations, with normal salt solution, with Kemp's double-current rectal tubes, are stated to stimulate the activity of the kidneys in a remarkable way.

II. HÆMATURIA

Etiology.—The following division may be made of the conditions in which hæmaturia occurs:

(1) Essential Hæmaturia.—How much basis there is for this group is a question and it seems doubtful whether the term should be retained. To make this diagnosis is to confess our inability to find any positive cause. There are some cases, usually in young adults, in which no cause can be found and in which operation gives no clue to the cause of the hæmorrhage. Some are due to varicosity of vessels in the papillæ. The subjects are usually under the age of thirty. The bleeding is spontaneous, often associated with pain, though in many cases the attacks are painless. The X-ray picture is negative, the hæmorrhage ceases of itself, and only in a few cases do the attacks recur with such frequency that the patient becomes anæmic. The condition has been referred to under Gull's name of "renal epistaxis" in previous editions. It is rarely serious, and many cases recover spontaneously, in others nephrotomy stops the tendency to bleeding, though why it should do so is difficult to say. The outlook is good (see Hale White, *Q. J. M.*, 1911).

(2) General Diseases.—In the malignant specific fevers, in purpura, and occasionally in leukæmia. It may be caused by malaria.

(3) Renal Causes.—Acute congestion and inflammation, as in nephritis or pyelonephritis, or due to the effect of toxic agents, such as turpentine, carbolic acid, and cantharides. When the carbolic spray was in use many surgeons suffered from hæmaturia in consequence of this poison. Renal infarction, as in ulcerative endocarditis. New growths, in which the bleeding is usually profuse. In tuberculosis at the onset, when the papillæ are involved, there may be bleeding. Stone in the kidney is a frequent cause. Parasites: The *Filaria bancrofti* and *Bilharzia* cause a form of hæmaturia met with in the tropics. The echinococcus is rarely associated with hæmorrhage. It is sometimes met with in floating kidney and hydronephrosis. An unusual cause is the painful, villous tumor of the renal pelvis, of which Savory and Nash report a remarkable case and collected 49 others from the literature. It would be difficult to distinguish the condition from stone. Angioma and capillary nævi of the papillæ may cause bleeding.

(4) Affections of the Urinary Passages.—Stone in the ureter, tumors, polypi, tuberculosis, diverticula, or ulceration of the bladder, the presence of a calculus, parasites, and, very rarely, ruptured veins in the bladder. Bleeding from the urethra occasionally occurs in gonorrhœa and as a result of the lodgment of a calculus. In females it may be due to prolapse or tumor of the urethra. Recurring hæmaturia may be an early symptom in malignant disease of or an enlarged prostate.

(5) Traumatism.—Injuries may produce bleeding from any part of the urinary passages. By a fall or blow on the back the kidney may be ruptured, and this may be followed by very free bleeding; less commonly the blood comes from injury of the bladder or of the prostate. Blood from the urethra is frequently due to injury by the passage of a catheter, or sometimes to falls. Transient hæmaturia follows all operations on the kidney.

(6) Exercise.—After strenuous exercise or exposure to cold temporary hæmaturia may occur with blood casts, followed by transient albuminuria, in individuals who show no signs of nephritis.

Diagnosis.—This is usually easy. The color of the urine varies from a light smoky to a bright red, or it may have a dark porter color. The blood-corpuscles are readily recognized microscopically, either plainly visible and retaining their color, in which case they are usually crenated, or simply as shadows. In ammoniacal urine or urines of low specific gravity the hæmoglobin is rapidly dissolved from the corpuscles.

It is important to distinguish between blood coming from the bladder and from the kidneys. From the bladder the blood may be found only with the last portions of urine, or only at the termination of micturition. In hæmorrhage from the kidneys the blood and urine are intimately mixed. Clots are more commonly found in the blood from the kidneys, and may form moulds of the pelvis or of the ureter. When the seat of the bleeding is in the bladder, on washing out this organ, the water is more or less blood-tinged; but if the source of the bleeding is higher, the water comes away clear. In many instances it is difficult to settle the question by the examination of the urine alone, and the symptoms and the physical signs must also be taken into account. Cystoscopic examination of the bladder and catheterization of the ureters are aids in the diagnosis of doubtful cases. The recognition of the cause may be difficult. New growth, tuberculosis and calculus should always be considered.

III. HÆMOGLOBINURIA

This is characterized by the presence of blood-pigment in the urine. The blood-cells are absent or in insignificant numbers. The coloring matter is not hæmatin, as indicated by the old name, *hæmatinuria,* nor in reality always hæmoglobin, but most frequently methæmoglobin. The urine has a red or brownish-red, sometimes quite black, color, and usually deposits a very heavy brownish sediment. When the hæmoglobin occurs only in small quantities, it may give a lake or smoky color to the urine. Microscopic examination shows the presence of granular pigment, sometimes fragments of blood disks, epithelium, and very often darkly pigmented urates. The urine is also albuminous. The number of red blood corpuscles bears no proportion to the intensity of the color of the urine. Examined spectroscopically, there are either the two absorption bands of oxyhæmoglobin, which is rare, or more commonly, there are the three absorption bands of methæmoglobin, of which the one in the red near *C* is characteristic. There are two clinical groups.

Toxic Hæmoglobinuria.—This is caused by poisons which produce rapid dissolution of the blood corpuscles, such as potassium chlorate in large doses, pyrogallic acid, carbolic acid, arseniuretted hydrogen, carbon monoxide, naphthol, and muscarine; also the poisons of scarlet fever, yellow fever, typhoid fever, malaria, and syphilis. It has also followed severe burns. Exposure to excessive cold and violent muscular exertion are stated to produce hæmoglobinuria. A most remarkable toxic form occurs in horses, coming on with great suddenness and associated with paresis of the hind legs. Death may occur in a few hours or a few days. The animals are attacked only after being stalled for some days and then taken out and driven, particularly in cold weather. The form of hæmoglobinuria from cold and exertion is extremely rare. No instance of it, even in association with frost-bites, came under our observation in Canada. Blood transfused from one mammal into another causes dissolution of the corpuscles with the production of hæmoglobinuria; and, lastly, there is the *epidemic hæmoglobinuria* of the newborn, associated with jaundice, cyanosis, and nervous symptoms.

Paroxysmal Hæmoglobinuria.—This rare disease is characterized by the occasional passage of bloody urine, in which the coloring matter only is present. It is more frequent in males than in females, and occurs chiefly in adults. It seems specially associated with cold and exertion, and has often been brought on, in a susceptible person, by the use of a cold foot-bath. It occurs in persons subject to Raynaud's disease, and the relation between these two affections is extremely close; some hold that they are manifestations of one and the same disorder. Druitt, the author of the well-known Surgical Vade-mecum, has given a graphic description of his sufferings, which lasted for many years, and were accompanied with local asphyxia and local syncope. The connection, however, is not very common. The relation of hæmoglobinuria to malaria has been considered. *Syphilis* is present in some cases. In a case reported by Brem after fifteen injections of arsphenamine, the hæmoglobinuria disappeared.

The attacks may come on suddenly after exposure to cold or as a result of mental or bodily exhaustion. They may be preceded by chills and pyrexia. In other instances the temperature is subnormal. There may be vomiting and diarrhœa. Pain in the lumbar region is not uncommon. The hæmoglobinuria rarely persists for more than a day or two—sometimes, indeed, not for a day. There are instances in which, even in a single day, there have been two or three paroxysms, and in the intervals clear urine has been passed. Jaundice has been present in a number of cases. The disease is rarely if ever fatal.

Much has been done to clear up the nature of this remarkable disease by the studies of Eason, Donath, Landsteiner, Hoover and Stone, and Moss. Briefly, the blood serum of these patients contains a complex hæmolysin, a potential toxin, capable of dissolving the patient's own corpuscles and those of other individuals. It is an amboceptor component of the hæmolysin, not the complement, that is peculiar, and this amboceptor differs "from other known hæmolytic amboceptors in that it will unite with the red blood-corpuscles only at a low temperature in the presence of complement, and furthermore in that it is capable of bringing about the solution of the patient's own cells (auto-hæmolytic action), and those of other members of the group to which the patient belongs, as well as the cells of members of other groups" (Moss). Atmospheric cold and congestion of the peripheral vessels, as in Raynaud's disease, will reduce the temperature of the blood sufficiently to permit of the union of the amboceptor and corpuscles, and hæmolysis occurs when the blood passes to the internal organs.

Treatment.—The essential treatment must depend on the cause. In all forms of hæmaturia rest is essential. In that produced by renal calculi the recumbent posture may suffice to check the bleeding. Full doses of acetate of lead and opium should be tried, then calcium lactate and epinephrin. Cold may be applied to the loins or dry cups in the lumbar region. Incision of the kidney has cured the so-called essential hæmaturia.

The treatment of paroxysmal hæmoglobinuria is unsatisfactory. Amyl nitrite will sometimes cut short or prevent an attack (Chvostek). During the paroxysm the patient should be kept warm and given hot drinks. If there is a syphilitic history active treatment should be given. In a warm climate the attacks are much less frequent. It is possible that an antitoxin may be obtained to neutralize the hæmolytic amboceptor of the disease.

IV. ALBUMINURIA

"Reasons drawn from the urine are as brittle as the urinal" is a dictum of Thomas Fuller peculiarly appropriate in connection with this subject.

The presence of albumin in the urine, formerly regarded as indicative of nephritis, is now recognized as occurring under many circumstances without the existence of serious organic change in the kidney. Two groups of cases may be recognized—those in which the kidneys show no coarse lesions, and those in which there are evident anatomical changes.

Albuminuria without Coarse Renal Lesions.—(*a*) FUNCTIONAL, SO-CALLED PHYSIOLOGICAL ALBUMINURIA.—In a normal condition of the kidney only the water and the salts are allowed to pass from the blood. When albuminous substances transude there is probably disturbance in the nutrition of the epithelium of the capillaries of the tuft, or of the cells surrounding the glomerulus. This statement is still in dispute, and many hold that there is a physiological albuminuria which may follow muscular work, the ingestion of food rich in albumin, violent emotions, cold bathing, and dyspepsia. On one point all agree, that the cause must be something unusual and excessive, as a very hard tramp, a football match, a race, etc. The presence of albumin in the urine, in any form and under any circumstance, may be regarded as indicative of change in the renal or glomerular epithelium, a change, however, which may be transient, slight, and unimportant, depending upon variations in the circulation or upon the irritating effects of substances taken with the food or temporarily present, as in febrile states.

Albuminuria of adolescence and cyclic albuminuria, in which the albumin is present only at certain times during the day—*orthostatic albuminuria*—are interesting forms. A majority of the cases occur in young persons—boys more commonly than girls—and the condition is often discovered accidentally. These are often the children of neurotic parents, and have well-marked vasomotor instability. Some cases last only during puberty, some throughout life. The condition is very common, particularly in young men in training—the athletic albuminuria to which Collier has called attention. Of 156 men in training 130 had albumin in the urine. Erlanger and Hooker have shown that the albumin is excreted only during periods with low pulse pressure. The urine, as a rule, contains only a very small amount of albumin, but in some instances large quantities are present. The most striking feature is the variability. It may be absent in the morning and present only after exertion; or it may be greatly increased after taking food, particularly proteins. Even the change to the upright position (orthostatic) may suffice to cause it, and in such cases there may be tension on the renal veins by increase of the lumbar curve, since it has been shown that a spinal jacket will prevent the appearance of the albumin. Support of a movable kidney may stop it. The quantity of urine may be but little, if at all, increased, the specific gravity is usually normal, and the color may be high. Occasionally hyaline casts may be found, and in some instances there has been transient glycosuria. As a rule, the pulse is not of high tension and the second aortic sound is not accentuated.

Various forms of this affection have been recognized by writers, such as neurotic, dietetic, cyclic, intermittent, and paroxysmal—names which indicate the characters of the different varieties.

Goodhart, from a study of the after history of more than 250 cases, holds that albuminuria of the adolescent has no sinister effect on health or upon duration of life, and that with due circumspection such cases ought not to be excluded from the advantages of life insurance. This is a very important statement from a man who has made a special study of the subject.

In a few cases the albumin is persistent, the amount is larger, though it may vary from day to day, the pulse tension is increased, and these are probably indications of organic changes in the kidney.

(*b*) Febrile Albuminuria.—Pyrexia, by whatever cause produced, may cause slight albuminuria. The presence of the albumin is due to slight changes in the glomeruli induced by the fever, such as cloudy swelling, which can not be regarded as an organic lesion. It is extremely common, occurring in pneumonia (in about 70 per cent. of our cases), diphtheria, typhoid fever (about 60 per cent. of our cases), malaria, especially the æstivo-autumnal type, and even in the fever of acute tonsillitis. The amount of albumin is slight, and it usually disappears from the urine with the cessation of the fever. Hyaline and even epithelial casts accompany the condition.

(*c*) Hæmic Changes.—Purpura, scurvy, chronic poisoning by lead or mercury, syphilis, leukæmia, and profound anæmia may be associated with slight albuminuria. Abnormal ingredients in the blood, such as bile pigment, may cause the passage of small amounts of albumin.

The transient albuminuria of pregnancy may belong to this hæmic group, although in a majority of such cases there are changes in the renal tissue. Albumin may be found sometimes after the inhalation of ether or chloroform.

(*d*) Nervous System.—In many morbid conditions of the nervous system, albumin may be present in the urine, and there are instances in young nervous persons which are not easy to separate from the so-called orthostatic forms. In brain tumors, following epileptic attacks, in various types of meningitis, albumin has been present. In meningeal hæmorrhage, as pointed out by Guillain, the albumin may be very abundant, 5 to 20 grams in the litre.

Albuminuria with Definite Lesions of the Urinary Organs.—(*a*) Congestion of the kidney, either active, such as follows exposure to cold and is associated with the early stages of nephritis, or passive, due to obstructed outflow in disease of the heart or lungs, or to pressure on the renal veins by the pregnant uterus or tumors.

(*b*) Organic disease of the kidneys—acute and chronic, nephritis, amyloid and fatty degeneration, suppurative nephritis, and tumors.

(*c*) Affections of the pelvis, ureters, bladder, and prostate, when associated with the formation of pus or hæmaturia.

(*d*) *Hereditary Familial Albuminuria and Hæmorrhagic Nephritis.*—Families have been described by Guthrie, and by Kendell and Hurst, in which through two and three generations members of the family have had albuminuria, high blood pressure, occasional hæmaturia or sometimes only microscopic blood, from early childhood. Some of the patients died early from uræmia; others lived to adult life. Hypertension and cardio-vascular features have been present in some cases.

Albumosuria.—Albumose, peptone, and globulin are occasionally found in the urine, but are of very slight clinical significance. They are found in many febrile diseases, in chronic suppuration, and whenever protein materials are undergoing autolysis, as in pneumonia, acute yellow atrophy, and during the involution of the uterus.

Myelopathic albumosuria, *"Kahler's disease,"* is characterized by multiple myelomata with persistent excretion of what is known as the Bence-Jones body, a protein discovered by him in 1848. Some believe that it is not a proteose but a higher protein of endogenous origin derived either from the tumor cells of a myeloma or from the abnormal synthesis of a body protein. Males above forty years of age are usually affected. The Bence-Jones body appears rarely with other tumors of the bones. The myeloma is a true tumor, the cells of which resemble the plasma rather than the myelocytes of the bone marrow (Christian). In a case seen with Hamburger the persistent albumosuria led to the diagnosis of multiple myelomata before any bone tumors could be felt. The disease runs a fatal course. The simplest reaction is the white precipitate formed on adding nitric acid to the urine; when boiled it disappears, to reappear on cooling. As in one of Bradshaw's cases, the urine may be of a milky white color when passed.

Prognosis.—Febrile albuminuria is transient, and in a majority of the cases depending upon hæmic causes the condition disappears and leaves the kidneys intact. A trace of albumin in a man over forty, with or without a few hyaline casts, is not of much significance, except as an indication that his kidneys, like his hair, are beginning to turn "gray" with age. In many instances the discovery is a positive advantage, as the man is made to realize, perhaps for the first time, that he has been living carelessly. The question was discussed from this standpoint in a paper with the paradoxical title "On the Advantages of a Trace of Albumin and a Few Tube-casts in the Urine of Men over Fifty Years of Age" (*N. Y. Med. Jour.*, vol. lxxiv). The persistence of a slight amount of albumin in young men without increased arterial tension is less serious, as even after continuing for years it may disappear. The outlook in the so-called cyclic albuminuria has been discussed.

Practically in all cases the presence of albumin indicates a change of some sort in the glomeruli, the nature, extent, and gravity of which it is difficult to estimate; so that other considerations, such as the presence of tube-casts, increased tension, the general condition of the patient, and the influence of digestion upon the albumin, must be carefully considered.

The physician is often consulted as to the relation of albuminuria and life assurance. As his function is to protect the interests of the company, he should reject all cases in which albumin occurs in the urine, except in young persons with transient albuminuria. Naturally, companies lay great stress upon the presence of albumin, but in the most fatal malady with which they have to deal—chronic interstitial nephritis—the albumin is often absent or transient, even when the disease is well developed. After the fortieth year, from a standpoint of life insurance, the state of the arteries and the blood pressure are more important than the condition of the urine.

V. BACTERIURIA

Described first by Roberts in 1881, much attention has been paid to it and its importance recognized both as a secondary and a primary affection. The secondary form is best illustrated by the common bacilluria of typhoid fever. In the cases in which there is no recognizable cause or primary focus, the colon bacillus, streptococci, and the gonococcus are the commonest organisms. The bacilli may come directly from the blood, as in typhoid fever, and probably multiply in the urinary passages, or they may come from a focus of infection anywhere from Bowman's capsule to the prostate.

Clinically there are two groups of cases, the bacilluria pure and simple and the bacilluric cystitis or pyelitis. In the former there may be no symptoms; the urine may have a slight haziness due to the enormous number of organisms, but there is no pus. In the other there are signs of inflammatory reaction in the urinary passages and there is pus. Usually with the *Bacillus coli* infection the urine is acid, with the staphylococcus alkaline and often with marked phosphaturia. The cases are often very intractable. Without cystitis or pyelitis there may be no symptoms, but in too many instances there are all the aggravated phenomena of these two affections. Many cases clear up rapidly with hexamine. Vaccine therapy has been extensively used but not with very good results.

VI. PYURIA

(*Pus in the Urine*)

Causes.—(*a*) Pyelitis and Pyelonephritis.—In large abscesses of the kidney, pyonephrosis, the pus may be intermittent, while in calculus and tuberculous pyelitis the pyuria is usually continuous, though varying in intensity. In cases due to the colon or tubercle bacillus the urine is acid, in those due to the proteus bacillus alkaline, while in the staphylococcus cases the urine is either less acid than normal, or alkaline. In the pyelitis and pyelonephritis following cystitis the urine is alkaline or acid, depending upon the infecting micro-organism; more mucus, frequent micturition, and a previous bladder history are aids in diagnosis. H. Cabot points out that if the fresh urine shows cocci in abundance, with a small amount of albumin, few red blood cells, many leucocytes or a little pus, and the renal function near normal, it is probably a coccus infection and mostly in the cortex. If there are many bacilli, little albumin, much pus and greatly decreased renal function it is probably a colon bacillus infection with the first effect on the convoluted tubes and the lesion of the pelvis secondary.

(*b*) CYSTITIS.—The urine is usually acid, especially in women, since the colon bacillus is a very common cause of these infections. The pus and mucus are more ropy, and triple phosphate crystals are found in the freshly passed urine in the alkaline infections. Pus may come from the prostate.

(*c*) URETHRITIS, particularly gonorrhœa. The pus appears first, is in small quantities, and there are signs of local inflammation.

(*d*) In LEUCORRHŒA the quantity of pus is usually small, and large flakes of vaginal epithelium are numerous. In doubtful cases, when leucorrhœa is present, the urine should be withdrawn through a catheter.

(*e*) RUPTURE OF ABSCESSES INTO THE URINARY PASSAGES.—In such cases as pelvic or perityphlitic abscess there have been previous symptoms of pus formation. A large amount is passed within a short time, then the discharge stops abruptly or rapidly diminishes within a few days.

Pus gives to the urine a white or yellowish-white appearance. On settling, the sediment is sometimes ropy, the supernatant fluid usually turbid. In cases due to urea-decomposing microbes (proteus bacillus, various staphylococci) the odor may be ammoniacal even in fresh urine. The pus cells are usually well formed when the pus comes from the bladder; the protoplasm is granular, and often shows many translucent processes.

The only sediment likely to be confounded with pus is that of the phosphates; but it is whiter and less dense, and is distinguished immediately by microscopic examination or by the addition of acid. With the pus there is always more or less epithelium from the bladder and pelves of the kidneys, but since in these situations the forms of cells are practically identical, they afford no information as to the locality from which the pus has come.

The treatment is considered under the conditions in which pyuria occurs.

VII. CHYLURIA—NON-PARASITIC

This is a rare affection, occurring in temperate regions and unassociated with the *Filaria bancrofti*. The urine is of an opaque white color; it resembles milk closely, is occasionally mixed with blood (hæmatochyluria), and sometimes coagulates into a firm, jelly-like mass. In other instances there is at the bottom of the vessel a loose clot which may be distinctly blood tinged. The turbidity seems to be caused by numerous minute granules—more rarely oil droplets similar to those of milk. In Montreal a dissection in a case of thirteen years' duration showed no trace of parasites. The urine may be much more milky shortly after taking food, and the recumbent posture increases the milkiness. In one case the urine only became chylous in the bladder, and Hertz found obstruction of the thoracic duct and a communicating ruptured lymphatic vessel in the bladder.

VIII. LITHURIA

The general relations of uric acid have been considered under gout.

Occurrence in the Urine.—The uric acid occurs in combination chiefly with ammonium and sodium, forming the acid urates. In smaller quantities are the potassium, calcium, and lithium salts. The uric acid may be separated from its bases and crystallizes in rhombs or prisms, which are usually of a deep red color, owing to the staining of the urinary pigments. The sediment is granular and the crystals look like grains of Cayenne pepper. It is very important not to mistake a deposit of uric acid for an excess. The deposition of numerous grains in the urine within a few hours after passing is more likely to be due to conditions which diminish the solvent power than to increase in the quantity. Of the conditions which cause precipitation of the uric acid Roberts gives the following: "(1) High acidity; (2) poverty in mineral salts; (3) low pigmentation; and (4) high percentage of uric acid." The grade of acidity is probably the most important element.

In health the amount of uric acid excreted bears a fairly constant ratio to the urea eliminated. According to von Noorden, the average ratio is 1 to 50, while the average ratio of the nitrogen of uric acid to the total nitrogen eliminated in the urine is 1 to 70. In several cases of gout Futcher found that in the intervals between acute attacks the uric acid was reduced to a much greater extent than the urea, so that the ratio of the former to the latter often varied between 1 to 300 up to (in one case) 1 to 1,500, a return to about the normal proportions occurring during the acute attacks.

More common is the precipitation of amorphous urates, forming the so-called brick-dust deposit, which has a pinkish color, due to urinary pigment. It is composed chiefly of the acid sodium urates. It occurs particularly in very acid urine of a high specific gravity. As the urates are more soluble in warm solutions, they frequently deposit as the urine cools. Here, too, the deposition does not necessarily, indeed usually does not, mean an excessive excretion, but the existence of conditions favoring the deposit.

Treatment.—Meat, fish, tea and coffee should be excluded from the diet and the patient should drink water freely. Alkalies and salicylic acid may be given.

IX. OXALURIA

The discovery of calcium oxalate crystals in the urine by Donné in 1838 led to the description of the so-called oxalic-acid diathesis. It is claimed that all the oxalic acid found in the urine is taken into the body with the food (Dunlop). In health none, or only a trace, is formed in the body. The amount fluctuates with the quantity of food taken, and is usually below 10 milligrams daily (H. Baldwin). It seems to be formed in the body when there is an absence of free hydrochloric acid in the gastric juice, and in connection with excessive fermentation in the intestines. It never forms a heavy deposit, but the crystals—usually octahedral, rarely dumb-bell-shaped—collect in the mucous cloud and on the sides of the vessel.

When in excess and present for any considerable time, the condition is known as *oxaluria,* the chief interest of which is in the fact that the crystals may be deposited before the urine is voided, and form a calculus. It is held by many that there is a special diathesis associated with its presence in excess and manifested clinically by dyspepsia, particularly the nervous form, irritability, depression of spirits, lassitude, and sometimes marked hypochondriasis. There may be in addition neuralgic pains and the general symptoms of neurasthenia. The local and general symptoms are probably dependent upon some disturbance of metabolism of which the oxaluria is one of the manifestations. It is a feature also in many gouty persons, and in the condition called lithæmia.

Treatment.—Water should be taken freely. In the diet the following should be avoided: spinach, rhubarb, cranberries, asparagus, radish, horse-radish, grapes and currants.

X. CYSTINURIA

This rare condition, a sort of chemical malformation (Garrod), is of clinical importance because cystin is very sparingly soluble and calculi may be formed, renal or vesical. It is strongly hereditary and has been traced through three generations. The quantity excreted is about 0.5 gram per diem, and the excretion persists for years, or even for life, without causing disturbance of health. Cystin is one of the amino-acid fragments of the protein molecule, and its excretion is one of the unexplained errors of protein metabolism. In the urinary sediment the colorless hexagonal crystals of cystin are readily detected.

Treatment.—This involves a decreased production of cystin by reducing the amount of protein in the diet or an increased solubility in the urine by giving sodium bicarbonate (90 to 150 grains, 6 to 10 gms. a day).

XI. PHOSPHATURIA

The phosphoric acid is excreted from the body in combination with potassium, sodium, calcium, and magnesium, forming two classes, the alkaline phosphates of sodium and potassium and the earthy phosphates of lime and magnesia. The amount of phosphoric acid (P_2O_5) excreted in the twenty-four hours varies, according to Hammarsten, between 1 and 5 grams, with an average of 2.5 grams. It is derived mainly from the phosphoric acid taken in the food, but also in part as a decomposition product from nuclein, protagon, and lecithin. Of the alkaline phosphates, those in combination with sodium are the most abundant. The alkaline phosphates of the urine are more abundant than the earthy phosphates.

Of the *earthy phosphates,* those of lime are abundant, of magnesium scanty. In urine which has undergone ammoniacal fermentation, either in- or outside the body, there is in addition the ammonio-magnesium or triple phosphate, which occurs in triangular prisms or in feathery or stellate crystals. The earthy phosphates occur as a sediment in the urine when the alkalinity is due to a fixed alkali, or under certain circumstances the deposit may take place within the bladder, and then the phosphates are passed at the end of micturition as a whitish fluid, popularly confounded with spermatorrhœa. Study of the cases with symptoms of neurasthenia and a phosphate sediment in the fresh urine indicates an abnormality in the calcium metabolism, an absolute increase of this with a decrease of the phosphoric acid. The calcium phosphate may be precipitated by heat and produce a cloudiness which may be mistaken for albumin, but is dissolved upon making the urine acid. This is frequent in persons suffering from dyspepsia or debility of any kind. The phosphates may be in great excess, rising in the twenty-four hours to from 7 to 9 grams (Teissier), whereas the normal amount is not more than 2.5 grams. Lastly, the phosphates may be deposited in urine which has undergone decomposition, in which the carbonate of ammonia from the urea combines with the magnesium phosphates, forming the triple salt. This is seen in *cystitis,* due to a urea decomposing microbe.

The clinical significance of an excess of phosphates, to which the term *phosphaturia* is applied, has been much discussed. A deposit does not necessarily mean an excess, to determine which a careful analysis of the twenty-four hours' secretion should be made. It has long been thought that there is a relation between the activity of the nerve tissues and the output of phosphoric acid; but the question can not yet be considered settled. The amount is increased in wasting diseases, such as tuberculosis, acute yellow atrophy of the liver, leukæmia, and severe anæmia, whereas it is diminished in acute diseases and during pregnancy.

Teissier, of Lyons, in 1876, described a condition to which he gave the name of "essential phosphaturia," and it has been called "phosphatic diabetes," the symptoms of which are polyuria, thirst, emaciation, and a great increase in the excretion of phosphates, which rise to as much as 7 to 9 grams a day. The condition sometimes simulates true diabetes very closely, even to the pruritus and dry skin. In a remarkable case of this kind, under observation for several years, Barker studied the metabolism and found it normal for carbohydrates, but the organic phosphorus percentage was high; the chief abnormality was an abnormally large amount of organic acids, so that chemically the condition was suggestive of an acidosis.

XII. INDICANURIA

The substance in the urine which has received this name is the indoxyl-sulphate of potassium, in which form it appears in the urine and is colorless. When concentrated acids or strong oxidizing agents are added to the urine, this substance is decomposed and the indigo set free. It is present only in small quantities in healthy urine. It is derived from the indol, a product formed in the intestine by the decomposition of the albumin under the influence of bacteria. When absorbed, this is oxidized in the tissues to indoxyl, which combines with the potassium sulphate, forming indican.

It is a common condition met with accidentally in persons of good health or with slight digestive complaints. It is not specially associated with constipation (Allen Jones). In gall-stone attacks, in hyperchlorhydria, in recurring appendicitis, in wasting diseases, in peritonitis, and in empyema it is usually present. In a few cases it is constantly present and in excess. Barr found only 32 such cases among 2,092 patients, and in these the symptoms did not suggest an "intestinal auto-intoxication," nor did lacto-bacillary treatment have the slightest influence on the condition.

Indican has occasionally been found in calculi. Though, as a rule, the urine is colorless when passed, there are instances in which decomposition has taken place within the body, and a blue color has been noticed immediately after the urine was voided. Sometimes, too, in alkaline urine on exposure there is a bluish film on the surface. Methylene blue, a coloring matter for candy, etc., must be excluded.

XIII. MELANURIA

Black urine may be dark when passed or may become so later. In the following conditions melanuria may occur: (1) Jaundice. Only in very chronic cases of deeply bronzed icterus do we see the urine quite dark, due to the presence of large quantities of biliverdin. (2) Hæmaturia and hæmoglobinuria. Here it is an exaggeration of the smoky tint due to the presence of blood. (3) Hæmatoporphyrinuria, to be considered later. (4) Melanuria, in which the urine has, as a rule, the normal color when passed, and on standing becomes black as ink. In some instances it is black when passed. Melanuria of this type only occurs with the presence of melanotic tumors. (5) Alkaptonuria. (6) Indicanuria. When rich in indoxyl sulphate the urine is brown in color, or becomes so after standing, due to the oxidation products of indol. This is by far the most common cause of black urine, and in any disease leading to an abundant secretion of indican, as in intestinal obstruction, etc., black urine may be passed. As Garrod suggests, it is probable that the black urine in cases of tuberculosis is of an allied nature. (7) After certain articles of diet and drugs. Some dark colored vegetable pigments, as in black cherries, plums and bilberries, cause darkening of the urine. Resorcin may do the same. Carboluria is by no means uncommon, and was frequently seen in the days of the antiseptic spray. It has been ascribed to hydrochinone formed from phenol. Naphthalene, creosote, and the salicylates may cause darkening of the urine, or even blackness.

XIV. ALKAPTONURIA

"Alkaptonuria is not the manifestation of a disease, but is rather of the nature of an alternative course of metabolism, harmless and usually congenital and lifelong" (Garrod). Of 40 known examples, 19 occurred in seven families, and several were the offspring of first cousins (Garrod). There are two points of clinical interest. The alkapton urine reduces Fehling's solution, and diabetes may be suggested, but it does not ferment, and it is optically inactive. The linen may be stained by the urine, which in some cases is dark when passed. In 1866 Virchow recorded a case of blackening of the cartilages and ligaments—ochronosis, which is considered elsewhere.

XV. PNEUMATURIA

Gas may be passed with the urine—1. After mechanical introduction of air in vesical irrigation or cystoscopic examination in the knee-elbow position. 2. As a result of the introduction of gas forming organisms in catheterization or other operation. Glycosuria has been present in a majority of the cases.

The yeast fungus, the colon bacillus, and the *Bacillus aërogenes capsulatus* have been found. 3. In cases of vesico-enteric fistula.

In gas production within the bladder the symptoms are those of a mild cystitis, with the passage of gas at the end of micturition, sometimes with a loud sound. The diagnosis is readily made by causing the patient to urinate in a bath or by plunging the end of the catheter under water.

XVI. OTHER SUBSTANCES

Lipuria.—Fat in the urine, or lipuria, occurs, first, without disease of the kidneys, as in excess of fat in the food, after the administration of cod liver oil, in fat embolism occurring after fractures, in the fatty degeneration in phosphorus poisoning, in prolonged suppuration, as in tuberculosis and pyæmia, in the lipæmia of diabetes mellitus; secondly, with disease of the kidneys, as in the fatty stage of chronic nephritis, in which fat casts are sometimes present, and, according to Ebstein, in pyonephrosis; and, thirdly, in the affection known as chyluria. The urine is usually turbid, but there may be fat drops as well, and fatty crystals have been found. In a few rare instances calculi composed of fat and coated with phosphates have been found.

Lipaciduria is applied to the condition in which there are volatile fatty acids in the urine, such as acetic, butyric, formic, and propionic acid.

Ketonuria.—The occurrence of *acetone, diacetic acid,* and *β-oxybutyric acid* has been considered under Diabetes.

Choluria and **glycosuria** are considered under jaundice and diabetes.

Hæmatoporphyrin occasionally occurs in the urine. It was first recognized by Hoppe-Seyler. Nencki and Sieler determined its exact formula, and the former demonstrated that the only chemical difference between hæmatin and hæmatoporphyrin is that the latter is simply hæmatin free from iron. It has been found in the urine in pulmonary tuberculosis, pleurisy with effusion, rheumatic fever, lead poisoning, and intestinal hæmorrhages. This pigment has been found very frequently after the administration of sulphonal, and sometimes imparts a very dark color to the urine.

V. URÆMIA

Definition.—A toxæmia from renal insufficiency developing in the course of nephritis or in conditions associated with anuria. The nature of the poison is in doubt.

Theories of Uræmia.—The chief views are: (*a*) That it is due to the accumulation in the blood of body poisons which should be excreted by the kidney. (*b*) That it is a disturbance of the normal kidney metabolism. Brown-Séquard suggested that the kidney had an internal secretion, to the disturbance of which it is thought that the symptoms of uræmia may be due. Rose Bradford's experiments show how profoundly the kidneys influence the body metabolism, particularly that of the muscles. If more than two-thirds of the total kidney weight is removed, there is an extraordinary increase in the production of urea and of the nitrogenous bodies of the creatin class. (*c*) Uræmia has been attributed to nephrolysins but the evidence is not convincing.

(*d*) The old view of Traube that the symptoms of uræmia, particularly the coma and convulsions, are due to localized œdema of the brain. (*e*) *Acidosis* has been suggested but while it may be associated, it is not an important cause and not always present. It seems probable that the causes vary in different patients.

Foster describes three forms of uræmia, but the majority of cases are not uncomplicated. 1. Retention type. In this there is a simple retention of urinary nitrogenous waste—a urinary poisoning. 2. Cerebral œdema type. In this there is defective water and salt excretion with a resulting cerebral œdema. 3. Toxic or epileptiform type. In this toxæmia is a marked feature, the result of abnormal metabolism. The first two represent a failure of excretion of water, salt and nitrogenous material. The third may show these but also an element foreign to normal metabolism, which causes toxæmia, and Foster has isolated a toxic base which causes convulsive seizures in animals. As regards the effect of urea itself Hewlett has shown that urea in the blood in amounts over 150 mg. per 100 c. c. produces symptoms like some of those seen in uræmia.

Symptoms.—Clinically, we may recognize latent, acute, and chronic forms. The latent form has been considered under the section on anuria. Acute uræmia may arise in any form of nephritis. It is more common in the post-febrile varieties. Bradford thinks that it is specially associated with a form of contracted white kidney in young subjects. Chronic forms of uræmia are more frequent in the arterio-sclerotic and granular kidney. For convenience the symptoms of uræmia may be described under cerebral, dyspnœic, and gastro-intestinal manifestations.

Among the CEREBRAL symptoms of uræmia may be described:

(*a*) *Mania.*—This may come on abruptly in an individual who has shown no previous indications of mental trouble, and who may not be known to have nephritis. In one case of this kind the patient became suddenly maniacal and died in six days. More commonly the delirium is less violent, but the patient is noisy, talkative, restless, and sleepless.

(*b*) *Delusional Insanity* (*Folie Brightique*).—Cases are by no means uncommon, and excellent clinical reports have been issued on the subject from several of the asylums, particularly by Bremer, Christian, and Alice Bennett. Delusions of persecution are common and the patients may commit suicide. The condition is of interest medico-legally because of its bearing on testamentary capacity. Profound melancholia may also supervene.

(*c*) *Convulsions.*—These may come on unexpectedly or be preceded by pain in the head and restlessness. The attacks may be general and identical with those of ordinary epilepsy, though the initial cry may not be present. The fits may recur rapidly, and in the interval the patient is usually unconscious. Sometimes the temperature is elevated, but more frequently it is depressed, and may sink rapidly after the attack. Local convulsions may occur in most characteristic form in uræmia. A remarkable sequence of the convulsions is blindness—*uræmic amaurosis*—which may persist for several days. This, however, may occur apart from the convulsions. It usually passes off in a day or two. There are, as a rule, no ophthalmoscopic changes. Sometimes uræmic deafness supervenes, and is probably also a cerebral manifestation. It may also occur in connection with persistent headache, nausea, and other gastric symptoms.

(*d*) *Coma.*—Unconsciousness invariably accompanies the general convulsions, but a coma may develop gradually without any convulsive seizures. Frequently it is preceded by headache, and the patient gradually becomes dull and apathetic. In these cases there may have been no previous indications of renal disease, and unless the urine is examined the nature of the case may be overlooked. Twitchings of the muscles occur, particularly in the face and hands, but there are many cases of coma in which the muscles are not involved. In some of these cases a condition of torpor persists for weeks or even months. The tongue is usually furred and the breath very foul and heavy.

(*e*) *Local Palsies.*—In the course of chronic nephritis hemiplegia, aphasia or monoplegia may come on spontaneously or follow a convulsion, and post mortem no gross lesions of the brain be found, but only a localized or diffused œdema. These cases, which are not very uncommon, may simulate almost every form of organic paralysis of cerebral origin.

(*f*) Of other cerebral symptoms, HEADACHE is important. It is most often occipital and extends to the neck. It may be an early feature and associated with giddiness. Other nervous symptoms of uræmia are intense itching of the skin, numbness and tingling in the fingers, and cramps in the muscles of the calves, particularly at night. An erythema may be present.

URÆMIC DYSPNŒA is classified by Palmer Howard as follows: (*a*) Continuous dyspnœa; (*b*) paroxysmal dyspnœa; (*c*) both types alternating; and (*d*) Cheyne-Stokes breathing. The attacks of dyspnœa are most commonly nocturnal; the patient may sit up, gasp for breath, and show great distress. Acidosis plays a part in some cases. Occasionally the breathing is noisy and stridulous. The Cheyne-Stokes type may persist for weeks or months. One patient, up and about, could feed himself only in the apnœa period. Though usually of serious omen and occurring with coma and other symptoms, recovery may follow even after persistence for a long period.

The GASTRO-INTESTINAL manifestations often set in with abruptness. Uncontrollable vomiting may come on and its cause be quite unrecognized. The attacks may be preceded by nausea and associated with diarrhœa. The diarrhœa may come on without the vomiting; sometimes it is profuse and associated with a catarrhal or diphtheritic inflammation of the colon.

A special URÆMIC STOMATITIS has been described in which the mucosa of the lips, gums, and tongue is swollen and erythematous. The saliva may be decreased, and there is difficulty in swallowing and in mastication. The tongue is usually very foul and the breath heavy and fetid. A cutaneous erythema may occur and a remarkable urea "frost" on the skin.

FEVER is not uncommon in uræmic states, and may occur with the acute nephritis, with the complications, and as a manifestation of the uræmia itself.

Very many patients with chronic uræmia succumb to terminal infections—acute peritonitis, pericarditis, pleurisy, meningitis, or endocarditis.

Diagnosis.—Blood analyses are of great value, both for diagnosis and prognosis. Non-protein nitrogen above 120 mgms., urea nitrogen above 80 mgms., uric acid above 4 mgms., and creatinine above 4 mgms. for 100 c. c. of blood point to the retention type. In the "œdema form" there may not be any increase. The test of the functional capacity of the kidney by the use of phenol-sulphonephthalein is of value both in differential diagnosis and in giving warning of impending uræmia. In uræmia the elimination of phthalein is nil or only a faint trace in two hours. In patients with chronic nephritis in whom the elimination in two hours is below 10 per cent. there is grave danger of uræmia.

Uræmia may be confounded with:

(*a*) Cerebral lesions, such as hæmorrhage, meningitis, or even tumor. In apoplexy, so commonly associated with nephritis and hypertension, the sudden loss of consciousness, particularly if with convulsions, may simulate uræmia; but the mode of onset, the existence of complete hemiplegia, with conjugate deviation of the eyes, suggest hæmorrhage. There are cases of uræmic hemiplegia or monoplegia which can not be separated from those of organic lesion and which post mortem show no trace of coarse disease of the brain. In some of these cases it is quite impossible to distinguish between the two conditions. So, too, cases of meningitis, in a condition of deep coma, with slight fever, furred tongue, but without localizing symptoms, may readily be confounded with uræmia.

(*b*) With certain infectious diseases. Uræmia may persist for weeks or months and the patient lies in a condition of torpor or even unconsciousness, with a heavily coated, perhaps dry, tongue, muscular twitchings, a rapid feeble pulse, with slight fever. This not unnaturally suggests the existence of one of the infectious diseases. Cases of the kind are not uncommon, and have been mistaken for typhoid fever and miliary tuberculosis.

(*c*) Uræmic coma may be confounded with poisoning by alcohol or opium. In opium poisoning the respiration is slow and the pupils contracted; in alcoholism they are more commonly dilated. In uræmia they are not constant; they may be either widely dilated or of medium size. The examination of the eye grounds should be made to determine the presence or absence of albuminuric retinitis. The urine should be examined. The odor of the breath sometimes gives an important hint. The condition of the heart and arteries should also be taken into account. Sudden uræmic coma is more common in chronic interstitial nephritis. The character of the delirium in alcoholism is sometimes important, and the coma is not so deep as in uræmia or opium poisoning. It may for a time be impossible to determine whether the condition is due to uræmia, profound alcoholism, or hæmorrhage into the pons Varolii.

And, lastly, in connection with sudden coma, it is to be remembered that insensibility may occur after prolonged muscular exertion, as after running a ten-mile race. In some instances unconsciousness has come on rapidly with stertorous breathing and dilated pupils. Cases have occurred under conditions in which sun-stroke could be excluded; and Poore considers that the condition is due to the too rapid accumulation of waste products in the blood, and to hyperpyrexia from suspension of sweating.

The treatment will be considered under Chronic Nephritis.

VI. ACUTE NEPHRITIS

Definition.—Acute diffuse nephritis, due to infection or to the action of toxic agents upon the kidneys. In all instances changes exist in the epithelial, vascular, and intertubular tissues, which vary in intensity in different forms: hence writers have described a tubular, a glomerular, and an acute interstitial nephritis.

Etiology.—The following are the principal causes of acute nephritis:

(1) Cold. Exposure to cold and wet is a common cause and determines, in all probability, an acute infection.

(2) The toxins of the acute infections, particularly scarlet fever. Many cases are due to streptococcus infection, secondary to some form of infection, as in the tonsils. An acute hæmatogenous infection may cause a very severe nephritis. It is evident that all grades of severity may occur. Syphilis is a factor in some cases. In exudative erythema and purpuric affections acute nephritis is not uncommon.

(3) *Epidemic nephritis.*—Described first during the American Civil War and noted by Italian observers, it prevailed widely during the recent war (Trench nephritis).

(4) Toxic agents, such as turpentine, mercury, potassium chlorate, and carbolic acid, may cause an acute congestion which sometimes terminates in nephritis. Alcohol probably never excites an acute nephritis.

(5) Pregnancy, in which the condition is probably due to toxic products as yet undetermined.

(6) Acute nephritis occurs occasionally in connection with extensive lesions of the skin, as in burns or in chronic skin-diseases, and also after trauma. It may follow operations on the kidney.

Poisons damage different portions of the kidney, corrosive sublimate the epithelium of the capsules and of the convoluted tubules of the adjacent first division, uranium chiefly the spiral portion of the convoluted tubes and Henle's loops, chromium the proximal and middle division of the convoluted and collecting tubules. It is not easy to correlate the experimental nephritis with the types of spontaneous nephritis in man. The experimental form has been studied with a view to determine the action of diuretics but without very positive results, except that in animals with experimental nephritis certain diuretics seem to shorten the duration of life.

Morbid Anatomy.—The kidneys may present to the naked eye in mild cases no evident alterations. When seen early in more severe forms the organs are congested, swollen, dark, and on section may drip blood. Bright's original description is as follows:

"The kidneys, . . . stripped easily out of their investing membrane, were large and less firm than they often are, of the darkest chocolate color, interspersed with a few white points, and a great number nearly black; and this, with a little tinge of red in parts, gave the appearance of a polished fine-grained porphyry or greenstone. . . . On (section) these colors were found to pervade the whole cortical part; but the natural striated appearance was not lost, and the external part of each mass of tubuli was particularly dark

. . . a very considerable quantity of blood oozed from the kidney, showing a most unusual accumulation in the organ."

In other instances the surface is pale and mottled, the capsule strips off readily, and the cortex is swollen, turbid, and of a grayish red color, while the pyramids have an intense beefy red tint. The glomeruli in some instances stand out plainly, being deeply swollen and congested; in other instances they are pale.

The histology may be thus summarized: (*a*) *Glomerular changes.* The tufts suffer first, and there is either an acute intracapillary glomerulitis, in which the capillaries become filled with cells and thrombi, or involvement of the epithelium of the tuft and of Bowman's capsule, the cavity of which contains leucocytes and red blood-corpuscles.

(*b*) The *alterations in the tubular epithelium* consist in cloudy swelling, fatty change, and hyaline degeneration. In the convoluted tubules, the accumulation of altered cells with leucocytes and blood-corpuscles causes the enlargement and swelling of the organ.

(*c*) *Interstitial changes.* In the milder forms a simple inflammatory exudate—serum mixed with leucocytes and red blood-corpuscles—exists between the tubules. In severer cases areas of small celled infiltration occur about the capsules and between the convoluted tubes.

Symptoms.—The onset is usually sudden, and, when the nephritis follows cold, dropsy may be noticed within twenty-four hours. After fevers the onset is less abrupt, but the patient gradually becomes pale and a puffiness of the face or swelling of the ankles is first noticed. In children there may be convulsions at the outset. Chilliness or rigors initiate the attack in a limited number of cases. Pain in the back, nausea, and vomiting may be present. The fever is variable. Many cases in adults have no rise in temperature. In young children with nephritis from cold or scarlet fever the temperature may, for a few days, range from 101° to 103°.

The most characteristic symptoms are the *urinary changes.* There may at first be suppression; more commonly the urine is scanty, highly colored, and contains blood, albumin, and tube casts. The quantity is reduced and only 4 or 5 ounces may be passed in twenty-four hours; the specific gravity is high—1.025, or more; the color varies from a smoky to a deep porter color, but is seldom bright red. On standing there is a heavy deposit; microscopically there are blood corpuscles, epithelium from the urinary passages, and hyaline, blood, and epithelial tube casts. The albumin is abundant, forming a curdy, thick precipitate. The largest amounts of albumin are seen in the early acute nephritis of syphilis, in which it may reach 8.5 per cent. The total excretion of urea is reduced, though the percentage is high.

Œdema is an early and marked symptom. In cases of extensive dropsy effusion may take place into the pleuræ and peritoneum. There are cases of scarlatinal nephritis in which the dropsy of the extremities is trivial and effusion into the pleuræ extensive. The lungs may become œdematous. In rare cases there is œdema of the glottis. Epistaxis may occur or cutaneous ecchymoses may develop in the course of the disease.

The pulse may be hard, the tension increased, and the second sound in the aortic area accentuated. The blood pressure may be very variable. Occasionally dilatation of the heart comes on rapidly and may cause sudden death. The skin is dry and it may be difficult to induce sweating.

Uræmic symptoms occur in a limited number of cases, either at the onset with suppression, more commonly later in the disease. Ocular changes are not so common in acute as in chronic nephritis, but hæmorrhagic retinitis may occur and occasionally papillitis.

The *course* varies considerably. The description just given is of the form which most commonly follows cold or scarlet fever. In many of the febrile cases dropsy is not a prominent symptom, and the diagnosis rests rather with the examination of the urine. Moreover, the condition may be transient and less serious. In other cases there may be hæmaturia and pronounced signs of interference with the renal function. The most intense acute nephritis may exist without anasarca. In *scarlatinal* nephritis, in which the glomeruli are most seriously affected, suppression of the urine may be an early symptom, the dropsy is apt to be extreme, and uræmic manifestations are common. Acute nephritis in children, however, may set in very insidiously and be associated with transient or slight œdema, and the symptoms may point rather to affection of the digestive system or to brain disease.

Diagnosis.—It is very important to bear in mind that the most serious involvement of the kidneys may be manifested only by slight œdema of the feet or puffiness of the eyelids, without impairment of the general health. On the other hand, from the urine alone a diagnosis can not be made with certainty, since simple cloudy swelling and circulatory changes may cause a similar condition of urine. The first indication of trouble may be a uræmic convulsion. This is particularly the case in the acute nephritis of pregnancy, and it is a good rule for the practitioner invariably to ask that during pregnancy the urine should be sent regularly for examination.

In nephritis from cold and in scarlet fever the symptoms are usually marked and the diagnosis is rarely in doubt. As already mentioned, every case in which albumin is present should not be called acute nephritis, not even if tube casts be present. Thus the common febrile albuminuria, although it represents the first link in the chain of events leading to acute nephritis, should not be placed in the same category. The most frequent error is to regard *acute exacerbations* in chronic nephritis as primary acute attacks. The history, the condition of the heart and vessels, the blood pressure, and the eye grounds are important points in recognizing the existence of former nephritis.

There are occasional cases of acute nephritis with anasarca, in which albumin is either absent or present only as a trace, but these are rare. Tube casts are usually found, and the absence of albumin is rarely permanent. The urine may be reduced in amount.

The character of the casts is of use in the diagnosis of the form of nephritis, but scarcely of such value as has been stated. The hyaline and granular casts are common to all varieties. The blood and epithelial casts, particularly those made up of leucocytes, are most common in the acute cases.

Prognosis.—The outlook varies somewhat with the cause. Recoveries in the form following exposure to cold are much more frequent than after scarlatinal nephritis. In younger children the mortality is high, amounting to at least one-third of the cases. Serious symptoms are low arterial tension, the occurrence of uræmia, and effusion into the serous sacs. The persistence of the dropsy after the first month, intense pallor, and a large amount of albumin indicate the possibility of the disease becoming chronic. For some months after the disappearance of the dropsy there may be traces of albumin and a few tube casts. If the nephritis is due to a focus of infection which can be removed the outlook is naturally better.

In scarlatinal nephritis, if the progress is favorable, the dropsy diminishes in a week or ten days, the urine increases, the albumin lessens, and by the end of a month the dropsy has disappeared and the urine is nearly free. In very young children the course may be rapid, and the urine may be free from albumin in the fourth week. Other cases are more insidious, and though the dropsy may disappear, the albumin persists in the urine, the anæmia is marked, and the condition becomes chronic, or, after several recurrences of the dropsy, improves and complete recovery takes place.

Prophylaxis.—Care in the infectious diseases which may be complicated by nephritis is important. Proper treatment of foci of infection, especially the tonsils, is of value. Care should be taken not to give any drugs which may irritate the kidney.

Treatment.—The patient should be in bed and remain there until all traces of the disease have disappeared or until there is no hope of complete recovery. A period of three months should be allowed for this. The presence of red blood cells in the urine is an indication for absolute rest. As sweating plays such an important part in the treatment, it is well, if possible, to accustom the patient to blankets. He should also be clad in thin Canton flannel.

The *diet* should consist of milk or butter-milk, gruels made of arrow-root or oat-meal, barley water, and fruit juices. It is sometimes better to confine the patient to a strictly milk diet for a few days. Cream and lactose may be added. As convalescence is established, bread and butter, lettuce, water cress, grapes, oranges, and other fruits may be given. Meats should be used very sparingly. As there is marked retention of the chlorides, which seem to bear a relation to the dropsy, salt should be withheld.

The *fluid* intake must be governed by the condition. With œdema it is well to restrict the total intake to 1000 or 1500 c. c. Otherwise the patient may drink freely of alkaline mineral waters, ordinary water, or lemonade. A useful drink is a dram of cream of tartar in a pint of boiling water, to which may be added the juice of half a lemon and a little sugar. Taken when cold, this is a pleasant diluent drink. Alkaline drinks are useful if there is acidosis. Fluid may be given by the bowel or by saline infusion if it is not well taken by mouth.

No remedies, so far as known, control directly the changes going on in the kidneys. The indications are: (1) To give the excretory function of the kidney rest by utilizing the skin and the bowels, in the hope that the natural processes may effect a cure; (2) to meet symptoms as they arise.

In a case of scarlet fever it may occasionally be possible to avert an attack, the premonitory symptoms of which are marked increase in the arterial tension and the presence of blood coloring matter in the urine (Mahomed). An active saline cathartic may completely relieve this condition.

At the onset, when there is pain in the back or hæmaturia, the Paquelin cautery or the dry cups give relief. Warm poultices are often grateful. In cases which set in with suppression of urine these measures should be adopted, and in addition the hot bath with subsequent pack, copious diluents, and a free purge. The dropsy is best treated by hydrotherapy—either the hot bath, the wet pack, or the hot-air bath. In children the wet pack is usually satisfactory. It is applied by wringing a blanket out of hot water, wrapping the child in it, covering this with a dry blanket, and then with a rubber cloth. In this the child may remain for an hour. It may be repeated daily. In the case of adults, the hot air bath or the vapor bath may be conveniently given by allowing the vapor or air to pass from a funnel beneath the bed clothes, which are raised on a low cradle. More efficient, as a rule, is a hot bath of from fifteen or twenty minutes, after which the patient is wrapped in blankets. The sweating produced by these measures is usually profuse, rarely exhausting, and in a majority of cases the dropsy can be relieved in this way. There are some cases in which the skin does not respond to the baths, and if the symptoms are serious, particularly if uræmia supervenes, pilocarpine may be used. The latter may be given hypodermically, in doses of from a sixth to an eighth of a grain (0.01 to 0.008 gm.) in adults, and from a twentieth to a twelfth of a grain (0.003 to 0.005 gm.) in children of from two to ten years.

The *bowels* should be kept open by a morning saline purge; in children the fluid magnesia is readily taken; in adults the sulphate of magnesia may be given by Hay's method, in concentrated form, in the morning, before anything is taken into the stomach. In nephritis it not infrequently causes vomiting. The compound powder of jalap (gr. xx, 1.3 gm.) or, if necessary, elaterin (gr. 1/20, 0.003 gm.) may be used. If the dropsy is not extreme, the urine not very concentrated, and uræmic symptoms are not present, the bowels should be kept loose without active purgation. If these measures fail to reduce the dropsy and it has become extreme, the skin may be punctured with a lancet or drained by a fine aspirator needle and the fluid allowed to flow through rubber tubing into a vessel beneath the bed. If the dyspnœa is marked, owing to pressure of fluid in the pleuræ, aspiration should be performed. In some instances the ascites is extreme and may require paracentesis. If uræmic convulsions occur, the intensity of the paroxysms may be limited by the use of chloroform; to an adult a pilocarpine injection should be at once given, and from a robust, strong man 20 ounces of blood may be withdrawn. In children the loins may be dry cupped, the wet pack used, and a brisk purgative given. Bromide of potassium and chloral sometimes prove useful. Vomiting may be relieved by ice and by restricting the amount of food.

As to the use of *diuretics* in acute nephritis the best diuretic is water, which may be taken freely with citrate of potash, if the kidneys can excrete it. Digitalis should be given only when the myocardial condition requires it.

For the persistent *albuminuria,* we have no remedy of the slightest value. Nothing indicates more clearly our helplessness in controlling kidney metabolism than inability to meet this common symptom.

For the *anæmia* associated with acute nephritis iron should be employed but not until the acute symptoms have subsided. In the adult it may be used in the form of the perchloride in increasing doses, as convalescence proceeds. In children, the syrup of the iodide of iron or the syrup of the phosphate of iron are useful preparations. Tyson urged caution in the too free use of iron in kidney disease. In convalescence care should be taken to guard the patient against cold. The diet should still consist chiefly of milk and a return to mixed food should be gradual. A change of air is often beneficial, particularly a residence in a warm, equable climate.

VII. CHRONIC NEPHRITIS

In nephritis there are two principal departures from normal: (1) The kidney lets out material which should be kept in (e. g. albumin) and (2) keeps in material which should be passed out. The first represents the significant urinary findings, the second the changes in the blood and body fluids.

A clinical classification of chronic nephritis offers many difficulties. A pathological classification deals with end results and can not be applied at the bedside. In all forms we deal with a diffuse process, involving epithelial, interstitial and glomerular tissue. A functional diagnosis is of great value but the function of the kidney may be influenced by factors outside the kidney itself. As regards an etiological classification there is more opportunity for this in acute nephritis than in the chronic forms in which it is only possible in a small proportion of cases and does not take us very far in estimating the present condition. Two main forms may be recognized. (1) Those termed chronic interstitial—the "dry" form, in which there is a retention of nitrogenous products in the blood, often ending in uræmia, and (2) the chronic parenchymatous—the "wet" form, in which there is retention of water and salt with resulting œdema. There are many intermediate forms and the terms mentioned may be regarded as describing the cases at each end of a series with every grade of variation between. The tendency is to consider the occurrence of hypertension and œdema with the result of the functional tests as designating a symptom-complex rather than a distinct disease. The most useful tests in estimating the kidney function are: (1) The phthalein test. (2) The determination of the urea nitrogen, uric acid and creatinine content of the blood with the estimation of the index of urea excretion (Ambard, McLean). (3) The two-hour test in which the patient is given full diet with fluid at mealtime only. The urine is collected every two hours from 8 a. m. to 10 p. m. and from 10 p. m. to 8 a. m. The important points are the lowering of the maximum specific gravity, the fixation of specific gravity and an increase in the night urine. (4) The response to the action of a diuretic.

The amyloid kidney is usually spoken of as a variety of nephritis, but in reality it is a degeneration which may accompany any form of nephritis.

I. CHRONIC PARENCHYMATOUS NEPHRITIS

Etiology.—In many cases the disease follows an acute nephritis, but more frequently than is usually stated the disease has an insidious onset and occurs independently of any acute attack. Continued bacterial septicæmia, secondary to a focal infection, is probably the most important cause. The fevers may play an important rôle in certain cases. Rosenstein, Bartels, I. E. Atkinson, and Thayer have laid stress upon malaria as a cause. The use of alcohol is believed to lead to this form of nephritis. In chronic suppuration, syphilis, and tuberculosis a diffuse nephritis is not uncommon, sometimes associated with amyloid disease. Males are rather more subject to the affection than females. It is met with most commonly in young adults, and is by no means infrequent in children as a sequence of scarlatinal nephritis.

Morbid Anatomy.—Several varieties have been recognized. The *large white kidney* of Wilks, in which the organ is enlarged, the capsule is thin, and the surface white with the stellate veins injected, is not common in America. On section the cortex is swollen and yellowish white in color, and often presents opaque areas. The pyramids may be deeply congested. On microscopic examination the epithelium is granular and fatty, and the tubules of the cortex are distended, and contain tube casts. Hyaline changes are present in the epithelial cells. The glomeruli are large, the capsules thickened, the capillaries show hyaline changes, and the epithelium of the tuft and of the capsule is extensively altered. The interstitial tissue is everywhere increased, though not to an extreme degree.

The second variety results from gradual increase in the connective tissue and subsequent shrinkage, forming what is called the *small white kidney* or the pale granular kidney. It is doubtful whether this is always preceded by the large white kidney. Some observers hold that it may be a primary independent form. The capsule is thickened and the surface rough and granular. On section the resistance is greatly increased, the cortex is reduced and presents numerous opaque white or whitish yellow foci, consisting of accumulations of fatty epithelium in the convoluted tubules. This combination of contracted kidney with areas of marked fatty degeneration has been given the name of small granular fatty kidney. The interstitial changes are marked, many glomeruli are destroyed, the degeneration of epithelium in the convoluted tubules is widespread, and the arteries are greatly thickened.

Belonging to this chronic tubal nephritis is a variety known as the *chronic hæmorrhagic nephritis,* in which the organs are enlarged, yellowish white in color, and in the cortex are many brownish red areas, due to hæmorrhage into and about the tubes. In other respects the changes are identical with those in the large white kidney.

Symptoms.—Following an acute nephritis, the disease may present, in a modified way, the symptoms of that affection. In many cases it sets in insidiously, and after an attack of dyspepsia or a period of failing health and loss of strength the patient becomes pale, and puffiness of the eyelids or swollen feet are noticed in the morning.

The symptoms are as follows: The urine is, as a rule, diminished in quantity, averaging 500 c. c. It has a dirty yellow, sometimes smoky, color, and is turbid from the presence of urates. On standing, a heavy sediment falls, in which are found numerous tube casts of various forms and sizes, hyaline, both large and small, epithelial, granular, and fatty casts. Leucocytes are abundant; red blood cells are frequently met with, and epithelium from the kidneys and pelves. The albumin is abundant and may be from 4 to 6 per cent. It is more abundant in the urine passed during the day. The specific gravity may be high in the early stages—from 1.020 to 1.025, even 1.040—though in the later stages it is lower. The urea is always reduced in quantity. As the patient improves from 5 to 6 litres of urine a day may be voided.

Dropsy is a marked and obstinate symptom of this form. The face is pale and puffy, and in the morning the eyelids are œdematous. The anasarca is general, and there may be involvement of the serous sacs. In these chronic cases associated with large white kidney there is often a distinctive appearance in the face; the complexion is pasty, the pallor marked, and the eyelids are œdematous. The dropsy is peculiarly obstinate. Epstein suggests that "the loss of protein incurred by the blood serum through the continuous albuminuria causes a decrease in the osmotic pressure of the blood, which favors the absorption or inhibition and retention of fluid by the tissues." With this there is a great increase in the lipoid content of the blood—lipoidæmia. Uræmic symptoms are common, though convulsions are perhaps less frequent than in interstitial nephritis.

The tension of the pulse may be increased; the vessels ultimately become stiff and the heart hypertrophied, though there are instances of this form in which the heart is not enlarged. The aortic second sound may be accentuated. Retinal changes, though less frequent than in the chronic interstitial nephritis, occur in a considerable number of cases.

Gastro-intestinal symptoms are common. Vomiting is frequently a distressing and serious symptom, and diarrhœa may be profuse. Ulceration of the colon may prove fatal and is common in the tropics in association with malarial and other forms of nephritis.

The *functional* tests may show great variations. In many cases the greatest change is in the ability to secrete water and salt, in others the reduction in function is more general and the phthalein excretion may be much reduced. In some cases there is hyperpermeability.

It is sometimes impossible to determine, even by the most careful examination of the urine or by analysis of the symptoms, whether the condition of the kidney is that of the large white or of the small white form. In cases, however, which have lasted for several years, with the progressive increase in the renal connective tissue and the cardio-vascular changes, the clinical picture may approach, in certain respects, that of the contracted kidney. The urine is increased, with low specific gravity. It is often turbid, may contain traces of blood, the tube casts are numerous and of every variety of form and size, and the albumin is abundant. Dropsy is usually present, though not so extensive as in the early stages.

Prognosis.—This is extremely grave. In a case which has persisted for more than a year recovery rarely takes place. Death is caused either by great effusion with œdema of the lungs, by uræmia, or by secondary inflammation of the serous membranes. Occasionally in children, even when the disease has persisted for two years, the symptoms disappear and recovery takes place. The frequency of acute exacerbations adds to the uncertainty of prognosis. A marked decrease in the kidney function is of grave omen.

Treatment.—Much the same treatment should be carried out as in acute nephritis. Rest need not be absolute if the general condition permits of some exertion. The dropsy should be treated by hot baths and a salt-free diet. Iron preparations should be given when there is marked anæmia but the pallor of the face may not be a good index of the blood condition. The acetate of potash, digitalis, and diuretin are useful in increasing the flow of urine. Basham's mixture given in plenty of water is often beneficial.

Diet.—In line with the views held by Epstein the effort should be to increase the protein content of the blood and reduce the excessive amount of lipoid. This must be done largely by a high protein and fat poor diet, with a moderate amount of carbohydrates. He gives 120 to 240 gm. of protein, 20 to 40 gm. of fat and 150 to 300 gm. of carbohydrate. The fluid intake is from 1200 to 1500 c. c. and the amount of salt is reduced to a minimum. The foods are lean veal and ham, egg white, oysters, gelatine, lima beans, split and green peas, rice, oatmeal, mushrooms, bananas, skimmed milk, coffee, tea and cocoa. The amount of fluid intake must in many cases be decided by results. The Karrell diet consists in giving 200 c. c. of milk at 8 a. m., 12 noon, and 4 and 8 p. m., and nothing more. After a week, a soft egg with bread may be added and the diet gradually increased but the intake of fluid should be kept at 800 c. c. a day for some time. Some patients with marked dropsy do well with this, but in others it is advisable to increase the amount of fluid.

II. CHRONIC INTERSTITIAL NEPHRITIS

(*Contracted Kidney; Arterio-sclerotic Kidney; Senile Kidney*)

Etiology and Morbid Anatomy.—Sclerosis of the kidney is met with (*a*) as a sequence of the large white kidney, forming the secondary contracted kidney; (*b*) as a primary independent affection, the red granular kidney; (*c*) as a sequence of arterio-sclerosis; and (*d*) as a senile change.

(*a*) SECONDARY FORM.—The small white kidney, as it is called, has already been described as a sequel to chronic parenchymatous nephritis.

(*b*) In the PRIMARY FORM, known also as the red granular kidney, the organ is smaller than in the secondary interstitial nephritis, the capsule is very adherent, the granulations small, the organ of a reddish brown color, the cysts numerous, the arteries very sclerotic, and the cortex greatly reduced in volume. The chief reason for calling this primary is that one can find no history of previous renal disease. Some families show the disease in many members for several generations. Syphilis, alcohol, and overeating are mentioned as contributory causes. Lead is a rare cause in America but a more common cause in parts of England. It is by no means always easy to differentiate between the secondary and the primary forms. As a rule, the former is paler and not so small. Of 174 cases of this form which came to autopsy, in 79 the combined weight of the kidneys was about 300 grams, in 57 cases 200 to 300 grams, in 30 cases 150 to 200 grams, and below 150 grams in 8 cases (Emerson). Unilateral nephritis is extremely rare, not occurring once in the series.

(*c*) ARTERIO-SCLEROTIC KIDNEY.—This is not necessarily a contracted kidney. The organ is very hard, red, and often heavier than normal. Of the cases, studied by Emerson, in 61 per cent. the combined weight was above 300 grams, and in only 6 per cent. was it below 200 grams. The surface may be smooth or the capsule only slightly thickened and adherent, tearing the substance very little as it is stripped off. In other cases the atrophy is in spots, affecting certain vascular districts, so that there is a large, sunken, deep red patch on the surface, or one pole of the kidney is shrunken, or the process is general in both kidneys, but the resulting contraction gives a warty rather than a granular surface.

(*d*) In the SENILE FORM, met with in the aged, the organs are reduced in size, the capsules thickened and adherent, the pelvic fat much increased, both cortical and pyramidal portions uniformly wasted, and the arteries of the kidney substance very prominent.

Almost invariably associated with chronic interstitial nephritis are general arterio-sclerosis and hypertrophy of the heart. The changes in the arteries will be described elsewhere. In the red granular kidney the left ventricle is specially hypertrophied, but in all forms the heart is greatly enlarged. In many cases the disease is latent, and the patients die of apoplexy or of acute uræmia. In the arterio-sclerotic form death is more commonly cardiac, and the condition of the kidneys may be entirely overlooked.

The disease is really one which involves the *cardiovascular-renal system*. Much discussion has taken place as to the association of hypertrophy of the heart and sclerosis of the blood-vessels with the renal changes. A complete solution of the problems has scarcely yet been offered. Briefly, there are two views—the mechanical and the chemical. Dating from the time of Bright it was thought that the heart had greater difficulty in driving the blood through the capillary system. Traube held that the obliteration of a large number of capillary territories in the kidney raised the arterial pressure and in this way led to hypertrophy of the heart. In explanation of the muscular hypertrophy of the walls of the smaller arteries George Johnson introduced the view of a stop-cock action of these vessels under the influence of irritating ingredients in the blood. The mechanical view was thus put by Cohnheim. The activity of the circulation through the kidneys at any moment does not depend upon the need of these organs for blood, but solely upon the amount of material for the urinary secretion existing in the blood. When parts of both kidneys have undergone atrophy, the blood flow in the parts remaining must be as great as it would have been to the whole of the organs, had they been intact; but in order that such a quantity of blood should pass through the restricted capillary area now open to it an excessive pressure is necessary. This can be brought to bear only by the exertion of an increased force on the part of the left ventricle with the maintenance of a corresponding resistance in all other arterial territories. In this way both the high arterial pressure and the cardio-vascular changes are explained.

The chemical view supposes the production (*a*) by the kidneys, (*b*) by the supra-renal glands, of certain pressor substances. So far as the kidney is concerned, the observations are by no means in accord. In chronic interstitial nephritis there is often hyperplasia of the cortical substance of the suprarenals, and some have claimed to have discovered in the blood of chronic nephritics an increase in the pressor substances, an adrenalinæmia. Through their influence, from one or both of these sources, the blood-pressure is raised, with the sequence of hypertrophy of the heart and sclerosis of the arteries.

Symptoms.—Many cases are latent, and are not recognized until the occurrence of one of the serious or fatal complications. Even an advanced grade of contracted kidney may be compatible with great mental and bodily activity.

There may have been no symptoms whatever to suggest to the patient the existence of a serious malady. In other cases the general health is disturbed. The patient complains of lassitude, is sleepless, has to get up at night to micturate; the digestion is disordered, the tongue is furred; there are complaints of headache, failing vision, and breathlessness on exertion.

So complex and varied is the clinical picture that it will be best to consider the symptoms under the various systems.

URINARY SYSTEM.—In the *small contracted kidney* polyuria is common. Frequently the patient has to get up two or three times during the night to empty the bladder, and there is increased thirst. It is for these symptoms occasionally that relief is sought. And yet in many cases with very small kidneys this feature has not been present. A careful study of the urine and the anatomical condition showed that no close parallelism could be made between the weight of the kidney, its appearance, and the urine it secreted before death. Of 174 cases with autopsy, in almost a third the renal changes were so slight that the nephritis was not mentioned as a part of the clinical diagnosis (Emerson). The color of the urine is a light yellow, and the specific gravity ranges from 1.005 to 1.012. Persistent low specific gravity is one of the most constant and important features. Traces of albumin are found, but may be absent at times, particularly in the early morning urine. It may be apparent only with the more delicate tests. The sediment is scanty, and in it a few hyaline or granular casts are found. The quantity of the solid constituents of the urine is, as a rule, diminished, though in some instances the urea may be excreted in full amount. In attacks of dyspepsia or bronchitis, or in the later stages when the heart fails, the quantity of albumin may be greatly increased and the urine diminished. Occasionally blood occurs in the urine; and there may be hæmaturia (S. West). Slight leakage, represented by the constant presence of a few red cells, may be present early in the disease and persist for years. In the *arterio-sclerotic form* the quantity of urine is normal, or reduced rather than increased; the specific gravity is normal or high, the color of the urine is good, and there are hyaline and finely granular casts. The amount of albumin varies with the food and exercise, and is usually much in excess of that seen with the contracted kidneys, and does not show so often the albumin free intervals of that form, also it is more common to find albumin without casts, while in the contracted kidney casts may occur without albumin.

The functional findings are very variable in different stages. They are of value in determining the approach of uræmia. As the studies of Janeway showed, in the majority of cases death is not from renal insufficiency but from cardiac failure or cerebral vascular disease. Functional tests are of value in deciding whether myocardial or renal insufficiency is the more important factor.

CIRCULATORY SYSTEM.—The pulse is hard, the tension increased, and the vessel wall, as a rule, thickened. A distinction must be made between increased tension and thickening of the arterial wall. The tension may be plus in a normal vessel, but in chronic nephritis it is more common to have increased tension in a stiff artery.

A pulse of increased tension has the following characters: It is hard and incompressible, requiring a good deal of force to overcome it; it is persistent, and in the intervals between the beats the vessel feels full and can be rolled beneath the finger. These characters may be present in a vessel the walls of which are little, if at all, increased in thickness. To estimate the latter the pulse wave should be obliterated in the radial, and the vessel wall felt beyond it. In a perfectly normal vessel the arterial coats, under these circumstances, can not be differentiated from the surrounding tissue; whereas, if thickened, the vessel can be rolled beneath the finger. Persistent *high blood pressure* is one of the earliest and most important symptoms of interstitial nephritis. During the disease the pressure may rise to 250 mm. or 300 mm. With dropsy and cardiac dilatation the pressure may fall, but not necessarily. The cardiac features are equally important, though often less obvious. Hypertrophy of the left ventricle occurs to overcome the resistance offered in the arteries. The enlargement of the heart ultimately becomes more general. The apex is displaced downward and to the left; the impulse is forcible and may be heaving. In elderly persons with emphysema the displacement of the apex may not be evident. The first sound at the apex may be duplicated; more commonly the second sound at the aortic cartilage is accentuated. The sound in extreme cases may have a bell-like quality. In many cases a systolic murmur develops at the apex, as a result of relative insufficiency. It may be loud and transmitted to the axilla. Finally the hypertrophy fails, the heart becomes dilated, gallop rhythm is present, and the general condition is that of chronic myocardial failure. In the arterio-sclerotic form the picture may be cardiac from beginning to close—dyspnœa and signs of dilated heart.

Blood.—The estimation of the urea N, uric acid and creatinin is particularly important, an increase meaning retention. The urea N (normal 12-15 mg. per 100 c. c.) is increased to 15-50 mgs. in chronic nephritis and 80-300 in uræmia. Uric acid (normal 1-2.5) is increased to 4 in chronic nephritis and 4-15 in uræmia. Creatinin (normal 1-2.5) is increased to 3 in chronic nephritis and from 3 to 5 in uræmia. These findings are important in diagnosis and prognosis. It is a question which of these is the most useful. Persistent low urea content in the blood, in the absence of œdema, is evidence against renal disease. As the uric acid is the most difficult to excrete some regard its estimation as particularly useful in the absence of gout. In the immediate prognosis the creatinin estimation is important. Amounts from 3 to 5 mg. per 100 c. c. of blood are unfavorable and if above 5 mg. an early termination may be expected.

Respiratory System.—Sudden œdema of the glottis may occur. Effusion into the pleuræ or sudden œdema of the lungs may prove fatal. Acute pleurisy and pneumonia are not uncommon. Bronchitis is a frequent accompaniment, particularly in the winter. Sudden attacks of dyspnœa, particularly at night, are not infrequent. This is often a uræmic symptom or due to acidosis but is sometimes cardiac. Cheyne-Stokes breathing may be present, most commonly toward the close, but the patient may be walking about and even attending to his occupation.

Acidosis.—The majority of advanced cases show some degree of acidosis, which is often severe and hastens a fatal issue.

Digestive System.—Dyspepsia and loss of appetite are common. Severe and uncontrollable vomiting may be the first symptom. This is usually regarded as a manifestation of uræmia, but it may occur without any other indications, and may prove fatal without any suspicion that chronic nephritis was present. Severe and even fatal diarrhœa may develop. The tongue may be coated and the breath heavy and urinous.

Nervous System.—Various cerebral manifestations have been mentioned under uræmia. Headache, sometimes of the migraine type, may be an early and persistent feature of chronic nephritis. A morning headache which wakes the patient early and lasts until midday is not uncommon. In hypertension mental work often causes headache. Cerebral hemorrhage is closely related to interstitial nephritis and may take place into the meninges or the cerebrum. It is usually associated with marked changes in the vessels. Neuralgias, in various regions, are not uncommon.

Special Senses.—Troubles in vision may be the first symptom. It is remarkable in how many cases the condition is diagnosed first by the ophthalmic surgeon. The flame shaped retinal hæmorrhages are the most common. Less frequent is diffuse retinitis or papillitis. Sudden blindness may supervene without retinal changes—uræmic amaurosis. Diplopia is a rare event. Recurring conjunctival and palpebral hæmorrhages are fairly common, particularly in the arterio-sclerotic form. Auditory troubles are by no means infrequent and ringing in the ears, with dizziness, is not uncommon. Various forms of deafness may occur.

Skin.—Œdema is not common in interstitial nephritis. Slight puffiness of the ankles may be present, but in a majority of the cases dropsy does not supervene. When extensive, it is almost always the result of gradual failure of the hypertrophied heart. The skin is often dry and pale, and sweats are not common. In some instances the sweat may deposit a white frost of urea on the surface of the skin. Eczema is a common accompaniment of chronic interstitial nephritis. Tingling of the fingers or numbness and pallor—the dead fingers—are not, as some suppose, in any way peculiar to nephritis. Intolerable itching of the skin may be present, and cramps in the muscles are by no means rare.

Hæmorrhages are not infrequent, particularly epistaxis. Severe and widespread purpura is a not uncommon terminal event and the primary disease may not be recognized. Broncho-pulmonary hæmorrhages may occur. Ascites is rare except in association with cirrhosis of the liver.

Diagnosis.—The autopsy often discloses the true nature of the disease, one of the many intercurrent affections of which may have proved fatal. The early stages of interstitial nephritis are difficult to recognize. In a patient with increased pulse tension (particularly if the vessel wall is sclerotic), with the apex beat of the heart dislocated to the left, the second aortic sound ringing and accentuated, the urine abundant and of low specific gravity, with a trace of albumin and an occasional hyaline or granular cast, the dignosis of interstitial nephritis may be safely made. Of all the indications, that offered by the pulse is the most important. Persistent high tension with thickening of the arterial wall in a man under fifty means that serious mischief has already taken place, that cardio-vascular changes are certainly, and renal most probably, present. In the arterio-sclerotic cases the history is of the "strenuous life"—work, alcohol, tobacco, Venus—and not of an infection or of lead or gout. The urine is not of persistently low specific gravity, there may be little or no albumin except in intercurrent attacks; the symptoms are cardiac rather than renal or cerebral; the ocular changes are hæmorrhagic, not the true albuminuric retinitis. Primary hypertension should be distinguished and in this the functional tests are of value.

Prognosis.—Chronic nephritis is an incurable affection, and the anatomical conditions on which it depends are quite as much beyond the reach of medicines as wrinkled skin or gray hair. However, it is compatible with the enjoyment of life for many years, and it is now recognized that increased tension, thickening of the arterial walls, and polyuria with a small quantity of albumin, neither doom a man to death within a short time nor necessarily interfere with the pursuits of an active life so long as proper care be taken. Patients with high tension and a little albumin in the urine with hyaline casts may live for ten, twelve, or even fifteen years. Serious indications are the occurrence of uræmic symptoms, dilatation of the heart, the onset of serous effusions, the onset of Cheyne-Stokes breathing, marked acidosis, persistent vomiting, and diarrhœa. The functional tests and blood analysis give valuable information and are material aids in prognosis.

Treatment.—Patients without local indications or in whom the condition has been accidentally discovered should so regulate their lives as to throw the least possible strain upon heart, arteries, and kidneys. A quiet life without mental worry, with gentle but not excessive exercise, and residence in an equable climate, should be recommended. In addition they should be told to keep the bowels open, the skin active by a daily tepid bath with friction, and the urinary secretion free by drinking daily a definite amount of either distilled water or some pleasant mineral water. Alcohol should be strictly prohibited. Tea and coffee are allowable.

The diet should be light and nourishing, and the patient should be warned not to eat excessively, and not to take meat more than once a day. Care in food and drink is probably the most important element in the treatment of early cases. A patient in good circumstances may be urged to go away during the winter months, or, if necessary, to move altogether to a warm equable climate, like that of Southern California. There is no doubt of the value in these cases of removal from the changeable, irregular weather which prevails in the temperate regions from November until April.

At this period medicines are not required unless for certain special symptoms. Patients derive much benefit from an annual visit to certain mineral springs, such as Poland, Bedford, Saratoga, in America, and Vichy and others in Europe. Mineral waters have no curative influence upon chronic nephritis; they simply help the interstitial circulation and keep the drains flushed. In this early stage, when the patient's condition is good, the tension not high, and the quantity of albumin small, medicines are not indicated, since no remedies are known to have the slightest influence upon the progress of the disease. Sooner or later SYMPTOMS arise which demand treatment. Of these the following are the most important:

(*a*) *Hypertension.*—It is to be remembered that a certain increase of tension is not only necessary but unavoidable in chronic nephritis, and probably the most serious danger is too great lowering of the tension. The happy medium must be sought between such heightened tension as throws a serious strain upon the heart and risks rupture of the vessels and the low tension which, under these circumstances, is specially liable to be associated with serous effusions. In cases with persistent high tension the diet should be light, an occasional saline purge should be given, and sweating promoted by means of hot air or the hot bath. A few days in bed on milk diet is sometimes useful. An occasional venesection helps some patients.

(*b*) More or less *anæmia* is present in advanced cases, and is best met by the use of iron.

(*c*) *Myocardial insufficiency.*—The patient should be allowed to assume the most comfortable position but rest should be as complete as possible. The diet should be greatly restricted and it is often wise to give no food for a day. Then milk (750 to 1000 c. c. a day) may be allowed. Later it is well to give food in small amounts with frequent feedings. The total intake of fluids must depend somewhat on the presence of œdema. With this the amount of fluid should not be over 1500 c. c. and salt withheld as far as possible. Free purgation is indicated, for which calomel or elaterin (gr. 1/20, 0.003 gm.) and salines may be used. With marked dilatation of the heart, venesection is advisable unless the patient is anæmic. Digitalis is indicated and a high blood pressure is not a contraindication to its use. Full doses should be employed and with a good preparation it matters little in which form it is given. In severe cases it is well to give it intramuscularly or administer one dose of strophanthin and follow this with digitalis. Of other preparations, theobromine (gr. v, 0.3 gm.), diuretin (gr. xv, 1 gm.), and theocin (gr. iii, 0.2 gm.) may be tried. None has an effect equal to digitalis.

(*d*) *Vaso-dilators.*—The giving of these is not indicated for the purpose of reducing pressure but they are often of service in relieving symptoms, especially headache, dizziness and dyspnœa. Nitroglycerine may be given beginning with gr. 1/100 (0.00065 gm.) and increasing till an effect is produced. Sodium nitrite is often more useful in doses of gr. ½-ii (0.03-0.12 gm.). Erythrol tetranitrate has a more prolonged effect. The dose of the vasodilator should be that which produces an effect.

(*e*) *Uræmic Symptoms.*—Even before marked manifestations are present there may be extreme restlessness, mental wandering, a heavy, foul breath, and a coated tongue. Headache is not often complained of, though intense frontal headache may be an early symptom of uræmia. In this condition, too, the patient may complain of palpitation, feelings of numbness, and sometimes nocturnal cramps. For these symptoms the saline purgatives should be ordered, and hot baths, so as to induce copious sweating. Water should be given freely, by mouth, by the drop method by the bowel, and by subcutaneous injection if necessary. Grandin states that irrigation of the bowel with hot water is most useful. If signs of acidosis are present, sodium bicarbonate (ʒ i, 4 gm., a day) should be given. For the uræmic convulsions, if severe, inhalations of chloroform may be used. If the patient is robust and full-blooded, from 12 to 20 ounces of blood should be removed. Lumbar puncture is often useful and can be done without hesitation. The patient should be freely sweated, and if the convulsions tend to recur chloral may be given, either by the mouth or per rectum, or, better still, morphia. Uræmic coma must be treated by active purgation, and sweating should be promoted by the use of pilocarpine or the hot bath. For the restlessness and delirium morphia is indispensable. Since its recommendation in uræmic states by Stephen MacKenzie, this remedy has been used extensively and is of great value in these cases. It is of special value in the dyspnœa and Cheyne-Stokes breathing of advanced arterio-sclerosis with chronic uræmia.

SURGICAL TREATMENT.—Edebohls introduced the operation of decapsulation of the kidneys in order to establish new vascular connections, and so influence the nutrition of the organs. There is probably a small group of suitable cases—the subacute and chronic forms which follow acute infections—in which the outlook is hopeless from medical treatment.

VIII. AMYLOID DISEASE

Amyloid (lardaceous or waxy) degeneration of the kidneys is simply an event in the process of chronic nephritis, most commonly in the chronic parenchymatous nephritis following fevers, or of cachectic states. It has no claim to be regarded as one of the varieties of nephritis. The affection of the kidneys is generally a part of a widespread amyloid degeneration occurring in prolonged suppuration, as in disease of the bone, in syphilis, tuberculosis, and occasionally leukæmia, lead poisoning, and gout. It varies curiously in frequency in different localities.

The amyloid kidney is large and pale, the surface smooth, and the venæ stellatæ well marked. On section the cortex is large and may show a peculiar glistening, infiltrated appearance, and the glomeruli are very distinct. The pyramids, in striking contrast to the cortex, are of a deep red color. A section soaked in dilute tincture of iodine shows spots of a walnut or mahogany brown color. The Malpighian tufts and the straight vessels may be most affected. In lardaceous disease the kidneys are not always enlarged but may be normal in size or small, pale, and granular. The amyloid change is first seen in the Malpighian tufts, and then involves the afferent and efferent vessels and the straight vessels. It may be confined entirely to them. In later stages the tubules are affected, chiefly the membrane, rarely, if ever, the cells themselves.

Symptoms.—The renal features alone may not indicate the presence of this degeneration. Usually the associated condition gives a hint of the nature of the process. The urine, as a rule, shows important changes; the quantity is increased, and it is pale, clear, and of low specific gravity. The albumin is usually abundant, but it may be scanty, and in rare instances absent. Possibly the variations in the situation of the amyloid changes may account for this, since albumin is less likely to be present when the change is confined to the vasa recta. In addition to ordinary albumin globulin may be present. The tube casts are variable, usually hyaline, often fatty or finely granular. Occasionally the amyloid reaction can be detected in the hyaline casts. Dropsy is present in many instances, particularly when there is much anæmia or profound cachexia. It is not an invariable symptom, and there are cases in which it does not develop. Diarrhœa is a common accompaniment.

Increased arterial tension and cardiac hypertrophy are not usually present, except in those cases in which amyloid degeneration occurs in the secondary contracted kidney; under which circumstances there may be uræmia and retinal changes, which, as a rule, are not met with in other forms.

Diagnosis.—By the condition of the urine alone it is not possible to recognize amyloid changes in the kidney. Usually, however, there is no difficulty, since the disease comes on in association with syphilis, prolonged suppuration, disease of the bone, or tuberculosis, and there is evidence of enlargement of the liver and spleen. A suspicious circumstance is the existence of polyuria with a large amount of albumin in the urine and few casts, or when, in these constitutional affections, a large quantity of clear, pale urine is passed, even without the presence of albumin.

The prognosis depends rather on the condition with which the nephritis is associated. As a rule it is grave.

IX. PYELITIS

(Consecutive Nephritis; Pyelonephritis; Pyonephrosis)

Definition.—Inflammation of the pelvis of the kidney and the conditions which result from it.

Etiology.—Pyelitis in almost all cases is induced by bacterial invasion and multiplication, rarely by the irritation of various substances such as turpentine. Normally the kidney can eliminate without harm to itself, apparently, various bacteria carried to it by the blood-current from some focus of infection; and it probably becomes infected only when its resistance is lowered, as a result of some general cause, as anæmia, malnutrition, or intercurrent disease, or of some local cause, as nephritis, displacement, congestion due to pressure of neoplasms upon the ureter, twisted ureter (Dietl's crisis), or of operation, or when the number or virulence of the micro-organisms is increased. These same factors probably play an important rôle also in the other common causes of pyelitis, ascending infection from an infected bladder (cystitis), and tuberculous infection. Other causes described are various fevers, cancer, hydatids, the ova of certain parasites, cold, and overexertion. Calculus seems not to be a common cause. It is a not uncommon complication of pregnancy (French).

Morbid Anatomy.—In the early stages of pyelitis the mucous membrane is turbid, somewhat swollen, and may show ecchymoses or a grayish pseudomembrane. The urine in the pelvis is cloudy, and, on examination, numbers of epithelial cells are seen.

In the calculous pyelitis there may be only slight turbidity of the membrane, which has been called by some catarrhal pyelitis. More commonly the mucosa is roughened, grayish in color, and thick. Under these circumstances there is almost always more or less dilatation of the calyces and flattening of the papillæ. Following this condition there may be (*a*) extension of the suppurative process to the kidney itself, forming a pyelonephritis; (*b*) a gradual dilatation of the calyces with atrophy of the kidney substance, and finally the production of the condition of pyonephrosis, in which the entire organ is represented by a sac of pus with or without a thin shell of renal tissue. (*c*) After the kidney structure has been destroyed by suppuration, if the obstruction at the orifice of the pelvis persists, the fluid portions may be absorbed and the pus become inspissated, so that the organ is represented by a series of sacculi containing grayish, putty like masses, which may become impregnated with lime salts.

Tuberculous pyelitis usually starts upon the apices of the pyramids, and may at first be limited in extent. Ultimately the condition produced may be similar to that of calculous pyelitis. Pyonephrosis is quite as frequent a sequence, while the transformation of the pus into a putty-like material impregnated with salts, forming the so-called scrofulous kidney, is even commoner.

The pyelitis consecutive to cystitis is generally bilateral, and the kidneys are sometimes involved, forming the so-called *surgical kidneys*—acute suppurative nephritis. There are lines of suppuration extending along the pyramids, or small abscesses in the cortex, often just beneath the capsule; or there may be wedge shaped abscesses. The pus organisms either pass up the tubules or, as Steven has shown, through the lymphatics.

Symptoms.—The forms associated with the fevers rarely cause any symptoms, even when the process is extensive. In mild grades there is pain in the back or there may be tenderness on deep pressure over the kidney. The urine, turbid and containing pus cells, some mucus, and occasional red blood-cells, is acid or alkaline, depending on the infecting microbe; usually the albuminuria is of higher grade comparatively than the pyuria.

Before the condition of pyuria is established there may be attacks of pain on the affected side (not reaching the severe agony of renal colic), rigors, high fever, and sweats. Under these circumstances the urine, which may have been clear, becomes turbid or smoky from the presence of blood, and may contain large numbers of mucous cells and transitional epithelium.

The statement is not infrequently made that the epithelium in the urine in pyelitis is distinctive and characteristic. This is erroneous, as may be readily demonstrated by comparing scrapings of the mucosa of the renal pelvis and of the bladder. In both the epithelium belongs to what is called the transitional variety, and in both regions the same conical, fusiform, and irregular cells with long tails are found, and yet in pyelitis more of these tailed cells occur, for in cystitis one must often search long for them.

When the pyelitis, whether calculous or tuberculous, has become chronic and discharges, the symptoms are:

(*a*) *Pyuria.*—The pus is in variable amount, and may be intermittent. Thus, as is often the case when only one kidney is involved, the ureter may be temporarily blocked, and normal urine is passed for a time; then there is a sudden outflow of the pent up pus and the urine becomes purulent. Coincident with this retention, a tumor mass may be felt on the side affected. The pus has the ordinary characters, but the transitional epithelium is not so abundant at this stage and comes from the bladder or from the pelvis of the healthy side. Occasionally, in rapidly advancing pyelonephritis, portions of the kidney tissue, particularly of the apices of the pyramids, may slough away and appear in the urine; or solid cheesy moulds of the calyces are passed. Casts from the kidney tubules are sometimes present. The reaction of the urine depends upon the infecting microbe, whether the condition is unilateral or bilateral, and whether the bladder is also infected, when vesical irritability and frequent micturition may be present. Polyuria is usually present in the chronic cases.

(*b*) Intermittent *fever* associated with rigors is usually present in cases of suppurative pyelitis. The chills may recur at regular intervals, and the cases are often mistaken for malaria. Owen-Rees called attention to the frequent occurrence of these rigors, which form a characteristic feature of both calculous and tuberculous pyelitis. Ultimately the fever assumes a hectic type and the rigors may cease.

(*c*) The general condition of the patient often indicates prolonged suppuration. There is more or less wasting with anæmia and a progressive failure of health. Secondary abscesses may develop and the clinical picture becomes that of pyæmia. In some instances, particularly of tuberculous pyelitis, the clinical course may resemble that of typhoid fever. There are instances of pyuria recurring, at intervals, for many years without impairment of the bodily vigor. Some of the chronic cases have practically no discomfort.

(*d*) Physical examination usually reveals tenderness or a definite swelling on the affected side, which may vary much in size and attain large dimensions if the kidney becomes enormously distended, as in pyonephrosis.

(*e*) Occasionally nervous symptoms, which may be associated with dyspnœa, supervene, or the termination may be in a curious toxæmia or by coma, not unlike that of diabetes. These have been attributed to the absorption of the decomposing materials in the urine, whence the so-called ammoniæmia. A form of paraplegia has been described in connection with some cases of abscess of the kidney, but whether due to a myelitis or to a peripheral neuritis has not been determined.

In suppurative nephritis following cystitis, the patient complains of pain in the back, the fever becomes high, irregular, and associated with chills, and in acute cases a typhoid state may precede the fatal event.

Diagnosis.—Between the tuberculous and the calculous forms of pyelitis it may be difficult or impossible to distinguish, except by the detection of tubercle bacilli in the pus. The examination for bacilli should be made systematically, and in suspicious cases intraperitoneal injections of guinea-pigs should also be made. From perinephric abscess pyonephrosis is distinguished by the more definite character of the tumor, the absence of œdematous swelling in the lumbar region, and, most important of all, the history. The urine, too, in perinephric abscess may be free from pus. There are cases, however, in which it is difficult indeed to make a satisfactory diagnosis.

Suppurative pyelitis and cystitis are apt to be confounded. The two conditions may coexist and prove puzzling, but the history, the higher relative grade of albuminuria in pyelitis, the polyuria, the mode of development, the local signs in one lumbar region, and the absence of pain in the bladder should be sufficient to differentiate the affections. By the cystoscope, it may be definitely determined whether the pus comes from the kidneys or from the bladder.

In the diagnosis of pyelitis from pyelonephritis, the functional test is important; this is normal in pyelitis and reduced in pyelonephritis.

Much may be done with X-ray examinations to determine the condition of the pelves of the kidneys. When an opaque solution is injected by the ureteral catheter a shadow is cast giving a very accurate outline of the pelvis of the organ.

Prognosis.—Cases coming on during the fevers usually recover. In the chronic cases the appearance of toxæmia is of grave omen. Tuberculous pyelitis may terminate favorably by inspissation of the pus and conversion into a putty-like substance with deposition of lime salts. With pyonephrosis the dangers are increased. Perforation may occur into the peritoneum, the patient may be worn out by the hectic fever, or amyloid disease may develop.

Treatment.—Fluids should be taken freely, particularly the alkaline mineral waters, to which potassium citrate may be added.

The treatment of the calculous form will be considered later. Practically there are no remedies which have much influence upon the pyuria. Some of the urinary antiseptics seem to be of value, especially in the acute cases. Hexamine should be given in full doses (gr. xv, 1 gm., three or four times a day); watch should be kept for signs of irritation and the dose reduced if they appear. Lavage of the pelvis of the kidney has been much employed. Vaccine therapy is sometimes of value. Tonics should be given, a nourishing diet, and milk and butter-milk may be taken freely. When the tumor has formed or even before it is perceptible, if the symptoms are serious and severe, the kidney should be explored, and, if necessary, nephrotomy or nephrectomy should be performed.

X. HYDRONEPHROSIS

Definition.—Dilatation of the pelvis and calyx of the kidney with atrophy of its substance, caused by the accumulation of non-purulent fluids, the result of obstruction.

Etiology.—The condition may be congenital, owing to some abnormality in the ureter or urethra. The tumor produced may be large enough to retard labor. Sometimes it is associated with other malformations. There is a condition of moderate dilatation, apparently congenital, which is not connected with any obstruction in the ducts. In some instances there has been contraction or twisting of the ureter, or it is inserted into the kidney at an acute angle or at a high level. In adult life the condition may be due to lodgment of a calculus, or to a cicatricial stricture following ulcer.

New growths, such as tubercle or cancer, may induce hydronephrosis; more commonly by pressure upon the ureter from without, particularly tumors of the ovaries and uterus. Occasionally cicatricial bands compress the ureter. Obstruction within the bladder may result from cancer, hypertrophy of the prostate, and in the urethra from stricture. It is stated that slight grades of hydronephrosis have been found in patients with excessive polyuria.

In whatever way produced, when the ureter is blocked the secretion accumulates in the pelvis and infundibula. Sometimes acute inflammation follows, but more commonly the slow, gradual pressure causes atrophy of the papillæ with gradual distention and wasting of the organ. In acquired cases from pressure, even when dilatation is extreme, there may usually be seen a thin layer of renal structure. In the most extreme stages the kidney is represented by a large cyst, which may perhaps show on its inner surface imperfect septa. The fluid is thin and yellowish in color, and contains traces of urinary salts, urea, uric acid, and sometimes albumin. The secretion may be turbid from admixture with small quantities of pus.

Total occlusion does not always lead to a hydronephrosis, but may be followed by atrophy of the kidney. It appears that when the obstruction is intermittent or not complete the greatest dilatation is apt to follow. The sac may be enormous, and cause a large abdominal tumor. The condition has even been mistaken for ascites. Enlargement of the other kidney may compensate for the defect. Hypertrophy of the left side of the heart usually follows.

Symptoms.—When small, it may not be noticed. The congenital cases when bilateral usually prove fatal within a few days; when unilateral, the tumor may not be noticed for some time. It increases progressively and has all the characters of a tumor in the renal region. In adult life many of the cases, due to pressure by tumors, as in cancer of the uterus and enlargement of the prostate, etc., give rise to no symptoms.

In *intermittent* hydronephrosis the tumor suddenly disappears with the discharge of a large quantity of clear fluid; the sac gradually refills, and the process may be repeated for years. In these cases the obstruction is unilateral; a cicatricial stricture exists, or a valve is present in the ureter, or the ureter enters the upper part of the pelvis. Many of the cases are in women and associated with movable kidney.

The examination of the abdomen shows, in unilateral hydronephrosis, a tumor occupying the renal region. When of moderate size it is readily recognized, but when large it may be confounded with ovarian or other tumors. In young children it may be mistaken for sarcoma of the kidney or of the retroperitoneal glands, the common cause of abdominal tumor in early life. The large hydronephrotic sac is frequently mistaken for ovarian tumor. The latter is, as a rule, more mobile, and rarely fills the deeper portion of the lumbar region so thoroughly. The ascending colon can often be detected passing over the renal tumor, and examination per vaginam, particularly under ether, will give important indications as to the condition of the ovaries. The fluid of the renal cyst is clear, or turbid from the presence of cell elements, rarely colloid in character; the specific gravity is low; albumin and traces of urea and uric acid are usually present; and the epithelial elements in it may be similar to those found in the pelvis of the kidney. In old sacs, however, the fluid may not be characteristic, since the urinary salts disappear, but in one case of several years' duration oxalates of lime and urea were found.

Perhaps the greatest difficulty is offered by the condition of hydronephrosis in a movable kidney. Here, the history of sudden disappearance of the tumor with the passage of a large quantity of clear fluid is a point of great importance in the diagnosis. In those rare instances of an enormous sac filling the entire abdomen, and sometimes mistaken for ascites, the character of the fluid might be the only point of difference. The tumor of pyonephrosis may be practically the same in physical characteristics. Fever is usually present, and pus is often found in the urine. In these cases, when in doubt, an exploratory operation should be done.

The outlook depends much upon the cause. When single, the condition may never produce serious trouble, and the intermittent cases may persist for years, and finally disappear. Occasionally the cyst ruptures into the peritoneum, more rarely through the diaphragm into the lung. The sac may discharge spontaneously through the ureter and the fluid never reaccumulate. In bilateral hydronephrosis there is danger of uræmia and blocking of the ureter on the sound side by calculus has been followed by uræmia. And, lastly, the sac may suppurate, and the condition change to one of pyonephrosis.

Treatment.—Cases of intermittent hydronephrosis which do not cause serious symptoms should be let alone. It is stated that, in sacs of moderate size, the obstruction has been overcome by massage, but, if practised, it should be done with great care. When the sac reaches a large size aspiration may be performed and repeated if necessary. Puncture should be made in the flank, midway between the ilium and the last rib. If the fluid reaccumulates and the sac becomes large, it may be incised and drained, or, as a last resort, the kidney may be removed. In women a carefully adapted pad and bandage will sometimes prevent the recurrence of an intermittent hydronephrosis.

XI. NEPHROLITHIASIS

(*Renal Calculus*)

Definition.—The formation in the kidney or in its pelvis of concretions, by the deposition of certain of the solid constituents of the urine.

Etiology and Pathology.—In the kidney substance itself the separation of the urinary salts produces a condition to which, unfortunately, the term infarct has been applied. Three varieties may be recognized: (1) The uric acid infarct, usually met with at the apices of the pyramids in new born children and during the first weeks of life. The priapism and attacks of crying in the new-born have been attributed to the passage of these infarcts; (2) the sodium urate infarct, sometimes associated with ammonium urate, which forms whitish lines at the apices of the pyramids and is met with chiefly, but not always, in gouty persons; and (3) the lime infarcts, forming very opaque white lines in the pyramids, usually in old people.

In the pelvis and calyces concretions of the following forms occur: (*a*) Small gritty particles, *renal sand,* ranging in size from the individual grains of the uric acid sediment to bodies 1 or 2 mm. in diameter. These may be passed in the urine for long periods without producing any symptoms, since they are too fine to be arrested in their downward passage.

(*b*) Larger concretions, ranging in size from a small pea to a bean, and either solitary or multiple in the calyces and pelvis. It is the smaller of these calculi which, in their passage, produce the attacks of renal colic. They may be rounded and smooth, or present numerous irregular projections.

(*c*) The dendritic form of calculus. The orifice of the ureter may be blocked by a Y-shaped stone. The pelvis itself may be occupied by the concretion, which forms a more or less distinct mould. These are the remarkable *coral calculi,* which form in the pelvis complete moulds of infundibula and calyces, the latter even presenting cup-like depressions corresponding to the apices of the papillæ. Some of these casts in stone of the renal pelvis are as beautifully moulded as Hyrtl's corrosion preparations.

Chemically the varieties of calculi are: (1) Uric acid and urates, forming the renal sand, the small solitary, or the large dendritic stones. They are very hard, the surface is smooth, and the color reddish. The larger stones are usually stratified and very dense. Usually the uric acid and the urates are mixed, but in children stones composed of urates alone may occur. Uric acid calculi are rare.

(2) Oxalate of lime, which forms mulberry-shaped calculi, studded with points and spines. They are often very dark in color, intensely hard, and are a mixture of oxalate of lime and uric acid. These comprise the great majority of renal calculi.

(3) Phosphatic calculi are composed of the calcium phosphate and the ammonio-magnesium phosphate, sometimes mixed with a small amount of calcium carbonate. The phosphatic salts are often deposited about the uric acid or calcium oxalate stones.

(4) Rare forms of calculi are made up of cystine, xanthine, carbonate of lime, indigo, and urostealith.

The mode of formation of calculi has been much discussed. They may be produced by an excess of a sparingly soluble abnormal ingredient, such as cystine or xanthine. Ord suggests that albumin, mucus, blood, and epithelial threads may be the starting point of stone. The demonstration of organisms in the centre of renal calculi renders it probable that in many cases the nucleus of the stone is an agglutinated mass of bacteria.

Renal calculi are most common in the early and later periods of life. They are moderately frequent in the United States, but there do not appear to be special districts, corresponding to the "stone counties" in England. Men are more often affected than women. Sedentary occupations seem to predispose to stone.

The effects are varied. It is by no means uncommon to find a dozen or more stones of various sizes in the calyces without any destruction of the mucous membrane or dilatation of the pelvis. A turbid urine fills the pelvis, in which there are numerous cells from the epithelial lining. There are cases of this sort in which, apparently, the stones may go on forming and are passed for years without seriously impairing the health and without inconvenience, except the attacks of renal colic. Still more remarkable are the cases of coral like calculi, which may occupy the entire pelvis and calyces without causing pyelitis, but which gradually lead to more or less induration of the kidney. The most serious effects are when the stone excites a suppurative pyelitis and pyonephrosis. Of 140 kidneys containing stones removed at the Mayo clinic, 9 were cancerous (Correll).

Symptoms.—Patients may pass gravel for years without having an attack of renal colic, and a stone may never lodge in the ureter. In other instances, the formation of calculi goes on year by year and the patient has recurring attacks such as have been so graphically described by Montaigne in his own case. A patient may pass enormous numbers of calculi. A patient may pass a single calculus, and never be troubled again. The large coral calculi may excite no symptoms. In a remarkable specimen of the kind, presented to the McGill Medical Museum by J. A. Macdonald, the patient, a middle-aged woman, died suddenly with uræmic symptoms. There was no pyelitis, but the kidneys were sclerotic.

Renal colic ensues when a stone enters the ureter, or follows an acute pyelitis. An attack may set in abruptly without apparent cause, or may follow a strain in lifting. It is characterized by agonizing pain, which starts in the flank of the affected side, passes down the ureter, and is felt in the testicle and along the inner side of the thigh. The pain may also radiate through the abdomen and chest, and be very intense in the back. In severe attacks nausea and vomiting follow and the patient is collapsed. Perspiration breaks out upon the face and the pulse is feeble and quick. A chill may precede the outbreak, and the temperature may rise as high as 103°. No one has more graphically described an attack of "the stone" than Montaigne, who was a sufferer for many years: "Thou art seen to sweat with pain, to look pale and red, to tremble, to vomit well-nigh to blood, to suffer strange contortions and convulsions, by starts to let tears drop from thine eyes, to urine thick, black, and frightful water, or to have it suppressed by some sharp and craggy stone, that cruelly pricks and tears thee." From personal experience the senior author can describe three sorts of pain in an attack of renal colic: (*a*) A constant localized, dull pain, the area of which could be covered on the skin of the back in the renal region by a penny piece, and which could be imitated exactly by deep firm pressure on a superficial bone. (*b*) Paroxysms of pain radiating in the course of the ureter or into the flank, and as they increase accompanied by sweating, fainting, and nausea. (*c*) Flushes or rushes of hot pain at intervals, often momentary, usually passing to the back, less often toward the groin. Dozens of these flushes relieved the monotony of (*b*). The symptoms persist for a variable period. In short attacks they do not last longer than an hour; in other instances they continue for a day or more, with temporary relief. Micturition is frequent, occasionally painful, and the urine, as a rule, is bloody. There are instances in which a large amount of clear urine is passed, probably from the other kidney. In rare cases the secretion of urine is completely suppressed, even when the kidney on the opposite side is normal, and death may occur from uræmia. This most frequently happens when the second kidney is extensively diseased, or when only a single kidney exists. Orchitis may follow an attack.

After the attack of colic has passed there is more or less aching on the affected side, and the patient can usually tell from which kidney the stone has come. Examination during the attack is usually negative. Very rarely the kidney becomes palpable. Tenderness on the affected side is common. In very thin persons it may be possible, on examination of the abdomen, to feel the stone in the ureter; or the patient may complain of a grating sensation.

When the calculi remain in the kidney they may produce very definite and characteristic symptoms, of which the following are the most important:

(*a*) *Pain,* usually in the back, which is often no more than a dull soreness, but which may be severe and come on in paroxysms. It is usually on the side affected, but may be referred to the opposite kidney, and there are instances in which the pain has been confined to the sound side. It radiates in the direction of the ureter, and may be felt in the scrotum or even in the penis. Vesical irritability is common. Pains of a similar nature may occur in movable kidneys or be referred in prostatic disease, and surgeons have incised the kidney for stone and found none. In an instance in which pain was present for a couple of years the exploration revealed only a contracted kidney.

(*b*) *Hæmaturia.*—Although this occurs most frequently when the stone becomes engaged in the ureter, it may also come on when the stones are in the pelvis. The bleeding is seldom profuse, as in cancer, but in some instances may persist for a long time. It is aggravated by exertion and lessened by rest. Frequently it only gives to the urine a smoky hue. The urine may be free for days, and then a sudden exertion or a prolonged ride may cause smokiness, or blood may be passed in considerable quantities.

(*c*) *Pyelitis.*—(1) There may be attacks of severe pain in the back, not amounting to actual colic, which are initiated by a heavy chill followed by fever, in which the temperature may reach 104° or 105°, followed by profuse sweating. The urine, which has been clear, may become turbid and smoky and contain blood and abundant epithelium from the pelvis. Attacks of this description may recur at intervals for months or years, and be mistaken for malaria, unless special attention is paid to the urine and to the existence of the pain in the back. This renal intermittent fever, due to the presence of calculi, is analogous to the hepatic intermittent fever, due to gall-stones, and in both it is important to remember that the most intense paroxysms may occur without any evidence of suppuration.

(2) More frequently the symptoms of purulent pyelitis, which have already been described, are present; pain in the renal region, recurring chills, and pus in the urine, with or without indications of pyonephrosis.

(*d*) *Pyuria.*—There are instances of stone in the kidney in which pus occurs continuously or intermittently in the urine for many years.

Patients with stone in the kidney are often robust, high livers, and gouty. Attacks of dyspepsia are not uncommon, or they may have severe headaches.

Diagnosis.—The X-ray picture is rarely at fault, and specialists in this department are becoming more and more skillful, so that mistakes are now rare. Renal may be mistaken for intestinal colic, particularly if the distention of the bowels is marked, or for biliary colic. The situation and direction of the pain, the retraction and tenderness of the testicle, the occurrence of hæmaturia, the vesical irritability and the altered character of the urine are distinctive features. Attention may again be called to the fact that attacks simulating renal colic are associated with movable kidney and disease of the prostate or even, it has been supposed, with the accumulation of the oxalates or uric acid in the pelvis of the kidney. The diagnosis between a stone in the kidney and stone in the bladder is not always easy, though in the latter the pain is particularly about the neck of the bladder, and not limited to one side. It is stated that differences occur in the symptoms produced by different sorts of calculi. The large uric acid calculi less frequently produce severe symptoms. On the other hand, as the oxalate of lime is a rougher calculus, it is apt to produce more pain (often of a radiating character) and to cause hæmorrhage. In both these forms the urine is acid. The phosphatic calculi are stated to produce the most intense pain, and the urine is commonly alkaline.

Treatment.—In the attacks of renal colic great relief is experienced by the hot bath, which is sometimes sufficient to relax the spasm. When the pain is very intense morphia should be given hypodermically and inhalations of chloroform may be necessary until the effects of the anodyne are manifest. Local applications are sometimes grateful—hot poultices, or cloths wrung out of hot water. The patient may drink freely of hot lemonade, soda water, or barley water. Occasionally change in posture or inversion will give great relief. Surgical interference should be considered in all cases, especially when the stone is large or the associated pyelitis severe.

In the intervals the patient should, as far as possible, live a quiet life, avoiding sudden exertion of all sorts. The essential feature in the treatment is to keep the urine abundant and, in the uric acid or uratic cases, alkaline. The patient should drink daily a large quantity of mineral water* or distilled water, which is just as satisfactory. The aching pains in the back are often greatly relieved by this treatment. Many patients find benefit from a stay at Saratoga, Bedford, Poland, or other mineral springs in the United States, or at Vichy or Ems in Europe.

If a stone has been passed its composition should be determined so that proper treatment can be carried out to prevent the further formation of stones if possible. For the uric acid stones, which are rare, an alkaline urine is advisable, but for the oxalate and phosphatic stones an acid reaction should be maintained. In case of oxalate calculi foods containing oxalic acid should be avoided. The most important are tea, coffee, cocoa, pepper, rhubarb, spinach, beetroot, beans, currants and figs. For the uric acid calculi the diet is that indicated in gout.

XII. TUMORS OF THE KIDNEY

These are benign and malignant. Of the benign tumors, the most common are the small nodular *fibromata* which occur frequently in the pyramids, and occasionally *lipoma, angioma,* or *lymphadenoma.* The *adenomata* may be congenital; small nodules of aberrant adrenal tissue are not uncommon.

Malignant growths—*cancer* or *sarcoma*—may be either primary or secondary. The sarcomata are either alveolar sarcoma or the remarkable form containing striped muscular fibres—rhabdomyoma. The most common and important renal tumor is the *hypernephroma,* growing in or upon the organ from the adrenal tissue—the aberrant "rests" of Grawitz. Of 163 cases only 6 were extra-renal (Ellis). They may be small and in the renal cortex or form large tumors with extensive metastases, particularly in the lungs. Most of the so-called carcinomas and alveolar sarcomas of the kidney are really hypernephromata. About 6 per cent. of cases of new growth are associated with calculi.

The tumors attain a very large size, and almost fill the abdomen. In children they may be enormous. They grow rapidly, are often soft, and hæmorrhage frequently takes place into them. In the sarcomata, invasion of the pelvis or of the renal vein is common. The rhabdomyomata rarely form very large tumors, and death occurs shortly after birth. In one case a child at the age of three years and a half died suddenly of embolism of the pulmonary artery and tricuspid orifice by a fragment of the tumor, which had grown into the renal vein.

In association with hypernephroma of the adrenal cortex precocious development of the external genitals has been noted, with in many instances overgrowth of the body, growth of hair on the face, and development of the

* Some of these, if we judge by the laudatory reports, are as potent as the waters of Corsena, declared by Montaigne to be "powerful enough to break stones."

breasts, with menstruation in girls. It seems probable that the tumor of the adrenal cortex stimulates the secretion and has indirect effects upon the other glands controlling metabolism.

Symptoms.—The following are the most important: (*a*) *Hæmaturia* in one-half the cases, which may be the first indication. The blood is fluid or clotted, and there may be very characteristic moulds of the pelvis of the kidney and of the ureter, which are rare except in cancer. Cancer elements may sometimes be recognized in the urine.

(*b*) *Pain* is an uncertain symptom. In several of the largest tumors which have come under our observation there has been no discomfort from beginning to close. When present, it is of a dragging, dull character, situated in the flank and radiating down the thigh. The passage of the clots may cause great pain. In one case the growth was at first upward, and the symptoms for some months were those of pleurisy.

(*c*) Progressive emaciation. The loss of flesh is usually marked and advances rapidly. There may, however, be a very large tumor without emaciation.

Physical Signs.—In almost all instances tumor is present. When small and on the right side, it may be very movable; in some instances, occupying a position in the iliac fossa, it has been mistaken for ovarian tumor. The large growths fill the flank and gradually extend toward the middle line, occupying the right or left half of the abdomen. Inspection may show two or three hemispherical projections corresponding to distended sections of the organ. In children the abdomen may reach an enormous size and the veins are prominent and distended. On bimanual palpation the tumor is felt to occupy the lumbar region and can usually be lifted slightly from its bed; in some cases it is very movable, even when large; in others it is fixed, firm, and solid. The respiratory movements have but slight influence upon it. Rapidly growing renal tumors are soft, and on palpation may give a sense of fluctuation. A point of considerable importance is the fact that the colon crosses the tumor, and can usually be detected without difficulty.

Diagnosis.—In children very large abdominal tumors are either renal or retroperitoneal. The retroperitoneal sarcoma (Lobstein's cancer) is more central, but may attain as large a size. If the case is seen only toward the end, a differential diagnosis may be impossible; but, as a rule, the sarcoma is less moveable. It is to be remembered that these tumors may invade the kidney. On the left side an enlarged spleen is readily distinguished, as the edge is very distinct and the notch or notches well marked; it descends during respiration, and the colon lies behind, not in front of it. On the right side growths of the liver are occasionally confounded with renal tumors: but such instances are rare, and there can usually be detected a zone of resonance between the upper margin of the renal tumor and the ribs. Late in the disease this is not possible, for the renal tumor is in close union with the liver. Metastases should be searched for, especially in the lungs.

A malignant growth in a movable kidney may be very deceptive and may simulate cancer of the ovary or myoma of the uterus. The great mobility upward of the renal growth and the negative result of examination of the pelvic viscera are the reliable points.

When the growth is small and the patient in good condition removal of the organ may be undertaken, but the percentage of cases of recovery is very small, only 5.4 per cent. (G. Walker).

XIII. CYSTIC DISEASE OF THE KIDNEY

The following varieties of cysts are met with:

Small Cysts.—These are described in connection with chronic nephritis, and result from dilatation of obstructed tubules or of Bowman's capsules. There are cases very difficult to classify, in which the kidneys are greatly enlarged and very cystic in middle-aged or elderly persons, and yet not so large as in the congenital form.

Solitary Cysts.—Solitary cysts, ranging in size from a marble to an orange, or even larger, are occasionally found in kidneys which present no other changes. In exceptional cases they may form tumors of considerable size. Newman operated on one which contained 25 ounces of blood. They, too, in all probability, result from obstruction.

Polycystic Kidneys.—In the polycystic kidneys, the greatly enlarged organs, weighing even as much as six pounds, are represented by a conglomeration of cysts, varying in size from a pea to a marble. Little or no renal tissue may be noticeable, although in microscopic sections it is seen that a considerable amount remains in the interspaces. The cysts contain a clear or turbid fluid, sometimes reddish brown or even blackish in color, and may be of a colloidal consistence. Albumin, blood crystals, cholesterin, with triple phosphates and fat drops, are found in the contents. Urea and uric acid are rarely present. The cysts are lined by a flattened epithelium. They occur in the fetus, and sometimes are of such a size as to obstruct labor. In the adult they are usually bilateral, and there is every reason to believe that they begin in early life and increase gradually. Indeed, a progressive growth has been noticed (Alfred King). They may be found in connection with cystic disease of the liver and other organs. It is difficult to account for the origin of this remarkable condition, which some regard as a defect of development rather than a pathological change, and point to the association in the fetal cases of other anomalies, as imperforate anus. Others believe the condition to be a new growth—a sort of mucoid endothelioma.

It is interesting to note that several members of a family may be affected. In one instance mother and son were the subjects of the disease.

Symptoms.—Of a series of cases seen in adults the condition was recognized during life in the majority. The features are characteristic.

(*a*) *Bilateral tumors* in the renal regions, which may increase in size under observation. They may cause great enlargement of the upper zone of the abdomen. The colon and stomach are in front of the tumors, on the surface of which in thin subjects the cysts may be palpable or even visible. While both kidneys are, as a rule, involved, one may be much smaller than the other.

(*b*) *Hæmaturia,* which may recur at intervals for years.

(*c*) The signs of a *chronic interstitial nephritis*—(1) pallor or muddy complexion; in rare instances a bronzing of the skin; (2) sclerosis of the arteries; (3) hypertrophy of the heart with accentuated second sound; (4)

urine abundant, of low specific gravity, with albumin, and hyaline and granular tube casts, and in one case cholesterin crystals. Death occurs from uræmia or the cardio-vascular complications of chronic nephritis. A rare event is rupture of a cyst with the formation of a perinephric abscess and peritonitis. The skin may be much pigmented.

Operation, by exposing the kidney and draining the cysts, has been successful. When the condition is unilateral the kidney has been removed and the patients have remained well for years.

Other Varieties.—Occasionally the kidneys and liver present numerous small cysts scattered through the substance. The spleen and the thyroid also may be involved, and there may be congenital malformation of the heart. The cysts in the kidney are small, and neither so numerous nor so thickly set as in the conglomerate form, though in these cases the condition is probably the result of some congenital defect. There are cases, however, in which the kidneys are very large. It is more common in the lower animals than in man. Instances of it occur in the hog; in one case the liver weighed 40 pounds, and was converted into a mass of simple cysts. The kidneys were less involved. Charles Kennedy found references to 12 cases of combined cystic disease of the liver and kidneys.

The echinococcus cysts have been described under the section on parasites. Paranephric cysts (external to the capsule) are rare; they may reach a large size.

XIV. PERINEPHRIC ABSCESS

Suppuration in the connective tissue about the kidney may follow (1) blows and injuries; (2) the extension of inflammation from the pelvis of the kidney, the kidney itself, or the ureters; (3) rupture of a septic infarct in the kidney; (4) perforation of the bowel, most commonly the appendix, in some instances the colon; (5) extension of suppuration from the spine, as in caries, or from the pleura, as in empyema; (6) as a sequel of the fevers, particularly in children.

Post mortem the kidney is surrounded by pus, particularly at the posterior part, though the pus may lie altogether in front, between the kidney and the peritoneum. Usually the abscess cavity is extensive. The pus is often offensive and may have a distinctly fæcal odor from contact with the large bowel. It may burrow in various directions and burst into the pleura and be discharged through the lungs. A more frequent direction is down the psoas muscle, when it appears in the groin, or it may pass along the iliacus fascia and appear at Poupart's ligament. It may perforate the bowel or rupture into the peritoneum; sometimes it penetrates the bladder or vagina.

Post mortem we occasionally find a condition of *chronic perinephritis* in which the fatty capsule of the kidney is extremely firm, with numerous bands of fibrous tissue, and is stripped off from the proper capsule with the greatest difficulty. Such a condition probably produces no symptoms.

Symptoms.—There may be intense pain, aggravated by pressure, in the lumbar region. In other instances the onset is insidious, without pain in the renal region; on examination signs of deep seated suppuration may be detected. On the affected side there is usually pain, which may be referred to the neighborhood of the hip joint or to the joint itself, or radiate down the thigh and be associated with the retraction of the testis. The patient lies with the thigh flexed, so as to relax the psoas muscle, and in walking throws, as far as possible, the weight on the opposite leg. He also keeps the spine immobile, assumes a stooping posture in walking, and has great difficulty in voluntarily adducting the thigh (Gibney).

There may be pus in the urine if the disease has extended from the pelvis or the kidney, but in other forms the urine is clear. When pus has formed there are usually chills with irregular fever and sweats. On examination, deep seated induration is felt between the last rib and the crest of the ilium. Bimanual palpation may reveal a distinct tumor mass. Œdema or puffiness of the skin is frequently present.

Diagnosis.—The diagnosis is usually easy; when doubt exists the aspirator needle should be used. We can not always differentiate the primary forms from those due to perforation of the kidney or of the bowel. This, however, makes but little difference, for the treatment is identical. It is usually possible by the history and examination to exclude diseases of the vertebra. In children hip-joint disease may be suspected, but the pain is higher, and there is no fullness or tenderness over the hip-joint itself. In left-sided abscess with the fluoroscope, on quickly moving the patient, a wave can be seen in the fluid (Fussell and Pancoast).

Treatment.—The treatment is clear—early, free, and permanent drainage.

SECTION IX

DISEASES OF THE BLOOD-FORMING ORGANS

I. ANÆMIA

Anæmia, a reduction of the amount of blood as a whole or of its corpuscles, or of certain of its constituents, may be due to failure in the manufacture, to increase in the consumption, or to a loss, sudden or gradual, as in hæmorrhage. Anæmia may be local, confined to certain parts, or general, involving the entire body.

LOCAL ANÆMIA

Tissue irrigation with blood is primarily from the heart, but provision is made for variations in the supply, according to the needs of a part. The sluices are worked by the stop-cock action of the arteries, which contract or expand under vaso-motor influence, central and peripheral. If the sluices of one large district are too widely open, so much blood may enter that other important regions have not enough to keep them at work. Local anæmia of the brain, causing swooning, ensues when the mesenteric channels, capable of holding all the blood of the body, are wide open. Emotional stimuli, reflex from pain, etc., removal of pressure, as after tapping in ascites, may cause this. Possibly many of the nervous and other symptoms in enteroptosis are due to the relative anæmia of the cerebral and spinal systems, owing to the persistent overfilling of the mesenteric reservoir. We know little of local anæmia of the various organs, but functional disturbance in the liver, kidneys, pancreas, heart, etc., may result from a permanently low pressure in the local blood "mains." Anæmia from spasm of the arterial walls is seen in Raynaud's disease, which usually affects the peripheral vessels, causing local syncope of the fingers, but it may occur in the visceral vessels, particularly of the brain, and cause temporary hemiplegia, aphasia, etc.

Pseudo-anæmia is common. Pallor may exist with a normal or even a plus blood count and color index. The transient pallor in nausea and after a drinking bout is a vaso-motor affair. In aortic insufficiency, in lead-workers, in the morphia habitué, the skin may be permanently pale. The skin of the face may be unusually thick or the capillaries poorly developed, as in sedentary workers in contrast to the ruddy complexion of country people. The Latin races are paler than the Anglo-Saxons. There are healthy and strong individuals with a permanent pallor and normal corpuscles and hæmoglobin.

GENERAL ANÆMIA—CLASSIFICATION

The general anæmias may be divided into the secondary or symptomatic and the primary or essential.

Acute Secondary Anæmia

Etiology.—In rupture of a large vessel, or of an aneurism, in the peptic ulcer, or in injury to blood vessels the loss of three or four pounds of blood may prove fatal. Seven and a half pounds may be shed into one cavity (rupture of an aneurism into the pleura). A patient with hæmatemesis lost ten pounds of blood in one week, and yet recovered from the immediate effects. Even after the severest traumatic hæmorrhage the blood count is rarely so low as in certain forms of hæmolytic anæmia. Thus in the case of hæmatemesis just mentioned the red blood-corpuscles were 1,390,000 per c. mm.

Symptoms.—Dyspnœa, rapid action of the heart, and faintness are the prominent symptoms of an acutely produced anæmia. There is marked pallor of the skin and mucous membranes, the pulse is jerking, the vessels throb, particularly the abdominal aorta, and the pistol shot sound is heard over them, the temperature is low, the patient feels giddy and faint and has noises in the ears. If the bleeding continues there may be nausea, vomiting, and, with the rapid loss of large quantities of blood, convulsions. Examination shows a great diminution of the red blood-corpuscles, often below two millions per c. mm. The hæmoglobin is proportionately lower, giving a color index of about 0.8. Irregularity in the red blood-corpuscles is seen; nucleated red corpuscles, usually normoblasts, appear early; the leucocytes are increased, usually the multi-nuclear neutrophiles. The process of regeneration goes on with great rapidity; the watery and saline constituents are readily restored by absorption; the albuminous elements are quickly renewed, but it may take weeks or months for the red blood-corpuscles to reach the normal standard. In a case of purpura the red blood-corpuscles fell between the 20th and 30th April to below two millions, and the leucocytes rose to 12,000. It was not until July that the red blood-corpuscles reached four million, and the blood was not normal until September. The hæmoglobin is restored more slowly than the corpuscles.

In repeated hæmorrhages the picture depends upon the interval between the losses of blood. If long enough to allow of complete regeneration each time the total amount of blood lost may be very great. Ehrlich mentions the case of a patient with hæmoptysis who lost 20 kilograms of blood in 6½ months. If, however, the intervals are short, so that complete recovery from each loss of blood is not possible, a chronic anæmia is soon induced with a very watery plasma, a low color index, and lymphocytosis.

Secondary Anæmia

Etiology.—There are many causes, the most important of which are:

(*a*) *Inanition.*—This may be brought about by defective food supply, or by conditions which interfere with the proper reception and preparation of the food, as in cancer of the œsophagus and chronic dyspepsia. The reduction in mass may be extreme, but the plasma suffers proportionately more than the corpuscles, which, even in the wasting of cancer of the œsophagus, may not be reduced more than one-half to three-fourths. The reduction in the plasma may be so great that the corpuscles show a relative increase.

(*b*) *Infections.*—In many acute fevers anæmia is produced, which may persist after the infection has subsided. We see this particularly in typhoid fever, rheumatic fever, sepsis, and malaria. Certain animal parasites, as the hookworm, and bothriocephalus, cause a profound anæmia.

(*c*) *Intoxications.*—Inorganic poisons, such as lead, mercury, arsenic; organic poisons, as the toxins of various fevers; and certain autogenous poisons occurring in chronic affections, such as nephritis and jaundice.

An interesting type of toxic anæmia is caused by arseniuretted hydrogen gas in submarines due to the slow action of gas evolved from the metallic portion of the battery plates. Of thirty cases studied by Dudley, the chief symptoms were dyspnœa, albuminuria, puffiness of the face with conjunctivitis, jaundice and mild neuritic symptoms. The anæmia was never extreme, i. e. below two millions, the color index was, as a rule, high with numerous megaloblasts.

(*d*) *Hæmorrhage.*—This, if repeated, may cause severe anæmia. This is particularly shown in cases of persistent bleeding from hæmorrhoids.

(*e*) Long continued drain upon the system, as in chronic suppuration, prolonged lactation, and in rapidly growing tumors of all sorts.

Symptoms.—Loss of bodily and mental vigor with loss of weight and obvious anæmia are the important features. The patient tires easily, the appetite is poor, digestion often faulty, palpitation is complained of, and there may be feelings of faintness, and, as the anæmia progresses, swelling of the feet. There is not infrequently slight fever. Petechiæ on the skin are not uncommon, and retinal hæmorrhages may occur. The blood picture is distinctive. The red blood-corpuscles are reduced, but rarely below two millions per c. mm. The hæmoglobin is relatively lower than the red cells, thus with 70 per cent. of red cells there may be only 40 per cent. of hæmoglobin, a low color index. The red blood-corpuscles are irregular in shape, nucleated forms may be present, and the leucocytes are usually increased in number.

Treatment.—The traumatic cases do best, and with plenty of good food and fresh air the blood is readily restored. In severe cases transfusion should be done. The extraordinary rapidity with which the normal percentage of red blood-corpuscles is reached without any medication whatever is an important lesson. The cause of the hæmorrhage should be sought and the necessary indications met. The large group depending on the drain on the albuminous materials of the blood, as in nephritis, suppuration, and fever, is difficult to treat successfully, and so long as the cause keeps up it is impossible to restore the normal blood condition. The anæmia of inanition requires plenty of nourishing food. When dependent on organic changes in the gastro-intestinal mucosa not much can be expected from either food or medicine. In the toxic cases due to mercury and lead the poison must be eliminated and a nutritious diet given with full doses of iron. In a great majority of these cases there is deficient blood formation, and the indications are briefly three: plenty of food, an open-air life, and iron. As a rule, it makes but little difference what form of the drug is administered. In the majority of cases Blaud's mass (gr. v-x, 0.3-0.6 gm.) does well. In some cases the citrate of iron hypodermically (gr. ii, 0.12 gm.) is advisable if there is gastric disturbance. In severe forms the patient should be at rest in bed and in the open air, if possible.

PRIMARY OR ESSENTIAL ANÆMIA

1. *Chlorosis*

Definition.—An anæmia of unknown cause, occurring in young girls, characterized by a marked diminution of the hæmoglobin with cardio-vascular and sometimes nervous symptoms.

Etiology.—It is a disease of girls, more often of blondes than of brunettes. It is doubtful if males are ever affected. The age of onset is between the fourteenth and seventeenth years; under the age of twelve cases are rare. Recurrences, which are common, may extend into the third decade. There exists a lowered energy in the blood-making organs, associated in some way with the evolution of the sexual apparatus in women. Possibly the internal secretion of the ovaries is at fault and some think the adrenals.

The disease is most common among the ill-fed, overworked girls of large towns, who are confined all day in close, badly lighted rooms, or have to do much stair-climbing. Cases occur, however, under the most favorable conditions of life, but not often in country-bred girls, as Maudlin sings in the *Compleat Angler.* Lack of proper exercise and of fresh air and the use of improper food are important factors. Emotional and nervous disturbances may be prominent—so prominent that certain writers have regarded the disease as a neurosis. De Sauvages speaks of a *chlorose par amour.* Newly arrived Irish girls were very prone to the disease in Montreal. The "corset and chlorosis" expresses O. Rosenbach's opinion. Menstrual disturbances are not uncommon, but are probably a sequence, not a cause, of chlorosis. Constipation has been assigned as a cause. The incidence of the disease is decreasing rapidly in the United States.

Symptoms.—(*a*) General.—The symptoms are those of anæmia. The subcutaneous fat is well retained or even increased in amount. The complexion is peculiar; neither the blanched aspect of hæmorrhage nor the muddy pallor of grave anæmia, but a curious yellow green tinge, which has given to the disease its name, and its popular designation, the green sickness. Occasionally the skin shows areas of pigmentation, particularly about the joints. The color may be deceptive, as the cheeks may have a reddish tint, particularly on exertion (chlorosis rubra). The subjects complain of breathlessness and palpitation, and there may be a tendency to fainting—symptoms which often lead to the suspicion of heart or lung disease. Puffiness of the face and swelling of the ankles may suggest nephritis. The disposition often changes, and the girl becomes low-spirited and irritable. The eyes have a peculiar brilliancy and the sclerotics are of a bluish color.

(*b*) Special Features.—*Blood.*—The drop as expressed looks pale. Johann Duncan, in 1867, first called attention to the fact that the essential feature was not a great reduction in the number of the corpuscles, but a quantitative change in the hæmoglobin. The corpuscles themselves look pale. In 63 consecutive cases examined by Thayer the average number per cubic millimetre of the red blood-corpuscles was 4,096,544, or over 80 per cent., whereas the percentage of hæmoglobin for the total number was 42.3 per cent. There may be all the physical characteristics and symptoms of a profound anæmia with the number of the blood-corpuscles nearly at the normal standard. No other form of anæmia presents this feature, at least with the same constancy and in the same degree. The importance of the reduction in the hæmoglobin depends upon the fact that it is the iron-containing elements of the blood with which in respiration the oxygen enters into combination. This marked diminution has also been determined by chemical analysis of the blood. In severe cases the red cells may be extremely irregular in size and shape—poikilocytosis. The color is noticeably pale and the deficiency may be seen either in individual corpuscles or in the blood itself. Nucleated red corpuscles (normoblasts) may be found in severe cases. The leucocytes may show a slight increase; the average in the 63 cases above referred to was 8,467 per cmm. The lymphocytes are usually normal; the blood platelets may be increased.

(*c*) Gastro-intestinal Symptoms.—The appetite is capricious, and patients may have a longing for unusual articles, particularly acids. In some instances they eat all sorts of indigestible things, such as chalk or even earth. Distress after eating and even cardialgic attacks may be present. Constipation is a common symptom. The stomach may be found vertically placed; sometimes the organ is dilated. The motor power is usually well retained. Enteroptosis with palpable right kidney is not uncommon.

(*d*) Circulatory Symptoms.—Palpitation of the heart may be the most distressing symptom. The transverse dulness may be increased. A systolic murmur is heard at the apex or at the base; more commonly at the latter, but in extreme cases at both. A diastolic murmur is rarely heard. The systolic murmur is usually loudest in the second left intercostal space, where there is sometimes a distinct pulsation. On the right side of the neck over the jugular vein a continuous murmur may be heard. The pulse is usually full and soft. Visible impulse is present in the veins of the neck, as noted by Lancisi. Pulsation in the peripheral veins is sometimes seen.

Thrombosis in the veins may occur, most commonly in the femoral, but occasionally in the cerebral sinuses. In 86 cases the veins of the legs were affected in 48, the cerebral sinuses in 29 (Lichtenstern). The chief danger in thrombosis of the extremities is pulmonary embolism, which occurred in 13 of 52 cases collected by Welch.

Fever is not uncommon. Chlorotic patients suffer frequently from headache and neuralgia, which may be paroxysmal. The hands and feet are often cold. Dermatographia is common. Hysterical manifestations are not infrequent. Menstrual disturbances are very common—amenorrhœa or dysmenorrhœa. With the improvement in the blood condition this function is usually restored.

Diagnosis.—The green sickness, as it is sometimes called, is in many instances recognized at a glance. The well-nourished condition of the girl, the peculiar complexion, which is most marked in brunettes, and the white or bluish sclerotics are very characteristic. A special danger exists in mistaking the apparent anæmia of the early stage of pulmonary tuberculosis for chlorosis. The palpitation of the heart and shortness of breath frequently suggest heart-disease, and the œdema of the feet and general pallor cause the cases to be mistaken for nephritis. In the great majority of cases the characters of the blood readily separate chlorosis from other forms of anæmia.

Treatment.—This affords one of the most brilliant instances—of which we have but three or four—of the specific action of a remedy. Apart from the action of quinine in malarial fever, and of arsenic, mercury and iodide of potassium in syphilis, there is no other drug the beneficial effects of which we can trace with the accuracy of a scientific experiment. It is a minor matter *how* the iron cures chlorosis. In a week we give to a case as much iron as is contained in the entire blood, as even in the worst case of chlorosis there is rarely a deficit of more than 2 grams of this metal.

In chlorosis, there is an increase in the red blood-corpuscles under the influence of iron, and the red cells may rise above normal. The increase in the hæmoglobin is slower and the maximum percentage may not be reached for a long time. There is no better form than Blaud's pills. During the first week one pill (gr. v, 0.3 gm.) is given three times a day; in the second week, two pills; in the third week, three pills, three times a day. An important feature in the treatment is to persist in the use of iron for at least three months, and, if necessary, subsequently to resume it in smaller doses, as recurrences are so common. The diet should consist of good, easily digested food. Special care should be directed to the bowels, and if constipation is present a saline purge should be given each morning. The dyspeptic symptoms may be relieved by alkalies. Dilute hydrochloric acid is often useful. Rest in bed is important in severe cases.

2. *Pernicious or Addisonian Anæmia*

Definition.—A recurring and usually fatal anæmia caused by hæmolytic agents and characterized by an embryonic type of hæmatopoiesis.

History.—Addison, after whom the disease should be called, gave the first accurate account (1855). Channing described cases of severe anæmia in the puerperal state. The writings of Gusserow and Biermer in the early seventies did much to awaken interest in the disease. The studies of Pepper (Secundus), H. C. Wood, and Palmer Howard made the disease familiar to American and Canadian physicians.

Distribution.—It is a widespread disease, the incidence of which in any community is a good deal a matter of keenness on the part of the practitioners (Cabot). It appears to be increasing.

Etiology.—The figures here quoted are from Cabot's analysis of some 1,200 cases given in his article in our "System of Medicine." It is a disease of middle life; a great majority—922—occurred over the age of 36. The youngest patient we have seen was a boy of ten years. Two or three cases may occur in one family, as a father and two girls.

The cause remains obscure, the nature and origin of the hæmolysins are unknown. Bunting has produced a very similar blood condition in animals by injecting ricin. The bothriocephalus anæmia is stated to be due to a lipoid body that may be extracted from the worm. Hæmolytic bodies have been extracted from the intestinal mucosa, but it has not been shown that they are specific. Oral sepsis and intestinal toxæmia have been brought forward and supported by many arguments (Hunter) but there must be something in addition. Naturally in the present endocrine craze hypersplenism has been invoked. Moffitt calls attention to the similarity of the disease to a protozoal infection—the remission, the nervous lesions, and the beneficial effects of arsenic.

In the horse there is a form of anæmia due to the presence of the larvæ of the *Œstrus equi,* a common parasite in the stomach (the infectious anæmia of the French). Anæmia may be produced experimentally by extracts of these larvæ, and apparently also when these extracts are freed from the hæmolytic lipoids with which the anæmia of the bothriocephalus is associated.

Nervous shock has appeared to be a factor in a few cases.

Sex.—It is twice as common in males, but under the age of 30 women are more often affected.

Among other factors in cases with the blood picture resembling the Addisonian anæmia are:—

Pregnancy and Parturition.—The anæmia may (1) come on during pregnancy or (2) follow delivery, without any special loss of blood, or (3) be an acute septic anæmia. There were 18 in Cabot's series of 1,200 cases.

Intestinal Parasites.—Anæmia of a severe and even pernicious type may be associated with the bothriocephalus or the hook-worm.

Hæmorrhage.—Anæmia after hæmorrhage is usually of the secondary type, but in every series of cases of Addison's anæmia will be found a few with a history of bleeding piles, epistaxis or loss of blood from other sources.

We have not got much beyond the position of Addison, who characterized the disease which he was describing as "a general anæmia occurring without any discoverable cause whatever; cases in which there had been no previous loss of blood, no existing diarrhœa, no chlorosis, no purpura, no renal, splenic, myasmatic, glandular, strumous, or malignant disease."

Pathology.—The body is rarely emaciated. A lemon tint of the skin is present in a majority of the cases. The muscles often are intensely red in color, like horse flesh, while the fat is light yellow. Hæmorrhages are common on the skin and serous surfaces. The heart is usually large, flabby, and empty. In one instance only 2 drams of blood were found in the right heart, and between 3 and 4 in the left. The muscle substance of the heart is intensely fatty, and of a pale, light yellow color. In no affection do we see more extreme fatty degeneration. The lungs show no special changes. The stomach in many instances is normal, but in some cases of fatal anæmia the mucosa is extensively atrophied. The liver may be enlarged and fatty. The iron is in excess, a striking contrast to the condition in cases of secondary anæmia. It is deposited in the outer and middle zones of the lobules.

The spleen shows no important changes. In one of Palmer Howard's cases the organ weighed only 1 ounce and 5 drams. The iron pigment is usually in excess. The lymph glands may be of a deep red color (hæmo-lymph gland). The amount of iron pigment is increased in the kidneys, chiefly in the convoluted tubules. The bone-marrow is usually red, lymphoid in character, showing great numbers of nucleated red corpuscles, especially the larger forms called by Ehrlich gigantoblasts. There are cases in which the bone-marrow shows no signs of activity—*aplastic anæmia.*

Spinal cord lesions were present in 84 per cent. of the post mortems collected by Cabot, a sclerosis chiefly of the posterior columns in the cervical region. Foci of a similar nature occur in the brain both in the gray and white matter (Woltman).

Symptoms.—The combination of pallor with good nutrition is a striking feature. As a rule there is very slight loss in weight and the fat is well preserved, in contrast to most of the secondary anæmias, with which wasting is associated. The description given by Addison is masterly: "It makes its approach in so slow and insidious a manner that the patient can hardly fix a date to the earliest feeling of that languor which is shortly to become so extreme. The countenance gets pale, the whites of the eyes become pearly, the general frame flabby rather than wasted, the pulse perhaps large, but remarkably soft and compressible, and occasionally with a slight jerk, especially under the slightest excitement. There is an increasing indisposition to exertion, with an uncomfortable feeling of faintness or breathlessness in attempting it; the heart is readily made to palpitate; the whole surface of the body presents a blanched, smooth, and waxy appearance; the lips, gums, and tongue seem bloodless, the flabbiness of the solids increases, the appetite fails, extreme languor and faintness supervene, breathlessness and palpitations are produced by the most trifling exertion or emotion; some slight œdema is probably perceived about the ankles; the debility becomes extreme—the patient can no longer rise from bed; the mind occasionally wanders; he falls into a prostrate and half-torpid state, and at length expires; nevertheless, to the very last, and after a sickness of several months' duration, the bulkiness of the general frame and the amount of obesity often present a most striking contrast to the failure and exhaustion observable in every other respect."

A surprising fact is that there are patients with extreme anæmia who are remarkably vigorous. One may see patients with a count of about two million red cells who insist that they are able to do everything as usual except for a little shortness of breath.

The appearance of the patient is usually very characteristic. The combination of a lemon-yellow tint of the skin with retention of the fat gives a very suggestive picture. Sometimes the tint is icteroid. In rare cases there is a white, anæmic pallor, and in a third group a brownish tinge of the skin (which is sometimes associated with leucoderma) deep enough to suggest Addison's disease. Muscular weakness, palpitation, headache, dyspnœa, vertigo, and œdema of the feet are common in this as in other types of anæmia.

Gastro-intestinal symptoms are not uncommon. Paroxysms of pain in the stomach with or without diarrhœa may occur in crises. In fully one-half of the cases diarrhœa occurs at some time during the course. The hydrochloric acid is usually greatly diminished or absent, and there may be complete achylia. A sore mouth and tongue, a feature to which attention was called especially by William Hunter, has not been common in our experience. There may be marked glossitis and ulceration. Pyorrhœa alveolaris may be said to be present in all cases, and the teeth are often very bad.

Complaint of palpitation and disturbance of the heart is common. Slight dilatation is common; murmurs are rarely missed, generally hæmic and basic. Apex diastolic murmurs may occur without valve lesions. Extraordinary throbbing of the arteries may occur, so that aneurism may be suspected; the pulse may be collapsing. Œdema is common, usually in the feet, sometimes in the hands. The urine is usually of low specific gravity, pale, and with diminished pigments. Sometimes, as pointed out by Hunter and Mott, it is of a deep sherry color, due to great excess of urobilin. Increase of urobilin and urobilinogen in the urine and stools is a constant finding, and the presence of these substances in the urine in the absence of signs of biliary or hepatic disease is suggestive of pernicious anæmia. The amount is of some value in the immediate prognosis.

Nervous System.—The more carefully the cases are investigated the greater the frequency of nervous lesions. Numbness and tingling are common and sometimes there are marked neuritic pains. Multiple neuritis may be a feature of the disease or due to arsenic. There are three groups of cases:

(*a*) The patient may have had no special symptoms pointing to involvement of the nervous system, but post mortem well marked lesions of the cord are found.

(*b*) With the anæmia there are signs of spinal cord lesions, a postero-lateral sclerosis, with spastic features and increased reflexes, or the picture may be rather of the tabetic type—lightning pains, girdle sensation, areas of anæsthesia, loss of the reflexes.

(*c*) There is a remarkable group carefully described by Risien Russell, Batten, and Collier, in which the nervous symptoms, usually those of a postero-lateral sclerosis, precede the anæmia.

As the disease progresses there may be great depression, sometimes delusions, but mental symptoms, as a rule, are not marked.

Hæmorrhages are not uncommon, chiefly in the form of small petechiæ. Retinal hæmorrhages are frequent. Optic neuritis is rare.

Blood.—The total quantity is much diminished. The drop may look of good color, but it is abnormally fluid. The red blood-corpuscles are greatly diminished; the average count in 81 cases, when they came under observation, was 1,575,000 per c. mm. There is no other disease which so often reduces the number of red blood-corpuscles below two millions per c. mm. In 12 per cent. of our cases the count was under one million. The lowest count on record is in a patient of Quincke's, 143,000 per c. mm.

The hæmoglobin, though quantitatively reduced, is relatively high. The color index is over 1 and may be 1.5. Marked irregularity in size and shape of the red cells with many large forms is a special feature. The macrocytes measure 8, 10 or even 15 μ. On the other hand, there are a great many very small red corpuscles—microcytes, from 2 to 6 μ in diameter, and of a deep red color. The irregularity in shape is remarkable. Some are elongated, rod-like, others pyriform; one end of the corpuscle may be of normal shape, while the other is extended like the neck of a bottle. Stippling of the red blood-corpuscles is common with dark blue or blackish discoloration—the so-called polychromatophilia. Mitochondria, small bodies of a lipoid nature, may be seen in the red cells.

Nucleated red blood-corpuscles are constantly present, varying very much in numbers from day to day. There are two types—normoblasts of the average size, and the megaloblasts, which are much larger. There are frequently intermediate forms between these two groups. These nucleated red cells vary extraordinarily in different cases, and there may be what have been called blood crises, in which a large number of the nucleated reds appear. In one such crisis there were 14,388 normoblasts, 460 intermediates, and 138 megaloblasts per c. mm. These crises are sometimes followed by gains in the blood count, but they may be terminal events, and not specially indicative of active blood regeneration.

The leucocytes are generally normal or diminished in number. Polynuclear cells are rarely reduced. Occasionally there is a marked increase in the small mononuclear forms. Myelocytes are frequently present, even up to

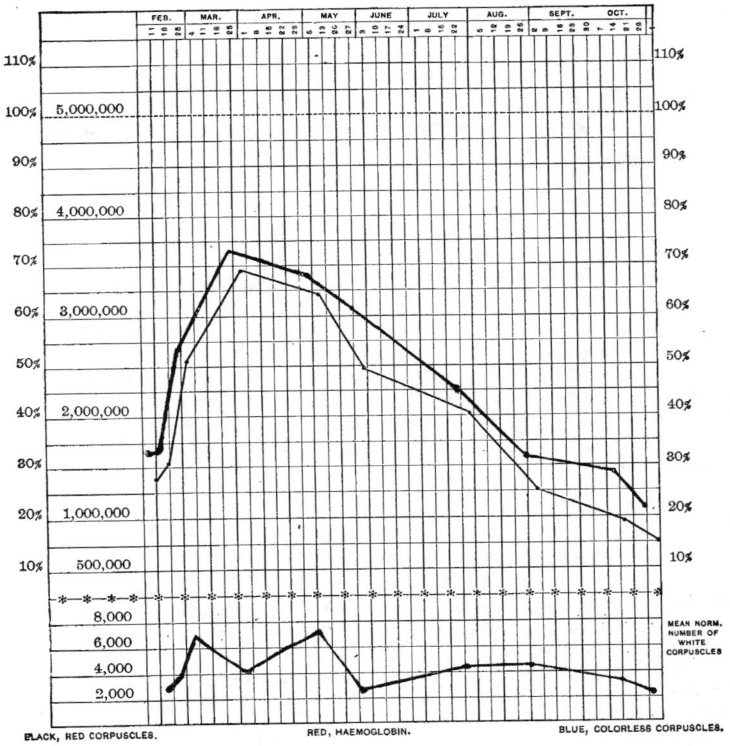

Chart XV.—Pernicious Anæmia

8 and 10 per cent. Blood-platelets are usually low; counts of 100,000 and less are not uncommon (Pratt).

Chart XV shows the blood condition in a case during nine months.

The metabolism has been the subject of many studies. A pathological destruction of proteins is usually present but a positive nitrogen balance may be maintained by forced feeding (Mosenthal).

Aplastic Anæmia.—A certain number of cases of primary anæmia run a rapid and progressive course, without remissions; and death occurs within a few weeks or months from the beginning of the attack. Post mortem, instead of an active hyperplasia of the bone marrow, there is atrophy or aplasia. To these cases the term "aplastic anæmia" has been given. It is a sub-type of pernicious anæmia with identical clinical features, except that it runs a more rapid course, is met with in younger persons, the color index may be low, hæmorrhages are more common, there may be leucopenia, and erythroblasts are usually absent. The hæmorrhages may be very severe, and some of the cases are of a pronounced purpuric type.

The diagnosis is only certain after an examination of the bones, when it is found that the marrow of the long bones is fatty, and even the red marrow may have disappeared from the short bones.

Prognosis and Course.—The disease may run a very acute course. In a patient of Finley's in Montreal the fatal termination occurred within ten days of the onset of the symptoms. The course may be from six to twelve weeks, but, as a rule, it is a chronic malady with remarkable remissions. It is rare to meet with a case in which recovery does not take place from the first attack. The number of remissions varies from two or three to five or six. In 524 cases analyzed by Cabot for this special point, 296 had one remission, 118 two, 65 three, 21 four, and 24 five. The duration of the remission may be from three months to four years. In 81 cases treated in the Hopkins Hospital death occurred in 27 while under observation. The average duration in these cases was about a year.

The ultimate prognosis in a great majority of cases is bad; only one case in our series appears to have recovered completely, another was alive and in good health six years after the last attack, and a third four years after. In Cabot's series there were ten cases which had lasted seven years or more, but there were only 6 out of the 1,200 cases analyzed which he regarded as having completely recovered.

Diagnosis.—Few diseases are more readily recognized at sight. There is something very characteristic about the general appearance of a patient with Addisonian anæmia, and nowadays practitioners are much more alert, and the disease is better known. The lemon colored tint of the skin may suggest jaundice; the anæmia, puffy face, swollen ankles, and albumin in the urine, nephritis; the pigmentation, Addison's disease; the shortness of breath and palpitation, heart disease; the pallor and gastric symptoms, cancer of the stomach. The retention of fat, the insidious onset, the absence of signs of local disease, and the blood features are the important diagnostic points. In a doubtful case the evidences of changes in the cord should be looked for; if present they are an important aid. From cancer of the stomach pernicious anæmia is distinguished by the absence of wasting, the high color index of the blood, the lower corpuscular count, and by the marked improvement in the first attacks under proper treatment.

Treatment.—There are five essentials: first, a diagnosis; secondly, rest in bed for weeks or even months, if possible (thirdly) in the open air; fourthly, all the good food the patient can take; fifthly, arsenic; Fowler's solution in increasing doses, beginning with ♏ iii or v (0.2 to 0.3 c. c.) three times a day, and increasing ♏ i each week until the patient takes ♏ xv (1 c. c.) three times a day. Other forms of arsenic may be tried, as sodium cacodylate or atoxyl hypodermically. Atoxyl can be given in doses of gr. ss (0.032 gm.) every five days, and the amount gradually increased. Arsphenamine in small doses (0.2 gm.) at short intervals has apparently been useful in some cases. It is generally helpful to give dilute hydrochloric acid in full doses, twice after each meal. Accessories are oil inunctions; bone-marrow, which has the merit of a recommendation by Galen; in some cases iron seems to do good. Care should be taken of the mouth and teeth, and mouth infection thoroughly treated. Focal infection anywhere should receive proper treatment. Gastric lavage and irrigations of the colon are useful in some cases.

Splenectomy has been done in a number of cases, but it is well to be cautious in judging of its value. Some patients have been helped for a time, but it is not proved that permanent benefit results.

Transfusion is again in vogue, and with a much improved technique. In patients with a rapidly falling count a transfusion may start improvement. The transfusion may be repeated three or four times at intervals of ten days or two weeks. It is important to use a homologous blood. Bloomfield's study (1918) seems to show that, even with the new methods, results are not more satisfactory than in the hands of the men who first practised it in the seventies.

II. LEUKÆMIA

Definition.—A disease characterized by a permanent increase in the leucocytes of the blood, associated with hyperplasia of the leucoblastic tissues.

History.—In October, 1845, Hughes Bennett recorded a case of "suppuration of the blood with enlargement of the spleen and liver," and he afterward gave the disease the name of "leukocythæmia." A month later Virchow described a similar condition of "white blood" to which he gave the name of "leukæmia." In 1870 Neumann determined the importance of the changes in the bone marrow. The work of Ehrlich enabled us to classify the cases according to the blood changes.

Varieties.—The whole hæmatopoietic system—marrow, spleen, and lymph glands—is involved. Formerly we spoke of three different groups—the splenic, lymphatic, and medullary, but we now recognize that the leucoblastic hyperplasia may begin in any part of the blood-glandular system, marrow, lymph glands, and probably in the spleen. The differences in the types depend upon the dominance of the lymphoid or the myeloid process, so that we now divide the cases roughly into two great groups: (1) the myelocytic or myeloid, corresponding to the spleno-medullary type, and (2) the lymphoid, which represents the lymphatic variety. Some cases not fitting accurately into either are spoken of as "atypical" or "transitional" forms.

The relation to *pregnancy* is interesting. Conception is rare during the course. The disease may begin during pregnancy and progress rapidly. In Cameron's case (Montreal) the grandmother, mother and brother had symptoms suggestive of leukæmia. During pregnancy the disease was first noted when her sixth child was three months old and he died of leukæmia at the sixth month. She was leukæmic through her seventh pregnancy and was delivered with a red cell count of one million and the white blood count 1:10. The child became purpuric and died on the fourth day with the red cell count normal and the leucocytes about 35,000. Another child aged 8 had leukæmia also.

I. Myeloid Leukæmia.—*Etiology.*—The acute cases resemble an infection. The cause remains unknown. The disease may be a myeloma. Multiple cases have been reported in a family. The disease is not very rare. There were 24 cases in the Johns Hopkins Hospital in fifteen years. It is not more frequent in malarial regions.

It is rather more common in males than in females, and between the 30th and 50th years. The youngest of our patients was a child of eight months.

It has followed a blow. Patients may have had a tendency to hæmorrhage, but, as a rule, the disease appears in fairly healthy persons without any recognizable cause.

Morbid Anatomy.—Dropsy is sometimes present. There may be a condition of polyæmia; the heart and veins are distended with large blood-clots. In one case the weight of blood in the heart chambers alone was 620 grams. There may be remarkable distention of the portal, cerebral, pulmonary, and subcutaneous veins. The blood is usually clotted, and the enormous increase in the leucocytes gives a pus like appearance to the coagula, so that it has happened more than once, as in Virchow's memorable case, that on opening the right auricle the observer at first thought he had cut into an abscess. The coagula have a peculiar greenish color, somewhat like the fat of a turtle and so intense as to suggest the color of chloroma. The fibrin is increased. Charcot's octahedral crystals may separate from the blood after death.

In the myelitic form the spleen is greatly enlarged, the capsule may be thickened, and the vessels at the hilus enlarged. The weight may range from 2 to 18 pounds. The organ is in a condition of chronic hyperplasia. It cuts with resistance, has a uniformly reddish brown color, and the Malpighian bodies are invisible. Grayish white, circumscribed, lymphoid tumors may occur throughout the organ, contrasting strongly with the reddish brown matrix. Instead of a fatty tissue, the medulla of the long bones may resemble the consistent matter which forms the core of an abscess, or it may be dark brown in color. There may be hæmorrhagic infarctions. There may be much expansion of the shell of bone with localized swellings.

Leukæmic enlargements in the solitary and agminated glands of Peyer may occur and leukæmic growths have been found in the stomach, omentum and peritoneum. The thymus may be enlarged in the acute cases. The liver may be greatly enlarged, due to a diffuse leukæmic infiltration or to definite growths. There are rarely changes of importance in the lungs. In 159 cases collected by Gowers there were 13 instances of leukæmic nodules in the liver and 10 in the kidneys. Tumors of the skin are rare.

Symptoms.—Anæmia is not a necessary accompaniment of all stages of the disease; the subjects may look very healthy and well. The onset is insidious, and, as a rule, the patient seeks advice for progressive enlargement of the abdomen and shortness of breath, or the pallor, palpitation, and other symptoms of anæmia. Bleeding at the nose is common. Gastro-intestinal symptoms may precede the onset. Occasionally the first symptoms are of a very serious nature. In one case a boy played lacrosse two days before the onset of the final hæmatemesis; and in another case a girl, who had, it was supposed, only a slight chlorosis, died of fatal hæmorrhage from the stomach before any suspicion had been aroused as to the true condition.

The gradual increase in the volume of the *spleen* is the most prominent feature in a majority of the cases. Pain and tenderness are common, though the progressive enlargement may be painless. A creaking fremitus may be felt on palpation. The enlarged organ extends downward to the right, and may be felt just at the costal edge, or when large it may extend as far over as the navel. In many cases it occupies fully one half of the abdomen, reaching to the pubes below and extending beyond the middle line. As a rule, the edge, in some the notch or notches, can be felt distinctly. Its size varies greatly from time to time. It may be perceptibly larger after meals. A hæmorrhage or free diarrhœa may reduce the size. The pressure of the enlarged organ may cause distress after eating; in one case it caused fatal obstruction of the bowels. On auscultation a murmur may sometimes be heard over the spleen, and Gerhardt described a pulsation in it.

The long bones are tender; leukæmic tumors are rare but there may be localized swellings, particularly on the ribs, which are tender and yield to firm pressure.

The pulse is usually rapid, soft, compressible, but often full in volume. The veins may be very large and full, and pulsation in those of the hand and arm is common. There are rarely any cardiac symptoms. The apex beat may be lifted an interspace by the enlarged spleen. Toward the close œdema may occur in the feet or general anasarca. Hæmorrhage is common. There may be most extensive purpura, or hæmorrhagic exudate into pleura or peritoneum. Epistaxis is the most frequent form. Hæmoptysis and hæmaturia are rare. Bleeding from the gums may be present. Hæmatemesis proved fatal in two of our cases, and in a third a large cerebral hæmorrhage rapidly killed.

Local gangrene may develop, with signs of intense infection and high fever. There are very few pulmonary symptoms. The shortness of breath is due, as a rule, to the anæmia. Toward the end there may be œdema of the lungs or pneumonia. The gastro-intestinal symptoms are rarely absent. Nausea and vomiting are early features in some cases, and diarrhœa may be very troublesome, even fatal. Intestinal hæmorrhage is not common. There may be a dysenteric process in the colon. Jaundice rarely occurs. Ascites may be a prominent symptom, probably due to the presence of the splenic tumor. A leukæmic peritonitis also may be present, due to new growths in the membranes.

The nervous system is not often involved. Facial paralysis has been noted. Headache, dizziness, and fainting spells are due to anæmia. The patients are usually tranquil. Coma may follow cerebral hæmorrhage. Paraplegia may be due to pressure of a leukæmic tumor on the cord.

There is a peculiar *retinitis,* due chiefly to the extravasation of blood, but there may be aggregations of leucocytes, forming small leukæmic growths. Optic neuritis is rare. Deafness has frequently been observed; it may appear early and possibly is due to hæmorrhage. Features suggestive of Ménière's disease may come on suddenly, due to leukæmic infiltration or hæmorrhage into the semi-circular canal.

The urine presents no constant changes. The uric acid is always in excess. *Priapism,* a curious symptom, is present in many cases, and may be the first symptom. It may persist for weeks. The cause is thrombosis of the veins in some cases.

Fever was present in two-thirds of our series. Periods of pyrexia may alternate with prolonged intervals of freedom. The temperature may range from 102° to 103° F.

Blood.—In all forms of the disease the diagnosis must be made by the examination of the blood, as it alone offers distinctive features.

The striking change is an increase in the leucocytes. The average in our series was 298,700 per c. mm., and the average ratio to the red cells was 1 to 10. Counts above 500,000 per c. mm. are common, and they may rise above 1,000,000 per c. mm. The proportion of white to red cells may be 1 to 5, or may even reach 1 to 1. There are instances on record in which the number of leucocytes has exceeded that of the red corpuscles.

The increase is in all the forms. The polynuclear neutrophiles make up from 30 to 50 per cent.; both the small and the large lymphocytes are increased; the eosinophiles and the mast cells show both a percentage and absolute increase. The abnormal cells, the myelocytes, range from 30 to 50 per cent. Normoblasts and megaloblasts are common. There is no anæmia at first. The red cell count may be normal, but sooner or later anæmia comes on, and the count may fall to 2,000,000 per c. mm. The color index is usually low. The blood platelets are increased. Charcot-Leyden crystals may separate from the clots and the hæmoglobin shows a remarkable tendency to crystallize.

ALEUKÆMIC INTERVALS.—It has long been known that the white cells may fall to normal or even below. In a case in the Johns Hopkins Hospital, the leucocytes diminished from 500,000 per c. mm. on Jan. 26 to 6,000 on Feb. 16, and throughout the greater part of March were as low as 2,000 per c. mm. This followed the use of arsenic. With this the spleen may or may not reduce. The same may occur spontaneously, but has been frequently seen following the benzol, radium and X-ray treatment. The question arises whether it is always possible in the aleukæmic intervals to diagnose the disease from the examination of the blood. In some cases the films are normal. These aleukæmic phases are not rare but unfortunately are only transitory.

II. LYMPHOID LEUKÆMIA.—Less common, this occurs in acute and chronic forms.

A. ACUTE LYMPHATIC LEUKÆMIA (acute lymphadenosis) is the most terrible of all blood diseases. It occurs in younger persons and more frequently in males. In onset and course the disease resembles an acute infection. Swelling of the tonsils, ulcerative angina, stomatitis, fever, hæmorrhages and a rapid anæmia are the dominant features. Dyspnœa, nausea, vomiting, and diarrhœa are not uncommon. Some cases resemble fulminant purpura, and cutaneous hæmorrhages may be present before the patient feels ill. The glands of the neck enlarge and usually other groups, but death may occur without marked adenitis. The spleen is usually palpable, rarely very large. Hæmorrhages from the mucous membranes and into the serous sacs are common. The course is rapid, and death may occur within a week of onset; more often in from three to six weeks. Remissions may occur and a case beginning acutely may linger for three or four months.

Leukæmia cutis, most common in this form, is characterized by nodular tumors in the skin, which may break down rapidly, hæmorrhages, pigmentation of the skin, and fever. The spleen and lymph glands may be little, if at all, enlarged.

The *blood picture* in the acute form may give the only data for diagnosis. The anæmia is rapid with the usual changes in the blood cells. The leucocytes are increased but less as a rule than in the myeloid forms. Counts of 100,000-200,000 per c. mm. are frequent and the count may rise to above 1,000,000. The distinctive feature is the predominance of large lymphocytes, usually over 90 per cent. Atypical blood pictures may be met with—a mixed small and large lymphocytosis, macrolymphocytes and their variants.

The enlargement of the spleen and lymph glands is less marked than in the myeloid form. Lymphoid swellings in the mouth, throat and intestines are common, and small tumors may be widely scattered on the serous membranes, skin, in the lungs, and even in the nervous system. The bone marrow is deep red, but the changes depend much on the duration of the disease.

B. Chronic Lymphatic Leukæmia (chronic lymphadenosis) is less common. Its existence has been denied, but cases of three, five, ten and thirteen years' duration have been reported. A patient of W. H. Draper's of New York seen ten years after the onset had a sheaf of blood counts from every clinician of note in Europe and the United States. There was no anæmia, the leucocytes were 242,000 per c. mm., the superficial lymph glands were enlarged and the spleen of moderate size.

It occurs in older persons, rarely, if ever, in children; the general health may be very good and the only inconvenience felt is from the bunches of enlarged glands. The spleen is rarely very large; the mesenteric and retroperitoneal groups may form big tumors. After lasting two or more years acute symptoms may come on—fever, hæmorrhages, stomatitis, tonsillitis. Pigmentation of the skin, itching with urticaria and lymphomas may be present, giving a skin picture very like that of Hodgkin's disease. The blood shows at first little or no anæmia. The leucocytes are usually above 100,000 per c. mm. and very high counts are common. The small lymphocytes predominate up to 90-95 per cent. The large forms are rare until the late stages when anæmia supervenes and the other elements show little or no change.

Atypical Leukæmias.—(1) Mixed leukæmias, in part myeloid and in part lymphoid; but in nearly all cases of the ordinary spleno-medullary leukæmia a certain percentage of lymphocytes is present, which toward the end may be materially increased.

(2) *Cases with atypical blood changes*, such as a very high percentage of eosinophiles, or a condition with a very high proportion of plasma cells.

(3) *Chloroma* is an atypical lymphoid leukæmia in which the lymphatic tumors have a greenish color. It is more common in children. Exophthalmos is frequent owing to tumor formation in the orbit. The tumor growths occur chiefly in the skull, the orbit, the long bones, and throughout the viscera. The typical picture of this distribution may be present without the green tint of chloroma. The nature of the pigment is unknown.

(4) In a few rare instances a condition of leukæmia has been found without changes in the blood-making organs.

(5) *Leukanæmia.*—This term was invented by Leube to describe a condition showing features both of leukæmia and severe anæmia. The cases are now regarded as a myeloid leukæmia with severe anæmia. Glandular enlargement is usually present; the onset may be like the acute types of leukæmia, and the blood picture either of the lymphoid or of the myeloid type.

Diagnosis.—The recognition of the acute forms may be difficult, particularly those which begin with marked angina and cutaneous hæmorrhages. It may not be until a blood examination is made or the glands enlarge that suspicion is aroused. The chronic forms are easily recognized. The enlarged spleen at once suggests a blood count, upon which alone the diagnosis rests. The diagnosis may be made by the ophthalmic surgeon. In the lymphatic form, too, the diagnosis rests with the blood examination. One has to recognize that there are certain cases of sepsis with marked lymphocytosis, in which the white blood-corpuscles may reach 30,000 or 40,000 per c. mm. When the regional lymph glands are involved this may raise a doubt. Cabot gives an instance of a child in whom after pneumonia and whooping-cough there was a leucocytosis of 94,000 per c. mm. It is important to remember that in the ordinary myelitic forms under treatment with arsenic or with X-rays the increase of leucocytes may disappear, but the differential count may still be characteristic.

Prognosis.—Recovery in leukæmia is practically unknown. The acute cases die within three months; the chronic forms last from six months to four or five years. The chronic lymphatic form is the most protracted.

Association with Other Diseases.—Tuberculosis is not uncommon. Dock collected 27 cases, in none of which did the tuberculosis show any special influence. Intercurrent infections as influenza, erysipelas, or sepsis may have a remarkable effect upon the disease. In a case reported by Dock, after an attack of influenza the leucocytes fell from 367,000 to 7,500 per c. mm. A course of antistreptococcic serum may do the same.

Treatment.—Fresh air, good diet, and abstention from mental worry and care are the important general indications. The *indicatio morbi* can not be met. There are certain remedies which have an influence upon the disease.

Of these arsenic is the best. Fowler's solution can be begun in doses of three drops and increased to the limit of tolerance or sodium cacodylate given by injection. *Benzol* has been extensively used but should be given with caution and discontinued if there is a drop in the red cell count. If the number of leucocytes decreases steadily, the drug should be discontinued when the number falls to 25,000. The dose is ʒ i (4 c. c.) per day given in capsules with olive oil. The *X-rays,* while not curative, add to the duration of life. They should not be used in the acute forms. The exposure should be over the long bones at first and care should be taken to watch for any signs of toxæmia. *Radium* has been successful in a considerable number of cases. Both it and the X-rays usually cause a marked drop in the leucocytes. Either may be used with arsenic or benzol administration. Removal of the spleen has been done after radium treatment but the value of this is doubtful. Recurrence is to be expected after any treatment.

III. HODGKIN'S DISEASE

Definition.—A disease characterized by enlargement of the lymph-glands with progressive anæmia and a fatal termination.

Anatomically there is an increase in the adenoid tissue of the glands, proliferation of the endothelial cells, formation of mononuclear and multinuclear giant cells, the presence of eosinophiles, and thickening of the fibrous reticulum.

History.—In 1832 Hodgkin recorded a series of cases of enlargement of the lymphatic glands and spleen. From the motley group that Hodgkin described, Wilks picked out the disease and called it *anæmia lymphatica.* Other names that have been given to it are *adénie* by Trousseau, *pseudo-leukæmia* by Cohnheim, and *generalized lymphadenoma.*

Etiology.—A widely spread disease in Europe and America, a majority of the cases occur in young adults, and more frequently in males than in females. Twins and sisters have been known to be attacked. The cause is unknown. Certain features suggest an acute infection: the rapid course of some cases, the association with local irritation in the mouth and tonsils, the frequency with which the disease starts in the cervical glands, the gradual extension from one gland group to another, and the recurring exacerbations of fever. Bunting and Yates described a diphtheroid organism with which they produced in the monkey a chronic lymphadenitis clinically resembling Hodgkin's disease. Possibly the disease is a spirillosis—in favor of which are the presence of eosinophilia, so characteristic of infection with animal parasites, the presence of eosinophilic cells in the glands, and the influence of arsenic on the disease. Sternberg suggested that the disease was a special form of tuberculosis; but the histological changes are quite characteristic, tubercle bacilli are not present in uncomplicated cases, the tuberculin test may be negative, and when present the tuberculosis appears to be a terminal infection.

Morbid Anatomy.—The superficial lymph glands are found most extensively involved, and from the cervical groups they form continuous chains uniting the mediastinal and axillary glands. The masses may pass beneath the pectoral muscles and even beneath the scapulæ. Of the internal glands, those of the thorax are most often affected, and the tracheal and bronchial groups may form large masses. The trachea and the aorta with its branches may be completely surrounded; the veins may be compressed, rarely the aorta itself. The masses perforate the sternum and invade the lung deeply. The retroperitoneal glands may form a continuous chain from the diaphragm to the inguinal canals. They may compress the ureters, the lumbar and sacral nerves, and the iliac veins. They may adhere to the broad ligament and the uterus and simulate fibroids. At an early stage the glands are soft and elastic; later they may become firm and hard. Fusion of contiguous glands does not often occur, and they tend to remain discrete, even after attaining a large size. The capsule may be infiltrated, and adjacent tissues invaded. On section the gland presents a grayish white semi-translucent appearance, broken by intersecting strands of fibrous tissue; there is no caseation of necrosis unless a secondary infection has occurred.

The spleen is enlarged in 75 per cent. of the cases; in young children the enlargement may be great, but the organ rarely reaches the size of the spleen in ordinary leukæmia. In more than half of the cases lymphoid growths are present. The marrow of the long bones may be converted into a rich lymphoid tissue. The lymphatic structures of the tonsillar ring and of the intestines may show marked hyperplasia. The liver is often enlarged, and may present scattered nodular tumors, which may also occur in the kidneys.

Histology.—The studies of Andrewes and of Dorothy Reed show a very characteristic microscopic picture—proliferation of the endothelial and reticular cells, with the formation of lymphoid cells of uniform size and shape, and characteristic giant cells, the so-called lymphadenoma cells, containing four or more nuclei. Eosinophiles are always present, and proliferation of the stroma leads to fibrosis of the gland. The difference between the soft and hard forms depends largely upon the stage. When tuberculosis occurs as a secondary infection the two processes may be readily distinguished.

Symptoms.—A tonsillitis may precede the onset. Enlargement of the cervical glands is usually an initial symptom; it is rare to find other superficial groups or the deeper glands attacked first. Months or even several years may elapse before the glands in the axillæ and groin become involved. During what may be called the first stage the patient's general condition is good; then anæmia comes on, not marked at first, but usually progressive. In the majority of cases the spleen is enlarged, but it never reaches the dimension of the leukæmic organ. There may be very little pain until the internal glands become involved. With swelling of the mediastinal glands there are cough, dyspnœa, and often intense cyanosis, with all the signs of intrathoracic tumor. There may be moderate fever. Bronzing of the skin may occur. apart altogether from the use of arsenic. Pruritus may be a very depressing symptom, and boils and ecthymatous blebs may occur. The leucocytes show no characteristic changes. There may be a moderate eosinophilia and, as the anæmia progresses, nucleated red corpuscles appear, and toward the end there are instances of a great increase in the lymphocytes. As the disease progresses there is marked emaciation with great asthenia, and sometimes anasarca. This represents the common clinical course, but there are many variations, among which the following are the most common:

(*a*) An ACUTE FORM has been described. In one case beginning, like so many cases of lymphatic leukæmia, with angina, the whole course was less than ten weeks. Ziegler mentions two cases of death within a month.

(*b*) LOCALIZED FORM.—The enlargement may be localized to certain groups, those in the neck, the groin, the retroperitoneum, or the thorax. Some of these cases present great difficulty in diagnosis, particularly when there are febrile paroxysms with very slight involvement of the external groups. The disease may be confined to one region for a year or more before there is any extension. The localized mediastinal group often presents a very remarkable picture—pressure signs, pain, orthopnœa—and, unless there are other groups involved, or enlargement of the spleen, it may be impossible to make the diagnosis during life.

(*c*) WITH RELAPSING PYREXIA.—To this remarkable type Pel and afterward Ebstein called attention. MacNalty made a careful study of this syndrome, which is one of the most remarkable in medicine. The relapsing pyrexia may occur in cases with involvement of the internal glands alone, or, more frequently, with a general involvement of all the groups. "Following on a period of low pyrexia, or of normal or subnormal temperature, there is a steady rise occupying two or four days to a maximum, which may reach 105°. For about three days the temperature remains at a high level, and then there is a gradual fall by lysis occupying about three days, and the temperature then becomes sub-normal" (MacNalty). An afebrile period of ten days or two weeks then occurs, to be followed by another bout of fever. This may be repeated for many months. In one case the pyrexia lasted for exactly fourteen days for many successive paroxysms. During the fever the glands swell and may become hot and tender. This febrile type may occur in connection with involvement of the internal glands alone. In one patient whose cervical glands had been thoroughly removed there were typical Pel-Ebstein paroxysms, and we could find no enlarged glands, internal or external.

(*d*) LATENT TYPE.—In his monograph Ziegler called attention to the importance of this form, in which anæmia, fever, and constitutional symptoms may be present with enlargement of the internal glands. In one case of this type the retroperitoneal glands alone were involved. Symmers reported an instance in which the glands and the hilus of the liver were attacked.

(*e*) SPLENOMEGALIC FORM.—Enlargement of the spleen is present in a large proportion of cases of Hodgkin's disease. Whether or not there is a type involving the spleen alone without the lymph glands is still a question. Formerly, under the name pseudo-leukæmia of Cohnheim, many cases of simple enlargement of the spleen with or without anæmia were spoken of as *pseudo-leukæmia splenica.* It is not improbable that the disease may originate in the lymphoid tissue of the spleen, and cases have been reported by Ziegler, Symmers, Warrington, and others. It must be very difficult to distinguish such cases clinically from the early stages of Banti's disease.

(*f*) LYMPHOGRANULOMATOSIS.—The skin lesions may be in the form of a true lymphogranulomatosis, which is rare, or show a wide variety of changes. Among these are: pruritus, urticaria, œdema, petechiæ and marked pigmentation.

(*g*) LYMPHADENIA OSSIUM has been described—cases in which there have been multiple bone tumors of the bone marrow and of the periosteum with enlargement of the glands and spleen. How far these should be grouped with Hodgkin's disease seems very doubtful.

Diagnosis.—(*a*) TUBERCULOSIS.—In the case of enlargement of the glands on one side of the neck beginning in a young person, it is often not easy to determine whether the disease is tuberculosis or beginning Hodgkin's disease. Two points should be decided. First, one of the small glands of the affected side should be excised and the structure carefully studied. The histological changes in Hodgkin's disease differ markedly from those in tuberculosis. Secondly, tuberculin should be used if the patient is afebrile. In early tuberculosis of the glands of the neck the reaction is prompt and decisive. In the later stages, when many groups of glands are involved and cachexia well advanced, the tuberculin reaction may be present in Hodgkin's disease, but even then the histological changes are distinctive. Other points to be noted are the tendency in the tuberculous adenitis to coalescence of the glands, adhesion to the skin, with suppuration, etc., and the liability to tuberculosis of the lung or pleura. There is a type of generalized tuberculous adenitis which occurs particularly in negroes and simulates Hodgkin's disease with enlargement of the gland groups in the neck, arms and axilla, never perhaps so much as in Hodgkin's disease, but firm, elastic masses. There is irregular remittent fever, not with periods of apyrexia, the course may be protracted, and at autopsy only the internal and external lymph glands may be found involved.

(*b*) Leukæmia.—The blood examination gives the diagnosis at once, as Hodgkin's disease presents only a slight leucocytosis. A difficulty arises only in those instances of leukæmia in which the leucocytes gradually decrease or the number for a time becomes normal. Histologically there are striking differences between the structure of the glands in the two conditions.

(*c*) Lympho-sarcoma.—Clinically the cases may resemble Hodgkin's disease very closely, and in the literature the two diseases have been confounded. The glands, as a rule, form larger masses, the capsules are involved, and adjacent structures are attacked, but this may be the case in Hodgkin's disease. Pressure signs in the chest and abdomen are much more common in lympho-sarcoma. But the most satisfactory mode of diagnosis is examination of sections of a gland. The blood condition, the type of fever, etc., need a more careful study in this group of cases.

Course.—There are acute cases in which the enlargements spread rapidly and death follows in a few months. As a rule, the disease lasts for two or three years. Remarkable periods of quiescence may occur, in which the glands diminish in size, the fever disappears, and the general condition improves. Even a large group of glands may almost completely disappear, or a tumor mass on one side of the neck may subside while the inguinal glands are enlarging. Usually a cachexia with anæmia and swelling of the feet precedes death. A fatal event may occur early from great enlargement of the mediastinal glands.

Treatment.—When the glands are small and limited to one side of the neck, operation should be advised; even when both sides of the neck are involved, if there are no signs of mediastinal growth, operation is justifiable. The course of the disease may be delayed, even if cure does not follow.

Radium or the X-rays do good in selected cases. Certainly the glands have been reduced in size, but there is no proof of a complete cure. Other local treatment of the glands seems to do but little good.

Arsenic is the only drug which has a positive value and in some cases the effects on the glands are striking. It may be given in the form of Fowler's solution in increasing doses. Recoveries have been reported (?). Ill effects from the larger doses are rare. Peripheral neuritis followed the use of ℥ iv, ʒ j, ♏ xviij during a period of less than three months. Quinine and iron are useful as tonics. For the pressure pains morphia should be given.

IV. PURPURA

Strictly speaking, purpura is a symptom, not a disease; but under this term are conveniently arranged a number of affections characterized by extravasations of the blood into the skin. In the present state of our knowledge a satisfactory classification can not be made. W. Koch groups all forms, including hæmophilia, under the designation *hæmorrhagic diathesis,* believing that intermediate forms link the mild purpura simplex and the most intense purpura hæmorrhagica. For a full discussion of the subject see Pratt's article in our "System of Medicine," Vol. IV.

The purpuric spots vary from 1 to 3 or 4 mm. in diameter. When small and pin-point-like they are called petechiæ; when large, they are known as ecchymoses. At first bright red in color, they become darker, and gradually fade to brownish stains. They do not disappear on pressure.

The following is a provisional grouping of the cases:

Symptomatic Purpura.—(*a*) Infectious.—In pyæmia, septicæmia, and malignant endocarditis (particularly in the last affection) ecchymoses may be very abundant. In typhus fever the rash is always purpuric. Measles, scarlet fever, and more particularly small-pox and cerebro-spinal fever, have each a variety characterized by an extensive purpuric rash.

(*b*) Toxic.—The virus of snakes produces extravasation of blood with great rapidity—a condition carefully studied by Weir Mitchell. Certain medicines, particularly copaiba, quinine, belladonna, mercury, ergot, and the iodides occasionally, are followed by a petechial rash. Purpura may follow the use of comparatively small doses of iodide of potassium. A fatal event may be caused by a small amount, as in a case reported by Stephen Mackenzie of a child who died after a dose of 2½ grains. An erythema may precede the hæmorrhage. It is not always a simple purpura, but may be an acute febrile eruption of great intensity. Workers with benzol, which is used as a solvent for rubber, may be attacked with severe purpura. Cases such as those reported by Selling have been in connection with the coating of tin cans, while the Swedish cases occurred in connection with the manufacture of bicycle tires. Under this division, too, comes the purpura so often associated with jaundice.

(*c*) Cachectic.—Under this heading are best described the instances of purpura which occur in the constitutional disturbance of cancer, tuberculosis, Hodgkin's disease, nephritis, scurvy, and in the debility of old age. In these cases the spots are usually confined to the extremities. They may be very abundant on the lower limbs and about the wrists and hands. This constitutes, probably, the commonest variety of the disease, and many examples of it can be seen in the wards of any large hospital.

(*d*) Neurotic.—One variety is met with in cases of organic disease. It is the so-called myelopathic purpura, which is seen occasionally in tabes dorsalis, particularly following attacks of the lightning pains and, as a rule, involving the area of the skin in which the pains have been most intense. Cases have been met with in acute and transverse myelitis, and occasionally in severe neuralgia. Another form is the remarkable hysterical condition in which stigmata, or bleeding points, appear upon the skin.

(*e*) Mechanical.—This variety is most frequently seen in venous stasis of any form, as in the paroxysms of whooping cough, in epilepsy and about tight bandages.

Arthritic Purpura.—This form is characterized by involvement of the joints. It is usually known, therefore, as "rheumatic," though in reality the evidence upon which this view is based is not conclusive. Of 200 cases of purpura analyzed by Stephen Mackenzie, 61 had a history of rheumatism. It seems more satisfactory to use the designation arthritic. Three groups of cases may be recognized:

(*a*) Purpura Simplex.—A mild form, often known as *purpura simplex*, seen most commonly in children, in whom, with or without articular pain, a crop of purpuric spots appears upon the legs, less commonly upon the trunk and arms. As pointed out by Graves, this form may be associated with diarrhœa. The disease is seldom severe. There may be loss of appetite, and slight anæmia. Fever is not, as a rule, present, and the patients get well in a week or ten days. Usually regarded as rheumatic, and certainly associated, in some instances, with rheumatic manifestations, yet in a majority of the patients the arthritis is slighter than in rheumatic fever and no other manifestations are present. The average duration is six weeks, but there are chronic cases lasting a year or more.

(*b*) Purpura (Peliosis) Rheumatica (*Schönlein's Disease*).—This remarkable affection is characterized by multiple arthritis and an eruption which varies greatly in character, sometimes *purpuric*, more commonly associated with *urticaria* or with *erythema exudativum*. The purpuric spots are of small size and appear in successive crops. The disease is most common in males between the ages of twenty and thirty. It not infrequently sets in with sore throat, a fever from 101° to 103°, and articular pains. The rash, which makes its appearance first on the legs or about the affected joints, may be a simple purpura or may show ordinary urticarial wheals. In other instances there are nodular infiltrations, not to be distinguished from erythema nodosum. The combination of wheals and purpura, the *purpura urticans*, is very distinctive. Much more rarely vesication is met with, the so-called *pemphigoid purpura*. The amount of œdema is variable; occasionally it is excessive. These are the cases which have been described as *febrile purpuric œdema*. The temperature range, in mild cases, is not high, but may reach 102° or 103° F.

The urine is sometimes reduced in amount and may be albuminous. The joint affections are usually slight, though associated with much pain, particularly as the rash comes out. Relapses may occur and the disease may return at the same time for several years in succession.

The diagnosis of Schönlein's disease offers no difficulty. The association of multiple arthritis with purpura and urticaria is very characteristic.

Schönlein's peliosis is thought by most writers to be of rheumatic origin, and certainly many of the cases have the characters of ordinary rheumatic fever, *plus* purpura. By many, however, it is regarded as a special affection, of which the arthritis is a manifestation analogous to that which occurs in hæmophilia and scurvy. The frequency with which sore throat precedes the attack, and the occasional occurrence of endocarditis or pericarditis, are certainly very suggestive of true rheumatism.

The cases usually do well, and a fatal event is extremely rare. The throat symptoms may persist and give trouble. In some instances necrosis and sloughing of a portion of the uvula has followed.

Visceral Lesions in Purpura.—In any form of purpura, in the erythemas, and in urticaria *visceral* lesions may occur. (*a*) Gastro-intestinal crises, pain, vomiting, melæna, and diarrhœa. The attacks have often been mistaken for appendicitis or for intussusception, and at operation the condition has been found to be an acute sero-hæmorrhagic infiltration of a limited area of the stomach or bowel. Identical attacks occur in angio-neurotic œdema. These crises may occur for years in children before an outbreak of purpura or urticaria gives a clue to their nature. (*b*) Enlargement of the spleen is usually present in these cases. (*c*) Albuminuria and acute nephritis may occur and form the most serious complication, of which seven cases in the series died (*Am. J. Med. Sc.*, Jan., 1904). The combination of purpura with colic is usually spoken of as Henoch's purpura.

Chronic Purpura.—For years patients may have outbreaks of purpura without serious symptoms. One patient was practically never free from spots somewhere on the skin for thirty-three years, during which time she had had several severe attacks of nose-bleed, during which the purpura increased greatly. Another patient had recurring purpura on the legs for many years, with great pigmentation and thickening of the skin. There is a form of in-

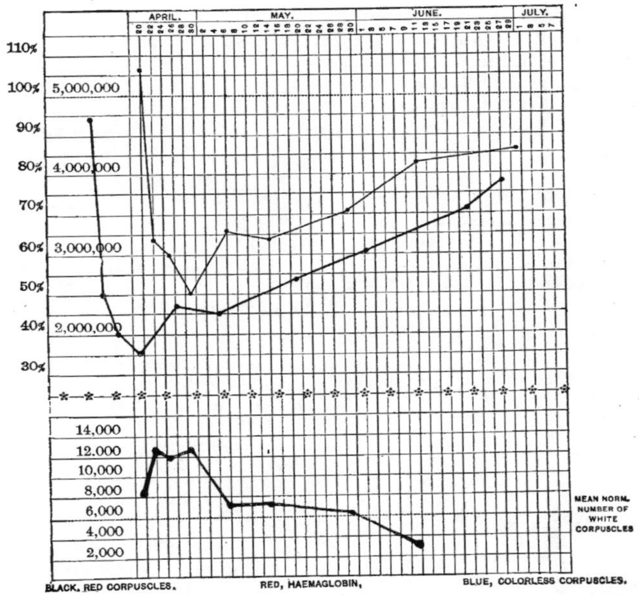

CHART XVI.—THE RAPIDITY WITH WHICH ANÆMIA IS PRODUCED IN PURPURA HÆMORRHAGICA, AND THE GRADUAL RECOVERY.

termittent purpura with attacks over long series of years, as long as twenty, sometimes only on the skin, at other times with involvement of the mucous membranes (Elsner).

Purpura Hæmorrhagica.—Under this heading may be considered cases of very severe purpura with hæmorrhages from the mucous membranes. The affection, known as the *morbus maculosus* of Werlhof, is most common in young and delicate individuals, particularly in girls; but the disease may attack adults in full vigor. After a few days of weakness and debility, purpuric spots appear on the skin and rapidly increase in number and size. Bleeding from the mucous surfaces sets in, and the epistaxis, hæmaturia, and hæmoptysis may cause profound anæmia. Death may take place from loss of blood, or from hæmorrhage into the brain. Slight fever usually accompanies the disease. In favorable cases the affection terminates in from ten days to two weeks, but the average duration is two months and there are chronic forms which persist for years. There are instances of purpura hæmorrhagica of great malignancy, which may prove fatal within twenty-four hours —*purpura fulminans.* This form is most common in children, is characterized chiefly by cutaneous hæmorrhages, and death may occur before any bleeding takes place from the mucous membranes.

In the *diagnosis* of purpura hæmorrhagica it is important to exclude scurvy, which may be done by the consideration of the previous health, the circumstances under which the disease occurs, and by the absence of swelling of the gums. The malignant forms of the fevers, particularly small-pox and measles, are distinguished by the prodromes and the higher temperature. As regards the special blood features, the blood plates are markedly decreased, there is prolonged bleeding time and a non-retractile soft blood clot. In the other purpuras the blood plates are normal. The special points in the diagnosis from hæmophilia are considered under that disease. The possibility of mistaking the acute forms of leukæmia for purpura should be kept in mind.

Treatment.—In symptomatic purpura attention should be paid to the conditions under which it occurs, and measures should be employed to increase the strength and to restore a normal blood condition. Tonics, good food, and fresh air meet these indications. The patient should always be at rest in bed. In the simple purpura of children, or that associated with slight articular trouble, arsenic in full doses should be given. No good is obtained from the small doses, but the Fowler's solution should be pushed freely until physiological effects are obtained. In peliosis rheumatica the sodium salicylate may be given, but with discretion. It does not seem to have any special control over the hæmorrhages.

Aromatic sulphuric acid (♏ xv-xxx, 1-2 c. c.) may be given three times a day, but oil of turpentine is perhaps the best remedy, in 10 or 15-minim (1 c. c.) doses three or four times a day. The calcium salts, preferably the lactate, may be given in doses of 15 grains (1 gm.) three or four times a day for a few days. In bleeding from the mouth, gums, and nose the inhalation of carbon dioxide, irrigations with 2-per-cent. gelatin solution, and epinephrine should be tried. The last remedy has often acted promptly. The treatment of the severe forms is the same as that given in hæmophilia. The intramuscular injection of 20-40 c. c. of citrated blood is the most useful measure in severe cases.

HÆMORRHAGIC DISEASES OF THE NEW-BORN

Syphilis Hæmorrhagica Neonatorum.—The child may be born healthy, or there may be signs of hæmorrhage at birth. Then in a few days there are extensive cutaneous extravasations and bleeding from the mucous surfaces and from the navel. The child may become deeply jaundiced. The post mortem shows numerous extravasations in the internal organs and extensive syphilitic changes in the liver and other organs.

Epidemic Hæmoglobinuria (*Winckel's Disease*).—Hæmoglobinuria in the new-born, which occasionally occurs in epidemic form in lying-in institutions, is a very fatal affection, which sets in usually about the fourth day after birth. The child becomes jaundiced, and there are marked gastro-intestinal symptoms, with fever, jaundice, rapid respiration, and sometimes cyanosis. The urine contains albumin and blood coloring matter—methæmoglobin. The disease has to be distinguished from the simple icterus neonatorum, with which there may sometimes be blood or blood coloring matter in the urine. The post mortem shows an absence of any septic condition of the umbilical vessels, but the spleen is swollen, and there are punctiform hæmorrhages in different parts. Some cases have shown marked acute fatty degeneration of the internal organs—the so-called Buhl's disease.

Morbus Maculosus Neonatorum.—Apart from the common visceral hæmorrhages, the result of injuries at birth, bleeding from one or more of the surfaces is a not uncommon event in the new-born, particularly in hospital practice. Forty-five cases occurred in 6,700 deliveries (C. W. Townsend). The bleeding may be from the navel alone, but more commonly it is general. Of Townsend's 50 cases, in 20 the blood came from the bowels, in 14 from the stomach, in 14 from the mouth, in 12 from the nose, in 18 from the navel, in 3 from the navel alone. The bleeding begins within the first week, but in rare instances is delayed to the second or third. Thirty-one of the cases died and 19 recovered. The disease is usually of brief duration, death occurring in from one to seven days. The temperature is often elevated. The nature of the disease is unknown. As a rule, nothing abnormal is found post mortem. The general and not local nature of the affection, its self limited character, the presence of fever, and the greater prevalence of the disease in hospitals suggest an infectious origin (Townsend). The bleeding may be associated with intense hæmatogenous jaundice. Not every case of bleeding from the stomach or bowels belongs in this category. Ulcers of the œsophagus, stomach, and duodenum have been found in the new-born. The child may draw the blood from the breast and subsequently vomit it.

Treatment.—The most useful measure is the intramuscular injection of fresh or citrated human blood in amounts of 20-40 c. c. This should be repeated every four to eight hours if the hæmorrhage continues.

V. HÆMOPHILIA

Definition.—A disease characterized by deficiency in the thromboplastic substances, thereby rendering the individual liable to severe and recurring hæmorrhages. The defect is hereditary, confined to the male sex but transmitted by the female alone.

History.—Our knowledge of this remarkable condition dates from 1803, when John C. Otto, a Philadelphia physician, published "an account of an hæmorrhagic disposition occurring in certain families," and first used the word "bleeder." The works of Grandidier and of Wickham Legg give full clinical details, and the monograph of Bulloch and Fildes (Dulan & Co., London, 1911) presents in extraordinary detail every aspect of the disease.

Distribution.—A majority of the cases have been reported from Germany, Switzerland, and the United States. Jews are supposed to be more prone to the disease, but this Bulloch doubts, and he discredits the negro cases.

SEX.—Bulloch and Fildes claim to have established the fact of immunity in females, denying the authenticity of all the published cases (19). "In none of the families of bleeders . . . do we find any unequivocal evidence of abnormality in the women, that is to say, any abnormality beyond what might be expected in any collection of females taken at random."

INHERITANCE.—Otto pointed out in his original paper that while the females do not themselves bleed they alone transmit the tendency. Of 171 recorded instances of transmission, 160 conform to the "law of Nasse" that the disease is transmitted by the unaffected female—"the conductor" (Bulloch and Fildes). They explain the 11 exceptions, and conclude that the disease is not capable of being propagated through a male. Hæmophilia without demonstrable inheritance is very rare. It is the best illustration in man of sex-limited inheritance, the mechanism of which has been worked out so beautifully by Morgan and his pupils in Drosophilia.

Pathogenesis.—The blood looks normal. Delay in the coagulation time, up to 30 or even 40 minutes, and imperfect clot formation are the outstanding features. In contrast to purpura hæmorrhagica the platelets are normal. The essential defect is a congenital inability to produce a proper thrombin, through the agency of which the fibrinogen is converted into fibrin. Sahli first suggested that the disease was due to a deficiency in the thrombokinase. "It may be classed as one of the ferment-deficiency diseases, with a strong hereditary association similar to other ferment-deficiency diseases such as cystinuria, alkaptonuria, etc." (Vines). The deficiency is relative, not absolute, and is on the organic side of the clotting mechanism, and not in the inorganic side, e. g., due to lack of calcium salts. One of the difficulties in explaining the bleeding in hæmophilia is the fact that the hæmorrhage continues in spite of the presence of clots in and about the wound. Addis believes that a higher amount of thrombokinase is required to produce rapid clotting in hæmophilic than in normal blood. In a wound, coagulation may occur only in those parts, as at the side, where the concentration of this material is highest; but the clot itself prevents the addition of further quantities of the thrombokinase from the tissues, and when the quantity of thrombin set free from the primary clot is insufficient completely to coagulate the blood in the centre of the wound, the bleeding may continue indefinitely.

Symptoms.—"The cardinal symptoms are three in number . . . an *inherited* tendency in *males* to *bleed*" (Bulloch and Fildes). A trifling injury, of no moment in a normal person, determines a hæmorrhage, which has no tendency to stop, but the blood trickles or oozes until death follows or there is spontaneous arrest. The bleeding may be external, internal, or into joints. A majority of the attacks may be traced to trauma but spontaneous bleeding may occur. The liability is first noticed in children and persists to adult life, gradually diminishing and eventually disappearing. Tooth extraction is a very common cause. Epistaxis is a frequent occurrence, heading the list in Grandidier's series of 334 cases. Other localities were: mouth 43, stomach 15, bowels 36, urethra 16, lungs 17, and a few instances of bleeding from the tongue, finger-tips, tear papilla, eyelids, external ear, vulva, navel, and scrotum. Trivial operations, as circumcision, have been followed by fatal hæmorrhage. Abdominal colic, due to bleeding into the intestinal wall, may occur as in Henoch's purpura. The patient may be admitted to hospital for appendicitis.

Hæmarthrosis, due to bleeding from the synovial membrane, and periarticular bleedings are common. The knee is most commonly attacked, and the affection has been mistaken for tuberculosis. König distinguishes three stages —hæmarthrosis, panarthritis, and deformity.

Eugenics.—The women of bleeder families should not marry or marrying, they should not bear children. Males may marry safely.

Diagnosis.—The monograph by Bulloch and Fildes should be read by all who value accuracy of observation and of investigation. Forms of bleeding are so common that it is a simple matter to construct a pedigree showing an inherited "hæmorrhagic diathesis." It is essential for the diagnosis that the individual should have been more or less subject to bleeding from various parts throughout his life. "No solitary hæmorrhage, however inexplicable, should, in our opinion, be regarded as hæmophilia; it is necessary to show that the individual has been repeatedly attacked, if not from birth, from infancy" (Bulloch and Fildes). There is no laboratory method by which we can determine the deficiency of the organic ferment on which the bleeding depends.

In the diagnosis from purpura hæmorrhagica the following points are important. In hæmophilia puncture of the skin rarely causes hæmorrhage, in purpura it usually does; the blood plates are normal in hæmophilia, much reduced in purpura; the coagulation time is prolonged in hæmophilia (but not constantly so; it may be normal in the intervals between attacks), normal or nearly so in purpura; the "bleeding time" is not prolonged in hæmophilia, much prolonged in purpura; in hæmophilia the blood clot retracts normally but not in purpura; the application of a tourniquet to the upper arm is without result in hæmophilia but in purpura results in the formation of petechiæ on the forearm. As regards heredity, it is well to remember that there are cases of hereditary purpura, some being found in hæmophiliac families.

Treatment.—Rational treatment consists in an attempt to supply the missing substance by the injection of serum or transfusion. A most useful measure is the subcutaneous or intramuscular injection of fresh or citrated human blood in doses of 20 to 40 c. c. Previous testing is not necessary. Fresh blood or serum from animals, such as the horse or rabbit, is also effective given subcutaneously in the same dosage. The injection should be repeated every twelve hours while necessary. The use of fresh anti-diphtheritic serum may be effectual. With obstinate bleeding and severe anæmia transfusion should be done. For surface hæmorrhage, compression should be employed combined with the application of various substances, as a sterile solution of gelatine (2 per cent.), epinephrine (1 to 1000), cocaine (5 per cent.), or fresh blood or serum. The last has been injected into or around the wound with advantage. Hæmophilia should be excluded before any surgical operation is done. The males in hæmophiliac families should be protected from injury and active games forbidden.

VI. ERYTHRÆMIA

(*Vaquez' Disease, Polycythæmia Vera*)

Definition.—A symptom-complex characterized by cyanosis, polycythæmia and splenic enlargement. It seems probable that it is not a definite specific disease but a syndrome with a varied etiology and pathology. Lucas (1912) in a study of the subject pointed out the difficulty of distinguishing between primary and secondary polycythæmia. Warthin has drawn attention to "Ayerza's Disease or Syndrome" in which the features mentioned above were associated with syphilitic disease of the pulmonary arteries. It may be that erythæmia will prove to be a condition always secondary to various causes. In the cases with pulmonary arterio-sclerosis the resulting changes are regarded as compensatory.

Pathology.—We see polycythæmia as a secondary condition in high altitudes, and in stasis of the blood in congenital heart disease and in emphysema of the lungs. The high altitude hyperglobulism is compensatory to lack of oxygen in the air, and there is an increased activity of the bone marrow. In erythræmia proper an increased activity of the bone marrow is present. The splenic enlargement is a secondary result of increased blood formation and destruction. In the cases with pulmonary arterio-sclerosis there is marked right heart hypertrophy.

Symptoms.—The three cardinal features are a change in the appearance of the patient, enlargement of the spleen, and polycythæmia. The superficial blood vessels, capillaries, and veins look full, so that the skin is always congested, in warm weather of a brick red color, in cold weather cyanosed. The engorgement of the face may be extreme, extending to the conjunctivæ, and in the cold the cyanosis of the face and hands may be as marked as any that is ever seen. There is often marked vasomotor instability, the hand becoming deeply engorged when held down, and rapidly anæmic when held up.

The spleen is usually enlarged, but not to the great extent of leukæmia. It may vary in size from time to time. It is hard, firm, and painless.

The total bulk of blood is enormously increased, and the ratio of corpuscles to plasma is high. The polycythæmia ranges from 7 to 12 or even 13 millions of red corpuscles per c. mm. As a rule, they are normal in appearance and shape; nucleated red blood-corpuscles may be present, the hæmoglobin ranging from 130 to 160 per cent., but the color index is relatively low. Moderate leucocytosis is the rule with a high percentage of mononuclears in some cases; a few myelocytes may be present. The specific gravity is high.

Of other symptoms the most common are incapacity for work, headache, flushing, and giddiness. Constipation is common, and albuminuria is usually present. The blood pressure may be high; occasionally there may be hæmorrhages into the skin and from the mucous membranes. Recurring ascites, probably in association with the splenic tumor, is present in some cases.

Christian has emphasized the frequency of nervous symptoms, among which are headache, dizziness, paræsthesias, paresis and paralysis. Disturbances of vision are common. In some cases the symptoms suggest brain tumor. In early stages circulatory disturbance is probably responsible; later cerebral hæmorrhage or thrombosis occurs.

Morris reported three cases with the general appearance of the disease and with slight enlargement of the spleen, but without polycythæmia. Geisböck described a variety, *polycythæmia hypertonica,* with increased tension, arteriosclerosis, and nephritis.

In the form called "Ayerza's Disease" or "cardiacos negros" there is headache, vertigo, somnolence, cyanosis, dyspnœa, cough, hæmoptysis, and polycythæmia. There is a pulmonary stage lasting for some years followed by the "cardiacos negros" stage lasting for two to five years, with marked enlargement of the right heart. The X-ray plate shows the shadow of the dilated pulmonary artery.

Diagnosis.—The triad of features above referred to are sufficient in the absence of congenital heart disease, emphysema, and forms of cyanosis associated with poisoning by coal tar products. In a few rare cases the polycythæmia has been associated with tuberculosis of the spleen.

Prognosis.—The prognosis is bad for cure, but the condition may persist for years with reasonably good health. Cardiac failure, hæmorrhage, and recurring ascites have been the usual modes of death.

Treatment.—When there is much fullness of the head and vertigo, repeated bleedings have given relief. Inhalations of oxygen may be tried when the cyanosis is extreme. Saline purges and a diet low in purin and iron content are also helpful. Benzol is of value in some cases. It can be given in doses of ♏ xv (1 c. c.) three times a day and the dose increased even to ʒ i (4 c. c.). The blood count is a good guide for the proper dose. If syphilis is suspected active treatment should be given. The X-rays have done no good in our cases. Splenectomy should not be performed.

VII. ENTEROGENOUS CYANOSIS

(Methæmoglobinæmia and Sulphæmoglobinæmia)

Definition.—A form of permanent cyanosis due to changes in the composition of the hæmoglobin of the blood.

Etiology.—It has long been known that with the use of certain drugs changes were induced in the hæmoglobin. In poisoning by potassium chlorate methæmoglobinæmia occurs often with an active hæmolysis. Carbon monoxide, sulphuretted hydrogen, the coal-tar products, acetanilide, phenacetin, sulphonal, and trional may cause a chronic cyanosis. Stokvis brought forward evidence to show that certain cases of chronic cyanosis are associated with intestinal disturbances, and he gives this form the name "enterogenous." Some of the forms are associated with methæmoglobinæmia, others with sulphæmoglobinæmia. In a doubtful case, with absence of lesions of the heart or lungs, a spectroscopic examination of the blood will determine if the cyanosis is of this nature, and which of the two derivatives of hæmoglobin is causing it.

Methæmoglobinæmia.—Several of the patients have had chronic diarrhœa, in two associated with parasites. In Stokvis' case there was clubbing of the fingers without any recognizable cause. Gibson and Douglas obtained from the blood of their patient a pure culture of a colon organism and suggested the name "Microbic cyanosis." In connection with this observation it may be mentioned that methæmoglobinæmia has been met with in Winckel's disease, in one case of which the staphylococcus has been isolated from the blood. But a still more striking confirmation is Boycott's discovery of an infective methæmoglobinæmia in rats, caused by Gaertner's bacillus, which gives a remarkable bluish tint to the skin of white rats.

Sulphæmoglobinæmia.—The appearance of the patients is very much the same. They look very badly, even death-like, but feel comfortable, and there is no shortness of breath. The main complaints are cyanosis, constipation, weakness and headache. A nitrite-producing bacillus has been found in the saliva in some cases. Intestinal disturbances have been present in a number of cases, and Garrod suggests that it is a chronic poisoning by hydrogen sulphide, possibly absorbed from the intestines. In *treatment,* foci of infection should be treated, especially in the mouth, and the patient should be purged frequently.

SECTION X

DISEASES OF THE CIRCULATORY SYSTEM

A. DISEASES OF THE PERICARDIUM

I. PERICARDITIS

Pericarditis is the result of infective processes, primary or secondary, or arises by extension of inflammation from contiguous organs.

Etiology.—PRIMARY, so-called idiopathic, inflammation is rare; but it has been met with in children without any evidence of rheumatism or of any local or general disease. Certain of the cases are tuberculous.

Pericarditis from injury usually comes under the care of the surgeon in connection with the primary wound. The trauma may be from within, due to the passage of a foreign body—a needle, a pin, or a bone—through the œsophagus—a variety exceedingly common in cows and horses.

SECONDARY: (*a*) Occurs most frequently in connection with rheumatic fever. In our 330 cases of rheumatic fever (Johns Hopkins Hospital) pericarditis occurred in twenty—practically 6 per cent. The articular trouble may be slight or, indeed, the disease may be associated with acute tonsillitis in rheumatic subjects. Certain of the so-called idiopathic cases have their origin in an acute tonsillitis. The pericarditis may precede the arthritis. (*b*) In septic processes; in the acute necrosis of bone and in puerperal fever it is not uncommon. (*c*) In tuberculosis, in which the disease may be primary or part of a general involvement of the serous sacs or associated with extensive pulmonary disease. (*d*) In the fevers. Not infrequent after scarlet fever, it is rare in measles, small-pox, typhoid fever, and diphtheria. In pneumonia it is not uncommon, occurring in 31 among 665 cases (Chatard). In 184 post mortems there were 29 instances of pericarditis. It is most frequent in double pneumonia, and in our series with disease of the right side, if only one lung was involved. Pericarditis sometimes complicates chorea; it was present in 19 of 73 autopsies; in only 8 of these was arthritis present. (*e*) Terminal pericarditis. In gout, in chronic nephritis—*pericardite brightique* of the French—in arterio-sclerosis, in scurvy, in diabetes, and in chronic illness of all sorts a latent pericarditis is common and usually overlooked.

(*f*) *By Extension.*—In pneumonia it is most often met with in children and alcoholics. With simple pleurisy it is rare. In ulcerative endocarditis, purulent myocarditis, and in aneurism of the aorta pericarditis is occasionally found. It may also follow extension of the disease from the mediastinal glands, the ribs, sternum, vertebræ, and even from the abdominal viscera.

The ordinary pus cocci, the pneumococcus, and the tubercle bacillus are the chief organisms met with in acute pericarditis.

Pericarditis occurs at all ages. Cases have been reported in the fetus. In the new-born it may result from septic infection through the navel. Throughout childhood the incidence of rheumatic fever and scarlet fever makes it a frequent affection, whereas late in life it is most often associated with tuberculosis, nephritis, and gout. Males are somewhat more frequently attacked than females. The so-called epidemics of pericarditis have been outbreaks of pneumonia with this as a frequent complication.

ACUTE FIBRINOUS PERICARDITIS

This, the most common and benign form, is distinguished by the small amount of exudate which coats the surface in a thin layer and may be partial or general. In the mildest grades the membrane looks lustreless and roughened, due to a thin fibrinous sheeting, which can be lifted with the knife, showing beneath an injected or ecchymotic serosa. As the fibrinous sheeting increases in thickness the constant movement of the adjacent surfaces gives to it sometimes a ridge-like, at others a honeycombed appearance. With more abundant fibrinous exudation the membranes present an appearance resembling buttered surfaces which have been drawn apart. The fibrin is in long shreds, and the heart presents a curiously shaggy appearance—the hairy heart of old writers, *cor villosum*.

In mild grades the subjacent muscle looks normal, but in the more prolonged and severe cases there is myocarditis, and for 2 or 3 mm. beneath the visceral layer the muscle presents a pale, turbid appearance. Many of these acute cases are tuberculous and the granulations are easily overlooked in a superficial examination.

There is usually a slight amount of fluid entangled in the meshes of fibrin, but there may be very thick exudate without much serous effusion.

Symptoms.—Unless sought for there may be no objective signs, and for this reason it is often overlooked, and in hospitals the disease is relatively more common in the post mortem room than in the wards.

Pain is a variable symptom, not usually intense, and in this form rarely excited by pressure. It is more marked in the early stage, and may be referred either to the præcordia or to the region of the xiphoid cartilage. In some instances the pain is of an aggravated and most distressing character resembling angina. *Fever* is usually present, but it is not always easy to say how much depends upon the primary disease, and how much upon the pericarditis. It is as a rule not high, rarely exceeding 102.5° F. In rheumatic cases hyperpyrexia has been observed.

Physical Signs.—*Inspection* is negative; *palpation* may reveal the presence of a distinct fremitus caused by the rubbing of the roughened pericardial surfaces. This is usually best marked over the right ventricle. It is not always to be felt, even when the friction sound on auscultation is loud and clear. *Auscultation:* The friction sound, due to the movement of the pericardial surfaces upon each other, is one of the most distinctive of physical signs. It is double, corresponding to the systole and diastole; but the synchronism with the heart sounds is not accurate, and the to and fro murmur usually outlasts the time occupied by the first and second sounds. In rare instances the friction is single; more frequently it appears to be triple in character—a sort of canter rhythm. The sounds have a peculiar rubbing, grating quality, characteristic when once recognized, and rarely simulated by endocardial murmurs. Sometimes instead of grating there is a creaking quality—the *bruit de cuir neuf*—the new leather murmur of the French. The pericardial friction appears superficial, very close to the ear, and is usually intensified by pressure with the stethoscope. It is best heard over the right ventricle, the part of the heart most closely in contact with the front of the chest—that is, in the fourth and fifth interspaces and adjacent portions of the sternum. There are instances in which the friction is most marked at the base, over the aorta, and at the superior reflection of the pericardium. Occasionally it is best heard at the apex. It may be limited to a very narrow area, or transmitted up and down the sternum. There are, however, no definite lines of transmission as in endocardial murmurs. An important point is the variability of the sounds, both in position and quality; they may be heard at one visit and not at another. The maximum of intensity will be found to vary with position. Friction may be present with a thin, almost imperceptible, layer of exudate; on the other hand it may not be present with a thick, buttery layer. The rub may be entirely obscured by the loud bronchial râles in pneumonia, in which disease pericarditis is recognized clinically in about half the cases, only 13 in 31 cases in the Hopkins series.

Diagnosis.—There is rarely any difficulty in determining the presence of a dry pericarditis, for the friction sounds are distinctive. The double murmur of aortic insufficiency may simulate closely the to and fro pericardial rub. The constant character of the aortic murmur, the direction of transmission, the phenomena in the arteries, the blood pressure record, and the associated conditions should prevent this error.

Pleuro-pericardial friction is very common, and may be associated with endo-pericarditis, particularly in cases of pneumonia. It is frequent, too, in tuberculosis. It is best heard over the left border of the heart, and is much affected by the respiratory movement. Holding the breath or taking a deep inspiration may abolish it. The rhythm is not the simple to and fro diastolic and systolic, but the respiratory rhythm is superadded, usually intensifying the murmur during expiration and lessening it on inspiration. In tuberculosis of the lungs there are instances in which, with the friction, a loud systolic click is heard, due to the compression of a thin layer of lung and the expulsion of a bubble of air from a softening focus or from a bronchus.

And, lastly, it is not very uncommon, in the region of the apex beat, to hear a series of fine crepitant sounds, systolic in time, often very distinct, suggestive of pericardial adhesions, but heard too frequently for this cause.

Course and Termination.—Simple fibrinous pericarditis never kills, but it occurs so often in connection with serious affections that we have frequent opportunities to see all stages of its progress. In the majority of cases the inflammation subsides and the thin fibrinous laminæ gradually become converted into connective tissue, which unites the pericardial surfaces firmly together. A very thin layer may "clear" without leaving adhesions. In other instances the inflammation progresses, with increase of the exudation, and the condition is changed from a "dry" to a "moist" pericarditis, or the pericarditis with effusion. In some instances the simple plastic pericarditis becomes chronic, and great thickening of both visceral and parietal layers is gradually induced.

PERICARDITIS WITH EFFUSION

Etiology.—Commonly a direct sequence of the dry or plastic pericarditis, of which it is sometimes called the second stage, this form is found most frequently in association with rheumatic fever, tuberculosis, and septicæmia, and sets in usually with præcordial pain, with slight fever or a distinct chill. In children the disease may, like pleurisy, come on without local symptoms, and, after a week or two of failing health, slight fever, shortness of breath, and increasing pallor, the physician may find, to his astonishment, signs of extensive pericardial effusion. These latent cases are often tuberculous. W. Ewart called special attention to latent and ephemeral pericardial effusions, which he thinks are often of short duration and of moderate size, with an absence of the painful features of pericarditis.

Morbid Anatomy.—The effusion may be sero-fibrinous, hæmorrhagic, or purulent. The amount varies from 200 to 300 c. c. to 2 litres. In the cases of sero-fibrinous exudation the pericardial membranes are covered with thick, creamy fibrin, which may be in ridges or honeycombed, or may present long, villous extensions. The parietal layer may be several millimetres in thickness and form a firm, leathery membrane. The hæmorrhagic exudation is usually associated with tuberculous or cancerous pericarditis, or with the disease in the aged. The lymph is less abundant, but both surfaces are injected and often show numerous hæmorrhages. Thick, curdy masses of lymph are usually found in the dependent part of the sac. In many cases the effusion is really sero-purulent, a thin, turbid exudation containing flocculi of fibrin.

The pericardial layers are greatly thickened and covered with fibrin. When the fluid is pus, they present a grayish, rough, granular surface. Sometimes there are distinct erosions on the visceral membrane. The heart muscle in these cases becomes involved to a greater or less extent and, on section, the tissue, for a depth of from 2 to 3 mm., is pale and turbid, and shows evidence of fatty and granular change. Endocarditis coexists frequently, but rarely results from the extension of the inflammation through the wall of the heart.

Symptoms.—Even with copious effusion the onset and course may be so insidious that no suspicion of the true nature of the disease is aroused.

As in the simple pericarditis, *pain* may be present, either sharp and stabbing or as a sense of distress and discomfort in the cardiac region. It is more frequent with effusion than in the plastic form. Pressure at the lower end of the sternum usually aggravates it. *Dyspnœa* is a common and important symptom, one which, perhaps, more than any other, excites suspicion of grave disorder and leads to careful examination of heart and lungs. The patient is restless, lies upon the left side or, as the effusion increases, sits up in bed. Associated with the dyspnœa is in many cases a peculiarly dusky, anxious countenance. The pulse is rapid, small; sometimes irregular, and may present the characters known as *pulsus paradoxus,* in which during each inspiration the pulse beat becomes very weak or is lost. These symptoms are due, in great part, to the direct mechanical effect of the fluid within the pericardium which embarrasses the heart's action. Other pressure effects are distention of the veins of the neck, dysphagia, which may be a marked symptom, and irritative cough from compression of the trachea. Aphonia is not uncommon, owing to compression or irritation of the recurrent laryngeal as it winds round the aorta. In massive effusion the pericardial sac occupies a large portion of the antero-lateral region of the left side and the condition has frequently been mistaken for pleurisy. Even in moderate grades the left lung is somewhat compressed, an additional element in the production of the dyspnœa.

Great restlessness, insomnia, and in the later stages low delirium and coma are symptoms in the more severe cases. Delirium and marked cerebral symptoms are associated with the hyperpyrexia of rheumatic cases, but apart from the ordinary delirium there may be peculiar mental symptoms. The patient may become melancholic and show suicidal tendencies. In other cases the condition resembles closely delirium tremens. Sibson, who specially described the condition, states that the majority of such cases recover. Chorea may also occur, as was pointed out by Bright. Convulsions are rare but have occurred during paracentesis.

PHYSICAL SIGNS.—*Inspection.*—In children the præcordia bulges and with copious exudation the antero-lateral region of the left chest becomes enlarged. A wavy impulse may be seen in the third and fourth interspaces, or there may be no impulse visible. The intercostal spaces bulge somewhat and there may be marked œdema of the wall. The epigastrium may be more prominent. Perforation externally through a space is very rare. Owing to the compression of the lung, the expansion of the left side is greatly diminished. The diaphragm and left lobe of the liver may be pushed down and may produce a distinct prominence in the epigastric region.

Palpation.—A gradual diminution and final obliteration of the cardiac impulse is a striking feature in progressive effusion. The position of the apex beat is not constant. In large effusions it is usually not felt. In children as the fluid collects the pulsation may be best seen in the fourth space, but this may not be the apex itself. The pericardial friction may lessen with the effusion, though it often persists at the base when no longer palpable over the right ventricle, or may be felt in the erect and not in the recumbent posture. Fluctuation can rarely, if ever, be detected.

Percussion gives most important indications. The gradual distention of the pericardial sac pushes aside the margins of the lungs so that a large area comes in contact with the chest wall and gives a greatly increased percussion dulness. The form of this dulness is irregularly pear-shaped; the base or broad surface directed downward and the stem or apex directed upward toward the manubrium. There is a disproportionate extension of dulness upward and to the right, with dulness in the right fifth interspace extending one or two inches to the right of the sternum (Rotch's sign). Williamson could not verify this in an experimental study. In large effusions there may be impaired resonance in the left axilla, and Bamberger called attention to an area of dulness near the angle of the scapula with bronchial breathing, which may alter when the patient leans forward.

Auscultation.—The friction sound heard in the early stages may disappear when the effusion is copious, but often persists at the base or at the limited area of the apex. It may be audible in the erect and not in the recumbent posture. With the absorption of the fluid the friction returns. One of the most important signs is the gradual weakening of the heart sounds, which with the increase in the effusion may become so muffled and indistinct as to be scarcely audible. The heart's action is usually increased and the rhythm disturbed. Occasionally a systolic endocardial murmur is heard. Early and persistent accentuation of the pulmonary second sound may be present.

Important accessory signs in large effusion are due to pressure on the left lung. The antero-lateral margin of the lower lobe is pushed aside and in some instances compressed, so that percussion in the axillary region, in and just below the transverse nipple line, gives a modified percussion note, usually a dull tympany. Variations in the position of the patient may change this modified percussion area, over which on auscultation there is either feeble or tubular breathing. The left lobe of the liver may be pushed down.

Course.—Cases vary extremely in the rapidity with which the effusion takes place. In every instance, when a pericardial friction murmur has been detected, the practitioner should first outline with care—using the aniline pencil—the upper and lateral limits of cardiac dulness, secondly mark the position of the apex beat, and thirdly note the intensity of the heart sounds. In many instances the exudation is slight in amount, reaches a maximum within forty-eight hours, and then gradually subsides. In other instances the accumulation is more gradual and progressive, increasing for several weeks. To such cases the term *chronic* has been applied. The rapidity with which a sero-fibrinous effusion may be absorbed is surprising. The possibility of the absorption of a purulent exudate is shown by the cases in which the pericardium contains semi-solid grayish masses in all stages of calcification. With sero-fibrinous effusion, if moderate in amount, recovery is the rule, with inevitable union, however, of the pericardial layers. In some of the septic cases there is a rapid formation of pus and a fatal result may follow in three or four days. More commonly, when death occurs with large effusion, it is not until the second or third week and takes place by gradual asthenia.

Prognosis.—In the sero-fibrinous effusions the outlook is good, and a large majority of all the rheumatic cases recover. The purulent effusions are, of course, more dangerous; the septic cases are usually fatal, and recovery is rare in the slow, insidious tuberculous forms.

Diagnosis.—Probably no serious disease is so frequently overlooked. Post mortem experience shows how often pericarditis is not recognized, or goes on to resolution and adhesion without attracting notice. In a case of rheumatic fever, watched from the outset, with the attention directed daily to the heart, it is one of the simplest of diseases to diagnose; but when one is called to a case for the first time and finds perhaps an increased area of præcordial dulness, it is often very hard to determine with certainty whether or not effusion is present. The difficulty usually lies in distinguishing between dilatation of the heart and pericardial effusion. Although the differential signs are simple enough on paper, it is notoriously difficult in certain cases, particularly in stout persons, to say which of the conditions exists. The points which deserve attention are:

(*a*) The character of the impulse, which in dilatation, particularly in thin-chested people, is commonly visible and wavy. (*b*) The shock of the cardiac sounds is more distinctly palpable in dilatation. (*c*) The area of dulness in dilatation rarely has a triangular form; nor does it, except in cases of mitral stenosis, reach so high along the left sternal margin or so low in the fifth and sixth interspaces *without visible or palpable impulse.* An upper limit of dulness shifting with change of position speaks strongly for effusion. (*d*) In dilatation the heart sounds are clearer, often sharp or fetal in character; gallop rhythm is common, whereas in effusion the sounds are distant and muffled. (*e*) Rarely in dilatation is the distention sufficient to compress the lung and produce the tympanitic note in the axillary region, or flatness behind. (*f*) The X-ray picture may be very definite, and unlike any form of dilatation or hypertrophy of the heart.

The number of excellent observers who have acknowledged that they have failed sometimes to discriminate between these two conditions, and who have indeed performed paracentesis *cordis* instead of paracentesis *pericardii,* is perhaps the best comment on the difficulties.

Massive (1½ to 2-litre) exudations have been confounded with a pleural effusion and the pericardium has been tapped under the impression that the exudate was pleuritic. The dull tympany in the infrascapular region, the absence of well-defined movable dulness, and the feeble, muffled sounds are indicative points. Followed from day to day there is rarely much difficulty, but it is different when a patient seen for the first time presents a large area of dulness in the antero-lateral region of the left chest, and there is no to and fro pericardial friction murmur. Many of the cases have been regarded as encapsulated pleural effusions.

A special difficulty exists in recognizing the large exudate in pneumonia. The effusion may be very much larger than the signs indicate, and the involvement of the adjacent lung and pleura is confusing. In at least three cases in our series we should have tapped the sac; post mortem the effusion was more than a litre.

The nature of the fluid can not positively be determined without aspiration; but a fairly accurate opinion can be formed from the nature of the primary disease and the general condition of the patient. In rheumatic cases the exudation is usually sero-fibrinous; in septic and tuberculous cases it is often purulent from the outset; in senile, nephritic, and tuberculous cases the exudate may be hæmorrhagic.

Treatment.—The patient should have absolute quiet, mentally and bodily, so as to reduce the heart's action to a minimum. Drugs given for this purpose, such as aconite or digitalis, are of doubtful utility. Local bloodletting by cupping or leeches is advantageous in robust subjects, particularly in the cases of extension in pneumonia. The ice bag is of great value. It may be applied to the præcordia at first for an hour or more at a time, and then continuously. It reduces the frequency of the heart's action and seems to retard the progress of an effusion. Blisters are not indicated in the early stage. Morphia should be given for pain or severe distress.

When *effusion* is present, the following measures to promote absorption may be adopted: Blisters to the præcordia, a practice not so much in vogue now as formerly. It is surprising, however, in some instances, how quickly an effusion will subside on their application. Purges and iodide of potassium are of doubtful utility. The diet should be light, dry, and nutritious. The action of the kidneys may be promoted by the infusion of digitalis and potassium acetate.

When signs of serious impairment of the heart occur, as indicated by dyspnœa, small, rapid pulse, dusky, anxious countenance, paracentesis or incision of the pericardium should be performed. With the sero-fibrinous exudate, such as commonly occurs after rheumatism, aspiration is sufficient; but when the exudate is purulent, the pericardium should be freely incised and freely drained. The puncture may be made in the fourth or fifth interspace, outside the left nipple line. In large effusions the pericardium can be readily reached without danger by thrusting the needle upward and backward close to the costal margin in the left costo-xiphoid angle. The results of paracentesis of the pericardium have not been satisfactory. With an earlier operation in many instances and a more radical one in others—incision and free drainage, not aspiration, when the fluid is purulent—the percentage of recoveries will be greatly increased. Repeated tapping may be needed. One patient with tuberculous effusion, tapped three times, recovered completely and was alive three years afterward.

CHRONIC ADHESIVE PERICARDITIS

(*Adherent Pericardium, Indurative Mediastino-pericarditis*)

The remote prognosis in pericarditis is very variable. A large majority of these cases get well and have no further trouble, but in young persons serious results sometimes follow adhesions and thickening of the layers. As Sequira has pointed out, the danger is here directly in proportion to the amount of dilatation and weakening of the pericardium in consequence of the inflammation. The loss of the firm support afforded to the heart by the rigid fibrous bag in which it is inclosed is the important factor. There are two groups of cases of adherent pericardium.

(*a*) Simple adhesion of the peri- and epicardial layers, a common sequence of pericarditis, met with post mortem as an accidental finding. It is not necessarily associated with disturbance in the function of the heart, which in a large proportion of the cases is neither dilated nor hypertrophied.

(*b*) Adherent pericardium with chronic mediastinitis and union of the outer layer of the pericardium to the pleura and to the chest walls. This constitutes one of the most serious forms of cardiac disease, particularly in early life, and may lead to an extreme grade of hypertrophy and dilatation of the heart. The peritoneum may be involved with perihepatitis, cirrhosis, and ascites (Pick's disease).

Symptoms.—The symptoms of adherent pericardium are those of hypertrophy and dilatation of the heart, and later of cardiac insufficiency. G. D. Head in a careful study of 59 cases divides them into (1) a small silent group with no symptoms, (2) a larger group with all the features of cardiac disease, and (3) a group comprising 11 cases in his series in which the features were hepatic. To this last group much attention has been paid since Pick's description. The hepatic features dominate the picture and the diagnosis of cirrhosis of the liver is usually made. Recurring ascites is the special feature and one patient was tapped one hundred and twenty-one times. There is chronic peritonitis, with great thickening of the capsule of the liver and consequent contraction of the organ.

Diagnosis.—The following are important points in the diagnosis: *Inspection.*—A majority of the signs of value come under this heading. (*a*) The præcordia is prominent and there may be marked asymmetry, owing to the enormous enlargement of the heart. (*b*) The extent of the cardiac impulse is greatly increased, and may sometimes be seen from the third to the sixth interspaces, and in extreme cases from the right parasternal line to outside the left nipple. (*c*) The character of the cardiac impulse. It is undulatory, wavy, and in the apex region there is marked systolic retraction. (*d*) Diaphragm phenomena. John Broadbent called attention to a very valuable sign in adherent pericardium. When the heart is adherent over a large area of the diaphragm there is with each pulsation a systolic tug, which may be communicated through the diaphragm to the points of its attachment on the wall, causing a visible retraction. This has long been recognized in the region of the seventh or eighth rib in the left parasternal line, but Broadbent called attention to the fact that it was frequently best seen on the left side behind, between the eleventh and twelfth ribs. This is a valuable and quite common sign, and may sometimes be very localized. One difficulty is that, as A. W. Tallant pointed out, it may occur in thin chested persons with great hypertrophy of the heart. Sir William Broadbent called attention to the fact that owing to the attachment of the heart to the central tendon of the diaphragm this part does not descend with inspiration, during which act there is not the visible movement in the epigastrium. (*e*) Diastolic collapse of the cervical veins, the so-called Friedreich's sign, is not of much moment.

Palpation.—The apex beat is fixed, and turning the patient on the left side does not alter its position. On placing the hand over the heart there is felt a diastolic shock or rebound, which some have regarded as the most reliable of all signs of adherent pericardium.

Percussion.—The area of cardiac dulness is usually much increased. In a majority of instances there are adhesions between the pleura and the pericardium, and the limit of cardiac dulness above and to the left may be fixed and is uninfluenced by deep inspiration. This, too, is an uncertain sign, inasmuch as there may be close adhesions between the pleura and the pericardium and between the pleura and the chest wall, which at the same time allow a very considerable degree of mobility to the edge of the lung.

Auscultation.—The phenomena are variable and uncertain. In the cases in children with a history of rheumatism endocarditis has usually been present. Even in the absence of chronic endocarditis, when the dilatation reaches a certain grade, there are murmurs of relative insufficiency, which may be present not only at the mitral but also at the tricuspid and pulmonary orifices. Theodore Fisher called attention to the fact that there may be a well-marked presystolic murmur in connection with adherent pericardium. Occasionally the layers of the pericardium are united in places by strong fibrous bands, 5-7 mm. long by 3-5 mm. wide. In one such case Drasche heard a remarkable whirring, systolic murmur with a twanging quality.

The pulsus paradoxus, in which during inspiration the pulse-wave is small and feeble, is sometimes present, but it is not a diagnostic sign of either simple pericardial adhesion or of the cicatricial mediastino-pericarditis. Treatment has to be directed to the heart muscle and is largely that of myocarditis. *Cardiolysis,* Brauer's operation, has been helpful in a few cases. Four or five centimetres of the fourth, fifth, and sixth left ribs with a couple of centimetres of the corresponding cartilages are resected, by which means the heart's action is less embarrassed. It is a justifiable procedure in selected cases—in, for example, a child with a very large, tumultuously acting heart, with much bulging of the chest.

II. OTHER AFFECTIONS OF THE PERICARDIUM

Hydropericardium.—The pericardial sac contains post mortem a few cubic centimetres of clear, citron colored fluid. In connection with general dropsy, due to kidney or heart disease, more commonly the former, the effusion may be excessive, adding to the embarrassment of the heart and the lungs, particularly when the pleural cavities are the seat of similar transudation. There are rare instances in which effusion into the pericardium occurs after scarlet fever with few, if any, other dropsical symptoms. Hydropericardium is frequently overlooked.

In rare cases the serum has a milky character—chylopericardium.

Hæmopericardium.—This condition is met with in aneurism of the first part of the aorta, of the cardiac wall, or of the coronary arteries, and in rupture and wounds of the heart. Death usually follows before there is time for the production of symptoms other than those of rapid heart failure due to compression. In rupture of the heart the patient may live for many hours or even days with symptoms of progressive heart failure, dyspnœa, and the signs of effusion. In the pericarditis of tuberculosis, of cancer, of nephritis, and of old people the exudate is often blood stained.

Pneumopericardium.—This is an excessively rare condition, of which Walter James was able to collect only 38 cases in 1903. We have met with but one instance, from rupture of a cancer of the stomach. Perforation of the sac occurred in all but 5, in which the gas bacillus was the possible cause, as in Nicholl's case in which this organism was isolated. Seven cases were due to perforation of the œsophagus and eight to penetrating wounds from without. The physical signs are most characteristic. A tympany replaces the normal pericardial flatness. On auscultation there is a splashing, gurgling, churning sound, called by the French *bruit de moulin.* This was described in 19 of the cases collected by James. Of the 38 cases, 26 died.

Calcified Pericardium.—This remarkable condition may follow pericarditis, particularly the suppurative and tuberculous forms; occasionally it extends from the calcified valves. It may be partial or complete. Of 59 cases collected by A. E. Jones, in 38 there were no cardiac symptoms. Adherent pericardium was diagnosed in one case. Jones' careful study shows that the condition is usually latent and unrecognized.

B. DISEASES OF THE HEART

I. SYMPTOMATIC AND MECHANICAL DISORDERS

I. SYMPTOMATIC DISORDERS

Introduction.—There are a number of disturbances referred to the heart which cannot be termed diseases—the term symptom-complex is a better designation. They may occur without any sign of organic cardiac disease but frequently cause extreme distress to the individual. It is not possible to group them in any systematic way. In some there are only subjective sensations, in others these occur with objective findings. We should remember that back of subjective disorders there is some cause and the effort should always be made to find it. Disturbances in the nervous system and in the internal secretions, unrecognized myocardial disease and the effects of toxic agents are particularly important.

(1) **Heart consciousness.**—In health we are unconscious of the action of the heart. A not infrequent indication of debility or overwork is the consciousness of the cardiac pulsations which may be perfectly regular. It may be most evident when the patient is lying down. It is usually due to nervous fatigue, some form of debility or anæmia. Occasionally it is present with organic disease.

(2) **Cardiac pain.**—This may be referred to the whole præcordia or to local areas, most often about the apex or outside it. The area corresponds to the distribution of the eighth cervical to the fourth dorsal segments. A distinction should be made between aortic pain (aortitis, acute and chronic, some cases of angina pectoris, and aneurism) and cardiac pain. The former is usually felt over the upper part of the sternum and may be referred to the arms. It is important to secure an exact statement of the seat of pain. The influence of exertion, emotion, fear and excitement in causation is important. There are many causes for more or less persistent cardiac pain: (1) Myocarditis, in which the pain is sometimes described as a pressure. (2) Dilatation (3) Pericarditis. (4) Valvular disease, especially aortic. (5) Certain toxic influences, especially tobacco. (6) With the "Effort Syndrome." (7) Angina pectoris (some cases). (8) With digestive disturbances, especially distention. (9) In a large group in which no evidence of cardiac disease can be found and often termed "cardiac neurosis," which means little. This is common in women, especially at the menopause, and is especially marked in those who are "neurotic." Two forms are common: in one there is a dull more or less continuous pain and in the other sharp stabbing pains of short duration. Emotion is a frequent exciting cause. In many a definite disturbance of sensation can be found, usually near the apex.

The term "pseudo-angina pectoris," so frequently used, should be dropped from our terminology. It has no set meaning and is very variously employed. Some use it as synonymous with vaso-motor angina pectoris. The group includes cases in neurotic persons or in those who have used too much tobacco. The attacks have no necessary relation to exertion and may come on at night or when the patient is at rest; they are commoner in women and may occur at any age; and are not associated with demonstrable organic disease of the heart or aorta. The attacks may last for an hour or longer. It must not be forgotten that there are cases of mild angina pectoris. It is safer to regard doubtful cases as examples of this than to label them "pseudo-angina."

The *diagnosis* of pain is based on the patient's statement; the estimation of its severity can be made by observation. The recognition of its cause demands thorough study. Careful search should be made for organic vascular disease; always suspect this until its absence is proved. Particular attention should be given to the state of the nervous system. The source of pain mistakenly regarded as cardiac but due to disease elsewhere is usually recognized by a thorough examination.

The *treatment* must be based on accurate diagnosis. In the "nervous group," the meaning of the symptom should be explained and every effort made to correct the causal factors. The use of bromides is indicated until there is improvement in the general condition. A dose of aromatic spirit of ammonia or Hoffman's anodyne is often helpful.

(3) **"Effort syndrome," "neuro-circulatory asthenia," "disordered action of the heart," "irritable heart."**—The condition to which these terms are applied does not represent a specific disease but a combination of symptoms in which shortness of breath, fatigue, and vaso-motor disturbances are the principal features. The condition is not confined to soldiers; it occurs in civil life, and in females and children as well as in men. The subjects are usually of a sub-normal type physically and unable to do heavy physical work. The etiological factors are many. Infection plays a part, especially rheumatic fever, tonsillitis, influenza, focal infection, etc.; syphilis plays a very small part. Hyperthyroidism is a factor in a small percentage only. Disturbance of the central nervous system is important. Certain of the patients are of the visceroptotic build, with long thin bodies, and in them cardioptosis ("dropped heart") is relatively common. Stress and strain which they are unfitted to endure is a common determining factor in war.

Symptoms.—Shortness of breath, rarely at rest, but almost invariably on exertion, is the most frequent complaint, and is increased by effort, especially if hurried. With this goes severe fatigue and exhaustion, sometimes with tremor. *Pain* is common, usually præcordial or in the lower left costal region, and increased by exercise. Præcordial tenderness and disturbance of sensation may accompany it. Palpitation of the heart on exertion and excitement often occurs. Syncope is not uncommon. Giddiness is frequent and may occur with change in position or on exertion. Vaso-motor phenomena are common; the hands and feet are blue, there is profuse sweating, and dermographia is marked. The patients show a nervous "make-up," and are easily upset. The pulse rate is increased and responds quickly to exertion. The return to normal after exercise is slow. The blood pressure does not show any striking changes. The heart shows an absence of signs of myocardial disease. Care must be taken to recognize the condition in which an overacting "nervous" heart simulates mitral stenosis.

In *treatment* any suggestion of "heart disease" should be avoided, and every effort made to explain the condition. Search should be made for the etiology and a causal factor treated if possible, especially a focus of infection. The whole method of life should be reviewed and every effort made to improve the general health by proper exercise, bathing and good hygiene. Cardiac drugs are not needed but general tonics should be given if indicated.

(4) **Palpitation.**—In health we are unconscious of the action of the heart. One of the first indications of debility or overwork is the consciousness of the cardiac pulsations, which may, however, be perfectly regular and orderly. This is not palpitation. The term is properly limited to irregular or forcible action of the heart perceptible to the individual. The condition of extra-systole is present in many cases.

Etiology.—The expression "perceptible to the individual" covers the essential element in palpitation of the heart. The most extreme disturbance of rhythm may be unattended with subjective sensations of distress, and there may be no consciousness of disturbed action. On the other hand, there are cases in which complaint is made of the most distressing palpitation and sensations of throbbing, in which examination reveals a regularly acting heart, the sensations being entirely subjective. This symptom occurs in a large group of cases in which there is increased excitability of the nervous system. Palpitation may be a marked feature at the time of puberty, at the climacteric, and occasionally during menstruation. It is common in hysteria and neurasthenia, particularly in the form of the latter associated with dyspepsia. Emotions, such as fright, are common causes of palpitation. It may occur as a sequence of the acute fevers. Females are more liable to the affection than males.

In a second group the palpitation results from the action upon the heart of certain substances, such as tobacco, coffee, tea, and alcohol. And, lastly, palpitation may be associated with organic disease of the heart, either of the myocardium or valves. As a rule it is a purely nervous phenomenon, seldom associated with organic disease in which the most violent action and extreme irregularity may exist without a subjective element of consciousness of the disturbance. It occurs frequently with hyperthyroidism.

Symptoms.—In the mildest form, such as occurs during a dyspeptic attack, there are slight fluttering of the heart and a sense of what patients sometimes call "goneness." In more severe attacks the heart beats violently, its pulsations against the chest wall are visible, the rapidity of the action is much increased, the arteries throb forcibly, and there is a sense of great distress. In some instances the heart's action is not at all quickened. The most striking cases are in neurasthenic women, in whom the mere entrance of a person into the room may cause the most violent action of the heart and throbbing of the peripheral arteries. The pulse may be rapidly increased until it reaches 150 or 160. A diffuse flushing of the skin may appear at the same time. After such attacks there may be the passage of a large quantity of pale urine. In many cases of palpitation, particularly in young men, the condition is at once relieved by exertion.

The physical examination of the heart is usually negative. The sounds, the shock of which may be very palpable, are clear, ringing, and metallic, but not associated with murmurs. The second sound at the base may be accentuated. A murmur may sometimes be heard over the pulmonary artery or even at the apex in cases of rapid action in neurasthenia or in severe anæmia. The attacks may be transient, lasting only for a few minutes, or may persist for an hour or more. In some instances any attempt at exertion renews the attack. Sometimes in vigorous young adults who are upset nervously, especially after exertion or during excitement, the signs of mitral stenosis are simulated. There is a systolic shock preceded by a suggestion of a thrill. On auscultation it may be difficult to decide whether or not there is a short presystolic murmur. A short period of observation usually removes the uncertainty and the administration of amyl nitrite, which increases the murmur of mitral stenosis, is an aid. Organic murmurs are sometimes increased by pressure on the eyeballs.

The *diagnosis* should always include the conditions which are responsible. Nervous states (especially the anxiety neuroses and those due to disturbance in the sexual sphere), anæmia, gastro-intestinal disorders, and particularly the possible influence of the thyroid gland should be considered. In the condition termed *phrenocardia* there are palpitation, pain in the cardiac region or to the left of the apex, and respiratory disorder shown by frequent attempts to take a deep breath. There may be spasm of the diaphragm with cardioptosis.

The *prognosis* is usually good, though it may be extremely difficult to remove the conditions underlying the palpitation.

Treatment.—An important element is to get the patient's mind quieted and assure him that there is no actual danger. The mental element is often very strong. If an underlying cause can be found this should receive attention. In palpitation, before using drugs, it is well to try the effect of hygienic measures. As a rule, moderate exercise may be taken with advantage. Regular hours should be kept, and at least ten hours out of the twenty-four should be spent in the recumbent posture. A tepid bath may be taken in the morning, or, if the patient is weak and nervous, in the evening, followed by a thorough rubbing. Hot baths and the Turkish bath should be avoided. The dietetic management is important and it is best to prohibit alcohol, tea, and coffee absolutely. The diet should be light and the patient should avoid taking large meals. Articles of food known to cause flatulency should not be used. If a smoker, the patient should give up tobacco. Sexual excitement is particularly pernicious, and the patient should be warned specially on this point. The cases of palpitation due to excesses or to errors in diet and dyspepsia are readily remedied by hygienic measures.

A course of iron is often useful. Strychnia is particularly valuable, and is perhaps best administered as the tincture of nux vomica in large doses. Very little good is obtained from the smaller quantities. It should be given freely, 20 minims (1.3 c. c.) three times a day. If there is great rapidity of action, aconite may be tried. There are cases associated with sleeplessness and restlessness which are greatly benefited by the bromides. Digitalis is very rarely indicated, but in obstinate cases it may be tried with the nux vomica.

II. MECHANICAL DISORDERS OF THE HEART-BEAT

Normal Mechanism.—In the normal heart-beat there is contraction of the chambers in proper sequence due to a stimulus which originates in the sino-auricular node ("pacemaker") situated in the wall of the right auricle close to the mouth of the superior vena cava. This node originates orderly waves of contraction (72 per minute) which pass through the walls of the auricles to the ventricles by a special conduction path at the origin of which is a node (of Tawara) situated low down in the wall of the right auricle. From this the auriculo-ventricular bundle (of His) extends, dividing below to send branches to the two ventricles. These by further subdivisions supply the ventricular fibres. The stimulus to contraction requires a definite period for preparation and the interval is constant. "The muscular fibres of the heart possess the power of rhythmically creating a stimulus, of being able to receive a stimulus, of responding to a stimulus by contracting, of conveying the stimulus from muscle fibre to muscle fibre, and of maintaining a certain ill-defined condition called tone." (Gaskill.)

A. DISTURBANCES OF RATE

(1) **Tachycardia** (with normal mechanism).—The rapid action may be perfectly natural. There are individuals whose normal heart action is at 100 or even more per minute. Emotional causes, violent exercise, and fevers all produce great increase in the rapidity of the heart's action. The extremely rapid action which follows fright may persist for days or even weeks. Cases are not uncommon at the menopause.

There are cases in which it depends upon definite changes in the pneumogastrics or in the medulla. Cases have been reported in which tumor or clot in or about the medulla or pressure upon the vagi has been associated with rapid heart. Tachycardia occurs under many conditions, such as hyperthyroidism, mitral stenosis (apart from fibrillation), interference with the vagus (mediastinal tumor, etc.), post-febrile conditions, anæmia, the effect of certain drugs (belladonna, thyroid extract), nervous disturbance, toxic states (tobacco), etc. The tachycardia may persist for months or indefinitely, and there is serious interference with the amount of muscular exertion such persons can take; in addition there is a sense of weakness and sometimes fainting attacks. The diagnosis of the cause is essential and on this the treatment must be based.

(2) **Bradycardia** (True).—Slow action of the heart is sometimes normal and may be a family peculiarity. Napoleon is stated to have had a pulse of only 40 per minute.

In any case of slow pulse it is important first to make sure that the number of heart and arterial beats correspond. In many instances this is not the case, and with a radial pulse at 40 the cardiac pulsations may be 80, half the beats not reaching the wrist. The heart contractions, not the pulse wave, should be taken into account.

Physiological Bradycardia.—As age advances the pulse rate becomes slow. In the puerperal state the pulse may beat from 44 to 60 per minute, or may even be as low as 34. It is seen in premature labor as well as at term but the explanation is not clear. Slowness of the pulse is associated with hunger. Bradycardia depending on individual peculiarity is extremely rare.

Pathological Bradycardia is met with under the following conditions: (*a*) In convalescence from acute fevers. This is extremely common, particularly after pneumonia, typhoid fever, and diphtheria. It is most frequent in young persons and in cases which have run a normal course. (*b*) In diseases of the digestive system, such as chronic dyspepsia, ulcer or cancer of the stomach, and jaundice. (*c*) In diseases of the respiratory system. Here it is by no means so common, but it is seen not infrequently in emphysema. (*d*) In diseases of the circulatory system. Bradycardia is not common in diseases of the valves. It is most frequent in fatty and fibroid changes in the heart, but is not constant in them. (*e*) In diseases of the urinary organs. It occurs occasionally in nephritis and may be a feature of uræmia. (*f*) From the action of toxic agents. It occurs in uræmia, poisoning by lead, alcohol, and follows the use of tobacco, coffee, and digitalis. (*g*) In constitutional disorders, such as anæmia, chlorosis, and diabetes. (*h*) In diseases of the nervous system. Apoplexy, epilepsy, one stage of tuberculous meningitis, cerebral tumors, affections of the medulla, and diseases and injuries of the cervical cord may be associated with a slow pulse. In general paresis, mania, and melancholia it is not infrequent. (*i*) It occurs occasionally in affections of the skin and sexual organs, and in sunstroke, or in prolonged exhaustion from any cause.

Treatment.—For the bradycardia itself little can be done. The cause should receive attention.

B. DISTURBANCES OF RHYTHM AND FORCE

1. **Sinus Arrhythmia.**—This depends on changes in the control of the sino-auricular node in which the effect of vagus influence is important. It is frequently seen in connection with respiration, especially in deep breathing. The rate increases with inspiration and slows with expiration. This is common in young children and about the time of puberty, and is seen occasionally in adults. In other cases it may be responsible for attacks of faintness or syncope, sometimes with a slow rate and a low blood pressure. The occurrence of irregularity, also with slow pulse rate, and which has no order in its occurrence, is sometimes seen. It may occur after the administration of digitalis, in rheumatic myocarditis or with the bradycardia so common after pneumonia. The condition is not serious in any way.

Diagnosis.—This is usually clear. The irregularity is of the whole beat and the pulse and apex beat correspond. The occurrence with respiration is significant. Exercise, fever and atropine usually abolish this irregularity.

Treatment.—None is required and this condition should not be regarded as an indication for rest or lessened activity.

(2) **Extra-systole (Premature contraction).**—A common form of irregularity is that due to extra-systole, to understand which it must be remembered that to a stimulus strong enough to set up a contraction the heart answers with all the contractility of which it is capable at the moment (Bowditch's law of maximal contraction). A second property of the heart muscle is that it possesses a "refractory phase" in which normally it is not excitable, or answers only to very strong stimuli. Extra-systoles are caused by pathological impulses which may arise in the auricle or ventricle, rarely in the tissue between them. An extra impulse arising in the ventricle and causing it to contract anticipates the next regular impulse which arrives when the ventricle is in the "refractory phase" and hence it does not contract, so that this auricular impulse is wasted. Until the next regular impulse reaches the ventricle there will be the usual interval and hence the diastole is longer than normal. The period of disturbed rhythm is equal to two cycles of the usual

rhythm. If the pathological impulse arises in the auricle there is premature contraction of both the auricle and ventricle followed by a normal pause. The time of disturbance is not equal to two cycles of the usual rhythm. There is usually a disturbance of the fundamental rhythm.

The premature beat is not an efficient one and may not open the aortic valves. If it does the impulse may or may not reach the radial artery; if it does the pulse wave will be small and follow close on the preceding regular impulse. On auscultation two sounds are heard if the aortic valves are opened, otherwise only a first sound. Evidently there can be many variations in the sounds and character of the pulse. Graphic records are usually necessary to distinguish between the auricular and ventricular origin of premature contractions. If a murmur is present it may be absent or less loudly heard with the premature beat. Fever, exercise, a change in posture, and a rapid heart rate may cause the temporary disappearance of extra-systoles.

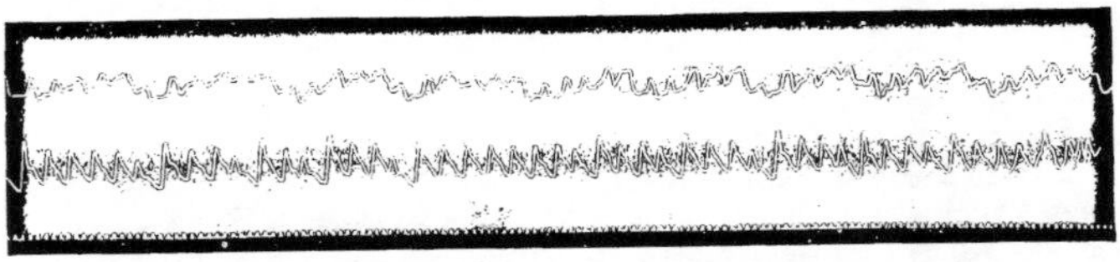

FIG. 1.—PREMATURE CONTRACTIONS OF VENTRICULAR ORIGIN.

The grouping of pulse beats shows the manner of production of bigeminal, trigeminal, and quadrigeminal pulses.

The irregularity, inequality, and intermission of the pulse as met with in every day experience are largely due to the occurrence of extra-systoles, which may present all sorts of combinations and groupings, depending upon whether the extra pulse beats are perceptible or not. And yet there may be no actual pathological change, and so far as the maintenance of the circulation is concerned the heart may be acting in a satisfactory manner. The subjective sensations vary greatly. In some the extra-systoles are not noticed but many complain of a variety of symptoms and especially of the pause with the succeeding strong contraction. Some patients are greatly disturbed by them.

Extra-systoles occur at all ages and under the most varied conditions but are most common in persons over fifty. There are several classes of cases. The arrhythmia may be a life-long condition. Without any recognizable disease, without any impairment of the action of the heart, there is permanent irregularity. This may be a peculiarity of the heart-muscle of the individual, who has extra-systole for the same reason—physiological but not well understood—as the dog and horse, in which animals this phenomenon is common. The late Chancellor Ferrier, of McGill University, who died at the age of eighty-seven, had an extremely irregular heart action for the last fifty years of his life. In debilitated and neurasthenic persons there may be an irritable weakness of the heart associated with extra-systole, and palpitation of a distressing character. In a second group toxic agents, as tobacco, tea, coffee, or the toxins of the infectious diseases are responsible. Digitalis may be a cause. Even reflexly, as in flatulent dyspepsia, extra-systoles may arise. Thirdly, a high blood pressure can set up extra-systoles; also change in posture. And, lastly, organic disease of the heart itself, especially myocardial.

The *significance* of premature contractions is not always easy to determine. They are often temporary, especially in young persons, but should not be regarded lightly. It is wiser to regard them as meaning some pathological change until the contrary is proved than to make light of them and recognize the error later. In those who have reached fifty years of age they may be the warning of serious myocardial damage. The patient seen to-day with extra-systoles may return with auricular fibrillation in two or three years.

Treatment.—This must depend on the other conditions found and not on the extra-systoles themselves. In nervous patients, bromide is indicated. The condition itself does not require digitalis.

(3) **Paroxysmal Tachycardia.**—This is characterized by paroxysmal attacks, beginning and ending abruptly, in which the heart rate increases to between 100 and 200 a minute (the common rate is between 110 and 190). The abnormal impulses arise from a new focus which may be in the auricle or ventricle, usually in the auricle. They represent "essentially a regular series of extra-systoles" (Lewis).

It may occur at any age but is most frequent in young adults, and more often in males. There may be definite myocardial disease but some patients show no sign of any lesion in the intervals. Naturally one is suspicious of some underlying factor (myocardial). Exertion, emotion or digestive disturbance may initiate an attack but in some cases no cause can be given. The duration of an attack varies from a few seconds to ten or more days.

The *symptoms* vary greatly with the duration and severity of the attack. A striking feature is the abrupt onset. In the very short attacks the patient may not be conscious of any disturbance or make any complaint. In more marked attacks there may be discomfort and palpitation, with weakness, sweating and gastric disturbance. Thoracic pain of varying distribution is common, sometimes with disturbance of sensation. If dilatation of the heart follows there are the symptoms associated with it. In the examination there may be little except the rapid heart and the general condition is often good. There may be marked pulsation in the veins of the neck. The heart rate should be determined by auscultation. The sounds are very short and sharp, like the fetal heart sounds. If there has been a previous murmur it may have disappeared. Enlargement of the heart, passive congestion of the lungs, sometimes with bloody sputum, cyanosis, œdema, and enlargement of the liver with abdominal tenderness may be found.

In *diagnosis* the history of previous attacks and of the onset of the present one is important. The cases of tachycardia of other etiology rarely cause doubt. The rapid rate with loss of compensation should not cause difficulty. Change in posture does not alter the rate in paroxysmal tachycardia. In cases of doubt a tracing is diagnostic.

The *outlook* is good but always has an element of uncertainty. In prolonged attacks with marked disturbance of the circulation there is always some danger. The condition of the heart between attacks and the behavior of the muscle during the attack are important points. As to the patient becoming free of the attacks, it is difficult to speak with any certainty. The condition is compatible with long life. The late H. C. Wood had a patient, aged eighty-seven, who had attacks at intervals for fifty years in which the pulse rate was usually 200. The taking of ice water or strong coffee arrested the attacks.

Treatment.—In an attack the patient should be quiet and in the position which gives him the greatest comfort. The diet should be liquid. If there is gastric disturbance, the giving of sedatives and alkalies may be useful. An ice bag applied over the præcordia often gives relief, if it does not stop the attack. The most diverse procedures may stop an attack, such as placing the head between the knees, being suspended with the head down, pressure on the vagus in the neck, or on the eye-balls, any sustained respiratory effort, the production of vomiting, the application of a tight abdominal binder, etc. The giving of strophanthin (gr. 1/250, 0.00026 gm.) or epinephrin (♏ x, 0.6 c. c. of a 1-10,000 solution) intravenously may be effectual. Chloral hydrate or morphia may be given to secure sleep. Any indicated symptomatic treatment should be given. Between attacks, any exciting cause should be avoided, the general health improved if possible, and attention paid to any gastro-intestinal disturbance. The wearing of an abdominal binder is sometimes useful.

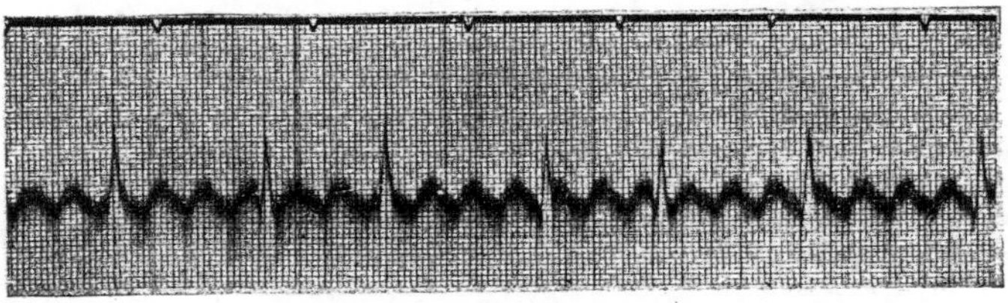

FIG. 2.—AURICULAR FLUTTER.

The curve shows a series of regular waves due to auricular contractions, interrupted by sharp spikes due to ventricular contractions. The ratio between auricular contractions and ventricular responses varies (2:1, 3:1 and 4:1) and averages 3:1. The slower ventricular rate is caused by a partial heart-block. The auricular rate is 210 per minute; the ventricular responses average 70.

(4) **Auricular Flutter.**—In this rather rare condition new impulses arise in the auricle, probably from a single focus, which cause it to beat rhythmically at a rate of 200 to 350 per minute. As Lewis says, this may not be readily distinguished from paroxysmal tachycardia but when the rate is over 200 special characteristics appear. Heart block is almost always present with it, the ventricular rate being half that of the auricle; 2:1 block is common but other ratios occur. The rate of the auricle is regular; the ventricle is usually regular but sometimes irregular. It is most frequent in advanced years, more common in males and usually associated with arterio-sclerosis and myocarditis.

The *symptoms* are fewer than might be expected and depend on the state of the muscle of the ventricle. There may be a complaint of palpitation and attacks of syncope. Occasionally the ventricle takes the auricular rate, with which the condition is very grave, but such attacks are usually of short duration. The recognition may be possible only by electrocardiographic tracings if the rate of the ventricle is not very rapid; otherwise a rate of 130 or over is very suggestive. The outlook is relatively good and is influenced by the state of the muscle and response to *treatment*. This consists in the use of digitalis or strophanthus in full doses. If disappearance of the flutter results, this is usually permanent.

(5) **Auricular Fibrillation.**—This common manifestation of cardiac irregularity is exceedingly important to recognize clinically. In the most pronounced form it is seen in the last stages of mitral stenosis, in which the pulse shows extreme irregularity, which, when once established, seldom returns to normal. A study of its features in this condition gave Mackenzie the clue to its explanation. He found that in certain cases the transition from regular to irregular pulse of this type occurred with suddenness, and that, whereas before the irregularity supervened the jugular pulse showed the normal features in the presence of auricular carotid and ventricular waves, with a marked presystolic murmur and thrill at the apex, after the irregularity was established, the auricular wave disappeared from the jugular pulse and the presystolic murmur from the apex. The inference drawn was that the right auricle

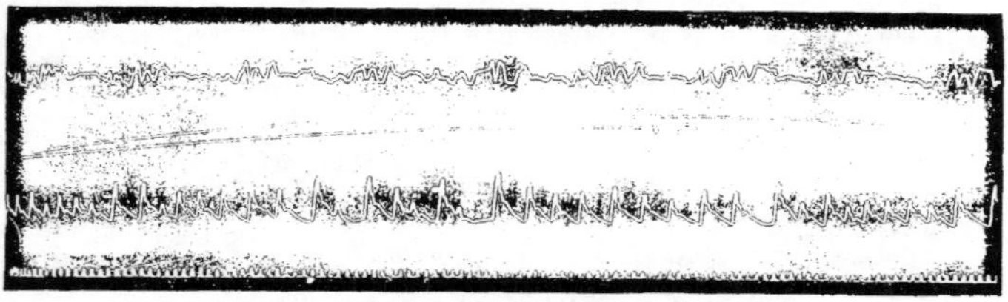

FIG. 3.—AURICULAR FIBRILLATION.

The altered rhythm, the variations in volume, and the rapid pulse rate are evident from the lower record (radial artery). The venous pulse record above shows fibrillary waves during ventricular diastole, with an absence of *a* waves produced by normally contracting auricles.

was so dilated as to prevent the formation of a normal auricular contraction. Complete proof of the cause of this condition has been supplied by Lewis, who found that patients with this irregularity showed in galvanometric tracings from the auricle numerous small and continuous waves, exactly similar to those obtained in the dog after fibrillation of the auricle has been induced by faradic stimulation of the appendix of the right auricle, or by ligation of the right coronary artery. The auricles do not contract normally but are in diastole with many fibrillary twitchings arising from pathological impulses originating in many areas. These impulses are probably identical with those which excite premature contractions. These numerous abnormal impulses come to the auricular-ventricular bundle but only some of them are able to pass and these reach the ventricle in an irregular fashion. Hence the contractions of the ventricle are disturbed and irregular. The state of the bundle determines how many impulses pass and hence the ventricular rate shows great variation. Heart-block and auricular fibrillation may occur together.

Auricular fibrillation forms a large proportion of the cases showing cardiac irregularity—about 40 per cent. (Lewis). Of etiological factors the most important is mitral stenosis, whether in the rheumatic form or that seen in women with no history of rheumatism. It is essentially a sign of marked myocardial disease. The average age of onset in those with a previous history of rheumatism is 30 to 40; in the non-rheumatic group it is between 50 and 60.

The *symptoms* depend largely on the associated conditions and are those of marked myocardial failure. The ventricular rate has some influence, as

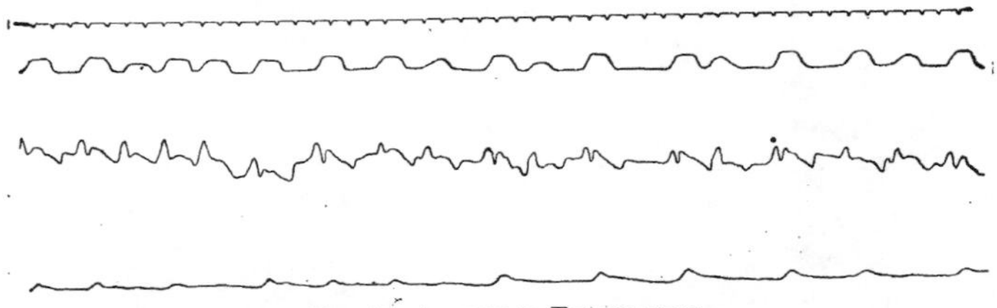

FIG. 4.—AURICULAR FIBRILLATION.

Several cardiac contractions at the apex (upper tracing) produced no pulsation at the wrist; others are so small as not to be felt. Synchronous counts at the apex and wrist for 10 seconds show 18 and 13 impulses respectively. The jugular shows only *c* and *v* waves, due to ventricular activity. Waves due to contraction of the auricles are absent, since they have ceased to act as efficient contracting chambers.

when it is very rapid (120-160), the distress and general symptoms of dilatation are more marked. The pulse is extremely irregular in every way and an irregular pulse with a rate over 120 is usually due to fibrillation. The more rapid the rate, the greater the irregularity. There is often a marked difference between the heart and pulse rate. The *diagnosis* is clear with a very rapid heart but when the rate is below 100 there may be slight difficulty until a careful study is made. Tracings remove any difficulty.

In *prognosis* the occurrence of fibrillation is always of grave omen. The condition is compatible with life for years but always means serious myocardial damage. The ventricular rate is of value, a persistent rate of 120 or over means a grave outlook and each increase in rate above this is more serious. The influence of treatment is of value in estimating the outlook.

Treatment.—For the general condition of the heart the problem is that of myocardial insufficiency, but for the fibrillation the remedy is digitalis, which acts by blocking the passage of many of the impulses from auricle to ventricle. The dosage is that which keeps the heart at the best possible rate, and must be decided for each patient. The dosage of digitalis depends somewhat on the severity of the condition; the present tendency is to give larger doses than formerly. In any case the object is to produce the required effect, whatever dose is required. Many of the patients should continue the use of digitalis permanently.

(6) **Heart-block** (Stokes-Adams Syndrome).—In the adult heart the auriculo-ventricular bundle of His is 18 mm. long, 2.5 mm. broad, and 1.5 mm. thick; it arises in the septum of the auricles below the foramen ovale and passes downward and forward through the trigonum fibrosum of auriculo-ventricular junction, where it comes into close relation with the mesial

leaflet of the tricuspid valve. Passing along the upper edge of the muscular septum, just where it joins with the posterior edge of the membranous septum, it radiates throughout the ventricles. If the function of the auriculo-ventricular bundle is impaired there may be a delay in the conduction of the impulse or it may be blocked completely. This may occur only with certain impulses (*partial heart-block*) or with all (*complete heart-block*). In the latter event the ventricles, released from the control of the normal pace-maker, assume their own rhythm (usually about 30 a minute).

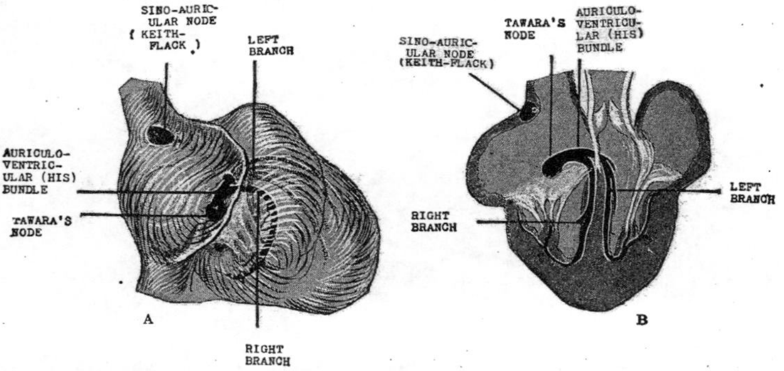

FIG. 5.—DIAGRAM SHOWING THE SINO-AURICULAR NODE AND THE AURICULAR BUNDLE. A, viewed from the right; B, cross section of the heart, viewed from the front. (Kindness of A. D. Hirschfelder.)

Etiology.—Heart-block may occur at any age depending on the cause. It is more common in males. It is not infrequent in infectious diseases, especially rheumatic fever, diphtheria and pneumonia, but occurs in many others. Syphilis is an important cause owing to the auriculo-ventricular bundle being affected in the myocardial involvement or by a gumma. Any form of myocarditis, acute or chronic, may be responsible. The action of digitalis in auricular fibrillation depends largely on its action on the impulses passing from auricle to ventricle and hence it is one of the causes of heart-block. The lesion in the bundle may be acute, usually in infections, or chronic, with fibrosis, gumma, etc.

The *symptoms* are variable, and depend to a considerable extent on the associated conditions. Some patients make little complaint but dizziness, weakness and fainting attacks are not uncommon. In the more severe forms the syncopal attacks are more frequent and severe. One variety is described under the Stokes-Adams syndrome. (It may be emphasized that this and heart-block are not synonymous terms.) The *signs* vary with the grade of block. An early manifestation may be reduplication of the first or second sound due to lengthening of the A-V interval which represents a delay in conduction. A dropped beat is easily recognized and if the ventricle is beating regularly at half the rate of the auricle (2:1 block) the pulse may be 40 to 50 a minute. Halving of the ventricular rate under digitalis therapy is always suggestive. It may be that the auricular rate can be counted by the pulsations in the veins of the neck. In *complete* block the ventricle beats at a rate below 35, and independently of the auricle. Faint sounds may be heard during the ventricular diastole, from auricular systoles. While the diagnosis can often be made from the physical signs, tracings render it certain. A block may occur in one of the branches of the bundle of His. Reduplication of the first sound may result. Electrocardiographic tracings are necessary for its recognition.

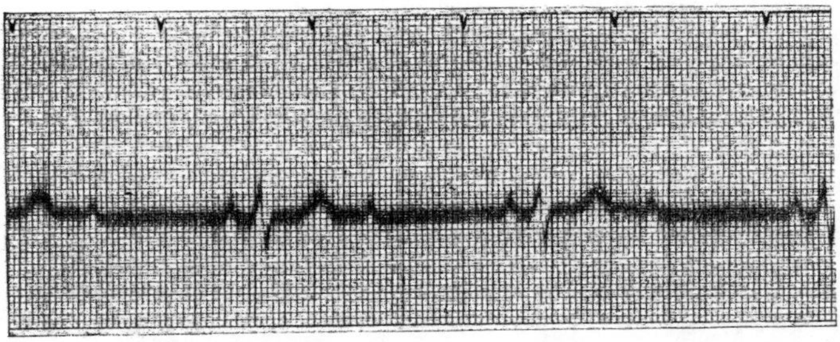

FIG. 6.—PARTIAL HEART-BLOCK WITH 2:1 RATIO; auricular rate 66, ventricular rate 33.

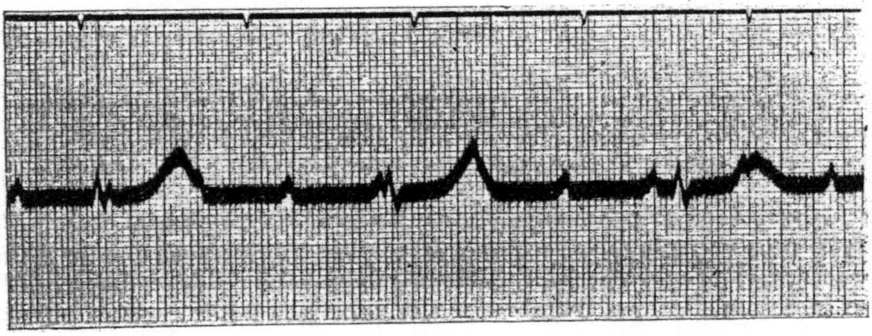

FIG. 7.—COMPLETE HEART-BLOCK.

The small blunt vertical waves (110 per minute) are due to auricular contraction; the diphasic sharply pointed wave and the large blunt wave which follows represent ventricular contractions (34 per minute). The contractions of the auricles and ventricles are independent of each other.

Stokes-Adams Syndrome.—Clinically this presents three features: (*a*) slow pulse, usually permanent, but sometimes paroxysmal, falling to 40, 20, or even 6 per minute; (*b*) cerebral attacks—vertigo of a transient character, syncope, pseudo-apoplectiform attacks or epileptiform seizures; (*c*) visible auricular impulses in the veins of the neck, as noted by Stokes—the beats varying greatly; a 2:1 or 3:1 rhythm is the most common. There are several groups of cases. It is usually a senile manifestation associated with arterio-sclerosis. The cases in young adults and middle aged men are often myocardial and of syphilitic origin. There is a neurotic group in which all the features may be present, and in which post mortem no lesions have been found (Edes and Councilman). In the attacks of slow pulse in this group the auricular as well as the ventricular rate may be slow and equal, the normal sequence of events being preserved; the origin of the condition is probably vagal. The outlook in this class of cases is good; in the others it is a serious disease and usually fatal, though it may last for many years. The cerebral attacks are due to anæmia of the brain or of the medulla in consequence of the imperfect ventricular action. In one of our cases Baetjer could see with the fluoroscope the more frequent contraction of the auricles.

The *prognosis* in the cases with acute infectious disease is usually good, with perhaps the exception of diphtheria and some cases of rheumatic fever. In the chronic forms the outlook is grave and sudden death is always possible. The syncopal and convulsive attacks are always serious. In some of the cases due to syphilis proper treatment may result in great improvement. In every case the state of the myocardium is important.

Treatment.—If a cause, such as syphilis, is found, the indications are evident. Acute heart-block demands absolute rest and treatment directed to the general cardiac condition. Digitalis should be given with care. In partial block it may increase the difficulty and yet the heart muscle may be aided by it. In complete block it may be more useful and it cannot increase the block. In partial heart-block the giving of atropine may be useful but rather in the cases due to acute infections than those with sclerotic processes. There is no special treatment for the syncopal attacks.

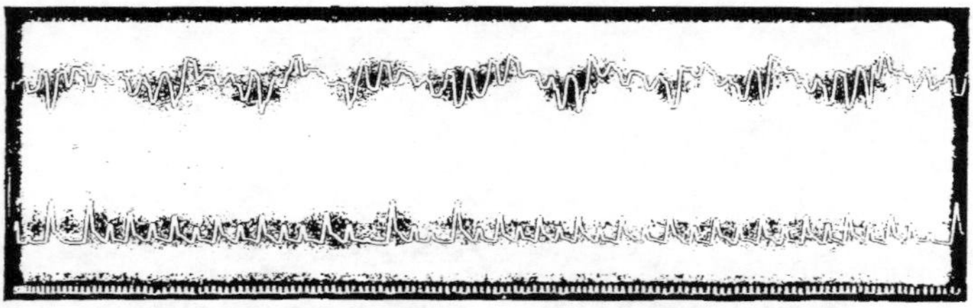

FIG. 8.—COMBINED ALTERNATION OF THE PULSE AND PREMATURE CONTRACTIONS.

The latter part of the record shows a pulse regular as to sequence, but alternating as to volume. In the first part this sequential regularity is irregularly interrupted by premature contractions of ventricular origin.

(7) **Alternation of the Heart.**—In this there is disturbance of the ventricular systole, so that larger and smaller amounts of blood are expelled by alternate contractions and consequently the pulse shows alternate large and small beats. It is suggested that a variable number of ventricular fibres contract and so vary the systoles. It is seen in conditions of very rapid heart rate, especially paroxysmal tachycardia, in which it has no special significance. Its occurrence when the heart rate is normal or nearly so has a very different and more serious meaning. It is observed in a variety of conditions in which marked circulatory disease is present, in severe infections, especially pneumonia, in uræmia, in lead poisoning, and in patients under the influence of digitalis. It occurs most often in advanced life and more in males. It is comparatively common but frequently overlooked.

The condition itself probably causes no *symptoms* but as it accompanies serious circulatory diseases, the features of these are present, such as dyspnœa, anginal pain, etc. It should be searched for in cases of hypertension, angina pectoris, myocarditis and when extra-systoles are present. It may be more evident after exertion, with the patient standing or after holding the breath. The variations may be felt by the finger but tracings give the most certain evidence of its presence. The difference in systolic pressure between the large and small beats may be an aid. Comparison with the heart rate distinguishes it from a dicrotic pulse. Excluding the cases of tachycardia and usually those due to digitalis, the *significance* of alternation is always serious. This applies particularly to the cases in which it is continuous, but in all it should be regarded as an evidence of great danger. Sudden death is comparatively common. The *treatment* is that of the underlying condition and special emphasis should be placed on rest, thorough and prolonged.

II. AFFECTIONS OF THE MYOCARDIUM

I. HYPERTROPHY

Varieties.—The heart enlarges to meet a demand for extra work, either general, as in the strain of athletics (the hypertrophy of work), or special to combat a deficiency of cardiac structure, such as a damaged valve. There are two forms, one in which the cavity or cavities are of normal size, and the other in which the cavities are enlarged and the walls increased in thickness (eccentric hypertrophy). The so-called concentric hypertrophy in which there is diminution of the size of the cavity with thickening of the walls is, as a rule, a post mortem change. The enlargement may affect the entire organ, or one side, or only one chamber. Naturally, as the left ventricle does the chief work the change is most frequently found here. Though its production is assisted by adequate nutrition, hypertrophy may appear even under conditions of starvation, given otherwise healthy organs. In the debilitated the limits to which hypertrophy may progress are small.

Hypertrophy of the left ventricle alone, or with general enlargement of the heart, is brought about by—

Conditions affecting the heart itself: (*a*) Disease of the aortic valve; (*b*) mitral insufficiency; (*c*) pericardial adhesions; (*d*) sclerotic myocarditis; (*e*) disturbed innervation with overaction, as in exophthalmic goitre, and as a result of the action of alcohol, in the "beer heart." In all of these the work of the heart is increased. In the case of the valve lesions the increase is due to increased intraventricular pressure; in the case of the adherent pericardium and myocarditis, to direct interference with the symmetrical and orderly contraction of the chambers.

Conditions acting upon the blood-vessels: (*a*) General arterio-sclerosis, with or without renal disease, especially sclerosis of the aorta, the renal arteries, and the vessels of the splanchnic area; (*b*) all states of increased arterial tension induced by the contraction of the smaller arteries under the influence of certain toxic substances, which, as Bright suggested, "by affecting the minute capillary circulation, render great action necessary to send the blood through the distant subdivisions of the vascular system"; (*c*) prolonged muscular exertion, which enormously increases the blood pressure in the arteries; (*d*) narrowing of the aorta, as in congenital stenosis.

HYPERTROPHY OF THE RIGHT VENTRICLE is met with under the following conditions—

(*a*) *Lesions of the mitral valve,* either incompetence or stenosis, which act by increasing the resistance in the pulmonary vessels. (*b*) *Pulmonary lesions* with obliteration of any number of blood vessels within the lungs, as in emphysema or cirrhosis. (*c*) *Valvular lesions* on the right side occasionally cause hypertrophy in the adult, not infrequently in the fetus. (*d*) *Chronic valvular disease of the left heart and pericardial adhesions* are sooner or later associated with hypertrophy of the right ventricle.

In the auricles simple hypertrophy is never seen; there is always dilatation with hypertrophy. In the left auricle the condition develops in lesions at the mitral orifice, particularly stenosis. The right auricle hypertrophies when there is greatly increased blood pressure in the lesser circulation, whether due to mitral stenosis or pulmonary lesions. Narrowing of the tricuspid orifice is a rare cause.

Symptoms.—There may be no complaint attributable to the hypertrophy, and if associated with renal disease or arterio-sclerosis there may be a marked sense of well-being. If, however, the cardiac defect be not fully compensated, the patient may complain of slight giddiness, headache, a sense of palpitation in the thorax, and some dyspnœa on exertion.

In hypertrophy of the right auricle the venous pulsation in the neck may be more evident, and a tracing may show a marked increase in the size of the auricular wave. An increase in dulness to the right of the sternum in the third and fourth interspaces may be detected, and on very rare occasions a sound preceding that of the ventricle over that area. Hypertrophy of the right ventricle causes a slight bulging of the costal angle with a positive instead of a negative pulsation at this spot. The apex beat may be diffuse, as the enlarged right ventricle prevents the left ventricle from coming into contact with the chest wall. The venous pulsation in the neck is usually marked, and the first sound over the tricuspid area louder than normal. Hypertrophy of the left auricle, which is seldom marked and never unassociated with dilatation, may be detected occasionally by dulness toward the base of the left lung behind; it is easily diagnosed by the extension backward of the cardiac shadow in oblique illumination of the chest by the X-rays. Hypertrophy of the left ventricle is usually easy to diagnose. There is a forcible impulse at the apex beat, both visible and palpable. This impulse may cause a movement of a large area of the chest wall. The apex beat, if there be only slight dilatation, is usually displaced downward, and is found in the 6th and 7th spaces; but if the dilatation be marked, the apex beat becomes more diffuse and is found well outside the nipple line in the 4th, 5th, and 6th spaces. The first sound is usually marked and sometimes has a distinct booming sound. The second sound at the base is accentuated. The pulse is full and of high tension at the height of the ventricular impulse. The blood pressure is usually raised.

II. DILATATION

As with other hollow muscular organs, the size of the chambers of the heart varies greatly within normal limits. Dilatation may be an acute process and quite transitory, as after severe muscular effort, or it may be chronic, in which case it is associated with hypertrophy. Not always, however; there is an extraordinary heart in the McGill College Museum showing a parchment like thinning of the walls with uniform dilatation of all the chambers; in places in the right auricle and ventricle only the epicardium remains. Dilatation is pathological only when permanent. Increase in capacity means increased work and in consequence hypertrophy to meet the demand.

Etiology.—Two important causes combine to produce dilatation—increased pressure within the cavities and impaired resistance, due to weakening of the muscular wall—which may act singly, but are often combined. A weakened wall may yield to a normal distending force, the weakened wall being due either to structural change in the cardiac muscle or to a diminution of its natural tonus.

(*a*) Heightened endocardiac pressure results either from an increased quantity of blood to be moved or an obstacle to be overcome. It does not necessarily bring about dilatation; simple hypertrophy may follow, as in the early period of aortic stenosis, and in the hypertrophy of the left ventricle in nephritis.

The size of the cardiac chambers varies in health. With slow action of the heart the dilatation is complete and fuller than it is with rapid action. Moderate exertion in a normal heart, or even prolonged exertion in a well-trained heart, lessens the heart size, but in conditions of ill health dilatation occurs. Physiologically, the limits of dilatation are reached when the chamber does not empty itself during the systole. This may occur as an acute, transient condition in severe exertion in an untrained or feeble condition—during, for example, the ascent of a mountain.

There may be great dilatation of the right heart, as shown by the increased epigastric pulsation and increase in the cardiac dulness. The *safety valve* action of the tricuspid valves may come into play, relieving the lungs by permitting regurgitation into the auricle. With rest the condition is removed, but, if it has been extreme, the heart may suffer a strain from which it may recover slowly, or, indeed, the individual may never be able again to undertake severe exertion. In the process of training the getting wind, as it is called, is largely a gradual increase in the capability of the heart, particularly of the right chambers. A degree of exertion can be safely maintained in full training which would be quite impossible under other circumstances, because, by a gradual process of what we may call physical education, the heart has strengthened its reserve force—widened enormously its limit of physiological work. Endurance in prolonged contests is measured by the capabilities of the heart, which by increasing its tonus has increased its resistance to dilatation. We have no positive knowledge of the nature of the changes in the heart which occur in this process, but it must be in the direction of increased muscular and nervous energy. The large heart of athletes may be due to the prolonged use of their muscles, but no man becomes a great runner or oarsman who has not naturally a capable if not a large heart. Master McGrath, the celebrated greyhound, and Eclipse, the race horse, both famous for endurance rather than speed, had very large hearts.

Excessive dilatation during severe muscular effort results in *heart-strain.* A man, perhaps in poor condition, calls upon his heart for extra work during the ascent of a high mountain, and is at once seized with pain about the heart and a sense of distress in the epigastrium. He breathes rapidly for some time, is "puffed," as we say, but the symptoms pass off after a night's quiet. An attempt to repeat the exercise is followed by another attack, or an attack of cardiac dyspnœa may come on while at rest. For months such a man may be unfitted for severe exertion or he may be permanently incapacitated. In some way he has overstrained his heart and become "broken-winded." In such cases there was probably previous myocardial change. The "heart-shock" of Latham includes cases of this nature—sudden cardiac break-down during exertion, not due to rupture of a valve. It seems probable that sudden death during long continued efforts, as in a race, is sometimes due to overdistention and paralysis of the heart.

Acute dilatative heart weakness is seen in many conditions, as in Graves' disease, in paroxysmal tachycardia, in old myocardial cases following exertion, and in angina pectoris. There is usually a striking contrast between the wide and forcible cardiac impulse and the small, feeble, irregular pulse.

Dilatation occurs in all forms of *valve lesions.* In aortic insufficiency blood enters the left ventricle during diastole from the unguarded aorta and from the left auricle, and the quantity of blood at the termination of diastole subjects the walls to an extreme degree of pressure, under which they inevitably yield. In time they augment in thickness, and present the typical eccentric hypertrophy of this condition.

In mitral insufficiency blood which should have been driven into the aorta is forced into and dilates the auricle from which it came, and then in the diastole of the ventricle a large amount is returned from the auricle, and with increased force. In mitral stenosis the left auricle is the seat of greatly increased tension during diastole, and dilates as well as hypertrophies; the distention may be enormous. Dilatation of the right ventricle is produced by a number of conditions, which were considered under hypertrophy. All circumstances, such as mitral stenosis, emphysema, etc., which permanently increase the tension in the pulmonary vessels cause its dilatation.

The dilatation and hypertrophy of beer drinkers also comes in this group, as it is brought about gradually by increased endocardial pressure.

(*b*) Impaired nutrition of the heart walls may lead to a diminution of the resisting power so that dilatation readily occurs.

The loss of tone due to parenchymatous degeneration or myocarditis in fevers may lead to a fatal condition of acute dilatation. It is a recognized cause of death in scarlatinal dropsy (Goodhart), and may occur in rheumatic fever, typhus, typhoid, etc. The changes in the heart muscle which accompany acute endocarditis or pericarditis may lead to dilatation, especially in the latter disease. In anæmia, leukæmia, and chlorosis the dilatation may be considerable. In sclerosis of the walls the yielding is always where this process is most advanced, as at the left apex. Under any of these circumstances the walls may yield with normal blood pressure.

Pericardial adhesions are a cause of dilatation, and we generally find in cases with extensive and firm union considerable hypertrophy and dilatation. There is usually here some impairment of the superficial layers of muscle.

III. CARDIAC INSUFFICIENCY

Etiology.—With lessening of the muscular power of the heart the rapidity with which the blood circulates is diminished, and the tissues fail to receive their proper supply of oxygen and food, and to be adequately relieved of their waste products—this is cardiac failure. The same effect may be produced in another way. The amount of blood in the body is much less than the total capacity of the vascular bed, and an adequate blood supply is only kept up by a general constriction of arterioles which dam the blood in the arterial system, but if by any chance there is a general vaso-dilatation of the arterioles, especially those in the splanchnic area, the heart does not receive an amount of blood sufficient to supply the bodily needs, with the same effect on the organs as in certain forms of cardiac failure. This condition does not concern us here, but it must be mentioned to avoid the impression that all failure of the circulation means failure of the heart.

The failure in muscular power may affect any cavity singly or the whole heart. Weakness of the left ventricle fails to give proper filling of the arterial system and general anæmia of the tissues results. Failure of the left auricle means stasis in the lung vessels with deficient aeration of the blood, and a tendency to œdema of the lung or to effusion into the pleural cavity. Failure of the right auricle and ventricle gives cyanosis of the organs, dyspnœa at rest and on slight exertion, with stasis in the abdominal organs and œdema.

The *reserve* power with which the cardiac muscle is endowed disappears in heart failure. This reserve, greatest in youth, is increased by adequate nutrition, certain congenital endowments, and, apart from other defects, by hypertrophy. It is lessened by defects in the cardiac structure, gross or minute, by defective nutrition, by certain bacterial and other poisons, and with advancing years. We have at present no means of gauging this reserve power of the organ as a whole or in its different parts.

The failure may be sudden or slow, according to the kind and rapidity of the lesion which causes it. When the left ventricle fails the effect may vary from immediate death, through all forms of fainting, giddiness, sense of dissolution, to a mild sense of bodily or mental fatigue; when the right ventricle fails the effect varies from a sudden dyspnœa to a dyspnœa which comes on with slight exertion.

As to the actual condition in cardiac failure generally, it is by no means easy in all cases to say what has been the cause. The lesions to which the cardiac musculature is liable are described further on, yet there is a proportion of cases in which neither by post mortem examination nor careful microscopic search can the source of the failure be even suggested. It is well to bear in mind a suggestion made by Aschoff, namely, that in certain cases the failure is due not so much to the implication of the general musculature as to an affection of the conducting system and of the bundle of His with its ramifications.

The *blood pressure* in cardiac insufficiency shows no uniform figures. The systolic pressure may be high even in a failing heart. In serious degrees of myocardial affection it is usually low. In cases in which there has been a raised blood pressure, the maximum may be lower or higher than the normal for the patient. We must recognize that probably in early stages of failure the heart is stimulated to put forth increased energy at each beat, and that the maximum pressure at the height of the beat slightly over-compensates the circulatory defect.

ACUTE CARDIAC INSUFFICIENCY.—Causes: (*a*) Wounds of the heart, (*b*) spontaneous rupture or rupture of valves, (*c*) rapid effusion into the pericardium, (*d*) access of air to the chambers of the heart, as from operations at the root of the neck or after exposure to a high atmospheric pressure, (*e*) large thrombi quickly formed in a heart cavity, (*f*) sudden interference with the coronary circulation, especially the left coronary artery, (*g*) mechanical interference with the heart from pressure on the trachea or larynx, as in strangulation, (*h*) acute infections, such as diphtheria or pericarditis, (*i*) certain poisons, such as pilocarpine, cocaine, phosphorus, etc., (*j*) stimulation of the vagus nerve, its centre in the medulla, or its termination in the heart.

CHRONIC CARDIAC INSUFFICIENCY.—Causes: (*a*) Lesions of the heart muscle, which will be described in more detail. *All cardiac failure is muscular.* The myocardium may be insufficiently nourished, as in the starvation atrophy of new growths or in diabetes, or there may be recognizable lesions. One or more of the functions of the cardiac muscle may be interfered with without producing any changes that can be detected by the microscope, such as the failure associated with aortic disease. (*b*) Lesions of the valves. (*c*) Lesions affecting the vascular fields of the efferent arteries. Emphysema, chronic bronchitis, asthma, sclerosis of the lungs, chest deformities, and mitral disease produce an embarrassment of the right heart; atheroma of the aorta and arterio-sclerosis, especially of the splanchnic and renal area, produce failure of the left heart. (*d*) Over-exertion. (*e*) Certain poisons, such as alcohol (especially beer) and phosphorus. (*f*) Other causes, such as adherent pericardium and exophthalmic goitre.

Anatomical Basis of Cardiac Insufficiency.—I. LESIONS OF THE CORONARY ARTERIES.—A knowledge of the changes produced in the myocardium by disease of the coronary vessels gives a key to the understanding of many problems in cardiac pathology. The terminal branches of the coronary vessels are end arteries; that is, the communication between neighboring branches is through capillaries only. J. H. Pratt has shown that the vessels of Thebesius, which open from the ventricles and auricles into a system of fine branches and thus communicate with the cardiac capillaries and coronary veins, may be capable of feeding the myocardium sufficiently to keep it alive even when the coronary arteries are occluded. The blocking of one of these vessels by a thrombus or an embolus leads usually to a condition known as—

(*a*) *Anæmic necrosis,* or white infarct. When this does not occur the reason may be sought in (1) the existence of abnormal anastomoses, which by their presence take the coronary system out of the group of end arteries; or (2) the vicarious flow through the vessels of Thebesius and the coronary veins. The condition is most commonly seen in the left ventricle and in the septum, in the territory of distribution of the anterior coronary artery. The affected area has a yellowish white color, sometimes a turbid, parboiled aspect, at other times a grayish red tint. It may be somewhat wedge-shaped, more often it is irregular in contour and projects above the surface. Microscopically the changes are characteristic. The nuclei disappear from the muscle fibres or undergo fragmentation. Leucocytes wander in from the surrounding tissue and may suffer disintegration. At a later stage a new growth of fibrous tissue is found in the periphery of the infarct which ultimately may entirely replace the dead fibres. In some instances there is complete transformation, and a firm white patch of hyaline degeneration may appear in the centre of the area. Rupture of the heart may be associated with anæmic necrosis.

(*b*) The second important effect of coronary artery disease is seen in the production of *fibrous myocarditis.* This may result from the gradual transformation of areas of anæmic necrosis. More commonly it is caused by the narrowing of a coronary branch in a process of obliterative endarteritis. Where the process is gradual evidences of granulation tissue are often wanting, and any distinction between the necrotic muscle fibres and the new scar tissue is difficult to establish. J. B. MacCallum showed that the muscle fibres undergo a change the reverse of that of their normal development and lose their fibril bundles preliminary to their complete replacement by connective tissue. The sclerosis is most frequent at the apex of the left ventricle and in the septum, but may occur in any portion. In the septum and walls there are often streaks and patches which are only seen in carefully made serial sections. Hypertrophy of the heart is commonly associated with this degeneration. It is the invariable precursor of aneurism of the heart.

(*c*) *Sudden Death in Coronary Artery Disease.*—Complete obliteration of one coronary artery, if produced suddenly, is usually fatal. When induced slowly, either by arterio-sclerosis at the orifice of the artery at the root of the aorta or by an obliterating endarteritis in the course of the vessel, the circulation may be carried on through the other vessel. Sudden death is not uncommon, owing to thrombosis of a vessel which has become narrowed by sclerosis. *In medico-legal cases it is a point of primary importance to remember that this is one of the common causes of sudden death.* This condition should be carefully sought for, inasmuch as it may be the sole lesion, except a general, sometimes slight, arterio-sclerosis. In the most extreme grade one coronary artery may be entirely blocked, with the production of extensive fibroid disease, and a main branch of the other also may be occluded.

(*d*) *Septic Infarcts.*—In pyæmia the smaller branches of the coronary arteries may be blocked with emboli which give rise to infectious or septic infarcts in the myocardium in the form of abscesses, varying in size from a pea to a pin's head. These may not cause any disturbance, but when large they may perforate into the ventricle or into the pericardium, forming what has been called acute ulcer of the heart.

II. Acute Interstitial Myocarditis.—In some infectious diseases and in acute pericarditis the intermuscular connective tissue may be swollen and infiltrated with small round cells and leucocytes, the blood vessels dilated, and the muscle fibres the seat of granular, fatty, and hyaline degeneration. Occasionally, in pyæmia the infiltration with pus cells has been diffuse and confined chiefly to the interstitial tissue. Councilman has described this condition of the heart wall in gonorrhœa, and demonstrated the gonococcus in the diseased areas. The commonest examples are found in diphtheria, typhoid fever, and acute endocarditis, as shown by the studies of Romberg. The foci may be the starting points of patches of fibrous myocarditis.

III. Fragmentation and Segmentation.—This condition was described by Renaut and Landouzy in 1877, and has been carefully studied. Two forms are met with: 1. Segmentation. The muscle fibres have separated at the cement line. 2. Fragmentation. The fracture has been across the fibre itself, and perhaps at the level of the nucleus. Longitudinal division is unusual. Although the condition doubtless arises in some instances during the death agony, as in sudden death by violence, in others it would seem to have clinical and pathological significance. It is found associated with other lesions, fibrous myocarditis, infarction, and fatty degeneration. J. B. MacCallum distinguished a simple from a degenerative fragmentation. The first takes place in the normal fibre, which, however, shows irregular extensions and contractions. The second succeeds degeneration in the fibre. Hearts the seat of marked fragmentation are lax, easily torn, the muscle fibres widely separated, and often pale and cloudy.

IV. Parenchymatous Degeneration.—This is usually met with in fevers, or in connection with endocarditis or pericarditis, and in infections and intoxications generally. It is characterized by a pale, turbid state of the cardiac muscle, which is general, not localized. Turbidity and softness are the special features. It is the softened heart of Laennec and Louis. Stokes speaks of an instance in which "so great was the softening of the organ that when the heart was grasped by the great vessels and held with the apex pointing upward, it fell down over the hand, covering it like a cap of a large mushroom." Histologically, there is a degeneration of the muscle fibres, which are infiltrated to a various extent with granules which resist the action of ether, but are dissolved in acetic acid. Sometimes this granular change in the fibres is extreme, and no trace of the striæ can be detected. It is probably the effect of a toxic agent, and is seen in its most marked form in the lumbar muscles in cases of toxic hæmoglobinuria in the horse.

V. Fatty Heart.—Under this term are embraced fatty degeneration and fatty overgrowth.

(*a*) *Fatty degeneration* is a common condition, and mild grades are met with in many diseases. It is found in the failing nutrition of old age, wasting diseases, and cachectic states; in prolonged infectious fevers, in which it may accompany the parenchymatous change. In pernicious anæmia and in phosphorus poisoning the most extreme degrees are seen. Pericarditis is usually associated with fatty or parenchymatous changes in the superficial layers of the myocardium. Disease of the coronary arteries is a much more common cause of fibroid degeneration than of fatty heart. Lastly, in the hypertrophied ventricular wall in chronic heart-disease fatty change is by no means infrequent. This may be limited to the heart or be more or less general in the solid viscera. The diaphragm may also be involved, even when the other muscles show no special changes. There appears to be a special proneness to fatty degeneration in the heart muscle, which may be connected with its incessant activity. So great is its need of an abundant oxygen supply that it feels at once any deficiency, and is in consequence the first muscle to show nutritional changes.

Anatomically the condition may be local or general. The left ventricle is most frequently affected. If the process is advanced and general, the heart looks large and is flabby and relaxed. It has a light yellowish brown tint, or, as it is called, a faded leaf color. Its consistence is reduced and the substance tears easily. In the left ventricle the papillary columns and the muscle beneath the endocardium show a streaked or patchy appearance. Microscopically, the fibres are seen to be occupied by minute globules distributed in rows along the line of the primitive fibres (Welch). In advanced grades the fibres seem completely occupied by the minute globules.

(*b*) *Fatty Overgrowth.*—This is usually a simple excess of the normal subpericardial fat, to which the term *cor adiposum* was given by the older writers. In pronounced instances the fat infiltrates between the muscular substance and, separating the strands, may reach even to the endocardium. In corpulent persons there is always much pericardial fat. It forms part of the general obesity, and occasionally leads to dangerous or even fatal impairment of the contractile power of the heart. Of 122 cases analyzed by Forchheimer there were 88 males and 34 females. Over 80 per cent. occurred between the fortieth and seventieth years.

The entire heart may be enveloped in a thick sheeting of fat through which not a trace of muscle substance can be seen. On section the fat infiltrates the muscle, separating the fibres, and in extreme cases—particularly in the right ventricle—reaches the endocardium. In some places there may be even complete substitution of fat for the muscle substance. In rare instances the fat may be in the papillary muscles. The heart is usually much relaxed and the chambers are dilated. Microscopically the muscle fibres may show, in addition to the atrophy, marked fatty degeneration.

VI. Other Degenerations.—(*a*) *Brown Atrophy.*—This is a common change in the heart muscle, particularly in chronic valvular lesions and in the senile heart. When advanced the color of the muscles is a dark red brown, and the consistence is usually increased. The fibres present an accumulation of yellow brown pigment chiefly about the nuclei. (*b*) *Amyloid degeneration* is occasionally seen. It occurs in the intermuscular connective tissue and in the blood vessels, not in the fibres. (*c*) The *hyaline transformation of Zenker* may occur in prolonged fevers. The affected fibres are swollen, homogeneous, translucent, and the striæ are very faint. (*d*) *Calcareous degeneration* occasionally occurs in the myocardium, and the muscle fibres may be infiltrated with lime salts.

Symptoms of Cardiac Insufficiency.—The symptoms of left sided cardiac failure differ from those of the right side, and in each we may distinguish a number of types, which, however, merge gradually the one into the other. Failure of the left ventricle is seen in its severest forms in the abrupt death stroke of angina pectoris, in the sudden faints with sweats and heart pain of fatty or fibroid hearts, or in the fainting and convulsive attacks of Stokes-Adams disease. Less severe failure may be seen in athletes after a hard race, when vomiting and a feeling of dissolution are present—a type which is sometimes seen in angina, when it is liable to be mistaken for a gastro-intestinal upset. The milder degrees show themselves in an inability to take much exercise or to do much mental work without the sense of great fatigue. Sudden and slow types are also seen in failure of the right side. Subjected to a slight strain, great hyperpnœa and distress may come on, and one form of cardiac dyspnœa which attacks the patient at night is of this nature. The severer forms show an increasing inability to undergo slight extra exertion, such as mounting stairs, or hyperpnœa even when at rest in bed, in both of which there is usually some œdema of the feet, especially at night, if the patient is on his feet most of the day.

Grouped under their special systems the symptoms complained of by patients with cardiac failure are as follows: (*a*) Cardio-vascular system: Pain in the cardiac area or extending to the shoulders and down the arms, a sense of weight in the præcordium; palpitation is seldom complained of. (*b*) Respiratory system: Dyspnœa at rest or on exertion, or orthopnœa, Cheyne-Stokes respiration, cough, loss of voice from pressure of a dilated left auricle on the left recurrent laryngeal nerve, hæmoptysis (from lung infarcts). (*c*) Central nervous system; sleeplessness, mental symptoms, delusions, melancholia, and especially toward the end stupor and drowsiness. (*d*) Cyanosis, pallor, œdema, and occasionally purpura in the lower limbs. (*e*) Alimentary system: The stasis in the abdominal organs in right heart failure produces loss of appetite, indigestion, flatulence, vomiting, constipation, diarrhœa, abdominal pain, hæmorrhoids, etc. (*f*) Renal system: The urine is scanty, high colored, and contains a slight amount of albumin.

Physical examination of the heart may reveal an apex-beat which is feeble, outside the nipple line, diffuse, and whose maximum intensity is not easily localized. The pulsation may be marked on inspection and cover a very wide area; arterial pulsation in the neck in the left heart failure may be great; in right heart failure the jugular veins may be very dilated. On percussion the cardiac area may be much increased to the right or to the left, or both. On auscultation the sounds may be difficult to hear, or feebler than normal; murmurs, usually soft, may be present at both apex and base. Gallop rhythm may be present. The pulse may show great variations; marked failure may exist with a full bounding pulse; more usually it is feeble with diminished tension; it may be irregular, intermittent, slow, or rapid. No one sign or combination of signs is significant of cardiac failure. A heart may be insufficient and yet perhaps nothing can be detected by physical examination except feeble sounds and a low tension pulse.

The myocardial lesion is not always proportionate to the intensity of the symptoms. A patient may present enfeebled, irregular action and signs of dilatation with shortness of breath and œdema, and the post mortem show little or no change in the myocardium.

When *dilatation* occurs there are gallop rhythm, shortening of the long pause, and a systolic murmur at the apex. Shortness of breath on exertion is an early feature in many cases, and anginal attacks may occur. There is sometimes a tendency to syncope, and the patient may wake from sleep in the early morning with an attack of severe dyspnœa. These "spells" may be associated with nausea and may alternate with others in which there are anginal symptoms. These are the cases, too, in which for weeks there may be mental symptoms. The patient has delusions and may even become maniacal. Toward the close the type of breathing known as Cheyne-Stokes may occur. It was described in the following terms by John Cheyne, speaking of a case of fatty heart (Dublin Hospital Reports, vol. ii, p. 221, 1818): "For several days his breathing was irregular; it would entirely cease for a quarter of a minute, then it would become perceptible, though very low, then by degrees it became heaving and quick, and then it would gradually cease again: this revolution in the state of his breathing lasted about a minute, during which there were about thirty acts of respiration." It is seen much more frequently in arterio-sclerosis and uræmic states than in fatty heart.

Fatty overgrowth of the heart is a condition certain to exist in very obese persons. It produces no symptoms until the muscular fibre is so weakened that dilatation occurs. These patients may for years present a feeble but regular pulse; the heart sounds are weak and muffled, and a murmur may be heard at the apex. Attacks of dyspnœa are not uncommon, and the patient may suffer from bronchitis. The physical examination is often difficult because of the great increase in the fat, and it may be impossible to define the area of dulness.

Thrombosis of the *coronary arteries* occurs usually in middle-aged or elderly people. Their vessels are sclerotic, the blood pressure may be high and they may have had angina pectoris. The seizure is severe and lasts for some time if death does not occur suddenly. The *pain* is substernal or referred to the lower sternum or epigastrium. It may radiate to the arms or neck. If referred to the abdomen with signs of collapse, an acute abdominal condition may be suspected. Some of the deaths attributed to "acute indigestion" belong here. The heart is rapid, often irregular, sometimes dilated, the sounds feeble, and a friction rub may be heard. The pulse is weak and the blood pressure lowered. Pulmonary stasis or œdema, passive congestion of the kidney and general œdema may result. Death may result rapidly or after some hours. In thrombosis of the smaller branches recovery may follow.

Cardioptosis.—This is found in thin persons with visceroptosis. The heart is narrow, lies vertically and is low in position. It is found in the sub-normal type with arterial hypoplasia, a tendency to under-nutrition, and vaso-motor instability. Dilatation occurs readily, with any slight infection or disturbance, and is easily overlooked owing to the small size of the heart with which a normal extent of dulness represents enlargement. They respond quickly to rest and digitalis.

Functional Tests.—There are many of these, the principle being to have the patient perform certain exercises, such as hopping on one leg, bending over, etc., and then studying the circulatory response. The exercise chosen should be suitable for the age and habits of the patient. The extent of response (pulse rate, blood pressure) and the length of time it persists are important points. But every patient is constantly doing "functional tests" in his daily life, which careful inquiry should elicit.

We may group the cases of failure from myocardial diseases as follows:

(1) Those in which sudden death occurs with or without previous indications of heart-trouble. Sclerosis of the coronary arteries exists—in some instances with recent thrombus and white infarcts; in others, extensive fibroid disease; in others again, fatty degeneration. Many patients never complain of cardiac distress, but, as in the case of Chalmers, the celebrated Scottish divine, enjoy unusual vigor of mind and body.

(2) Cases in which there are cardiac arrhythmia, shortness of breath on

exertion, attacks of dyspnœa, sometimes anginal attacks, collapse symptoms with sweats and slow pulse, and occasionally marked mental symptoms.

(3) Cases with general arterio-sclerosis and hypertrophy and dilatation of the heart. They are robust men of middle age who have worked hard and lived carelessly. Dyspnœa, cough, and swelling of the feet are the early symptoms, and the patient comes under observation either with a gallop rhythm, embryocardia, or an irregular heart with an apex systolic mumur of mitral insufficiency. Recovery from the first or second attack is the rule. It is one of the most common forms of heart-disease.

Prognosis.—Each case must be judged on its own merits, special notice being taken of the age, probable origin, and anatomical basis of the insufficiency. With disturbance of rhythm the nature of this should be determined as this has an important bearing on the outcome. The outlook in affections of the myocardium occurring late in life is extremely grave. Patients recover, however, in a surprising way from the most serious attacks, particularly those of the third group.

Treatment.—Some patients never come under treatment; the first are the final symptoms. Other cases with well marked failure, if treated on general lines, recover quickly. Much more difficult is the management of those cases in which there is marked disturbance of function as heart-block, auricular fibrillation or alternation of the heart.

The following are the general methods in the treatment of cardiac failure:

(*a*) Rest.—Disturbed compensation may be completely restored by rest of the body. In some cases with œdema of the ankles, moderate dilatation of the heart, and irregularity of the pulse, rest in bed and a purge suffice, within a week or ten days, to restore the compensation.

(*b*) Diet.—In acute conditions it is usually well to limit this in amount, especially the fluids. With marked passive congestion liquid diet may be advisable; otherwise small amounts of simple food may be given at short intervals. In any case with dilatation it is well to limit the total daily intake of fluids to 1,500 c. c. A "dry diet" for a few days is sometimes useful.

(*c*) The relief of the embarrassed circulation.

(1) *By Venesection.*—In cases of dilatation, from whatever cause, in mitral or aortic lesions or distention of the right ventricle in emphysema, when signs of venous engorgement are marked and when there is orthopnœa with cyanosis, the abstraction of from 20 to 30 ounces of blood is indicated. This is the occasion in which timely venesection may save the patient's life. It is particularly helpful in the dilated heart of arterio-sclerosis.

(2) *By Depletion through the Bowels.*—This is particularly valuable when dropsy is present. The salines are to be preferred; before breakfast from half an ounce to an ounce and a half of Epsom salts may be given in concentrated form. This usually produces liquid evacuations. The compound jalap powder in half dram (2 gm.) doses, or elaterin (gr. 1/10 0.006 gm.) may be employed for the same purpose. Even when the pulse is very feeble cathartics are well borne, and they deplete the portal system rapidly and efficiently.

(3) *The Use of Remedies Which Stimulate the Heart.*—Of these by far the most important is digitalis, which was introduced into practice by Withering. The indication for its use is weakness of the heart muscle, most especially when auricular fibrillation is present; a contra-indication is a perfectly bal-

anced compensatory hypertrophy. Broken compensation in valvular disease, no matter what the lesion may be, is the signal for its use. It slows and at the same time increases the force of the contractions. It acts on the peripheral arteries, so that a steady and equable flow of blood is maintained in the capillaries, which, after all, is the prime aim and object of the circulation. High blood pressure is not a contra-indication to its use. The beneficial effects are best seen in cases of mitral disease with auricular fibrillation. On theoretical grounds it has been urged that its use is not so advantageous in aortic insufficiency, since it prolongs the diastole and leads to greater distention. This need not be considered, and digitalis is just as serviceable in this as in any other condition associated with progressive dilatation. It may be given as the tincture or the infusion. In cases of cardiac dropsy, from whatever cause, 15 minims (1 c. c.) of the tincture or half an ounce (15 c. c.) of the infusion may be given every three hours for two days, after which the dose may be reduced. The present tendency is to give larger doses. Some prefer the tincture, others the infusion; it is a matter of indifference if the drug is good. The urine of a patient taking digitalis should be carefully estimated each day. As a rule, when its action is beneficial, there is within twenty-four hours an increase in the amount; often the flow is very great. Under its use the dyspnœa is relieved, the dropsy gradually disappears, the pulse becomes firmer, fuller in volume, and sometimes, if it has been intermittent, less irregular.

Ill effects sometimes follow digitalis. There is no such thing as a cumulative action of the drug manifested by sudden symptoms. Toxic effects are seen in the production of nausea and vomiting. The pulse becomes irregular and small, and there may be two beats of the heart to one of the pulse, or alternation of the heart-beat. The urine is reduced in amount. These symptoms subside on the withdrawal of the digitalis, and are rarely serious. There are patients who take digitalis uninterruptedly for years, and feel palpitation and distress if the drug is omitted. There are many cases of auricular fibrillation in which the irregularity is not affected by the digitalis. When the compensation has been re-established the drug may be omitted. When there is dyspnœa on exertion and cardiac distress, from 5 to 10 minims (0.3 to 0.6 c. c.) three times a day may be advantageously given for prolonged periods, but the effects should be carefully watched. In cardiac dropsy digitalis should be used at the outset with a free hand. Small doses should not be given, but from the first half-ounce doses of the infusion every three hours, or from 15 to 20 minims of the tincture. In severe conditions and if there is vomiting it may be necessary to give digitalis or strophanthus intramuscularly. Some of the special fluid preparations of digitalis suitable for hypodermic use should be employed in doses of ♏15—30 (1-2 c. c.). There is some risk in giving these drugs intravenously and this method should be used only in a severe emergency.

Of other remedies strophanthus alone is of service, but as its effect is uncertain when given by mouth it should be administered by intramuscular injection. Doses of 10 to 15 minims (0.6 to 1 c. c.) of the tincture or strophanthin gr. 1/200 (0.00032 gm.) are given and repeated once or twice at intervals of twenty-four hours. The intramuscular is safer than the intravenous administration. Convallaria, caffeine, adonis vernalis and sparteine are recommended as substitutes for digitalis, but their inferiority is so manifest that their use is rarely indicated.

There are two valuable adjuncts in the treatment of myocardial disease—iron and strychnia. When anæmia is a marked feature iron should be given in full doses. Arsenic is an excellent substitute, and one or other, or both, should be administered in all instances of heart trouble when anæmia is present. Strychnia may be given alone or in combination with digitalis in 1 or 2 drop doses of the 1 per cent. solution, or hypodermically in doses of 1/40-1/10 gr. (0.0016 to 0.006 gm.).

Treatment of Special Symptoms.—(*a*) Dropsy.—The improved circulation under the influence of digitalis hastens the interstitial lymph flow and favors resorption of the fluid. Cathartics, by depleting the blood, promote the absorption of the fluid from the lymph spaces and the lymph sacs. These two measures usually suffice to rid the patient of dropsy. In some cases, however, it cannot be relieved, and the legs may be punctured by ordinary aspirating needles, with rubber tubing attached, which may be inserted and left for hours; they often drain away large amounts. If done with care, after a thorough cleaning, and if antiseptic precautions are taken, scarification is a serviceable measure. Canton flannel bandages may be applied on the œdematous legs. In case of marked hydrothorax or ascites tapping is advisable before digitalis is given.

(*b*) Dyspnœa.—The patients are usually unable to lie down and should have a comfortable bed-rest—if possible, one with lateral projections, so that in sleeping the head can be supported as it falls over. The shortness of breath is associated with dilatation, chronic bronchitis, or hydrothorax. The chest should be carefully examined, as hydrothorax is a common cause of shortness of breath. There are cases of mitral regurgitation with recurring hydrothorax, usually on the right side, which is relieved, week by week or month by month, by tapping. For the nocturnal dyspnœa, particularly when combined with restlessness, morphia is invaluable and may be given without hesitation. The value of the calming influence of opium in all conditions of cardiac insufficiency is not sufficiently recognized. There are instances of cardiac dyspnœa unassociated with dropsy, particularly in mitral valve disease, in which nitroglycerin or sodium nitrite is of great service, given in increasing doses. They are especially serviceable in the cases in which the pressure is high.

(*c*) Palpitation and Cardiac Distress.—In instances of great hypertrophy and in the throbbing which is so distressing in some cases of aortic insufficiency, aconite is of service in doses of from 1 to 3 drops every two or three hours. An ice bag over the heart is also of service. For the pains, which are often so marked in aortic lesions, iodide of potassium in 10-grain (0.6 gm.) doses, three times a day, or nitroglycerin may be tried. Small blisters are sometimes advantageous. It must be remembered that an important cause of palpitation and cardiac distress is flatulent distention of the stomach or colon, against which suitable measures must be directed.

(*d*) Gastric Symptoms.—The cases of cardiac insufficiency which do badly and fail to respond to digitalis are most often those in which nausea and vomiting are prominent features. The liver is often greatly enlarged in these cases; there is more or less stasis in the hepatic vessels, and but little can be expected of drugs until the venous engorgement is relieved. If the vomiting persists, it is best to stop food and give small bits of ice, small quantities of milk and lime water, and effervescing drinks. The bowels should be freely moved and drugs given hypodermically, if possible.

(*e*) Cough and Hæmoptysis.—The former is almost a necessary concomitant of cardiac insufficiency, owing to engorgement of the pulmonary vessels and more or less bronchitis. It is allayed by measures directed rather to the heart than to the lungs. Hæmoptysis in chronic valvular disease is sometimes a salutary symptom. An army surgeon, who was invalided during the American civil war on account of hæmoptysis, supposed to be due to tuberculosis, had for many years, in association with mitral insufficiency and enlarged heart, many attacks of hæmoptysis. He was sure that his condition was invariably better after an attack. It is rarely fatal, except in some cases of acute dilatation, and seldom calls for special treatment.

(*f*) Sleeplessness.—One of the most distressing features, even in the stage of compensation, is disturbed sleep. Patients may wake suddenly with throbbing of the heart, often in an attack of nightmare. Subsequently, when the compensation has failed, it is also a worrying symptom. The sleep is broken, restless, and frequently disturbed by frightful dreams. Sometimes a dose of the spirit of chloroform with spirit of camphor will give a quiet night. The compound spirit of ether, Hoffmann's anodyne, though very unpleasant to take, is frequently a great boon in the intermediate period when compensation has partially failed and the patients suffer from restless and sleepless nights. Paraldehyde and chloral hydrate are sometimes serviceable, but it is best, if these fail, to resort to morphia without hesitation.

(*g*) Renal Symptoms.—With broken compensation and lowering of the tension, the urinary secretion is diminished, and the amount may sink to 5 or 6 ounces in the day. Digitalis and strophanthus usually increase the flow. A brisk purge may be followed by augmented secretion. The combination in pill form of digitalis, squill, and calomel will sometimes prove effective when digitalis alone has failed. Diuretin in doses of 15 grains (1 gm.) four times a day is sometimes useful.

The diet in chronic cardiac diseases is often very difficult to regulate. Widal and others have shown that retention of the chlorides is an important factor in cardiac dropsy and heart failure. A milk diet, 2 litres a day, favors their elimination, and in the intervals between attacks a salt free diet as far as possible should be used. Starchy foods and all articles likely to cause flatulency should be forbidden.

In certain cases of weak heart, particularly when it is due to fatty overgrowth, the plans recommended by Oertel and by Schott are advantageous. They are invaluable methods in those forms of heart weakness due to intemperance in eating and drinking and defective bodily exercise. The Oertel plan consists of three parts: First, the reduction in the amount of liquid. This is an important factor in reducing the fat in these patients. It also slightly increases the density of the blood. Oertel allows daily about 36 ounces of liquid, which includes the amount taken with the solid food. Free perspiration is promoted by bathing (if advisable, the Turkish bath), or even by the use of pilocarpine.

The second important point in his treatment is the diet, which should consist largely of proteins. *Morning.*—Cup of coffee or tea, with a little milk, about 6 ounces altogether. Bread, 3 ounces. *Noon.*—Three to 4 ounces of soup, 7 to 8 ounces of roast beef, veal, game, or poultry, salad or a light vegetable, a little fish; 1 ounce of bread or farinaceous pudding; 3 to 6 ounces of fruit for dessert. No liquids at this meal, as a rule, but in hot weather 6 ounces of fluid may be taken. *Afternoon.*—Six ounces of coffee or tea, with as much water. As an indulgence an ounce of bread. *Evening.*—One or 2 soft-boiled eggs, an ounce of bread, perhaps a small slice of cheese, salad, and fruit; 10 to 12 ounces of fluid.

The most important element is graduated exercise, not on the level, but up hills of various grades. The distance walked each day is gradually lengthened. In this way the heart is systematically exercised and strengthened.

The Schott Treatment.—This consists in a combination of baths with exercises. The water has a temperature of from 82°-95° F., and is very richly charged with CO_2. The good effects are claimed to come from a cutaneous excitation, induced by the mineral and gaseous constituents of the bath, and a stimulation of the sensory nerves. There is no question that the bath, in suitable cases, will alter the position of the apex beat, and that it lessens the area of cardiac dulness. Artificial baths can be used with various strengths of sodium chloride and calcium chloride. The exercises, resistance gymnastics, consist in slow movements executed by the patient and resisted by the operator. The best cases for this treatment are those with myocardial weakness. For valvular heart diseases in the stage of broken compensation with dropsy, etc., and in marked arterio-sclerosis, it is not so suitable. The "neurotic heart" is often much benefited.

III. ENDOCARDITIS

Inflammation of the lining membrane of the heart is usually confined to the valves, so that the term is practically synonymous with valvular endocarditis. It occurs in two forms—*acute,* characterized by the presence of vegetations with loss of continuity or of substance in the valve tissues; *chronic,* a slow sclerotic change, resulting in thickening, puckering, and deformity.

I. ACUTE ENDOCARDITIS

This occurs in rare instances as a primary, independent affection; but in the great majority of cases it is an accident in various infective processes, so that in reality the disease does not constitute an etiological entity.

For convenience of description we speak of a simple or benign, and a malignant, ulcerative, or infective endocarditis, between which, however, there is no essential anatomical difference, as all gradations can be traced, and they represent but different degrees of intensity of the same process.

Etiology.—SIMPLE ENDOCARDITIS does not constitute a disease of itself, but is invariably found with some other affection. In 330 cases of rheumatic fever at the Johns Hopkins Hospital there were 110 cases of endocarditis. Bouillaud first emphasized the frequency of the association of simple endocarditis with rheumatic fever. Before him, however, the association had been noticed. Tonsillitis, which in some forms is regarded as a rheumatic affection, may be complicated with endocarditis. Of the specific diseases of childhood it is not uncommon in scarlet fever, while it is rare in measles and chicken-pox. In diphtheria simple endocarditis is rare. In small-pox it is not common. In typhoid fever it occurred six times among 1,500 cases.

In pneumonia both simple and malignant endocarditis are common. In 100 autopsies in this disease at the Montreal General Hospital there were 5 instances of the former. Among 61 cases of endocarditis studied bacteriologically in Welch's laboratory, pneumococci were found in 21 (Marshall). Of 517 fatal cases of acute endocarditis, 115 were in connection with pneumonia—22.3 per cent. (E. F. Wells). Acute endocarditis is by no means rare in pulmonary tuberculosis and was found in 12 cases in 216 post mortems.

In chorea simple warty vegetations are found on the valves in a large majority of all fatal cases, in 62 of 73 collected cases. There is no disease in which, post mortem, acute endocarditis has been so frequently found. And, lastly, simple endocarditis is met with in diseases associated with loss of flesh and progressive debility, as cancer, gout, and nephritis.

A very common form is that which occurs on the sclerotic valves in old heart-disease—the so-called recurring endocarditis.

Malignant or infective endocarditis is met with: (a) As a primary disease of the lining membrane of the heart or of its valves.

(*b*) As a secondary affection in pneumonia, in various specific fevers, in septic processes of all sorts, and most frequently of all as an infection on old sclerotic valves. In a majority of all cases it is a local process in an acute infection. Congenital lesions are very prone to the severer types of endocarditis, particularly affections of the orifice of the pulmonary artery and the margins of the imperfect ventricular septum (C. Robinson).

The existence of a primary endocarditis has been doubted; but there are instances in which persons previously in good health, without any history of affections with which endocarditis is usually associated, have been attacked by a severe infection. In one case death occurred on the sixth day and no lesions were found other than those of malignant endocarditis.

The simple endocarditis of rheumatic fever or of chorea rarely progresses into the malignant form. Of all acute diseases complicated with severe endocarditis pneumonia probably heads the list. Gonorrhœa is a much more common cause than has been supposed. The affection may complicate erysipelas, septicæmia (from whatever cause), and puerperal fever. Malignant endocarditis is very rare in tuberculosis, typhoid fever, diphtheria, dysentery, small-pox, and scarlet fever.

Morbid Anatomy.—Simple endocarditis is characterized by the presence on the valves or on the lining membrane of the chambers of minute vegetations, ranging from 1 to 4 mm. in diameter, with an irregular and fissured surface, giving to them a warty or verrucose appearance. Often these little cauliflower-like excrescences are attached by very narrow pedicles. They are more common on the left side of the heart than the right, and occur on the mitral more often than on the aortic valves. The vegetations are upon the line of closure of the valves—i. e., on the auricular face of the auriculo-ventricular valves, a little distance from the margin, and on the ventricular side of the sigmoid valves, festooned on either half of the valve from the corpora

Arantii. It is rare to see any swelling or macroscopic evidence of infiltration of the endocardium in the neighborhood of even the smallest of the granulations, or of redness, indicative of distention of the vessels, even when they occur upon valves already the seat of sclerotic changes, in which capillary vessels extend to the edges. With time the vegetations may increase greatly in size, but in simple endocarditis the size rarely exceeds that mentioned above. Hirschfelder has shown experimentally that they may form with great rapidity, even in a few hours.

The earliest vegetations consist of elements derived from the blood, and are composed of blood platelets, leucocytes, and fibrin in varying proportions. At a later stage they appear as small outgrowths of connective tissue. The transition of one form into the other can often be followed. The process consists of a proliferation of the endothelial cells and the cells of the subendothelial layer which gradually invade the fresh vegetation, and ultimately entirely replace it. The blood cells and fibrin undergo disintegration and are gradually removed. Even when the vegetation has been entirely converted into connective tissue it is often found at autopsy to be capped with a thin layer of fibrin and leucocytes.

Micro-organisms are generally, even if not invariably, found associated with the vegetations. They tend to be entangled in the granular and fibrillated fibrin or in the older ones to cap the apices.

Subsequent Changes.—(*a*) The vegetations may become organized and the valve restored to a normal state (?). (*b*) The process may extend, and a simple may become an ulcerative endocarditis. (*c*) The vegetations may be broken off and carried in the circulation to distant parts. (*d*) The vegetations become organized and disappear, but they initiate a nutritive change in the valve tissue which ultimately leads to sclerosis, thickening, and deformity. The danger in any case of simple endocarditis is not immediate, but remote, and consists in this perversion of the normal processes of nutrition which results in sclerosis of the valves.

A gradual transition from the simple to a more severe affection, to which the name malignant or ulcerative endocarditis has been given, may be traced. Practically in every case of ulcerative endocarditis vegetations are present. In this form the loss of substance in the valve is more pronounced, the deposition—thrombus formation—from the blood is more extensive, and the micro-organisms are present in greater number and often show increased virulence. Ulcerative endocarditis is often found in connection with heart valves already the seat of chronic proliferative and sclerotic changes.

In this form there is much loss of substance, which may be superficial and limited to the endocardium, or, what is more common, it involves deeper structures, and not very infrequently leads to perforation of a valve, the septum, or even of the heart itself. The affected valve shows necrosis, with more or less loss of substance; the tissue is devoid of preserved nuclei and presents a coagulated appearance. Upon it a mixture of blood platelets, fibrin and leucocytes enclosing masses of micro-organisms are found. The subjacent tissue often shows sclerotic thickening and always infiltration with exuded cells.

Parts Affected.—The following figures, taken from the Goulstonian lectures (Osler) give an approximate estimate of the frequency with which in 209 cases different parts of the heart were affected in malignant endocarditis:

Aortic and mitral valves together, in 41; aortic valves alone, in 53; mitral valves alone, in 77; tricuspid in 19; the pulmonary valves in 15; and the heart walls in 33. In 9 instances the right heart alone was involved, in most cases the auriculo-ventricular valves.

Mural endocarditis is seen most often at the upper part of the septum of the left ventricle. Next in order is the endocarditis of the left auricle on the postero-external wall. The vegetations may extend along the intima of the pulmonary artery into the hilum of the lung. A common result of the ulceration is the production of valvular aneurism. In three fourths of the cases the affected valves present old sclerotic changes. The process may extend to the aorta, producing extensive endarteritis with multiple acute aneurisms.

ASSOCIATED LESIONS.—The associated changes are those of the primary disease, those due to embolism, and the changes in the myocardium. In the endocarditis of septic processes there is the local lesion—an acute necrosis, a suppurative wound, or puerperal disease. In many cases the lesions are those of pneumonia, rheumatism, or other febrile processes.

The changes due to *embolism* constitute the most striking features, but it is remarkable that in some instances, even with endocarditis of a markedly ulcerative character, there may be no trace of embolic processes. The infarcts may be few in number—only one or two, perhaps, in the spleen or kidney—or they may exist in hundreds throughout various parts of the body. They may present the ordinary appearance of red or white infarcts of a suppurative character. They are most common in the spleen and kidneys, though they may be numerous in the brain, and in many cases are very abundant in the intestines. In right sided endocarditis there may be infarcts in the lungs. In many of the cases there are innumerable miliary abscesses. Acute suppurative meningitis was met with in 5 of 23 of the Montreal cases, and in over 10 per cent. of the 209 cases analyzed in the literature. Acute suppurative parotitis may occur. Lastly, as Romberg pointed out, the accompanying myocarditis plays an important rôle. The valvular insufficiency in an acute endocarditis is probably not due to the row of little vegetations, but to the associated myocarditis, which interferes with the proper closure of the orifice.

Bacteriology.—No distinction in the micro-organisms found in the two forms of endocarditis can be made. In both, cocci—streptococci, staphylococci, pneumococci, and gonococci—are the most frequent bacteria. More rarely, especially in the simple vegetative endocarditis, the bacilli of tuberculosis, typhoid fever, and anthrax have been encountered. The colon bacillus has also been found, and Howard described a case of malignant endocarditis due to an attenuated form of the diphtheria bacillus. Marshall in 61 cases found the pneumococci in 21, streptococci alone or with other bacteria in 26, staphylococcus pyogenes aureus in 12. The meningococcus may cause endocarditis. Combined infections are not uncommon. In the chronic infective form the *Streptococcus viridans* is a common organism (Libman).

As a rule no organisms are found in the simple endocarditis in many chronic diseases, as carcinoma, tuberculosis, nephritis, etc. They may have been present and died out, or the lesions may be caused by the toxins.

Symptoms.—Neither the clinical course nor the physical signs of SIMPLE ENDOCARDITIS are in any respect characteristic. The great majority of the cases are latent and there is no indication whatever of cardiac mischief. Endocarditis is frequently found post mortem in persons in whom it was not suspected during life. There are certain features, however, by which its presence is indicated with a degree of probability. The patient, as a rule, does not complain of any pain or cardiac distress. In a case of rheumatic fever, for example, the symptoms to excite suspicion would be increased rapidity of the heart, perhaps slight irregularity, and an increase in the fever, without aggravation of the arthritis. Rows of tiny vegetations on the mitral or on the aortic segments seem a trifling matter to excite fever, and it is difficult in the endocarditis of febrile processes to say definitely in every instance that an increase in the fever depends upon this complication; but a study of the recurring endocarditis—which is of the warty variety, consisting of minute beads on old sclerotic valves—shows that the process may be associated, for weeks or months, with slight fever ranging from 100° to 102½°. Palpitation may be a marked feature and is a symptom upon which certain authors lay great stress.

The *diagnosis* rests upon physical signs, which are notoriously uncertain. The presence of a murmur at one or other of the cardiac areas in a case of fever is often taken as proof of the existence of endocarditis—a common mistake which has arisen from the fact that a murmur is common to it and to a number of other conditions. At first there may be only a slight roughening of the first sound, which may gradually increase to a distinct murmur. The apex systolic bruit is probably more often the result of a myocarditis. It may not be present in the endocarditis of such chronic maladies as tuberculosis and carcinoma, since in them the muscle involvement is less common (Krehl). Reduplication and accentuation of the pulmonic second sound are frequently present.

It is difficult to give a satisfactory clinical picture of MALIGNANT ENDOCARDITIS because the modes of onset are so varied and the symptoms so diverse. Arising in the course of some other disease, there may be simply an intensification of the fever or a change in its character. In a majority of the cases there are present certain general features, such as irregular pyrexia, sweating, delirium, and gradual failure of strength.

Embolic processes may give special characters, such as delirium, coma, or paralysis from involvement of the brain or its membranes, pain in the side and local peritonitis from infarction of the spleen, bloody urine from implication of the kidneys, impaired vision from retinal hæmorrhage and suppuration, and even gangrene in various parts from the distribution of the emboli.

Two special types are recognized—the septic or pyæmic and the typhoid. In some the cardiac symptoms are most prominent, while in others the main symptoms are those of an acute affection of the nervous system.

The *septic type* is met with usually in connection with an external wound, the puerperal process, or an acute necrosis or gonorrhœa. There are rigors, sweats, irregular fever, and all of the signs of septic infection. The heart symptoms may be completely masked by the general condition, and attention called to them only on the occurrence of embolism. In many cases the features are those of a severe septicæmia, and the organisms may be isolated from the blood. Optic neuritis is not uncommon, and was present in 15 cases of chronic septic endocarditis examined by Faulkner, and in four of these recurrent retinal hæmorrhages were present.

The *typhoid type* is by far the most common and is characterized by a less irregular temperature, early prostration, delirium, somnolence, and coma, relaxed bowels, sweating, which may be of a most drenching character, petechial and other rashes, and occasionally parotitis. The heart symptoms may be completely overlooked, and in some instances the most careful examination has failed to discover a murmur.

Under the *cardiac group,* as suggested by Bramwell, may be considered those cases in which patients with chronic valve disease are attacked with marked fever and evidence of recent endocarditis. Many such cases present symptoms of the pyæmic and typhoid character and run a most acute course. In others there may be only slight fever or even after a period of high fever recovery takes place.

In what may be termed the *cerebral group* of cases the clinical picture may simulate a meningitis. There may be acute delirium or, as in three of the Montreal cases, the patient may be brought into the hospital unconscious.

Certain special symptoms may be mentioned. The fever is not always of a remittent type, but may be high and continuous. Petechial rashes are very common and render the similarity very strong to certain cases of typhoid and cerebro-spinal fever. In one case the disease was thought to be hæmorrhagic small-pox. Erythematous rashes are not uncommon. The sweating may be most profuse, even exceeding that which occurs in pulmonary tuberculosis and malaria. Diarrhœa is not necessarily associated with embolic lesions in the intestines. Jaundice has been observed, and cases are on record which were mistaken for acute yellow atrophy.

The heart symptoms may be entirely latent and are not found unless a careful search be made. Instances are recorded by careful observers in which the examination of the heart has been negative. Cases with chronic valve disease usually present no difficulty in diagnosis.

The course is varied, depending largely upon the nature of the primary trouble. Except in the disease grafted upon chronic valvulitis the course is rarely extended beyond five or six weeks. The most rapidly fatal case on record is described by Eberth, the duration of which was scarcely two days.

Subacute Bacterial Endocarditis.—Due particularly to the work of Libman we recognize that these cases are much more common than was supposed. Organisms of the *Streptococcus viridans* group are often found. A special feature is that the patients may become bacteria-free. The prominent features given by Libman are: (1) Marked progressive anæmia, (2) brown pigmentation of the face, (3) marked renal disease, (4) marked splenic enlargement and (5) endocarditic symptoms, such as fever, embolism, arthritis and petechiæ. The cardiac features may be (1) those of any form of valvular disease and (2) those due largely to embolism. The renal changes are especially in the glomeruli and are often embolic. Renal insufficiency is a common cause of death. The anæmia is of the secondary type and usually the leucocytes are normal or diminished. Tenderness over the sternum is a special feature and may be most marked in the bacteria-free stage. The course may be prolonged, the blood may become bacteria-free and some patients recover. In such cases the splenic enlargement may lead to an error in diagnosis.

Chronic Infective Endocarditis.—This is almost always engrafted on an old, sometimes an unrecognized, valve lesion. At first fever is the only symptom; in a few cases there have been chills at onset or recurring chills may arouse the suspicion of malaria. The patient may keep at work for months with a daily rise of temperature, or perhaps an occasional sweat. The heart features may be overlooked. The murmur of the old valve lesion may show no change, and even with the most extensive disease of the mitral cusps the heart's action may be little disturbed. For months—six, eight, ten, even thirteen!—fever and progressive weakness may be the only symptoms. These are the cases in which, with recurring chills, the diagnosis of malaria is made. With involvement of the aortic segments the signs of a progressive lesion are more common. Embolic features are not common, occurring only toward the close. Ephemeral *cutaneous nodes,* red raised painful spots on the skin of hands or feet and lasting a few days, rarely occur except in this form. Post mortem a remarkable vegetative endocarditis has been found, involving usually the mitral valves, sometimes with much encrusting of the chordæ tendineæ, and large irregular firm vegetations quite different to those of the ordinary ulcerative form. In some cases the aortic and tricuspid segments are involved, and the vegetations may extend to the walls of the heart.

Diagnosis.—In many cases this is very difficult; in others, with marked embolic symptoms, it is easy. From simple endocarditis it is readily distinguished, though confusion occasionally occurs in the transitional stage, when a simple is developing into a malignant form. The constitutional symptoms are of a graver type, the fever is higher, rigors are common, and septic symptoms occur. Perhaps a majority of the cases not associated with puerperal processes or bone disease are confounded with typhoid fever. A differential diagnosis may be impossible, particularly when we consider that in typhoid fever infarctions and parotitis may occur. The diarrhœa and abdominal tenderness may also be present, which with the stupor and progressive asthenia make a picture not to be distinguished from this disease. Points which may guide us are: The more abrupt onset in endocarditis, the absence of any regularity of the pyrexia in the early stage and the cardiac pain. Oppression and shortness of breath may be early symptoms in malignant endocarditis. Rigors, too, are not uncommon. There is a marked leucocytosis in infective endocarditis. Between pyæmia and malignant endocarditis there are practically no differential features, for the disease really constitutes an *arterial pyæmia* (Wilks). In the acute cases resembling malignant fevers the diagnosis of typhus, typhoid, cerebro-spinal fever, or even of hæmorrhagic smallpox may be made. The intermittent pyrexia, occurring for weeks or months, has led to the diagnosis of malaria, but this disease can be excluded by the blood examination. Blood cultures aid greatly in the diagnosis.

The cases usually terminate fatally. The instances of recovery are the subacute forms and the recurring endocarditis developing on old sclerotic valves in chronic heart disease.

Treatment.—We know no measures by which in rheumatic fever, chorea, or the eruptive fevers endocarditis can be prevented. As it is probable that many cases arise, particularly in children, in mild forms of these diseases, it is well to insist upon rest and quiet, and to bear in mind that of all complications an acute endocarditis, though in its immediate effects harmless, is perhaps the most serious. This statement is enforced by the observations of Sibson that on a system of absolute *rest* the proportion of cases of rheumatic fever attacked by endocarditis was less than of those who were not so treated. It is doubtful whether in rheumatic fever the salicylates have an influence in reducing the liability to endocarditis. Considering the extremely grave after results of simple endocarditis in children, the question arises whether it is possible to do anything to avert the onset of progressive sclerosis of the affected valve. Catŏn recommends a systematic plan of treatment: (1) Prolonged rest in bed for three months; (2) a series of small blisters over the heart; and (3) iodide of potassium in moderate doses for many months. If there is much vascular excitement aconite may be given and an ice bag placed over the heart. The treatment of malignant endocarditis is practically that of septicæmia—useless and hopeless in a majority of the cases. Blood cultures should be taken as soon as possible and a vaccine prepared. Horder and others have reported good results. Personally we have not seen a successful case.

II. CHRONIC ENDOCARDITIS

Definition.—A sclerosis of the valves leading to shrinking, thickening, and adhesion of the cusps, often with the deposition of lime salts, with shortening and thickening of the chordæ tendineæ, leading to insufficiency and to narrowing of the orifice. It may be primary, but is oftener secondary to acute endocarditis, particularly the rheumatic form.

Etiology.—It is a mistake to regard every case of sclerotic valve as a sequel to an acute endocarditis. It is long ago since Roy and Adami called attention to the possibility that sclerosis of the valve segments might be a sequel of high pressure. The preliminary endocarditis may be a factor in weakening the valve, the progressive thickening of which may be a direct consequence of the strain. As age advances the valves begin to lose their pliancy, show slight sclerotic changes and foci of atheroma and calcification. The poisons of the specific fevers may initiate the change. A very important factor in the case of the aortic valves is *syphilis.* The strain of prolonged and heavy muscular exertion may play a part. In the aortic segments it may be only the valvular part of a general arterio-sclerosis.

The *frequency* with which chronic endocarditis is met with may be gathered from the following figures: In the statistics, from 12,000 to 14,000 autopsies, reported from Dresden, Würzburg, and Prague, the percentage ranged from four to nine. The relative frequency of involvement of the various valves is thus given in the collected statistics of Parrot: The mitral orifice in 621, the aortic in 380, the tricuspid in 46, and the pulmonary in 11. This gives 57 instances in the right to 1,001 in the left heart.

Morbid Anatomy.—Vegetations in the form in which they occur in acute endocarditis are not present. In the early stage, the edge of the valve is a little thickened and perhaps presents a few small nodular prominences, which in some cases may represent the healed vegetations of the acute process. In the aortic valves the tissue about the corpora Arantii is first affected, producing a slight thickening with an increase in the size of the nodules. The substance of the valve may lose its translucency, and the only change noticeable be a grayish opacity and a slight loss of its delicate tenuity. In the auriculo-ventricular valves these early changes are seen just within the margin and here it is not uncommon to find swellings of a grayish red, somewhat infiltrated appearance, almost identical with the similar structures on the intima of the aorta in arterio-sclerosis. Even early there may be seen yellow or opaque white subintimal fatty degenerated areas. As the sclerotic changes increase, the fibrous tissue contracts and produces thickening and deformity of the segment, the edges of which become round, curled, and incapable of that delicate apposition necessary for perfect closure. An aortic valve, for instance, may be narrowed one fourth or even one third across its face, the most extreme grade of insufficiency being induced without any special deformity and without any narrowing of the orifice. In the auriculo-ventricular segments a simple process of thickening and curling of the edges of the valves, inducing a failure to close without forming any obstruction to the normal course of the blood-flow, is less common. Still, we meet with instances at the mitral orifice, particularly in children, in which the edges of the valves are curled and thickened, so that there is extreme insufficiency without any material narrowing of the orifice. More frequently, as the disease advances, the chordæ tendineæ become thickened, first at the valvular ends and then along their course. The edges of the valves at their angles are gradually drawn together and there is a narrowing of the orifice, leading in the aorta to more or less stenosis and in the left auriculo-ventricular orifice—the two sites most frequently involved—to constriction. Finally, in the sclerotic and necrotic tissues lime salts are deposited and may even reach the deeper structures of the fibrous rings, so that the entire valve becomes a dense calcareous mass with scarcely a remnant of normal tissue. The chordæ tendineæ may gradually become shortened, greatly thickened, and in extreme cases the papillary muscles are implanted directly upon the sclerotic and deformed valve. The apices of the papillary muscles usually show marked fibroid change.

In all stages the vegetations of simple endocarditis may be present, and the severer, ulcerative forms often attack these sclerotic valves.

Chronic *mural* endocarditis produces cicatricial like patches of a grayish white appearance which are sometimes seen on the muscular trabeculæ of the ventricle or in the auricles. It often occurs with myocarditis.

The endocarditis of the fetus is usually of the sclerotic form and involves the valves of the right more frequently than those of the left side.

IV. CHRONIC VALVULAR DISEASE

GENERAL INTRODUCTION

Effects of Valve Lesions.—The general influence on the work of the heart may be briefly stated as follows: The sclerosis induces insufficiency or stenosis, which may exist separately or in combination. The narrowing retards in a measure the normal outflow and the insufficiency permits the blood current to take an abnormal course. The result in the former case is difficulty in the expulsion of the contents of the chamber through the narrow orifice; in the other, the overfilling of a chamber by blood flowing into it from an improper source as in mitral insufficiency, when the left auricle receives blood both from the pulmonary veins and from the left ventricle. In both instances the effect is dilatation of a chamber, and to expel the normal amount of blood from a dilated chamber a relatively greater amount of energy is required, which by various adjustments the muscle is stimulated to do.

The cardiac mechanism is fully prepared to meet ordinary grades of dilatation which constantly occur during sudden exertion. A man, for instance, at the end of a hundred yard race has his right chambers greatly dilated and his reserve cardiac power worked to its full capacity. The slow progress of the sclerotic changes brings about a gradual, not an abrupt, insufficiency, and the moderate dilatation which follows is at first overcome by the exercise of the ordinary reserve strength of the heart muscle. Gradually a new factor is

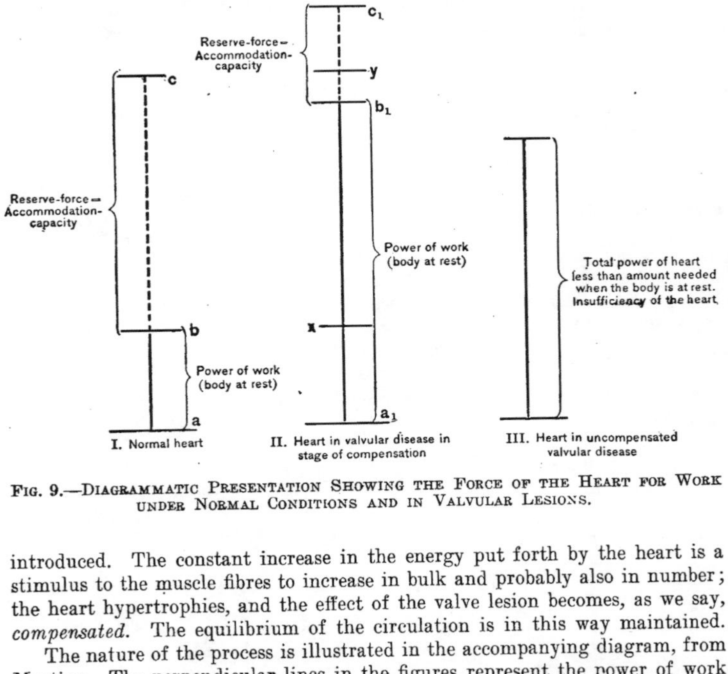

Fig. 9.—Diagrammatic Presentation Showing the Force of the Heart for Work under Normal Conditions and in Valvular Lesions.

introduced. The constant increase in the energy put forth by the heart is a stimulus to the muscle fibres to increase in bulk and probably also in number; the heart hypertrophies, and the effect of the valve lesion becomes, as we say, *compensated*. The equilibrium of the circulation is in this way maintained.

The nature of the process is illustrated in the accompanying diagram, from Martius. The perpendicular lines in the figures represent the power of work of the heart. While the muscle in the healthy heart (Diagram I) has at its disposal the maximal force, *a c*, it carries on its work under ordinary circumstances (when the body is at rest) with the force *a b* and *b c* is the reserve force by which the heart accommodates itself to greater exertion.

If there be a gross valvular lesion, the force required to do the ordinary work of the heart (at rest) becomes very much increased (Diagram II). But in spite of this enormous call for force, insufficiency of the muscle does not necessarily result, for the working force required is still within the limits of the maximal power of the heart, a_1 b_1 being less than a_1 c_1. The muscle accommodates itself to the new conditions by making its reserve force mobile. If nothing further occurred, this could not be permanently maintained, for there would be left over for emergencies only the small reserve force, b_1 y. Even when at rest the heart would be using continuously almost its entire maximal force. Any slight exertion requiring more extra force than that represented by the small value b_1 y (say the effort required on walking or on going upstairs) would bring the heart to the limit of its working power, and palpitation and dyspnœa would appear. Such a condition does not last long. The working power of the heart gradually increases. More and more exertion can be borne without causing dyspnœa, for *the heart hypertrophies*. Finally, a new, more or less permanent condition is attained, in that the hypertrophied heart possesses the maximal force, a_1 c_1. Owing to the increase in volume of the heart muscle, the total force of the heart is greater *absolutely* than that of the normal heart by the amount y c_1. It is, however, *relatively* less efficient, for its reserve force is much less than that of the healthy heart. Its capacity for accommodating itself to unusual calls upon it is accordingly permanently diminished.

Turning now to the disturbances of compensation, it is to be distinctly borne in mind that any heart, normal or diseased, can become insufficient whenever a call upon it exceeds its maximal working capacity. The liability to such disturbance will depend, above all, upon the accommodation limits of the heart—the less the width of the latter, the easier will it be to go beyond the heart's efficiency. A comparison of Diagrams I and II will immediately make it clear that the heart in valvular disease will much earlier become insufficient than the heart of a healthy individual. It is obvious that the heart in valvular disease, on account of its small amount of reserve force, has to do maximal or nearly maximal work far more frequently than does the normal heart. The power of the heart may become decreased to the amount necessary simply to carry on the work of the heart when the body is at rest, or it may cease to be sufficient even for this. The reserve force gained through the compensatory process may be entirely lost (Diagram III). If the loss be only temporary, the exhausted heart muscle quickly recovering, the condition is spoken of as a "disturbance of compensation." The term "loss of compensation" is reserved for the condition in which the disturbance is continuous.

AORTIC INSUFFICIENCY

Insufficiency of the aortic valves arises either from inability of the valve segments to close an abnormally large orifice or more commonly from disease of the segments themselves. This best-defined and most easily recognized of valvular lesions was first carefully studied by Corrigan, whose name it sometimes bears.

Etiology and Morbid Anatomy.—It is more frequent in males than in females, affecting chiefly men at the middle period of life. The ratio which it bears to other valve diseases has been given as from 30 to 50 per cent.

There are six groups of cases: I. Those due to *congenital malformation,* particularly fusion of two of the cusps—most commonly those behind which the coronary arteries are given off. It is probable that an aortic orifice may be competent with this bicuspid state of the valves, but a great danger is the liability of these malformed segments to sclerotic endocarditis. Of 17 cases all presented sclerotic changes, and the majority of them had, during life, the clinical features of chronic heart-disease.

II. The *endocarditic group.* Endocarditis may produce an acute insufficiency by ulceration and destruction of the valves; the aortic valves may be completely eroded away. The valvulitis of rheumatic fever, while more rarely aortic, is common enough, and the insufficiency is caused by nodular excrescences at the margins or in the valves, which may ultimately become calcified; more often it induces a slow sclerosis of the valves with adhesions, causing also some degree of narrowing.

III. *Syphilis.*—This is probably the most important cause, especially in young and middle aged patients. The spirochætes may be found in the valves. The process frequently involves the aorta also. In some cases it causes a localized process at the root of the aorta which may involve the valves secondarily or cause dilatation of the aortic ring with relative insufficiency. Some of the supposed cases of cure of syphilitic aortic endocarditis may be instances of the latter.

IV. The *arterio-sclerotic group.* A common cause of insufficiency is a slow, progressive sclerosis of the segments, resulting in a curling of the edges. It may be associated with general arterio-sclerosis. The condition of the valves is such as has been described in chronic endocarditis. It may be noted, however, how slight a grade of curling may produce serious insufficiency. Associated with the valve disease is, in a majority of cases, a more or less advanced arterio-sclerosis of the arch of the aorta, one serious effect of which may be a narrowing of the orifices of the coronary arteries. The sclerotic changes are often combined with atheroma which may exist at the attached margin of the valves without inducing insufficiency. In other instances insufficiency may result from a calcified spike projecting from the aortic attachment into the body of the valve, and so preventing its proper closure. Anatomically one can usually recognize the arterio-sclerotic variety by the smooth surface, the rounded edges, and the absence of excrescences.

V. Insufficiency may be induced by *rupture of a segment*—a very rare event in healthy valves, but not uncommon in disease, either from excessive effort during heavy lifting or from the ordinary strain on a valve eroded and weakened by ulcerative endocarditis.

VI. *Relative insufficiency,* due to dilatation of the aortic ring and adjacent arch, is not very frequent. It occurs in extensive arterial sclerosis of the ascending portion of the arch with great dilatation just above the valves. The valve segments are usually involved with the arterial coats, but the changes in them may be very slight. In aneurism just above the aortic ring relative insufficiency of the valve may be present.

It would appear from the careful measurements of Beneke that the aortic orifice, which at birth is 20 mm., increases gradually with the growth of the heart until at one and twenty it is about 60 mm. At this it remains until the age of forty, beyond which date there is a gradual increase in the size up to the age of eighty, when it may reach from 68 to 70 mm. There is thus at the period in which sclerosis of the valve is most common a physiological tendency toward the production of a relative insufficiency.

The insufficiency may be combined with various grades of narrowing, particularly in the endocarditic group. In a majority of the cases of the arterio-sclerotic form there is no stenosis. On the other hand, with aortic stenosis there is almost without exception some grade, however slight, of insufficiency.

Non-valvular insufficiency may occur when there is a stretching of the aortic ring in connection with dilatation of the ascending portion of the arch. Whether insufficiency occurs apart from this in dilatation of the left ventricle has been much discussed—a relative incompetency similar to that which occurs at the pulmonary orifice. Cases are reported in which transient diastolic murmurs have occurred with dilatation of the heart, of which Anders reported and collected corroborative cases. Some years ago J. B. MacCallum, whose untimely death was a great loss to science, described a sphincter-like band of muscle encircling the opening of the left ventricle into the aorta, and in these cases the relaxation of this ring muscle may be associated with insufficiency of the valve.

Effects.—The direct effect of aortic insufficiency is the regurgitation of blood from the artery into the ventricle, causing an overdistention of the cavity and a reduction of the blood column; that is, a relative anæmia in the arterial tree. The amount returning varies with the size of the opening. The double blood flow into the left ventricle causes dilatation of the chamber, and finally hypertrophy, the grade depending upon the lesion. In this way the valve defect is compensated, and, as with each ventricular systole a larger amount of blood is propelled into the arterial system, the regurgitation of a certain amount during diastole does not, for a time at least, seriously impair the nutrition of the peripheral parts. For a time at least there is little or no resistance offered to the blood flow from the auricle—the ventricle accommodates itself readily to the extra amount, and there is no disturbance in the lesser circulation. In acute cases, on the other hand, with rapid destruction of the segments, there may be the most intense dyspnœa and even profuse hæmoptysis. In this lesion dilatation and hypertrophy reach their most extreme limit. The heaviest hearts on record are described in connection with this affection. The so-called bovine heart, *cor bovinum,* may weigh 35 or 40 ounces, or even, as in a case of Dulles's, 48 ounces. The dilatation is usually extreme and is in marked contrast to the condition of the chamber in cases of pure aortic stenosis. The papillary muscles may be greatly flattened. The mitral valves are usually not seriously affected, though the edges may present slight sclerosis, and there is often relative insufficiency, owing to distention of the mitral ring. Dilatation and hypertrophy of the left auricle are common, and secondary enlargement of the right heart occurs in all cases of long standing. In the arterio-sclerotic group there is an ever present possibility of narrowing of the orifices of the coronary arteries or an extension of the sclerosis to their branches, leading to fibroid myocarditis. In the endocarditis cases the intima of the aorta may be perfectly smooth. The so-called dynamic dilatation of the arch is best seen in these cases. A young girl, whose case had been reported as one of aneurism, had forcible pulsation and a tumor which could be grasped above the sternum—post mortem the innominate artery did not admit the little finger and the arch was not dilated!

Although the coronary arteries, as shown by Martin and Sedgwick, are filled during the ventricular systole, the circulation in them must be embarrassed in aortic insufficiency. They must miss the effect of the blood pressure in the sinuses of Valsalva during the elastic recoil of the arteries, which surely aids in keeping the coronary vessels full. The arteries of the body usually present more or less sclerosis consequent upon the strain which they undergo during the forcible ventricular systole.

Symptoms.—The condition is often discovered accidentally in persons who have not presented any features of cardiac disease.

Headache, dizziness, flashes of light, and a feeling of faintness on rising quickly are among the earliest symptoms. Palpitation and cardiac distress on slight exertion are common. Long before any signs of failing compensation *pain* may be a marked feature. It is extremely variable in its manifestations. It may be of a dull, aching character confined to the præcordia but more frequently it is sharp and radiating, and transmitted up the neck and down the arms, particularly the left. Disease of the aorta is often responsible for the pain. Attacks of angina pectoris are more frequent in this than in any other valvular disease. Anæmia is common, much more so than in aortic stenosis or mitral affections.

As compensation fails more serious symptoms are shortness of breath and œdema of the feet. The attacks of dyspnœa are liable to come on at night, and the patient has to sleep with his head high or even in a chair. Cyanosis is rare. It is most commonly due to complicating valve disease, or it is stated that it may result from bulging of the septum ventriculorum and encroachment upon the right ventricle. Of respiratory symptoms cough is common, due to the congestion of the lungs or œdema. Hæmoptysis is less frequent than in mitral disease but there are cases in which it is profuse and believed to be due to tuberculosis of the lungs. General dropsy is not common, but œdema of the feet may occur early and is sometimes due to the anæmia, sometimes to the venous stasis, at times to both. Unless there is coexisting mitral disease, it is rare for the patient to die with general anasarca. Sudden death is frequent; more so than in other valvular diseases. As compensation fails the patient takes to bed and slight irregular fever, associated usually with a recurring endocarditis, is not uncommon toward the close. Embolic symptoms are not infrequent—pain in the splenic region with enlargement of the organ, hæmaturia, and in some cases paralysis. Distressing dreams and disturbed sleep are more common in this than in other forms of valvular disease.

Mental symptoms are often seen with this lesion or the patients may be irritable and difficult to manage; toward the close there may be delirium, hallucinations, and morbid impulses. It is important to bear this in mind, for patients occasionally display suicidal tendencies.

Physical Signs.—*Inspection* shows a wide area of forcible impulse with the apex beat in the sixth or seventh interspace, and perhaps as far out as the anterior axillary line. In young subjects the præcordia may bulge. There may be slight visible pulsation in the second right interspace, or, in some acute cases of insufficiency or ulcerative endocarditis, a couple of inches from the sternal margin. In very slight insufficiency there may be little or no enlargement. On *palpation* a thrill, diastolic in time, is occasionally felt, but is not common. The impulse is usually strong and heaving, unless in extreme dilatation, when it is wavy and indefinite. Occasionally two or three interspaces between the nipple line and sternum are depressed with systole as the result of atmospheric pressure. *Percussion* shows a great increase in the area of heart dulness, chiefly downward and to the left.

Auscultation.—A diastolic murmur is heard at the base of the heart and propagated down the sternum. It may be feeble or inaudible at the aortic cartilage, and is usually heard best at midsternum opposite the third costal cartilage or along the left border of the sternum as low as the ensiform cartilage. It is usually soft, blowing in quality, and is prolonged, or "long drawn," as the phrase is. It is produced by the reflux of blood into the ventricle. In some cases it is loudly transmitted to the axilla at the level of the fourth interspace, not by way of the apex. The second sound may be well heard or be replaced by the murmur, or with a dilated arch the second sound may have a ringing metallic or booming quality, and the diastolic murmur is well heard, or even loudest, over the manubrium.

The first sound may be clear at the base; more commonly there is a soft, short, systolic murmur. In the arterio-sclerotic group the systolic bruit is, as a rule, short and soft, while in the endocarditic group, in which the valve segments are united and often covered with calcified vegetations and excrescences, the systolic murmur is rough and may be accompanied by a thrill.

At the apex, or toward it, the diastolic murmur may be faintly heard propagated from the base. With full compensation the first sound is usually clear at the apex; with dilatation there is a loud systolic murmur of relative mitral insufficiency, which may disappear as the dilatation lessens.

Flint Murmur.—A second murmur at the apex, probably produced at the mitral orifice, is not uncommon, to which attention was called by the late Austin Flint. It is of a rumbling, echoing character, occurring in the middle or latter part of diastole, and limited to the apex region. It is similar to, though less intense than, the murmur of mitral stenosis, and may be associated with a palpable thrill. It is probably caused by the impinging of the regurgitant current from the aortic orifice on the large, anterior flap of the mitral valve, so as to cause interference with the entrance of blood at the time of auricular contraction. The condition is thus essentially the same as in a moderate mitral stenosis. This murmur is present in about half of the cases of uncomplicated aortic insufficiency (Thayer). It is very variable, disappearing and reappearing again without apparent cause. The sharp, first sound and abrupt systolic shock, so common in true mitral stenosis, are rarely present, while the pulse is characteristic of aortic insufficiency.

Arteries.—The examination of the arteries in aortic insufficiency is of great value. Visible pulsation is more commonly seen in the peripheral vessels in this than in any other condition. The carotids may be seen to throb forcibly, the temporals to dilate, and the brachials and radials to expand with each heart-beat. With the ophthalmoscope the retinal arteries are seen to pulsate. Not only is the pulsation evident, but the characteristic jerking quality is apparent. The throbbing carotids may lead to the diagnosis of aneurism. In many cases the pulsation can be seen in the suprasternal notch and the abdominal aorta may lift the epigastrium with each systole. In severe cases with great hypertrophy, particularly if anæmia is present, the vascular throbbing may be of an extraordinary character, jarring the whole front of the chest, causing the head to nod, and even the tongue may throb rhythmically. To be mentioned with this is the *capillary pulse,* met very often in aortic insufficiency, and best seen in the finger nails or by drawing a line upon the forehead, when the margin of hyperæmia on either side alternately blushes and pales. In extreme grades the face or the hand may blush visibly at each systole. It is met with also in profound anæmia, occasionally in neurasthenia, and in health in conditions of great relaxation of the peripheral arteries. Pulsation may also be present in the peripheral veins. On palpation the characteristic collapsing or Corrigan pulse is felt. The pulse wave strikes the finger forcibly with a quick jerking impulse, and immediately recedes or collapses. The characters of this are sometimes best appreciated by grasping the arm at the wrist and holding it up. The pulse may be retarded or delayed—i. e., there is an appreciable interval between the beat of the heart and the pulsation in the radial artery, which varies according to the extent of the regurgitation. Occasionally in the carotid artery the second sound is distinctly audible when absent at the aortic cartilage. Indeed, according to Broadbent, it is at the carotid that we must listen for the second aortic sound, for when heard it indicates that the regurgitation is small in amount, and is consequently a

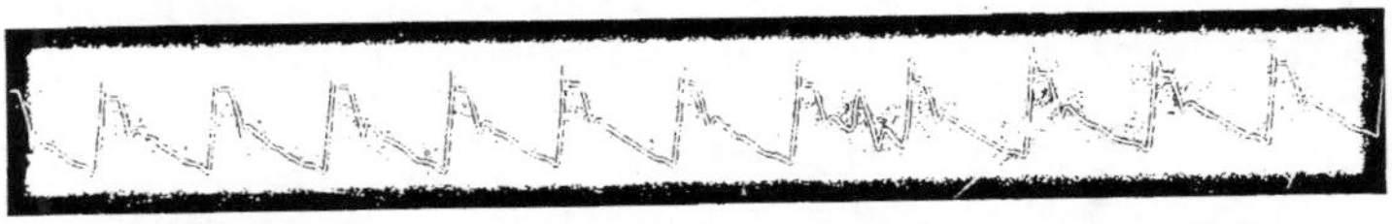

FIG 10.—PULSE TRACING IN AORTIC INSUFFICIENCY; AN EXTRA SYSTOLE IS SHOWN.

favorable prognostic element. In the larger arteries a systolic thud or shock may be heard and sometimes a double murmur. The systolic pressure is often high and the diastolic much decreased. The sphygmographic tracing is very characteristic. The high ascent, the sharp top, the quick drop in which the dicrotic notch and wave are very slightly marked.

The studies of Stewart and of W. G. MacCallum have shown that in aortic insufficiency the low position of the dicrotic notch in the descending arm of the pulse wave and the characteristic collapsing character of the pulse are not due, as was formerly supposed, to the regurgitation in the left ventricle, but to the dilatation of the peripheral arteries, which is a sort of protective adaptation under the vaso-motor influences.

Aortic insufficiency may be fully *compensated* for years. Persons do not necessarily suffer any inconvenience, and the condition is often found accidentally. So long as the hypertrophy equalizes the valvular defect there may be no symptoms and the individual may even take moderately heavy exercise without experiencing sensations of distress. The cases which last the longest are those in which the insufficiency follows endocarditis and is not a part of a general arterio-sclerosis. The age at the time of onset is a most important consideration, as in youth the lesion is not often from sclerosis, and the coronary arteries are unaffected. Coexistent lesions of the mitral valves tend to disturb compensation early. Pure aortic insufficiency is consistent with years of average health and with a tolerably active life.

With the onset of myocardial changes, with increasing degeneration of the arteries, particularly with a progressive sclerosis of the arch and involvement of the orifices of the coronary arteries, the compensation becomes disturbed.

The insufficiency of the circulation is seen first on the arterial side in occasional faintings, giddiness, or mental irritability and enfeeblement; later there may be mitral regurgitation and embarrassment of the right side of the heart with its usual features. In advanced cases the changes about the aortic ring may be associated with alterations in the cardiac nerves and ganglia and so introduce an important factor.

AORTIC STENOSIS

Narrowing or stricture of the aortic orifice is not nearly so common as insufficiency. The two conditions, as already stated, may occur together, however, and probably in almost every case of stenosis there is some leakage.

Etiology and Morbid Anatomy.—In the milder grades there is adhesion between the segments, which are so stiffened that during systole they cannot be pressed back against the aortic wall. The process of cohesion between the segments may go on without great thickening, and produce a condition in which the orifice is guarded by a comparatively thin membrane, on the aortic face of which may be seen the primitive raphes separating the sinuses of Valsalva. In some instances this membrane is so thin and presents so few traces of atheromatous or sclerotic changes that the condition looks as if it had originated during fetal life. More commonly the valve segments are thickened and rigid, and have a cartilaginous hardness. In advanced cases they may be represented by stiff, calcified masses obstructing the orifice, through which a circular or slit like passage can be seen. The older the patient the more likely it is that the valves will be rigid and calcified.

We may speak of a *relative stenosis* of the aortic orifice when with normal valves and ring the aorta immediately beyond is greatly dilated. A stenosis due to involvement of the aortic ring in sclerotic and calcareous changes without lesion of the valves is referred to by some authors. We have never met with an instance of this kind. A subvalvular stenosis, the result of endocarditis in the mitro-sigmoidean sinus, usually occurs as the result of fetal endocarditis. In comparison with aortic insufficiency, stenosis is rare. It is usually met with at a more advanced period of life than insufficiency, and the most typical cases of it are found associated with extensive calcareous changes in the arterial system in old men.

Owing to the obstruction the ventricle works against increased resistance and its walls become hypertrophied, usually at first with little or no dilatation. We see in this condition the most typical instances of concentric hypertrophy, in which, without much, if any, enlargement of the cavity, the walls are greatly thickened. The systole is prolonged, even as much as twenty-five per cent. There may be no changes in the other cardiac cavities if compensation is well maintained; but with its failure come dilatation, impeded auricular discharge, pulmonary congestion, and increased work for the right heart. The arterial changes are, as a rule, not so marked as in insufficiency, for the walls have not to withstand the impulse of greatly increased blood-wave with each systole. On the contrary, the amount of blood propelled through the narrow orifice may be smaller than normal, though when compensation is fully established the pulse wave may be of medium volume.

Symptoms.—PHYSICAL SIGNS.—*Inspection* may fail to reveal any area of cardiac impulse. Particularly is this the case in old men with rigid chest walls and large emphysematous lungs. Under these circumstances there may be a high grade of hypertrophy without any visible impulse. Even when the apex beat is visible, it may be, as Traube pointed out, feeble and indefinite. In many cases the apex is seen displaced downward and outward, and the impulse looks strong and forcible.

Palpation reveals in many cases a *thrill* at the base of the heart of maximum force in the aortic region. With no other condition do we meet with thrills of greater intensity. The apex beat may not be palpable under the conditions above mentioned, or there may be a slow, heaving, forcible impulse.

Percussion never gives the same wide area of dulness as in aortic insufficiency. The extent of it depends largely on the state of the lungs, whether emphysematous or not.

Auscultation.—A rough systolic murmur, of maximum intensity at the aortic cartilage, and propagated into the great vessels, is the most constant physical sign. One of the last lessons learned by the student is to recognize that a systolic murmur at the aortic area does not necessarily mean obstruc-

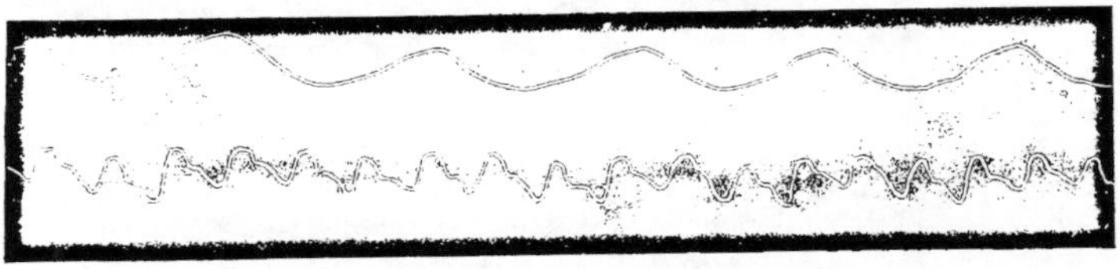

Fig. 11.—Pulse Tracing in Aortic Stenosis.

tion of the orifice. Roughening of the valves, or of the intima of the aorta, and hæmic states are much more frequent causes. In aortic stenosis the murmur often has a much harsher quality, is louder, and is more frequently musical than in the conditions just mentioned. When compensation fails and the ventricle is dilated and feeble, the murmur may be soft and distant. The second sound is rarely heard at the aortic cartilage, owing to the thickening and stiffness of the valve. A diastolic murmur is not uncommon, but in many cases it can not be heard. Occasionally, as noted by W. H. Dickinson, there is a musical murmur of greatest intensity in the region of the apex, due probably to a slight regurgitation at high pressure through the mitral valves. The pulse in pure aortic stenosis is small, usually of good tension, well sustained, regular, and perhaps slower than normal.

The condition may be latent for an indefinite period, as long as the hypertrophy is maintained. Early symptoms are those due to defective blood supply to the brain, dizziness, and fainting. Palpitation, pain about the heart, and anginal symptoms are not so marked as in insufficiency. With myocardial failure, relative insufficiency of the mitral valve is established, and the patient may present all the features of engorgement in the lesser and systemic circulations. Many of the cases in old people, without presenting any dropsy, have symptoms pointing rather to general arterial disease. Cheyne-Stokes breathing is not uncommon with or without uræmia.

Diagnosis.—With an extremely rough or musical systolic murmur of maximum intensity at the aortic region, hypertrophy of the left ventricle, a thrill, and a hard, slow pulse of moderate volume and fairly good tension, which in a tracing gives a curve of slow rise, a broad, well sustained summit and slow decline, a diagnosis of aortic stenosis can be made with some degree of certainty, particularly if the subject is an old man. Seldom is there difficulty in distinguishing the murmur due to anæmia, since it is rarely so intense and is not associated with a thrill or with marked hypertrophy of the left ventricle. In aortic insufficiency a systolic murmur is usually present, but has neither the intensity nor the musical quality, nor is it accompanied by a thrill. With roughening and dilatation of the aorta the murmur may be harsh or musical; but the existence of a second sound, accentuated and ringing in quality, is usually sufficient to differentiate this condition.

MITRAL INSUFFICIENCY

Etiology.—Insufficiency of the mitral valve ensues: (*a*) From changes in the segments whereby they are contracted and shortened, usually combined with changes in the chordæ tendineæ, or with more or less narrowing of the orifice. (*b*) As a result of changes in the muscular walls of the ventricle, either dilatation, so that the valve segments fail to close an enlarged orifice, or changes in the muscular substance, so that the segments are imperfectly coapted during the systole—*muscular insufficiency*. The common lesions producing insufficiency result from endocarditis, which causes a gradual thickening at the edges of the valves, contraction of the chordæ tendineæ, and union of the edges of the segments, so that in a majority of the instances there is not only insufficiency, but some grade of narrowing as well. Except in children, we rarely see the mitral leaflets curled and puckered without narrowing of the orifice. Calcareous plates at the base of the valve may prevent perfect closure of one of the segments. In long-standing cases the entire mitral structures are converted into a firm calcareous ring. From valvular insufficiency the other condition of muscular insufficiency must be carefully distinguished. It is met with in all conditions of extreme dilatation of the left ventricle, and also in weakening of the muscle in prolonged fevers and in anæmia.

Morbid Anatomy.—The effects of insufficiency of the mitral segment upon the heart and circulation are as follows: (*a*) The imperfect closure allows a certain amount of blood to regurgitate from the ventricle into the auricle, so that at the end of auricular diastole this chamber contains not only the blood which it has received from the lungs, but also that regurgitated from the left ventricle. This necessitates dilatation, and, as increased work is thrown upon it in expelling the augmented contents, hypertrophy as well.

(*b*) With each systole of the left auricle a larger volume of blood is forced into the left ventricle, which dilates and subsequently hypertrophies.

(*c*) During the diastole of the left auricle, as blood is regurgitated into it from the left ventricle, the pulmonary veins are less readily emptied. In consequence the right ventricle expels its contents less freely, and in turn becomes hypertrophied and dilated.

(*d*) Finally, the right auricle also is involved, its chamber is enlarged, and its walls are increased in thickness.

(e) The effect upon the pulmonary vessels is to produce dilatation both of the arteries and veins—often in long-standing cases, atheromatous changes; the capillaries are distended, and ultimately the condition of brown induration is produced. Perfect compensation may be effected, chiefly through the hypertrophy of both ventricles, and the effect upon the peripheral circulation may not be manifested for years, as a normal volume of blood is discharged from the left heart at each systole. The time comes, however, when, owing either to increase in the grade of the incompetency or to failure of compensation, the left ventricle is unable to send out its normal volume into the aorta. Then there are overfilling of the left auricle, engorgement in the lesser circulation, embarrassed action of the right heart, and congestion in the systemic veins. For years this somewhat congested condition may be limited to the lesser circulation, but finally the tricuspid valves become incompetent, and the systemic veins are engorged. This leads to the condition of cyanotic induration in the viscera and, when extreme, to dropsical effusion.

Muscular insufficiency, due to impaired nutrition of the mitral and papillary muscles, is rarely followed by such perfect compensation. There may be in acute destruction of the aortic segments an acute dilatation of the left ventricle with relative incompetency of the mitral segments, great dilatation of the left auricle, and intense engorgement of the lungs, under which circumstances profuse hæmorrhage may result. In these cases there is little chance for the establishment of compensation. In cases of hypertrophy and dilatation of the heart, without valvular lesions, the insufficiency of the mitral valve may be extreme and lead to great pulmonary congestion, engorgement of the systemic veins, and a condition of cardiac dropsy, which can not be distinguished by any feature from that of mitral insufficiency due to lesion of the valve itself. In chronic nephritis the left ventricle may gradually fail, leading, in the later stages, to relative insufficiency of the mitral valve, and the production of pulmonary and systemic congestion, similar to that induced by the most extreme grade of lesion of the valve itself. Adherent pericardium, especially in children, may lead to like results.

Symptoms.—During the development of the lesion, unless the insufficiency comes on acutely in consequence of rupture of the valve segment or of ulceration, the compensatory changes go hand in hand with the defect, and there are no subjective symptoms. So, also, in the stage of perfect compensation, there may be the most extreme grade of mitral insufficiency with enormous hypertrophy, yet the patient may not be aware of the existence of heart trouble, and may suffer no inconvenience except perhaps a little shortness of breath on exertion. It is only when the compensation has not been perfectly effected, or, having been so, is broken that the patients begin to be troubled. The symptoms may be divided into two groups:

(a) The minor manifestations while compensation is still good. Patients with extreme insufficiency often have a congested appearance of the face, the lips and ears have a bluish tint, and the venules on the cheeks may be enlarged—signs in many cases very suggestive. In long standing cases, particularly in children, the fingers may be clubbed, and there is shortness of breath on exertion. This is one of the most constant features in mitral insufficiency and may exist for years, even when the compensation is perfect. Owing to the somewhat congested condition of the lungs these patients have a tendency to attacks of bronchitis or hæmoptysis. There may also be palpitation of the heart. As a rule, however, in well balanced lesions in adults, this period of full compensation or latent stage is not associated with symptoms which call the attention to an affection of the heart, and with care the patient may reach old age in comparative comfort without being compelled to curtail seriously his pleasures or his work.

(*b*) Sooner or later comes a period of broken compensation, in which the most intense symptoms are those of venous engorgement. There are palpitation, weak, irregular action of the heart, and signs of dilatation. The irregularity may be due to extra-systoles or auricular fibrillation. Dyspnœa is an especial feature, and there may be cough. A distressing symptom is the cardiac "sleep-start," in which, just as the patient falls asleep, he wakes gasping and feeling as if the heart were stopping. There is usually slight cyanosis, and even a jaundiced tint to the skin. The most marked symptoms are those of venous stasis. The overfilling of the pulmonary vessels accounts in part for the dyspnœa. There is cough, often with bloody or watery expectoration, and the alveolar epithelium containing brown pigment-grains is abundant. Dropsical effusion usually sets in, beginning in the feet and extending to the body and the serous sacs. Right sided hydrothorax may recur and require repeated tapping. The urine is usually scanty and albuminous, and contains tube casts and sometimes blood corpuscles. With judicious treatment compensation may be restored and all the serious symptoms pass away. Patients usually have recurring attacks of this kind, and die with a general dropsy; or there is progressive dilatation of the heart. Sudden death in these cases is rare. Some cases of mitral disease—stenosis and insufficiency—reach what may be called the *hepatic stage,* when all the symptoms are due to the secondary changes in the liver.

Physical Signs.—*Inspection.*—In children the præcordia may bulge and there may be a large area of visible pulsation. The apex beat is to the left of the nipple, in some cases in the sixth interspace, in the anterior axillary line. A localized right ventricle impulse may sometimes be seen below the right costal border in the parasternal line. There may be a wavy impulse in the cervical veins, which are often full, particularly when the patient is recumbent.

Palpation.—A thrill is rare; when present it is felt at the apex, often in a limited area. The force of the impulse may depend largely upon the stage in which the case is examined. In full compensation it is forcible and heaving; when the compensation is disturbed, usually wavy and feeble.

Percussion.—The dulness is increased, particularly in a lateral direction. There is no disease of the valves which produces, in long standing cases, a more extensive transverse area of heart dulness. It does not extend so much upward along the left margin of the sternum as beyond the right margin and to the left of the nipple line.

Auscultation.—At the apex there is a systolic murmur which wholly or partly obliterates the first sound. It is loudest here, and has a blowing, sometimes musical character, particularly toward the latter part. The murmur is transmitted to the axilla and may be heard at the back, in some instances over the entire chest. There are cases in which, as pointed out by Naunyn, the murmur is heard best along the left border of the sternum. Usually at the apex the loudly transmitted second sound may be heard. Occasionally there is also a soft, sometimes a rough or rumbling presystolic murmur. As a rule, in cases of extreme mitral insufficiency from valvular lesion with great hypertrophy of both ventricles, there is heard only a loud blowing murmur during systole. A murmur of mitral insufficiency may vary a great deal according to the position of the patient. In cases of dilatation, particularly when dropsy is present, a soft systolic murmur due to tricuspid regurgitation may be heard at the ensiform cartilage and in the lower sternal region. An important sign is the accentuated pulmonary second sound, heard to the left of the sternum in the second interspace, or over the third left costal cartilage.

The *pulse,* during the period of full compensation, may be full and regular, often of low tension. Usually with the first onset of symptoms it becomes irregular, a feature which then dominates the case throughout. There may be no two beats of equal force or volume. Often after the disappearance of the symptoms of failure of compensation the irregularity of the pulse persists. This is usually due to auricular fibrillation.

The three important physical signs of mitral regurgitation are: (*a*) Systolic murmur of maximum intensity at the apex, propagated to the axilla and heard at the angle of the scapula; (*b*) accentuation of the pulmonary second sound; (*c*) evidence of enlargement of the heart, particularly increase in the transverse diameter, due to hypertrophy of both ventricles.

Diagnosis.—There is rarely any difficulty in the diagnosis of mitral insufficiency. The physical signs are characteristic and distinctive. Two points are to be borne in mind. First, a murmur, systolic in time, and of maximum intensity at the apex, and propagated even to the axilla, does not necessarily indicate mitral insufficiency. There is heard in this region a large group of what are termed accidental murmurs, the precise nature of which is doubtful. Some are cardio-respiratory.

Second, it is not always possible to say whether the insufficiency is due to lesion of the valve segment or to dilatation of the mitral ring and relative incompetency. Here neither the character of the murmur, the propagation, the accentuation of the pulmonary second sound, nor the hypertrophy assists in the differentiation. The history is sometimes of greater value than the examination. The cases most likely to lead to error are those of the so-called idiopathic dilatation and hypertrophy (in which the systolic murmur may be of the greatest intensity), and the instances of arterio-sclerosis with dilated heart. Balfour and others maintain that organic disease of the mitral leaflets sufficient to produce insufficiency is always accompanied with a certain degree of narrowing of the orifice, so that the only unequivocal proof of actual disease of the mitral valve is the presence of a presystolic murmur.

MITRAL STENOSIS

Etiology.—There are two groups of cases, one following an acute endocarditis, the other the result of a slow sclerosis of the valves without any history of rheumatic fever or other infection. It is much more common in women than in men—in 63 of 80 cases noted by Duckworth, while in 4,791 autopsies at Guy's Hospital during ten years there were 196 cases, of which 107 were females and 89 males (Samways). This is not easy to explain, but there are at least two factors to be considered. Rheumatic fever prevails more in girls than in boys and chorea has an important influence, occurring more frequently in girls and being often associated with endocarditis. In a surprising number of cases of what the French call *pure* mitral stenosis no recognizable etiological factor can be discovered. This has been regarded by some writers as favoring the view that they may be of congenital origin, but congenital affections of the mitral valve are notoriously rare. Whooping-cough, with its terrible strain on the heart-valves, may be accountable for certain cases. While met with at all ages, stenosis is certainly most frequent in young adult women.

Morbid Anatomy.—The valve segments and chordæ may be fused together, the result of repeated attacks of endocarditis. The condition varies a good deal, according to the amount of atheromatous change. In many cases the curtains are so welded together and the whole valvular region so thickened that the orifice is reduced to a mere chink—Corrigan's button-hole contraction. In non-endocarditic cases the curtains are not much thickened, but narrowing has resulted from gradual adhesion at the edges, and thickening of the chordæ tendineæ, so that from the auricle it looks cone like—the so-called funnel shaped variety. The instances in which the valve segments are slightly deformed, but in which the orifice is considerably narrowed, are regarded by some as possibly of congenital origin. Occasionally the curtains are in great part free from disease, but the narrowing results from large calcareous masses, which project into them from the ring. The involvement of the chordæ tendineæ is usually extreme, and the papillary muscles may be inserted directly upon the valve. In moderate grades of constriction the orifice will admit the tip of the index finger; in more extreme forms the tip of the little finger; and occasionally one meets with a specimen in which the orifice seems almost obliterated. The heart is not greatly enlarged, rarely weighing more than 14 or 15 ounces. Occasionally, in an elderly person, it may seem only slightly, if at all, enlarged, and again there are instances in which the weight may reach as much as 20 ounces. The left ventricle is sometimes small, and may look very small in comparison with the right ventricle, which forms the greater portion of the apex. In cases in which with the narrowing there is insufficiency the left ventricle may be moderately dilated and hypertrophied.

It is not uncommon at the examination to find white thrombi in the appendix of the left auricle. Occasionally a large part of the auricle is occupied by an ante-mortem thrombus. Still more rarely the remarkable *ball thrombus* is found, in which a globular concretion, varying in size from a walnut to a small egg, lies free in the auricle.

The left auricle discharges its blood with greater difficulty and in consequence dilates, and its walls reach three or four times their normal thickness. Although the auricle is by structure unfitted to compensate an extreme lesion, the probability is that for some time during the gradual production of stenosis the increasing muscular power of the walls counterbalances the defect. In 36 cases of well-marked stenosis Samways found the auricle hypertrophied in 26, dilatation coexisting in 14. Eventually the tension is increased in the pulmonary circulation and extra work thrown on the right ventricle, which gradually hypertrophies. Relative incompetency of the triscuspid and congestion of the systemic veins supervene.

Physical Signs.—*Inspection.*—In children the lower sternum and the fifth and sixth left costal cartilages are often prominent, owing to hypertrophy of the right ventricle. The apex beat may be ill defined. Usually it is not dislocated far beyond the nipple line, and the chief impulse is over the lower sternum and adjacent costal cartilages. Often in thin chested persons there is pulsation in the third and fourth left interspaces close to the sternum. When compensation fails, the impulse is much feebler, and in the veins of the neck there may be marked pulsation or the right jugular near the clavicle may stand out as a prominent tumor. In the later stage there is great enlargement with pulsation of the liver.

Palpation reveals in a majority of the cases a characteristic, well defined fremitus or thrill, which is best felt, as a rule, in the fourth or fifth interspace within the nipple line. It is of a rough, grating quality, often peculiarly limited in area, most marked during expiration, and terminates in a sharp, sudden shock, synchronous with the impulse. This most characteristic of physical signs is pathognomonic of narrowing of the mitral orifice, and is perhaps the only instance in which the diagnosis of a valvular lesion can be made by palpation alone. The cardiac impulse is felt most forcibly over the lower sternum and in the fourth and fifth left interspaces. The impulse is felt very high in the third and fourth interspaces, or in rare cases even in the second, and it has been thought that in the latter interspace the impulse is due to pulsation of the auricle. It is always the impulse of the conus arteriosus of the right ventricle; even in the most extreme grades of mitral stenosis there is never such tilting forward of the auricle or its appendix as would enable it to produce an impression on the chest wall.

Percussion gives an increase in the cardiac dulness to the right of the sternum and along the left margin; not usually a great increase beyond the nipple line, except in extreme cases.

Auscultation.—The findings are varied and a most puzzling combination of sounds and murmurs may be heard. In some cases to the inner side of the apex beat, often in a very limited region, there is heard a rough, vibratory or purring murmur, cumulative or crescendo in character, often of short duration, which terminates abruptly in the loud snapping first sound. By combining palpation and auscultation the purring murmur is found to be synchronous with the thrill and the loud shock with the first sound. The murmur may occupy the entire period of the diastole, or the middle or only the latter half, corresponding to the auricular contraction. A difference can often be noted between the first and second portions of the murmur, when it occupies the entire time. In some cases a soft diastolic murmur is heard after the second sound at the apex. This may increase and merge into the presystolic murmur. Often there is a peculiar rumbling or echoing quality, which in some instances is very limited and may be heard only over a single bell-space of the stethoscope. The administration of amyl nitrite may bring out the murmur more clearly. A rumbling, echoing presystolic murmur at the apex is heard in some cases of aortic insufficiency (Flint murmur), occasionally in adherent pericardium with great dilatation of the heart, and in upward dislocation of the organ. The Graham Steell murmur of relative pulmonary insufficiency may be heard in the pulmonic area.

A systolic murmur may be heard at the apex or along the left sternal border, often of extreme softness and audible only when the breath is held. Sometimes the systolic murmur is loud and distinct and is transmitted to the axilla. The second sound in the second left interspace is loudly accentuated, and often reduplicated. It may be transmitted far to the left and be heard with great clearness beyond the apex. In uncomplicated cases of mitral stenosis there are usually no murmurs audible at the aortic region, at which spot the second sound is less intense than at the pulmonary area. In advanced cases at the lower sternum and to the right a systolic tricuspid murmur is sometimes heard. With good compensation the second sound is heard at the apex; its disappearance suggests the approach of decompensation. Other points to be noted are the following: The usually sharp, snapping first sound which follows the presystolic murmur, the cause of which is by no means easy to explain. It can scarcely be a valvular sound produced chiefly at the mitral orifice, since it may be heard with great intensity in cases in which the valves are rigid and calcified. It has been suggested that it is a loud "snap" of the tricuspid valves caused by the powerful contraction of the greatly hypertrophied right ventricle. Broadbent thinks it may be due to the abrupt contraction of a partially filled left ventricle. The sound may be audible at a distance, as one sits at the bedside of the patient (Graves). In one patient the first sound was audible six feet, by measurement, from the chest wall.

These physical signs, it is to be borne in mind, are characteristic only of the stage in which compensation is maintained. The murmur may be soft, almost inaudible, and only brought out after exertion. Finally there comes a period in which, with the establishment of auricular fibrillation, the signs change. This is due to the absence of contraction of the auricle. Thus a short presystolic murmur may disappear as there is not the usual difference in pressure in the auricle and ventricle at the time when the auricle should be contracting. With the auricle paralyzed the murmur is more likely to be heard early in diastole. Difference in rate may cause marked changes in the time and character of the murmur.

Sometimes in the apex region a sharp first sound or gallop rhythm may be heard. The systolic shock may be present after the disappearance of the thrill and the characteristic murmur. If partial heart-block occurs a complicated set of signs results as the auricle is contracting more often than the ventricle. Under treatment, with gradual recovery of compensation, probably with increasing vigor of contraction of the right ventricle and left auricle, the presystolic murmur reappears. In cases seen at this stage the nature of the valve lesion may be entirely overlooked. *Auricular fibrillation* is the rule in the arrhythmia of mitral stenosis.

Stenosis of the mitral valve may for years be efficiently compensated by the hypertrophy of the right ventricle. Many persons with the characteristic signs of this lesion present no symptoms. They may for years be short of breath on going upstairs, but are able to pass through the ordinary duties of life without discomfort. The pulse is smaller in volume than normal, and very often irregular (auricular fibrillation). A special danger is the recurring endocarditis. Vegetations may be whipped off into the circulation and, blocking a cerebral vessel, may cause hemiplegia or aphasia, or both. This, unfortunately, is not an uncommon sequence in women. Patients with mitral stenosis may survive this accident for an indefinite period.

Pressure of the enlarged auricle on the left recurrent laryngeal nerve, causing paralysis of the vocal cord on the corresponding side, has been described and the diagnosis of aneurism of the arch of the aorta may be made. Fetterolf and Norris conclude that it is not due to the pressure of the left auricle directly, but to squeezing of the nerve between the pulmonary artery and the aortic arch, and that the paralysis is due to the neuritis so excited.

Failure of compensation brings in its train the group of symptoms which have been discussed under cardiac insufficiency. Briefly enumerated, they are: Rapid and irregular action of the heart, shortness of breath, cough, signs of pulmonary engorgement, and very frequently hæmoptysis. Attacks of this kind may recur for years. Bronchitis or a febrile attack may cause shortness of breath or slight blueness. Inflammatory affections of the lungs or pleura seriously disturb the right heart, and these patients stand pneumonia very badly. Many, perhaps a majority of, cases of mitral stenosis do not have dropsy. The liver may be greatly enlarged, and in the late stages ascites is not uncommon, particularly in children.

TRICUSPID VALVE DISEASE

Tricuspid Regurgitation.—Occasionally this results from acute or chronic endocarditis with puckering; more commonly the condition is one of relative insufficiency, and is secondary to lesions of the valves on the left side, particularly of the mitral. It is met with also in all conditions of the lungs which cause obstruction to the circulation, such as cirrhosis and emphysema, particularly in combination with chronic bronchitis. The symptoms are those of obstruction in the lesser circulation with venous congestion in the systemic veins, already described with mitral insufficiency. The signs are:

(*a*) Systolic regurgitation of the blood into the right auricle and the transmission of the pulse wave into the veins of the neck. If the regurgitation is slight or the contraction of the ventricle is feeble there may be no venous throbbing, but in other cases there is marked systolic pulsation in the cervical veins. It may be seen both in the internal and the external vein, particularly in the latter. Marked pulsation in these veins occurs only when the valves guarding them become incompetent. Slight oscillations are by no means uncommon, even when the valves are intact. The distention is sometimes enormous, particularly in the act of coughing, when the right jugular at the root of the neck may stand out, forming an extraordinarily prominent ovoid mass. Occasionally the regurgitant pulse wave may be widely transmitted and be seen in the subclavian and axillary veins, and even in the subcutaneous veins over the shoulder, or in the superficial mammary veins.

Regurgitant pulsation through the tricuspid orifice may be transmitted to the inferior cava, and so to the hepatic veins, causing a systolic distention of the liver. This is best appreciated by bimanual palpation, placing one hand over the fifth and sixth costal cartilages and the other in the lateral region of the liver in the mid-axillary line. The pulsation may be readily distinguished, as a rule, from the impulse from the ventricle or transmitted from the aorta.

(b) The second important sign is the occurrence of a systolic murmur of maximum intensity over the lower sternum. It is usually a soft, low murmur, often to be distinguished from a coexisting mitral murmur by differences in quality and pitch, and may be heard to the right as far as the axilla. Sometimes it is very limited in its distribution.

Together these two signs indicate tricuspid regurgitation. In addition, the percussion usually shows increase in the area of dulness to the right of the sternum, and the impulse in the lower sternal region is forcible. In the great majority of cases the symptoms are those of the associated lesions. In fibrosis of the lung and in chronic emphysema the failure of compensation of the right ventricle with insufficiency of the tricuspid not infrequently leads to gradual failure with cardiac dropsy.

Tricuspid Stenosis.—The condition is rare both clinically and anatomically, and it is not often recognized during life. Of 26,000 medical admissions in the Johns Hopkins Hospital there were only 8 with either clinical or post mortem diagnosis of this condition; and in a total of 3,500 autopsies, only 5 cases were found, all in females. Of a total of 195 collected cases, there were 141 females, 38 males, 16 sex unknown. In a majority of the cases—104—the mitral and tricuspid were affected together, in 14 the tricuspid alone, in 64 the tricuspid and aortic. A definite history of rheumatism was present in only 66 cases (Futcher).

The *diagnosis* is not often made; extreme cyanosis and dyspnœa are common, and toward the end the ordinary signs of cardiac failure. Among the important physical signs are presystolic pulsation in the jugular veins and in the enlarged liver. A presystolic thrill may be felt at the tricuspid area with a marked systolic shock. The cardiac dulness is greatly increased to the right, a rumbling presystolic murmur may be present over the lower sternum with an extension to the right border. This, with a very snappy first sound, great increase of dulness to the right, and chronic breathlessness with cyanosis, are the important features.

PULMONARY VALVE DISEASE

Murmurs in the region of the pulmonary valves are extremely common; lesions of the valves are exceedingly rare. Balfour has well called the pulmonic area the region of "auscultatory romance." A systolic murmur is heard here under many conditions—(1) very often in health, in thin chested persons, particularly in children, during expiration and in the recumbent posture; (2) when the heart is acting rapidly, as in fever and after exertion; (3) it is a favorite situation of the cardio-respiratory murmur; (4) in anæmic states; and (5) the systolic murmur of mitral insufficiency may be transmitted along the left sternal margin. Actual lesions of the pulmonary valves are rare.

Stenosis is almost invariably a congenital anomaly and constitutes one of the most important of the congenital cardiac affections. The valve segments are usually united, leaving a small, narrow orifice. In adults cases occasionally occur. The congenital lesion is commonly associated with patency of the ductus Botalli and imperfection of the ventricular septum. There may also be tricuspid stenosis. Acute endocarditis not infrequently attacks the sclerotic valves.

The physical *signs* are extremely uncertain. There may be a systolic murmur with a thrill heard best to the left of the sternum in the second intercostal space. This murmur may be very like a murmur of aortic stenosis, but is not transmitted into the vessels. Naturally the pulmonary second sound is weak or obliterated, or may be replaced by a diastolic murmur. Usually there is hypertrophy of the right heart.

Pulmonary Insufficiency.—This rare lesion was originally described by Morgagni. Pitt analysed 109 cases from the Guy's Hospital Reports, of which 60 had infectious endocarditis, 18 were due to a dilated pulmonary artery, 14 to pulmonary stenosis, 14 to aortic aneurism, 13 to abnormality in the number of the valves, and 6 unclassified. Pitt makes two groups, one with a rapid course, sometimes with definite symptoms pointing to the heart but the signs to general septicæmia. In the second group the cardiac symptoms are marked, dyspnœa, cough, etc., and the physical signs are definite.

The physical *signs* are those of regurgitation into the right ventricle, but, as a rule, it is difficult to differentiate the murmur from that of aortic insufficiency, though the maximum intensity may be in the pulmonary area. The absence of the vascular features of aortic insufficiency is the most suggestive feature. Both Gibson and Graham Steell called attention to the possibility of leakage through these valves in cases of great increase of pressure in the pulmonary artery, and to a soft diastolic murmur heard under these circumstances.

Combined Valvular Lesions.—Valvular lesions are seldom single or pure; combined lesions are more common. This is particularly the case in congenital disease. In young children mitral and aortic lesions, the result of rheumatic fever, are common. Pure mitral insufficiency and pure mitral stenosis may exist for years, but in time the tricuspid becomes involved. Aortic valve lesions are more commonly uncombined than mitral lesions. The added lesion may be hurtful or helpful. The stenosis which so often accompanies the endocarditic variety may lessen the regurgitation in aortic insufficiency; and a progressive narrowing of the mitral orifice may be beneficial in mitral regurgitation.

Prognosis in Valvular Disease.—The question is entirely one of efficient compensation. So long as this is maintained the patient may suffer no inconvenience, and even with the most serious forms of valve lesion the function of the heart may be little, if at all, disturbed.

Practitioners who are not adepts in auscultation and feel unable to estimate the value of the various heart murmurs should remember that the best judgment may be gathered from inspection and palpation. With an apex beat in the normal situation and a regular rhythm the auscultatory phenomena may be practically disregarded. The myocardium is more important than the valve.

A murmur *per se* is of little or no moment in determining the prognosis in any given case. There is a large group of patients who present no other symptoms than a systolic murmur heard over the body of the heart, or over the apex, in whom the left ventricle is not hypertrophied, the heart rhythm is normal, and who may not have had rheumatism. Among the conditions influencing prognosis are:

(*a*) AGE.—Children under ten are bad subjects. Compensation is well effected, and they are free from many of the influences which disturb compensation in adults. The coronary arteries are healthy and nutrition of the heart muscle can be readily maintained. Yet, in spite of this, the outlook in cardiac lesions in young children is usually bad. The valve lesion itself is apt to be rapidly progressive, and the limit of cardiac reserve force is early reached. There seems to be proportionately a greater degree of hypertrophy and dilatation. Among other causes of the risks of this period are insufficient food in the poorer classes, the recurrence of rheumatic attacks, and the existence of pericardial adhesions. The outlook in a child who can be carefully supervised and prevented from damaging himself by overexertion is better than in one who is constantly overtasking his circulation. The valvular lesions which occur at, or subsequent to, the period of puberty are more likely to be permanently and efficiently compensated. Sudden death from heart disease is very rare in children.

(*b*) SEX.—Women bear valve lesions, as a rule, better than men, owing partly to the fact that they live quieter lives, partly to the less common involvement of the coronary arteries, and to the greater frequency of mitral lesions. Pregnancy and parturition are disturbing factors, but are less serious than some writers would have us believe.

(*c*) VALVE AFFECTED.—The relative prognosis of the different valve lesions is difficult to estimate and each case must be judged on its own merits. *Aortic insufficiency* is unquestionably the most serious; yet for years it may be perfectly compensated. Favorable circumstances in any case are a moderate grade of hypertrophy and dilatation, the absence of all symptoms of cardiac distress, and the absence of extensive arterio-sclerosis and of angina. The prognosis rests largely with the condition of the coronary arteries. Rheumatic lesions of the valves, inducing insufficiency, are less apt to be associated with endarteritis at the root of the aorta; and in such cases the coronary arteries may escape for years. On the other hand, when aortic insufficiency is only a part of an arterio-sclerosis at the root of the aorta, the coronary arteries are almost invariably involved, and the outlook is much more serious. Sudden death is not uncommon, either from acute dilatation during exertion, or, more frequently, from blocking of one of the branches of the coronary arteries. The liability of this form to be associated with angina pectoris also adds to its severity. *Aortic stenosis* is comparatively rare, most common in middle aged or elderly men, and is, as a rule, well compensated. In Broadbent's series, in which autopsy showed definite aortic narrowing, forty years was the average age at death, and the oldest was but fifty-three.

In mitral lesions the outlook on the whole is more favorable than in aortic insufficiency. *Mitral insufficiency,* when well compensated, carries with it a better prognosis than mitral stenosis. Except aortic stenosis, it is the only lesion commonly met with in patients over three-score years. The cases which last the longest are those in which the valve orifice is more or less narrowed, as well as incompetent. There is, in reality, no valve lesion so poorly compensated and so rapidly fatal as that in which the mitral segments are gradually curled and puckered until they form a narrow strip around a wide mitral ring—a condition specially seen in children. There are cases of mitral insufficiency in which the defect is thoroughly balanced for thirty or even forty years, without distress or inconvenience. Even with great hypertrophy and the apex beat almost in the mid-axillary line the compensation may be most effective. Women may pass safely through repeated pregnancies, though here they are liable to accidents associated with the severe strain.

In *mitral stenosis* the prognosis is usually regarded as less favorable but our experience places this lesion almost on a level, particularly in women, with mitral insufficiency. It is found very often in persons in perfect health, who have had neither palpitation nor signs of heart-failure, and who have lived laborious lives. The figures given by Broadbent indicate that the date of death in mitral stenosis is comparatively advanced. Of 53 cases from the post mortem records of St. Mary's Hospital, thirty-three was the age for males, and thirty-seven or thirty-eight for females. These women pass through repeated pregnancies with safety. There are, of course, those too common accidents, the result of cerebral embolism, which are more likely to occur in this than in other forms.

Hard and fast lines can not be drawn in the question of prognosis in valvular disease. The outlook depends largely on the condition of the *myocardium,* which in large measure governs the situation. With evidence of muscular insufficiency the prognosis is always grave. The etiological factor is important, thus rheumatic fever or syphilis may have caused serious myocardial mischief. Every case must be judged separately, and all the circumstances carefully balanced. The development of auricular fibrillation, alternation of the heart, etc., must be taken into account. There is no question which requires greater experience and more mature judgment, and the most experienced are sometimes at fault. The following conditions justify a favorable prognosis: Good general health and good habits; no exceptional liability to rheumatic or catarrhal affections; origin of the valvular lesion independently of degeneration; existence of the valvular lesion without change for over three years; sound ventricles, of moderate frequency, and general regularity of action; the absence of serious forms of arrhythmia; sound arteries, with a normal tension: and freedom from pulmonary, hepatic, and renal congestion.

Treatment.—(*a*) Stage of Compensation.—Medicinal treatment is not necessary and is often hurtful. A very common error is to administer cardiac drugs, such as digitalis, on the discovery of a murmur or of hypertrophy. If the lesion has been found accidentally, it may be best not to tell the patient, but rather an intimate friend. Often it is necessary to be perfectly frank in order that the patient may take certain preventive measures. He should lead a quiet, regulated, orderly life, free from excitement and worry, and the risk of sudden death makes it imperative that the patient suffering from aortic disease should be specially warned against overexertion and hurry. An ordinary wholesome diet in moderate quantities should be taken; tobacco may be allowed in moderation, but alcohol should be interdicted or used in very small amount. Exercise should be regulated entirely by the feelings of the patient. So long as no cardiac distress or palpitation follows, moderate exercise will prove very beneficial. The skin should be kept active by a daily bath. Hot baths should be avoided and the Turkish bath forbidden. In the case of full-blooded, somewhat corpulent individuals, an occasional saline purge should be taken. Patients with valvular lesions should not go to very high altitudes. The act of coition has serious risks, particularly in aortic insufficiency. Knowing that the causes which most surely and powerfully disturb the compensation are overexertion, mental worry, and malnutrition, the physician should give suitable instructions in each case. As it is always better to have the coöperation of an intelligent patient, he should, as a rule, be told of the condition, but in this matter the physician must be guided by circumstances, and there are cases in which reticence is the wiser policy.

(*b*) Stage of Broken Compensation.—The break may be immediate and final, as when sudden death results from acute dilatation or from blocking of a branch of the coronary artery, or it may be gradual. Among the first indications are shortness of breath on exertion or attacks of nocturnal dyspnœa. These are often associated with impaired nutrition, particularly with anæmia, and a course of iron or change of air may suffice to relieve the symptoms.

Irregularity of the heart is not necessarily an indication of failing compensation but demands an accurate diagnosis of the cause. Serious failure of compensation is indicated by signs of dilatation, marked cyanosis, gallop rhythm, or certain forms of arrhythmia, with or without the existence of dropsy. These are dependent on the myocardium and the same measures are to be carried out as are indicated under treatment in cardiac insufficiency.

V. SPECIAL PATHOLOGICAL CONDITIONS

I. ANEURISM OF THE HEART

Aneurism of a valve results from acute endocarditis, which produces softening or erosion and may lead to perforation of the segment or to gradual dilatation of a limited area under the influence of the blood pressure. The aneurisms are usually spheroidal and project from the ventricular face of an aortic valve. They are much less common on the mitral segments. They frequently rupture and produce extensive destruction and insufficiency.

Aneurism of the walls results from the weakening due to chronic myocarditis, or occasionally follows acute mural endocarditis, which more commonly, however, leads to perforation. It has followed a stab wound, a gumma of the ventricle, and, according to some authors, pericardial adhesions. The left ventricle near the apex is usually the seat, this being the situation in which fibrous degeneration is most common. Of the 90 cases collected by Legg 59 were situated here. In the early stages the anterior wall of the ventricle, near the septum, sometimes even the septum itself, is slightly dilated, the endocardium opaque, and the muscular tissue sclerotic. In a more advanced stage the dilatation is pronounced and layers of thrombi occupy the sac. Ultimately a large rounded tumor may project from the ventricle and attain a size equal to that of the heart. Occasionally the aneurism is sacculated and communicates with the ventricle through a small orifice. The sac may be double, as in the cases of Janeway and Sailer. In the museum of Guy's Hospital there is a specimen showing the wall of the ventricle covered with aneurismal bulgings. Rupture occurred in 7 of the cases collected by Legg.

The *symptoms* are indefinite. Occasionally there is marked bulging in the apex region and the tumor may perforate the chest wall. In mitral stenosis the right ventricle may bulge and produce a visible pulsating tumor below the left costal border, which has been mistaken for cardiac aneurism. When the sac is large and produces pressure upon the heart itself, there may be a marked disproportion between the strong cardiac impulse and the feeble pulsation in the peripheral arteries.

II. RUPTURE OF THE HEART

This rare event is usually associated with fatty infiltration or degeneration of the heart-muscle. In some instances acute softening in consequence of embolism of a branch of the coronary artery, suppurative myocarditis, or a gummatous growth has been the cause. Of 100 cases collected by Quain, fatty degeneration was noted in 77. Two thirds of the patients were over sixty years of age. It may occur in infants. Schaps reports a case in an infant of four months associated with an embolic infarct of the left ventricle. Harvey, in his second letter to Riolan (1649), described the case of Sir Robert Darcy, who had distressing pain in the chest and syncopal attacks with suffocation, and finally cachexia and dropsy. Death occurred in one of the paroxysms. The wall of the left ventricle of the heart was ruptured, "having a rent in it of size sufficient to admit any of my fingers, although the wall itself appeared sufficiently thick and strong."

The rent may occur in any of the chambers, but is most frequent in the left ventricle on the anterior wall, not far from the septum. The accident usually takes place during exertion. There may be no preliminary symptoms, but without any warning the patient may fall and die in a few moments. Sudden death occurred in 71 per cent. of Quain's cases. In other instances there may be a sense of anguish and suffocation, and life may be prolonged for several hours. In a Montreal case, the patient walked up a steep hill after the onset of the symptoms, and lived for thirteen hours. A case is on record in which the patient lived for eleven days.

III. NEW GROWTHS AND PARASITES

Primary cancer or sarcoma is extremely rare. Secondary tumors may be single or multiple, and are usually unattended with symptoms, even when the disease is most extensive. In one case in the wall of the right ventricle a mass was found which involved the anterior segment of the tricuspid valve and partly blocked the orifice. The surface was eroded and there were numerous cancerous emboli in the pulmonary artery. In another instance the heart was greatly enlarged, owing to the presence of innumerable masses of colloid cancer the size of cherries. The mediastinal sarcoma may penetrate the heart, though it is remarkable how extensive the disease of the mediastinal glands may be without involvement of the heart or vessels.

Cysts in the heart are rare. They are found in different parts, and are filled either with a brownish or a clear fluid. Blood cysts occasionally occur.

The parasites have been discussed, but it may be mentioned here that both the *Cysticercus cellulosæ* and echinococcus cysts occur occasionally.

IV. WOUNDS AND FOREIGN BODIES

Wounds of the heart may be caused by external injuries, as stabs and bullet wounds, by foreign bodies passing from the gullet or œsophagus, or by puncture for therapeutic purposes.

(*a*) Bullet wounds of the heart are common. Recovery may take place, and bullets have been found encysted in the organ. Stab wounds are still more common. A medical student, while on a spree, passed a pin into his heart. The pericardium was opened, and the head of the pin was found outside of the right ventricle. It was grasped and an attempt made to remove it, but it was withdrawn into the heart and, it is said, caused the patient no further trouble (Moxon).

(*b*) Hysterical girls sometimes swallow pins and needles, which, passing through the œsophagus and stomach, are found in various parts of the body. A remarkable case is reported by Allen J. Smith of a girl from whom several dozen needles and pins were removed, chiefly from subcutaneous abscesses. Several years later she developed symptoms of chronic heart disease. At the post mortem needles were found in the tissues of the adherent pericardium, and between thirty and forty were embedded in the thickened pleural membranes of the left side.

(*c*) Puncture of the heart (cardiocentesis) has been recommended as a therapeutic procedure. The proceeding is not without risk. Hæmorrhage may take place from the puncture, though it is not often extensive. Sloane has urged its use in all cases of asphyxia and in suffocation by drowning and from coal gas. The successful case which he reports illustrates its stimulating action.

VI. CONGENITAL AFFECTIONS OF THE HEART

These have only a limited clinical interest, as in a large proportion of the cases the anomaly is not compatible with life, and in others nothing can be done to remedy the defect or even to relieve the symptoms.

The congenital affections result from interruption of the normal course of development or from inflammatory processes—endocarditis; sometimes from a combination of both.

General Anomalies.—Of general anomalies of development the following conditions may be mentioned: *Acardia,* absence of the heart, which has been met with in the monstrosity known by the same name; *double heart,* which has occasionally been found in extreme grades of fetal deformity; *dextrocardia,* in which the heart is on the right side, either alone or as part of a general transposition of the viscera; *ectopia cordis,* a condition associated with fission of the chest wall and of the abdomen. The heart may be situated in the cervical, pectoral, or abdominal regions. Except in the abdominal variety, the condition is very rarely compatible with extra-uterine life. Occasionally, as in a case reported by Holt, the child lives for some months, and the heart may be seen and felt beating beneath the skin in the epigastric region. This infant was five months old at the date of examination.

Anomalies of the Cardiac Septa.—The septa of both auricles and ventricles may be defective, in which case the heart consists of but two chambers, the *cor biloculare* or reptilian heart. In the septum of the auricles there is a very common defect, owing to the fact that the membrane closing the foramen ovale has failed at one point to become attached to the ring, and leaves a valvular slit which may admit the handle of a scalpel. Neither this nor the small cribriform perforations of the membrane are of any significance.

The *foramen ovale* may be patent without a trace of membrane closing it. In some instances this exists with other serious defects, such as stenosis of the pulmonary artery, or imperfection of the ventricular septum. In others the patent foramen ovale is the only anomaly, and in many instances it does not appear to have caused any embarrassment, having been found in persons who have died of various affections. The ventricular septum may be absent, the condition known as trilocular heart. Much more frequently there is a small defect in the upper portion of the septum, either in the situation of the membranous portion known as the "undefended space" or in the region just anterior to this. This is frequently associated with narrowing of the pulmonary orifice or of the conus arteriosus of the right ventricle.

Apart from the instances in association with narrowing of the orifice of the pulmonary artery, or of the conus, there are cases in which defect of the *membranous septum* is the only lesion, a condition not incompatible with long and fairly active life. The late Professor Brooks of the Johns Hopkins University knew from early manhood that he had heart trouble, but he accomplished an extraordinary amount of work, and lived to be about 60. Imperfect septum was the only lesion. The physical signs are fairly distinctive, with usually some evident enlargement of the heart, and a murmur described by Roger as follows: "It is a loud murmur, audible over a large area, and, commencing with systole, is prolonged so as to cover the normal tic-tac. It has its maximum, not at the base to the right, as in aortic stenosis, or to the left, as in pulmonary stenosis, but at the upper third of the præcordial region. It is central, like the septum, and from this central point gradually diminishes in intensity in every direction. The murmur does not vary at any time, and it is not conducted into the vessels." In some cases there is a distinct systolic intensification of this loud continuous murmur.

Anomalies and Lesions of the Valves.—Numerical anomalies of the valves are not uncommon. The semilunar segments at the arterial orifices are not infrequently increased or diminished in number. Supernumerary segments are more frequent in the pulmonary artery than in the aorta. Four, or sometimes five, valves have been found. The segments may be of equal size, but, as a rule, the supernumerary valve is small.

Instead of three there may be only two semilunar valves, or, as it is termed, the *bicuspid condition;* this is more frequent in the aortic valve. Of 21 instances only 2 occurred at the pulmonary orifice. Two of the valves have united, and from the ventricular face show either no trace of division or else a slight depression indicating where the union has occurred. From the aortic side there is usually to be seen some trace of division into two sinuses of Valsalva. There has been a discussion as to the origin of this condition, whether it is really an anomaly or due to endocarditis, fetal or post-natal. The combined segment is usually thickened, but the fact that this anomaly is met with in the fetus without a trace of sclerosis or endocarditis shows that it may, in some cases at least, result from a developmental error.

Clinically this is a very important congenital defect, owing to the liability of the combined valve to sclerotic changes. Except two fetal specimens, all of a series showed thickening and deformity, and in 15 of those reported death resulted directly or indirectly from the lesion (Osler).

The little fenestrations at the margins of the sigmoid valves have no significance; they occur in a considerable proportion of all bodies.

Anomalies of the auriculo-ventricular valves are not often met with.

Fetal endocarditis may occur either at the arterial or auriculo-ventricular orifices. It is nearly always of the chronic or sclerotic variety. Very rarely, indeed, is it of the warty or verrucose form. There are little nodular bodies, sometimes six or eight in number, on the mitral and tricuspid segments—the nodules of Albini—which represent the remains of fetal structures, and must not be mistaken for endocardial outgrowths. The little rounded, bead like hæmorrhages of a deep purple color, which are very common on the heart valves of children, are also not to be mistaken for the products of endocarditis. In fetal endocarditis the segments are usually thickened at the edges, shrunken, and smooth. In the mitral and tricuspid valves the cusps are found united and the chordæ tendineæ are thickened and shortened. In the semilunar valves all trace of the segments has disappeared, leaving a stiff membranous diaphragm perforated by an oval or rounded orifice. It is sometimes very difficult to say whether this condition has resulted from fetal endocarditis or is an error in development. In many instances the processes are combined; an anomalous valve becomes the seat of chronic sclerotic changes, and, according to Rauchfuss, endocarditis is more common on the right side of the heart only because the valves are here more often the seat of developmental errors.

Lesions at the Pulmonary Orifice.—*Stenosis* of this orifice is one of the commonest and most important of congenital heart affections. A slow endocarditis causes gradual union of the segments and narrowing of the orifice to such a degree that it admits only the smallest sized probe. In some of the cases the smooth membranous condition of the combined segments is such that it would appear to be the result of faulty development. In some instances vegetations occur. The condition is compatible with life for many years, and in a considerable proportion of the cases of congenital heart disease above the tenth year this lesion is present. With it there may be defect of the ventricular septum. Pulmonary tuberculosis is a very common cause of death. Obliteration or *atresia* of the pulmonary orifice is a less frequent but more serious condition than stenosis. It is associated with persistence of the ductus arteriosus, together with patency of the foramen ovale or defect of the ventricular septum with hypertrophy of the right heart. *Stenosis of the conus arteriosus* of the right ventricle exists in a considerable proportion of the cases of obstruction at the pulmonary orifice. At the outset a developmental error, it may be combined with sclerotic changes. The ventricular septum is imperfect, the foramen ovale usually open, and the ductus arteriosus patent. The lesions at the pulmonary orifice constitute the most important group of congenital cardiac affections. Of 631 instances of various congenital anomalies analyzed by Maude Abbott, 150 cases came under this category.

Congenital lesions of the aortic orifice are not very frequent. Rauchfuss collected 24 cases of stenosis and atresia; stenosis of the left conus arteriosus may also occur, a condition not incompatible with prolonged life. Ten of the 16 cases tabulated by Dilg were over thirty years of age.

Transposition of the large arterial trunks is a not uncommon anomaly. There may be neither hypertrophy, cyanosis, nor heart murmur.

Symptoms of Congenital Heart Disease.—Cyanosis occurs in over 90 per cent. of the cases, and forms so distinctive a feature that the terms "blue disease" and "morbus cæruleus" are practically synonyms for congenital heart-disease. The lividity in a majority of cases appears only within the first week of life, and may be general or confined to the lips, nose, and ears, and to the fingers and toes. In some instances there is in addition a general dusky suffusion, and in the most extreme grades the skin is almost purple. It may vary a good deal and may be intense only on exertion. The external temperature is low. Dyspnœa on exertion and cough are common symptoms. A great increase in the number of the red corpuscles has been noted. In a case of Gibson's there were above eight millions of red blood cells per c. mm. There may be nucleated red cells and great variation in size and shape. The children rarely thrive, and often display a lethargy of both mind and body. The fingers and toes are clubbed to a degree rarely met with in any other affection. The cause of the cyanosis has been much discussed. Morgagni referred it to the general congestion of the venous system due to obstruction. Morrison's analysis of 75 cases of congenital heart disease shows that closure of the pulmonary orifice with patency of the foramen ovale and the ventricular septum is the condition most frequently associated with cyanosis, and he concludes that the deficient aeration of the blood owing to diminished lung function is the most important factor. Another view, often attributed erroneously to William Hunter, was that the discoloration was due to the admixture in the heart of venous and arterial blood; but lesions may exist which permit of very free mixture without producing cyanosis. The question of the cause of cyanosis can not be considered as settled. Variot made the suggestion that the cause is not entirely cardiac, but is associated with disturbance throughout the whole circulatory system, and particularly a vaso-motor paresis and malaëration of the red blood corpuscles.

Diagnosis.—In the case of children, cyanosis, with or without enlargement of the heart, and the existence of a murmur, are sufficient, as a rule, to determine the presence of a congenital heart lesion. The cyanosis gives us no clew to the precise nature of the trouble, as it is a symptom common to many lesions and it may be absent in certain conditions. The murmur is usually systolic. It is not always present, and there are instances of complicated congenital lesions in which the examination showed normal heart sounds. In two or three instances fetal endocarditis has been diagnosed *in gravida* by the presence of a rough systolic murmur, and the condition corroborated subsequent to the birth of the child. Hypertrophy is present in a majority of the cases of congenital defect. The fatal event may be caused by abscess of the brain. For a full discussion of the subject the student is referred to the monograph of Dr. Maude Abbott in Vol. IV of our "System of Medicine." The conclusions of Hochsinger are as follows:

"(1) In childhood, loud, rough, musical heart murmurs, with normal or only slight increase in the heart dulness, occur only in congenital heart disease. The acquired endocardial defects with loud heart murmurs in young children are almost always associated with great increase in the heart dulness. In the transposition of the large arterial trunks there may be no cyanosis, no heart murmur, and an absence of hypertrophy.

"(2) In young children heart murmurs with great increase in the cardiac dulness and feeble apex beat suggest congenital changes. The increased dulness is chiefly of the right heart, whereas the left is only slightly altered. On the other hand, in the acquired endocarditis in children, the left heart is chiefly affected and the apex beat is visible; the dilatation of the right heart comes late and does not materially change the increased strength of the apex beat.

"(3) The entire absence of murmurs at the apex, with their evident presence in the region of the auricles and over the pulmonary orifice, is always an important element in differential diagnosis, and points rather to septum defect or pulmonary stenosis than to endocarditis.

"(4) An abnormally weak second pulmonic sound associated with a distinct systolic murmur is a symptom which in early childhood is only to be explained by the assumption of a congenital pulmonary stenosis, and possesses therefore an importance from a point of differential diagnosis which is not to be underestimated.

"(5) Absence of a palpable thrill, despite loud murmurs which are heard over the whole præcordial region, is rare except with congenital defects in the septum, and it speaks, therefore, against an acquired cardiac affection.

"(6) Loud, especially vibratory, systolic murmurs, with the point of maximum intensity over the upper third of the sternum, associated with a lack of marked symptoms of hypertrophy of the left ventricle, are very important for the diagnosis of a persistence of the ductus Botalli, and can not be explained by the assumption of an endocarditis of the aortic valve."

Escherich suggests that the systolic basic murmur heard sometimes in the newborn, particularly if premature, may originate in the ductus Botalli before its closure.

Treatment.—The child should be warmly clad and guarded from all circumstances liable to excite bronchitis. In the attacks of urgent dyspnœa with lividity blood should be freely let. Saline cathartics are also useful. Digitalis must be used with care; it is sometimes beneficial in the later stages. When the compensation fails, the indications for treatment are those of muscular insufficiency in acquired cardiac disease.

VII. ANGINA PECTORIS

(*Stenocardia, Breast Pang*)

Definition.—A disease characterized by paroxysmal attacks of pain, usually pectoral, associated with vascular changes.

History.—In 1768 Heberden described a "disorder of the breast," to which he gave the name of "Angina Pectoris." Before this date Morgagni and Rougnon had described cases. The association with coronary artery disease was early shown by Jenner. John Hunter died in an attack. The connection with aortitis as demonstrated by Corrigan and Allbutt, the recognition of extra-pectoral forms, and the introduction of nitrites in treatment by Lauder Brunton are the important contributions of the nineteenth century.

Etiology.—The disease is not uncommon; there were 1,062 deaths in England and Wales in 1916. In the United States the death rate is increasing; there were 5,914 deaths in the registration area in 1917.

It is a rare disease in hospitals; a case a year is about the average, even in the large metropolitan hospitals. It is a disease of the better classes, and a consultant in active work may see a dozen or more cases a year.

Age.—In our series of 300 cases there were, under 30, 9 cases; between 30 and 40, 42; between 40 and 50, 60; between 50 and 60, 93; between 60 and 70, 72; between 70 and 80, 20; above 80, 4.

Sex.—Women are rarely attacked. Of our cases 256 were men and 44 women.

Race.—As mentioned, the disease seems to be relatively more frequent in the United States. Jews are particularly prone, 42 of our 300 cases.

Occupation.—It is not an affection of the working classes. The life of stress and strain, particularly of worry, seems to predispose to it, and this is perhaps why it is so common in our profession. In our series of 300 cases there were 38 physicians, a large proportion. From John Hunter onward a long list of distinguished physicians have been its victims, among whom in recent years were Charcot, Nothnagel, and William Pepper.

Cardio-vascular Disease.—In persons under forty syphilis is an important feature, causing an aortitis, often limited to the root of the vessel. Whatever the cause, arterio-sclerosis predisposes to angina. A majority of the patients have sclerosis, many high blood pressure. Business men leading lives of great strain, and eating, drinking, and smoking to excess, form the large contingent of angina cases. Slight attacks may occur with high blood pressure alone.

Heredity.—The disease may occur in members of three generations, as in the Arnold family.

Imitative Features.—Outbreaks of angina-like attacks have been described. After the death of one member of a family from the disease, another may have somewhat similar attacks. Two of his physicians had angina after Senator Sumner's fatal attack. One of them died within two weeks; the other, a young man, recovered completely.

Pathology.—The lesions in 17 post mortems were as follows:

(*a*) *Coronary artery disease* was present in 13 cases. The orifices only may be involved in a sclerotic aortitis. In one case they were narrowed to admit only a bristle, while the vessels beyond were normal. Blocking of a branch with a fresh thrombus, or with an embolus, is not uncommon. During an attack an infarct may soften, with perforation of the ventricular wall. Obliterative endarteritis, *the* lesion of the disease, was present in 9 of the cases. In elderly subjects the coronary vessels may be calcified—the condition found by Jenner in John Hunter.

(*b*) *Aortitis* was present in four of the cases, in syphilitic subjects, all under 40 years of age. Corrigan first called attention to this lesion in angina, the great importance of which has been emphasized by Clifford Allbutt. It is usually limited to the supra-sigmoidal area.

(*c*) In a few instances no lesions have been found. In one case of the list a man aged 26 had attacks, which were regarded as functional, on and off for two years. Death occurred after a series of paroxysms. The aorta was small, otherwise there were no changes.

Pathogenesis.—No completely satisfactory explanation of the phenomena of the attack has yet been offered. It has been regarded as a neuralgia of the cardiac nerves, a cramp of the heart muscle, or of certain parts of it, or an expression of tension of the ventricular walls. The view of Clifford Allbutt that the pain is dependent on tension of the first portion of the aorta has much to recommend it. A similar pain occurs in dilatation of the aorta. In some ways the intermittent claudication theory of Allan Burns meets the case. This may be defined as a state in which an artery admits enough blood to a muscular structure for quiet work, but not enough for increased work, so that the contractile function of the muscle is disturbed and pain results. Burns remarked that ". . . If we can call into vigorous action a limb around which we have with moderate tightness applied a ligature, we find that then the member can only support its action for a very short time, for now the supply of energy and its expenditure do not balance each other. . . . A heart, the coronary arteries of which are cartilaginous or ossified, is nearly in a similar condition; it can, like the limb begirt with a moderately tight ligature, discharge its functions so long as its action is moderate and equal. Increase, however, the action of the whole body, and along with the rest that of the heart, and you will soon see exemplified the truth of what has been said."

Angina results from an alteration in the working of the muscle fibres of any part of the cardio-vascular system, whereby painful afferent stimuli are excited. Cold, emotion, or toxic agents interfering with the orderly action of the peripheral circulation increase the tension in the heart walls or in the larger central mains, causing strain and a type of contraction capable of exciting in the involuntary muscles painful afferent stimuli. In disturbance of this all-important Gaskellian function, in the stretching, in the alteration of the wall tension at any point, sufficient to excite a pain-producing resistance to this by the muscle elements, are to be sought an explanation of the phenomenon of the attack. Spasm, or narrowing of a coronary artery, or of one branch, may so modify the action of a section of the heart that it works with disturbed tension, and with stretching and strain sufficient to rouse painful sensations. Or the heart may be in the same state as the leg muscles of a man with intermittent claudication, working smoothly when quiet, but the instant an effort is made, or if a wave of emotion touches the peripheral vessels, the normal contraction is disturbed and a crisis of pain excited.

Symptoms.—Classified by the severity of the attacks, cases may be grouped in three categories:

(*a*) Mildest Form (*"Les Formes Frustes"* of the French).—There is a feeling of substernal tension, uneasiness, or distress, rising at times to positive pain, usually associated with emotion, sometimes with exertion, but soon passing off. There may be slight pallor, or a feeling of faintness. When rising to speak in public there may be a feeling of substernal tension—it is a common experience—which passes off. Muscular effort, as in climbing a hill or a stair, may bring on the sensation. In the high pressure life a man may experience for weeks or months this sense of substernal tension, not pain, and without accurate localization or radiation, and not increased by exercise or emotion. It is, as one patient expressed it, a "hot-box" indicating too great pressure and too high speed. It is away after the night's rest, and may disappear entirely when the "harness" is taken off.

(*b*) Mild Form (*Angina Minor*).—Pain in the heart of moderate severity with radiation to the arm is met with in nervous persons, in tobacco smokers, sometimes following the acute infections, particularly influenza. The attacks are brought on by emotion, more frequent in women, and never fatal. Often called pseudo, false, functional, or toxic angina, the difference in the character of the attacks may be one of degree only. The conditions under which the attacks come on are of greater importance than the nature of the attack itself. There may be marked vaso-motor disturbance, with cold, numb, and blue extremities, followed by præcordial pain and a feeling of faintness. In persons addicted to tea, coffee, and tobacco heart pain is not infrequent, sharp and shooting, associated with palpitation, or severe and truly anginal.

(*c*) Severe Angina (*Angina Major*).—The two special features in this group are the existence in a large proportion of all the cases of organic disease of heart or vessels and the liability to sudden death. An exciting cause of the attack can usually be traced; muscular effort is the most common. Mental emotion is a second potent cause. John Hunter used to say that "his life was in the hands of any rascal who chose to worry him," and his fatal attack occurred in a fit of anger. A third very common excitant is flatulent distention of the stomach. Many patients are very sensitive to cold, and the chill of getting out of bed or of a bath may bring on a paroxysm.

Phenomena of the Attack.—During exertion or intense mental emotion the patient is seized with an agonizing pain in the region of the heart and a sense of constriction, as if the heart had been seized in a vice. The pains radiate to the neck and down the arm, and there may be numbness of the fingers or in the cardiac region. The face is usually pallid and may assume an ashy gray tint, and not infrequently a profuse sweat breaks out over the surface. The paroxysm lasts from several seconds to a minute or two, during which, in severe attacks, the patient feels as if death were imminent. As pointed out by Latham, there are two elements in it, the pain—*dolor pectoris*—and the indescribable feeling of anguish and sense of imminent dissolution—*angor animi*. There are great restlessness and anxiety, and the patient may drop dead at the height of the attack or faint and pass away in syncope. The condition of the heart during the attack is variable; the pulsations may be uniform and regular. The pulse tension, however, is usually increased, but it is surprising, even in the cases of extreme severity, how slightly the character of the pulse may be altered. After the attack there may be eructations, or the passage of a large quantity of clear urine. The patient usually feels exhausted, and for a day or two may be badly shaken; in other instances in an hour or two the patient feels himself again. While dyspnœa is not a constant feature, the paroxysm is not infrequently associated with it; there is wheezing in the bronchial tubes, which may come on very rapidly, and the patient gets short of breath.

Death may occur in the first attack, as in the well known case of Thomas Arnold; or at the end of a series of attacks, the so-called *status angiosus*. Paroxysms may occur at intervals of a few weeks for a year or more before the fatal attack.

There is a chronic form represented by 12 cases in our series, in which attacks occur irregularly. John Hunter's first seizure was in 1773, and he had many in the 20 years before his death. Sometimes life is a terrible burden, as any emotion or effort may bring on an attack. And, lastly, after paroxysms of great severity recurring for months, or even for so long as two years, complete recovery takes place.

Extra-pectoral Features of Angina.—In the attack the pain usually radiates up the neck and down the left arm. As the studies of Mackenzie and Head have shown in disease of the heart and of the aorta, the pain is referred to the 1st, 2d, 3d, and 4th dorsal areas; and in angina it may be also in areas of the distribution of the 5th to the 9th dorsal nerves. The pain may begin in the left arm, or in the jaw, even in the front teeth, or in one testis. Sometimes the pain remains in these distant parts, and yet the attack presents, as noted by Heberden, all the features of angina. The attack may begin with agonizing pain in the left leg or in the left pectoral muscle. The entire features of the attack may be sub-diaphragmatic—the so-called *angina abdominis.* In at least twelve of our series the pains were abdominal, and, as first pointed out by Leared, gastralgia may be diagnosed.

The *pulmonary features* are remarkable. A condition like acute emphysema may come on, with wheezing and an inflated state of the lungs. Acute œdema may follow with the expectoration of large quantities of a thin, bloody fluid. The blood pressure, may be extraordinarily high—340 mm. Hg in one case. *Cerebral features* are not common, but unconsciousness may occur. Transient monoplegia, or hemiplegia and aphasia, may occur.

Prognosis.—In men under 40 syphilis must be suspected, and with appropriate treatment recovery may be complete (see the Lumleian Lectures (Osler), Lancet, 1910, I). In men in the 5th and 6th decades who have lived the high pressure life a change of habits may bring relief; but, as Walshe remarked, "the cardinal fact in real angina is its uncertainty." Even after attacks of the greatest severity recovery is possible. The circumstances that bring on an attack are important. Emotion is of the least importance. The angina of effort that follows any slight exertion is, as a rule, more serious than that which comes on spontaneously, or is excited by emotion; yet one patient who could never dress without having what he called "angor de toilette" lived for 11 years. The cardio-vascular condition is of the first importance in prognosis. Very high blood pressure, advanced arterio-sclerosis, valvular disease, signs of myocardial weakness are of serious import. It is to be remembered that a large proportion of all cases have no obvious signs of cardiac disease; and the coronary arteries may be extensively diseased with clear heart sounds and a good pulse. In women the forms of angina with marked vaso-motor disturbance as a rule do well, and when neurotic or hysterical manifestations are prominent the outlook is good.

There are three modes of dying in angina—one, as Walshe says, "is sudden, instantaneous, coeval with a single pang." The functions of life stop abruptly, and with a gasp all is over. Ventricular fibrillation may be the cause. In a second mode, following a series of attacks, the heart grows weaker and the patient dies in a progressive asthenia; while in a third there is a gradually induced cardiac insufficiency with dyspnœa.

Treatment.—Prolonged rest is important and every effort should be made to reduce anxiety and sources of irritation. Factors which induce an attack should be avoided. The diet should be simple and the bowels kept freely open. If there are any signs of myocardial insufficiency an occasional course of digitalis is advisable. Syphilitic cases require active treatment—arsphenamine in the subjects under 40, mercury and iodide of potassium in older persons. In the neurotic cases with a recognition of the basic disturbance in the vaso-motor system a rest cure and hydrotherapy are indicated. A persistent course of wet packs is often helpful. When high tension is present the nitrites may be given; and ergotin grs. ii (0.13 gm.) three times a day has a definite value in vaso-motor instability. In the severer types the treatment is concerned with the attack and with the general condition afterward. In the attack inhalation of nitrite of amyl, introduced by Lauder Brunton, may give instant relief. We see its benefit particularly in cases with widespread arterial constriction. In the recurring terrible paroxysms it may lose its effect, but many milder forms are relieved promptly, and it gives great comfort and confidence to the patient to carry the *perles*. Morphia should be used freely when amyl nitrite fails and when the attacks recur with great frequency. As Burney Yeo pointed out, angina patients are very resistant to this drug. Chloroform may have to be used, and is always helpful, never harmful. With a dusky cyanosis and asthma like breathing oxygen inhalations may be given.

For the general condition, if high tension is present, iodide of potassium and the nitrites in all forms are useful. The use of theobromine, advocated by Marchiafava, grs. xv (1 gm.) three times a day, is sometimes of benefit.

C. DISEASES OF THE ARTERIES

I. ARTERIO-SCLEROSIS

(*Arterio-capillary Fibrosis*)

The conception of arterio-sclerosis as an independent affection—a general disease of the vascular system—is due to Gull and Sutton.

Definition.—A condition of thickening of the arterial coats, with degeneration, diffuse or circumscribed. The process leads, in the larger arteries, to what is known as atheroma and to endarteritis deformans, and seriously interferes with the normal functions of various organs.

Etiology.—Among the important factors are the following:

(*a*) HYPERTENSION.—The blood pressure, the tension or force with which the blood circulates, depends upon five factors: The heart pump supplies the force; the elastic coats of the large arteries store and convert an intermittent into a continuous stream; the small arteries act as sluices or taps regulating the control to different parts; the capillary bed is the irrigation field over which the nutritive fluid is distributed; and the drainage system is represented by the veins and lymph channels.

Galen first grasped the fact that life depends upon the maintenance of a due pressure in these irrigation fields: "Many canals dispersed throughout all the parts of the body convey to them blood as those of a garden convey moisture, and the intervals separating those canals are wonderfully disposed by nature in such a way that they should neither lack a sufficient quantity of blood for absorption, nor be overloaded at any time with an excessive supply."

The blood pressure varies greatly in different individuals, and in the same individual under varying conditions. The normal blood pressure is from 120 to 130 mm. of mercury, but in persons over 50 it is very often from 140 to 160 mm. A permanent pressure above the latter figure may be called high, but there are great regional variations. Permanently low blood pressure may be met with in asthenia from any cause, in the various toxæmias of the infectious diseases, in adrenal insufficiency, and there are persons in apparently good health with chronic hypotension.

High tension is met with in many chronic diseases, in various forms of cardiac and renal disease, in lead poisoning, and in connection with general arterio-sclerosis. The relation to arterio-sclerosis has been much discussed. Briefly, there are three groups of cases: (1) First, the simple high tension without signs of arterial or renal disease—what Clifford Allbutt calls *hyperpiesia.* In this well recognized condition, met with in individuals otherwise healthy, the blood pressure is permanently high—above 180—but, so far as can be ascertained, there are no arterial, cardiac, or renal changes. It is difficult to exclude internal, not discernible alterations in the splanchnic and other vessels, since vascular disease may be very localized. But clinically the group is well defined and very important. The condition is met with most frequently in keen business men, who work hard, drink hard, and smoke hard.

The exact cause of this high tension we do not know. Some have attributed it to over-activity of the adrenals, but it is much more likely that the primary difficulty is somewhere in the capillary bed—in that short space in which the real business of life is transacted. However produced, the important point here is that this hypertension itself leads to arterio-sclerosis, which can be produced experimentally by the injection of epinephrin and other hypertensive substances.

(2) In the second group of cases the high tension is associated with an arterio-sclerosis with consecutive cardiac and renal disease.

(3) In the third group the high tension is secondary to forms of chronic nephritis in association with cardio-vascular disease.

(*b*) As an INVOLUTION PROCESS arterio-sclerosis is an accompaniment of old age, and is the expression of the natural wear and tear to which the tubes are subjected. Longevity is a vascular question, which has been well expressed in the axiom that "a man is only as old as his arteries." To a majority of men death comes primarily or secondarily through this portal. The onset of what may be called physiological arterio-sclerosis depends, in the first place, upon the quality of arterial tissue (vital rubber) which the individual has inherited, and secondly upon the amount of wear and tear to which he has subjected it. That the former plays a most important rôle is shown in the cases in which arterio-sclerosis sets in early in life in individuals in whom none of the recognized etiological factors can be found. Thus, for instance, a man of thirty may have the arteries of a man of sixty, and a man of forty may present vessels as much degenerated as they should be at eighty. Entire families sometimes show this tendency to early arterio-sclerosis—a tendency which can not be explained in any other way than that in the makeup of the machine bad material was used for the tubing. More commonly the arterio-sclerosis results from the bad use of good vessels.

(*c*) INTOXICATIONS.—Alcohol, lead, and gout play an important rôle in the causation of arterio-sclerosis, although the precise mode of their action is not yet very clear. They may act, as Traube suggests, by increasing the peripheral resistance in the smaller vessels and in this way raising the blood tension, or possibly, as Bright taught, they alter the quality of the blood and render more difficult its passage through the capillaries. The observations of Cabot throw doubt on the importance of alcohol as a factor. The poisons of the acute infections may produce degenerative changes in the media and adventitia. Thayer called attention to the frequency of arterial changes as a sequence of typhoid fever.

(*d*) SYPHILIS, one of the most important single causes, will be spoken of under morbid anatomy.

(*e*) OVEREATING.—This plays an important part in inducing arterio-sclerosis. George Cheyne's advice, quoted at page 441, was never more needed then by the present generation.

(*f*) STRESS AND STRAIN.—There are men in the fifth decade who have not had syphilis or gout, who have eaten and drunk with discretion, and in whom none of the ordinary factors are present—men in whom the arterio-sclerosis seems to come on as a direct result of a high pressure life.

(*g*) OVERWORK OF THE MUSCLES, which acts by increasing the peripheral resistance and by raising the blood pressure.

(*h*) RENAL DISEASE.—The relation between the arterial and kidney lesions has been much discussed, some regarding the arterial degeneration as secondary, others as primary. There are two groups of cases, one in which the arterio-sclerosis is the first change, and the other in which it is secondary to a primary affection of the kidneys.

Morbid Anatomy.—The affection is met with most frequently in the aorta and its main branches. It is comparatively less frequent in the mesenteric and rare in the pulmonary arteries. Several forms may be recognized:

(*a*) NODULAR.—The aorta presents in the early stages, from the ring to the bifurcation, numerous flat projections, yellowish or yellowish white in color, and situated particularly about the orifices of the branches. In the early stage these patches are scattered and do not involve the entire intima. In more advanced stages the patches undergo atheromatous changes. The matrial constituting the button undergoes softening and breaks up into granular material, consisting of molecular débris—the so-called atheromatous abscess. Klotz has called attention to the frequency of nodular endarteritis about the orifices of the intercostal arteries in young people, usually in association with acute infections.

(*b*) DIFFUSE ARTERIO-SCLEROSIS.—In this form, met with usually in middle-aged men, or younger persons, the affection is widespread throughout the arteries. In the aorta the media shows necrotic and hyaline changes, while the intima may be smooth or show very slight thickenings—scattered elevated areas of an opaque white color, some of which undergo atheromatous changes. The smaller arteries show thickening of the walls, due particularly to increase in the sub-endothelial connective tissue. The muscular coat may be at first hypertrophied, but later undergoes hyaline and calcareous changes. In this group the heart hypertrophies and fibrous myocarditis is often present. The aortic valves are opaque and sclerotic. The kidneys are sclerotic, may be increased in size, and are usually very firm. In places the surface may be rough, or present atrophied depressed areas of a deep red color.

(*c*) Senile Arterio-sclerosis.—In this the larger arteries are dilated and tortuous, the walls thin and stiff, and the smaller vessels, as the radials, converted into rigid tubes like pipe-stems. The intima of the aorta may be occupied by rough, calcareous plaques, with here and there fissures and loss of substance. There may be sub-endothelial softening with the formation of atheromatous ulcers on which thrombi may deposit; though, as a rule, there may be the most extreme calcification and roughness with erosions of the aorta without thrombus formation. In the smaller vessels, as the radials, there are degeneration and calcification of the media—the so-called Moncke-berg type.

The syphilitic arterio-sclerosis is usually a mesaortitis with definite characteristics. Macroscopically it may be limited in extent, localized at the root of the aorta, or about the orifice of an aneurism, or there is a band of an inch in width on some portion of the tube, while other parts of the aorta and its branches are normal. In other instances the intima is involved, not with the usual plaque-like areas of atheroma, but there are shallow depressions of a bluish tint, and short transverse or longitudinal puckerings, sometimes with a stellate arrangement; or the intima is pitted and scarred with small depressions and linear sulci. Microscopically the most important changes are found in the media and adventitia: (*a*) perivascular infiltration of the vasa vasorum; (*b*) small-celled infiltration in areas of the media, with (*c*) splitting, separation, and destruction of elastic fibres and the muscle cells. The intima over these areas may be perfectly normal, but it often shows signs of thickening with fatty degeneration and the production of hyaline. Similar changes have been described by Klotz in the larger blood vessels in cases of congenital syphilis. And, lastly, the specific nature of this mesaortitis has been determined by the detection of the spirochætes. Other forms affecting the smaller vessels have been referred to under syphilis.

Sclerosis of the pulmonary artery is met with in various conditions. (1) With high tension, particularly in emphysema and mitral disease, the sclerosis may be marked, the main branches may be dilated, and the valves thickened and incompetent. (2) Gummatous arteritis has been met with (Warthin). (3) Primary sclerosis is not uncommon in India (Leonard Rogers). Aneurismal dilatation may be present. Syphilis is a factor in some cases. Dyspnœa, cyanosis, polycythæmia, repeated hæmoptysis, angina with enlargement of the heart, and chronic passive congestion are features. Our South American colleagues call it "Ayerza's disease."

In many cases of arterio-sclerosis the condition is not confined to the arteries, but extends not only to the capillaries but also to the veins, and may properly be termed an *angio-sclerosis*.

Sclerosis of the veins—*phlebo-sclerosis*—is not at all an uncommon accompaniment of arterio-sclerosis. It is seen in conditions of heightened blood pressure, as in the portal system in cirrhosis of the liver and in the pulmonary veins in mitral stenosis. The affected vessels are usually dilated, and the intima shows, as in the arteries, a compensatory thickening, which is particularly marked in those regions in which the media is thinned. The new-formed tissue in the endophlebitis may undergo hyaline degeneration, and is sometimes extensively calcified. Without existing arterio-sclerosis the peripheral veins may be sclerotic, usually in conditions of debility, but not infrequently in young persons.

Symptoms.—INCREASED TENSION.—The pressure with which the blood flows in the arteries depends upon the degree of peripheral resistance and the force of the ventricular contraction. A high-tension pulse may exist with very little arterio-sclerosis; but, as a rule, when the condition has been persistent, the sclerosis and high tension are found together. On the other hand, a very *low* or *normal tension* may be present in extremely sclerotic vessels.

GENERAL SYMPTOMS.—The early symptoms are interesting. Stengel has called attention to the pallor, and there may be dyspeptic symptoms. It is remarkable with what rapidity the disease may progress. The peripheral arteries may stiffen and grow old in a couple of years.

The combination of heightened blood pressure, a palpable thickening of the arteries, hypertrophy of the left ventricle, and accentuation of the aortic second sound are signs pathognomonic of arterio-sclerosis. From this period of establishment the course may be very varied. For years the patient may have good health, and be in a condition analogous to that of a person with a well compensated valvular lesion. There may be no renal symptoms, or there may be the passage of a larger amount of urine than normal, with transient albuminuria, and now and then hyaline tube casts. The subsequent history is extraordinarily diverse, depending upon the vascular territory in which the sclerosis is most advanced, or upon the accidents which are so liable to happen, and the symptoms may be cardiac, cerebral, renal, etc. In some cases there is a rapid loss of weight.

(*a*) *Cardiac.*—Involvement of the coronary arteries may lead to various symptoms—thrombosis with sudden death, fibroid degeneration of the heart, aneurism of the heart, rupture, and angina pectoris. The last is not uncommon, and the organic variety is almost always associated with arterio-sclerosis. A second important group of cardiac symptoms results from the dilatation which finally gets the better of the hypertrophy. The patient presents all the symptoms of cardiac insufficiency and when he comes under observation for the first time the clinical picture is that of chronic valvular disease, and a loud blowing murmur at the apex may throw the practitioner off his guard. Many cases terminate in this way.

(*b*) The *cerebral* symptoms are varied and important, and embrace those of many degenerative diseases, acute and chronic (which follow sclerosis of the smaller branches), and cerebral hæmorrhage. Syphilis should always be considered in these cases. Transient hemiplegia, monoplegia, or aphasia may occur in advanced arterio-sclerosis. The attacks are very characteristic, often brief, lasting twenty-four hours or less. Recovery may be perfect. Recurrence is the rule, and a patient may have a score or more attacks of aphasia, or in a couple of years there may be half a dozen transient hemiplegic attacks or one or two monoplegias, or paraplegia for a day or two. These cases seem best explained on the view of transient spasm as suggested by Peabody. Vertigo occurs frequently, and may be simple, or associated with slow pulse and syncopal or epileptiform attacks—the Stokes-Adams syndrome.

(*c*) *Renal* symptoms supervene in a large number of the cases. A sclerosis, patchy or diffuse, is present in a majority of the cases at the time of autopsy, and the condition is practically that of contracted kidney. It is seen typically in the senile form, and not infrequently develops early in life as a direct sequence of the diffuse variety. It is often difficult to decide clinically (and the question is one upon which good observers might not agree in a given case) whether the arterial or the renal disease has been primary.

(*d*) *Abdominal Arterio-sclerosis.*—It is believed to be associated particularly with overeating and chronic overtaxing of the stomach and intestines. The condition is not uncommon, and the sclerosis of the splanchnic vessels may be advanced out of all proportion to that elsewhere. The symptoms are indefinite, sometimes resembling those of the ordinary neurosis with marked constipation, features that are by no means certainly associated with sclerosis; on the other hand, there is much more reason to connect the attacks of severe abdominal pain, the gastric crises of lead and of tabes with spasm of the vessels in this condition. There are cases of angina pectoris with abdominal pain which may be due to angiospasm of the sclerotic vessels.

(*e*) Among other events in arterio-sclerosis may be mentioned *gangrene* of the extremities, due either directly to endarteritis or to the dislodgment of thrombi. Sudden transient paralysis of the legs may occur.

(*f*) *Sclerosis of the Vessels of the Legs.*—The main symptom is pain in the legs, after walking for a few minutes or on walking fast, which may pull the patient "up short" or gradually reach a point at which motion is impossible. The patient rarely falls and after resting for a few minutes he can again walk. The attacks are similar to those of angina pectoris; as one intelligent man expressed it—"there is no difference in the sensation, it is only in the place." Cramp of the muscles may occur, and aggravate the pain, sometimes in paroxysms of very severe intensity, or nocturnal cramp may be troublesome. Numbness, tingling and sensations of cold are common, and when dependent the feet may become deeply congested. The posterior tibials and dorsal arteries of the feet may be felt as hard cords without pulsation and phlebosclerosis is common.

Intermittent lameness or claudication, the dysbasia angio-sclerotica of Erb, the crural angina of Walton, is associated with arterio-sclerosis. In the horse, in which the intermittent lameness was first described by Bouley, verminous aneurisms are present in the aorta or the iliac arteries. In man Charcot described the condition in 1856 in an old soldier who was not able to walk for more than a quarter of an hour without severe cramps in the legs. The post mortem showed a traumatic aneurism of one iliac artery. The loss of function and the pain in the muscles are due to the relative ischæmia. Of 127 cases there were only 7 in women (Erb). Hebrews seem more frequently affected. Syphilis, alcohol, and tobacco are common factors.

Thrombo-angeitis obliterans (Buerger) is an acute inflammatory lesion with occlusion thrombosis, probably due to infection. There is excruciating pain in the foot and leg, worse at night. The feet are blue and congested, and the skin clammy with decreased sensitiveness to heat and cold. There may be atrophy of the toes with dark colored skin and sometimes gangrene. Pulsation in the vessels of the affected leg is decreased or absent.

Treatment.—In the late stages the conditions must be treated as they arise in connection with the various viscera. In the early stages, before any local symptoms are manifest, the patient should be enjoined to live a quiet, well regulated life, avoiding excesses in food and drink. It is well to reduce the intake of salt. It is usually best to explain frankly the condition of affairs, and so gain his intelligent coöperation. Special attention should be paid to the state of the bowels and urine, and the secretion of the skin should be kept active by daily baths. Alcohol in all forms should be prohibited, and the food restricted to plain, wholesome articles. The use of mineral waters or a residence every year at one of the mineral springs is usually serviceable. If there has been a syphilitic history the persistent use of iodide of potassium is indicated; indeed, even in the non-syphilitic cases it seems to do good. It is best given in small doses, grains v to x (0.3 to 0.6 gm.). Whenever the blood pressure is high nitroglycerine or sodium nitrite may be given to relieve symptoms rather than with any hope of essentially influencing the disease. For intermittent claudication not much can be done. In the thrombo-angeitis obliterans small doses of thyroid extract may be given. Injections of 300-500 c. c. of salt solution subcutaneously may be tried.

In cases which come under observation for the first time with dyspnœa, slight lividity, and signs of cardiac insufficiency, venesection is indicated. In some instances, with very high tension, striking relief is afforded by the abstraction of 10 to 20 ounces of blood. Cardiac failure, renal symptoms, etc., require the usual treatment.

II. AORTITIS

Acute Aortitis.—This is much more common than is usually recognized. It may occur in the acute infections but most especially in septicæmia and rheumatic fever, particularly in children who have aortic endocarditis. Of greatest importance is its occurrence in syphilis.

Pathology.—The process may be diffuse or most evident in slightly raised areas which at first are soft and later harder and with a yellow tinge. The first portion of the arch is most often affected and this may involve the orifices of the coronary arteries. If the aorta was previously diseased, all stages of atheroma may be found.

Symptoms.—Pain is common, usually referred to the upper part of the sternum and sometimes radiating into the arms. There may be dyspnœa and a sense of thoracic oppression. In the syphilitic form, pain is the outstanding symptom. In the other forms the pain is merged in the symptoms of the primary condition, especially in the acute infections.

Signs.—There may be marked pulsation in the neck, especially in the suprasternal notch, where the aorta may be seen and felt, and in the first and second interspaces. There is dulness over the manubrium and in the first two interspaces, both to right and left. The second sound may have a musical bell-like quality, sometimes very characteristic. The *syphilitic* form as a rule shows in addition the signs of aortic insufficiency.

Diagnosis.—The main requisite is that the condition be kept in mind. It is unrecognized because not considered. If there is any doubt the X-ray examination should decide. A positive Wassermann reaction or other evidence of syphilis gives the diagnosis of this form.

Prognosis.—The condition in itself probably does not shorten life but may lead to permanent damage of the aortic orifice. In the syphilitic forms the degree of this depends greatly on early diagnosis and proper treatment.

The *treatment* is that of the etiological condition.

Chronic Aortitis.—(Dilatation of the Aorta).—This is a common condition, frequently overlooked. The diffuse dilatation is sometimes described under aneurism but deserves separate mention. It was first described by Hodgson in 1815 as "preternatural permanent enlargement of the cavity of an artery." It is often associated with aortic insufficiency, which the French term *maladie de Hodgson.*

Etiology.—It is much more common in males and the colored race shows a relatively high incidence. There are several special groups: (1) As a result of infection and acute aortitis a permanent dilatation remains. Two diseases are particularly concerned, rheumatic fever and syphilis. (2) As part of a general arterio-sclerosis in which the aorta is specially involved. The influence of syphilis and hard muscular work is important in this form. (3) In the aged it is common as part of an advanced arterial degeneration.

Pathology.—The extent of dilatation varies greatly and may involve only a portion of the arch, extend throughout the whole extent of the aorta or only to where the aorta passes through the diaphragm. The orifices and part of the vessels given off from the aorta may be involved in the dilatation. Thrombus formation in the aorta may occur. The aorta shows all grades of gross atheromatous change.

Symptoms.—There are several groups: (1) Latent cases, especially in the aged. (2) In many cases those due to associated cardiac disease predominate, with the features of myocardial insufficiency or of aortic insufficiency. (3) A group with features suggestive of angina pectoris, not surprising in view of the disease of the first part of the aorta. The pain may radiate down either arm or sometimes down both. The common complaints are of pain, dyspnœa, and cough.

Signs.—The neck may be full with distended veins and a collar of pulsation above the clavicles and sternum. Pulsation in the suprasternal notch is common. The manubrium may be lifted and pulsation in the upper two interspaces is often seen. The order of frequency is second right, second left, first right and first left interspace. This pulsation is usually diffuse and can rarely be felt distinctly. The aorta may be felt above the sternum or with the finger behind it. *Dulness* is very important, over the manubrium and adjoining interspaces. It is continuous with the heart dulness in most cases but not always. The width of the dulness in the first interspaces may be 8 to 14 cm. and the extent may vary from time to time. On *auscultation* the second sound often has an amphoric bell-like quality, which is diagnostic if present. The murmur of an associated aortic insufficiency may have the same quality. The blood pressure is low in the majority. Arterio-sclerosis is usually and aortic insufficiency (relative or permanent) often present. *The pressure signs* are practically the same as in aneurism, inequality of the pupils, laryngeal paralysis, tracheal tug, inequality of the radial pulses, and dysphagia.

Diagnosis.—The main point is to know of the condition and look for it. The diagnosis from aneurism or displacement of the aorta is difficult in a few cases; the X-ray examination will decide. The pain suggests angina pectoris but it is rarely so severe, often lasts for a considerable time, and is not often caused by exertion. In fact mild exertion often relieves the pain. Sweating is very rare.

Treatment.—A quiet even life with avoidance of strain, physical or mental, a limited diet, open bowels, and the treatment of symptoms are the main points. If syphilis is responsible, thorough treatment should be given but usually the damage is done and beyond repair. Vaso-dilators are useful for the pain.

III. ANEURISM

Definition.—A tumor containing fluid or solid blood in direct communication with the cavity of the heart, the surface of a valve, or the lumen of an artery.

History.—Galen knew external aneurism well, and in the second century A. D., Antyllos devised his operation of incising and emptying the sac inclosed between ligatures. Internal aneurism was recognized by Fernelius in the 16th century, and Vesalius was very familiar with it. Ambroise Paré suggested the relation of aneurism to syphilis, which was insisted upon in the great monograph of Lancisi in 1728. Morgagni in 1761 described very fully the symptoms and morbid anatomy. The modern views date from the studies of Helmstedter and Köster, who showed that the primary change was in the media. The researches of Eppinger, Thoma, and Welch emphasized the importance of these changes in the media, particularly as brought about by syphilis.

Classification.—The following classification may be adopted:

I. True aneurism (aneurisma verum or aneurisma spontaneum), in which one or more of the coats of the vessel form the wall of the tumor: (*a*) *Dilatation-aneurism*—(1) Limited to a certain portion of the vessel, fusiform, cylindroid; (2) extending over a whole artery and its branches—cirsoid aneurism. (*b*) *Circumscribed saccular aneurism,* which is the common form of aneurism of the aorta. (*c*) *Dissecting aneurism,* with splitting of the media, and occasionally with the formation of a new tube lined with intimal endothelium.

II. False aneurism, following a wound or the rupture of an artery, or of a true aneurism, causing a diffuse, or circumscribed, hæmatoma.

III. Arterio-venous aneurism, either with direct communication between an artery and vein, or with the intervention of a sac, varicose aneurism.

IV. Special forms, as the parasitic, erosion, traction, and mycotic.

Etiology.—Predisposing Causes.—*Age.*—Nearly one half of the deaths in England and Wales from aneurism in males occur between the ages of 30 and 45. In the young and in the very old the disease is rare, but it may occur at any age. Congenital aneurism has been described.

Sex.—Males are attacked much more frequently than females—5 to 1.

Race and Locality.—The disease is more common in Great Britain than on the Continent. Among about 19,000 post mortems at Vienna there were 230 cases of aneurism, while among 18,678 at Guy's Hospital there were 325 cases. It is more common in the negroes of the Southern States of America than among the whites. Of 345 admissions for aneurism to the medical wards of the Hopkins Hospital 132 were in colored and 213 in white patients—a ratio of 1 to 1.6, while the ratio of colored to white in the hospital at large was 1 to 5. In India aneurism is rare, though syphilis and arterial disease are common. Possibly, as Rogers suggests, the low blood pressure in the natives may have something to do with this comparative immunity.

Occupation.—Soldiers, sailors, draymen, iron and steel workers, and dock workers are particularly prone. In soldiers and sailors, who are peculiarly liable, the disease is in direct proportion to the prevalence of syphilis.

DETERMINING CAUSES.—These are three in number:

I. *The Acute Infections.*—In the specific fevers areas of degeneration are common in the aorta. Fortunately in most instances they are confined to the intima, but occasionally, as Thayer pointed out in typhoid fever, the changes may be in the media. *The* infection with which aneurism is especially connected is syphilis—a fact recognized in the eighteenth century by Lancisi and by Morgagni, and dwelt upon specially in 1876 by Francis H. Welch, of the British Army. All recent figures show a very high percentage of syphilis and it is rare not to find a positive Wassermann reaction in an aneurismal patient under fifty. The lesion, a mesaortitis, has been described under arterio-sclerosis. Other infections play a very minor rôle. With rheumatic fever, pneumonia, and septicæmia, the mycotic aneurism may be associated.

II. The second determining factor is *strain,* particularly the internal strain associated with sudden and violent muscular effort. The media is the protecting coat of the artery, and during a violent effort, as in lifting or jumping, laceration or splitting of the intima may occur over a weak spot. If small this leads to a local bulging of the media and the gradual production of a sac, or the tear of the intima may heal completely, or a dissecting aneurism may form. In other instances a widespread mesaortitis leads to a gradual, diffuse distention of the artery. This type of aneurism, frequently seen in the aged, may follow ordinary chronic atheroma.

III. *Occasional Causes.*—(*a*) Embolism: The emboli may consist of vegetations or calcified fragments from the valves. This form, often multiple, is met with in infective endocarditis, in which the emboli probably pass to the vasa vasorum, causing mesaortitis with weakening of the wall; but in the smaller vessels the aneurisms are caused by the direct lodgment of the emboli which infect and weaken the wall. (*b*) External Injury: A blow on the chest, a sudden fall, or the jar of an accident may cause a rupture of the intima over a weak spot in the aorta, with the production of a dissecting or sacculated aneurism. (*c*) External Erosion: A tuberculous focus may involve the wall of the aorta; or a bullet lodged near the wall of an artery may weaken it and be followed by aneurism. (*d*) In the horse there is a *parasitic aneurism* common in the mesenteric vessels, due to growth in them of the *Strongylus armatus.* (*e*) Thoma described a "traction" aneurism at the concavity of the arch at the point of insertion of the ductus Botalli.

Morbid Anatomy and Pathology.—NUMBER.—Usually there is one aneurism, but three or four or even a dozen may be present. Multiple cup-shaped tumors in the aorta are always syphilitic. The mycotic are usually multiple, and in the peripheral vessels there may be a dozen or more.

FORM.—There are two great types—one in which the lumen of the vessel is dilated, and the other in which a limited section of the wall gives way with the formation of a sac. Typical cylindrical and spindle shaped aneurisms are seen in the aorta and in the vessels of the second and third dimensions. The sacculated form is the more common. They are either flat, saucer-shaped, or cup-shaped, or sometimes beyond a very narrow orifice is a cylindrical tumor of variable size, from a pin's head in the smaller vessels, as in the brain, to a huge sac which may fill one half of the chest.

VESSELS AFFECTED.—Of a series of 551 cases studied by Crisp, the thoracic aorta was involved in 175, the abdominal aorta in 59, the femoral-iliac in 66, the popliteal in 137, the innominate in 20, the carotids in 25, subclavians in 23, axillary in 18. The other smaller vessels are rarely attacked. Of late years aneurism of the external vessels appears to have become much less frequent.

I. ANEURISM OF THE AORTA

A. Aneurism of the Thoracic Aorta.—For purposes of discussion this part of the vessel may be divided into the sinuses of Valsalva, ascending, transverse, and descending portions.

(*a*) ANEURISM OF THE SINUSES OF VALSALVA, a common and important variety, is met with most frequently in young syphilitic subjects. There may be pouching of one or of all three sinuses; the aortic ring is apt to be involved and one or more of the valves rendered incompetent. The special features are: (1) It is often latent, causing sudden death by perforation into the pericardium. (2) It is a medico-legal aneurism met with most frequently in coroner's cases. (3) Angina pectoris is not uncommon and may be the only symptom. (4) Aortic insufficiency is often associated with it. (5) In a majority of all cases syphilitic mesaortitis is present.

(*b*) ANEURISM OF THE ASCENDING ARCH.—Along the convex border aneurism frequently arises and may grow to a large size, either passing out into the right pleura or forward, pointing at the second or third interspace, eroding the ribs and sternum, and producing large external tumors. In this situation the sac may compress the superior vena cava, causing engorgement of the vessels of the head and arm; sometimes it compresses only the subclavian vein, and causes enlargement and œdema of the right arm. Perforation may take place into the superior vena cava, of which accident Pepper and Griffith collected 29 cases. In rare instances, when the aneurism springs from the concave side of the vessels, the tumor may appear to the left of the sternum. Large aneurisms in this situation may cause much dislocation of the heart, pushing it down and to the left, and sometimes compressing the inferior vena cava, and causing swelling of the feet and ascites. The right recurrent laryngeal nerve is often compressed. The innominate artery is rarely involved. Death commonly follows from rupture into the pericardium, the pleura, or into the superior cava; less commonly from rupture externally, sometimes from syncope.

(*c*) ANEURISM OF THE TRANSVERSE ARCH.—The direction of growth is most commonly backward, but the sac may grow forward, erode the sternum, and form a large tumor. The sac presents in the middle line and to the right of the sternum much more often than to the left, which occurred in only 4 of 35 aneurisms in this situation (O. A. Browne). Even when small and producing no external tumor it may cause marked pressure signs in its growth backward toward the spine, involving the trachea and the œsophagus, and giving rise to cough, often of a paroxysmal character, and dysphagia. The left recurrent laryngeal is often involved in its course round the arch. A small aneurism from the lower or posterior wall of the arch may compress a bronchus, inducing bronchorrhœa, gradual bronchiectasis, and suppuration in the lung—a process which not infrequently causes death in aneurism, and a condition which at the Montreal General Hospital we were in the habit of terming "aneurismal phthisis." Occasionally enormous aneurisms arise in this situation, and grow into both pleuræ, extending between the manubrium and the vertebræ; they may persist for years. The sac may be evident at the sternal notch. The innominate artery, less commonly the left carotid and subclavian, may be involved, and the radial or carotid pulse absent or retarded. Sometimes the thoracic duct is compressed.

The ascending and transverse portions of the arch are not infrequently involved together, usually without the branches; the tumor grows upward, or upward and to the right.

(*d*) ANEURISM OF THE DESCENDING PORTION OF THE ARCH.—It is not infrequently the traction aneurism of Thoma. The sac projects to the left and backward, and often erodes the vertebræ from the third to the sixth dorsal, causing great pain and sometimes compression of the spinal cord. Dysphagia is common. Pressure on a bronchus may induce bronchiectasis, with retention of secretions, and fever. A tumor may appear externally in the region of the scapula, and attain an enormous size. Death not infrequently occurs from rupture into the pleura, or the sac may grow into the lung and cause hæmoptysis.

(*e*) ANEURISM OF THE DESCENDING THORACIC AORTA.—This is the least common situation of aortic aneurism. The larger number occur close to the diaphragm, the sac lying upon or to the left of the bodies of the lower dorsal vertebræ, which are often eroded. It is frequently latent, in 3 of 14 cases (Osler), and is often overlooked; pulmonary and pleural symptoms are common. Pain in the back is severe; dysphagia is not infrequent. The sac may reach an enormous size and form a subcutaneous tumor in the left back.

Physical Signs.—INSPECTION.—A good light is essential; cases are often overlooked owing to a hasty inspection. The face is often suffused, the conjunctivæ injected, and veins of the chest and of one arm engorged. One pupil may be enlarged. In many instances inspection is negative. On either side of the sternum there may be abnormal pulsation, due to dislocation of the heart, to deformity of the thorax, or to retraction of the lung. Three sorts of pulsation may be seen in the chest: (1) A general shock, such as is seen in the violent throbbing of the heart or of an aneurism. In anæmia, in neurasthenia, and in great hypertrophy this widespread shock may suggest aneurism. (2) A diffuse impulse localized in a certain part of the chest, which may be caused by a deep-seated aneurism but which is met with also in tumors, in pulsating pleurisy, and in a few cases without evident cause (see "Modern Medicine," Vol. IV). (3) The punctate, heaving true aneurismal impulse which when of any extent is visibly expansile. It is seen most frequently above the level of the third rib to the right of the sternum, in the second left interspace, over the manubrium, and behind in the left interscapular region. When the innominate is involved the throbbing may be seen at the right sterno-clavicular joint and above it. An external tumor is present in many cases, projecting either through the upper part of the sternum or to the right, sometimes involving the sternum and costal cartilages on both sides, forming a swelling the size of a cocoanut or even larger. The skin is thin, often blood stained, or it may have ruptured, exposing the laminæ of the sac. The apex beat may be much dislocated, particularly when the sac is large. It is more commonly a dislocation from pressure than from enlargement of the heart itself.

Palpation.—The area and degree of pulsation are best determined by palpation. When the aneurism is deep seated and not apparent externally, the bimanual method should be used, one hand upon the spine and the other on the sternum. There may be only a diffuse impulse. When the sac has perforated the chest wall the impulse is, as a rule, forcible, slow, heaving, and expansile, and has the same qualities as a forcible apex beat. The resistance may be very great if there are thick laminæ beneath the skin; more rarely the sac is soft and fluctuating. The hand upon the sac, or on the region in which it is in contact with the chest wall, may feel a diastolic shock, often of great intensity, which forms one of the valuable physical signs of aneurism. A systolic thrill is sometimes present. The pulsation may sometimes be felt in the suprasternal notch.

Percussion.—The small and deep seated aneurisms are in this respect negative. In the larger tumors, as soon as the sac reaches the chest wall, there is produced an area of abnormal dulness, the position of which depends upon the part of the aorta affected. Aneurisms of the ascending arch grow forward and to the right, producing dulness on one side of the manubrium; those from the transverse arch produce dulness in the middle line, extending toward the left of the sternum, while aneurisms of the descending portion most commonly produce dulness in the left interscapular and scapular regions. The percussion note is flat and gives a feeling of increased resistance.

Auscultation.—Adventitious sounds are not always to be heard. Even in a large sac there may be no murmur. Much depends upon the thickness of the laminæ of fibrin. An important sign, particularly if heard over a dull region, is a ringing, accentuated second sound, a phenomenon rarely missed in large aneurisms of the aortic arch. A systolic murmur may be present; sometimes a double murmur, in which case the diastolic *bruit* is usually due to associated aortic insufficiency. The systolic murmur alone is of little moment in the diagnosis of aneurism. A continuous humming top murmur with systolic intensification is heard when the aneurism communicates with the vena cava or the pulmonary artery.

Among other physical signs of importance are retardation of the pulse in the arteries beyond the aneurism, or in those involved in the sac. There may, for instance, be a marked difference between the right and left radial, both in volume and time. The blood pressure on the two sides may be unequal. A physical sign of large thoracic aneurism is obliteration of the pulse in the abdominal aorta and its branches. Attention was called to this in a patient who was stated to have aortic insufficiency. There was a well-marked diastolic murmur, but in the femorals and in the aorta no trace of pulsation could be found, and not the slightest throbbing in the abdominal aorta or in the peripheral arteries of the leg. The circulation was, however, unimpaired in them and there was no dilatation of the veins. A careful examination of the patient's back showed what neither the patient nor any of his physicians had noticed, that he had a very large area of pulsation in the left scapular region. The sac probably was large enough to act as a reservoir annihilating the ventricular systole, and converting the intermittent into a continuous stream.

A remarkable condition suggestive of pneumothorax may be caused by compression of one bronchus by the sac (Newton Pitt). The air is inspired beyond the obstruction, but has difficulty in getting out, so that the lung is gradually distended, causing enlargement of the side with a hyperresonant note on percussion, and on auscultation absence of breath sounds. The X-ray picture may alone decide the diagnosis.

The *tracheal tugging,* a valuable sign in deep-seated aneurisms, was described by Surgeon-Major Oliver, who gave the following directions: "Place the patient in the erect position, and direct him to close his mouth and elevate his chin to almost the full extent; then grasp the cricoid cartilage between the finger and thumb, and use steady and gentle upward pressure on it, when, if dilatation or aneurism exists, the pulsation of the aorta will be distinctly felt transmitted through the trachea to the hand." The tug is usually felt more easily if the chin is held down. This is a sign of great value in the diagnosis of deep-seated aneurisms, though it may occasionally be felt in tumors and in the extreme dynamic dilatation of aortic insufficiency. It may be visible in the thyroid cartilage. The trachea may be pushed to one side.

Occasionally a systolic murmur may be heard in the trachea, as pointed out by David Drummond, or even at the patient's mouth, when opened. This is either the sound conveyed from the sac, or is produced by the air as it is driven out of the wind pipe during the systole. Feeble respiration in one lung is a common effect of pressure.

Symptoms.—Broadbent made the useful division of aneurisms of *symptoms* and aneurisms of *physical signs;* the former is more commonly seen when the transverse arch is involved, the latter when the ascending portion. There may be no symptoms. A man may present a tumor which has eroded the chest wall without pain or any discomfort but this is rare.

An important but variable feature in thoracic aneurism is *pain,* which is particularly marked in deep seated tumors. It is usually paroxysmal, sharp, and lancinating, often very severe when the tumor is eroding the vertebræ, or perforating the chest wall. In the latter case after perforation the pain may cease. Anginal attacks are not uncommon, particularly in aneurisms at the root of the aorta. Frequently the pain radiates down the left arm or up the neck, sometimes along the upper intercostal nerves. Superficial tenderness may be felt in the skin over the heart or over the left sternomastoid muscle. *Cough* results either from the direct pressure on the trachea, or is associated with bronchitis. The expectoration in these instances is abundant, thin, and watery; subsequently it becomes thick and turbid. Paroxysmal cough of a peculiar brazen, ringing character is a characteristic symptom in some cases, particularly when there is pressure on the recurrent laryngeal nerves, or the cough may have a peculiar wheezy quality—the "goose cough."

Dyspnœa, which is common in cases of aneurism of the transverse portion, is not necessarily associated with pressure on the recurrent laryngeal nerves, but may be due directly to compression of the trachea or the left bronchus. It may occur with marked stridor. Loss of voice and hoarseness are consequences of pressure on the recurrent laryngeal, usually the left, inducing either a spasm in the muscles of the left vocal cord or paralysis.

Paralysis of an abductor on one side may be present without any symptoms. It is more particularly, as Semon states, when the paralytic contractures supervene that the attention is called to laryngeal symptoms.

Hæmorrhage in thoracic aneurism may come from (*a*) the soft granulations in the trachea at the point of compression, in which case the sputum is blood tinged, but large quantities of blood are not lost; (*b*) from rupture of the sac into the trachea or a bronchus; (*c*) from perforation into the lung or erosion of the lung tissue. The bleeding may be profuse, rapidly proving fatal, and is a common cause of death. It may persist for weeks or months, in which case it is simply hæmorrhagic weeping through the sac, which is exposed in the trachea. In some instances, even after a very profuse hæmorrhage, the patient recovers and may live for years. A man with well-marked thoracic aneurism, who had several brisk hæmorrhages, died four years after, having in the meantime enjoyed average health. Death from hæmorrhage is relatively more common in aneurism of the third portion of the arch and of the descending aorta.

Difficulty of swallowing is a comparatively rare symptom, and may be due either to spasm or to direct compression. The sound should never be passed in these cases, as the œsophagus may be almost eroded and perforation of the sac has taken place.

Heart Symptoms.—Pain is often anginal in character, and is most common when the root of the aorta is involved. The heart is hypertrophied in less than one-half of the cases. The aortic valves are sometimes incompetent, either from disease of the segments or stretching of the aortic ring.

Among other signs, venous compression may involve one subclavian or the superior vena cava. A curious phenomenon in intrathoracic aneurism is the clubbing of the fingers and incurving of the nails of one hand, of which two examples were without any special distention or signs of venous engorgement. Tumors of the arch may involve the pulmonary artery, producing compression, or in some instances adhesion of the pulmonary segments and insufficiency of the valve; or the sac may rupture into the artery, which happened in two cases, producing instantaneous death.

Pupil Signs.—These may be due to, first, pressure on the sympathetic, which may cause dilatation of one pupil from irritation, contraction when the nerve is paralyzed. Flushing of the side of the face and ear, increased temperature, and sweating may be present. Secondly, as Ainley Walker and Wall have shown, the anisocoria is most frequently due to vascular conditions —with low blood pressure in one carotid the pupil on that side is dilated, with high pressure contracted, and in 26 cases of aneurism they found a relation between the state of the pupil and the arteries on the same side. Thirdly, in some cases the anisocoria is a syphilitic manifestation.

An X-ray examination should be made in all doubtful cases. The fluoroscope gives an accurate picture of the situation, the size, and the relation to the heart. Even a small sac may be seen. The diagnosis may rest upon it alone in cases in which scarcely a physical sign was present. Sailer and Pfahler have shown that a condition of tortuosity of the aorta, due to arterio-sclerosis, may exist, suggesting very strongly the presence of aneurism, particularly on examination with the fluoroscope.

The clinical picture of aneurism of the aorta is extremely varied. Many cases present characteristic symptoms and no physical signs, while others have well-marked physical signs and few or no symptoms.

Diagnosis.—Aneurism of the aorta may be confounded with: (*a*) The violent throbbing impulse of the arch in aortic insufficiency.

(*b*) *Simple Dynamic Pulsation.*—This is common in the abdominal aorta, but is rare in the arch. A case which came under the care of William Murray and Bramwell presented, without any pain or pressure symptoms, pulsation and dulness over the aorta. The condition gradually disappeared and was thought to be neurotic.

(*c*) Dilatation of the arch which has many of the features of aneurism. The X-ray examination may be required to decide the diagnosis.

(*d*) In curvature of the spine there may be great displacement of the aorta, so that it pulsates forcibly to the right of the sternum.

(*e*) *Solid Tumors.*—When the tumor projects externally and pulsates the difficulty may be considerable. In tumor the heaving, *expansile* pulsation is absent, and there is not that sense of force and power which is so striking in the throbbing of a perforating aneurism. There is not to be felt, as in aortic aneurism, the shock of the heart sounds, particularly the diastolic shock. Auscultatory sounds are less definite, as large aneurisms may occur without murmurs; and, on the other hand, murmurs may be heard over tumors. The greatest difficulty is in the deep seated thoracic tumors, and here the diagnosis may be impossible. The physical signs may be indefinite. The ringing aortic second sound is of great importance and is rarely, if ever, heard over tumor. Tracheal tugging is here a valuable sign. Pressure phenomena are less common in tumor. The general appearance of the patient in aneurism is much better than in tumor, in which there may be cachexia and enlargement of the glands in the axilla or in the neck. The result of the Wassermann reaction is of aid. Occasionally cancer of the œsophagus may simulate aneurism, producing pressure on the left bronchus.

(*f*) *Pulsating Pleurisy.*—In cases of *empyema necessitatis,* if the projecting tumor is in the neighborhood of the heart and pulsates, the condition may be mistaken for aneurism. The absence of the heaving, firm distention and of the diastolic shock would, with the history and the existence of pleural effusion, determine the nature of the case. If necessary, puncture may be made with a fine needle. In a majority of the cases of pulsating pleurisy the throbbing is diffuse and widespread, moving the whole side. The X-ray study is of value.

Prognosis.—The outlook is always grave. Life may be prolonged for some years, but the patients are in constant jeopardy. Spontaneous cure is not very infrequent in the small sacculated tumors of the ascending and thoracic portions. The cavity becomes filled with laminæ of firm fibrin, which become more and more dense and hard, the sac shrinks considerably, and finally lime salts are deposited in the old fibrin. The laminæ of fibrin may be on a level with the lumen of the vessel, causing complete obliteration of the sac. The cases which rupture externally, as a rule, run a rapid course, although to this there are exceptions; the sac may contract, become firm and hard, and the patient may live for five, or even for ten or twenty years. The cases which last longest are those in which a saccular aneurism has projected from the ascending arch. One patient in Montreal had been known to have aneurism for eleven years. The aneurism may be enormous, occupying a large area of the chest, and yet life be prolonged for many years. One of the most remarkable instances is the case of dissecting aneurism reported by Graham. The patient was invalided after the Crimean War with aneurism of the aorta, and for years was under the observation of J. H. Richardson, of Toronto, under whose care he died in 1885. The autopsy showed a healed aneurism of the arch, with a dissecting aneurism extending the whole length of the aorta, which formed a double tube.

Treatment.—In a large proportion of the cases this can only be *palliative.* Still in every instance measures should be taken which are known to promote clotting and consolidation within the sac. In any large series of cured aneurisms a considerable majority of the patients have not been known to be subjects of the disease, but the obliterated sac has been found accidentally at the post mortem.

The most satisfactory plan in early cases, when it can be carried out thoroughly, is the modified Valsalva method advised by Tufnell, of Dublin, the essentials of which are rest and a restricted diet. The rest should, as far as possible, be absolute. The reduction of the daily number of heart beats, when a patient is recumbent and without exertion, amounts to many thousands, and is one of the principal advantages of this plan. Mental quiet should also be enjoined. The diet advised by Tufnell is extremely rigid—for breakfast, 2 ounces of bread and butter and 2 ounces of milk or tea; dinner, 3 ounces of mutton and 3 of potatoes or bread and 4 ounces of claret; supper, 2 ounces of bread and butter and 2 ounces of tea. This low diet diminishes the blood volume and is thought also to render the blood more fibrinous. "Total per diem, 10 ounces of solid food and 8 ounces of fluid, and *no more.*" This treatment should be pursued for several months, but, except in persons of a good deal of mental stamina, it is impossible to carry it out for more than a few weeks at a time. It is a form of treatment adapted only to the saccular form, and in cases of large sacs communicating with the aorta by a comparatively small orifice the chances of consolidation are fairly good. Unquestionably rest and the restriction of the liquids are the important parts of the treatment, and a greater variety and quantity of food may be allowed with advantage. If this plan can not be thoroughly carried out, the patient should be advised to live a very quiet life, moving about with deliberation and avoiding all sudden mental or bodily excitement. The bowels should be kept regular, and constipation and straining carefully avoided. Of medicines, iodide of potassium is of great value. It may be given in doses of from 10 to 20 grains (0.6 to 1.3 gm.) three times a day. Larger doses are not necessary. The most striking effect of the iodide is the relief of pain. The evidence is conclusive that the syphilitic cases are more benefited by it than the non-syphilitic. All these measures have little value unless the sac is of a suitable form and size. The large tumors with wide mouths communicating with the ascending portion of the aorta may be treated on the most approved plans for months without the slightest influence other than reduction in the intensity of the throbbing. A patient with a tumor projecting into the right pleura remained on the most rigid Tufnell treatment for more than one hundred days, during which time he took potassium iodide faithfully. The pulsations were greatly reduced and the area of dulness diminished, and we congratulated ourselves that the sac was probably consolidating. Sudden death followed rupture into the pleura, and the sac contained only fluid blood, not a shred of fibrin. In cases in which the tumor is large, or in which there seems little prospect of consolidation, it is perhaps better to advise a man to go on quietly with his occupation, avoiding excitement and worry. Our profession has offered many examples of good work, thoroughly and conscientiously carried out, by men with aneurism of the aorta, who wisely preferred, as did the late Hilton Fagge, to die in harness.

Surgical Measures.—Consolidation may be promoted in the sac by the combination of wiring and electrolysis. Moore, in 1864, first wired a sac, putting in 78 feet of fine wire. Death occurred on the fifth day. Corradi proposed the combined method of wiring with electrolysis, which was first used by Burresi in 1879. H. A. Hare has done the operation 32 times without any accident. He emphasizes the importance of employing a gold platinum wire without too much spring (silver is not suitable), of using the positive pole in the aneurism and of not giving too strong a current (5 milliamperes at the beginning, gradually increased to 50, and then decreased to 5 again, the current being passed for about 50 minutes). In nearly all of Hare's patients there was marked benefit, the duration of which was variable. One patient lived for nine years. The decrease in the size of the aneurism is often marked but the relief of pain is the most striking feature. The most favorable cases are those in which the aneurism is sacculated, which can usually be determined by the X-rays. The sudden filling by clot of an aneurism of the cœliac axis of the superior mesenteric artery may result fatally from infarct of the intestine.

Other Conditions.—Pressure on veins causing engorgement, particularly of the head and arms, is sometimes promptly relieved by free venesection, and, at any time during the course of a thoracic aneurism, if attacks of dyspnœa with lividity supervene, bleeding may be resorted to with great benefit. In the final stages morphia is, as a rule, necessary. Dyspnœa, if associated with cyanosis, is best relieved by bleeding. Chloroform inhalations may be necessary. The question of tracheotomy sometimes comes up in the cases of urgent dyspnœa. If it can be shown by laryngoscopic examination that it is due to bilateral abductor paralysis the trachea may be opened, but this is extremely rare, and in nearly every instance the urgent dyspnœa is caused by pressure about the bifurcation. When the sac appears externally and grows large, an ice bag or a belladonna plaster may be applied to allay the pain but wiring with electrolysis is most useful for this. In some instances an elastic support may be used with advantage, and a physician with an enormous external aneurism in the right mammary region for many months obtained great relief by an elastic support, passing over the shoulder and under the arm of the opposite side.

The nitrites may be given if the blood pressure is high, but rest and diet, restriction of the fluids, and free purgation are usually more effectual than drugs in reducing blood pressure.

B. Aneurism of the Abdominal Aorta.—Of 233 cases collected by Nixon,

207 were in males, 26 in females; 121 were between the ages of twenty-five and forty-five. Nixon reports a case in a syphilitic girl of twenty. There were 16 cases among 16,000 admissions at the Johns Hopkins Hospital.

Pathology.—The sac is most common just below the diaphragm in the neighborhood of the cœliac axis. The tumor may be fusiform or sacculated, and it is sometimes multiple. Projecting backward, it erodes the vertebræ and may cause numbness and tingling in the legs and finally paraplegia, or it may pass into the thorax and burst into the pleura. More commonly the sac is on the anterior wall and projects forward as a definite tumor, which may be either in the middle line or a little to the left. The tumor may project in the epigastric region (which is most common), in the left hypochondrium, in the left flank, or in the lumbar region. When high up beneath the pillar of the diaphragm it may attain considerable size without being very apparent on palpation. When it ruptures into the retro-peritoneal tissues a tumor in the flank may be formed gradually, which enlarges with very little pulsation. It may be mistaken for a rapidly growing sarcoma or for appendicitis, and an operation may be performed.

The symptoms are chiefly pain, very often of a neuralgic nature, passing round to the sides or localized in the back, and more persistent and intense than in any other variety of aneurism. Gastric symptoms, particularly vomiting, may be early and deceptive features. Retardation of the pulse in the femoral artery is a very common symptom.

Diagnosis and Physical Signs.—Inspection may show marked pulsation in the epigastric region, sometimes a definite tumor. A thrill is not uncommon. The pulsation is forcible, expansile, and sometimes double when the sac is large and in contact with the pericardium. On palpation a *definite tumor can be felt.* Though usually fixed, the aneurism may be freely movable. If large, there is some degree of dulness on percussion, which usually merges with that of the left lobe of the liver. On auscultation, a systolic murmur is, as a rule, audible, and is sometimes best heard at the back. A diastolic murmur is occasionally present, usually very soft in quality. No pulsation, however forcible, no thrill, however intense, no murmur, however loud, justifies the diagnosis of abdominal aneurism unless there is a *definite tumor which can be grasped and which has an expansile pulsation.* Attention to this rule will save many errors. The *throbbing abdominal aorta* was well described by Morgagni and Laennec, and called by Allan Burns the "preternatural pulsation in the epigastrium." It is met with (a) in nervous women often associated with enteroptosis and pain, and sometimes, as Morgagni pointed out, with vomiting of blood. (*b*) In anæmia particularly after severe hæmorrhage, in which the throbbing may shake the patient and the bed. (*c*) In aortic insufficiency. (*d*) In sclerosis of the abdominal aorta. A common mistake is to regard this throbbing aorta as aneurism. The vessel may appear dilated and even may be grasped in the hand. Very frequently a tumor of the pylorus, of the pancreas, or of the left lobe of the liver is lifted with each impulse of the aorta and may be confounded with aneurism. The absence of the forcible expansile impulse and the examination in the knee elbow position, in which the tumor, as a rule, falls forward, and the pulsation is not then communicated, suffice for differentiation.

Prognosis.—The outlook is bad but a few cases heal spontaneously. Death may result from (*a*) complete obliteration of the lumen by clots; (*b*) compression paraplegia; (*c*) rupture (which occurred in 152 of the 233 cases in Nixon's series) either into the pleura, retroperitoneal tissues, peritoneum, or the intestines, most commonly into the duodenum; (*d*) embolism of the superior mesenteric artery, producing intestinal infarction.

The **treatment** is the same as in thoracic aneurism. When the aneurism is low down pressure has been successfully applied in a case by Murray, of Newcastle. It must be kept up for many hours under chloroform. The plan is not without risk, as patients have died from bruising and injury of the sac. Nine cases in our series were treated surgically. In two the wiring and electrolysis were followed by great improvement; one man lived for three years.

C. Dissecting Aneurism.—The majority of aneurisms of the aorta begin with a split or crack of the intima over a spot of syphilitic mesaortitis. Once this split has started the aorta may rupture in all its coats, or an aneurism may form at the site, or the fracture of the intima, though large and often circumferential, may heal; or the blood may extend between the coats, separating them for many inches, or in the entire extent, forming a dissecting aneurism; and, lastly, such a dissecting aneurism may heal perfectly.

Rupture of the Aorta is not very infrequent, as medico-legal work indicates. Usually there is agonizing pain with features of shock, and death may take place instantly; but in fully half of the cases there are two very characteristic stages, the first corresponding to the rupture of the inner coats, the second eight to ten hours, or as long as fifteen or sixteen days later, to fatal rupture of the external layer.

Dissecting aneurism is not very common. There were only two cases in 16 years at the Hopkins Hospital, where aneurism may be said to be exceptionally frequent. The primary split is most frequently in the arch, not far above the valves, and is in the form of a transverse, or vertical, clean cut incision, as if made with a razor. The extent of the separation of the coats is variable. If the adventitia is reached, rupture is certain to take place, as only the structures of the middle coat can resist for any time the pressure of the blood. The blood may pass for three or four or more inches, separating the media, and then burst internally or externally. In other cases the dissection reaches from the ascending arch to the bifurcation of the aorta, even passing down the iliac and femorals into the smaller vessels of the leg. The splitting of the coats may reach to all the subdivisions of the aorta. The symptoms are those spoken of under rupture; but a very remarkable condition may follow, leading to:

Healed Dissecting Aneurism.—The earlier observers of this remarkable condition regarded it as an anatomical anomaly of a double aorta. Adami collected 39 cases, in a majority of which there was no advanced disease of the aorta itself. The outer tube formed by the dissecting aneurism may extend the entire length of the aorta, occupying the full extent of the circumference. The most extraordinary feature is that the outer tube may present a perfectly smooth and natural appearance, and be lined with a new intima. The condition may last for many years.

II. ANEURISM OF THE BRANCHES OF THE ABDOMINAL AORTA

The **cœliac axis** is itself not infrequently involved in aneurism of the first portion of the abdominal aorta. Of its branches, the **splenic artery** is occasionally the seat of aneurism. This rarely causes a tumor large enough to be felt; sometimes, however, the tumor is of large size. In a case in a man, aged thirty, who had an illness of several months' duration, the severe epigastric pain and vomiting led to a diagnosis of gastric ulcer. There was a deep seated tumor in the left hypochondriac region, the dulness of which merged with that of the spleen. There was no pulsation, but it was thought on one occasion that a *bruit* was heard. The chief symptoms were vomiting, severe epigastric pain, occasional hæmatemesis, and finally severe hæmorrhage from the bowels. An aneurism of the splenic artery the size of a cocoanut was situated between the stomach above and the transverse colon below, and extended to the right as far as the level of the navel. The sac contained densely laminated fibrin. It had perforated the colon. Of 39 instances of aneurism on the branches of the abdominal aorta collected by Lebert, 10 were of the splenic artery.

Of aneurism of the **hepatic artery** Rolland collected 40 cases (1908), of which 24 were extra-hepatic. In Rolland's case there were three sacs—all intra-hepatic. Rupture took place in 32 cases—in 16 into the peritoneal cavity, in 13 into the bile passages. The sac is rarely large, but in the case of Wollmann's it was as large as a child's head. Cholelithiasis and duodenal ulcer are the conditions for which it is most likely to be mistaken. In Ross and Osler's case the liver was enlarged, with symptoms of pyæmia.

Aneurism of the **superior mesenteric artery** is not very uncommon. The diagnosis is scarcely possible from aneurism of the aorta. Plugging of the branches or of the main stem may cause infarction of the bowel.

Renal Artery.—Henry Morris collected 21 instances of aneurism, 12 of which arose from injury. Many of them were false. Pulsation and a *bruit* are not always present. Four cases were operated upon; three recovered. In a case of Keen's the tumor and the kidney were removed together.

Pulmonary Artery.—Primary aneurism of the trunk is very rare. The forms are: (*a*) Of the trunk and main branches Henschen to 1906 collected 42 cases; and Possett (1909) added nine. Most of the patients were in the third and fourth decades, and syphilis is the important factor. Warthin demonstrated spirochætes in atherosclerosis with aneurism. (*b*) Acute embolic aneurism, which may be multiple in connection with septic thrombi in the veins or endocarditis of the right side of the heart. (*c*) The small aneurisms in the walls of pulmonary cavities, already considered.

III. ARTERIO-VENOUS ANEURISM

In this form, known to Galen, but first accurately described by the great William Hunter, there is abnormal communication between an artery and a vein. When a tumor lies between the two it is known as *varicose aneurism;* when there is a direct communication without tumor the vein is chiefly distended and the condition is known as *aneurismal varix.*

While it may occur in the aorta, it is much more common in the peripheral arteries as a result of stab or gunshot wounds.

An aneurism of the ascending portion of the arch may open directly into the vena cava. Twenty-nine cases of this lesion were analyzed by Pepper and Griffith. Cyanosis, œdema, and great distention of the veins of the upper part of the body are the most frequent symptoms, and develop, as a rule, with suddenness. Of the physical signs a thrill is present in some cases. A continuous murmur with systolic intensification is of great diagnostic value. Thurnam (Medico-Chirurgical Transactions, 1840) gave the first accurate account of this murmur and of this characteristic type of cyanosis. There is only one condition with which it could be confounded, viz., the remarkable cyanosis of the upper part of the body which follows crushing accidents to the thorax. Perforation between the aorta and pulmonary artery causes very much the same symptoms. In a few cases an aneurism of the abdominal aorta perforates the inferior vena cava—œdema and cyanosis of the legs and lower half of the body, and the distinctive thrill and murmur are present.

In the *arterio-venous* aneurisms which follow stab and bullet wounds of the subclavian, axillary, carotid, femoral, and popliteal arteries the clinical features are most characteristic. First, the veins enlarge as the arterial blood flows under high pressure into them. The affected limb may be greatly swollen and in a young person may lengthen, and the growth of hair is increased. Secondly, a strong thrill is felt, of maximum intensity at the site of the aneurism, but sometimes to be felt at the most distant parts of a limb. Thirdly, the characteristic continuous murmur with systolic intensification is heard. In the external arteries the condition may persist for years before disability is caused by enlargement of the veins and swelling of the limb. Surgical treatment by a skilled operator is indicated.

Periarteritis Nodosa

An inflammatory lesion of the smaller arteries, beginning in the outer coats, with hyaline degeneration of the media, and formation of secondary aneurisms with thrombosis and rupture. The nodular syphilitic arteritis should not be included in this group. Described first by Kussmaul and Maier, it has been made the subject of special study of late years by Dickson, Longcope, Lamb, and Klotz. Some 42 cases are on record.

The *etiology* is uncertain. Most of the cases are in males of middle age and syphilis has been noted in a few cases. The disease appears to be a subacute infection with forms of staphylococci and streptococci (Klotz). The smaller arteries are involved, the branches of the cœliac axis, the mesenteric, the renal, hepatic, coronary, and more rarely those of the skin, lungs and brain. The nodular tumors vary in numbers from a dozen or more to many hundreds and are usually visible to the naked eye. They differ in structure from the other forms of nodular arteritis, the syphilitic and mycotic. The subcutaneous nodules present in eight cases led to the diagnosis in two.

The disease runs a course with mild fever, weakness, anæmia, muscular and joint pains, epigastric pain, vomiting, diarrhœa and purpura. Tonsillitis has not infrequently preceded the attack. The duration is from a few weeks to three or four months. Recovery has occurred.

SECTION XI

DISEASES OF THE DUCTLESS GLANDS

Introduction.—Disturbances in the endocrine glands may be due to hyper-, hypo- or dysfunction. The results may be shown in various ways: (1) the features caused by disturbance in the gland specially involved, (2) secondary disturbances in other endocrine glands, as they are all bound together, causing a polyglandular syndrome, and (3) involvement of the vegetative nervous system and, through this, widespread influence on many organs. There seem to be special relations between certain glands, which may take the form of inhibition or of stimulation. It is evident that the polyglandular syndromes may present very complex problems.

I. DISEASES OF THE SUPRARENAL BODIES AND CHROMAFFIN SYSTEM

Introduction.—Of the two parts of the suprarenal bodies, (1) the *medullary* belongs to what is known as the chromaffin system, which includes a similar tissue scattered in the sympathetic ganglia and the carotid glands, and (2) the cortex with an epithelial origin and belonging to the interrenal system. The chromaffin bodies produce an internal secretion, *epinephrin,* the chief function of which is to maintain the blood pressure and the sympathetic tonus, though this is disputed by some workers, *e. g.,* Vincent. In some way it also controls the pigment metabolism of the skin and possibly the muscular vigor. Disturbance in function of the medullary portion of the suprarenal bodies is known only through the remarkable disease described by Addison. Beyond this all is debatable, and much visionary. The function of the cortical part of the gland is unknown, but that it bears some relation to the sexual organs is shown by the sex anomalies that develop with tumors of these parts and by the enlargement during pregnancy. Hyperplasia of the cortex or tumor formation may be associated with precocious sexual development and hypoplasia with infantilism. The interrenal system produces *cholin* which lowers blood-pressure.

Glycosuria is caused by the injection of epinephrin, and in animals a form of arterio-sclerosis, probably due to the high blood pressure. Many theoretical conceptions have been entertained of the relation between a defect of the adrenal secretion and asthenic affections, and it is suggested that adrenal insufficiency plays an important rôle in acute infections, in tuberculosis, and many wasting diseases, with which it is interesting to note that increased pigmentation may be associated.

I. ADDISON'S DISEASE

Definition.—A disease characterized by muscular and vascular asthenia, gastro-intestinal disturbance, and pigmentation of the skin; due either to tuberculosis or atrophy of the adrenals, or to degenerative changes in the chromaffin system generally.

The recognition of the disease is due to Addison of Guy's Hospital, whose monograph on "The Constitutional and Local Effects of Disease of the Suprarenal Capsules" was published in 1855.

Etiology.—The disease is rare. Only 17 cases were seen in 21 years in the United States (Osler). In large clinics a year or more may pass without a case. Males are more frequently attacked than females. In Greenhow's analysis of 183 cases, 119 were males and 64 females. The majority of cases occur between the twentieth and fortieth years. A congenital case has been described, in which the child lived for eight weeks, and post mortem the adrenals were found to be large and cystic. In a few cases a blow on the abdomen or back has preceded the onset. A certain number of cases have been associated with Pott's disease. An increase in the disease in France was reported during the recent war.

Morbid Anatomy.—There is rarely emaciation or anæmia. Rolleston thus summarizes the condition of the suprarenal bodies in Addison's disease:

"1. The fibro-caseous lesion due to tuberculosis—far the commonest condition found. 2. Simple atrophy. 3. Chronic interstitial inflammation leading to atrophy. 4. Malignant disease invading the capsules, including Addison's case of malignant nodule compressing the suprarenal vein. 5. Blood extravasated into the suprarenal bodies. 6. No lesion of the suprarenal bodies themselves, but pressure or inflammation involving the semilunar ganglia.

"The first is the only common cause of Addison's disease. The others, with the exception of simple atrophy, may be considered as very rare."

The nerve-cells of the semilunar ganglia have been found degenerated and deeply pigmented, and the nerves sclerotic. The ganglia are not uncommonly entangled in the cicatricial tissue about the adrenals. The chromaffin cells in the sympathetic ganglia and in the abdominal plexuses generally disappear. The cases of extensive destruction of the glands without Addison's disease are explained by a persistence of the chromaffin structures elsewhere, while extensive involvement of the extra-capsular chromaffin system may itself be sufficient to cause the symptoms, the adrenals themselves being intact.

Few changes of importance are found in other organs. The spleen is occasionally enlarged; the thymus may be persistent and the lymph nodes and tonsils enlarged as in status lymphaticus. The other organs show only the alterations associated with a protracted illness.

Symptoms.—In the words of Addison, the characteristic symptoms are "anæmia, general languor or debility, remarkable feebleness of the heart's action, irritability of the stomach, and a peculiar change of color in the skin." The onset is, as a rule, insidious. The feelings of weakness usually precede the pigmentation. In other instances the gastro-intestinal symptoms, the weakness, and the pigmentation come on together. There are a few cases in which the whole process is acute, following a shock or some special depression. There are three important symptoms:

(*a*) Pigmentation of the Skin.—This, as a rule, first attracts the attention of the patient's friends. The grade of coloration ranges from a light yellow to a deep brown, or even black. In typical cases it is diffuse, but always deeper on the exposed parts and in the regions where the normal pigmentation is more intense, as the areolæ of the nipples and about the genitals; also wherever the skin is compressed or irritated, as by the waist-band. At first it may be confined to the face and hands. Occasionally it is absent. Patches showing atrophy of pigment, leucoderma, may occur. The pigmentation occurs on the mucous membranes of the mouth, conjunctivæ, and vagina but it is not distinctive as it has been found in chronic gastric disease and is common in the negro. A patchy pigmentation of the serous membranes has often been found. Over the diffusely pigmented skin there may be little mole like spots of deeper pigmentation, and upon the trunk, particularly on the lower abdomen, it may be "ribbed" like the sand on the seashore.

(*b*) Gastro-intestinal Symptoms.—The disease may set in with attacks of nausea and vomiting, spontaneous in character. Toward the close there may be pain with retraction of the abdomen, and even features suggestive of peritonitis. A marked anorexia may be present. The gastric symptoms are variable throughout the course; occasionally they are absent. Attacks of diarrhœa are frequent and come on without obvious cause.

(*c*) Asthenia, the most characteristic feature, may be manifested early as a feeling of inability to carry on the ordinary occupation, or the patient may complain constantly of feeling tired. The weakness is specially marked in the muscular and cardio-vascular systems. There may be an extreme degree of muscular prostration in an individual apparently well nourished, whose muscles feel firm and hard. The cardio-vascular asthenia is manifest in a feeble, irregular action of the heart, which may come on in paroxysms, in attacks of vertigo, or of syncope, in one of which the disease may prove fatal. The blood pressure is low, falling to 70 or 80 mm. of Hg. Headache is a frequent symptom; convulsions occasionally occur. Pain in the back may be an early and important symptom.

Anæmia, a symptom specially referred to by Addison, is not common. In a majority of the patients the blood count is normal. The sugar content of the blood has been found to be low in some cases. McMunn described an increase in the urinary pigments, and a pigment has been isolated of very much the same character as the melanin of the skin.

The mode of termination is by syncope, which may occur even early in the disease, by gradual progressive asthenia, or by the development of tuberculous lesions. A noisy delirium with urgent dyspnœa may precede the fatal event.

Diagnosis.—Pigmentation of the skin is not confined to Addison's disease. The following conditions may give rise to an increase in the pigment; some of which, *e. g.*, *a* and *b*, are due, as in Addison's disease, to disturbance in the chromaffin system.

(*a*) *Abdominal growths*—tubercle, cancer, or lymphoma. In tuberculosis of the peritoneum pigmentation is not uncommon.

(*b*) *Pregnancy,* in which the discoloration is usually limited to the face, the so-called *masque des femmes enceintes*. Uterine disease is a common cause of a patchy melasma.

(*c*) *Hæmochromatosis*, associated with cirrhosis of the liver, pigmentation of the skin, and diabetes.

(*d*) In overworked persons of constipated habit there may be a patchy staining of the face and forehead.

(*e*) The vagabond's discoloration, caused by the irritation of lice and dirt, may reach a high grade, and has been mistaken for Addison's disease.

(*f*) In rare instances there is deep discoloration of the skin in melanotic cancer, so general that it has been confounded with *melasma suprarenale*.

(*g*) In certain cases of *exophthalmic goitre* abnormal pigmentation occurs.

(*h*) In a few rare instances the pigmentation in *scleroderma* may be general and deep.

(*i*) In the face there may be an extraordinary degree of pigmentation due to innumerable small black comedones. If not seen in a very good light, the face may suggest argyria. Pigmentation of an advanced grade may occur in chronic ulcer of the stomach and in dilatation of the organ.

(*j*) *Argyria* has sometimes been mistaken for Addison's disease.

(*k*) *Arsenic* may cause a most intense pigmentation of the skin.

(*l*) With arterio-sclerosis and chronic heart-disease there may be marked melanoderma.

(*m*) In *pernicious anæmia* the pigmentation may be extreme, most commonly due to the prolonged administration of arsenic.

(*n*) There is a form of deep pigmentation, usually in women, which persists for years without any special impairment of health. The pigmentation is a little more leaden than is usual in Addison's disease.

(*o*) In *ochronosis* there may be a deep melanotic pigmentation of the face and hands.

(*p*) In von Recklinghausen's disease the pigmentation may be uniform and suggestive of adrenal disease.

In any case of unusual pigmentation these various conditions must be sought for; the diagnosis of Addison's disease is scarcely justifiable without the asthenia. In many instances it is difficult early in the disease to arrive at a definite conclusion. The occurrence of fainting fits, of nausea, and gastric irritability are important indications. As the lesion of the capsules is almost always tuberculous, in doubtful cases the tuberculin test may be used.

Prognosis.—The disease is usually fatal. The cases in which the bronzing is slight or does not occur run a more rapid course. There are occasionally acute cases which, with great weakness, vomiting, and diarrhœa, prove fatal in a few weeks. In a few cases the disease is much prolonged, even to six or ten years. In rare instances recovery has taken place, and periods of improvement, lasting many months, may occur.

Treatment.—When asthenia appears the patient should be confined to bed and sudden efforts and muscular exercise should not be allowed. Fatal syncope may occur at any time. For the debility arsenic and strychnia are useful; for the diarrhœa large doses of bismuth, and for the irritability of the stomach very simple diet and alkalies. The diet should be light and nutritious; sugar should be given freely. As the disease is nearly always tuberculous an open air treatment may be carried out. Tuberculin may be tried cautiously, particularly if the case is seen early.

Operation has been suggested. The lesion is usually localized, and it should not be a difficult matter to remove the diseased glands; but, so far as we know, in animals this is always a fatal procedure, and in any case, unless there were supernumerary adrenals and a considerable portion of the extra-capsular chromaffin intact, the operation would be useless.

Adrenal Therapy.—Evidently the relation of Addison's disease to the adrenals is not the same as that of myxœdema to the thyroid gland, in which the insufficiency is promptly relieved by the administration of thyroid preparations. The tuberculous nature of the lesions in most of the cases of Addison's disease is an obstacle, and there is usually widespread involvement of the sympathetic system. There is now a large series of cases treated with various preparations, but only a very few with satisfactory results. In only three of our patients was there marked improvement. In one, all the severer symptoms disappeared, the pigmentation cleared up, and the patient died subsequently of an acute infection, which apparently had nothing to do with the disease. The adrenals were found sclerotic but not tuberculous. The dried gland may be given in doses of from 5 to 20 grains (0.3 to 1.3 gm.) three times a day. Epinephrin may be used hypodermically in doses of ♏v-xv (0.3-1 c. c.) of the 1-1000 solution. The results should be watched carefully.

II. OTHER AFFECTIONS OF THE SUPRARENAL GLANDS

Lesions of the Adrenal Cortex.—Remarkable changes in the secondary sexual characters have been associated with tumors and other lesions of this part—the so-called suprarenal genital syndrome. Pseudo-hermaphroditism has been found in connection with hyperplasia of the cortex, as in a case in which the internal organs were those of a female but the external had male characters. The reverse may occur. Premature puberty, with the development of the secondary sexual characters, may appear as early as the fifth or sixth year. After puberty the presence of a tumor may lead to the remarkable condition known in women as virilismus or hirsutismus, in which a growth of hair occurs on the face, the voice becomes masculine, and the muscular strength may increase. Later, as the signs of tumor develop, there are emaciation, pigmentation, and mental changes.

Hyper- and Hypo-function of the Adrenals.—The state of our physiological knowledge is at present far too uncertain to make it worth while to discuss the clinical vagaries which have been grouped under the terms hyper- and hypo-epinephrinæmia. The suggestion of Sergent that the vaso-constrictor skin reflex, causing the "white line," is an evidence of adrenal insufficiency has not been generally supported but in some cases of asthenia and low blood pressure, which show the "white line," the response to the administration of epinephrin is prompt. That certain disturbances come under these headings can not be doubted but much experimental work and many observations are necessary before they can be accurately stated.

Hæmorrhage.—Acute hæmorrhagic adrenalitis presents a picture somewhat resembling acute pancreatitis—a sudden onset with pain, vomiting, profound prostration and death within a few days. In other cases convulsions occur or the patient falls into a typhoid state with profound asthenia. In children the disease may be associated with purpura, both cutaneous and visceral.

Tumors.—Both carcinoma and sarcoma have been described. They are apt to undergo fatty degeneration and hæmorrhage, so that they may form very large cysts. In children excessive development of the genitals with hair and fat has been found, as noted by Bullock and Sequeira, who collected a number of cases. On this account a suggestion has been made that the adrenal cortex has an hormonic internal secretion which influences sexual development. Robert Hutchison described a remarkable syndrome in children of adrenal tumor, exophthalmos, and cranial tumors; and William Pepper (tertius) described a form characterized by rapid growth, diffuse involvement of the liver, and great distention of the abdomen without ascites or jaundice.

Carotid Glands.—Situated at the bifurcation of the carotid arteries, these bodies, each about the size of a grain of wheat, belong to the chromaffin group. Their function is unknown. They are of interest as the seat of tumors, benign at first but which may become malignant, at the level of the top of the thyroid cartilage.

II. DISEASES OF THE THYMUS GLAND

The thymus in structure has little resemblance to the other ductless glands, with the exception of the epiphysis cerebri, and must be classed as an epithelial rather than as a lymphoid organ (Pappenheimer).

At birth the thymus gland weighs about 12 grams; from the first to the fifth year about 23 grams; from the sixth to the tenth year about 26 grams; from the eleventh to the fifteenth year about 37½ grams, and from the sixteenth to the twentieth year about 25½ grams, after which it undergoes a gradual atrophy (Hammar). Involution not taking place, a "persistent thymus" remains.

The function of the gland is not known. There is an obscure relationship between the thymus and the sexual glands. After castration N. Patton found persistency and hypertrophy of the gland. A disturbance of the normal development of the bones, particularly in ossification, also occurs (Basch) and there is an increase in the excitability of the nerves. The nature of the internal secretion is unknown. Many experiments have been made with extract from the gland, but without definite results.

I. HYPERTROPHY OF THE THYMUS

The size of the gland varies so greatly that it is not easy to define the limits between persistency and enlargement. Between the manubrium sterni and the vertebral column in an infant of eight months the distance is only 2.2 cm. (Jacobi), so that it is easy to understand how an enlarged gland may induce what Warthin calls "thymic tracheostenosis." There would appear to be, as this author suggests, three groups of cases:

(*a*) Thymic stridor, either congenital or developing soon after birth, varying in intensity and aggravated by crying and coughing.

(*b*) Thymic asthma, sometimes known as Kopp's or Miller's asthma, is an exaggerated and more persistent form of the stridor. While much dispute exists as to this form, there can be no doubt as to its occurrence, as there are cases in which complete relief has followed removal of the gland. Olivier collected 39 cases of thymectomy with 24 recoveries.

(*c*) Lastly, in some cases sudden death has occurred, usually in connection with the condition of lymphatism about to be described.

Persistence of the gland has been met with in many affections, such as Graves' disease, Addison's disease, acromegaly, myasthenia gravis, rickets, etc. Many observers regard the association of an enlargement with Graves' disease as more than accidental and as a sort of compensatory process.

II. ATROPHY OF THE THYMUS

This is met with accidentally in children who show no special pathological changes, especially as Ruhräh has shown, in marasmus and the chronic wasting disorders of children. Of other morbid conditions, hæmorrhages are not uncommon. Mediastinal tumors may originate in the remnants of the thymus; dermoid tumors and cysts have also been met with; tuberculosis and syphilis of the gland are occasionally seen. The condition described by Dubois in congenital syphilis, in which there are fissure like cavities in the gland filled with a purulent fluid, is probably post mortem softening.

III. STATUS THYMICO-LYMPHATICUS

(*Lymphatism*)

Definition.—A combination of constitutional anomalies among which are hyperplasia of the lymphoid tissues and of the thymus, hypoplasia of the cardio-vascular system, and peculiarities of configuration.

Formerly the condition was regarded as specially important in young children, but it is found both in children and adults. In Bellevue Hospital, 457 cases were found among 5,652 autopsies (8 per cent.). Of these only 92 were below the age of twenty years (Symmers). The cases in adults have received much attention and present a definite picture.

The results of the condition are various; among them are: (1) The liability to sudden death. This may be from several causes. (*a*) Anaphylaxis. Necrosis occurs in the lymphoid tissues with resulting sensitization. With further necrosis a fatal attack may result. (*b*) Cerebral hæmorrhage. The hypoplastic arteries rupture easily, as from slight trauma, which is a point of medico-legal importance. (*c*) In young children sudden death may result from pressure of the enlarged gland ("thymic death"), but this is probably very rare. (2) Increased susceptibility to acute infections and decreased resistance to them. This applies particularly to endocarditis, pneumonia, cerebro-spinal fever and sepsis. (3) In women there is increased danger in childbirth. (4) Psychical Instability. The subjects form a considerable proportion of cases of drug addiction and suicide.

Pathology.—Symmers describes two forms—status lymphaticus and recessive status lymphaticus. The former shows well-developed changes in the lymphoid tissues and occurs at an age when these structures are active. The recessive form shows atrophic changes in the lymphoid structures which vary with the time of involution. Of 249 cases, 118 were instances of status lymphaticus, 89 of the recessive form and 42 were border-line cases, tending toward recession. In the status lymphaticus form the thymus was hyperplastic, the average weight being about 25 gm. No instance was found of death being due to pressure from the thymus. Histologically the thymus showed hyperplasia, which may be extreme. Necrotic changes were marked in the lymph nodes and this was especially marked in the case of sudden death from slight causes. This is regarded by Symmers as being in close relation to anaphylaxis.

Symptoms.—Children with lymphatism are often fat, may be anæmic and flabby but are usually regarded as in good health. The tonsils are enlarged and adenoids are present. They have little resistance to infections and are easily upset by trifling ailments. They are often subject to nasal catarrh, mouth breathing is common, and vaso-motor changes are frequent. The blood may show a marked lymphocytosis. The enlarged thymus may be shown by dulness over the upper sternum and to each side of it which shifts upward with extreme retraction of the head (Boggs). There may be bulging or the gland may be felt in the episternal notch. The X-ray shadow may be distinct. In these cases there may be attacks, often after a fit of temper or a crying spell, in which the child shows noisy breathing, stridor and cyanosis. Respiration may stop for some seconds or death may occur.

After puberty the condition is easily recognized. In males the main points are (1) A slender thorax, rounded arms and thighs, and a suggestion of the feminine type. (2) A soft delicate skin. (3) A scanty growth of hair on the face; especially on the upper lip and chin, and in the axillæ, with the pubic hair showing the feminine distribution. (4) The external genitals may be poorly developed; some are cryptorchids. (5) The cervical and axillary glands may be palpable. In females the main features are (1) A slender thorax and extremities. (2) A soft delicate skin. (3) Scanty axillary and pubic hair. (4) Hypoplasia of the genital organs.

Diagnosis.—Suspected cases should be carefully examined before trifling operations. The enlargement of the superficial glands of the tonsillar tissues and of the spleen is easily determined. The adult forms are readily recognized from the general characteristics.

Treatment.—In children it is well to reduce the sugar and starch in the diet to a minimum, giving skim milk, eggs, meat, green vegetables and fruits. A general tonic treatment with iron and arsenic should be given. A large thymus causing compression may require removal but treatment by the X-ray is often successful. In the adult forms there is no special treatment.

III. DISEASES OF THE THYROID GLAND

I. CONGESTION

At puberty, in girls, often at the onset of menstruation, the gland enlarges; in certain women the neck becomes fuller at each menstruation, and it was an old idea that the gland enlarged at or after defloration. The slight enlargement at puberty may persist for months and cause uneasiness, but, as a rule, it disappears completely. From mechanical causes, as tight collars or repeated crying, the gland may swell for a short time. Slight enlargement is common in acute infections.

II. THYROIDITIS

Etiology.—Inflammation of the gland, which is nearly always secondary to some infection, may be simple or purulent. It is most frequent in typhoid fever, small-pox, measles, pneumonia, rheumatic fever, and mumps. Epidemics of thyroiditis have been reported. It is a rare disease in ordinary hospital practice, and did not occur in our series of 1,500 cases of typhoid fever.

Symptoms.—The whole gland may be involved, or only one lobe. There are swelling, pain on pressure, redness over the affected part, and, when suppuration occurs, softening or fluctuation. Often the acute inflammation subsides spontaneously. Myxœdema has followed destruction of the entire gland by acute suppuration.

A remarkable sclerotic thyroiditis has been described by Riedel and is sometimes called after his name. It is important, as, in the rapidity of its evolution and in the production of a diffuse tumor involving the whole gland, the clinical picture may resemble cancer. The gland becomes firmly fixed to the surrounding parts and serious effects may be produced by compression of the trachea and the recurrent laryngeal nerves. The cut section of the gland is white and smooth, and shows a dense fibrous tissue.

III. TUMORS OF THE THYROID

Of these the most important are: (*a*) Infective granulomata—tuberculosis, actinomycosis, and syphilis. Cases are very rare. Tuberculosis may be mistaken for exophthalmic goitre. Swelling of the gland has been seen in recent syphilitic infection, and gummata may occur in the congenital form. (*b*) Adenomata, simple or malignant. The latter may cause extensive metastases, as in the case reported by Haward, in which tumors resembling thyroid tissue occurred in the lungs and various bones. (*c*) Cancer and sarcoma, which are rare, have a surgical interest.

IV. ABERRANT AND ACCESSORY THYROIDS

In various places, from the root of the tongue to the arch of the aorta, fragments of thyroidal tissue have been found. These aberrant portions of the gland are very apt to enlarge and undergo cystic degeneration. In the mediastinum they may form large tumors, and in the pleura an accessory cystic thyroid may occupy the upper portion, and a case was reported by F. A. Packard, in which the cystic gland filled nearly the entire side. The so-called lingual thyroid is not uncommon, varying in size from a hemp seed to a pea, usually free in the deep muscles of the tongue, or attached to the hyoid bone. When enlarged the *lingual goitre* may form a tumor of considerable size. The true thyroid gland has been absent, and removal of the lingual goitre has been followed by myxœdema.

V. GOITRE

(Struma, Bronchocele)

Definition.—A chronic enlargement of the thyroid gland, of unknown origin, occurring sporadically or endemically.

Distribution.—Goitre in the United States is perhaps most common in the region of the Great Lakes. In an investigation in Michigan, Dock found a large number of cases and the disease is not uncommon in Lower Canada. In England it is common in certain regions; the Thames valley, the Dales, Derbyshire, Sussex, and Hampshire. It is very prevalent about Oxford and the upper Thames valley. In Switzerland, in the mountains of Germany and Austria, the mountainous districts of France, and in the Pyrenees the disease is very prevalent. In regions of Central Asia, in the Abyssinian mountains, and in the Himalayas there are many foci of the disease.

Etiology.—The disease is rarely congenital except in very goitrous districts. Cases are most common at or about puberty, and the tendency diminishes after the twentieth year. Women are much more frequently attacked than men, in a proportion of 6 or 8 to 1.

In its endemic form the disease occurs at every latitude and in every altitude, in valleys and in plains, and in various climates. It seems to be much less prevalent by the seashore.

The cause is obscure. The water in goitrous districts is hard, rich in lime and magnesia, poor in iodine, and (so Rédin affirms of the Swiss waters) with a high degree of radio-activity. Others speak of a "miasma" of the soil which gets into the drinking water. McCarrison in Kashmir found that the specific agent could be killed by boiling the water and that it did not pass a Berkefeld filter. He produced goitre in himself and in others by the daily consumption of the residue of the filter, but the residue when boiled was harmless. The disease was transmitted to goats who drank water contaminated by goitre patients. There are "goitre springs" and "goitre wells." These and other facts strongly suggest a specific organism; and this view is supported by the remarkable outbreaks of acute goitre in schools, lasting for a few months and disappearing. In one such outbreak 161 boys among 350 and 245 girls among 381 were attacked (Guillaume).

Morbid Anatomy.—Usually the whole gland is involved, but one lobe only may be attacked. When the enlargement is uniform, and the appearance of the gland natural, it is spoken of as parenchymatous goitre; when the blood vessels are very large, vascular goitre. In both forms there is an increase in the colloid material of the follicles. Degenerations of various kinds are common, particularly cystic, in which there are many large and small cavities with colloid contents. In some of these cystic forms there are papillary ingrowths into the alveoli. Sometimes the cysts contain blood and extensive hæmorrhages occur in the gland.

Symptoms.—When small a goitre is not inconvenient, but when large pressure symptoms may cause the patient to seek relief. The windpipe may be flattened from pressure, usually of an enlarged isthmus, or it is narrowed by circular compression. The symptoms are more or less marked stridor and cough, which may persist for years without special aggravation. They may be present with very large glands, or with the small encircling goitre, or with the goitre which passes deeply beneath the sternum. Pressure on the recurrent nerves may cause attacks of dyspnœa, particularly at night, and the voice may be altered. Pressure on the vagus is not common. Sometimes there is difficulty in swallowing, and the veins of the neck may be compressed. The heart is often involved, either from pressure on the vagi, or there is dilatation associated with dyspnœa. This is sometimes spoken of as the "goitre heart" in contra-distinction to the cardiac condition in Graves' disease.

Prognosis.—Many cases in the young get well; too often in goitrous districts the tumor persists. It may disappear on leaving the district. Many cases get well without medical treatment, but when pressure symptoms occur surgery gives relief.

Treatment.—In goitrous districts the drinking water should be boiled. Simple goitre can be prevented by small doses of iodine. Iodine in some form is used extensively, and often is curative. Its effect is to stimulate the gland to healthy action. In young people 2 to 5 grains (0.13 to 0.3 gm.) of potassium or sodium iodide may be given daily. Iodine injections into the gland are not advisable. Iodine may be applied externally as an ointment (5 per cent.). The X-rays have been tried with success. When the gland is large, surgical measures are indicated.

VI. HYPOTHYROIDISM

(*Cretinism and Myxœdema*)

Definition.—A constitutional affection due to the loss of function of the thyroid gland, characterized clinically by a myxœdematous condition of the subcutaneous tissues and mental failure, and anatomically by atrophy of the thyroid gland.

History.—As early as 1859 Schiff had noted that in the dog removal of the gland was followed by certain symptoms. Gull described "A cretinoid change in women," and in the eighties the observations of Ord and other English physicians separated a well defined clinical entity called "myxœdema."

Kocher (in 1883) reported that 30 of his first 100 thyroidectomies had been followed by a very characteristic picture, to which he gave the name "cachexia strumipriva," an observation which had already been made in the previous year by the Reverdins, who also had recognized the relation of this change to the disease known as "myxœdema." The researches of Horsley, and the investigation of the Committee of the Clinical Society of London, made it clear that the changes following complete removal of the gland, cachexia strumipriva, myxœdema, and the sporadic cretinism, were one and the same disease, due to the loss of the function of the thyroid gland. Schiff and Horsley demonstrated that animals could be saved by the transplantation of the glands. Lastly came the discovery of George Murray and Howitz that feeding with the thyroid extract replaced the gland function, and cured the disease. The first patient given thyroid by Murray in 1891 died in 1919, aged 74, from heart disease. The activitv of the gland is connected with the metabolism of iodine.

Kendall has isolated the active principle which he terms thyroxin and which contains 65 per cent. of iodine. It is an amino-acid which enters into reaction and is regenerated so that it can repeat the process. It acts as does thyroid extract in myxœdema. There is a quantitative relation between thyroxin and the rate of basal metabolism.

The outcome of a host of researches has been the recognition of the enormous importance of the internal secretion of the gland, which is essential for normal growth in childhood, and has a marked influence on metabolism. It stimulates both vegetative nervous systems.

Clinical Forms.—There are three groups of cases—cretinism, myxœdema proper, and operative myxœdema. To Felix Semon is due the credit of recognizing that these were one and the same condition and all due to loss of function of the thyroid gland.

CRETINISM.—Two forms are recognized—the sporadic and the endemic. In the *sporadic* form the gland may be congenitally absent, or is atrophied after one of the specific fevers, or the condition develops with goitre. The disease is not very uncommon; the histories of 58 cases were collected in a few years in the United States and Canada (Osler). It is more common in females than in males—35 in the series.

Morbid Anatomy.—Absence of the gland, or complete fibrous atrophy, is the common condition. Goitre with any trace of gland tissue is rare. In the sporadic form sometimes the hypophysis and thymus have been found enlarged. Arrest of development, a brachycephalic skull in the endemic, and a dolichocephalic in the sporadic form, are the chief skeletal changes.

Symptoms.—In the congenital cases the condition is rarely recognized before the infant is six or seven months old. Then it is noticed that the child does not grow so rapidly and is not bright mentally. The tongue looks large and hangs out of the mouth. The hair may be thin and the skin very dry. Usually by the end of the first year and during the second year the signs become very marked. The face is large, looks bloated, the eyelids are puffy and swollen; the alæ nasi are thick, the nose looks depressed and flat. Dentition is delayed, and the teeth which appear decay early. The abdomen is swollen, the legs are thick and short, and the hands and feet are undeveloped and pudgy. The face is pale and sometimes has a waxy, sallow tint. The fontanelles remain open; there is muscular weakness, and the child can not support itself. In the supraclavicular regions there are large pads of fat. The child does not develop mentally and may lapse into imbecility.

In cases in which the atrophy of the gland follows a fever the condition may not come on until the fourth or fifth year, or later. This is really, as Parker determined, a juvenile myxœdema. In a few of the sporadic forms cretinism develops with an existing goitre. It may retard development, bodily and mental, without ever progressing to complete imbecility.

ENDEMIC CRETINISM.—This occurs wherever goitre is very prevalent, as in parts of Switzerland, Savoy, Tyrol, and the Pyrenees. It formerly prevailed in parts of England. The clinical features are the same as in the sporadic form, stunted growth and feeble mind, plus goitre. To some poison in the water—mineral or organic—the thyroid changes have been attributed, but whatever the toxic agent may be, it is the interference with the function of the gland that leads to the cretinous change in the body.

The *diagnosis* is very easy after one has seen a case, or good illustrations. Infants a year or so old sometimes become flabby, lose their vivacity, or show a protuberant abdomen, and lax skin with slight cretinoid appearance. These milder forms, as they have been termed, are probably due to transient functional disturbance in the gland.

Myxœdema of Adults (*Gull's Disease*).—Women are much more frequently affected than men—in a ratio of 6 to 1. The disease may affect several members of a family, and it may be transmitted through the mother. In some instances there has been first the appearance of exophthalmic goitre. Though most common in women, it seems to have no special relation to menstruation or pregnancy; the symptoms of myxœdema may disappear during pregnancy or may develop post partum. Myxœdema and exophthalmic goitre may occur in sisters. It is not so common in America as in England. In sixteen years only 10 cases were seen in Baltimore, 7 of which were in the hospital. C. P. Howard collected 100 American cases, of which 86 were in women. The symptoms, as given by Ord, are marked increase in the general bulk of the body, a firm, inelastic swelling of the skin, which does not pit on pressure; dryness and roughness, which tend with the swelling to obliterate in the face the lines of expression; imperfect nutrition of the hair; local tumefaction of the skin and subcutaneous tissues, particularly in the supraclavicular region. Perspiration is often much decreased. The physiognomy is altered in a remarkable way: the features are coarse and broad, the lips thick, the nostrils broad and thick, and the mouth is enlarged. Over the cheeks, sometimes the nose, there is a reddish patch. There is a striking slowness of thought and of movement. The memory becomes defective, the patients grow irritable and suspicious, and there may be headache. In some instances there are delusions and hallucinations, leading to a final condition of dementia. The gait is heavy and slow. The temperature may be below normal. The patients often suffer in cold weather. The functions of the heart, lungs, and abdominal organs are normal. Hæmorrhage sometimes occurs. Albuminuria is sometimes present, more rarely glycosuria. Death is usually due to some intercurrent disease, most frequently tuberculosis (Greenfield). The thyroid gland is diminished in size and may become completely atrophied and converted into a fibrous mass. The subcutaneous fat is abundant, and in one or two instances a great increase in the mucin has been found. The larynx is also involved.

The basal metabolism is reduced 20 to 40 per cent. below the normal.

The course is slow but progressive, and extends over ten or fifteen years. A condition of acute and temporary myxœdema may develop in connection with enlargement of the thyroid in young persons. Myxœdema may follow exophthalmic goitre. In other instances the symptoms of the two diseases have been combined. In one case a young man became bloated and increased in weight enormously during three months, then had tachycardia with tremor and active delirium, and died within six months of the onset of the symptoms.

Operative Myxœdema; Cachexia Strumipriva.—Horsley showed that complete removal of the thyroid in monkeys was followed by the production of a condition similar to that of myxœdema and sometimes associated with spasms or tetanoid contractures, and followed by apathy and coma. An identical condition sometimes follows extirpation of the thyroid in man. The disease follows only a certain number of total and a much smaller proportion of partial removals of the thyroid gland. Of 408 cases, in 69 the operative myxœdema occurred (Kocher). If a small fragment of the thyroid remains, or if there are accessory glands, which in animals are very common, the symptoms do not develop. Operative myxœdema is very rare in America. A few years ago only two cases were found, one of which, McGraw's, referred to in previous editions of this work, has since been cured.

The *diagnosis* of myxœdema is easy, as a rule. The general aspect of the patient—the subcutaneous swelling and the pallor—suggests nephritis, which may be strengthened by the discovery of tube casts and of albumin in the urine; but the solid character of the swelling, the exceeding dryness of the skin, the yellowish white color, the low temperature, the loss of hair, and the dull, listless mental state should suffice to differentiate the conditions. In mild cases the result of thyroid administration may be an aid in diagnosis. In dubious cases not too much stress should be laid upon the supraclavicular swellings. There may be marked fibro-fatty enlargements in this situation in healthy persons, the supraclavicular pseudo-lipomata of Verneuil.

Hypothyroidism should be considered in children who are dull and backward, in women who have symptoms suggesting a premature menopause, in obesity, and in those with constipation the cause for which is obscure.

Treatment.—The patients suffer in cold and improve greatly in warm weather. They should therefore be kept at an even temperature, and should, if possible, move to a warm climate during the winter months. Repeated warm baths with massage are useful. Our art has made no more brilliant advance than in the cure of these disorders due to disturbed function of the thyroid gland. That we can to-day rescue children otherwise doomed to helpless idiocy—that we can restore to life the hopeless victims of myxœdema—is a triumph of experimental medicine for which we are indebted very largely to Victor Horsley and his pupil Murray. Transplantation of the gland was first tried; then Murray used an extract subcutaneously. Hector Mackenzie in London and Howitz in Copenhagen introduced the method of feeding. We now know that the gland is efficacious in a majority of all the cases of myxœdema in infants or adults. It makes little difference how the gland is administered. The dried gland is the most convenient. It is well to begin with the Thyroideum siccum U. S. P. 1 grain (0.065 gm.) three times a day. The dose may be increased gradually until the patient takes 10 or 15 grains (0.6 gm. to 1 gm.) in the day. Care should be taken to be sure of the strength of the preparation which is given. In many cases there are no unpleasant symptoms; in others there are irritation of the skin, restlessness, rapid pulse, and delirium; in rare instances tonic spasms, the condition to which the term *thyroidism* is applied. The results, as a rule, are most astounding—unparalleled by anything in the whole range of curative measures. Within six weeks a poor, feeble-minded, toad-like caricature of humanity may be restored to mental and bodily health. Loss of weight is one of the first and most striking effects; one patient lost over 30 pounds within six weeks. The skin becomes moist, the urine is increased, the perspiration returns, the temperature rises, the pulse rate quickens, and the mental torpor lessens. Ill effects are rare. Two or three cases with old heart lesions have died during or after the treatment; in one a temporary condition of Graves' disease was induced.

The treatment, as Murray suggests, must be carried out in two stages—one, early, in which full doses are given until the cure is effected; the other, the permanent use of small doses sufficient to preserve the normal metabolism. In the cases of cretinism it seems to be necessary to keep up the treatment indefinitely as relapse may follow the cessation of the use of the extract.

VII. HYPERTHYROIDISM; EXOPHTHALMIC GOITRE

(Graves', Basedow's, or Parry's Disease)

Definition.—A disease characterized by goitre, exophthalmos, tachycardia, and tremor, associated with a perverted or hyperactive state of the thyroid gland and increased activity of the vegetative nervous system.

A distinction should be made between hyperthyroidism and Graves' disease. Not all the cases of over-activity of the gland go on to exophthalmic goitre, but it is probable that the possibility of this progress exists. It may be difficult to classify some of the borderline cases.

Historical Note.—In the posthumous writings of Caleb Hillier Parry (1825) is a description of 8 cases of Enlargement of the Thyroid Gland in Connection with Enlargement or Palpitation of the Heart. In the first case, seen in 1786, he also described the exophthalmos: "The eyes were protruded from their sockets, and the countenance exhibited an appearance of agitation and distress, especially in any muscular movement." The Italians claim that Flajani described the disease in 1800. Moebius states that his original account is meagre and inaccurate, and bears no comparison with that of Parry. If the name of any physician is to be associated with the disease, undoubtedly it should be that of the distinguished old Bath physician. Graves described the disease in 1835 and Basedow in 1840.

Etiology.—*Age.*—In Sattler's collection of 3,477 cases only 184 were under the age of sixteen. *Sex*—In England and America the proportion of females is greatly in excess, as much probably as 20 to 1, but in Sattler's collected cases the ratio was 5.4 to 1, which would indicate marked differences in different countries.

The exciting factors are probably varied. The acute infections, local infections, thyroiditis, profound nervous disturbance, worry, mental shock, a severe fright, and changes in the vegetative nervous system, may be responsible.

A strong *family predisposition* may exist and five or six members may be affected.

Pathology.—The essential change consists in increased activity of the gland, which enlarges as a result of hyperplasia and shows increased vascularity. The normal colloid is greatly reduced or absent. The epithelial cells of the follicles show proliferation and the lymph-adenoid tissue is increased. These changes may occur only in limited areas of the gland tissue. The enlargement occasionally results in mechanical disturbance. The increased secretion causes definite results: (1) There is a great increase in metabolism; (2) other endocrine glands are affected, and (3) the vegetative nervous system is stimulated. The active principle—thyroxin—has been isolated by Kendall. In many cases there is enlargement of the thymus, which may play a part in the lymphocytosis usually found (30-60 per cent.) with decrease in the neutrophiles. Myxœdema may develop in the late stages, and there are transient œdema and in a few cases scleroderma, which indicate that the nutrition of the skin is involved.

Anatomical Changes.—In rare instances the thyroid gland has been stated to be normal. In the majority of cases there is active hyperplasia of the gland, with enlarged and newly formed follicles, and an increase in the lymphoid tissue of the gland stroma. Involuntary and regressive changes are common; the hyperplasia may cease and the gland returns to the colloid state. Finally, in certain cases, atrophy of the cell elements takes place.

The iodine content of the gland bears a direct relationship to the amount of colloid; the gland in hyperplasia has the lowest percentage, the pure colloid glands the highest.

Symptoms.—Acute and chronic forms may be recognized. In the acute form the disease may arise with great rapidity. In a patient of J. H. Lloyd's, of Philadelphia, a woman, aged thirty-nine, who had been considered perfectly healthy, but whose friends had noticed that for some time her eyes looked rather large, was suddenly seized with intense vomiting and diarrhœa, rapid action of the heart, and great throbbing of the arteries. The eyes were prominent and the thyroid gland was much enlarged and soft. The gastro-intestinal symptoms continued, the pulse became more rapid, the vomiting was incessant, and the patient died on the third day of the illness. The acute cases show marked toxæmia but are not always associated with delirium.

More frequently the onset is gradual and the disease is chronic. There are four characteristic symptoms—tachycardia, exophthalmos, enlargement of the thyroid, and tremor.

Tachycardia.—Rapid heart action is the most constant phenomenon. The pulse rate at first may be not more than 95 or 100, but when the disease is established it may be from 140 to 160, or even higher. The increase is most marked in the sympathicotonic cases. Irregularity is not common, except toward the close. In a well developed case the visible area of cardiac pulsation is much increased, the action is heaving and forcible, and the shock of the heart sounds is well felt. The large arteries at the root of the neck throb forcibly. There is visible pulsation in the peripheral arteries. The capillary pulse is readily seen, and there are few diseases in which one may see at times with greater distinctness the venous pulse in the veins of the hand. The throbbing pulsation of the arteries may be felt even in the finger tips. Vascular erythema is common—the face and neck are flushed and there may be a widespread erythema of the body and limbs. Murmurs are usually heard, a loud apex systolic and loud bruits at the base and over the manubrium. The heart sounds may be very intense. In rare instances they may be heard at some distance from the patient; according to Graves, as far as four feet. Attacks of acute dilatation may occur with dyspnœa, cough, and a frothy bloody expectoration.

Exophthalmos.—A characteristic facial aspect is given by the staring expression, caused in part by protrusion of the eyeballs, but more particularly by retraction of the lids exposing the scleræ. The exophthalmos, which may be unilateral, usually follows the vascular disturbance. The protrusion may become very great and the eye may even be dislocated from the socket, or both eyes may be destroyed by panophthalmitis. The vision is normal. Graefe noted that when the eyeball is moved downward the upper lid does not follow it as in health. This is known as Graefe's sign. The palpebral aperture is wider than in health, owing to spasm or retraction of the upper lid. The patient winks less frequently than in health (Stellwag's sign). There is marked tremor of the lids and they contract spasmodically in advance of the elevating eyeball. Moebius called attention to the lack of convergence of the two eyes. The majority of the eye signs are autonomic in origin. Changes in the pupils and in the optic nerves are rare. Pulsation of the retinal arteries is common.

Enlargement of the thyroid is the rule. It may be general or in only one lobe, and is rarely so large as in ordinary goitre. It may be absent. The swelling is firm, but elastic. There are rarely pressure signs. The vessels are usually much dilated, and the whole gland may be seen to pulsate. A thrill may be felt on palpation and on auscultation a systolic murmur. A double murmur is common and is pathognomonic (Guttmann).

Tremor is the fourth cardinal symptom, and was really first described by Basedow. It is involuntary, fine, about eight to the second. It is of great importance in the diagnosis of the early cases.

Other features are anæmia, emaciation, and slight fever. The blood shows lymphocytosis. Attacks of vomiting and diarrhœa may occur. The latter may be very severe and distressing, recurring at intervals. The greatest complaint is of the forcible throbbing in the arteries, often accompanied with unpleasant flushes of heat and profuse perspirations. An erythematous flushing is common. Pruritus may be a severe and persistent symptom. Multiple telangiectases have been described. Solid, infiltrated œdema is not uncommon and may be transitory. A remarkable myxœdematous state may supervene. Pigmentary changes are common and may be patchy or generalized. The coexistence of scleroderma and Graves' disease has been frequently noticed. Irritability of temper, change in disposition, and great mental depression occur. An important complication is acute mania, in which the patient may die in a few days. Weakness of the muscles is not uncommon, particularly a feeling of "giving way" of the legs. If the patient holds the head down and is asked to look up without raising the head, the forehead remains smooth and is not wrinkled, as in a normal individual (Joffroy). A feature of interest noted by Charcot is the great diminution in the electrical resistance, which may be due to the saturation of the skin with moisture owing to the vaso-motor dilatation (Hirt). Bryson noted that the chest expansion may be greatly diminished. The emaciation may be extreme. Glycosuria and albuminuria are not infrequent and true diabetes may occur.

The *basal metabolism* (minimal heat production) shows a marked increase and this is an important aid in diagnosis. In very severe cases the increase may be 75 per cent. or over, in severe cases 50 to 75 per cent., and in milder forms from 20 to 50 per cent.

The course is usually chronic, lasting several years. After persisting for six months or a year the symptoms may disappear. There are remarkable instances in which the symptoms have come on with great intensity, following fright, and have disappeared again in a few days.

Prognosis.—Statistics are misleading as only the severe cases come under hospital treatment. Sattler estimates the mortality at 11 per cent. In Hale White's series it was 84 in 214 cases. In the hands of competent surgeons the mortality from operation is low and the results are excellent.

Diagnosis.—The typical cases are easily recognized but the difficulty comes with the partially developed forms and hyperthyroidism. The patient should be kept at rest and carefully studied. If the giving of thyroid extract (gr. i-ii, 0.06-0.12 gm.) or iodine for a few days increases the symptoms and pulse rate, it is significant. The test of Goetsch which consists in the response to the injection of epinephrin (0.5 c. c.) is sometimes of value. An increase in the pulse rate and blood-pressure and aggravation of the general symptoms are the important points. It may aid in the diagnosis from early tuberculosis which may show features suggestive of hyperthyroidism. Certain signs should suggest the possibility of hyperthyroidism: (1) tachycardia, (2) rapid emaciation without evident cause, (3) diarrhœa without evident cause, (4) lymphocytosis, and (5) a neurasthenic condition otherwise difficult to explain. Increase in the basal metabolism is very important.

Treatment.—It is usually well to try medical treatment before surgery is considered. Halfway measures should not be considered; the patient should be in bed, at absolute rest and excitement and irritation avoided. Any causes of worry should be corrected if possible. Long hours of sleep should be secured by sedatives if necessary. Any focus of infection should be treated. Tobacco, alcohol, tea and coffee should be forbidden. In the diet, milk, buttermilk and foods prepared with milk should figure largely. Cereals, eggs, butter, bread or toast, vegetables and fruits may be given. Meat broths and meat are not to be given; small amounts of chicken may be taken occasionally. Water should be taken freely, best as distilled water, but, if not available, boiled water. An icebag should be applied over the heart. Of internal remedies, belladonna, ergot and sodium phosphate seem helpful in some cases. The application of the X-rays is sometimes useful and is worth a trial.

Surgical Treatment.—Operation is indicated, (1) when there are compression signs, (2) when there is no gain under a proper trial of medical treatment and (3) when medical treatment causes improvement but there is not complete recovery. Severe toxæmia is usually a contra-indication to surgery. Removal of part of the thyroid gland offers the best hope of permanent cure. It is remarkable with what rapidity all the symptoms may disappear after partial thyroidectomy. A second operation may be necessary in severe cases. Tying of the arteries may be enough. Excision of the superior cervical ganglia of the sympathetic has one beneficial result, viz., the production of slight ptosis, which obviates the staring character of the exophthalmos.

IV. DISEASES OF THE PARATHYROID GLANDS

The parathyroid bodies occur, as a rule, in two pairs on either side of the lateral lobes of the thyroid gland; small ovoid structures from 6 to 8 mm. in length. They have an internal secretion supplementing that of the thyroid gland and controlling calcium metabolism. Following their removal in animals there are twitching, spasms of the voluntary muscles, gradual paralysis with dyspnœa, and death from exhaustion. These sometimes disappear when a saline extract of the parathyroid is injected into a vein, or if the parathyroid glands are fed or transplanted. The association of tetany with the disturbance of the function of the parathyroid seems definitely established. MacCallum has shown the importance of the function of these glands in controlling calcium metabolism, and it is possible that in impoverishment of the tissues in this ingredient is to be sought the cause of the great excitability of the nervous system and of tetany.

These studies have thrown great light upon various spasmodic disorders of children, and some have gone so far as to embrace such conditions as laryngismus, infantile convulsions, and tetany under the term "spasmophilia." These glands have also hormonic relations, as yet not thoroughly understood, with the other ductless glands, and have some influence on carbohydrate metabolism. The experimental association of the glands with tetany is sufficient warrant for treating this disease here, though some regard the relationship to spontaneous tetany as doubtful.

TETANY

Definition.—Hyperexcitability of the neuro-muscular system with bilateral chronic or intermittent spasms of the muscles of the extremities. There are definite changes in the calcium metabolism, possibly due to disturbance in the functions of the parathyroid glands.

Etiology.—It occurs in epidemic form, particularly in the spring, the so-called "rheumatic" tetany, sometimes with slight fever and behaves like an acute infection. It may occur in, or follow, the infections, typhoid fever, measles, etc. In medical wards it is not uncommon. Of 8 cases reported by C. P. Howard, 4 were associated with dilatation of the tomach, 2 with hyperacidity, 1 with chronic diarrhœa, and 1 with lactation. In adults the gastro-intestinal group is the most common. It may follow successive pregnancies—the "nurse's contracture" of Trousseau.

In children it is common with rickets (so much so that many regard it as a feature of the disease) and in gastro-intestinal affections of artificially fed infants associated with wasting. Laryngo-spasm and child crowing are usually manifestations of tetany.

The fact that tetany may follow removal of the thyroid (tetania strumipriva) led to the experimental studies showing a supposed relationship of the disease to the parathyroid gland. Removal of these bodies is followed by tetany, and in animals transplantation of living parathyroids cures experimental tetany; indeed, there are cases of human tetany that have been cured by transplantation. Where no disease of the glands has been found a parathyroid insufficiency is assumed.

The relation of the disease to *calcium metabolism* has been studied by W. G. MacCallum and others, and the hyperexcitability of the nervous system is thought to be due to excessive loss of the lime salts. On the other hand Noel Paton believes that the error in metabolism is an intoxication caused by guanidin compounds. That there is a striking reduction in the calcium content of the blood in tetany as shown by MacCallum has been confirmed by Howland and Marriott in clinical cases (falling from the normal 10 to 11 mgms. per 100 c. c. to an average of 5.6 mgms.); but these writers conclude that the cause of the calcium deficiency is not yet explained and that the parathyroid theory lacks confirmation.

Morbid Anatomy.—Atrophy, hæmorrhages, adenomas, cysts and inflammations have been found in the parathyroids, but the glands have been found normal in fatal cases.

Symptoms.—The tonic spasms occur chiefly in the upper extremities; the arms are flexed across the chest with the hands in the so-called "obstetric" position, the proximal phalanges flexed, the middle and distal extended with the thumb contracted in the palm. The legs are extended with plantar flexion of the feet and toes. The muscles of the face are not so often involved, but there may be trismus and spasm of the muscles of expression.

Laryngo-spasm may occur with noisy inspiration. The spasms may last only for a few hours or the condition may persist for days or weeks, recurring in paroxysms. Contracture of the back muscles is rare; occasionally there are general convulsions. There is not often pain. The pulse may be quickened and the temperature raised. Disturbance of sensation is rare. In chronic cases, the skin looks tense or drawn, there may be œdema, the hair falls out, and the teeth may subsequently show defects in the enamel. Perinuclear cataract may follow a prolonged attack.

Certain additional features are present:

Trousseau's sign is thus described by him—"So long as the attack is not over, the paroxysm may be reproduced at will. This is effected by simply compressing the affected parts, either in the direction of their principal nerve trunks, or over their blood vessels so as to impede the arterial or venous circulation." The spasm is really caused by pressure on the nerves. It may be elicited months, or even years, after an attack. It is not always present.

Chvostek's phenomenon depends on an increased excitability of the motor nerves. A slight tap on the facial will throw the muscles into spasm, sometimes only limited groups. It is sometimes seen in debilitated children who have not had tetany.

Erb's phenomenon is due to increased electrical excitability of the motor nerves. In normal infants a cathodal opening contraction is not caused by a current of less than 5 milliamperes; contraction is obtained in tetany with much less. Anodal hyperexcitability is also present, especially in latent tetany, but it may occur in normal infants and in other conditions.

Diagnosis.—The disease is readily recognized. Between the attacks, or even long after, the signs just described may be obtained. The common carpopedal spasm of debilitated infants is regarded by some as mild tetany. The predisposing factors, gastro-intestinal disease, thyroidectomy, pregnancy, etc., should be borne in mind. There is rarely any difficulty in differentiating tetanus, epilepsy or functional cramps.

Prognosis.—Post-operative cases may prove fatal. Death in the gastro-intestinal forms is usually from the primary conditions. Recovery is the rule in children.

Treatment.—In children the condition with which the tetany is associated should be treated. Baths and cold sponging are recommended and often relieve the spasm as promptly as in child-crowing. Bromide of potassium may be tried. In severe cases chloroform inhalations may be given. Massage, electricity, and the spinal icebag have also been used with success. Cases, however, may resist all treatment, and the spasms recur for many years. The thyroid extract should be tried.

Calcium therapy has proved very efficacious in doses of gr. v-xv (0.3-1 gm.) of the lactate every three or four hours. The symptoms are promptly relieved, but the drug must be continued for some weeks.

In gastric tetany, especially when due to dilatation of the stomach, the mortality is high, and recovery without operative interference is rare. Regular, systematic lavage with large quantities of saline or mildly antiseptic solutions is sometimes beneficial.

V. DISEASES OF THE PITUITARY BODY

The hypophysis cerebri consists of two lobes, (*a*) an anterior lobe, originating from the roof of the pharynx and composed of large granular epithelial cells arranged in columns surrounded by large venous spaces into which their secretion discharges; and (*b*) a smaller posterior lobe which arises from the floor of the third ventricle and is composed (1) of a central neuroglial portion (pars nervosa) and (2) an investment of epithelial cells (pars intermedia). The secretion of the posterior lobe is supposed by some to find its way into the cerebro-spinal fluid.

Complete experimental removal of the gland is fatal (Paulesco). Partial removal leads, in young animals, to a stunting of growth, to adiposity and failure of sexual development, in adult animals to adiposity and genital dystrophy (Cushing).

Modern knowledge of the functions of the gland began with the studies of Marie on its relation to acromegaly and gigantism. Then Schäfer and Oliver discovered that injection of an extract of the gland caused a rise in blood pressure. Since these observations an enormous amount of work has been done, and we now appreciate the remarkable influence of this small structure upon the processes of development and metabolism. Briefly, the anterior lobe influences growth and development, and is necessary to life; the posterior lobe influences the metabolism of the carbohydrates and fats.

Disturbances in the function of the pituitary gland are not clearly grouped into the effects of deficiency and excess, though one can differentiate states of hyper- and hypopituitarism. The hypophysis appears to be closely related to other glands of internal secretion and involvement of any member of the series causes a readjustment in the activity of the others. Owing to the situation of the gland it is very liable to feel the effect of pressure from neighboring or even distant lesions, so that disturbance of function may be due not only to a primary involvement, but to secondary compression. As a result of experimental work and clinical studies Cushing prefers to group the conditions associated with disturbance of the function of the gland under the term "dyspituitarism" and recognizes a number of groups:

(*a*) Cases of tumor growth showing signs of distortion of neighboring structures, and the constitutional effects of altered glandular activity. The X-rays show changes in the configuration of the pituitary fossa; there are pressure signs on the adjacent cranial nerves, bi-temporal hemianopia, optic atrophy, and oculomotor palsies. Uncinate fits are not unusual. Epistaxis is common and cerebro-spinal rhinorrhœa may occur. The constitutional effects vary from primary over-activity to glandular under-activity.

(*b*) Cases in which the neighborhood manifestations are pronounced but the constitutional features are slight. The characteristic regional signs of tumor are marked, but there may be slight or very transient evidence of disturbed glandular activity, perhaps only disturbed carbohydrate metabolism with adiposity.

(*c*) Cases in which the neighborhood manifestations are absent or slight, though the glandular symptoms are unmistakable. The gland is not so large as to cause regional symptoms. There are skeletal changes either of over- or undergrowth. Disturbance of carbohydrate metabolism is a matter of modified posterior lobe activity, whether occurring as a lowering of the assimilation limit, so often associated with the early stages of acromegaly, or a great increase in tolerance, as characterizes all grades of hypopituitarism. In posterior lobe insufficiency there is a tendency to the deposition of fat, subnormal temperature, drowsiness, slow pulse, dry skin, loss of hair, and an extraordinary high tolerance for sugars. Most cases of acromegaly fall in this group and show at first evidences of hyperpituitarism, and later of insufficiency. In the adult, adiposity, high sugar tolerance, subnormal temperature, psychic manifestations, and sexual infantilism of the reversive type indicate hypopituitarism and may exist without the regional symptoms of tumor.

(*d*) Hypophysial symptoms may be shown by patients with internal hydrocephalus from any cause, probably by interference with the passage of the posterior lobe secretion into the cerebro-spinal fluid, and this obstructive dyspituitarism may result from any lesion, inflammatory or neoplastic, in the neighborhood of the third ventricle.

These are the most important of the groups to which Cushing refers, but there are also cases with manifestations indicating involvement of other internal secretions together with that of the hypophysis, and a large group in which transient hypophysial symptoms occur, as, in pregnancy, cranial injuries and infectious diseases.

It is quite clear that disturbances in the function of the pituitary gland may lead to remarkable changes in growth; *hyperpituitarism* may lead to gigantism, when the process antedates ossification of the epiphyses—the Launois type; to acromegaly when it is of later date; *hypopituitarism* to adiposity, with skeletal and sexual infantilism when the process originates in childhood—the Fröhlich type; to adiposity and sexual infantilism of the reversive type when originating in the adult.

Much has been done to clear the subject, but much remains, particularly to clear up the relations of the various types of infantilism which have been described—the Lorain, the Brissaud, the pancreatic, the intestinal—to the different internal secretions. One condition merits separate consideration, that differentiated clearly by Marie and known as acromegaly. (The student is referred to Hastings Gilford's "Disorders of Post-natal Growth," to Vincent's "Innere Secretion," *Ergeb. d. Phys.*, IX and X, and to Cushing's work, "The Pituitary Gland and Its Disorders," J. B. Lippincott Co., 1912.)

ACROMEGALY

Definition.—A dystrophy characterized by increase in size of the face and extremities associated with perverted function of the anterior lobe of the pituitary gland.

The essence of the disease is a dystrophy of hypophysial origin (Marie), which, if it antedates ossification of the epiphyses, leads to gigantism, and in the adult leads to over-growth of the skeleton and other changes which we know as acromegaly.

Etiology.—It is a rare disease, and rather more frequent in women. It affects particularly persons of large size. Twenty per cent. of acromegalics are above six feet in height when the symptoms begin, and fully 40 per cent. of giants are acromegalics (Sternberg). Trauma, the infections, and emotional shock have preceded the onset of the disease.

Pathology.—Practically all of the cases show changes in the pituitary gland, hyperplasia, adenoma, fibroma, or sarcoma, causing distention of the sella turcica and, in the late stages, pressure on surrounding structures; the symptoms are in part due to disturbance of the function of the gland, and in part to the pressure on the adjacent parts.

The bones show the most striking changes; there is a general enlargement of the extremities, but the skeleton on the whole is more or less affected. The enlargement, due to a periosteal growth, is most evident in the hands and feet. The bones of the face are always involved. The orbital arches, frontal prominences, zygoma, malar, and nasal bones are all increased in size, the lower jaw is elongated, thickened, and the teeth separated. The X-ray picture shows very characteristic changes in the sella turcica. The skin and subcutaneous tissues are thickened and the hypertrophy is seen in the soft parts of the face as well.

The brain has been found large, but the most important changes are those due to pressure at the base. The internal organs have been found enlarged, and in Osborne's case the heart weighed 2 lbs. 9 oz.

Symptoms.—When the pituitary gland is involved in tumor growth, which is the common condition in acromegaly, the symptoms may be grouped into those due to the mechanical effects and those associated with perversion of the secretion of the gland.

(*a*) Regional Symptoms.—Headache is common, usually frontal, and often very severe. Somnolence has been noted in many cases, and may be the first symptom. Ocular features occur in a large proportion of the cases, bitemporal hemianopia, optic atrophy, and, in the late stages, pressure on the third nerve and the abducens. One eye only may be affected. Exophthalmos may occur. Deafness is not infrequent. Irritability of temper, marked change in the disposition, great depression, and progressive dementia have been noted. Epistaxis and rhinorrhœa may be present.

(*b*) Symptoms due to the perversion of the internal secretion itself form the striking features of the disease. The patient's friends first notice a gradual increase in the features, which become heavy and thick; or the patient himself may notice that he takes a larger size of hat, or with the progressive enlargement of the hands a larger size of gloves. The enlargement of the extremities does not interfere with their free use.

The hypertrophy is general, involving all the tissues, and gives a curious spadelike character to the hands. The lines on the palms are much deepened. The wrists may be enlarged, but the arms are rarely affected. The feet are involved like the hands and are uniformly enlarged. The big toe, however, may be much larger in proportion. The nails are usually broad and large, but there is no curving, and the terminal phalanges are not bulbous. The joints may be painful and neuralgia is common. The head increases in volume, but not as much in proportion as the face, which becomes much elongated and enlarged in consequence of the increase in the size of the superior and inferior maxillary bones. The latter in particular increases greatly in size, and often projects below the upper jaw. The alveolar processes are widened and the teeth are often separated. The soft parts also increase in size, and the nostrils are large and broad. The eyelids are sometimes greatly thickened, and the ears enormously hypertrophied. The tongue in some instances becomes greatly enlarged. Late in the disease the spine may be affected and the back bowed—kyphosis. The bones of the thorax may slowly and progressively enlarge. With this gradual increase in size the skin of the hands and face may appear normal. Sometimes it is slightly altered in color, coarse, or flabby, but it has not the dry, harsh appearance of the skin in myxœdema. The muscles are sometimes wasted.

Also associated with disturbance of the function of the gland is the diabetes noticed in many cases, which is common in the early stages; in the advanced stages there is an extraordinary high tolerance for sugar. Symptoms on the part of other ductless glands are common. Goitre is of frequent occurrence. Myxœdema or a flabby obesity may occur late. Amenorrhœa is an early symptom in women. Impotence is common in advanced cases in men.

Treatment.—The use of extracts of the gland has been extensively tried but with practically no results. Surgical treatment has been carried out in a number of cases, the chief indication being to give relief to the local pressure symptoms when there is marked glandular enlargement. Partial removal of the growth or the evacuation of a cyst under favorable circumstances may save the optic nerves from complete pressure atrophy.

VI. DISEASES OF THE PINEAL GLAND

"That there is a small gland in the brain in which the soul exercises its functions more particularly than in the other parts" was the opinion of Descartes; and for more than two and a half centuries this was the type of our knowledge of the functions of the pineal gland. What we know now is derived chiefly from clinical cases. But the nature of the internal secretion is unknown; Barker, indeed, believes that the pressure exerted by tumors of the gland may explain the symptoms.

Disease of the gland, usually tumor, may cause (1) pressure symptoms, due to internal hydrocephalus, (2) focal symptoms, due to involvement of the cranial nerves, particularly those of the eyes, (3) features believed to be due to disturbance of the internal secretion, as premature puberty, carbohydrate tolerance, obesity and increase in the growth of hair.

VII. DISEASES OF THE SEX GLANDS

The endocrine part of the testicle is represented by the *interstitial cells* of Leydig and of the ovary by the interstitial cells and the cells of the corpus luteum. The secretions influence the development of the secondary sexual characters. *Hyperfunction* causes premature sexual development in both sexes. *Hypofunction* is shown (1) in eunuchs, in whom there is complete loss of the glands, and (2) in eunochoids, in whom there is insufficiency of the glands. In eunuchs there is lack of genital development, the body is large and fat, there is scanty growth of hair, and the psychical state is altered. In females whose ovaries are removed after puberty the features of the artificial menopause appear. Eunochoids differ according as the insufficiency occurred before or after puberty. There is usually involvement of other glands, especially the pituitary, with a polyglandular syndrome. The individuals are usually tall and fat with absence of secondary sexual characters. The genitals show hypoplasia and sterility, with disturbance of the sexual function, is the rule. In treatment, various combinations of glandular extracts may be used, especially testicular and pituitary in the male and ovarian in the female.

VIII. INFANTILISM

Definition.—A disturbance in growth characterized by persistence of infantile characters and a general retardation of development, bodily and mental.

Etiology.—It is not possible to make a satisfactory classification of the causes or of the cases of infantilism—in some no cause is evident, in others the failure in development has followed obvious disease, and there are cases directly dependent upon loss of some internal secretion.

I. Cachectic infantilism is by no means uncommon, as any serious chronic malady may delay sexual development. For example, the children affected with *hookworm* disease may reach the age of 20 or older before the change from the infantile to the adult state. *Syphilis* is a very common cause. In regions in which *malaria* is very prevalent delayed sexual development is not uncommon in children, and we see it not infrequently in cases of congenital heart disease. There is also a toxic infantilism due to the slow and prolonged action of alcohol and tobacco.

II. Idiopathic Infantilism (*So-called Lorain Type*).—"In this variety the figure is so small that, at first sight, it looks like that of a child. When the patient is stripped, however, his outlines are seen to be those of an adult, and not those of childhood. The head is proportionately small, and the trunk well formed; for the shoulders are broad compared to the hips, and the bony prominences and the muscles stand out distinctly. We have before us a miniature man (or woman, as the case may be), and not one who has retained the characteristics of childhood beyond the proper time. There is, indeed, no growth of facial, pubic or axillary hair, yet the genital organs, though small, are well shaped and quite large enough for the size of the body. The intelligence in both sexes is generally normal" (John Thomson).

The cause of this form is probably associated with perversion of the pituitary secretions. It has also been called an "angioplastic infantilism," in the belief that it was due to a defect of development of the vascular system.

III. The Hormonic Type.—Here we are on safer ground, as we know definitely of several varieties directly dependent upon disturbance of the internal secretions. The most important of these are:

(*a*) Thyroidal or Cretinoid Infantilism.—This has been described.

(*b*) The Fröhlich type, dystrophia adiposo-genitalis, associated with a tumor of the pituitary region, is characterized by great obesity and genital hypoplasia. The symptoms are due to a secretory deficit, for they are capable of experimental reproduction by partial glandular extirpation in animals (Cushing). There are adult and infantile types, just as there are in myxœdema; in the former the individual becomes fat and the sexual organs revert to the preadolescent state. The *Brissaud type* is in all probability due to hypopituitarism. A round, chubby face, under-developed skeleton, prominent abdomen, large layer of fat over the whole body, rudimentary sexual organs, no growth of hair except on the head, and absence of the second dentition, are some of the prominent features of this form, which Brissaud attributed to hypothyroidism, but which appears more likely to be due to dyspituitarism.

(*c*) Pancreatico-intestinal Type.—Bramwell, Herter, Freedman, and others have reported cases of infantilism associated with intestinal changes. Bramwell thought the pancreas was at fault, and his cases improved remarkably under treatment with pancreatic extract. In Herter's case there were looseness of the bowels, often fatty stools, and a change in the flora of the intestine with a rise in the ethereal sulphates in the urine.

IV. Progeria.—Under this term Hastings Gilford described a condition in children of incomplete development (infantilism) with premature decay. The facial appearance, the attitude, the loss of hair, wasting of the skin, are those of old age, and post mortem extensive fibroid changes are found, particularly in the arteries and kidneys. The condition is probably associated with unknown changes in the internal secretions.

IX. DISEASES OF THE SPLEEN

I. GENERAL REMARKS

Though a ductless gland, the spleen is not known to have an internal secretion, and its functions are as yet ill understood. It is not an organ essential to life. In the fetus it takes part in the formation of the red blood corpuscles, and as it contains hæmatoblasts, it is possible that in the adult this function may be exercised to some extent, particularly in cases of severe anæmia.

Hæmolysis is generally believed to be its special function, a view—not held by all physiologists—based upon the presence of a large percentage of organic compounds of iron, the deposit in the organ of blood pigments in various diseases, the presence of many macrophages containing red blood corpuscles, and upon the evidence, after removal of the spleen, of compensatory hæmolysis in many newly formed hæmo-lymph glands (Warthin).

Removal of the spleen, an operation practised by the ancients in the belief that it improved the wind of runners, is not, as a rule, followed by serious effects. There may be slight eosinophilia and temporary anæmia, and later there is usually slight leucocytosis, with relative increase of the lymphocytes.

In infections the organ enlarges and micro-organisms are present in large numbers. It has been supposed to play some part in the processes of immunity and phagocytosis goes on actively in the organ. In experimental anæmia caused by various hæmolytic agents the spleen enlarges, and in these conditions Bunting and Norris found evidence of vicarious blood formation. Chronic splenomegaly may be present with little disturbance of health.

II. MOVABLE SPLEEN

Movable or wandering spleen is seen most frequently in women the subjects of enteroptosis. It may be present without signs of displacement of other organs. It may be found accidentally in individuals who present no symptoms whatever. In other cases there are dragging, uneasy feelings in the back and side. All grades are met with, from a spleen that can be felt completely below the margin of the ribs to a condition in which the tumor-mass impinges upon the pelvis; indeed, the organ has been found in an inguinal hernia! In the large majority of all cases the spleen is enlarged. Sometimes it appears that the enlargement has caused relaxation of the ligaments; in other instances the relaxation seems congenital, as movable spleens have been found in different members of the same family. Possibly traumatism may account for some of the cases. Apart from the dragging, uneasy sensations and the worry in nervous patients, wandering spleen causes very few serious symptoms. Torsion of the pedicle may produce a serious condition, leading to great swelling of the organ, high fever, or even to necrosis. A young woman was admitted to H. A. Kelly's ward with a tumor supposed to be ovarian, but which proved to be a wandering, moderately enlarged spleen. She was transferred to the medical ward, where she had suddenly great pain in the abdomen, a large swelling in the left flank, and much tenderness. Halsted operated and found an enormously enlarged spleen in a condition of necrosis. He laid it open freely, and large necrotic masses of spleen tissue discharged for some time. She made a good recovery.

The *diagnosis* of a wandering spleen is usually easy unless the organ becomes fixed and is deformed by adhesions and perisplenitis. The shape and the sharp margin with the notches are the points to be specially noted.

The *treatment* is important. Occasionally the organ may be kept in position by a properly adapted belt and a pad under the left costal margin. Removal of the displaced organ has been advised and carried out in many cases, and is not a very serious operation. It is, however, as a rule unnecessary. In two cases of enlarged spleen, with great mobility, causing much discomfort and uneasiness, Halsted completely relieved the condition by replacing the spleen, packing it in position with gauze, and allowing firm adhesions to take place. More than eighteen months after the operation the organ had remained in position.

III. RUPTURE OF THE SPLEEN

This is of interest in connection with the spontaneous rupture in cases of acute enlargement during typhoid fever or malaria, which is very rare. Rupture of a malarial spleen may follow a blow, a fall, or exploratory puncture. In India and in Mauritius rupture of the spleen is stated to be common. Fatal hæmorrhage may follow puncture of a swollen spleen with a hypodermic needle. Occasionally the rupture results from the breaking of an infarct or of an abscess. The symptoms are those of hæmorrhage into the peritoneum, and the condition demands immediate laparotomy.

IV. INFARCT CYSTS AND TUBERCULOSIS OF THE SPLEEN

Emboli in the splenic arteries causing *infarcts* may be infective or simple and are seen most frequently in ulcerative endocarditis and septic conditions. Infarcts may also follow the formation of thrombi in the branches of the splenic artery in cases of fever. They are not very infrequent in typhoid. In a few instances the infarcts have followed thrombosis in the splenic veins. They are chiefly of pathological interest. Infarct of the spleen may be suspected in cases of septicæmia or pyæmia when there are pain in the splenic region, tenderness on pressure, and slight swelling of the organ; a well-marked friction rub is occasionally heard. Occasionally in the infective infarcts large *abscesses* are formed, and in rare instances the whole organ may be converted into a sac of pus.

Tumors of the spleen, hydatid and other *cysts* of the organ, and *gummata* are rare conditions of anatomical interest. In Hodgkin's disease the organ may be enlarged and smooth, or irregular from the presence of nodular tumors.

Cysts are rare; the senior author saw but two, one an echinococcus, and the other a double cyst of the hilus. The latter probably arise from a hæmatoma subcapsular or in the hilus. They have been successfully removed. Very small cysts are not infrequent in connection with polycystic disease of the liver and the kidneys. A dermoid cyst has been described. The diagnosis of cysts is not often made; the mass is usually irregular in the region of the spleen, but the splenic outlines are marked. In the case with two cysts at the hilus, the tumor was very movable and irregular, and operation was urged on the grounds of mechanical discomfort, and increase in size. Musser collected notes of 21 operations, all successful, in cysts of this sort.

Primary tuberculosis is rare. Winternitz collected 51 cases in 1912. In some cases the symptoms resemble those of an acute infection, with pain in the splenic region and enlargement of the organ. In the chronic cases there is progressive enlargement of the spleen, often with cyanosis and sometimes with polycythæmia. Splenectomy has been successful in some cases.

V. PRIMARY SPLENOMEGALY WITH ANÆMIA

(*Splenic Anæmia, Banti's Disease*)

Definition.—A primary disease of the spleen of unknown origin, characterized by progressive enlargement, attacks of anæmia, a tendency to hæmorrhage, and in some cases a secondary cirrhosis of the liver, with jaundice and ascites. That the spleen itself is the seat of the disease is shown by the fact that complete recovery follows its removal.

History.—The name "splenic anæmia" was applied to a group of cases by

Griesinger in 1866. H. C. Wood, in 1871, described cases as the splenic form of pseudo-leukæmia. The real study of the disease was initiated by Banti in 1883. In France the condition was called "primitive splenomegaly," and many different types have been described. Here we shall deal only with the form referred to in the definition as splenic anæmia and Banti's disease.

Etiology.—In the majority of cases the enlargement of the spleen comes on without any recognizable cause. In a few cases malaria has been present, but in the greater number the first thing noticed has been the mechanical inconvenience of the big spleen. Males are more frequently attacked than females. It is a disease of young and middle life, the majority of cases occurring before the fortieth year. Some hold that syphilis is important in the etiology. It is also met with in young children. Some of the cases of infantile splenic anæmia of von Jaksch and of the Italian writers belong to this disease.

Morbid Anatomy.—The spleen is greatly enlarged, coming perhaps next to the size of the leukæmic organ. It is very firm, the capsule is thickened, the texture of the gland very tough and firm, and the whole in a state of advanced fibrosis. Banti described a proliferation of the endothelial cells of the venous sinuses of the pulp. The blood vessels in the neighborhood of the spleen may be very large, particularly the vasa brevia, and the splenic vein itself and the portal vein may be enormously dilated, and show atheroma and calcification. The lymphatic glands are not involved. Hyperplasia of the bone marrow has been found, but no other changes of special importance.

The cases of the Gaucher type, primitive endothelioma of the spleen, do not belong in this group.

Symptoms.—The disease is extraordinarily chronic; eight of our cases had a longer duration than ten years. Usually the first feature to attract attention is:

Splenomegaly.—The enlargement is uniform, smooth, painless, usually reaches to the navel, very often to the anterior superior spine, and the organ may occupy the whole of the left half of the abdomen. It may exist for years without any symptoms other than the inconvenience caused by the distention of the abdomen. Following an infarct pain may be present.

Anæmia.—Sooner or later the patients become anæmic. The attack may develop with rapidity, and in children a severe and even fatal form may follow in a few weeks. More commonly the pallor is gradual and the patient may come under observation for the first time with swelling of the feet, shortness of breath, and all the signs of advanced anæmia. The blood picture is that of a secondary anæmia with a very low color index and a marked leucopenia. The red blood corpuscles may fall as low as two million and in an average of a series of uncomplicated cases the leucocyte count was under 3,500 per c. mm. There are no special changes in the differential count. Following a severe hæmorrhage there may be a rise in the leucocytes. Some patients have permanent slight anæmia of the secondary type; others remain very well except for recurring attacks of anæmia, of great severity, which may be independent of hæmorrhage.

Hæmorrhages.—Bleeding, usually hæmatemesis, may be a special feature of the disease and occur at intervals for many years. One of our patients had recurring attacks for twelve years, and one at the London Hospital for fifteen years (Hutchison). In such cases the diagnosis of ulcer of the stomach may be made. The bleeding may be of great severity. On several occasions one of our patients was brought into the hospital completely exsanguine; in two the hæmorrhage proved directly fatal; in a third the hæmorrhage proved fatal ten days after a successful removal of the spleen. The bleeding comes, as a rule, from œsophageal varices. Malæna may be present. Hæmaturia and purpura may occur.

Ascites.—Usually a terminal event, it may be due to the enlarged spleen itself or to secondary cirrhosis of the liver. When due to the liver, it is associated with slight jaundice.

Jaundice.—Icterus has been a rare symptom in our cases. Enlargement of the spleen may persist for many years without any consecutive change in the liver. One patient with splenomegaly and repeated hæmorrhages had more than twelve years of good health after splenectomy. Slight jaundice may persist for years, sometimes with enlargement of the liver, in others with distinct reduction in its volume, and in either case with a progressive cirrhosis—the features to which Banti called special attention.

Course.—It is extraordinarily chronic. Some cases never progress to the stage of Banti's disease. A patient may for ten or twelve years have a large spleen causing no inconvenience, then an attack of anæmia may occur, from which recovery gradually takes place; or the first symptom may be ascites or a severe hæmorrhage from the stomach. As a rule, the anæmia becomes more or less chronic, with marked exacerbations, and in the later stages cirrhosis of the liver with jaundice and ascites develops.

Diagnosis.—Here may be mentioned a series of forms of splenomegaly which differ essentially from splenic anæmia.

Splenomegaly with Acholuric Hæmolytic Jaundice.—This type, first described by Minkowski and sometimes called after his name, is usually a familial form, often hereditary. It is consistent with good health throughout life, and there may be no symptoms. Characteristic features are: (*a*) its familial form; (*b*) chronic enlargement of the spleen; (*c*) good health; (*d*) chronic slight jaundice; (*e*) presence of urobilin in the urine, but absence of bile pigment. In a few instances gall stone colic has been present, due to small calculi. The red blood corpuscles have an increased fragility, the cause of which is unknown, but this is an essential feature. In the familial form good health is the rule, but in the acquired form the patient often becomes anæmic and is very ill. Cures have been reported after splenectomy.

Splenomegaly of the Gaucher Type (*Primary Endothelioma*).—This familial disease was described by Gaucher in 1882. It shows splenomegaly, moderate anæmia, leucocytes normal or low, and a brown or yellowish brown pigmentation of the skin. The liver is enlarged but there is no jaundice. The spleen contains large endothelial cells. Splenectomy may be beneficial but is not always curative.

Splenomegaly with Primary Pylethrombosis.—Cases have been reported of enlarged spleen in connection with phlebitis of the splenic and portal veins, and such cases closely resemble Banti's disease. The spleen is very large and there are jaundice and ascites with moderate anæmia. The recognition of the pylethrombosis is only made post mortem.

Hepatic Splenomegaly.—Three varieties of cirrhosis of the liver may lead to great enlargement of the spleen with anæmia and a symptom-complex resembling that of splenic anæmia.

(*a*) *Alcoholic Cirrhosis.*—With recurring hæmorrhages, a consecutive anæmia, ascites, and an unusually large spleen, the condition may simulate closely the last stage of splenic anæmia. The history, particularly the late appearance of the hepatic changes, may be the most important point. In the cases in which we have been in doubt the difficulty has arisen from an imperfect history and from the presence of recurring hæmorrhages.

(*b*) *Syphilitic Cirrhosis.*—Great enlargement of the spleen may occur with hepatic syphilis, congenital or acquired. Toward the close the picture is similar to Banti's disease—slight jaundice, ascites, big spleen, recurring hæmorrhages, and marked anæmia. Syphilis may cause marked enlargement without involvement of the liver.

(*c*) In a few cases of hypertrophic cirrhosis, as in Hanot's form and in hæmochromatosis, the spleen may be greatly enlarged, and when ascites and hæmorrhages occur, the clinical picture may be like that of splenic anæmia.

Splenomegaly in Pernicious Anæmia.—Sometimes the spleen is greatly enlarged, reaching to the navel, but, as a rule, the blood findings enable one to make the diagnosis.

Tropical Splenomegaly.—Kala-azar can be distinguished by the presence of the Leishman-Donovan bodies in the spleen. There are big spleens with anæmia in the Tropics which are not Kala-azar, and the experience of some of the physicians in Cairo indicates that some of these are of the ordinary splenic anæmia type, in which removal of the organ cures the disease.

The cause of the enlarged spleen in leukæmia and erythræmia is determined by the blood examination; in Hodgkin's disease, carcinoma, amyloid disease and infective endocarditis, other features usually prevent error.

Treatment.—There is only one means of radical cure—removal of the spleen. This should be done as early as possible, but if there is severe anæmia the usual treatment for this should be given and the effort made to improve the blood condition before operation. When marked hepatic changes have occurred, operation is usually contra-indicated. In the cases too far advanced for operation the treatment is that of any severe anæmia and with cirrhosis of the liver and ascites the usual measures should be adopted. If there is any evidence of syphilis active treatment for that should be given.

SECTION XII

DISEASES OF THE NERVOUS SYSTEM

A. GENERAL INTRODUCTION

The Neurone.—ITS STRUCTURE.—The nervous system is a combination of units called neurones, each composed of a receptive cell body and of conductors—namely, protoplasmic processes or dendrites, and the axis-cylinder process or axone. The dendrites conduct impulses toward the cell body (cellulipetal conduction) and the axones conduct them away from the cell (cellulifugal conduction). Depending upon whether the axones conduct impulses in a direction away from or toward the cerebrum they are called efferent or afferent. The axis-cylinder process gives off at varying intervals lateral branches called collaterals, running at right angles, and these, and finally the axis-cylinder process itself, split up at their terminations into many fine fibres, forming the end brushes. These, known as arborizations, surround the body of one or more of the many other cells, or interlace with their protoplasmic processes. Thus, the terminals of the axone of one neurone are related to the dendrites and cell bodies of other neurones by contact or by concrescence.

FUNCTION OF THE NEURONE.—The function of the neurone is to conduct nervous impulses. Reduced to its simplest form, the mode of action may be represented by two cells, one of which, reacting to the environment, conducts impulses inward, whereas the other, awakened by this afferent impulse, conducts an impulse outward. This reflex response Marshall Hall showed to be the fundamental principle of action of the nervous system. The environment acts on the afferent neurones through special sense organs, so that a variety of afferent impulses, olfactory, visual, auditory, gustatory, tactile, painful, thermic, muscular, visceral, and vascular, may be originated. The efferent neurones convey impulses outward to non-nervous tissues, to the skeletal, visceral, and vascular muscles and to the secretory glands, whose activities are thus augmented or inhibited. The most important reflex centres lie in the bulbo-spinal axis. The situation of the vascular and respiratory centres in the bulb makes it the vital centre of the body. In the spinal cord the location of many reflex centres, particularly those for the muscle tendons and for some of the viscera, is represented in the table on page 891. The visceral mechanism is almost wholly regulated by the bulbo-spinal axis, and its reactions are usually unperceived. In conditions of disease the visceral reflexes may "rise into consciousness," and at such times referred pains and areas of tenderness are produced in the skin-fields of the spinal segments corresponding to the centre for registration of the visceral reflex.

DEGENERATION AND REGENERATION OF THE NEURONE.—The nutrition of the neurone depends upon the condition of the cell body, and this in turn upon the activity of the nucleus. If the cell is injured the processes degenerate, or the processes separated from the cell degenerate. Though the nerve cells cease to multiply soon after birth, they nevertheless retain remarkable powers of growth and repair. Injury to the cell body may not be recovered from, but if the axone be severed and degeneration take place in consequence, it may under favorable circumstances be replaced by sprouts from the central stump, and its function be regained. Even the peripheral section, independently of the cell body, may have the power of regeneration. It is probable, however, that both factors play a part in the regeneration—namely, the down growth of the axone from the central end of the divided nerve as well as the changes in the periphery, which are most marked in the cells of the sheath of Schwann.

Cell Systems.—The cell bodies of the neurones are collected more or less closely together in the gray matter of the brain and spinal cord and in the ganglia of the peripheral nerves. Their processes, especially the axis-cylinder processes, run for the most part in the white tracts of the brain and spinal cord and in the peripheral nerves. In this way the different parts of the central nervous system are brought into relation with each other and with the rest of the body. Furthermore, the axis-cylinder processes arising from cells subserving similar functions are collected together into bundles or tracts, and though in many cases the course of these tracts and the functions which they possess are extremely complicated and as yet have not been completely unravelled, nevertheless some of them are simple and fairly well understood. By the study of degenerations resulting from injury or from the toxins of certain diseases which possess an affinity for one or another of these individual tracts or systems, it has been possible to trace the course of certain of them. Fortunately for the clinician, the best understood and the simplest system in its arrangement is that which conveys motor impulses from the cortex to the periphery—the so-called pyramidal tract.

The Motor System.—Motor impulses starting in the left side of the brain cause contractions of muscles on the right side of the body, and those from the right side of the brain in muscles of the left side of the body. Leaving out of consideration some few exceptions, it may be stated as a general rule that the motor path is crossed, and that the crossing takes place in the upper segment (Figs. 12 and 13). Every muscular movement, even the simplest, requires the activity of many neurones. In the production of each movement special neurones are brought into play in a definite combination, and acting in this combination specific movement is the result. In other words, all the movements of the body are represented in the central nervous system by combinations of neurones—that is, they are localized. Muscular movements are localized in every part of the motor path, so that in cases of disease of the nervous system a study of the motor defect often enables one to fix upon the site of the process, and it would be hard to over-estimate the importance of a thorough knowledge of such localization. A voluntary motor impulse starting from the brain cortex must pass through at least two neurones before it can reach the muscles, and we therefore speak of the motor tract as being composed of two segments—an upper and a lower.

The Lower Motor Segment.—The neurones of the lower segment have

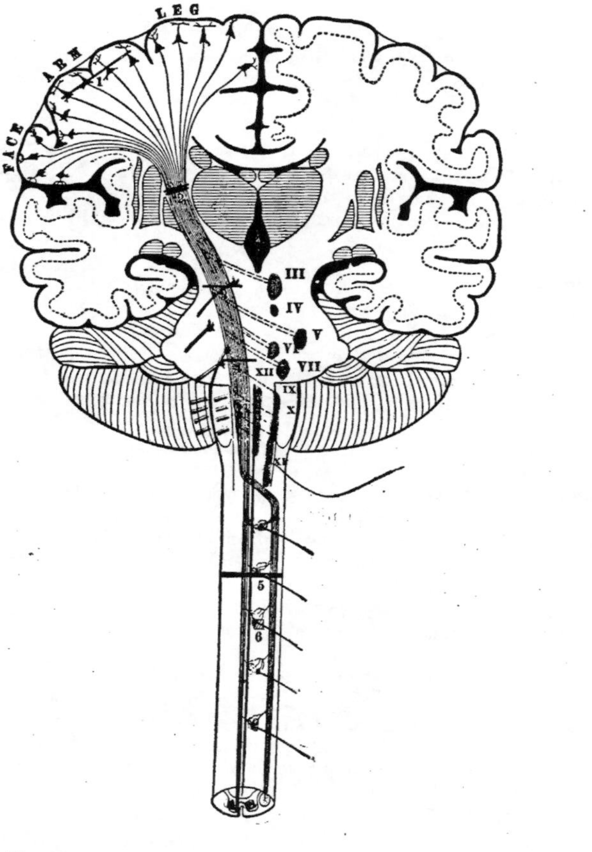

FIG. 12.—DIAGRAM OF MOTOR PATH FROM LEFT BRAIN.

The upper segment is black, the lower red. The nuclei of the motor cerebral nerves are shown in red on the right side; on the left side the cerebral nerves of that side are indicated. A lesion at 1 would cause upper segment paralysis in the arm of the opposite side—cerebral monoplegia; at 2, upper segment paralysis of the whole opposite side of the body—hemiplegia; at 3, upper segment paralysis of the opposite face, arm, and leg, and lower segment paralysis of the eye muscles on the same side—crossed paralysis; at 4, upper segment paralysis of opposite arm and leg, and lower segment paralysis of the face and the external rectus on the same side—crossed paralysis; at 5, upper segment paralysis of all muscles below lesion, and lower segment paralysis of muscles represented at level of lesion—spinal paraplegia; at 6, lower segment paralysis of muscles localized at seat of lesion—anterior poliomyelitis. (Van Gehuchten, modified.)

the cell bodies and their protoplasmic processes in the different levels of the ventral horns of the spinal cord and in the motor nuclei of the cerebral nerves. The axis-cylinder processes of the lower motor neurones leave the spinal cord in the ventral roots and run in the peripheral nerves, to be distributed to all the muscles of the body, where they end in arborizations in the motor end plates. These neurones are direct—that is, their cell bodies, their processes, and the muscles in which they end are all on the same side of the body.

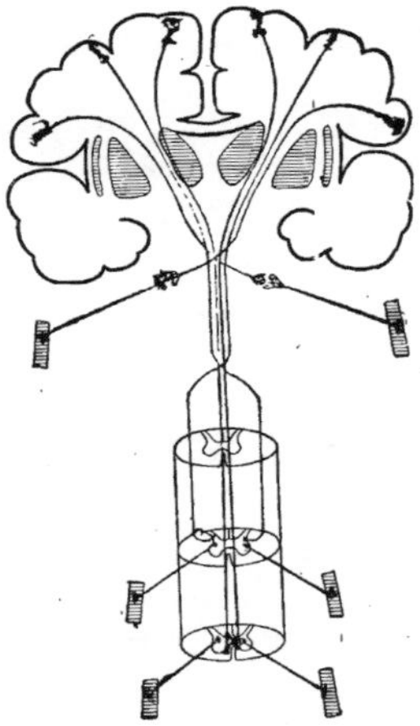

FIG. 13.—DIAGRAM OF MOTOR PATH FROM EACH HEMISPHERE, SHOWING THE CROSSING OF THE PATH, WHICH TAKES PLACE IN THE UPPER SEGMENT BOTH FOR THE CRANIAL AND SPINAL NERVES. (Van Gehuchten, colored.)

The ventral roots of the spinal cord are collected, from above down, into small groups, which, after joining with the dorsal roots of the same level of the cord, leave the spinal canal between the vertebræ as the spinal nerves. That part of the cord from which the roots forming a single spinal nerve arise is called a segment, and corresponds to the nerve which arises from it and not to the vertebra to which it may be opposite. With the exception of the cervical region, in which all the nerve roots but the eighth emerge from above the vertebræ, the roots of each segment for the remainder of the cord leave the spinal canal below the vertebra of corresponding number, and consequently, owing to the fact that during growth the bony canal lengthens much more than the cord itself, the more tailward one goes the greater is the discrepancy in position between each spinal segment and its particular vertebra. This must be borne in mind when determining upon the site of a lesion known to occupy a given segment, for it may lie far above the vertebra of like number and name. A chart has been prepared from numerous measurements by Reid showing the level of the various segments of the cord in relation to the spines of the vertebræ. The axis-cylinder processes which go to make up any one peripheral nerve do not necessarily arise from the same segment of the spinal cord; in fact, most peripheral nerves contain processes from several often quite widely separated segments. Most of the long striped muscles, furthermore, having originated in the embryo from more than one myatome, are innervated from more than one segment.

Our knowledge of the localization of the muscular movements in the gray matter of the lower motor segment is far from complete, but enough is known to aid materially in determining the site of a spinal lesion. The following table, in which is included for each of the spinal segments the centres of representation for the more important skeletal muscles, the main reflex centres, and the main location of the segmental skin-field, has been prepared from the studies of Starr, Edinger, Wichmann, Sherrington, Bolk, and others (pages 891, 892 and 893).

THE UPPER MOTOR SEGMENT AND MOTOR AREAS OF THE CORTEX.—The cell bodies of the upper motor neurones are found in the brain cortex lying for the most part in a strip anterior to the fissure of Rolando, and it is in this region that we find the movements of the body again represented.

True motor responses are elicited only by stimulation *anterior* to the Rolandic fissure; practically no point over the ascending frontal convolution fails to respond to stimulation. There is but slight extension of the motor cortex on to the paracentral lobule of the mesial surface of the brain. Movements are obtainable not only from the exposed part of the convolution, but also from its hidden surface to the very depths of the Rolandic sulcus. There is an area of representation for the trunk between the centres for the leg and arm, and also for the neck between those of the arm and face. The superior and inferior genua are the landmarks which indicate the situation of these small areas of representation for trunk and neck. These results have in large measure been confirmed by Cushing by unipolar electrical stimulation of the human cortex. From above down the motor areas occur in the following order: leg, trunk, arm, neck, head (Fig. 14). Those of the leg and arm occupy the upper half of the convolution, and that for the head, including movements of the face, jaws, tongue, and larynx, the lower half.

The speech centres are indicated in the diagram (Fig. 14) in accordance with the generally accepted views: that for motor speech occupies the posterior part of the left third frontal or Broca's convolution. It is a disputed point whether or not there is a separate centre presiding over the movements employed in writing. Some have assumed such a centre to be present in the second frontal convolution as indicated on the diagram. The conjugate movement of head and eyes to the opposite side has commonly been found in apes to follow stimulation of the external surface of the frontal lobe. Similarly movements of the eyes may be elicited from the occipital cortex, but probably none of these reactions are comparable to the more simple movements through the pyramidal tract which follow stimulation of the ascending frontal convolution.

The axis-cylinder processes of the upper motor neurones after leaving the gray matter of the motor cortex pass into the white matter of the brain and form part of the corona radiata. They converge and pass between the basal ganglia in the internal capsule. Here the motor axis-cylinders are collected into a compact bundle—the pyramidal tract—occupying the knee and anterior

LOCALIZATION OF THE FUNCTIONS IN THE SEGMENTS OF THE SPINAL CORD

SEGMENT.	STRIPED MUSCLES.	REFLEX.	SKIN-FIELDS (CF. FIGS. 18 AND 19).
I, II and III C.	Splenius capitis. Hyoid muscles. Sterno-mastoid. Trapezius. Diaphragm (C III–V). Levator scapulæ (C III–V).	Hypochondrium (?). Sudden inspiration produced by sudden pressure beneath the lower border of ribs (diaphragmatic).	Back of head to vertex. Neck (upper part).
IV C.	Trapezius. Diaphragm. Levator scapulæ. Scaleni (C IV–T I). Teres minor. Supraspinatus. Rhomboid.	Dilatation of the pupil produced by irritation of neck. Reflex through the sympathetic (C IV–T I).	Neck (lower part to second rib). Upper shoulder.
V C	Diaphragm. Teres minor. Supra and infra spinatus (C V–VI). Rhomboid. Subscapularis. Deltoid. Biceps. Brachialis anticus. Supinator longus (C V–VII). Supinator brevis (C V–VII). Pectoralis (clavicular part). Serratus magnus.	Scapular (C V–T I). Irritation of skin over the scapula produces contraction of the scapular muscles. Supinator longus and biceps. Tapping their tendons produces flexion of forearm.	Outer side of shoulder and upper arm over deltoid region.
VI C.	Teres minor and major. Infraspinatus. Deltoid. Biceps. Brachialis anticus. Supinator longus. Supinator brevis. Pectoralis (clavicular part). Serratus magnus (C V–VIII). Coraco-brachialis. Pronator teres. Triceps (outer and long heads). Extensors of wrist (C VI–VIII).	Triceps. Tapping elbow tendon produces extension of forearm. Posterior wrist. Tapping tendons causes extension of hand (C VI–VII).	Outer side of forearm, front and back. Outer half of hand (?).
VII C.	Teres major. Subscapularis. Deltoid (posterior part). Pectoralis major (costal part). Pectoralis minor. Serratus magnus. Pronators of wrist. Triceps. Extensors of wrist and fingers. Flexors of wrist. Latissimus dorsi (C VI–VIII).	Scapulo-humeral. Tapping the inner lower edge of scapula causes adduction of the arm. Anterior wrist. Tapping anterior tendons causes flexion of wrist (C VII–VIII).	Inner side and back of arm and forearm. Radial half of the hand.

Localization of the Functions in the Segments of the Spinal Cord (*Continued*)

Segment.	Striped Muscles	Reflex.	Skin-Fields (cf. Figs. 18 and 19).
VIII C.	Pectoralis major (costal part). Pronator quadratus. Flexors of wrist and fingers. Latissimus. Radial lumbricales and interossei.	Palmar. Stroking palm causes closure of fingers.	Forearm and hand, inner half.
I T.	Lumbricales and interossei. Thenar and hypothenar eminences (C VII–T I).		Upper arm, inner half.
II to XII T.	Muscles of back and abdomen. Erectores spinæ (T I–LV). Intercostals (T I–T XII). Rectus abdominis (T V–T XII). External oblique (T V–XII). Internal oblique (T VII–L I). Transversalis (T VII–L I).	Epigastric. Tickling mammary region causes retraction of epigastrium (T IV–VII). Abdominal. Stroking side of abdomen causes retraction of belly (T IX–XII).	Skin of chest and abdomen in oblique dorso-ventral zones. The nipple lies between the zone of T IV and T V. The umbilicus lies in the field of T X.
I L.	Lower part of external and internal oblique and transversalis. Quadratus lumborum (L I–II). Cremaster. Psoas major and minor (?).	Cremasteric. Stroking inner thigh causes retraction of scrotum (L I–II).	Skin over lowest abdominal zone and groin.
II L.	Psoas major and minor. Iliacus. Pectineus. Sartorius (lower part). Flexors of knee (Remak). Adductor longus and brevis.		Front of thigh.
III L.	Sartorius (lower part). Adductors of thigh. Quadriceps femoris (L II–L IV). Inner rotators of thigh. Abductors of thigh.	Patellar tendon. Tapping tendon causes extension of leg. "Knee-jerk."	Front and inner side of thigh.
IV L.	Flexors of knee (Ferrier). Quadriceps femoris. Adductors of thigh. Abductors of thigh. Extensors of ankle (tibialis anticus). Glutei (medius and minor).	Gluteal. Stroking buttock causes dimpling in fold of buttock (L IV–V).	Mainly inner side of thigh and leg to ankle.
V L.	Flexors of knee (ham-string muscles) (L IV–S II). Outward rotators of thigh. Glutei. Flexors of ankle (gastrocnemius and soleus) (L IV–S II). Extensors of toes (L IV–S I). Peronæi.		Back of leg, and part of foot.

LOCALIZATION OF THE FUNCTIONS IN THE SEGMENTS OF THE SPINAL CORD (*Continued*)

SEGMENT.	STRIPED MUSCLES.	REFLEX.	SKIN-FIELDS (CF. FIGS. 18 AND 19).
I to II S.	Flexors of ankle (L V–S II). Long flexor of toes (L V–S II). Peronæi. Intrinsic muscles of foot.	Foot reflex. Extension of Achilles tendon causes flexion of ankle (S I–II). Ankle-clonus. Plantar. Tickling sole of foot causes flexion of toes or extension of great toe and flexion of others.	Back of thigh, leg and foot; outer side.
III to V S.	Perineal muscles. Levator and sphincter ani (S I–III).	Vesical and anal reflexes.	Skin over sacrum and buttock. Anus. Perineum. Genitals.

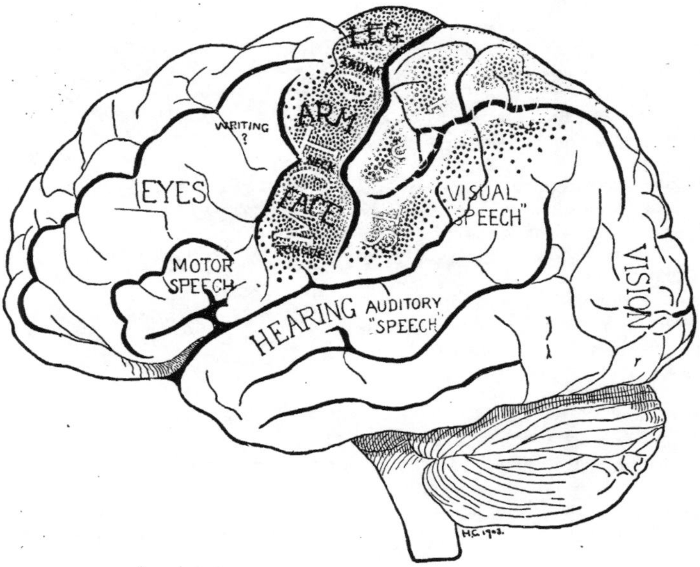

FIG. 14.—DIAGRAMMATIC REPRESENTATION OF CORTICAL LOCALIZATION IN THE LEFT HEMISPHERE, SHOWING THE SPEECH CENTRES.

The motor areas determined by unipolar faradic excitation of the anthropoid cortex (Sherrington and Grünbaum) are here shown stippled in red and lie anterior to the Rolandic fissure. The sensory areas presumably lie posterior to this fissure and are roughly indicated in blue without accurate delineation. Lying as it does on the upper surface of the hemisphere, the leg area should not be visible on a lateral view such as is given here.

two-thirds of the posterior limb of the internal capsule. The order in which the movements of the opposite side of the body are represented at this level, as learned from experimental observations on apes, is given in Fig. 15.

After passing through the internal capsule the fibres of the pyramidal tract leave the hemisphere by the crus, of which they occupy about the middle three-fifths (Fig. 16). The movements of the tongue and lips are represented nearest the middle line.

As soon as the tract enters the crus, some of its axis-cylinder processes leave it and cross the middle line to end in arborizations about the ganglion cells in the nucleus of the third nerve on the opposite side; and in this way, as the pyramidal tract passes down, it gives off at different levels fibres which end in the nuclei of all the motor cerebral nerves on the opposite side of the body. Some fibres, however, go to the nuclei of the same side. From the crus the pyramidal tract runs through the pons and forms in the medulla oblongata the pyramid, which gives its name to the tract. At the lower part of the medulla, after the fibres going to the cerebral nerves have crossed the middle line, a large proportion of the remaining fibres cross, decussating with those from the opposite pyramid, and pass into the opposite side of the spinal cord, forming the crossed pyramidal tract of the lateral column (fasciculus cerebro-spinalis lateralis) (Fig. 17, 1). The smaller number of fibres which do not at this time cross descend in the ventral column of the same side, forming the direct pyramidal tract, or Türck's column (fasciculus cerebro-spinalis ventralis) (Fig. 17, 2).

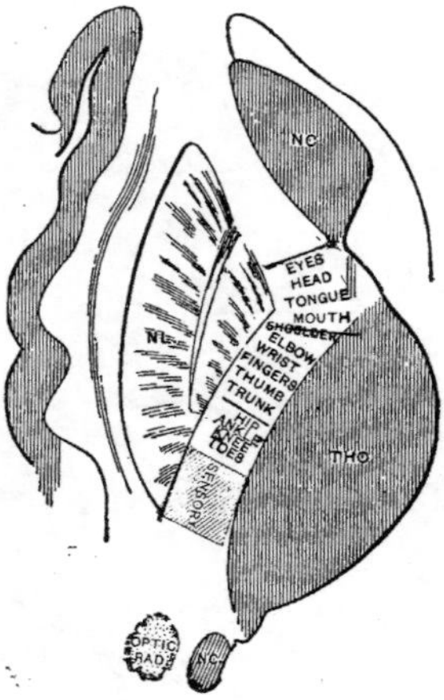

FIG. 15.—DIAGRAM OF MOTOR AND SENSORY REPRESENTATION IN THE INTERNAL CAPSULE.

NL., Lenticular nucleus. NC., Caudate nucleus. THO., Optic thalamus. The motor paths are red and black, the sensory are blue.

At every level of the spinal cord axis-cylinder processes leave the crossed pyramidal tract to enter the ventral horns and end about the cell bodies of the lower motor neurones. The tract diminishes in size from above downward. The fibres of the direct pyramidal tract cross at different levels in the ventral white commissure, and also, it is believed, end about cells in the ventral horns on the opposite side of the cord. This tract usually ends about the middle of the thoracic region of the cord.

The Sensory System.—The path for sensory conduction is more complicated than the motor path, and in its simplest form is composed of at least three sets of neurones, one above the other. The cell bodies of the lowest neurones are in the ganglia on the dorsal roots of the spinal nerves and the ganglia of the sensory cerebral nerves. These ganglion cells have a special form, having apparently but a single process, which, soon after leaving the cell, divides in a T-shaped manner, one portion running into the central nervous system and the other to the periphery of the body. Embryological and comparative anatomical studies have made it seem probable that the peripheral sensory fibre, the process which conducts toward the cell, represents the protoplasmic processes, while that which conducts away from the cell is the axis-cylinder process. In the peripheral sensory nerves we have, then, the

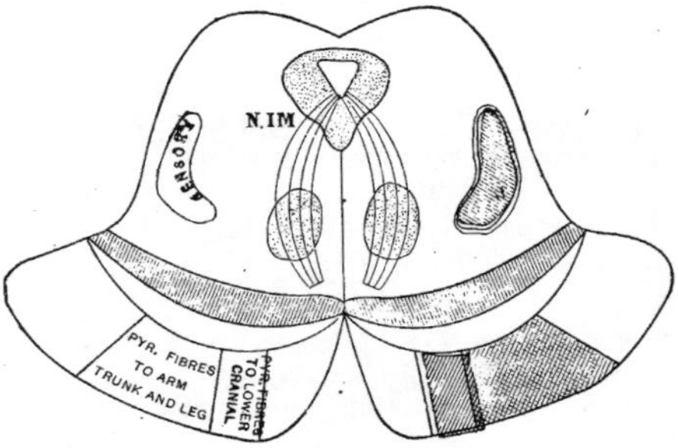

FIG. 16.—DIAGRAM OF MOTOR AND SENSORY PATHS IN CRURA.

dendrites of the lower sensory neurones. These start in the periphery of the body from their various specialized end organs. The axis-cylinder processes leave the ganglia and enter the spinal cord by the dorsal roots of the spinal nerves. After entering the cord each axis-cylinder process divides into an

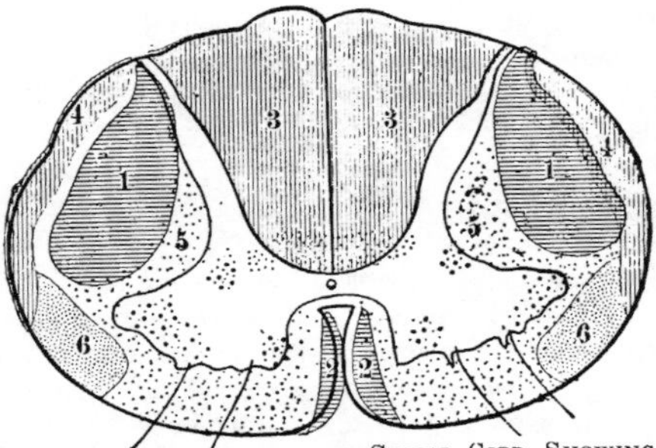

FIG. 17.—DIAGRAM OF CROSS-SECTION OF THE SPINAL CORD, SHOWING MOTOR, RED, AND SENSORY, BLUE, PATHS.

1, Lateral pyramidal tract. 2, Ventral pyramidal tract. 3, Dorsal columns. 4, Direct cerebellar tract. 5, Ventro-lateral ground bundles. 6, Ventro-lateral ascending tract of Gowers. (Van Gehuchten, colored.)

ascending and a descending branch, which run in the dorsal fasciculi. The descending branch runs but a short distance, and ends in the gray matter of the same side of the cord. It gives off a number of collaterals, which also end in the gray matter. The ascending branch may end in the gray matter soon after entering, or it may run in the dorsal fasciculi as far as the medulla, to end about the nuclei there. In any case it does not cross the middle line. The lower sensory neurone is direct.

The cells about which the axis-cylinder processes and their collaterals of the lower sensory neurone end are of various kinds. They are known as sensory neurones of the second order. In the first place, some of them end about the cell bodies of the lower motor neurones, forming the path for reflexes. They also end about cells whose axis-cylinder processes cross the middle line and run to the opposite side of the brain. In the spinal cord these cells are found in the different parts of the gray matter, and their axis-cylinder processes run in the opposite ventro-lateral ascending tract of Gowers (Fig. 15, 6) and in the ground bundles (fasciculus lateralis proprius and fasciculus ventralis proprius).

In the medulla the nuclei of the dorsal fasciculi (nucleus fasciculi gracilis and nucleus fasciculi cuneati) contain for the most part cells of this character. Their axis-cylinder processes, after crossing, run toward the brain in the medial lemniscus or bundle of the fillet; certain of the longitudinal bundles in the formatio reticularis also represent sensory paths from the spinal cord and medulla toward higher centres. The fibres of the medial lemniscus or fillet do not, however, run directly to the cerebral cortex. They end about cells in the ventro-lateral portion of the optic thalamus, and the tract is continued on by way of another set of neurones, which send processes to end in the cortex of the posterior central and parietal convolutions. This is the most direct path of sensory conduction, but by no means the only one. The peripheral sensory neurones may also end about cells in the cord whose axones run but a short distance toward the brain before ending again in the gray matter, and the path, if path it can be called, is made up of a series of these superimposed neurones. The gray matter of the cord itself is also believed to offer paths of sensory conduction. All these paths reach the tegmentum and optic thalamus, and thence are distributed to the cortex along with the other sensory paths. There may also be paths of sensory conduction through the cerebellum by way of the direct cerebellar tract and Gowers' bundle.

From this short summary it is evident that the possible paths for the conduction of afferent impulses are many, and become more complex as the various tracts approach the brain where our knowledge of them is somewhat indefinite. The anatomical arrangement of the two lower orders of sensory neurones is, however, sufficiently well understood to be of great clinical value. We have seen in the case of the motor neurones that the distribution of the peripheral nerves to the muscles, owing largely to the interlacing into plexuses of the neurones from the various spinal units, is quite different from that of the ventral roots themselves, and the same rule holds true for the peripheral nerve and dorsal root distribution for the cutaneous areas. The *cutaneous* fields corresponding to the peripheral nerves are well known, and although our knowledge of the exact site and outline of some of the *segmental* skin-fields, represented by the dorsal roots, is less accurately established, nevertheless they are sufficiently well understood to be of aid in determining the segmental level of spinal cord and of dorsal root lesions. Information concerning the topography in the adult of these skin units or dermatomes has been obtained from various sources; from morphological studies; from anatomical dissections; from physiological experimentation, particularly in Sherrington's hands; from the study of anæsthesias in clinical cases after traumatic injuries to the cord, and from Head's studies of the distribution of the cutaneous lesions in herpes zoster, and of the areas of referred pain and tenderness in visceral disease. The diagrams on pages 898 and 899 embody the results of many of these observations.

The cutaneous sensory impressions are in man conducted toward the brain, probably on the opposite side of the cord—that is, the path crosses to the opposite side soon after entering the cord. Muscular sense, on the other hand, is conducted on the same side of the cord in the fasciculus of Goll, to cross above by means of the axones of sensory neurones of the second order in the medulla.

Sensory Areas of the Brain.—There are probably two sensory centres—one in the optic thalamus, the other in a considerable area of the cerebral cortex. The thalamus plays a three-fold part. Here all the afferent paths terminate; secondly, it contains a mass of gray matter which forms the centre for certain fundamental elements of sensation, particularly those capable of evoking pleasure and discomfort and consciousness of changes of state. Thirdly, in the lateral part of the thalamus is the centre through which the cortex influences the essential thalamic centre, controlling and checking its activity. On their way from the periphery to the cortex afferent impulses pay toll to the co-ordinate mechanisms of the spinal cord and the cerebellum. At the thalamic junction they are re-grouped to act upon the two terminal centres. One of these, the essential organ of the optic thalamus, responds to all those elements which evoke consciousness of an internal change in state, more particularly pleasure and discomfort. Sensory impulses, then, pass by way of the internal capsule to the cortex, and in the main five groups of sensory impulses are distributed in this way: (1) those underlying postural recognition, and the appreciation of passive movement and weight; (2) the impulses underlying the recognition of tactile differences; (3) those upon which depends the recognition of size and space; (4) those which enable us to localize the spot stimulated; and (5) thermal impulses (Head and Holmes).

These afferent materials are combined in the cortex with each other and with other sense impressions in intellectual processes. The cortical area concerned is that situated between the pre-central fissure and the occipital lobe.

The paths for the conduction of the stimuli which underlie the special senses are given in the section upon the cerebral nerves, and it is only necessary here to refer to what is known of the cortical representation of these senses.

Visual impressions are localized in the occipital lobes. The primary visual centre is on the mesial surface in the cuneus, especially about the calcarine fissure, and here are represented the opposite visual half-fields. Some authors believe that there is another higher centre on the outer surface of the occipital lobe, in which the vision of the opposite eye is chiefly represented. However this may be, most authors hold that the angular gyrus of the left hemisphere is a part of the brain in which are stored the memories of the meaning of letters, words, figures, and, indeed, of all seen objects. This is designated as the visual speech centre on the diagram (Fig. 14).

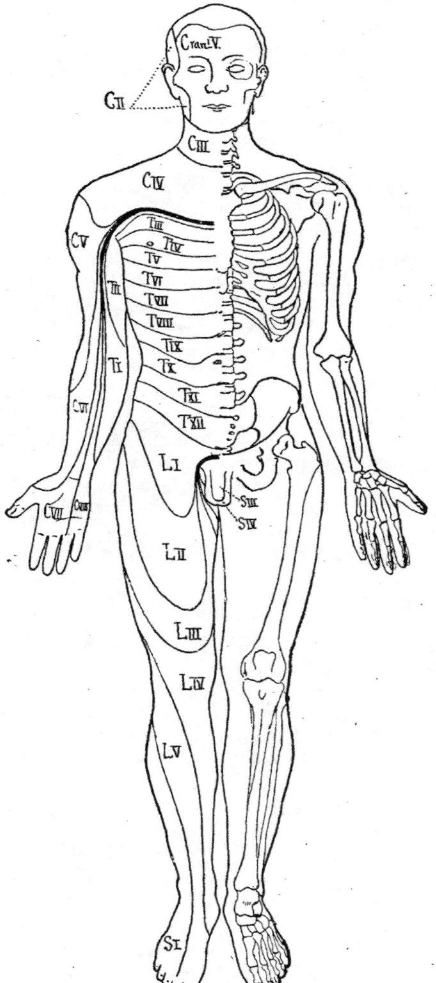

Fig. 18.—Anterior Aspect of the Segmental Skin Fields of the Body, Combined from the Studies of Head, Kocher, Starr, Thorburn, Edinger, Sherrington, Wichmann, Seiffer, Bolk, Cushing, and Others.

Heavy lines represent levels of fusion of dermatomes and the preaxial and postaxial lines of the limbs.

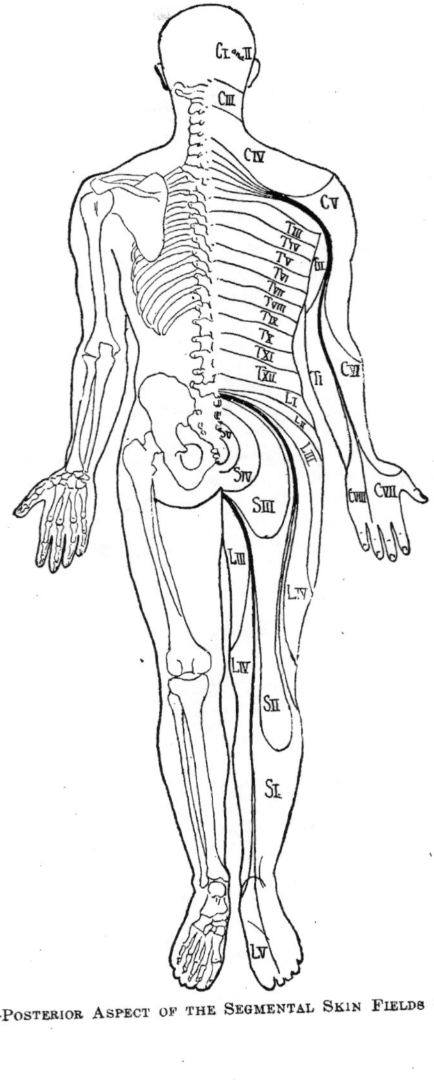

FIG. 19.—POSTERIOR ASPECT OF THE SEGMENTAL SKIN FIELDS OF THE BODY.

Auditory impressions are localized for the most part in the first temporal convolution and the transverse temporal gyri, and it is in this region in the left hemisphere that the memories of the meanings of heard words and sounds are stored. Musical memories are localized somewhat in front of those for words. The cortical centres for smell include a part of the base of the frontal lobe, the uncus, and perhaps the gyrus hippocampi. The centres for taste are supposed to be situated near those for smell, but we possess as yet no definite information about them.

Topical Diagnosis.—The successful diagnosis of the position of a lesion in the nervous system depends upon a careful examination into all the symptoms present, and then endeavoring with the help of anatomy and physiology to determine the place, a disturbance at which might produce these symptoms. The abnormalities of motion are usually the most important localizing symptoms, both on account of the ease with which they can be demonstrated, and also because of the comparative accuracy of our knowledge of the motor path.

Lesions in any part of the motor path cause disturbances of motion. If destructive, the function of the part is abolished, and as the result there is *paralysis.* If, on the other hand, the lesion is an irritative one, the structures are thrown into abnormal activity, which produces *abnormal muscular contraction.* The character of the paralysis or of the abnormal muscular contraction varies with lesions of the upper and lower segment, the variations depending, first, upon the anatomical position of the two segments; and, secondly, upon the symptoms which are the result of secondary degeneration in each of the segments.

(*a*) Lesions of the Lower or Spino-muscular Segment.—*Destructive Lesions.*—The nutrition of all parts of a neurone depends upon their connection with its healthy cell body; if the cell body be injured, its processes undergo degeneration, or if a portion of a process be separated from the cell body, that part degenerates along its whole length. This so-called secondary degeneration plays a very important rôle in the symptomatology.

In the lower motor segment the degeneration not only affects the axis-cylinder processes which run in the peripheral nerves, but also the muscle fibres in which the axis-cylinder processes end. The degeneration of the nerves and muscles is made evident, first by the muscles becoming smaller and flabby, and, secondly, by change in their reaction to electrical stimulation. The degenerated nerve gives no response to either the galvanic or the faradic current, and the muscle does not respond to faradic stimulation, but reacts in a characteristic manner to the galvanic current. The contraction, instead of being sharp, quick, lightning-like, as in that of a normal muscle, is slow and lazy, and is often produced by a weaker current, and the anode-closing contraction may be greater than the cathode-closing contraction. This is the *reaction of degeneration,* but it is not always present in the classical form. The essential feature is the slow, lazy contraction of the muscle to the galvanic current, and when this is present the muscle is degenerated.

The myotatic irritability, or muscle reflex, and the muscle tonus depend upon the integrity of the reflex arc, of which the lower motor segment is the efferent limb, and in a paralysis due to lesion of this segment the muscle reflexes (tendon reflexes) are abolished and there is a diminished muscular tension.

Lower segment paralyses have for their characteristics degenerative atrophy with the reaction of degeneration in the affected muscles, loss of their reflex excitability, and a diminished muscular tension. These are the general characteristics, but the anatomical relations of this segment also give certain peculiarities in the distribution of the paralyses which help to distinguish them from those which follow lesions of the upper segment, and which also aid in determining the site of the lesion in the lower segment itself. The cell bodies of this segment are distributed in groups, from the level of the peduncles of the brain throughout the whole extent of the spinal cord to its termination opposite the second lumbar vertebra, and their axis-cylinder processes run in the peripheral nerves to every muscle in the body; so that the component parts are more or less widely separated from each other, and a local lesion causes paralysis of only a few muscles or groups of muscles, and not of a whole section of the body, as is the case where lesions affect the upper segment. The muscles which are paralyzed indicate whether the disease is in the peripheral nerves or spinal cord; for the muscles are represented differently in the peripheral nerves and in the spinal cord. Sensory symptoms, which may accompany the paralysis, are often of great assistance in making a local diagnosis. Thus, in a paralysis with the characteristics of a lesion of the lower motor segment, if the paralyzed muscles are all supplied by one nerve, and the anæsthetic area of the skin is supplied by that nerve, it is evident that the lesion must be in the nerve itself. On the other hand, if the muscles paralyzed are not supplied by a single nerve, but are represented close together in the spinal cord, and the anæsthetic area corresponds to that section of the cord (see table), it is equally clear that the lesion must be in the cord itself or in its nerve roots.

Irritative Lesions of the Lower Motor Segment.—Lesions of this segment cause comparatively few symptoms of irritation. The fibrillary contractions which are so common in muscles undergoing degeneration are probably due to stimulation of the cell bodies in their slow degeneration, as in progressive muscular atrophy, or to irritation of the axis-cylinder processes in the peripheral nerves, as in neuritis. Lesions which affect the motor roots as they leave the central nervous system may cause spasmodic contractions in the muscles supplied by them. Certain convulsive paroxysms, of which laryngismus stridulus is a type, and to which the spasms of tetany also belong, are believed to be due to abnormal activity in the lower motor centres. These are the "lowest level fits" of Hughlings Jackson. Certain poisons, as strychnia and that of tetanus, act particularly upon these centres.

The lower motor segment may be involved in all diseases involving the peripheral nerves in cerebral and spinal meningitis, in injuries, in hæmorrhages and tumors of the medulla and cord or their membranes, in lesions of the gray matter of the segment, in anterior poliomyelitis, progressive muscular atrophy, bulbar paralysis, ophthalmoplegia, syringomyelia, etc.

(*b*) Lesions of the Upper Motor Segment.—*Destructive lesions* cause paralysis, as in the lower motor segment, and here again the secondary degeneration which follows the lesion gives to the paralysis its distinctive characteristics. In this case the paralysis is accompanied by a *spastic* condition, shown in an exaggeration of muscle reflex and an increase in the tension of the muscle. It is not accurately known how the degeneration of the pyramidal fibres causes this excess of the muscle reflex. The usual explanation is that under normal circumstances the upper motor centres are constantly exerting a restraining influence upon the activity of the lower centres, and that when the influence ceases to act, on account of disease of the pyramidal fibres, the lower centres take on increased activity, which is made manifest by an exaggeration of the muscle reflex.

The neurones composing each segment of the motor path are to be considered as nutritional units, and therefore the secondary degeneration in the upper segment stops at the beginning of the lower. For this reason the muscles paralyzed from lesions in the upper segment do not undergo degenerative atrophy, nor do they show any marked change in their electrical reactions.

The separate parts of the upper motor segment lie much more closely together than do those of the lower segment, and therefore a small lesion may cause paralysis in many muscles. This is more particularly true in the internal capsule, where all the axis-cylinder processes of this segment are collected into a compact bundle—the pyramidal tract. A lesion in this region usually causes paralysis of most of the muscles on the opposite side of the body—that is, hemiplegia. The pyramidal tract continues in a compact bundle, giving off fibres to the motor nuclei at different levels; a lesion anywhere in its course is followed by paralysis of all the muscles whose spinal centres are situated below the lesion. When the disease is above the decussation, the paralysis is on the opposite side of the body; when below, the paralyzed muscles are on the same side as the lesion. Above the internal capsule the path is somewhat more separated, and in the cortex the centres for the movements of the different sections of the body are comparatively far apart, and a sharply localized lesion in this region may cause a more limited paralysis, affecting a limb or a segment of a limb—the cerebral monoplegias; but even here the paralysis is not confined to an individual muscle or group of muscles, as is commonly the case in lower segment paralysis (see Fig. 12 and explanation).

To sum up, the paralyses due to lesions of the upper motor segment are widespread, often hemiplegic; the paralyzed muscles are spastic (the tendon reflexes exaggerated), they do not undergo degenerative atrophy, and they do not present the degenerative reaction to electrical stimulation.

Irritative Lesions of the Upper Motor Segment.—Our knowledge of such lesions is confined for the most part to those acting on the motor cortex. The abnormal muscular contractions resulting from lesions so situated have as their type the localized convulsive seizures classed under *Jacksonian* or cortical epilepsy, which are characterized by the convulsion beginning in a single muscle or group of muscles and involving other muscles in a definite order, depending upon the position of their representation in the cortex. For instance, such a convulsion, beginning in the muscles of the face, next involves those of the arm and hand, and then the leg. The convulsion is usually accompanied by sensory phenomena and followed by a weakness of the muscles involved.

A majority of lesions of the motor cortex are both destructive and irritative—i. e., they destroy the nerve cells of a certain centre, and either in their growth or by their presence throw into abnormal activity those of the surrounding centres.

The upper motor segment is involved in nearly all the diseases of the brain and spinal cord, especially in injuries, tumors, abscesses, and hæmorrhages; transverse lesions of the cord; syringomyelia, progressive muscular atrophy, bulbar paralysis, etc. One lesion often involves both the upper and the lower motor segments, and there is paralysis in the different parts of the body, with the characteristics of each. Such a combination enables us in many cases to make an accurate local diagnosis.

Lesions in the optic path and in the different speech centres also give localizing symptoms, which should always be looked for.

(*c*) Lesions of the Sensory Path.—Here again the lesion may be either irritative or destructive. *Irritative lesions* cause abnormal subjective sensory impression—paræsthesia, formication, a sense of cold or constriction, and pain of every grade of intensity. The character of the sensory symptoms gives very little indication as to the position of the irritating process. Intense pain is, as a rule, a symptom of a lesion in the peripheral sensory neurones, but it may be caused by a disease of the sensory path within the central nervous system.

The exact distribution of symptoms gives more accurate data, for if they are confined to the distribution of a peripheral nerve or of a spinal segment the indication is plain. If one side of the body is more or less completely affected, the lesion is somewhere within the brain, etc.

Destructive Lesions.—A complete destruction of the sensory paths from any part of the body would of course deprive that part of sensation in all its qualities. This occurs most frequently from injury to the peripheral sensory neurones within the peripheral nerves, and the area of anæsthesia depends upon the nerve injured. Complete transverse lesion of the cord causes complete anæsthesia below the injury.

Unilateral lesions of the cord, medulla, dorsal part of the pons, tegmentum, thalamus, internal capsule, and cortex cause disturbances of sensation on the *opposite* side of the body; here again the extent of the defect more than its character helps us to determine the position of the lesion. Hemianæsthesia involving the face as well as the rest of the body can only occur above the place where the sensory paths from the fifth nerve have crossed the middle line on their way to the cortex. This is in the upper part of the pons. From this point to where they leave the internal capsule the sensory paths are in fairly close relation, and are at times involved in a very small lesion. Above the internal capsule the paths diverge quickly, and for this reason only an extensive lesion can involve them all, and in lesions of this part we are more apt to have the sensory disturbances confined to one or another region of the body. Unilateral lesions of the thalamus, pons, medulla, and cord usually cause sensory disturbances on the same side of the body, as well as those on the opposite side. These are due to the involvement of the sensory paths as they enter the central nervous system at or a little below the site of the lesion and before the axones of the sensory neurones of the second order have crossed the middle line. The area of disturbed sensation on the same side is limited to the distribution of one or more spinal segments and often indicates accurately the position and extent of the diseased process. As a rule, destructive lesions of the central nervous system do not involve all the paths of sensory conduction, and the loss of sensation is not complete. It is often astonishing how very slight the sensory disturbances are which result from an extensive lesion. Sensation may be diminished in all of its qualities, or, what is more common, certain qualities may be affected while others are normal. Thus, the sense of pain and temperature may be lost while that of touch remains normal, as is often the case in diseases of the spinal cord, or there may be simply a loss of the muscular sense and of the stereognostic sense (the complex sensory impression which enables one to recognize an object placed in the hand), as occurs frequently from lesions of the cortex. Occasionally pain sensation persists with loss of tactile and thermic sensations. Almost every other combination has been described. It is the *distribution* more than the character of the sensory defect that is of importance, and often the distribution gives but uncertain indication of the position of the lesion. The combination of the sensory defect with different forms of paralysis gives the most certain diagnostic signs.

Sympathetic Nervous System (Involuntary, Vegetative, Visceral, Autonomic).—This system innervates the pupils, non-striped muscles, glands, viscera, heart and blood vessels, and genital organs. It is outside the control of the will but can be influenced by the central nervous system, especially by emotional stimuli.

This involuntary or vegetative nervous system consists of two parts which are distinct anatomically and antagonistic physiologically.

1. Sympathetic proper (thoracico-lumbar).
2. Para-sympathetic (*a*) cranio-bulbar and (*b*) sacral.

There is some confusion in the use of the term "autonomic" which was applied by Langley to the whole vegetative system, but is also used to designate the para-sympathetic alone.

The fibres of the sympathetic proper arise from cells in the intermedio-lateral region of the cord (preganglionic), pass by the anterior roots to end in ganglia which in turn send fibres (postganglionic) to the terminations in smooth muscle, the heart, blood vessels, sweat glands, secreting glands, etc. The receptor (afferent) elements are concerned with visceral sensations and referred visceral pain. The excitor (efferent) elements form synapses in the ganglia and in this way one fibre may stimulate a number of cells. From these cells the postganglionic fibres pass directly to their destinations. The ganglia act as "distributing stations" and form a series in front of the vertebral column, one on each side. In the neck there are three ganglia in each chain, connected with the cord through the first and second thoracic roots. In the thoracic, lumbar and sacral regions there is a ganglion for each nerve root.

The para-sympathetic system (often termed autonomic or system of the "extended vagus") has the ganglia placed more peripherally. In the *cranio-bulbar* portion, fibres pass from the mid-brain to the ciliary ganglion, constricting the pupil, from the medulla secretory fibres go to the submaxillary glands and by the vagus inhibitory fibres go to the heart, constrictor to the bronchi, motor to the œsophagus, stomach and intestines, and secretory to the stomach and intestines. The vagus nerve is the most important constituent of the para-sympathetic system. From the sacral portion by the pelvic nerve fibres go to the descending colon, rectum, anus, bladder and genital system. The vegetative system has three plexuses, cardiac, solar and hypogastric, which receive fibres from both systems.

When the sympathetic and para-sympathetic supply the same structure, their influences are antagonistic. Thus the sympathetic dilates the pupil, the other contracts it; the sympathetic increases the heart rate, the other slows it; the sympathetic inhibits the movements of the gastro-intestinal tract, the other increases them. In conditions of health there is a balance between the two systems. To describe the resulting condition when this balance is disturbed the term sympathicotonia and vagotonia are employed, depending on which system is over-active. In the diagnosis of this the effects of certain drugs are important. Thus the sympathetic system is stimulated by epinephrin (1 c. c. of 1-1000 solution) with resulting tremor, rigor, a sense of cold, glycosuria and a rise in blood pressure. The para-sympathetic system is stimulated by pilocarpine (gr. 1/20-1/6, 0.003-0.01 gm.) with resulting salivation, nausea, sweating, flushing and a fall in blood pressure. Atropine (gr. 1/100-1/50, 0.00065-0.001 gm.) paralyses the para-sympathetic system with resulting dryness of the mouth and throat, palpitation and oppression.

Clinically among the features of vagotonia are small pupils, salivation, flushing, sweating, clammy hands and feet, dermographia, bradycardia, irregularity of respiration, hyperacidity, cardio- and pylorospasm, spastic constipation, and sphincter contraction. Among those of sympathicotonia are, dilated pupils, prominence of the eyes, dryness of the mouth and dry skin. Actually it is found that many patients show features suggestive of disturbance in both systems. Some show vagotonia at one time and sympathicotonia later. The sympathetic system stands in close relation to the endocrine glands and its stimulation may cause increased activity of the adrenal and thyroid glands particularly.

B. SYSTEM DISEASES

I. INTRODUCTION

There are certain diseases of the nervous system which are confined, if not absolutely, still in great part, to definite tracts (combinations of neurones) which subserve like functions. These tracts are called *systems,* and a disease which is confined to one of them is a *system disease.* If more than one system is involved, the process is called a combined system disease. Just what diseases should be classed under these names has given rise to much discussion but to very little agreement. We can not speak positively; our knowledge is not sufficiently accurate, either in regard to the exact limits of the systems themselves, or to the nature and extent of the morbid process in the several diseases.

It may be said that the nervous system is composed of two great systems of neurones, the afferent or sensory system and the efferent or motor system, and the connections between them. (See General Introduction.)

Tabes dorsalis is a disease confined at its onset to the afferent system, and progressive muscular atrophy is one of the efferent system. Several theories have been advanced to explain why a disease should be limited to a definite system of neurones. One view is based upon the idea that in certain individuals one or the other of these systems has an innate tendency to undergo degeneration; another assumes that neurones with a similar function have a similar chemical construction (which differs from that of neurones with a different function), and this is taken to explain why a poison circulating in the blood should show a selective action for a single functional system of neurones.

II. DISEASES OF THE AFFERENT OR SENSORY SYSTEM

I. TABES DORSALIS

(*Locomotor Ataxia; Posterior Spinal Sclerosis*)

Definition.—An affection characterized clinically by sensory disturbances, incoördination, trophic changes, and involvement of the special senses, particularly the eyes. Anatomically there are found degenerations of the root fibres of the dorsal columns of the cord, of the dorsal roots, and at times of the spinal ganglia and peripheral nerves. Degenerations have been described in the brain, particularly the cortex cerebri, in the ganglion cells of the cord, and in the endogenous fibres of the dorsal columns.

Etiology.—It is a widespread disease, more frequent in cities than in the country. The relative proportion may be judged from the fact that of 16,562 cases in the neurological dispensary of the Johns Hopkins Hospital there were 201 cases of tabes. Males are attacked more frequently than females, the proportion being nearly 10 to 1. The disease is not very uncommon in the negro in the United States. It is a disease of adult life, the great majority of cases occurring between the thirtieth and fiftieth years. There are a good many cases of the existence of the disease in both husband and wife, and a few in which the children were also affected. Occasionally cases are seen in young men, and it may occur in children with congenital syphilis. Syphilis is *the* important cause. There is evidence which suggests that certain strains of the Treponema are particularly likely to attack the nervous system. The interval between the syphilitic infection and the first symptoms of tabes is variable. Five to fifteen years is the period in one-half the cases. Intervals from two to twenty-five years occur.

Morbid Anatomy and Pathology.—Posterior spinal sclerosis, although the most obvious gross change, is not an adequate description. The dorsal fibres are of two kinds, those with their cell bodies outside the cord in the spinal ganglia, the so-called exogenous, or root fibres, and those which arise from cells within the cord, the endogenous fibres. These two sets occupy fairly well-determined regions, and a study of early cases of tabes has shown that it is the exogenous or root fibres that are first affected. The fibres of the dorsal roots enter the cord in two divisions, an external and an internal; the former is composed of fibres of small calibre, which, in the cord, make up Lissauer's tract, and occupy the space between the apex of the dorsal cornua and the periphery of the cord, and really do not form part of the dorsal columns. They are short, soon entering the gray matter, and do not seem to be affected, or only slightly so, in early cases.

The larger fibres enter the cord by the internal division, just medial to the cornua, in what is known as the root entry zone. Some enter the gray matter of the spinal cord almost directly and others after a longer course, while still others run in the cord to the medulla, to end in the nuclei of the dorsal columns. As the fibres of every spinal nerve enter the cord between the dorsal cornua and the nerve fibres which have entered lower down, the fibres from each root are successively pushed more and more toward the median line, and so in the cervical cord the fasciculi of Goll are largely composed of long fibres derived from the sacral and lumbar roots.

That it is the coarse dorsal root fibres which are first affected in tabes is generally admitted, but there is much divergence of opinion as to the character and location of the initial process.

Nageotte calls attention to the frequency of a transverse, interstitial neuritis of the dorsal roots just after they have left the ganglia and are still surrounded by the dura, and he believes that it is this neuritis which is the primary lesion. Obersteiner and Redlich laid stress on the presence of inflammation of the pia mater over the dorsal aspect of the cord, which involves the root fibres as they pass through. They point out that it is just here that the dorsal roots are most vulnerable, for at this point—that is, while surrounded by the pia—they are almost completely devoid of their myelin sheaths. Changes in the blood-vessels of the cord, of the pia, and of the nerve roots have been described in early tabes, and Marie and Guillain advanced the belief that the changes in the cord are due to syphilis of the posterior lymphatic system which is confined to the dorsal columns of the cord, the pia mater over them, and the dorsal roots. For them the changes in the nervous system are only apparently radicular or systemic.

With the Marchi stain, degeneration of the root fibres in the root-entry zone is a constant finding in early cases. This change is radicular in the sense that it varies in intensity with the different roots and is most marked in the sacral and lumbar regions. The degeneration is not found in the dorsal roots, but begins within the cord just beyond where the root fibres lose their neurolemma and their myelin sheaths. Degenerated fibres may be traced into the dorsal gray matter and among the ganglion cells of the columns of Clarke. The long columns which ascend the cord also degenerate.

In more advanced cases, there are degeneration of the dorsal roots and some alteration of the cells in the spinal ganglia. The fibres distal to the ganglia are practically normal, although at times the sensory fibres, at the periphery of a limb, show degeneration. Within the cord, the exogenous fibres are diseased as already described; there is also degeneration in the endogenous system of fibres. Optic atrophy is frequently found. The other cranial nerves, especially the fifth with its ganglion, have been found degenerated.

The disease occasionally spreads beyond the sensory system in the cord, and in advanced cases the cells in the ventral horns may be degenerated in association with muscular atrophy. Mott very generally found more or less marked changes in the pyramidal fibres; these he believed to be evidence of changes in the cerebral cortex. Degeneration of the cortex may exist, but even when mental symptoms are absent, or very mild, similar though slight changes have been described, just as in general paresis, without marked tabetic symptoms, there may be degeneration of the dorsal columns. The close association of tabes and general paresis will be considered later.

Symptoms.—For convenience, these are considered under three stages—the incipient or preataxic, the ataxic and the paralytic.

INCIPIENT STAGE.—The onset differs very widely in the different cases, and mistakes in diagnosis are often made early in the disease. The following are the most characteristic initial symptoms:

Pains, usually of a sharp stabbing character; hence, the term lightning pains. They last for only a second or two and are most common in the legs or about the trunk, and tend to follow dorsal root areas. They dart from place to place. At times they are associated with a hot burning feeling and often leave the affected area painful to pressure, and occasionally herpes may follow. The intensity of the pain varies from a sore, burning feeling of the skin to a pain so intense that, were it not for momentary duration, it would exceed human endurance. They occur at irregular intervals, and are prone to follow excesses or to come on when health is impaired. When typical, these pains are practically pathognomonic. Gastric and other crises may occur. Paræsthesia may be among the first symptoms—numbness of the feet, tingling, etc—and at times a sense of constriction about the body.

Ocular Symptoms.—(*a*) Optic atrophy. This occurs in about 10 per cent. of the cases, and is often an early and even the first symptom. There is a gradual loss of vision, which in a large majority of cases leads to total blindness. This appears to be secondary to a syphilitic meningitis. (*b*) Ptosis, which may be double or single. (*c*) Paralysis of the external muscles of the eye. This may be of a single muscle or occasionally of all the muscles of the eye. The paralysis is often transient, the patient merely complaining that he saw double for a certain period. (*d*) Argyll-Robertson pupil, in which there is loss of the iris reflex to light but contraction during accommodation. The pupils are often very small—spinal myosis.

Bladder Symptoms.—The first warning which the patient has may be a difficulty in emptying the bladder. Incontinence of urine occurs only at a later stage. Decrease in sexual desire and power may be an early symptom.

Trophic Disturbances.—These usually occur later, but at times they are early symptoms, and it is not very infrequent to have one's attention called to the trouble by a perforating ulcer or a characteristic Charcot's joint.

Loss of the Deep Reflexes.—This early and most important symptom may occur years before the development of ataxia. Even alone it is of great moment, since it is very rare to meet with individuals in whom the knee and ankle jerks are normally absent. The combination of loss of either of these with one or more of the symptoms mentioned above, especially with the lightning pains and ptosis or Argyll-Robertson pupil, is practically diagnostic.

These reflexes gradually decrease, and one may be lost before the other, or disappear first in one leg.

These initial symptoms may persist for years without the development of incoördination. The patient may look well and feel well, and be troubled only by occasional attacks of lightning pains or of one of the other subjective symptoms. Progressive nerve deafness and paralysis of the vocal cords, with the laryngeal muscles paralyzed or paretic, may occur. The disease may never progress beyond this stage, and when optic atrophy develops early and leads to blindness, ataxia rarely, if ever, supervenes, an antagonism noted by many authors.

Ataxic Stage.—*Motor Symptoms.*—The ataxia, which comes on gradually, is believed to be due to a disturbance or loss of the afferent impulses from the muscles, joints, and deep tissues. A disturbance of the muscle sense itself can usually be demonstrated. One of the first indications is inability to get about readily in the dark or to maintain equilibrium when washing the face with the eyes shut. When the patient stands with the feet together and the eyes closed, he sways and has difficulty in maintaining his position (Romberg's symptom), and he may be quite unable to stand on one leg. He does not start off promptly at the word of command. On turning quickly he is apt to fall. He has more difficulty in descending than ascending stairs. Gradually the characteristic ataxic gait develops. The normal man walks by faith, the tabetic by sight. The patient, as a rule, walks with a stick, the eyes are directed to the ground, the body is thrown forward, and the legs are wide apart. In walking, the leg is thrown out violently, the foot is raised too high and is brought down in a stamping manner with the heel first, or the whole sole comes in contact with the ground. Ultimately the patient may be unable to walk without the assistance of two canes. This gait is very characteristic, and unlike that seen in any other disease. The incoördination is not only in walking, but in the performance of other movements. If the patient is asked, when in the recumbent posture, to touch one knee with the other foot, the irregularity of the movement is very evident. Incoördination of the arms is less common, but usually develops in some grade. It may in rare instances exist before the incoördination of the legs. It may be tested by asking the patient to close his eyes and to touch the tip of the nose or the tip of the ear with the finger, or with the arms thrust out to bring the tips of the fingers together. The incoördination may be noticed early by a difficulty in buttoning the collar or performing one of the routine acts of dressing.

One of the most striking features is that with marked incoördination there is but little loss of muscular power. The grip of the hands may be strong and firm, the power of the legs may be unimpaired, and their nutrition, except toward the close, may be unaffected.

There is a remarkable muscular relaxation (*hypotonia*) which enables the joints to be placed in positions of hyperextension and hyperflexion. It gives sometimes a marked backward curve to the legs.

Sensory Symptoms.—The lightning pains may persist. They vary greatly in different cases. Some patients are rendered miserable by the frequent occurrence of the attacks; others escape altogether. In addition, common symptoms are tingling, pins and needles, particularly in the feet, and areas of hyperæsthesia or of anæsthesia. The patient may complain of a change in the sensation in the soles of the feet, as if cotton was interposed between the floor and the skin. Sensory disturbances occur less frequently in the hands. Objective sensory disturbances can usually be demonstrated, and, indeed, almost every variety of sensory disturbance of tactile, pain and temperature sense has been described. Bands of a moderate grade of anæsthesia about the chest are not uncommon; they are apt to follow the distribution of spinal segments. The most marked disturbances are usually found on the legs. Retardation of the sense of pain is common, and a pin prick on the foot is first felt as a simple tactile impression, and the sense of pain is not perceived for a second or two or may be delayed for as much as ten seconds. The pain felt may persist. A curious phenomenon is the loss of the power of localizing the pain. For instance, if the patient is pricked on one limb he may say that he feels it on the other (allocheiria), or a pin prick on one foot may be felt on both feet. Pruritus may occur over the areas affected by the pains. The muscular sense, which is usually affected early, becomes much impaired and the patient no longer recognizes the position in which his limbs are placed. This may be present in the preataxic stage.

Reflexes.—The loss of the knee and ankle jerks is one of the earliest symptoms but occasionally they are retained, and anatomically it has been shown that in these cases the lumbar segments were little if at all involved. The skin reflexes may at first be increased, but later are usually involved with the deep reflexes. The oculo-cardiac reflex is often absent.

Special Senses.—The eye symptoms noted above may be present, but, as mentioned, ataxia is rare with optic atrophy. Deafness may occur, due to lesion of the auditory nerve. There may also be attacks of vertigo. Olfactory symptoms are rare.

W. B. Swift has drawn attention to a voice sign which consists in ataxic speech with "a slovenly indistinct enunciation that shows partially in the vowels but predominantly in the consonants." Suggested tests are "e" (as in ell), "t," "journals" and "Time and tide wait for no man."

Visceral Symptoms.—Among the most remarkable sensory disturbances are the *tabetic crises,* severe paroxysms of pain referred to various viscera; thus, ocular, laryngeal, gastric, nephritic, rectal, urethral, and clitoral crises have been described. The most common are the gastric and laryngeal. Gastric crises may occur early and persist as the most prominent feature. Starr found them as the first symptom 18 times in 450 cases. The onset is usually sudden, with severe pain in the epigastrium, radiating to the back and behind the sternum. Vomiting follows the pain, and may be quite independent of food. Hæmatemesis may occur, not necessarily due to ulcer. Pallor, sweating, cold extremities, and a small pulse are associated, and in rare instances death occurs in collapse. The blood pressure may be very high, as reported by Barker, and it seems not improbable that the condition is associated with angiospasm in the territory of the gastric and mesenteric vessels. The X-ray examination shows spasmodic contractions of the stomach. No special change may be found at autopsy. In the laryngeal crises there may be true spasm with dyspnœa and noisy inspiration. A patient may die in the attack. There are also nasal crises, associated with sneezing fits.

The contrary condition may occur, that is absence of pain from visceral lesions, as rupture of a gastric ulcer, and render diagnosis very difficult.

The *sphincters* are frequently involved. Early in the disease there may be a retardation or hesitancy in making water. Later there is retention, and cystitis may occur. Unless great care is taken the inflammation may extend to the kidneys. Constipation is extremely common. Later the sphincter ani is weakened. The sexual power is usually lost in the ataxic stage.

Trophic Changes.—Skin rashes, such as herpes, œdema, or local sweating, may occur in the course of the lightning pains. Alteration in the nails may occur. A perforating ulcer may develop on the foot, usually beneath the great toe. A perforating buccal ulcer has also been described. Onychia may prove very troublesome.

Arthropathies (Charcot's Joints).—Anatomically there are: (1) enlargement of the capsule with thickening of the synovial membranes and increase in the fluids; (2) slight enlargement of the ends of the bones, with slight exostoses; (3) a dull velvety appearance of the cartilages, with atrophy in places. The knees are most frequently involved. The spine is affected in rare instances. Recurring trauma is an important element in the causation, but trophic disturbances have a strong influence. A striking feature is the absence of pain. Suppuration may occur, also spontaneous fractures. *Atrophy* of the muscles, usually a late manifestation, may be localized and associated with neuritis or due to involvement of the ventral horns.

Aneurism is found in as high as 20 per cent. of some series, and aortic insufficiency is common. Both are associated syphilitic manifestations.

Cerebral Symptoms.—Hemiplegia may develop at any stage of the disease, more commonly when it is well advanced. It may be due to hæmorrhagic softening from disease of the vessels, to progressive cortical changes or rarely to coarse syphilitic disease. The lost knee jerk may return on the affected side. Hemianæsthesia is sometimes present.

Cerebro-Spinal Fluid.—The examination of this is of great value; the findings are:

(1) *Cell Content.*—Lymphocytosis is found in about 90 per cent., the number of cells usually being between 40 and 60, and rarely over 100. The higher counts are found when irritative symptoms are marked. With an arrest of the process the counts are lower. (2) *Globulin.* This is positive in 90-95 per cent. In old quiescent cases there may be no increase. (3) *Wassermann reaction.* This is nearly always positive but may be negative in quiescent cases. The blood Wassermann test is positive in about 70 per cent. (4) *Colloidal Gold reaction.* This is present in 85-90 per cent. and is useful in diagnosing tabes from paresis. If a paretic curve is given in a patient with signs of tabes it points to the possible development of paresis subsequently.

Paralytic Stage.—After persisting for an indefinite number of years the patient gradually becomes bedridden and paralyzed. In this condition he is likely to be carried off by some intercurrent affection, such as pyelo-nephritis, pneumonia, or tuberculosis.

Course.—A patient may remain in the preataxic stage for an indefinite period; and the loss of knee-jerk and the atrophy of the optic nerves may be the sole indications of the disease. In such cases incoördination rarely develops. In a majority of cases the progress is slow, and after six or eight years, sometimes less, the ataxia is well marked. The symptoms may vary a good deal; thus, the pains, which may have been excessive at first, often lessen. The disease may remain stationary for years; then exacerbations occur and it makes rapid progress. Occasionally the process seems to be arrested. There are instances of what may be called acute ataxia, in which, within a year or even less, the incoördination is marked, and the paralytic stage may develop within a few months. The disease itself rarely causes death, and after becoming bedridden the patient may live for fifteen or twenty years.

Diagnosis.—In the initial stage the lightning pains are distinctive. The association of progressive atrophy of the optic nerves with loss of knee-jerk is characteristic. The early ocular palsies are of the greatest importance. A squint, ptosis, or the Argyll-Robertson pupil may be the first symptom, and may exist with the loss only of the knee-jerk. Loss of the knee-jerk alone, however, does occasionally occur in healthy individuals. The Wassermann reaction and a study of the spinal fluid are of help in doubtful cases.

The diseases most likely to be confounded with tabes dorsalis are: (*a*) Peripheral Neuritis.—The steppage gait of arsenical, alcoholic, or diabetic paralysis is quite unlike that of tabes. There is a paralysis of the feet, and the leg is lifted high in order that the toes may clear the floor. The use of the word *ataxia* in this connection should not be continued. In the rare cases in which the muscle sense nerves are particularly affected and in which there is true ataxia, the absence of the lightning pains and eye symptoms and the history will suffice to make the diagnosis clear. In diphtheritic paralysis the early loss of the knee-jerk and the associated eye symptoms may suggest tabes, but the history, the existence of paralysis of the throat, and the absence of pains render a diagnosis easy.

(*b*) Combined Sclerosis.—Marked incoördination with spastic paralysis is characteristic of the condition which Gowers termed ataxic paraplegia. In a majority of the cases this is distinguished also by the absence of pains and eye symptoms, but it may be a manifestation of the cord lesions in tabo-paralysis.

(*c*) Cerebral Disease.—In diseases of the brain involving the afferent tracts ataxia is at times a prominent symptom. It is usually unilateral or limited to one limb; this, with the history and the associated symptoms, excludes tabes.

(*d*) Cerebellar Disease.—The cerebellar incoördination has only a superficial resemblance to that of tabes, and is more a disturbance of equilibrium than a true ataxia; the knee-jerk is usually present, there are no lightning pains, no sensory disturbances; while, on the other hand, there are headache, optic neuritis, and vomiting.

(*e*) Acute syphilitic affections involving the dorsal columns of the cord may be associated with incoördination and resemble tabes very closely.

(*f*) General Paresis.—Though of identical origin and often associated, it is of great practical importance to determine, if possible, whether the type is to be spinal or cerebral, for when this is established, it does not often change. The difficulty arises in the premonitory stage, when ocular changes and abnormalities of sensation and the deep reflexes may be the only symptoms. Any alteration in the mental characteristics is of the utmost significance.

Loss of the deep reflexes and lightning pains speak for tabes; active reflexes, with ocular changes, especially optic atrophy, are suggestive of paresis.

(*g*) VISCERAL CRISES and NEURALGIC SYMPTOMS may lead to error, and in middle-aged men with severe, recurring attacks of gastralgia it is always well to bear in mind the possibility of tabes, and to make a careful examination of the eyes and of the knee-jerk.

Prognosis.—Complete recovery can not be expected, but arrest of the process is not uncommon and a marked amelioration is frequent. Optic-nerve atrophy, one of the most serious events in the disease, has this hopeful aspect—that incoördination rarely follows and the progress of the spinal symptoms may be arrested. On the other hand, mental symptoms are more likely to follow. The optic atrophy itself is occasionally checked. On the whole, the prognosis in tabes is bad. There is more hope that in very early cases coming on soon after infection the course may be arrested. Death is usually from some cardio-vascular complication; next in frequency from tuberculosis and pneumonia.

Treatment.—To arrest the progress and to relieve, if possible, the symptoms are the objects which the practitioner should have in view. A quiet, well-regulated method of life is essential. It is not well, as a rule, for a patient to give up his occupation so long as he is able to keep about and perform ordinary work, provided there is no evident mental change. Tabetics have for years conducted large businesses, and there have been several notable instances in our profession of men who have risen to distinction in spite of the existence of this disease. Care should be taken in the diet, particularly if gastric crises have occurred. Excesses of all sorts, more particularly *in baccho et venere,* should be carefully avoided. A man in the pre-ataxic stage should not marry.

To secure arrest of the disease many remedies have been employed.

In the specific treatment the object should be to secure a normal spinal fluid if possible. It is well to begin with small doses of arsphenamine intravenously (0.2-0.3 gm.) once a week for six weeks. Then a course of mercury should be given by inunction or injection, followed by arsphenamine again. If this results in improvement in the spinal fluid it may be kept up at intervals with periods of rest in between. If there is no change or only slight gain the intraspinal treatment with auto-arsphenaminized serum may be used. The number of injections can be decided by the findings in the spinal fluid. This treatment should be carried out persistently. In some cases the giving of mercury in full doses by inunction followed by a spinal puncture in which as much serum is withdrawn as possible has proved of benefit. The use of mercurial serum has been helpful in some cases. Iodide of potassium can be given in addition in full dosage.

For the pains, complete rest in bed and counter-irritation to the spine (either blisters or the thermo-cautery) may be employed. The severe spells which come on particularly after excesses of any kind are often promptly relieved by a hot bath or by a Turkish bath. For the severe recurring attacks of lightning pains spinal cocainization may be tried. Cannabis indica is sometimes useful. Suppositories of codein (gr. 1, 0.06 gm.) and extract of belladonna (gr. ½, 0.03 gm.) may give relief. In the severe paroxysms of pain hypodermics of morphia or of cocaine must be used. The use of morphia should be postponed as long as possible. Electricity is of very little benefit. For the severe attacks of gastralgia morphia is also required. Gastro-enterostomy has been performed, the solar plexus has been stretched, and the dorsal spinal nerve roots of the seventh, eighth, ninth, and tenth have been divided with good results. The laryngeal crises are rarely dangerous. An application of cocaine may be made during the spasm, or a few whiffs of chloroform or nitrite of amyl may be given. In all cases of tabes with increased arterial tension the prolonged use of nitroglycerin, given until the physiological effect is produced, is of great service in allaying the neuralgic pains and diminishing the frequency of the crises. Its use must be guarded when there is aortic insufficiency. The special indication is increased tension. The bladder symptoms demand constant care. When the organ can not be perfectly emptied the catheter should be used, and the patient may be taught its use and how to keep it thoroughly sterilized.

Frenkel's method of re-education often helps the patient to regain to a considerable extent the control of the voluntary movements which he has lost. By this method the patient is first taught, by repeated systematic efforts, to perform simple movements; from this he goes to more and more complex movements. The treatment should be directed and supervised by a trained teacher, as the result depends upon the skill of the teacher quite as much as upon the perseverance of the patient.

II. GENERAL PARESIS AND TABO-PARALYSIS

It is undoubted that most cases of tabes run their course with practically no mental symptoms, and that cases of general paresis may never present symptoms that suggest tabes. For practical purposes we are forced to keep the distinction clearly in mind, and for this reason it seems best to consider them separately. There is, however, a group of cases in which the symptoms of the two diseases are associated in every combination for which the name "tabo-paralysis" is used.

General Paresis

Definition.—A chronic meningo-encephalitis caused by the spirochæte of syphilis, often associated with other local changes leading to mental disturbances and finally to dementia and paralysis.

Etiology.—The average interval from the syphilitic infection is twelve years. Males are affected much more frequently than females. It occurs chiefly between the ages of thirty and fifty-five, although it may begin in childhood as the result of congenital syphilis. An overwhelming majority of the cases are in married people, and not infrequently both husband and wife are affected, or one has paresis and the other tabes. Statistics show that it is more common in the lower classes of society, but in America in general medical practice the disease is certainly more common in the well-to-do classes.

Morbid Anatomy.—The dura is often thickened, and its inner surface may show the various forms of hypertrophic pachymeningitis. The pia is cloudy, thickened, and adherent to the cortex. The cerebro-spinal fluid is increased in the meningeal spaces, especially in the meshes of the pia, and at times to such an extent as to resemble cysts. The brain is small, and weighs less than normal. The convolutions are atrophied, especially in the anterior and middle lobes. In acute cases the brain may be swollen, hyperæmic, and œdematous. The brain cortex is usually red, and, except in advanced cases, it may not be atrophied, the atrophy of the hemispheres being at the expense of the white matter. The lateral ventricles are dilated to compensate for the atrophy of the brain, and the ependyma may be granular. The fourth ventricle is more constantly dilated, with granulations of its floor covering the calamus scriptorius, a condition seldom seen in any other affection.

In many cases changes are present in the spinal cord and peripheral nerves. There are the typical tabetic changes. There may be degeneration of the pyramidal systems of fibres secondary to the cortical changes. Most commonly there is a combination of these two processes. Foci of hæmorrhages, and softening dependent upon coarse vascular changes, are not infrequently found, but are not typical of the disease.

There are various views as to the nature of the changes. The vascular theory is that from an inflammatory process starting in the sheaths of the arterioles there is a diffuse parenchymatous degeneration with atrophic changes in the nerve cells and neuroglia. The syphilitic toxin causes degeneration in the nervous tissues with secondary changes in the neuroglia and vascular systems. The spirochætes are found in the brain tissue and rarely in the cord.

Symptoms.—PRODROMAL STAGE.—Irritability, inattention to business amounting sometimes to indifference or apathy, and sometimes a *change in character,* marked by acts which may astonish the friends and relatives, are usually the first indications. There may be unaccountable fatigue after moderate physical or mental exertion. Instead of apathy or indifference there may be an extraordinary degree of physical and mental restlessness. The patient is continually planning and scheming, or may launch into extravagances and speculation of the wildest character. A common feature at this period is the display of an unbounded egoism. He boasts of his personal attainments, his property, his position in life, or of his wife and children. Following these features are important indications of moral perversion, manifested in offences against decency or the law, many of which acts have about them a suspicious effrontery. Forgetfulness is common, and may be shown in inattention to business details and in the minor courtesies of life. At this period there may be no motor phenomena. The onset is usually insidious, although cases are reported in which epileptiform or apoplectiform seizures were the first symptoms. Attacks of hemicrania, like ophthalmic migraine, may occur. Among the early motor features are tremor of the tongue and lips in speaking, slowness of speech and hesitancy with mixing of syllables or letters. Inequality of the pupils, temporary paresis of the eye muscles with diplopia, the Argyll-Robertson pupil, optic atrophy, and changes in the deep reflexes, may precede the occurrence of mental symptoms for years.

SECOND STAGE.—This is characterized in brief by mental exaltation or excitement and a progress in the motor symptoms. "The intensity of the excitement is often extreme, acute maniacal states are frequent; incessant restlessness, obstinate sleeplessness, noisy, boisterous excitement, and blind, uncalculating violence especially characterize such states" (Lewis). It is at this stage that the delusion of grandeur becomes marked and the patient believes himself to be possessed of countless millions or to have reached the most exalted sphere possible in profession or occupation. This expansive delirium is, however, not characteristic of general paresis. Besides, it does not always occur, but in its stead there may be marked melancholia or hypochondriasis, or, in other instances, alternate attacks of delirium and depression.

The facies has a peculiar stolidity, and in speaking there is marked tremulousness of the lips and facial muscles. The tongue is also tremulous, and may be protruded with difficulty. The speech is slow, interrupted, and blurred. Writing becomes difficult on account of unsteadiness of the hand. Letters, syllables, and words may be omitted. The subject matter of the patient's letters gives valuable indications of the mental condition. In many instances the pupils are unequal, irregular, sluggish, sometimes large. Important symptoms in this stage are apoplectiform seizures and paralysis. There may be slight syncopal attacks in which the patient turns pale and may fall. Some of these are *petit mal.* In the apoplectiform seizure the patient falls suddenly, becomes unconscious, the limbs are relaxed, the face is flushed, the breathing stertorous, the temperature increased, and death may occur. Epileptic seizures are more common than the apoplectiform. There may be a definite aura. The attack usually begins on one side and may not spread. There may be twitchings either in the facial or brachial muscles. Typical Jacksonian epilepsy may occur. Recurring attacks of aphasia are not uncommon, and paralysis, either monoplegic or hemiplegic, may follow these epileptic seizures, or may come on with great suddenness and be transient. In this stage the gait becomes impaired, the patient trips readily, has difficulty in going up or down stairs, and the walk may be spastic or occasionally tabetic. This paresis may be progressive. The deep reflexes are usually increased, but may be lost. Bladder or rectal symptoms gradually develop. The patient becomes helpless, bedridden, and completely demented, and unless care is taken may suffer from bedsores. Death occurs from exhaustion or some intercurrent affection. The spinal cord features may come on with or precede the mental troubles. There are cases in which one is in doubt for a time whether the symptoms indicate tabes or general paresis, and it is well to bear in mind that every feature of pre-ataxic tabes may exist in the early stage of general paresis.

Cerebro-Spinal Fluid.—The findings are as follows: (1) *Cell content.* A lymphocytosis is present in 98-100 per cent. and the average content is 30-60 cells. (2) *Globulin.* This is practically always positive. (3) *Wassermann reaction.* This is positive in nearly every case and usually there is a strong reaction with small amounts. The blood reaction is positive in 98-100 per cent. (4) *Colloidal Gold reaction.* This is nearly always positive in 98-100 per cent., with a typical paretic curve.

Tabo-paralysis

Emphasis has been laid on the identity of the processes underlying tabes and general paresis, the spinal cord in the first case receiving the full force of the attack, and the brain in the second. It is suggested that stress determines the location of the process; men whose occupations require much bodily exercise are apt to have tabes, while those whose activities are largely mental would suffer from paresis. Usually when the cord symptoms are pronounced the symptoms from the brain remain in abeyance, and the reverse is also true. There are exceptions, and cases of well marked tabes may later show the typical symptoms of paresis, but even then the ataxia, if it is not of too high a grade, may improve.

Optic atrophy, when it occurs in the pre-ataxic stage of tabes, usually indicates that the ataxia will never be pronounced, but unfortunately it is frequently followed by the occurrence of mental symptoms. Mott states that about 50 per cent. of his asylum cases of tabo-paralysis had preceding optic atrophy. Its occurrence is therefore of grave significance. The mental symptoms may be delayed for many years.

Made up of a combination of features of the two conditions, the *symptom complex* of tabo-paralysis varies greatly. It may begin as tabes with lightning pains, bladder symptoms, Argyll-Robertson pupil, loss of the deep reflexes, etc., to have the mental symptoms added later; or, on the other hand, cord symptoms may come on after the patient has shown marked mental changes. The symptoms from the first may be so combined that the name tabo-paralysis is at once applicable. Absent knee-jerks, ocular palsies, or pupillary symptoms may precede the breakdown for many years, but none of them have so grave a significance in regard to the mental state as has optic atrophy. Other types of alienation may interrupt the course of tabes, and the mistake must not be made of regarding them all as general paresis.

Diagnosis.—The recognition of general paresis in the earliest stage is extremely difficult, as it is often impossible to decide that the slight alteration in conduct is anything more than one of the moods or phases to which most men are at times subject. The following description by Folsom is an admirable presentation of the diagnostic characters of the early stage of the disease: "It should arouse suspicion if, for instance, a strong, healthy man, in or near the prime of life, distinctly not of the 'nervous,' neurotic, or neurasthenic type, shows some loss of interest in his affairs or impaired faculty of attending to them; if he becomes varyingly absent-minded, heedless, indifferent, negligent, apathetic, inconsiderate, and, although able to follow his routine duties, his ability to take up new work is, no matter how little, diminished; if he can less well command mental attention and concentration, conception, perception, reflection, judgment; if there is an unwonted lack of initiative, and if exertion causes unwonted mental and physical fatigue; if the emotions are intensified and easily change, or are excited readily from trifling causes; if the sexual instinct is not reasonably controlled; if the finer feelings are even slightly blunted; if the person in question regards with a placid apathy his own acts of indifference and irritability and their consequences, and especially if at times he sees himself in his true light and suddenly fails again to do so; if any symptoms of cerebral vaso-motor disturbances are noticed, however vague or variable."

There are cases of *cerebral syphilis* which closely simulate general paresis. The mode of onset is important, particularly since paralytic symptoms are usually early in syphilis. The affection of the speech and tongue is not present. Epileptic seizures are more common and more liable to be cortical or Jacksonian in character. The expansive delirium is rare. While symptoms of general paresis are not common in connection with the development of gummata or definite gummatous meningitis, there are, on the other hand, instances of paresis following closely upon the syphilitic infection. Post mortem in such cases there may be nothing more than a general arterio-sclerosis and diffuse meningo-encephalitis, which may present nothing distinctive, but the lesions may be caused by the spirochæte. Cases also occur in which typical syphilitic lesions are combined with the ordinary lesions of general paresis. There are certain forms of lead encephalopathy which resemble general paresis, and, considering the association of plumbism with arterio-sclerosis, it is not unlikely that the anatomical substratum of the disease may result from this poison. *Tumor* may sometimes simulate progressive paresis, but in the former the signs of general increase of the intracranial pressure are usually present. The findings in the spinal fluid are important aids.

Cytodiagnosis.—The study of the cerebro-spinal fluid is an important diagnostic measure, particularly in tabes and paresis. Spinal lymphocytosis is the rule and is usually associated with a marked globulin reaction—the normal fluid containing at most minute traces, and a negligible number of formed elements. It is the expression of a subacute or chronic inflammatory process, just as polymorphonuclear leukocytosis is characteristic of an acute process. It is the syphilitic triad—tabes, paresis, and cerebro-spinal lues—which is suggested by lymphocytosis in the spinal fluid. Positive reactions, cytological and chemical, are among the earliest somatic signs, and may clear up obscure cases of tabes and paresis, just at the time when diagnosis is most difficult.

Prognosis.—The disease rarely ends in recovery. As a rule the progress is slowly downward and the case terminates in a few years, although it is occasionally prolonged ten or fifteen years.

Treatment.—Specific treatment has been disappointing on the whole, particularly by the intra-spinal method, and some authorities regard it as contraindicated. Certainly some patients are harmed by it but in such a hopeless condition there is some justification for taking the risk. The treatment is practically the same as in tabes dorsalis. Careful nursing and the orderly life of an asylum are necessary in a great majority of the cases. For sleeplessness and the epileptic seizures bromides may be used. Prolonged remissions, which are not uncommon, are often erroneously attributed to the action of remedies. Active treatment in the early stage by wet-packs, cold to the head, and systematic massage has been followed by temporary improvement.

III. DISEASES OF THE EFFERENT OR MOTOR TRACT

I. PROGRESSIVE (CENTRAL) MUSCULAR ATROPHY

(*Poliomyelitis Anterior Chronica; Amyotrophic Lateral Sclerosis; Progressive Bulbar Paralysis*)

Definition.—A disease characterized by a chronic degeneration of the motor tract, usually of the whole, but at times limited to the lower segment. Associated with it is a progressive atrophy of the muscles, with more or less spastic rigidity.

Three affections, as a rule described apart, belong together in this category: (*a*) Progressive muscular atrophy of spinal origin; (*b*) amyotrophic lateral sclerosis; and (*c*) progressive bulbar paralysis. A slow atrophic change in the motor neurones is the anatomical basis, and the disease involves, in many cases, the cortical, bulbar, and spinal centres. There may be simple muscular atrophy with little or no spasm, or progressive wasting with marked spasm and great increase in the reflexes. In others, there are added symptoms of involvement of the motor nuclei in the medulla—a glosso-labio-laryngeal paralysis; while in others, again, with atrophy (especially of the arms), a spastic condition of the legs and bulbar phenomena, tremors develop and signs of cortical lesion. These various stages may be traced in the same case.

For convenience, bulbar paralysis is considered separately, and *progressive muscular atrophy* and *amyotrophic lateral sclerosis* are taken together.

History.—The disease is known as the Aran-Duchenne type of progressive muscular atrophy and as Cruveilhier's palsy, after the French physicians who early described it. Luys and Lockhart Clarke first demonstrated that the cells of the ventral horns of the spinal cord were diseased. Charcot separated two types—one with simple wasting of the muscles, due, he believed, to degeneration confined to the ventral horns (and to this he restricted the name progressive muscular atrophy—type, Aran-Duchenne); the other, in which there was spastic paralysis of the muscles followed by atrophy. As the anatomical basis for this he assumed a primary degeneration of the pyramidal tracts and a secondary atrophy of the ventral horns. To this he gave the name of amyotrophic lateral sclerosis. There is but little evidence, however, to show that any such sharp distinction can be made between these two diseases, and Leyden and Gowers regard them as identical.

Etiology.—The cause is unknown. It is more frequent in males than in females and affects adults, usually after the thirtieth year, though occasionally younger persons are attacked. Cases of progressive muscular atrophy under twenty five years of age belong as a rule to the dystrophies. Cold, wet, exposure, fright, and mental worries are mentioned as possible causes. Certain cases follow injury. The Werdnig-Hoffman type is a familial affection and does not belong here. The spastic form may develop late in life—after seventy—as a senile change.

Morbid Anatomy.—The essential anatomical change is a slow degeneration of the motor path, involving particularly the lower motor neurones. The upper neurones are also involved, either first, simultaneously, or at a later period. Associated with the degeneration in the cells of the ventral horns there is a degenerative atrophy of the muscles. The following are the important anatomical changes: (*a*) The gray matter of the cord shows the most marked alteration. The large ganglion cells of the ventral horns are atrophied, or, in places, have entirely disappeared, the neuroglia is increased, and the medullated fibres are much decreased. The fibres of the ventral nerve-roots passing through the white matter are wasted. (*b*) The ventral roots outside of the cord are also atrophied. (*c*) The muscles affected show degenerative atrophy, and the inter-muscular branches of the motor nerves are degenerated. (*d*) The degeneration of the gray matter is rarely confined to the cord, but extends to the medulla, where the nuclei of the motor cerebral nerves are found extensively wasted. (*e*) In a majority of all the cases there is sclerosis in the ventro-lateral white tracts, the lateral pyramidal tracts particularly are diseased, but the degeneration is not confined to them, but extends into the ventro-lateral ground bundles. The direct cerebellar and the ventro-lateral ascending tracts are spared. The degeneration in the pyramidal tracts extends toward the brain to different levels, and in several cases has been traced to the motor cortex, the cells of which have been found degenerated. In the medulla the medial longitudinal fasciculus has been found diseased. (*f*) In those cases in which no sclerosis has been found in the pyramidal tracts there has been a sclerosis of the ventro-lateral ground bundle (short tracts).

Symptoms.—Irregular pains may precede the onset of the wasting. The hands are usually first affected, and there is difficulty in performing delicate manipulations. The muscles of the ball of the thumb waste early, then the interossei and lumbricales, leaving marked depressions between the metacarpal bones. Ultimately the contraction of the flexor and extensor muscles and the extreme atrophy of the thumb muscles, the interossei, and lumbricales produce the claw-hand—*main en griffe* of Duchenne. The flexors of the forearm are usually involved before the extensors. In the shoulder-girdle the deltoid is first affected; it may waste even before the other muscles of the upper extremity. The trunk muscles are gradually attacked; the upper part of the trapezius long remains unaffected. Owing to the feebleness of the muscles which support it, the head tends to fall forward. The platysma myoides is unaffected and often hypertrophies. The arms and the trunk muscles may be much atrophied before the legs are attacked. The face muscles are attacked late. Ultimately the intercostal and abdominal muscles may be involved, the wasting proceeds to an extreme grade, and the patient may be actually "skin and bone," and, as "living skeletons," the cases are not uncommon in "museums" and "side-shows." Deformities and contractures result, and lordosis is almost always present. A curious twitching of the muscles (fibrillation) is common and may occur in muscles which are not attacked. It is a most important symptom, but is not a characteristic feature. The irritability of the muscles is increased. Sensation is unimpaired, but the patient may complain of numbness and coldness of the affected limbs. The galvanic and faradic irritability of the muscles progressively diminishes and may become extinct, the galvanic persisting for the longer time. In cases of rapid wasting and paralysis the reaction of degeneration may be obtained. The excitability of the nerve trunks may persist after the muscles have ceased to respond. The loss of power is usually proportionate to the wasting.

Amyotrophic Spastic Form.—The foregoing description applies to the group of cases in which the atrophy and paralysis are flaccid—*atonic,* as Gowers called it. In other cases, those which Charcot described as amyotrophic lateral sclerosis, spastic paralysis precedes the wasting. The reflexes are greatly increased. It is one of the rare conditions in which a jaw clonus may be obtained. The most typical condition of spastic paraplegia may be produced. On starting to walk, the patient seems glued to the ground and makes ineffectual attempts to lift the toes; then four or five short, quick steps are taken on the toes with the body thrown forward; and finally he starts off, sometimes with great rapidity. Some of the patients can walk up and down stairs better than on the level. The wasting is never so extreme as in the atonic form, and the loss of power may be out of proportion to it. The sphincters are unaffected. Sexual power may be lost early. A flaccid atrophic paralysis with increased reflexes is the common finding. The differences depend upon the relative extent of the involvement of the upper and lower motor segments and the time of the involvement of each. The condition may be unilateral.

As the degeneration extends upward an important change takes place from the occurrence of bulbar symptoms, which may, however, precede the spinal manifestations. The lips, tongue, face, pharynx, and larynx may be involved. The lips may be affected and articulation impaired for years before serious symptoms occur. In the final stage there may be tremor, the memory fails, and a condition of dementia supervenes.

Diagnosis.—Progressive (central) muscular atrophy begins, as a rule, in adult life, without hereditary or family influences (the early infantile form being an exception), and usually affects first the muscles of the thumb, and gradually involves the interossei and lumbricales. Fibrillary contractions are common, electrical changes occur, and the deep reflexes are usually increased. These characteristics are usually sufficient to distinguish it from the other forms of muscular wasting. It is well to remember that the earliest and most marked indication of *cervical rib* may be atrophy of the small muscles of the hand.

In *syringomyelia* the symptoms may be similar to those in the spastic form of muscular atrophy. The sensory disturbances in the former disease, as a rule, make the diagnosis clear, but when these are absent or but little developed it may be very difficult or impossible to distinguish the diseases.

Treatment.—The disease is incurable. The downward progress is slow but certain, though in a few cases a temporary arrest may take place. Arsenic and hypodermic injections of strychnine may be tried. Systematic massage is useful in the spastic cases.

Bulbar Paralysis (*Glosso-labio-laryngeal Paralysis*)

When the disease affects the motor nuclei of the medulla first or early, it is called bulbar paralysis, but it has practically no independent existence, as the spinal cord is sooner or later involved.

Symptoms.—The disease begins with slight defect in the speech, and difficulty in pronouncing the dentals and linguals. The paralysis starts in the tongue, and the superior lingual muscle gradually becomes atrophied, and finally the mucous membrane is thrown into transverse folds. In the process of wasting the fibrillary tremors are seen. Owing to the loss of power in the tongue, the food is with difficulty pushed back into the pharynx. The saliva also may be increased, and is apt to accumulate in the mouth. When the lips become involved the patient can neither whistle nor pronounce the labial consonants. The mouth looks large, the lips are prominent, and there is constant drooling. The food is masticated with difficulty. Swallowing becomes difficult, owing partly to the regurgitation into the nostrils, partly to the involvement of the pharyngeal muscles. The muscles of the vocal cords waste and the voice becomes feeble, but the laryngeal paralysis is rarely so extreme as that of the lips and tongue.

The **course** is slow but progressive. Death may result from an aspiration pneumonia, sometimes from choking, more rarely from involvement of the respiratory centres. The mind usually remains clear. The patient may become emotional. In a majority of the cases the disease is only part of a progressive atrophy, either simple or associated with a spastic condition. In the later stage of amyotrophic lateral sclerosis the bulbar lesions may paralyze the lips long before the pharynx or larynx becomes affected.

The **diagnosis** is readily made, either in the acute or chronic form. The involvement of the lips and tongue is usually well marked, while that of the palate may be long deferred. In *pseudo-bulbar paralysis* bilateral disease of the motor cortex in the lower part of the ascending frontal convolution, or about the knee of the internal capsule may interfere with the supranuclear paths, causing paralysis of the lips and tongue and pharynx, which closely simulates a lesion of the medulla. Sometimes the symptoms appear on one side, but they may develop suddenly on both sides. Bilateral lesions have usually been found, but the disease may be unilateral. There is arteriosclerosis and the bulbar features are usually sequels of hemiplegic attacks.

Acute bulbar paralysis may be due to (*a*) hæmorrhagic or embolic softening in the pons and medulla; (*b*) acute inflammatory softening, analogous to polio-myelitis, occurring occasionally as a post-febrile affection. It has occasionally followed diphtheria, and occurred after severe electric shocks of high voltage. It usually comes on very suddenly, hence the term apoplectiform. The symptoms may correspond closely to those of an advanced case of chronic bulbar paralysis. The sudden onset and the associated symptoms make the diagnosis easy. In these acute cases there may be loss of power in one arm, or hemiplegia, sometimes alternate hemiplegia, with paralysis on one side of the face and loss of power on the other side of the body. (*c*) In polio-myelitis there are cases with acute bulbar symptoms.

II. SPASTIC PARALYSIS OF ADULTS

(*Primary Lateral Sclerosis*)

Definition.—A gradual loss of power with spasm of the muscles of the body, the lower extremities being first and most affected, unaccompanied by muscular atrophy, sensory disturbance, or other symptoms. A systemic degeneration of the pyramidal tracts is assumed.

Symptoms.—The general symptoms of spastic paraplegia in adults are very distinctive. The patient complains of feeling tired, of stiffness in the legs, and perhaps of pains of a dull aching character in the back or in the calves. There may be no definite loss of power, even when the spastic condition is well established. In other instances there is definite weakness. The stiffness is felt most in the morning. In a well developed case the gait is most characteristic. The legs are moved stiffly and with hesitation, the toes drag and catch against the ground, and, in extreme cases, when the ball of the foot rests upon the ground a distinct clonus develops. The legs are kept close together, the knees touch, and in certain cases the adductor spasm may cause cross-legged progression. On examination, the legs may at first appear tolerably supple, perhaps flexed and extended readily. In other cases the rigidity is marked, particularly when the limbs are extended. The spasm of the adductors of the thigh may be so extreme that the legs are separated with the greatest difficulty. In cases of this extreme rigidity the patient usually loses the power of walking. The nutrition is well maintained, the muscles may be hypertrophied. The reflexes are greatly increased. The slightest touch upon the patellar tendon produces an active knee-jerk. The rectus clonus and the ankle clonus are easily obtained. In some instances the slightest touch may throw the legs into violent clonic spasm, the condition to which Brown-Séquard gave the name of spinal epilepsy. The superficial reflexes are also increased. The arms may be unaffected for years, but occasionally they become weak and stiff at the same time as the legs.

The course of the disease is progressively downward. Years may elapse before the patient is bedridden. Involvement of the sphincters, as a rule, is late; occasionally it is early. The sensory symptoms rarely progress, and the patients may retain their general nutrition and enjoy excellent health. Ocular symptoms are rare.

Diagnosis.—The diagnosis, so far as the clinical picture is concerned, is readily made, but it is often very difficult to determine accurately the nature of the underlying pathological condition. A history of syphilis is present in many of the cases. Cases which have run a fairly typical clinical course upon coming to autopsy have been found to have been due to very different conditions—transverse myelitis, multiple sclerosis, cerebral tumor, etc. General paresis may begin with symptoms of spastic paraplegia, and Westphal believed that it was only in relation to this disease that a primary sclerosis of the pyramidal tracts ever occurred. In any case the diagnosis of primary systemic degeneration of the pyramidal tract is, to say the least, doubtful.

Treatment.—Not much can be done to check the progress. Division of the posterior nerve roots is permissible when the motor weakness is due chiefly to spasticity. A number of cases have been operated upon successfully. The same practice has been followed in the spasticity with bilateral athetosis.

III. SECONDARY SPASTIC PARALYSIS

Following any lesion of the pyramidal tract there may be a spastic paralysis; thus, in a transverse lesion of the cord, whether the result of slow compression (as in caries), chronic myelitis, the pressure of tumor, chronic meningo-myelitis, or multiple sclerosis, degeneration takes place in the pyramidal tracts, below the point of disease. The legs soon become stiff and rigid, and the reflexes increase. Bastian has shown that in compression paraplegia if the transverse lesion is complete, the limbs may be flaccid, without increase in the reflexes—*paraplégie flasque* of the French. The condition of the patient in these secondary forms varies very much. In chronic myelitis or in multiple sclerosis he may be able to walk about, but with a characteristic spastic gait. In the compression myelitis, in fracture, or in caries, there may be complete loss of power with rigidity.

It may be difficult or even impossible to distinguish these cases from those of primary spastic paralysis. Reliance is to be placed upon the associated symptoms; when these are absent no definite diagnosis as to the cause of the spastic paralysis can be given.

Syphilitic Spinal Paralysis.—Erb described a symptom group under the term syphilitic spinal paralysis. The points upon which he laid stress are a very gradual onset with a development finally of the features of a spastic paresis; the tendon reflexes are increased, but the muscular rigidity is slight in comparison with the exaggerated deep reflexes. There is rarely much pain, and the sensory disturbances are trivial, but there may be paræsthesia and the girdle sensation. The bladder and rectum are usually involved, and there is sexual failure or impotence. And, lastly, improvement is not infrequent. A majority of instances of spastic paralysis of adults not the result of slow compression of the cord are associated with syphilis and belong to this group.

C. HEREDITARY AND FAMILIAL DISEASES

I. THE MUSCULAR DYSTROPHIES

(*Dystrophia muscularis progressiva,* Erb. *Primary Myopathy*)

Definition.—Muscular wasting, with or without an initial hypertrophy, beginning in various groups of muscles, usually progressive in character, and dependent on primary changes in the muscles themselves or the neuro-muscular endings.

Etiology.—No factor other than heredity is known, which may show itself by true heredity—the disease occurring in two or more generations—or several members of the same generation may be affected. Members of the same family may be attacked through several generations: as many as 20 or 30 cases have been described in five generations. Males, as a rule, are more frequently affected than females. In families, persons of the same sex are usually attacked, but unaffected females may transmit the disease. In Erb's cases 44 per cent. showed no heredity. The disease usually sets in before puberty, but the onset may be as late as the twentieth or twenty-fifth year, or in some instances even later.

Pathology.—At first the muscle fibres hypertrophy, and become round; the nuclei increase, and the fibres may become fissured. At the same time there is a slight increase in the connective tissue. Sooner or later the fibres begin to atrophy, and the nuclei become greatly increased. Vacuoles and fissures appear, and the fibres become completely atrophic, the connective tissue increasing with deposition of fat to such an extent as to cause hypertrophic lipomatosis—pseudo-hypertrophy. The different stages of these changes may be found in a single muscle at the same time.

The nervous system has very generally been found to be without demonstrable lesions, but in certain cases changes in the cells of the ventral horns have been described.

Changes in the *pineal gland,* producing shadows, have been demonstrated by the X-rays, from which very naturally it is suggested that the disease is due to a disturbance in the internal secretions.

Symptoms.—Clumsiness in the movements of the child is the first symptom noticed and on examination certain muscles or groups of muscles seem to be enlarged, particularly those of the calves. The extensors of the leg, the glutei, the lumbar muscles, the deltoid, triceps and infraspinatus, are the next most frequently involved, and may stand out with great prominence. The muscles of the neck, face, and forearm rarely suffer. Sometimes only a portion of a muscle is involved. With this hypertrophy of some muscles there is wasting of others, particularly the lower portion of the pectorals and the latissimus dorsi. The attitude when standing is very characteristic. The legs are far apart, the shoulders thrown back, the spine is greatly curved, and the abdomen protrudes. The gait is waddling and awkward. In getting up from the floor the position assumed, so well known now through Gowers' figures, is pathognomonic. The patient first turns over in the all-fours position and raises the trunk with his arms; the hands are then moved along the ground until the knees are reached; then with one hand upon a knee he lifts himself up, grasps the other knee, and gradually pushes himself in the erect posture, as it has been expressed, by climbing up his legs. The striking contrast between the feebleness of the child and the powerful looking pseudo-hypertrophic muscles is very characteristic. The enlarged muscles may, however, be relatively very strong.

The course is slow, but progressive. Wasting proceeds and finally all traces of the enlarged condition of the muscles disappear. At this late period distortions and contractions are common. The muscles of the shoulder-girdle are nearly always affected early, causing a symptom upon which Erb lays great stress. With the hands under the arms, when one endeavors to lift the patient, the shoulders are raised to the level of the ears, and one gets the impression as though the child were slipping through. These "loose shoulders" are very characteristic. The abnormal mobility of the shoulder blades gives them a winged appearance, and makes the arms seem much longer than usual when they are stretched out.

There are no sensory symptoms. The atrophic muscles do not show the reaction of degeneration except in extremely rare instances.

Clinical Forms.—A number of types have been described, depending upon the age at onset, the muscles first affected, the occurrence of hypertrophy, heredity, etc., but there is no sharp division between the forms. The following are the more important:

1. *The pseudo-hypertrophic of Duchenne,* most common in childhood and in family groups. The hypertrophy of the muscles is the striking feature, whether a true hypertrophy or a lipomatosis. There is also a juvenile type with atrophy, affecting chiefly the shoulder girdles and upper arms. Isolated cases occur in adults.

II. *The facio-scapulo-humeral type* of Landouzy-Dejerine. The face is first involved, causing the myopathic facies, the lips prominent, the upper one projecting, the eyes cannot be closed, nor the forehead wrinkled, the smile is transverse, from inaction of the levators of the lip. Later the shoulder-girdle muscles are involved, the scapulæ are winged, the upper arms wasted, and lastly, the thigh muscles. With all this there may be no hypertrophy, though often, if carefully sought, there will be found areas of enlargement—the so-called muscle balls. This form may begin in adults.

III. *The thigh-muscle type* of Leyden, Moebius, and Zimmerlin, in which the disease starts in the extensors of the thighs which are deeply involved before other groups of upper arms and trunk are attacked.

In all forms, when the muscles of the trunk become involved, there is flattening of the chest and the peculiar *"wasp-waist"* described by Marie.

Diagnosis.—The muscular dystrophies can usually be distinguished readily from the other forms of muscular atrophy.

(*a*) In the cerebral atrophy loss of power usually precedes the atrophy.

(*b*) Progressive (central) muscular atrophy begins in the small muscles of the hand, the reaction of degeneration is present and fibrillary twitchings occur in both the atrophied and non-atrophied muscles. The central atrophies come late in life, the dystrophies, as a rule, early. In the progressive muscular dystrophies heredity plays an important rôle. In the rare cases of early infantile spinal muscular atrophy occurring in families the symptoms are so characteristic of a central disease that the diagnosis presents no difficulty.

(*c*) In the neuritic muscular atrophies, due to lead or to trauma, seen for the first time at a period when the wasting is marked there is often difficulty, but the absence of family history and the distribution are important features. Moreover, the paralysis is out of proportion to the atrophy. Sensory symptoms may be present.

(*d*) Progressive neural muscular atrophy. Here heredity is also a factor, and the disease usually begins in early life, but the distribution of atrophy and paralysis, which is at first confined to the periphery of the extremities, helps to distinguish it from the dystrophies.

Prognosis.—The outlook in the primary muscular dystrophies is bad. The wasting progresses uniformly, uninfluenced by treatment.

Treatment.—Erb holds that by electricity and massage the progress is occasionally arrested. The general health should be carefully looked after, moderate exercise allowed, friction of the muscles with oil, and when the patient becomes bedfast, as is inevitable sooner or later, care should be taken to prevent contractures in awkward positions.

II. FAMILIAL SPINAL MUSCULAR ATROPHY

(*Werdnig-Hoffman*)

A rare disease which may be hereditary as well as occurring in a family without disease in the ascendants. Anatomically there is marked degeneration of the anterior horns in the spinal cord, of the anterior roots, and less marked changes in the peripheral nerves, with widespread atrophy of the muscular fibres. While in many cases the disease resembles muscular dystrophy, anatomically it appears to be a progressive central muscular atrophy. It presents a close similarity to Amyotonia Congenita (Oppenheim's Disease). The onset is early, even before walking. The proximal muscles of the limbs and the muscles of the trunk are first involved. There is no pseudo-hypertrophy. Fibrillary tremors may be present. The disease is progressive, sometimes with great rapidity, and death usually occurs before the sixth year.

III. PROGRESSIVE NEURAL MUSCULAR ATROPHY

(*Peroneal type and hypertrophic type—Charcot-Marie-Tooth*)

The peroneal type, described first by Charcot, Marie, and Tooth, is a hereditary and familial disease beginning in childhood, affecting first the muscles of the peroneal group, leading to club-foot, either *pes equinus* or *pes equino-varus*.

The pathology is not clear: the disease seems to occupy a position intermediate between central muscular atrophy and the muscular dystrophies, resembling the latter in the early onset and familial character, and the former in the occurrence of fibrillary twitchings, the presence of electrical changes and the implication of the small muscles of the hand. Anatomically sclerosis of the posterior columns, atrophy of the cells of the anterior horns and alterations of the peripheral nerves have been found.

The disease may begin in the hands, but as a rule the upper limbs are not affected until after the legs, and then the trouble starts in the small muscles of the hand, so that claw-foot and claw-hand are very striking features. Disturbances of sensation are common. Fibrillary twitchings also occur; the deep reflexes are lost in the paralysed muscles. The essential feature is implication of the distal with normal proximal portions of the limbs, which gives a very characteristic picture. There is great decrease of the electrical excitability. Ocular symptoms are rare; occasionally there is atrophy of the optic nerves. The disease should be suspected in cases of acquired double club-foot.

IV. PROGRESSIVE INTERSTITIAL HYPERTROPHIC NEURITIS

Definition.—A familial disease beginning, as a rule, in infancy with a combination of the symptoms of tabes and muscular atrophy. Anatomically there is sclerosis of the posterior columns of the cord with interstitial hypertrophic neuritis.

It was first described by Dejerine and Sottas, and, though rare, a good many families have been reported, one by Marie in which seven children were affected.

Pathology.—The spinal cord lesions resemble those of tabes, and result from degeneration of the posterior nerve roots. The hypertrophy of the nerves is of a type that occurs in no other form of disease. The connective tissue sheaths are greatly thickened, and there is widespread parenchymatous degeneration.

Symptoms.—These begin in early life and are: (*a*) Incoördination very like that of tabes dorsalis, only as the disease progresses the gait is steppage; (*b*) sensory disturbances, sometimes pains which are fulgurant in character; (*c*) muscular atrophy, limbs and face, in the former chiefly distal, in the latter resembling a myopathy. The feet are usually in the varus position, kypho-scoliosis is also present. (*d*) Ocular symptoms are marked—myosis (Argyll-Robertson sign). (*e*) Added to this, the peripheral nerves are hypertrophied, sometimes double the normal size, smooth and not painful, those of the lower limbs being chiefly involved. The optic and olfactory nerves escape.

V. HEREDITARY ATAXIA

(*Friedreich's Ataxia*)

Definition.—A familial disease occurring late in childhood characterized by locomotor and static ataxia, speech disturbances and nystagmus, and anatomically by degeneration of the postero-lateral and spino-cerebellar tracts. In 1863 Friedreich first reported six cases.

Etiology.—It is a family disease affecting brothers and sisters. The 143 cases analysed by Griffiths occurred in 71 unrelated families. Males are most frequently attacked, 86 to 57 in Griffiths' series. Direct inheritance is rare, noted only in 33 cases. The onset is usually before puberty, but may be as late as the 25th year. The cause is unknown. Various influences in the parents, such as consanguinity, alcoholism, and syphilis have been reported. The disease belongs to Gower's abiotrophies, an inherited weakness, lack of vitality in certain sections of the nervous system, leading to early degeneration.

Morbid Anatomy.—Both cord and cerebellum have been reported smaller than usual. The posterior meninges may be thickened. The important change is a complete sclerotic degeneration of the postero-lateral tracts forming the most typical example of combined degeneration. The sclerosis of Burdach's tract is less complete, as a rule, than that of Goll's. Gowers' tract and the direct cerebellar are always involved. Dejerine and Letulle suggest that the disease differs from ordinary spinal sclerosis and is a gliosis due to developmental errors.

Symptoms.—The incoördination begins in the legs, and the gait is swaying, irregular, and more like that of a drunken man without the characteristic stamping gait of the true tabes. Romberg's sign may or may not be present. The ataxia of the arms occurs early and is very marked; the movements are almost choreiform, irregular and somewhat swaying. In making any voluntary movement the action is overdone, the prehension is clawlike, and the fingers may be spread or overextended just before grasping an object. The hand frequently moves about an object for a moment, and then suddenly pounces upon it. There are irregular, swaying movements of the head and shoulders. There is present in many cases what is known as static ataxia, that is to say, ataxia of quiet action. It occurs when the body is held erect or when a limb is extended—irregular, oscillating movements of the head and body or of the extended limb.

Sensory symptoms are not usually present. The deep reflexes are lost early in the disease, and, next to the ataxia, this is the most constant and important symptom. Babinski's sign may be present at first. The skin reflexes are normal, and the pupil reflex is not affected.

Nystagmus is a characteristic symptom. Atrophy of the optic nerve rarely occurs. Disturbance of speech is common. It is usually slow and scanning; the expression is often dull; the mental power is, as a rule, maintained, but late in the disease becomes impaired. A striking feature is early deformity of the feet, a *talipes equinus,* so that the patient walks on the outer edge of the feet. The big toe is flexed dorsally on the first phalanx. Scoliosis is very common.

Trophic lesions are rare. As the disease advances, paralysis comes on and may ultimately be complete. Some of the patients never walk.

Diagnosis.—This is not difficult when several members of a family are affected. The onset in childhood, the curious form of incoördination, the loss of knee-jerks, the early talipes equinus, the position of the great toe, scoliosis, the nystagmus, and scanning speech make up an unmistakable picture. With hereditary chorea it has certain similarities, but usually this disease does not set in until after the 30th year.

The affection lasts for many years and is incurable. Care should be taken to prevent contractures.

VI. HEREDITARY CEREBELLAR ATAXIA (*Marie*)

Though resembling Friedreich's ataxia, it differs in—(1) Beginning late in life (after twenty); (2) the ataxia is more purely cerebellar; (3) the knee-jerks are retained, sometimes increased; (4) there is no talipes or scoliosis; and (5) ocular palsies are common. In L. F. Barker's study of two cases in the family (24 cases in all) recorded by Sanger Brown, there was congenital hypoplasia of the cerebellum and cord with degeneration of the spino-cerebellar paths and slight degeneration of the pyramidal tracts. He regards it as the cerebellar type of Friedreich's ataxia.

VII. HEREDITARY SPASTIC PARAPLEGIA

Definition.—A familial, abiotrophic disease, involving chiefly the pyramidal tracts. It is sometimes hereditary.

Etiology.—It begins in children usually after the seventh year; the onset may be delayed until the twentieth: three or four members of a family may be attacked, boys more often than girls in the proportion of 88 to 51 (Deléarde and Minet). In some families in which the disease has been hereditary, the females have escaped. Mild cases in a family may exist with increase of the reflexes as the only symptom.

Pathology.—The spinal degeneration is chiefly in the pyramidal tracts of the lumbar and lower thoracic regions. In the late stages the lesions may be those of a combined sclerosis with involvement of the direct cerebellar tracts. Newmark's studies show imperfect development of the cord (agenesia) as an important factor.

Symptoms.—Early exaggeration of the knee-jerks may precede any paralysis or weakness: gradually there are spasticity and Babinski's sign, with contractures and paralysis. It is important to rule out the cases with mental features and Little's disease. The paralysis may extend to the upper limbs, and eyes and speech are involved. In others again there is atrophy of the muscles, and the picture is not unlike amyotrophic lateral sclerosis, or a disseminated sclerosis. Very different pictures may be presented by affected children in the same family.

VIII. CHRONIC HEREDITARY CHOREA

(*Huntington's Chorea*)

Definition.—A hereditary disease characterized by irregular movements, disturbance of speech and progressive mental deterioration.

History.—In 1863 Lyon described it as chronic hereditary chorea. In 1872 George Huntington, whose father, grandfather, and great-grandfather had treated cases, gave in three brief paragraphs its salient features—heredity, the late onset, and the mental changes. The disease is more common in the United States than in Europe. Davenport has studied the four great family complexes of eastern Long Island, southwestern Connecticut, south-central Connecticut, and eastern Massachusetts "which show nearly 1000 cases of Huntington's chorea, and yielding the remarkable results that practically all can be traced back to some half-dozen individuals, including three (probable) brothers who migrated to America in the XVIIth century."

Inheritance.—It never skips a generation. The age of onset does not appear to vary, averaging from thirty-five to thirty-eight. The mental type is usually hyperkinetic. Among 3000 persons related to the 962 cases studied by Davenport, there were many other nervous disorders—epilepsy in 39, infantile convulsions in 19, and feeble-mindedness in 73.

Pathology.—There is marked destruction of the smaller ganglion cells of the globus pallidus system which have a coördinating and inhibitory control over the larger motor cells. When this is lost chorea results (Hunt). The large cell system of the globus pallidus stands in relation to the paralysis agitans syndrome and the small cell system to the chorea syndrome. The other findings are varied. Meningeal thickening and atrophy of the cortex, with a loss of cells, have been present in some cases. Arterio-sclerotic changes are common in older subjects.

Symptoms.—Difficulty in performing delicate actions with the hands, as in writing, or in buttoning a shirt collar, may be the earliest indication, or there are slight involuntary movements of the head and face. When well established, the movements are slower than in Sydenham's chorea, irregular and incoördinate. The face muscles are early involved, causing involuntary grimaces. The gait is irregular and swaying, not unlike that of a drunken man. The speech is slow and the syllables blurred. The reflexes, not altered at first, are later increased. Certain biotypes have been observed by Davenport. Thus the tremors may be absent and the mental condition present, or the muscular movements may be present without mental defects. The chorea may not progress and the onset may be early in life. He found family differences in all these points.

The mental changes may come early, outbreaks of temper and excitement are common, alternating with periods of depression. Usually a progressive failure of the mental powers leads to complete dementia. Dreading a terrible fate, it is not surprising to hear of suicide in certain members of the families.

Little or nothing can be done to arrest the progress of the disease.

Prevention.—Davenport's study shows how much more serious the disease is than we had hitherto thought. It is transmitted through males and females, and Davenport states that there is no evidence of any abstention from or selection against marrying in the members of the large group of hereditary choreas studied by him. There is no efficient treatment.

IX. PROGRESSIVE LENTICULAR DEGENERATION

(*Wilson's Disease*)

Definition.—A familial, not hereditary, disease usually coming on early in life, characterized by tremor and spasticity with bilateral changes in the lenticular nuclei and cirrhosis of the liver.

Described by Wilson in 1912, it is apparently the same condition which Gowers designated tetanoid chorea and resembles the pseudo-sclerosis of Westphal and Strümpell. As to pathogenesis Wilson suggests the selective action of some toxin possibly due to the hepatic cirrhosis. The lenticular nuclei show degeneration with cavitation and atrophy. The process may extend more widely to the internal capsule, motor cortex and pyramidal tracts. The cirrhosis of the liver is marked and of a mixed type.

The features are involuntary choreiform movements, muscular rigidity, spasticity, and painful muscular contractions. When the patient grasps an object he may have difficulty in relaxing his hold. There is difficulty in speech and swallowing, muscular weakness, and contractures with progressive emaciation. There may be emotional disturbances and mental weakness. The hepatic cirrhosis does not seem to have caused any symptoms or signs in the reported cases. A curious annular brownish-green pigmentation of the cornea has been noted in a few cases. The disease is progressive with a course in acute cases of a few months and in chronic forms of four to seven years. There is no specific treatment.

X. PERIODIC PARALYSIS

Definition.—A recurring paralysis, lasting from a few hours to a few days, affecting members of the same family, with abolition of the faradic excitability of both muscles and nerves. Death may occur in an attack.

History.—After a few scattered references in literature, the disease was accurately described in 1885 by Westphal and Oppenheim. Family groups then began to be recognized, and now a large number of cases have been studied.

Etiology.—The majority have occurred in groups. Holtzapple reported seventeen cases in four generations. Many members of this family suffered from migraine. Transmission is either through the male or female; the disease may skip a generation. Sporadic cases occur.

Pathology.—Nothing definite is known. Winternitz could find no organic lesions in two fatal cases in the family reported by Holtzapple. Naturally autointoxication has been suggested, and extensive researches into metabolism have been made. Diminution of creatinin excretion has been determined. In some respects the disease is similar to Myasthenia gravis, in which there are attacks of transient paralysis. Westphal regarded the disease as a vasomotor neurosis associated with migraine, which was such a striking feature in Holtzapple's cases. Temporary collapse of the vessels is met with in this condition, and Holtzapple suggests that this may occur in the anterior horns.

Symptoms.—The clinical picture is similar in all recorded cases. The paralysis involves, as a rule, the arms and legs, but may be general below the neck. It comes on in healthy persons without apparent cause, and often during sleep. At first there may be weakness of the limbs, a feeling of weariness and sleepiness, but rarely with sensory symptoms. The paralysis, beginning in the legs, to which it may be confined, is usually complete within the first twenty-four hours. The neck muscles are sometimes involved, and occasionally those of the tongue and pharynx. The cerebral nerves and the special senses are, as a rule, unaffected. The temperature is normal or subnormal, and the pulse slow. The deep reflexes are diminished, sometimes abolished, and the skin reflexes may be enfeebled. The faradic excitability of both muscles and nerves is reduced or abolished. Improvement begins within a few hours or a day or two, the paralysis disappearing completely and the patient becoming perfectly well. The attacks usually recur at intervals of one to two weeks, but they may return daily. They generally cease after the fiftieth year. There may be signs of acute dilatation of the heart during the attack.

Treatment.—Potassium citrate in full doses may shorten or abort an attack.

XI. AMAUROTIC FAMILY IDIOCY

(*Tay-Sachs' Disease*)

Definition.—A family disease of infancy characterized by lack of mental development, progressive muscular weakness, and macular changes in the retina.

History.—In 1881 Waren Tay reported a group of cases characterized by muscular weakness, macular lesions, and death before the age of two years. B. Sachs extended our knowledge of the disease, a comparatively rare one, about 100 cases being reported to 1917 (Naville).

Etiology.—Among familial diseases it is unique in the limitation to one race—the Hebrew, and almost exclusively to the Polish branch. No other factor is known; syphilis is excluded. A dominant Mendelian character is present as 50 per cent. of the children are usually affected and 100 per cent. of the same sex. The cause is unknown. Sachs believes that the children are born with a nervous system so inadequate to meet the demands that the cells, after performing their function for a few years or months, undergo complete degeneration. The disease comes into the category of Gowers' abiotrophies.

Pathology.—There is marked agenesia of the brain, with degenerative changes in the large pyramidal cells, and swelling of the dendrites. The degenerative changes are widely spread throughout the gray matter of the brain, the cord, and the spinal ganglia (Schaffer). The retinal changes are due to a similar degeneration in the ganglion cells.

Symptoms.—Healthy at birth, and to the third or fourth month, the child then begins to be listless, moving the limbs very little, and as time goes on, is not able to hold up the head or sit up. The muscles are flaccid, rarely spastic. Examination of the fundus shows a cherry-red spot in the region of the macula. Within a year a hitherto well-developed baby becomes marantic, completely blind, and death occurs as a rule before the end of the second year. The disease must be distinguished from the ordinary diplegias and paraplegias. It is not always easy as spasticity may be present, but the retinal changes are distinctive.

A juvenile form occurring between the eighth and the twelfth year associated with blindness, but no macular changes, has been reported, and not in the Hebrew race. It is doubtful whether this is the same disease. Related to the Tay-Sachs disease is the remarkable familial macular degeneration without dementia in which the disease starts about puberty.

XII. MYOCLONIC EPILEPSY

Definition.—A familial disorder, beginning in childhood with epilepsy, chiefly nocturnal, and followed by myoclonic attacks and progressive dementia.

Etiology.—A majority of the cases have occurred in family groups and often in degenerate stock. Single cases may occur in normal families. Nothing is known of the causation; Lundborg suggests a thyroid origin.

Pathology.—The changes found in the brain cortex have been those of chronic epilepsy and dementia.

Symptoms.—The onset, in childhood, is with nocturnal epilepsy, which in a year or two is followed by myoclonia, sometimes preceded by tremor. All the voluntary muscles are involved in short, quick, clonic spasms, which progressively increase in intensity. The child may at first have good and bad days, the latter following, as a rule, nights with severe epileptic seizures. The myoclonia grows worse and the patient falls into a state of dementia. The severe myoclonia attacks lead up to genuine epileptic seizures. There is a strong psychic feature which is intensified if the patient knows he is watched; bright lights, sounds, and handling the muscles have the same effect (Lundborg). The familial character and the nocturnal epilepsy separate it from the essential myoclonia of Friedreich.

D. DISEASES OF THE MENINGES

I. DISEASES OF THE DURA MATER

(*Pachymeningitis*)

1. Pachymeningitis Externa.—Cerebral.—Hæmorrhage often occurs as a result of fracture. Inflammation of the external layer of the dura is rare. Caries of the bone, either extension from middle-ear disease or due to syphilis, is the principal cause. In the syphilitic cases there may be a great thickening of the inner table and a large collection of pus between the dura and the bone.

Occasionally the pus is infiltrated between the two layers of the dura mater or may extend through and cause a dura-arachnitis.

The *symptoms* of external pachymeningitis are indefinite. In the syphilitic cases there may be a small sinus communicating with the exterior. Compression symptoms may occur with or without paralysis.

Spinal.—An acute form may occur in syphilitic affections of the bones, in tumors, and in aneurism. The symptoms are those of a compression of the cord. A chronic form is more common, and is a constant accompaniment of tuberculous caries of the spine. The internal surface of the dura may be smooth, while the external is rough and covered with caseous masses. The entire dura may be surrounded, or the process may be confined to the ventral surface.

2. Pachymeningitis Interna.—This occurs in three forms: (1) Pseudo-membranous, (2) purulent, and (3) hæmorrhagic. The first two are unimportant. Pseudo-membranous inflammation of the lining membrane of the dura is not usually recognized, but a characteristic example of it came under observation as a secondary process in pneumonia. Purulent pachymeningitis may follow an injury, but is more commonly the result of extension from inflammation of the pia. It is remarkable how rarely pus is found between the dura and arachnoid membranes.

3. **Hæmorrhagic Interna Pachymeningitis.**—CEREBRAL FORM.—This remarkable condition, first described by Virchow, is very rare in general medical practice. During ten years no case came to autopsy at the Montreal General Hospital. On the other hand, in the post-mortem room of the Philadelphia Hospital, which received material from a large almshouse and asylum, the cases were not uncommon, and within three months there were four characteristic examples, three of which came from the medical wards. The frequency in asylum work may be gathered from the fact that in 1,185 post mortems at the Government Hospital for the Insane, Washington, to June 30, 1897, there were 197 cases with "a true neo-membrane of internal pachymeningitis" (Blackburn). Of these cases, 45 were chronic dementia, 37 were general paresis, 30 senile dementia, 28 chronic mania, 28 chronic melancholia, 22 chronic epileptic insanity, 6 acute mania, and 1 case imbecility. Forty-two of the cases were in persons over seventy years of age.

It has also been found in profound anæmia and other diseases of the blood and of the blood vessels, and has followed the acute fevers—typhoid fever in a child (Barker). The lesion has been found in badly nourished cachectic children (Herter).

Pathology.—Virchow's view that the delicate vascular membrane precedes the hæmorrhage is undoubtedly correct. Practically we see one of three conditions: (*a*) subdural vascular membranes, often of extreme delicacy; (*b*) simple subdural hæmorrhage; (c) a combination of the two, vascular membrane and blood clot. Certainly the vascular membrane may exist without a trace of hæmorrhage—simply a fibrous sheet of varying thickness, permeated with large vessels, which may form beautiful arborescent tufts. On the other hand, there are instances in which the subdural hæmorrhage is found alone, but it is possible that in some of these at least the hæmorrhage may have destroyed all trace of the vascular membrane. In some cases a series of laminated clots are found, forming a layer from 3 to 5 mm. in thickness. Cysts may occur within this membrane. The source of the hæmorrhage is probably the dural vessels. Huguenin and others hold that the bleeding comes from the vessels of the pia mater, but certainly in the early stage there is no evidence of this; on the other hand, the highly vascular subdural membrane may be seen covered with the thinnest possible sheeting of clot, which has evidently come from the dura. The subdural hæmorrhage is usually associated with atrophy of the convolutions, and it is held that this is one reason why it is so common in the insane, especially in dementia paralytica and dementia senilis. We meet with the condition also in various cachectic conditions in which cerebral wasting is as common and almost as marked as in cases of insanity. König found in 135 cases of hæmorrhagic pachymeningitis that 23 per cent. accompanied tuberculosis.

The *symptoms* are indefinite, or there may be none at all, especially when the hæmorrhages are small or have occurred very gradually, and the diagnosis can not be made with certainty. Headache has been a prominent symptom in some cases, and when the condition exists on one side there may be hemiplegia. The most helpful signs for diagnosis, indicating that the hæmorrhage in an apoplectic attack is meningeal, are (1) those referable to increased intracranial pressure (slowing and irregularity of the pulse, vomiting, coma, contracted pupils, reacting to light slowly or not at all) and (2) paresis and paralysis, gradually increasing in extent, accompanied by symptoms which point to a *cortical* origin. Extensive bilateral disease may, however, exist without any symptoms whatever.

The *spinal fluid* may be bloody but this is not always the case. It is not a little curious that coma may come on and be the chief feature when anatomically the condition is a laminated hæmatoma evidently of long standing.

Spinal Form.—The spinal *pachymeningitis interna,* described by Charcot and Joffroy, involves chiefly the cervical region (*P. cervicalis hypertrophica*). The space between the cord and the dura is occupied by a firm, concentrically arranged, fibrinous structure, which is seen to have arisen within, not outside of, the dura mater. It is a condition anatomically identical with the hæmorrhagic pachymeningitis interna of the brain. The etiology is unknown; syphilis has existed in a few cases. The cord is usually compressed; the central canal may be dilated—hydromyelus—and there are secondary degenerations. The nerve roots are involved in the growth and are damaged and compressed. The extent is variable. It may be limited to one segment, but more commonly involves a considerable portion of the cervical enlargement. Some cases present a characteristic group of symptoms. There are intense neuralgic pains in the course of the nerves whose roots are involved. They are chiefly in the arms and in the cervical region, and vary greatly in intensity. There may be hyperæsthesia with numbness and tingling; atrophic changes may develop, and there may be areas of anæsthesia. Gradually motor disturbances appear; the arms become weak and the muscles atrophied, particularly in certain groups, as the flexors of the hand. The extensors, on the other hand, remain intact, so that the condition of claw-hand is gradually produced. The grade of the atrophy depends much upon the extent of involvement of the cervical nerve roots, and in many cases the atrophy of the muscles of the shoulders and arms becomes extreme. The condition is one of cervical paraplegia, with contractures, flexion of the wrist, and typical *main en griffe.* Usually before the arms are greatly atrophied there are the symptoms of what the French writers term the second stage—namely, involvement of the lower extremities and the gradual production of a spastic paraplegia, due to secondary changes in the cord.

The disease runs a chronic course, lasting, perhaps, two or more years. In a few instances, in which symptoms pointed definitely to this condition, recovery has taken place. The disease is to be distinguished from amyotrophic lateral sclerosis, syringomyelia, and tumors. From the first it is separated by the marked severity of the initial pains in the neck and arms; from the second by the absence of the sensory changes characteristic of syringomyelia. From certain tumors it is very difficult to distinguish; in fact, the fibrinous layers form a tumor around the cord.

The condition known as *hæmatoma* of the dura mater may occur at any part of the cord, or, in its slow, progressive form—pachymeningitis hæmorrhagica interna—may be limited to the cervical region and produce the symptoms just mentioned. It is sometimes extensive, and may coexist with a similar condition of the cerebral dura. Cysts may occur filled with hæmorrhagic contents.

II. DISEASES OF THE PIA MATER

(*Acute Cerebro-spinal Leptomeningitis*)

Etiology.—Under cerebro-spinal fever and tuberculosis the two most important forms of meningitis have been described. Other conditions with which meningitis is associated are : (1) *The acute fevers,* more particularly pneumonia, erysipelas, and septicæmia; less frequently small-pox, typhoid fever, scarlet fever, measles, influenza, etc. (2) *Injury or disease of the bones of the skull.* In this group by far the most frequent cause is necrosis of the petrous portion of the temporal bone in chronic otitis. (3) *Extension from disease of the nose.* Meningitis has followed perforation of the skull in sounding the frontal sinuses, suppurative disease of these sinuses, and necroses of the cribriform plate. As mentioned under cerebro-spinal fever, the infection is thought to be possible through the nose. (4) As a *terminal infection* in chronic nephritis, arterio-sclerosis, heart disease, and the wasting diseases of children.

The following etiological table of the chief acute forms of meningitis may be useful to the student:

ACUTE LEPTOMENINGITIS.	Primary.	1. Of cerebro-spinal fever.	(*a*) Sporadic. (*b*) Epidemic.	Meningococcus.
		2. Pneumococcic.	Meninges involved alone or in a general pneumococcus or streptococcus infection.	Pneumococcus.
		3. Streptococcic.		Streptococcus.
	Secondary.	1. Tuberculous	....	Bacillus tuberculosis.
		2. Pneumococcic.	(*a*) Secondary to pneumonia, endocarditis, etc. (*b*) Secondary to disease or injury of cranium or its fossæ.	Pneumococcus.
		3. Pyogenic.	(*a*) Following local disease of cranium or a local infection elsewhere. (*b*) Terminal infection in various chronic maladies.	Various forms of staphylococci and streptococci.
		4. Miscellaneous acute infections.	In typhoid fever, influenza, diphtheria, gonorrhœa, anthrax, actinomycosis, and other acute diseases.	Typhoid bacillus, influenza bacillus, diphtheria bacillus, gonococcus, etc.

Morbid Anatomy.—The basal or cortical meninges may be chiefly attacked. The degree of involvement of the spinal meninges varies. In the form associated with pneumonia and ulcerative endocarditis the disease is bilateral and usually limited to the cortex. In extension from disease of the ear it is often unilateral and may be accompanied with abscess or with thrombosis of the sinuses. In the non-tuberculous form in children, in the meningitis of chronic nephritis, and in cachectic conditions the base is usually involved. In the cases secondary to pneumonia the effusion beneath the arachnoid may be very thick and purulent, completely hiding the convolutions. The ventricles also may be involved, though in these simple forms they rarely present the distention and softening which are so frequent in the tuberculous meningitis. For a more detailed description the student is referred to the sections on cerebro-spinal fever and tuberculous meningitis.

Symptoms.—Cortical meningitis is not to be recognized by any symptoms or set of symptoms from a condition which may be produced by the poison of many of the specific fevers. In the cases of so-called cerebral pneumonia, unless the base is involved and the nerves affected, the disease is unrecognizable, since identical symptoms may be produced by intense engorgement of the meninges. In typhoid fever, in which meningitis is very rare, the twitchings, spasms, and retraction of the neck are almost invariably associated with cerebro-spinal congestion, not with meningitis.

A knowledge of the *etiology* gives a very important clue. Thus, in middle-ear disease the development of high fever, delirium, vomiting, convulsions, and retraction of the head and neck would be extremely suggestive of meningitis or abscess. *Headache,* which may be severe and continuous, is the most common symptom. While the patient remains conscious this is usually the chief complaint, and even when semicomatose he may continue to groan and place his hand on his head. In the fevers, particularly in pneumonia, there may be no complaint of headache. Delirium is frequently early, and is most marked when the fever is high. Photophobia is often present. *Convulsions* are less common in simple than in tuberculous meningitis. In the simple meningitis of children they may occur. Epileptiform attacks which come and go are highly characteristic of direct irritation of the cortex. Rigidity and spasm or twitchings of the muscles are more common. Stiffness and retraction of the muscles of the neck are important symptoms; but they are not constant, and are most frequent when the inflammation is extensive on the meninges of the cervical cord. There may be trismus, gritting of the teeth, or spastic contraction of the abdominal muscles. Vomiting is a common symptom in the early stages, particularly in basilar meningitis. Constipation is usually present. In the late stages the urine and fæces may be passed involuntarily. Optic neuritis is rare in the meningitis of the cortex, but is not uncommon when the base is involved. Marked hyperæsthesia is common.

Important symptoms are due to lesions of the nerves at the base. Strabismus or ptosis may occur. The facial nerve may be involved, producing slight paralysis, or there may be damage to the fifth nerve, producing anæsthesia and, if the Gasserian ganglion is affected, trophic changes in the cornea. The pupils are at first contracted, subsequently dilated, and perhaps unequal. The reflexes in the extremities are often accentuated at the beginning of the disease; later they are diminished or entirely abolished. Herpes is common, particularly in the epidemic form.

Fever is present, moderate in grade, rarely rising above 103°. In the non-tuberculous leptomeningitis of debilitated children and in nephritis there may be little or no fever. The pulse may be increased in frequency at first, though this is unusual. One of the striking features is the slowness of the pulse in relation to the temperature, even in the early stages. Subsequently it may be irregular and still slower. The very rapid emaciation which often occurs is doubtless to be referred to a disturbance of the cerebral influence upon metabolism. Kernig's sign has been described under cerebro-spinal fever. There may be a concomitant reflex of one leg when passive flexion is made of the other or when the neck is bent forward there is flexion of the legs both at the knees and hips or of all four extremities (Brudzinski's sign). Lumbar puncture is exceedingly valuable for diagnosis. The sugar in the spinal fluid is reduced or absent. A turbid fluid usually indicates an acute non-tuberculous meningitis. At first the fluid may be only opalescent. A close relationship exists between the severity of the symptoms, the height of the pyrexia, and the degree of turbidity (Connal). As a rule a preponderance of polynuclear leucocytes is present with the meningococcus or the pyogenic organisms; a mononuclear exudate is characteristic of tuberculosis or polio-myelitis. In tuberculous meningitis the fluid is usually clear; in only one of 69 cases was it opalescent (Connal).

Treatment.—There are no remedies which in any way control the course of acute meningitis. An ice-bag should be applied to the head. Absolute rest and quiet should be enjoyed. When disease of the ear is present, a surgeon should be called early, and if there are symptoms of meningo-encephalitis which can in any way be localized trephining should be practised. An occasional saline purge will do more to relieve the congestion than blisters and local depletion. Warm baths should be given every three hours. Recovery may follow in the primary pneumococcus and streptococcus forms (Netter). Large doses of iodide of potassium and mercury are recommended by some authors. Hexamine in doses of 60 grains (4 gm.) daily may be tried, as Crowe has shown that it is excreted in the cerebro-spinal fluid and controls the growth of organisms in the meninges.

Lumbar puncture, as a therapeutic measure, is of great value, relieving the headache and sometimes reducing the fever.

The posterior basic meningitis of Gee, Lees, and Barlow is the sporadic form of cerebro-spinal fever and has been already described.

Meningism.—Sometimes spoken of as the syndrome of Dupré, this is a condition in which there are symptoms of meningitis, but post mortem the characteristic pathological changes are not present. It is practically the condition described formerly as meningeal irritation, and is seen most frequently in the acute fevers of children, particularly in pneumonia and typhoid fever, sometimes in alcoholism and in middle-ear disease. Lumbar puncture usually gives a large amount of clear fluid, sterile, and sometimes showing a slight increase in the number of cells.

Chronic Leptomeningitis.—This is rarely seen apart from syphilis or tuberculosis, in which the meningitis is associated with the growth of the granulomata in the meninges and about the vessels. The symptoms in such cases are extremely variable, depending entirely upon the situation of the growth. The epidemic meningitis may run a very chronic course, but of all forms the posterior basic may be the most protracted, as cases have been described with a duration of a year or more. Quincke's *meningitis serosa* is considered with hydrocephalus.

E. MENINGO-MYELO-ENCEPHALITIS

I. ACUTE POLIO-MYELITIS

(Heine-Medin Disease)

Definition.—An acute infection characterized anatomically by widespread lesions of the nervous system, with special localization in many of the cases in the anterior horns of the gray matter in the spinal cord—hence the common name, polio-myelitis anterior.

History.—In 1840 von Heine separated this type from other forms of paralysis and in 1887 Medin called attention to its occurrence in widespread epidemics, which have been specially studied in Sweden by Wickham, Harbitz, and others. Within the past thirteen years serious outbreaks have occurred in many parts of the United States and Canada. The incidence of the disease has also increased in Great Britain and on the Continent of Europe, while in Sweden and Norway and parts of Austria the disease has assumed epidemic proportions. In New York City in 1907-8 there were about 2,000 cases, with a mortality of 6 to 7 per cent.; in 1916 in the U. S. registration area there were 7,130 deaths and 1,182 in 1917.

Etiology.—In its epidemic behavior the disease resembles closely cerebro-spinal fever. Sporadic cases occur in all communities and under at present unknown conditions increase at times to epidemic proportions. It prevails in the late summer and autumn.

Age is an important predisposing element; a majority of all cases occur in children in the first dentition. The more prevalent the epidemic form the greater the proportion of young adults attacked. Males and females are about equally attacked.

The degree of contagiousness from person to person is slight, and in this the disease resembles cerebro-spinal fever and pneumonia.

The *organism* has been isolated by Flexner and his co-workers. The colonies consist of globular bodies averaging 0.15 to 0.3 micron in size. Monkeys inoculated with the twentieth generation of the culture developed typical experimental polio-myelitis. The infective agent is present in the brain and spinal cord, in the naso-pharyngeal secretions and in the blood. The disease is inoculable into monkeys and may be transmitted from one animal to another. It has been transmitted also by intracerebral injection of an emulsion made from flies which had fed on the spinal cord of a monkey dead of the disease. An important point is that the virus passes from the central nervous system in the monkey to the nasal mucosa and vice versa, and the application of the virus to this part is a ready means of inoculation. It has also been found in the tonsils and pharyngeal mucosa of children. The path of invasion is apparently by the upper respiratory tract.

So far as we know, the disease is transmitted either directly by contact or by the intervention of carriers. The distribution is more independent of sanitary conditions than in the common children's diseases.

Morbid Anatomy.—The lesions are widespread in the nervous system. We can no longer regard it as an affection limited to the anterior horns of the gray matter of the spinal cord, but a widespread polio-myelo-encephalo-meningitis.

Swelling of the spleen and a marked general hyperplasia of the lymphoid apparatus have been found. The cerebro-spinal fluid is usually increased but clear. The pia mater is hyperæmic and moist, but without exudate. Cases in which the cerebral symptoms have been pronounced show swelling and flattening of the convolutions, with hyperæmia of the gray matter and here and there small hæmorrhages. The changes in the spinal cord are very characteristic. The meninges are moist, the pia is hyperæmic, sometimes with small capillary hæmorrhages. On section the cut surface bulges, the gray matter is hyperæmic, appearing as a reddened H, or the redness is limited to the anterior horns, which may show spots of hæmorrhage. These changes may be localized to the swellings of the cord or extend throughout its entire extent.

Microscopically there is small-celled infiltration about the vessels of the meninges, most marked in the lumbar and cervical swellings. The infiltration extends into the fissures of the cord and follows the blood-vessels. The amount of meningeal implication is much more intense than is indicated macroscopically. In the cord itself the smaller blood-vessels are distended, hæmorrhages occur in the gray matter, there is marked perivascular infiltration, chiefly of lymphocytes, which collect about the vessels, forming definite foci. Sometimes the majority of the cells are polynuclear leucocytes. The ganglion cells, usually those of the anterior horns, degenerate and gradually disappear, changes probably secondary to the acute vascular alterations. Hyperæmia, œdema and infiltration are marked. In the fatal cases there are changes in the medulla and pons of much the same nature, but the ganglion cells rarely show such widespread destruction.

Symptoms.—The incubation period is from 3 to 10 days. In the pre-paralytic stage naso-pharyngeal symptoms are common. F. R. Fraser notes among the pre-paralytic symptoms, fever, drowsiness or heaviness, irritability, twitchings and jerkings, and gastro-intestinal symptoms. In 72 of 90 cases there was stiffness of the neck and back, and general tenderness (hyperæsthesia) on handling is not at all uncommon. More commonly a child who has gone to bed well awakens in the morning with the paralysis and slight fever. Prodromal symptoms are more common in the epidemic form.

The studies of recent years have shown a number of well-characterized types, of which the following are the most important:

(*a*) Abortive Form.—In epidemics, just as in cerebro-spinal fever, there are cases of illness with the general symptoms of infection, and indications of cerebro-spinal irritation, but without any motor disturbances. The symptoms pass away and the nature of the trouble remains doubtful, nor would suspicion be aroused were it not for the existence of other cases. It is interesting to note that Anderson and Frost have shown the presence of specific immune bodies in the blood of these cases.

(*b*) Common Polio-myletic or Spinal Form.—There is paresis before the paralysis or the paralysis is abrupt in its onset, reaches its maximum in a very short time, showing the irregularity and lack of symmetry which is characteristic. The legs are involved much more often than the arms. Paralysis of the trunk muscles occurs often. One or both arms may be affected, or one arm and one leg, or both legs, or it may be the right leg and left arm, or vice versa. In the arm the paralysis is rarely complete, the upper-arm muscles may be most affected or the lower-arm group; muscles acting functionally together, with centres near each other in the spinal cord, are paralyzed together. Careful examination usually shows some degree of weakness to be more widespread than appears at first sight. Disturbances of sensation are common. In this type the bladder and rectum are rarely involved.

(*c*) Progressive Ascending Form.—A certain number of cases, particularly in epidemics, run a course similar to Landry's paralysis, with which, no doubt, some of them have been confounded. The disease begins in the legs with the usual initial symptoms, the paralysis extends upward, involving the arms and the trunk, and death may occur with bulbar symptoms from the third to the fifth day. In the Swedish epidemic of 1905 of the 159 cases which died within the first two weeks, 45 presented this type.

(*d*) Bulbar Form.—It has long been known that occasionally in the ordinary spinal paralysis of children the cerebral nerves are involved, but in the epidemic form the disease may begin with paralysis of the ocular, facial, lingual, or pharyngeal muscles. The patient has fever, and the local picture depends upon the extent and distribution of the lesions in the medulla and pons. In the 1905 Swedish epidemic there were 34 cases in which the cerebral nerves were alone involved, and in the New York epidemic this localization was not very uncommon. A fatal result may follow extension of the bulbar symptoms.

(*e*) Meningitic Form.—This is important, as the cases simulate closely and are apt to be mistaken for cerebro-spinal fever. The picture is one of an acute meningitis—headache, pain and stiffness in the neck, vomiting, pain and rigidity in the back, drowsiness and unconsciousness. The disease may begin with the paralytic features and subsequently show the meningeal complications. Convulsions and Kernig's sign may be present. A serious difficulty is that the two diseases may prevail together, and only the careful examination of the cerebro-spinal fluid may give a differential diagnosis.

(*f*) Cerebral Form.—Here the picture is that which we have learned to recognize as the acute encephalitis or polio-encephalitis of children, a description of which we owe to von Strümpell. The disease sets in suddenly, with fever, vomiting and convulsions, followed by paralysis of one side of the body or one limb. Many of the patients die, others recover and present the usual after-picture of the cerebral hemiplegia of children. A large proportion of the cases of this disease probably represent this type of the sporadic form of acute infectious polio-myelo-encephalitis.

(*g*) Polyneuritic Form.—Many cases of the ordinary type and a majority of the sporadic form are painless. It is one of the features of the epidemic form that the patients complain much more of pain. This is particularly the case in a form which simulates a polyneuritis. There is loss of the tendon reflexes and disturbance of sensation. There is pain in the affected limbs, particularly on movement, with tenderness on pressure along the nerves and on pressing the muscles; the paralysis may extend like neuritis, involving chiefly the peripheral extensor muscle groups, and be followed by rapid wasting.

(*h*) Transverse Myelitic Form.—Following slight fever and indisposition, the features may be those of a transverse myelitis, a complete flaccid paraplegia. Of two cases of this type in young adults, in one recovery was complete, and in the other with a very small amount of residual paralysis.

Anomalous forms and symptoms are common during an epidemic. The muscles of respiration may be involved early, the diaphragm alone may be paralyzed, or the intercostals or the muscles of the palate and pharynx. Involvement of the facial muscles, usually a slight weakness, may be present, but in 5 out of 90 cases studied by F. R. Fraser the facial muscles alone were involved. In one instance ptosis was the only paralytic symptom on admission. Remarkable types may occur quite unlike the classical picture. In one case there was paralysis of one side of the soft palate with slight fever; the serum of this patient protected a monkey from intra-cerebral injection of the polio-myelitic virus. There may be slight fever with general spasticity of the muscles and tremor or rigidity of the muscles with coma.

Spinal Fluid.—This usually shows increase both in amount and pressure; it may be clear or slightly hazy. There is an increase in the number of cells, which may be from 15 or 20 up to 1200 per c. mm. The largest number are usually mononuclears; occasionally there is a larger number of polynuclears found early. The albumin and globulin are usually slightly or moderately increased. Fehling's solution is generally reduced as promptly as by the normal fluid. The Wassermann reaction may be the only means of diagnosing the condition from syphilis.

Course.—After the acute features have subsided there is little change for two or three weeks, after which improvement begins. This may continue for two or three months. The residual paralysis is usually less than seemed probable at first. The atrophy becomes evident in a few weeks from the onset of the attack. The affected limbs show less development as the patient grows older, and the deformity is usually most marked in the leg. The reaction of degeneration is present in the atrophied muscles. Early in the course the muscles lose the faradic response.

Diagnosis.—In the ordinary spinal sporadic cases there is rarely any difficulty. An important point to remember is that in periods of epidemic prevalence the disease presents an extraordinary number of clinical types. Some cases run a course like an acute infection, others have the picture of Landry's paralysis, in others again meningeal symptoms predominate, or there may be hyperæsthesia and pain, with the picture of a polyneuritis.

It seems not improbable that some obscure cases of meningitis are really instances of sporadic poliomyelitis. The same may be said of the acute encephalitis in children causing hemiplegia. The extraordinary complexity of the symptoms makes the diagnosis very difficult, so that the examination of the spinal fluid is important.

The diagnosis from peripheral neuritis may be very difficult; in both the paralysis is of the legs, with wasting, loss of reflexes, and the bladder and rectum may be involved. Loss of the vibrating sensation tested with a large tuning fork is more common in peripheral neuritis, and later the electrical changes and the action of degeneration may be distinctive.

Prognosis.—The mortality varies greatly in different epidemics. It was 27 per cent. in New York City in 1916. The fatal cases are usually of the ascending, bulbar and meningeal types. As regards the muscles, complete loss of response to faradism means severe atrophy. If it is never completely lost the outlook is good and even extensive paralyses may disappear. The prognosis for the paralysis is not easy to determine. Formerly, we thought it almost the rule that residual paralysis would remain if any large number of muscle groups were involved, but cases of very severe and widespread involvement may recover gradually and completely.

Prophylaxis.—The disease has been made notifiable. The patient should be isolated, the discharges and articles used by patients and nurses carefully disinfected, and special care should be taken of the nasal and pharyngeal discharges. It does not seem necessary to enforce a quarantine against those who come into relation with the patients, but the throat and nose of such persons should be disinfected with a menthol spray. There is some warrant for the administration of prophylactic doses of hexamine.

Treatment.—Hexamine may be given in doses of gr. v to xv (0.3 to 1 gm.).

When the fever is high the general treatment is that of an acute infection. The serum of those who have recovered has been used, possibly with benefit if given early. Sedatives for the pain may be given. Lumbar puncture has been advised, and if the pressure is found to be high it should be repeated. The intraspinous injection of epinephrine has been tried but without much effect. The affected limb should be wrapped in cotton wool, and placed in the position of least strain, and, if there is much pain, local sedative applications may be used. In the meningeal type of the disease warm baths and hot packs will be helpful. In the early stages it is well not to attempt to do much to the muscles, but within ten days careful massage may be practised, using either lanolin or sweet oil. Strychnine hypodermically has been extensively used, but how far it has any influence may be questioned. It should not be given early. Electricity may be used and it has a value in keeping up the nutrition of the muscles. The faradic current should be employed if there is response, if not, the galvanic. The damage always looks to be much worse than it really is, as many of the symptoms depend on meningeal and vascular changes which undergo resolution. Fatigue is harmful and should be guarded against for many months.

The muscle itself as a factor has been emphasized by William MacKenzie of Melbourne (Brit. Med. Jour. 1915, i) as biologically it is all important in treatment. The disease really destroys muscle adjustments, and one of the first things to do is to place the muscle at physiological rest in the zero position, in which it is itself relaxed, and both its own action, and that of its opponent prevented. Massage, he urges, should not be given too early, until, for example, the patient can elevate the upper limb when sitting up, and the heel when lying on the back. Persistent gradual re-education of the muscles yields remarkable results. Passive movements may be used and with toys a child may be encouraged to use the muscles of any group which still act. The treatment of residual deformities is a question of orthopædic surgery.

II. EPIDEMIC ENCEPHALITIS

(*Encephalitis lethargica; Epidemic stupor; Epidemic polio-encephalitis; Infective encephalitis*)

Definition.—An infectious disease, with protean manifestations, chiefly in the central nervous system, characterised by lethargy, paralysis of the cranial nerves (usually the third), and in some cases, spinal and neuritic features.

History.—There are records of outbreaks suggesting this disease in 1712 in Germany and in 1890 in parts of southern Europe (to which the name Nona was given). Cases occurred in Austria in 1917 and in England in the spring of 1918 with unusual cerebral features, a drowsiness passing into lethargy, progressive muscular weakness, and ophthalmoplegia. At first these were regarded as cases of botulism. The disease was widely spread, only a few cases occurring in each locality, sometimes two or three in the same house. The disease was recognized in the United States about the end of 1918.

Etiology.—Males and females are attacked in about equal numbers. In striking contrast to polio-myelitis, the disease is more common after the age of twenty. Of 100 cases of each disease analysed by James, 39.6 per cent.

of the encephalitis patients were over the age of twenty, while 79.2 per cent. of the polio-myelitis patients were under this age. Of the encephalitis patients, 15 per cent. were above the age of fifty. It is important to note that during this outbreak there was no increase of cases of polio-myelitis, either general or in the neighborhoods where the encephalitis prevailed. The nature of the virus has not been determined; the disease apparently has been successfully transmitted to monkeys.

Pathology.—In 40 cases investigated by Macintosh, the changes were chiefly in the upper part of the pons and in the basal nuclei, consisting of peri-vascular infiltration, with large and small mononuclear lymphocytes, chiefly those of small and medium size. The areas of extra-vascular infiltration may form actual foci visible to the naked eye. A striking feature was the absence of destruction of the ganglion cells so characteristic of polio-myelitis. The Noguchi-Flexner bodies, found in polio-myelitis, have not been found. Cortical lesions, such as occur in Strümpell's *polio-encephalitis superior,* have not been found, nor were there extensive lesions of the gray matter, though Marinesco found changes in the cells of Purkinje. Altogether the anatomical lesions are like those found in rabies and sleeping sickness. The spinal cord lesions have been very slight. Comparing the lesions with those in acute polio-myelitis, there is some similarity.

The disease is apparently distinct from the acute *encephalitis superior* of Strümpell. Whatever the etiology may be, the outbreak presents new features. All agree that similar clinical features had not been seen, at any rate, in such numbers. The question is complicated by the occurrence of many cases in soldiers of an acute febrile disease with the features of polyneuritis, but occasionally with bulbar and cerebral symptoms, and anatomical changes not unlike those present in *endemic encephalitis* and in polio-myelitis. Some of these are only special localizations of polio-myelitis. The lethargy may be toxic but is possibly mechanical due to interruption of stimuli in the thalamus, which is frequently involved.

Clinical Features.—The clinical picture is new, particularly the combination of lethargy with third nerve and facial paralysis, and perhaps weakness of the extremities. MacNulty groups the clinical forms into: (1) Cases with general features but without localizing signs. (2) Cases with third nerve paralysis. (3) Cases with facial paralysis. (4) Cases with spinal manifestations. (5) Cases with polyneuritic manifestations. In 2, 3, 4 and 5 there are general disturbances of the central nervous system. (6) Cases with mild or transient manifestations (so-called "abortive" cases). To these should be added cases of paralysis of other nerves than those mentioned.

The incubation period is variable and uncertain. Prodromal symptoms range from a few hours to a week, and are chiefly headache, lethargy, stiffness in the back, diffuse pains, and catarrhal features. Among the early symptoms conjunctivitis is noted, and tonsillitis with headache and giddiness.

Lethargy, present in 80 per cent. of the cases, comes on as a rule gradually, occasionally very suddenly, and is sometimes not more than a stupor and heaviness, from which the patient can easily be roused, the so-called "anergic apathy," but in others it is a much deeper stupor, passing into coma. Ocular palsies occur early, with diplopia and double ptosis. Combined with the stupor, this makes a very characteristic picture. The fever ranges from 100°

to 104°, and rarely lasts more than four or five days to a week. It may drop at the end of three or four days and then recur. There is nothing peculiar in the pulse rate or respiration. As the disease progresses, the patient presents a dull apathetic look. The wrinkles are smoothed, the muscles of the face may be moved with great difficulty, or there may be definite bilateral facial paralysis. The pupils are dilated, perhaps unequal, with complete third nerve paralysis. The arms are flexed, and catalepsy is not uncommon. When roused the patient may answer simple questions intelligently. Active delirium may be present. One patient in the fourth week of the disease had violent mania and then recovered rapidly. The speech may be blurred and difficult; this depends on the degree of involvement of the facial muscles. Tremors, twitchings, and marked choreiform movements may occur, and persist long into convalescence.

Sensory disturbances are rare. There may be pain, particularly on pressure of the muscles, and there is sometimes hyperæsthesia. Paralysis of the arms and legs may occur, either alone or with bulbar involvement. As a rule, the reflexes are normal, except when there is paraplegia; the knee-jerks may be abolished for a time. Sphincter features are sometimes present. Dysphagia has been recorded in a number of cases.

The general features may be present without local paralysis, which seems more common in children. Other cases present the third nerve paralysis alone or with facial paralysis, or facial paralysis on one side or both with general weakness of the extremities. There are cases with early ataxia combined with ocular paralysis. Lastly, a certain number of cases (seven in MacNulty's series), all in adults, showed signs of polyneuritis in addition to the bulbar features. Mild or abnormal types, with slight lethargy, slight ataxia, headache and transient facial paralysis are rare. One patient had unusual drowsiness with an ataxia so marked that he was thought to be drunk. He was not ill enough to be in bed, and the symptoms passed off within ten days.

Signs suggestive of meningeal involvement are rare. The cerebro-spinal fluid is, as a rule, clear with 10 to 20 cells per c. mm. (rarely 100 cells), the globulin little, if at all, increased. Mononuclear and polymorphonuclear cells are found.

The duration is variable, from two to ten or twelve weeks. Out of 168 cases 37 died, the majority with bulbar features. Of sequels the most serious are residual palsies which resemble those of polio-myelitis. Muscular tremors or definite athetosis may persist.

Diagnosis.—Typical cases offer no difficulty. Special watch should be kept for the cranial paralysis which in mild cases may be of short duration. The following conditions deserve mention: (1) Polio-myelitis. The similarity may be marked but the spinal fluid usually shows more marked changes in this disease. (2) Psychoses characterized by stupor, lethargy or catalepsy. (3) Tuberculous meningitis in which the spinal fluid findings are not characteristic. (4) Acute syphilitic meningo-encephalitis and endarteritis. (5) Botulism. (6) Cerebral hæmorrhage or thrombosis may be simulated by some cases of encephalitis. (7) Status epilepticus. (8) Uræmia. (9) Other forms of encephalitis.

Treatment.—The patient should be isolated and carefully nursed, care being taken to avoid bed sores; nasal and rectal feeding may be required and special care should be taken to keep the mouth and throat clean. Lumbar puncture often relieves the headache. Drugs are not indicated.

F. MYELITIS

I. ACUTE MYELITIS

Etiology.—Acute myelitis affecting the cord in a limited or extended portion—the gray matter chiefly, or the gray and white matter together, is met with: (*a*) As an independent affection following exposure to cold, or exertion, and leading to rapid loss of power with the symptoms of an acute ascending paralysis. Some of these cases are unusually widespread acute forms of polio-myelitis. There is also an acute hæmorrhagic form with high fever (Burley), the relation of which to other forms is uncertain. (*b*) As a sequel of the infectious diseases, such as small-pox, typhus, measles, and gonorrhœa. (*c*) As a result of traumatism, either fracture of the spine or very severe muscular effort. Concussion without fracture may produce it, but this is rare. Acute myelitis, for instance, scarcely ever follows railway accidents. (*d*) In diseases of the bones of the spine, either caries or cancer. This is a more common cause of localized acute transverse myelitis than of the diffuse affection. (*e*) In disease of the cord itself, such as tumors and syphilis; in the latter, either in association with gummata, in which case it is usually a late manifestation; or it may follow within a year or eighteen months of the primary affection.

Morbid Anatomy.—In localized acute myelitis affecting white and gray matter, as met with after accident or an acute compression, the cord is swollen, the pia injected, the consistence greatly reduced, and on incising the membrane an almost diffluent material may escape. In less intense grades, on section at the affected area, the distinction between the gray and white matter is lost, or is extremely indistinct. There are cases with the appearances of an acute hæmorrhagic myelitis.

Symptoms.—(*a*) Acute Diffuse Myelitis.—This form is in the epidemic polio-myelitis, or occurs in connection with syphilis or one of the infectious diseases, or is seen in a typical manner in the extension from injuries or from tumor. The onset, though scarcely so abrupt as in hæmorrhage, may be sudden; a person may be attacked on the street and have difficulty in getting home. In some instances, the onset is preceded by pains in the legs or back, or a girdle sensation is present. It may be marked by chills, occasionally by convulsions; fever is usually present from the beginning—at first slight, but subsequently it may become high.

The *motor* functions are rapidly lost, sometimes as quickly as in Landry's ascending paralysis. The paraplegia may be complete, and, if the myelitis extends to the cervical region, there may be impairment of motion, and ultimately complete loss of power in the upper extremities as well. The sensation is lost, but there may at first be hyperæsthesia. The *reflexes* in the initial stage are increased, but in acute central myelitis, unless limited in extent to the thoracic and cervical regions, the reflexes are usually abolished. The rectum and bladder are paralyzed. Trophic disturbances are marked; the muscles waste rapidly; the skin is often congested, and there may be localized sweating. The temperature of the affected limbs may be lowered. Acute bed-sores may occur over the sacrum or on the heels, and sometimes a multiple arthritis is present. In these acute cases the general symptoms become greatly aggravated, the pulse is rapid, the tongue becomes dry; there is delirium, the fever increases, and may reach 107° or 108° F.

The course of the disease is variable. In very acute cases death follows in from five to ten days. The cases following the infectious diseases, particularly the fevers and sometimes syphilis, may run a milder course.

The *diagnosis* of this variety is rarely difficult. In common with the acute ascending paralysis of Landry, and with certain cases of multiple neuritis, it presents a rapid and progressive motor paralysis. From the former it is distinguished by more marked involvement of sensation, trophic disturbances, paralysis of bladder and rectum, rapid wasting, electrical changes, and fever. From acute cases of *multiple neuritis* it may be more difficult to distinguish, as the sensory features may be marked, though there is rarely, if ever, in multiple neuritis complete anæsthesia; the wasting, moreover, is more rapid in myelitis. The bladder and rectum are rarely involved—though in exceptional cases they may be—and, most important of all, the trophic changes, the development of bullæ, bed-sores, etc., are not seen in multiple neuritis.

(*b*) Acute Transverse Myelitis.—The symptoms naturally differ with the situation of the lesion.

(1) Acute transverse myelitis in the *thoracic region*, the most common situation, produces a very characteristic picture. The symptoms of onset are variable. There may be initial pains or numbness and tingling in the legs. The paralysis may set in quickly and become complete within a few days; but more commonly it is preceded for a day or two by sensations of pain, heaviness, and dragging in the legs. The paralysis of the lower limbs is usually complete, and if at the level, say, of the sixth thoracic vertebra, the abdominal muscles are involved. Sensation may be partially or completely lost. At the onset there may be numbness, tingling, or even hyperæsthesia in the legs. At the level of the lesion there is often a zone of hyperæsthesia. A girdle sensation may occur early, and when the lesion is in this situation it is usually felt between the ensiform and umbilical regions. The reflexes are variable. There may at first be abolition; subsequently, those which pass through the segments lower than the one affected may be exaggerated and the legs may take on a condition of spastic rigidity. It does not always happen, however, that the reflexes are increased here, for in a total transverse lesion of the cord they are usually entirely lost, as pointed out by Bastian. That this is not due to the preliminary shock is shown by the fact that the abolition may be permanent. The muscles become extremely flabby, waste, and lose their faradic excitability, and the sphincters lose their tone. The temperature of the paralyzed limbs is variable. It may at first rise, then fall and become subnormal. Lesions of the skin are not uncommon, and bed-sores are apt to form. There is at first retention of urine and subsequently spastic incontinence. If the lumbar centres are involved, there are vesical symptoms from the outset. The urine is alkaline in reaction and may rapidly become ammoniacal. The bowels are constipated and there is usually incontinence of

fæces. Some writers attribute the cystitis associated with transverse myelitis to disturbed trophic influence.

The course of complete transverse myelitis depends upon its cause. Death may result from extension. Segments of the cord may be completely and permanently destroyed, in which case there is persistent paraplegia. The pyramidal fibres below the lesion undergo the secondary degeneration, and there is an ascending degeneration of the dorsal median columns. If the lower segments of the cord are involved the legs may remain flaccid. In some instances a transverse myelitis of the thoracic region involves the ventral horns above and below the lesion, producing flaccidity of the muscles, with wasting, fibrillary contractions, and the reaction of degeneration. More commonly, however, in the cases which last many months there is more or less rigidity of the muscles with spasm or persistent contraction of the flexors of the knee.

(2) *Transverse Myelitis of the Cervical Region.*—If the lesion is at the level of the sixth or seventh cervical nerves, there is paralysis of the upper extremities, more or less complete, sometimes sparing the muscles of the shoulder. Gradually there is loss of sensation. The paralysis is usually complete below the point of lesion, but there are rare instances in which the arms only are affected, the so-called cervical paraplegia. In addition to the symptoms already mentioned there are several which are more characteristic of transverse myelitis in the cervical region, such as the occurrence of vomiting, hiccough, and slow pulse, which may sink to 20 or 30, pupillary changes—myosis—sometimes attacks of dysphagia, dyspnœa, or syncope.

Treatment of Acute Myelitis.—In the rapidly advancing form due either to a diffuse inflammation in the gray matter or to transverse myelitis, the important measures are scrupulous cleanliness, care and watchfulness in guarding against bed-sores, and the avoidance of cystitis. In an acute onset in a healthy subject the spine may be cupped. Counter-irritation is of doubtful advantage. Chapman's ice-bag is sometimes useful. No drugs have the slightest influence upon an acute myelitis, except in subjects with well-marked syphilis, in which case mercury and potassium iodide should be given energetically. Tonic remedies, such as quinine, arsenic, and strychnia, may be used in the later stages. When the muscles have wasted, massage is beneficial in maintaining their nutrition. The patient should make every effort to perform muscular movements himself and thus aid improvement. Electricity should not be used in the early stages. It is of no value in the transverse myelitis in the thoracic region with retention of the nutrition in the muscles of the leg.

II. ACUTE ASCENDING (LANDRY'S) PARALYSIS

Definition.—An acute ascending flaccid paralysis without the anatomical changes of polio-myelitis or polyneuritis. Whether or not there is a disease conforming to this definition, after excluding the neuritic and myelitic cases, remains to be determined.

Etiology and Pathology.—The disease occurs most commonly in males between the twentieth and thirtieth years. It has followed the specific fevers and various organisms have been isolated. There is a form of the epidemic polio-myelitis which has an acute course and a clinical picture similar to Landry's paralysis. It has been suggested that this disease always represents the sporadic variety. Spiller in a rapidly fatal case found destructive changes in the peripheral nerves and corresponding alterations in the cell bodies of the ventral horns. He suggests that the toxic agent acts on the lower motor neurones as a whole, and that possibly the reason why no lesions were found in some of the cases is that the more delicate histological methods were not used. The view that it is a functional disorder is supported by the study of cases in which no lesion has been found.

Symptoms.—Weakness of the legs, gradually progressing, often with tolerable rapidity, is the first symptom. In some cases within a few hours the paralysis of the legs becomes complete. The muscles of the trunk are next affected, and within a few days, or even less in more acute cases, the arms are also involved. The neck muscles are next attacked, and finally the muscles of respiration, deglutition, and articulation. The reflexes are lost, but the muscles neither waste nor show electrical changes. The sensory symptoms are variable; in some cases tingling, numbness, and hyperæsthesia have been present. In the more characteristic cases sensation is intact and the sphincters are uninvolved. Enlargement of the spleen has been noted. Bulbar symptoms may be early and there are cases in which the picture has been of acute *descending* paralysis. The course of the disease is variable. It may prove fatal in less than two days. Other cases persist for a week or for two weeks. In a large proportion of the cases the disease is fatal. One patient was kept alive for 41 days by artificial respiration (C. L. Greene).

Diagnosis.—The diagnosis is difficult, particularly from certain forms of multiple neuritis, and if we include in Landry's paralysis the cases in which sensation is involved distinction between the two affections is impossible. We apparently have to recognize the existence of a rapidly advancing motor paralysis without involvement of the sphincters, without wasting or electrical changes in the muscles, without trophic lesions, and without fever—features sufficient to distinguish it from either the acute central myelitis or the polio-myelitis anterior. It is doubtful, however, whether these characters always suffice to enable us to differentiate the cases of multiple neuritis. The cases of acute polio-myelitis with the picture of an acute ascending paralysis should not be difficult to recognize during the progress of an epidemic.

III. DEGENERATIVE MYELITIS

I. COMBINED POSTERO-LATERAL SCLEROSIS

(Ataxic Paraplegia (Gowers); Subacute Ataxic Paraplegia (Russell, Batten and Collier); Primary Combined Sclerosis (J. J. Putnam); Toxic Combined Sclerosis.)

Definition.—A disorder with symptoms referable to degeneration of the posterior and lateral columns of the cord, occasionally occurring without obvious cause, but most commonly an associated lesion of the cachexias, anæmias, chronic toxæmias and prolonged sub-infections.

Etiology.—Excluding syphilis, the cause no doubt of many of the cases in male adults which we formerly called ataxic paraplegia, and excluding multiple sclerosis, the cause of many of the cases described in women, there are two groups:

I. A rare and doubtful *Primary Combined Sclerosis* in which in adult males without lues or obvious cause the symptoms of ataxia and spastic paraplegia are present.

II. The Secondary Combined Sclerosis associated with:

(a) Chronic ill-health in women, as in the form described by J. J. Putnam.

(b) Anæmia, as described by Russell, Batten and Collier.

(c) The toxæmias—ergot, lead and pellagra.

(d) The cachexias—cancer, tuberculosis, diabetes, etc.

The *anatomical* features, a degenerative myelitis, are a sclerosis of the dorsal columns, which is not more marked in the lumbar region and not specially localized in the root zone of the cuneate fasciculi. The involvement of the lateral columns is diffuse, not always limited to the pyramidal tracts, and there may be an annular sclerosis.

Symptoms.—The patient complains of a tired feeling in the legs, not often of actual pain. The sensory symptoms of true tabes are absent. An unsteadiness in the gait gradually comes on with progressive weakness. The reflexes are increased from the outset, and there may be well marked ankle clonus. Rigidity of the legs comes on slowly, but it is rarely extreme as in the uncomplicated cases of lateral sclerosis. From the onset incoördination is a well characterized feature, and the difficulty of walking in the dark, or swaying when the eyes are closed, may, as in true tabes, be the first symptom to attract attention. In walking the patient uses a stick, keeps the eyes fixed on the ground, the legs far apart, but the stamping gait, with elevation and sudden descent of the feet, is not often seen. The incoördination may extend to the arms. Sensory symptoms are rare, but Gowers called attention to a dull, aching pain in the sacral region. The sphincters usually become involved. Eye symptoms are rare. Late in the disease mental symptoms may occur, similar to those of general paresis.

In the *secondary* variety there may be few or no symptoms in patients long bed-ridden (Lichtheim, Bramwell). In Putnam's group, in which 30 of 51 were women, paræsthesia was an early and permanent feature, and the same occurs in the anæmic and cachectic forms. When fully developed there are (1) muscular hypotony, (2) loss of the knee-jerks, and (3) ataxia, due to involvement of the posterior columns; or (1) muscular hypertony, (2) exaggerated deep reflexes and positive Babinski sign, and (3) motor weakness due to degeneration of the pyramidal tracts (L. F. Barker). In the late stages the bladder and rectum may be involved. Pupil changes are rare. It is a curious thing that a severe anæmia may follow, not precede, the signs of cord disease.

Diagnosis.—Syphilis in middle aged adults must be excluded and disseminated sclerosis, which may cause a similar clinical picture. The spastic-ataxic gait is a marked feature.

Treatment.—This offers little beyond general measures. Any primary condition should receive the treatment indicated.

"Central Neuritis."—This name has been given by Scott to a disease in adults occurring in Jamaica, which perhaps belongs here. The early features are inflammation of the eyes, and later changes in the mouth followed by diarrhœa or marked changes in the nervous system. In the latter the first symptoms are sensory disturbances in the feet and legs, followed by incoordination and loss of control over the legs. The knee-jerks are absent. Death usually occurred from inanition with diarrhœa and true paralysis does not occur. In those who recovered there is disturbance of vision, deafness and a peculiar steppage gait. Histologically the nervous system showed general changes, perivascular infiltration, degeneration and fibrosis. The disease suggests some form of toxæmia. The term "central neuritis" was given by Adolf Meyer to a "parenchymatous systemic degeneration, mainly in the nervous system," found in alcoholic, senile and cachectic states, and in depressive psychoses at the time of involution. The features are fever, diarrhœa, emaciation, twitching and rigidity of the extremities, and changed reflexes. Mentally there is an anxious agitation with delirium or stupor.

II. SENILE SPASTIC PARALYSIS

Unlike the Deacon's "Wonderful One-Hoss Shay," the wear and tear incident to daily use tells more on one part of the machine than another. Like Dean Swift "Some go at the top first, others in their legs, others again in both simultaneously." While the whole nervous system may show decay—"the golden bowl broken and the silver cord loosened"—an early sign of old age is the lessening of the control over the muscles, evidenced by tremor and inability to perform the finer movements with the same precision. The gait becomes tottering, the steps uncertain, and at last the use of the legs is lost for purposes of walking, though every muscle group may be put in action. Or one may watch the gradual onset of a spastic paraplegia—a progressive weakness of legs with spasticity and greatly increased reflexes. The steps are short, the feet not lifted from the ground, and the gait uncertain; yet in many cases the strength of the muscles is maintained, and the patient may "keep on his legs" for years. The sphincters are not, as a rule, affected. Arteriosclerosis is usually present and in premature senility the vessels of the legs may be very stiff and the dorsal arteries of the feet obliterated. Typical intermittent claudication may precede the paraplegia.

IV. COMPRESSION OF THE SPINAL CORD

(*Compression Myelitis*)

Definition.—Interruption of the functions of the cord by slow compression.

Etiology.—Caries of the spine, new growths, aneurism, and parasites are the important causes of slow compression. Caries, or Pott's disease, as it is usually called, after the surgeon who first described it, is in a majority of instances tuberculous and associated with angular curvature. The involvement of the cord is due to pachymeningitis externa, to abscess, or in rare cases to direct spicules of bone. There may be a tuberculous pachymeningitis without caries. The paraplegia in Pott's disease without any spinal deformity is difficult to recognize, and is usually associated with pressure of tuberculous material inside the dura. The paraplegia may be due to a secondary myelitis. In a few cases it is due to syphilis and occasionally to extension of disease from the pharynx. It is most common in early life, but may occur after middle age. It may follow trauma. Compression may result from aneurism of the thoracic aorta or the abdominal aorta, in the neighborhood of the cœliac axis. Malignant growths frequently cause a compression paraplegia. A retroperitoneal sarcoma or the growths of Hodgkin's disease may invade the vertebræ. More commonly the involvement is secondary to scirrhus of the breast. Of parasites, the echinococcus and the cysticercus may occur in the spinal canal.

Symptoms.—These may be considered as they affect the bones, the nerves, and the cord.

VERTEBRAL.—In malignant diseases and in aneurism erosion of the bodies may take place without producing deformity of the spine. Fatal hæmorrhage may follow erosion of the vertebral artery. In caries, on the other hand, it is the rule to find more or less deformity, amounting often to angular curvature. The compression of the cord, however, is rarely if ever the direct result of this bony kyphosis but is due to thickening of the dura and the presence of caseous and inflammatory products between this membrane and the bodies of the diseased vertebræ. The spinous processes of the affected vertebræ are tender on pressure, and pain follows jarring movements or twisting of the spine. There may be extensive tuberculous disease without much deformity, particularly in the cervical region. In the case of aneurism or tumor pain is a constant and agonizing feature.

NERVE-ROOT SYMPTOMS.—These result from compression of the nerve roots as they pass out between the vertebræ. In caries, even when the disease is extensive and the deformity great, radiating pains from compression involvement of the roots are rare. Pains are more common in cancer of the spine secondary to that of the breast, and in such cases may be agonizing. There may be acutely painful areas—the *anæsthesia dolorosa*—in regions of the skin which are anæsthetic to tactile and painful impressions. Trophic disturbances may occur, particularly herpes. Pressure on the ventral roots may give rise to wasting of the muscles supplied by the affected nerves. This is most noticeable in disease of the cervical or lumbar regions.

CORD SYMPTOMS.—(*a*) *Cervical Region.*—The caries may be between the axis and the atlas or between the latter and the occipital bone. In such instances a retropharyngeal abscess may be present, giving rise to difficulty in swallowing. There may be spasm of the cervical muscles, the head may be fixed, and movements may either be impossible or cause great pain. In a case of this kind in the Montreal General Hospital movement was liable to be followed by transient, instantaneous paralysis of all four extremities, owing to compression of the cord. In one of these attacks the patient died.

In the lower cervical region there may be signs of interference with the cilio-spinal centre and dilatation of the pupils. Occasionally there is flushing of the face and ear of one side of unilateral sweating. Deformity is not so common, but healing may take place with the production of a callus of enormous breadth, with complete rigidity of the neck.

(*b*) *Thoracic Region.*—The deformity is here more marked and pressure symptoms are more common. The time of onset of the paralysis varies very much. It may be an early symptom, even before the curvature is manifest, and it is noteworthy that Pott first described the disease that bears his name as "a palsy of the lower limbs which is frequently found to accompany a curvature of the spine." More commonly the paralysis is late, occurring many months after the curvature. The paraplegia is slow in its development; the patient at first feels weak in the legs or has disturbance of sensation, numbness, tingling, pins and needles. The girdle sensation may be marked, or severe pains in the course of the intercostal nerves. The legs are frequently drawn up, sometimes in spasm, the reflex spinal automatism. Motion is, as a rule, more quickly lost than sensation. The paraplegia is usually of the spastic type, with exaggeration of the reflexes. Bastian's symptom—abolition of the reflexes—is rarely met with in compression from caries as the transverse nature of the lesion is rarely complete. The paraplegia may persist for months, or even for more than a year, and recovery still be possible.

(*c*) *Lumbar Region.*—In the lower dorsal and lumbar regions the symptoms are practically the same, but the sphincter centres are involved and the reflexes are not exaggerated.

(*d*) *Old Lesions of Cord.*—Following trauma in Pott's disease the dura may be much thickened, the cord narrowed and embedded in cicatricial tissue.

Diagnosis.—The X-ray picture is of first importance. Caries is by far the most frequent cause of slow compression of the cord, and when there are external signs the recognition is easy. There are cases in which the exudation in the spinal canal between the dura and the bone leads to compression before there are any signs of caries, and if the root symptoms are absent it may be extremely difficult to arrive at a diagnosis. Persistent lumbago is a symptom of importance in masked Pott's disease, particularly after injury. Brown-Séquard's paralysis is more common in tumor and in injuries than in caries. Pressure on the nerve roots, too, is less frequent in caries than in malignant disease. The cervical form of pachymeningitis also produces a pressure paralysis. Following removal of the breast for carcinoma, at intervals of a year to ten or more years, recurrence in the vertebræ may cause pressure on the spinal nerves or on the cord itself. There may be no local recurrence. Neuralgic pains in the neck or back, or in the course of the sciatic, often associated with obscure nervous symptoms, suggesting hysteria, may be present for months before any signs of paralysis or of recurrence elsewhere. The persistence of the pains and their intensity should always arouse suspicion. Finally paraplegia may come on, not often with deformity, and the pains may be of terrible intensity, well deserving the name *paraplegia dolorosa.*

Treatment.—In compression by aneurism or metastatic tumors the condition is hopeless. In the former the pains are often not very severe, but in the latter morphia is always necessary. On the other hand, compression by caries is often successfully relieved even after the paralysis has persisted for a long period. When caries is recognized early, rest and support to the spine by various methods may do much to prevent the onset of paraplegia. When paralysis has occurred, rest with extension gives the best hope of recovery. It is to be remembered that restoration may occur after compression of the cord has lasted for many months, or even more than a year. Cases have been cured by recumbency alone, enforced for weeks or months; the extradural and inflammatory products are absorbed and the caries heals. In earlier days brilliant results were obtained in these cases by suspension, a method introduced by J. K. Mitchell in 1826, and pursued with remarkable success by his son, Weir Mitchell. In recent years the suspension methods in the erect posture have been largely superseded by those of hyperextension during recumbency with the application of plaster jackets to hold the body and spine immovable in the improved position. Forcible correction of the deformity under anæsthesia as sometimes advocated is not to be recommended; but the gentler partial corrections, perhaps repeated several times with a few weeks' interval, often lead to a rapid disappearance of paralyses through lessening of the deformity of the vertebræ. In protracted cases, after these methods have been given a fair trial, laminectomy may be advisable, and has in many instances been successful in relieving paralyses when bloodless methods have failed. In old traumatic lesions operation may be indicated for severe nerve-root pains. The general treatment of caries is that of tuberculosis.

G. DIFFUSE SCLEROSES

General Remarks.—The supporting tissue of the central nervous system is the neuroglia, derived from the ectoderm, with distinct morphological and chemical characters. The meninges are composed of true connective tissue derived from the mesoderm, a little of which enters the brain and cord with the blood-vessels. The neuroglia plays the chief part in pathological processes within the central nervous system, but changes in the connective tissue elements may also be important. A convenient division of the cerebro-spinal scleroses is into degenerative, inflammatory, and developmental forms.

The *degenerative scleroses* comprise the largest and most important subdivision, in which provisionally the following groups may be made: (*a*) The common secondary Wallerian degeneration which follows when nerve fibres are cut off from their trophic centres; (*b*) toxic forms, among which may be placed the scleroses from lead and ergot, and, most important of all, the scleroses of the dorsal columns, due in a large proportion of cases to syphilis; (*c*) the sclerosis associated with change in the smaller arteries and capillaries, met with as a senile process in the convolutions.

The *inflammatory scleroses* embrace a less important and less extensive group, comprising secondary forms which follow irritative inflammation about tumors, foreign bodies, hæmorrhages, and abscess. Possibly a similar change may follow the primary, acute encephalitis, which Strümpell holds is the initial lesion in the cortical sclerosis so commonly found post mortem in infantile hemiplegia.

The *developmental scleroses* are believed to be of a purely neurogliar character, and embrace the new growth about the central canal in syringomyelia and, according to French writers, the sclerosis of the dorsal columns in Friedreich's ataxia.

MULTIPLE (INSULAR: DISSEMINATED) SCLEROSIS

Definition.—A chronic affection of the brain and cord, characterized by localized areas in which the nerve elements are more or less replaced by neuroglia. This may occur in the brain or cord alone, more commonly in both.

ETIOLOGY.—It is most common in young persons and in females. Several members in a family may be attacked. It is much less common in the United States than in Great Britain; only 91 cases among 12,000 patients (Collins) against 159 among 2568 cases in three years at the National Hospital, London. The etiology is obscure; trauma, fatigue, cold, exposure, intoxications and infections have all been mentioned. The essential nature of the process has been much discussed—the result of the action of a toxic agent on the sheaths and axis cylinders, with secondary proliferation of the glia, a primary interstitial process, a multiple gliosis in which congenital influences play a part, a primary vascular disorder with secondary changes in the nervous and interstitial tissues, are among the prevailing views.

MORBID ANATOMY.—The sclerotic areas are widely distributed through the white and gray matter. The patches are most abundant in the neighborhood of the ventricles, and in the pons, cerebellum, basal ganglia and the medulla. The cord may be only slightly involved or there may be very many areas throughout its length. The cervical region is apt to be most affected. The nerve roots and the branches of the cauda equina are often attacked. There is a degeneration of the medullary sheaths, with the persistence for some time of the axis-cylinders which are thought by some to be new formed nerve fibres. There is marked proliferation of the neuroglia, the fibres of which are denser and firmer. Secondary degeneration, although relatively slight, does occur.

SYMPTOMS.—The onset is slow and the disease is chronic. The patients are often emotional or even hysterical. Attacks of transient paralysis, suggestive of hysteria, may precede the onset. Feebleness of the legs with irregular pains and stiffness are among the early symptoms. Indeed, a common clinical picture is that of spastic paraplegia. The following are the most important features:

(*a*) *Volitional or Intention Tremor.*—There is no weakness of the arms, but on attempting to pick up an object there is a trembling or rapid oscillation. A patient may be unable to lift even a glass of water to the mouth. The tremor may be marked in the legs, and in the head, which shakes as he walks. When the patient is recumbent the muscles may be perfectly quiet. On attempting to raise the head from the pillow, trembling at once comes on. (*b*) *Scanning Speech.*—The words are pronounced slowly and separately, or the individual syllables may be accentuated. This staccato or syllabic utterance is a common feature. (*c*) *Nystagmus,* a rapid oscillatory movement of both eyes, is more common in multiple sclerosis than any other affection of the nervous system.

Sensation is unaffected in the majority of the cases. Optic atrophy may occur early, but is usually partial, rarely leading to complete blindness. The sphincters, as a rule, are unaffected until the last stages. Mental debility is not uncommon. Remarkable remissions occur in the course of the disease, in which for a time all the symptoms may improve. Vertigo is common, and there may be sudden apoplectiform attacks, such as occur in general paresis. The presence of the extensor plantar reflex (Babinski sign) and the absence of the abdominal reflexes are common.

The symptoms, on the whole, are extraordinarily variable, corresponding to the very irregular distribution of the nodules.

DIAGNOSIS.—For the early diagnosis the three important symptoms are—loss of abdominal reflexes, weakness of the abdominal muscles and pallor of the temporal sides of the optic disks (L. F. Barker). Volitional tremor, scanning speech, and nystagmus form a characteristic symptom-group, but this classical triad is less common than the irregular forms which are very apt to escape recognition. Paralysis agitans, certain cases of general paresis, and occasionally hysteria may simulate the disease very closely. Of all organic diseases of the nervous system disseminated sclerosis in its early stages is that which is most commonly taken for hysteria (Buzzard, Sr.). The points to be relied upon in the differentiation are, in order of importance, optic atrophy, the nystagmus, the bladder disturbances, when present, and the volitional tremor. The tremor in hysteria is not volitional but the diseases may co-exist. Unilateral cases are recorded. If the case is not seen until near the end the diagnosis may be impossible.

Pseudo-sclerosis—the Westphall-Strümpell disease—is a rare condition simulating multiple sclerosis and not often distinguished from it during life. Mental changes are more pronounced, the tremor is more exaggerated, the nystagmus not always present, and the gait more ataxic. It sets in earlier, sometimes in the first decade, and in a majority of the cases no lesions have been found post mortem.

The PROGNOSIS is unfavorable. Ultimately, the patient, if not carried off by some intercurrent affection, becomes bedridden. In 200 cases the average duration was twelve years; 3 recovered (Bramwell).

TREATMENT.—No known treatment has any influence on the progress of sclerosis of the brain. Neither the iodides nor mercury have the slightest effect, but a prolonged course of arsenic may be tried. Avoidance of fatigue, physical and mental, is important. In acute stages there should be absolute rest. Benefit has resulted from opening the spinal canal (Elsberg).

Miliary sclerosis is a term which has been applied to several different conditions. Gowers mentions a case in which there were grayish red spots at the junction of the white and gray matters, and in which the neuroglia was increased. There is also a condition in which, on the surface of the convolutions, there are small nodular projections, varying from a half to five or more millimetres in diameter.

Diffuse sclerosis, which may involve an entire hemisphere, or a single lobe, in which case the term *sclérose lobaire* has been applied to it by the French. It is not an important condition in general practice, but occurs most frequently in idiots and imbeciles. In extensive cortical sclerosis of one hemisphere the ventricle is usually dilated. The symptoms of this condition depend upon the region affected. There may be a considerable extent of sclerosis without symptoms or much mental impairment. In a majority of cases there is hemiplegia or diplegia with imbecility or idiocy.

Tuberose Sclerosis.—Described by Bourneville in feeble-minded children, and regarded as a pathological curiosity, the researches of Vogt, Wolback, Fowler and Dickson and others have shown it to be a definite type of disease, which may sometimes be recognized clinically. Imbecility and epilepsy are present, without, as a rule, paralysis. Anatomically there are remarkable tuberous tumors, embedded in the cortex cerebri, ranging in size from a pea to a walnut, white in color, and of a stony hardness. There is an overgrowth of the neuroglia and of large ganglionic cells. A remarkable peculiarity, which sometimes enables the disease to be recognized, is the occurrence of congenital tumors in other organs, heart, kidneys and skin. Adenoma sebaceum of the face, small, closely-set growths about the nose and cheeks, often with a vascular matrix, is the most common. Renal tumors were found in 19 of 29 cases.

H. DIFFUSE AND FOCAL DISEASES OF THE SPINAL CORD

I. TOPICAL DIAGNOSIS

From the symptoms presented by a spinal cord lesion it is possible to determine more or less accurately not only the level but also the transverse extent of the segmental involvement. The effects of an injury or of disease may be circumscribed and involve the gray matter of the segment or the tracts running through it; it may be more extensive and involve the cord in a given level in its entire transverse extent; finally, there are cases in which only one lateral half of the cord is implicated. It is well for the student to have a definite routine to follow in making his examinations, for each factor may be helpful in determining the site and character of the lesion. Some of the more important points to observe are the following: (1) *subjective sensations,* particularly the character and seat of pain, if any be present, such as the radiating pains of dorsal root compression; (2) the patient's *attitude,* as the position of the arms in cervical lesions, the character of the respiration, whether diaphragmatic, etc.; (3) *motor symptoms,* the groups of paralyzed muscles and their electrical reaction; (4) the *sensory symptoms,* including tests for tactual, thermic, and painful impressions, for muscle sense, bone sensation, etc.; (5) the condition of the *reflexes,* both the tendon and the skin reflexes as well as those of the pupil, the bladder and rectum, etc.; (6) the surface temperature and condition of moisture or dryness of the skin, which gives an indication of *vaso-motor* paralysis. The table on pages 891-893 and the figures on pages 898 and 899 will be useful while making an examination.

Focal Lesions.—A lesion involving a definite part of the gray matter destroying the cell bodies of the lower motor neurones and leading to degeneration of their axis-cylinder processes, is accompanied by a loss of power to perform certain definite movements. Thus in anterior polio-myelitis the only symptom may be a flaccid paralysis, and the seat of the lesion is revealed by the muscles involved. If from injury or disease a lesion involves more than the gray matter and, for example, if the neighboring fibres of the pyramidal tract be affected there may be in addition a spastic paralysis of the muscles whose centres lie in the lower levels of the cord. The degree of such a paralysis depends upon the intensity of the lesion of the pyramidal tract and may vary from a slight weakness in dorsal flexion of the ankle to an absolute paralysis of all the muscles below the lesion. Again, if the afferent tracts are affected sensory symptoms may be added to the motor palsy. There may be disturbances of pain and temperature sense alone or touch also may be affected. This, however, is rare except in serious lesions. The upper border of disturbed sensation often indicates most clearly the level of the disease, especially when this is in the thoracic region where the corresponding level of motor paralysis is not easily demonstrated. It is unusual for cutaneous anæsthesia in organic lesions of the cord to extend above the level of the second rib and the tip of the shoulder, for this represents the lower border of the skin-field of the fourth cervical (see sensory charts), and as the chief centre for the diaphragm lies in this segment, a lesion at this level sufficiently serious to cause sensory disturbances would probably occasion motor paralyses as well and would entirely shut off the movements necessary for respiration. The demonstrable upper border of the anæsthetic field may not quite reach that which represents the level of the lesion. This is due to the functional overlapping of the segmental skin-fields (Sherrington) and applies more to touch than to pain and temperature. There is often a narrow zone of hyperæsthesia above the anæsthetic region.

Complete Transverse Lesions.—When the transverse lesion is total and the lower part of the cord is cut off entirely from above, there is complete sensory and motor paralysis to the segmental level of the injury, and the tendon reflexes, whose centres lie below, are lost instead of being exaggerated, as they are apt to be in case the lesion is a focal one. The symptomatology of total transverse lesions is thus given by Collier. (1) Total flaccid paralysis of muscles below the level of the lesion. (Spastic paralysis indicates that the lesion is incomplete.) (2) Permanent abolition of the knee-jerk and other deep reflexes supplied by the lower segments of the cord (Bastian's symptom). (3) A rapid wasting of the paralyzed muscles with a loss of the faradic excitability. (4) The sphincters lose their tone and there is dribbling of urine. (5) There is total anæsthesia to the level of the lesion (the zone of hyperæsthesia is rarer). (6) The only sign of self-action remaining is in the occasional presence, though in reduced degree, of certain skin reflexes such as the plantar reflex with its dorsal flexor response in the great toe.

Unilateral Lesions (*Brown-Séquard Paralysis*).—The motor symptoms, which follow lesions limited to one lateral half of the cross section of the spinal cord, are confined to one side of the body; they are on the same side as the lesion. At the level of the lesion, owing to destruction of cell bodies of the lower system of neurones, there will be found flaccid paralysis and atrophy of those muscles whose centres of innervation happen to lie at this level. Owing to degeneration of the pyramidal tract, the muscles whose centres be at lower levels are also paralyzed, but they retain their normal electrical reactions, become spastic, and do not atrophy to any great degree.

The *sensory* symptoms are peculiar. On the side of the lesion corresponding to the segment or segments of the cord involved there is a zone of anæsthesia to all forms of sensation. Below this there is no loss in the perception of pain, temperature, or touch. Indeed, hyperæsthesia has been described. Muscle sense is disturbed, and the ability to appreciate the size, consistency, weight, and shape of an object. On the side opposite to the lesion and nearly up to its level there is complete loss of perception for pain and temperature and there may be some dulling of tactile sense as well.

The following table, slightly modified from Gowers, illustrates the distribution of these symptoms in a complete semi-lesion of the cord:

Cord

Zone of cutaneous hyperæsthesia. Zone of cutaneous anæsthesia. Lower segment type of paralysis with atrophy.	Lesion.	
Upper segment type of paralysis. Hyperæsthesia of skin. Muscular sense and allied sensations impaired. Reflex action first lessened and then increased. Surface temperature raised.		Muscular power normal. Loss of sensibility of skin to pain and temperature. Muscular sense normal. Reflex action normal. Temperature same as that of above lesion.

It is common in syphilitic diseases of the cord, tumors and stab-wounds, and is not infrequently associated with syringomyelia and hæmorrhages into the cord. It is only in exceptional cases, of course, that the lesion is absolutely limited to the hemi-section of the cord and the symptoms consequently may vary somewhat in degree.

Lesions of the Conus Medullaris and Cauda Equina.—The chief lesions of this region are (1) fractures and dislocations, (2) myelitis, (3) tumors, (4) gunshot wounds, and (5) neuritis of the nerves of the cauda.

1. Conus Alone.—It may be in the seat of a tumor or a focal myelitis or hæmorrhage, and it has been damaged in a lumbar puncture. The features are characteristic—paralysis of the rectum and bladder, with the "riding-breeches anæsthesia" of the perineum, scrotum, penis, and postero-internal aspects of the thighs. There is less pain than in caudal lesions and the disturbance of sensation is bilateral.

2. The Epiconus may be involved alone, leading to degenerative atrophy of the muscles innervated by the sacral plexus, particularly the peronei and the glutei. "If the lesion be limited to the grey matter of the epiconus, the Achilles reflex is abolished, but the knee-jerk can be elicited and the sphincters remain unaffected" (Barker).

3. Cauda Equina.—An unusual number of cases have followed bullet and shell wounds in the late war. The picture varies with the level of the lesion, from complete paralysis of all the muscles of the legs with anæsthesia, including the genitals, but if below the second sacral roots, there is no paralysis of the lower limbs, but there is the typical saddle-shaped anæsthesia. The caudal lesions are more often unilateral, and the neuralgic pains are more severe.

Of tumors of the cauda mention must be made of the diffuse giant tumors described by Collins and Elsberg, with well marked caudal and conus symptoms. There is also a remarkable *neuritis* in which the caudal roots are swollen and the nerves degenerated, in association with a high grade of local arteriosclerosis. The symptoms in the five cases reported by Kennedy and Elsberg were pain, sphincter involvement, and sensory changes in the sacral roots. A similar neuritis has been described in the horse.

II. AFFECTIONS OF THE BLOOD VESSELS

I. CONGESTION

Apart from actual myelitis, we rarely see congestion of the spinal cord, and, when we do, it is usually limited either to the gray matter or to a definite portion of the organ. The white matter is rarely found congested, even when inflamed. The gray matter often has a reddish pink tint, but rarely a deep reddish hue, except when myelitis is present. If we know little anatomically of congestion of the cord, we know less clinically, for there are no features in any way characteristic of it.

II. ANÆMIA

So, too, with this state. There may be extreme grades without symptoms. In chlorosis, for example, there are rarely symptoms pointing to the cord, and there is no reason to suppose that such sensations as heaviness in the limbs and tingling are especially associated with anæmia.

Profound anæmia follows ligature of the aorta. Within a few moments after the application of the ligature paraplegia came on (Herter). Paralysis of the sphincters occurred, but less rapidly. Observations made by Halsted on occlusion of the abdominal aorta in dogs have shown that paraplegia occurs in a large percentage of cases, many of which, however, may recover as the collateral circulation is established. In the fatal cases Gilman found extensive alterations in the cell bodies of the lower part of the cord with degenerations. This is of interest in connection with the occasional rapid development of a paraplegia after profuse hæmorrhage, usually from the stomach or uterus. It may come on at once or at the end of a week or ten days, and is probably due to an anatomical change in the nerve elements similar to that produced in Herter's experiments. The degeneration of the dorsal columns of the cord in pernicious anæmia has been described.

III. EMBOLISM AND THROMBOSIS

Blocking of the spinal arteries by emboli rarely occurs. Thrombosis of the smaller vessels in connection with endarteritis plays an important part in many of the acute and chronic changes in the cord.

IV. ENDARTERITIS

It is remarkable how frequently in persons over fifty the arteries of the spinal cord are found sclerotic. The following forms may be met with: (1) A nodular peri-arteritis or endarteritis associated with syphilis and sometimes with gummata of the meninges; (2) an arteritis obliterans, with great thickening of the intima and narrowing of the lumen, involving chiefly the medium and larger-sized arteries. Miliary aneurisms or aneurisms of the larger vessels are rarely found in the spinal cord. Attacks of transient paraplegia may be due to spasm or other changes in the vessels of the cord. In the remarkable neuritis of the cauda equina described by Kennedy and Elsberg there is marked sclerosis of the arteries.

V. HÆMORRHAGE INTO THE SPINAL MEMBRANES; HÆMATORACHIS

In meningeal apoplexy, as it is called, the blood may lie between the dura mater and the spinal canal—extra-meningeal hæmorrhage—or within the dura mater—intra-meningeal hæmorrhage.

Extra-meningeal hæmorrhage occurs usually as a result of traumatism. The exudation may be extensive without compression of the cord. The blood comes from the large plexuses of veins which may surround the dura. The rupture of an aneurism into the spinal canal may produce extensive and rapidly fatal hæmorrhage.

Intra-meningeal hæmorrhage is a less frequent result of trauma, but in general is perhaps rather more common. It is rarely extensive from causes acting directly on the spinal meninges themselves. Scattered hæmorrhages are not infrequent in the acute infectious fevers, and there may be much extravasation in malignant small-pox. It may be into the theca alone and along the spinal nerve roots. Bleeding may occur also in death from convulsive disorders, such as epilepsy, tetanus, and strychnia poisoning, and has been recorded with difficult parturition and in purpura. The most extensive hæmorrhages occur in cases in which the blood comes from rupture of an aneurism at the base of the brain, either of the basilar or vertebral artery. In ventricular apoplexy the blood may pass from the fourth ventricle into the spinal meninges. In cranial fractures, particularly those of the base of the skull, the resultant hæmorrhage almost always finds its way into the subarachnoid space about the cord and may be demonstrated by the withdrawal of bloody fluid by a lumbar puncture. The procedure is of considerable diagnostic value. On the other hand, hæmorrhage into the spinal meninges may possibly ascend into the brain.

Symptoms.—The symptoms in moderate grades may be slight and indefinite. The spinal features suggest lumbar puncture and the nature of the fluid, flowing under pressure, determines the presence of hæmorrhage. In the non-traumatic cases the hæmorrhage may either come on suddenly or after a day or two of uneasy sensations along the spine. As a rule, the onset is abrupt, with sharp pain in the back and symptoms of irritation in the course of the nerves. There may be muscular spasms, or paralysis may come on suddenly, either in the legs alone or both in the legs and arms. In some instances the paralysis develops more slowly and is not complete. There are no signs of cerebral disturbance. The clinical picture varies. If the hæmorrhage is in the lumbar region, the legs alone are involved, the reflexes may be abolished, and the action of the bladder and rectum is impaired. If in the thoracic region, there is more or less complete paraplegia, the reflexes are usually retained, and there are signs of disturbance in the thoracic nerves, such as girdle sensations, pains, and sometimes eruption of herpes. In the cervical region the arms as well as the legs may be involved; there may be difficulty in breathing, stiffness of the muscles of the neck, and occasionally pupillary symptoms. In a case of influenza-pneumonia in the recent epidemic there was bilateral spastic rigidity associated with extensive hæmorrhage into the theca spinalis and along the nerve roots. There was no free blood in the canal. Branson reports two cases, probably influenza, with bloody fluid (40-50 c. c.)

withdrawn under considerable pressure. The spinal symptoms were slight and both patients recovered.

The prognosis depends much upon the cause of the hæmorrhage. Recovery may take place in the traumatic cases and in those associated with the infectious diseases.

VI. HÆMORRHAGE INTO THE SPINAL CORD; HÆMATOMYELIA

Most frequently a result of traumatism, intraspinal hæmorrhage is naturally more common in males and during the active period of life. Cases have been known to follow cold or exposure; it occurs also in tetanus and other convulsive diseases, and hæmorrhage may be associated with tumors, with syringomyelia or myelitis. A direct injury to the spine from blows or from falls is by far the most common cause. Acute flexure of the neck, often without attendant fracture or dislocation of the vertebræ, is the most common form of accident. There were many such cases during the war. The level of the lesion, for this reason, is most frequently in the lower cervical region.

Anatomical Condition.—The extent of the hæmorrhage may vary from a small focal extravasation to one which finds its way in columnar fashion a considerable distance up and down the cord. The bleeding primarily takes place into the gray matter, and this as a rule suffers most, but the surrounding medullated tracts may be thinned out and lacerated.

Symptoms.—As one side of the cord is usually involved more than the other, the Brown-Séquard syndrome is common. The symptoms are sudden in onset, and leave the patient with hyperæsthesia and a paralysis which becomes spastic and is most marked on one side, while anæsthesia, chiefly to pain and temperature, is most marked on the opposite side of the body. Often a most distressing hyperæsthesia, usually a "pins and needles" sensation, may be present for many days, but there is rarely any acute pain of the radiating or root type. As hæmatomyelia is most frequent in the lower cervical region, in addition to the symptoms just mentioned a brachial type of palsy is commonly seen, with flaccid and atrophic paralysis of the muscles innervated from the lowest cervical and first thoracic segments. The hæmorrhage may occur in segments farther down the cord, the lumbar enlargement being affected next in frequency to the lower cervical. The segmental level of the paralysis necessarily would vary accordingly.

The condition may prove rapidly fatal, particularly if the extravasation is bilateral and extends high enough in the cord to involve the centres for the diaphragm. More frequently there is a more or less complete recovery with a residual palsy of the upper extremity and a partial anæsthesia, corresponding to the level of the lesion, and some spasticity of the leg.

Diagnosis.—The diagnosis of the traumatic cases is comparatively easy, and it is important to recognize them, as they are often needlessly subjected to operation under the belief that they are instances of acute compression. The residual symptoms in old cases may closely simulate those seen in syringomyelia.

Treatment.—Absolute rest is important and the patient should be disturbed as little as possible. Special care must be given the skin to prevent bed-sores and to the bladder to prevent cystitis. Treatment of the paralyzed parts should not be begun for six weeks after the hæmorrhage, when electricity, gentle massage, and passive movements are indicated.

III. TUMORS OF THE SPINAL CORD AND ITS MEMBRANES

I. SYRINGOMYELIA (GLIOMA, GLIOMATOSIS)

Definition.—A gliosis about the central canal, either forming a local tumor, or more often a diffuse growth associated with cavity formations, extending lengthwise, and sometimes communicating with the central canal.

Dilatation of the central canal—hydromyelus—which must be distinguished from syringomyelia, is met with as a congenital anomaly; only in a few instances do the cavity formations of syringomyelia represent the distended canal itself.

Morbid Anatomy.—The cervical and dorsal regions are the usual seat. There are: (1) either a diffuse gliosis or at one level a definite tumor from which the growth extends for some inches, causing enlargement of the cord: (2) Tube like cavities, extending for a variable distance, usually in the dorsal aspect and sometimes involving only one cornu. The processes leading to the formation of the cavities are various, such as hæmorrhage and thrombotic degenerations, evidences of which may be present. The wall of the tubes may be smooth and lined with ependymal cells. (3) Degenerative changes in other parts of the cord due to pressure.

Symptoms.—Men are more often affected, 133 of 190 cases collected by Schlesinger. A familiar type has been described. The disease begins, as a rule, before the thirtieth year. The symptoms vary with the seat and extent of the disease. A typical case beginning in the lower cervical region presents the following features: (1) Lower motor neurone involvement, with a progressive atrophy of the muscles of the hands and arms, and sometimes fibrillary tremors, so that the Aran-Duchenne disease is suspected. The typical claw-hand may exist. As the disease progresses, there is degeneration of the pyramidal tracts with a spastic paraplegia, so that the picture suggests amyotrophic lateral sclerosis.

(2) Sensory changes; (a) pains of the nerve-root type, chiefly in the arms; (b) the syringomyelic dissociation of sensation, in which the sense of touch is retained, while those of heat and of pain are lost. The muscular sense is not disturbed. The loss of temperature sense may be early, and a patient's fingers may be burnt by cigarettes or even charred.

(3) Trophic changes, as destructive whitlows, with atrophy of the terminal phalanges (Morvan's disease), vaso-motor swelling of the hands, sweating, and arthropathies, which latter occur in about 10 per cent. of the cases. While this is the common and readily recognized form, there may be no disturbance of sensation for years, only the amyotrophic type of paralysis; there may be general anesthesia to pain and temperature, with very little motor disturbance; and there is a form with bilateral spastic diplegia.

Marked scoliosis may be present, a feature not easily explained. The analgesia and loss of thermic sense are due to involvement of the peri-ependymal gray matter and the posterior horns. The tactile sensations travel in the postero-lateral regions of the cord which are rarely involved.

The *diagnosis* is easy in well pronounced cases, but when the motor features predominate, it may not be possible to distinguish the disease from amyotrophic muscular paralysis. With the widespread anæsthesia hysteria is simulated; while the combination of anæsthesia and loss of the finger tips may suggest leprosy. In a few instances the gliosis extends to the medulla with the production of bulbar symptoms.

Treatment.—In a few cases the X-rays have appeared to give relief to the pains and stiffness.

II. TUMORS OF THE MENINGES

A majority of all growths are extra-medullary, and originate on the dura or pia in the blood vessels or on the nerve-roots. Schlesinger's tabulation of 400 cases shows that the growths in order of frequency are tubercle, fibroma and syphiloma. Rarer forms are lipoma, psammoma, neuroma, myxoma and angioma. A few cases of aneurism and echinococcus cyst have been reported. The nature, rate of growth, size and situation are the important factors.

Symptoms.—There are two groups: (1) *Irritation*—sensory and motor. Pressure on the posterior roots causes pain, unilateral or bilateral, at the level of the distribution of the nerves. Hyperæsthesia with a sense of burning is common. In the cervical region the sympathetic fibres may be involved. Only in a few cases are sensory features absent. Motor irritation due to pressure on the anterior roots and on the antero-lateral columns causes spontaneous spasms of the muscles, rarely of the arms, but very often of the legs, and they constitute the most important *single* symptom in tumor involving the cord. Suddenly, without the patient's knowledge, the legs are drawn up, sometimes in pain, the thighs flexed on the abdomen, the legs on the thighs and foot, and especially the big toe on the ankle. It is a reflex of spinal automatism similar to that described by Sherrington in the decerebrated animal. It is the "defensive" reflex of Babinski, but Sherrington's term is preferable. It may be excited by stimulating the skin of the leg or foot, but the important point is the automatic type of the reflex and its significance as a sign of pressure irritation on the cord, at any stage early or late of the process.

(2) *Compression.*—Anæsthesia may occur in the region of distribution of the nerve-root or roots involved; atrophy of the muscles may follow pressure on the anterior roots. Pressure on the cord itself may produce the symptoms of a hemi-lesion with a typical Brown-Séquard syndrome. Gradually, after months or even years, the compression is complete with a spastic paraplegia and all the features of a spinal automatism. All stages from nerve-root irritation to a total transverse lesion may be followed through a period of months or years, and this sequence of events carefully studied is one of the most valuable helps in diagnosis.

The situation of the growth is determined by the root-levels involved, and it is to be remembered that the tendency is usually to locate it below the actual situation. The X-rays are often of great value in determining the nature of the pressure, particularly in excluding disease of the vertebræ.

Spinal Fluid.—From a study of five cases and a hundred collected from the literature, Sprunt and Walker describe two forms of xanthrochromia, in one of which the color is due to dissolved hæmoglobin, the fluid does not coagulate, and the amount of globulin is small. This is more common with brain tumor. In a larger group the fluid is clear yellow, coagulates, and has a large amount of globulin and no hæmoglobin—the so-called Froin syndrome; and is a compression sign, associated with the isolation of a lumber cul-de-sac, in which the fluid stagnates. It suggests spinal tumor or intra-dural inflammation.

Lumbar puncture may give a clear normal fluid. The leucocytes may be increased, and the chief interest is the occurrence of xanthrochromia.

Diagnosis.—When constant and severe root pains are associated with a progressive paralysis, the diagnosis may be easily made. Caries may cause identical symptoms, but the radiating pains are rarely so severe. Cervical meningitis simulates tumor very closely, and in reality produces identical effects, but the very slow progress and the bilateral character from the outset may be sufficient to distinguish it. Syphilitic meningo-myelitis may resemble tumor very closely and present radiating pains, a sense of constriction, and progressive paralysis. Syringomyelia may give a similar picture. A radiogram may be of diagnostic aid in case the vertebræ are infiltrated by the growth. The nature of the tumor can rarely be indicated with precision. With a marked syphilitic history gumma may be suspected, or, with coexisting tuberculous disease, a solitary tubercle.

Treatment.—It is difficult to say which rouses the greater admiration—the brilliant diagnosis of the clinician or the technique of the physiological surgeon, the combination of which enabled Gowers and Horsley to remove, for the first time, and with permanent success, a tumor of the spinal cord. The report of this case should be read to his class by every teacher of neurology (Medico-Chir. Soc. Trans., London, LXXI, 1888). In syphiloma recovery is possible, even after complete paraplegia. The only hopeful cases are the isolated growths springing from the membranes, and the operation has been followed by an ever increased percentage of recovery.

I. DIFFUSE AND FOCAL DISEASES OF THE BRAIN

I. TOPICAL DIAGNOSIS

In many regions disease may exist without causing symptoms—the so-called *silent areas*. Other areas at once give symptoms. These are the cortical motor centres and the associated sensory centres, the speech centres, the centres for the special senses, and the tracts which connect these cortical areas with each other and with other parts of the nervous system.

The following is a brief summary of the effects of lesions from the cortex to the spinal cord:

The Cerebral Cortex.—(*a*) *Destructive lesions* of the motor cortex cause *paralysis* in the muscles of the opposite side of the body. The paralysis is at first flaccid, later spastic, the extent depending upon that of the lesion. It is apt to be limited to the muscles of the head or of an extremity, giving rise to the cerebral monoplegias. One group of muscles may be more affected than others, especially in lesions of the highly differentiated area for the upper extremity. It is uncommon to find all the muscle groups of an extremity equally involved in cortical monoplegia. In small bilateral symmetrical lesions monoplegia of the tongue may result without paralysis of the face. A lesion may involve centres lying close together or overlapping one another, thus producing associated monoplegias—e. g., paralysis of the face and arm, or of the arm and leg, but not of the face and leg without involvement of the arm. Very rarely the whole motor cortex is involved, causing paralysis of the opposite side—cortical hemiplegia.

Adjoining and posterior to the motor area is the region of the cortex in which the impulses concerned in general bodily sensation (cutaneous sensibility, muscle sense, visceral sensations) first arrive (the somæsthetic area). Combined with the muscular weakness there is usually some disturbance of sensations, particularly of those of the muscular sense. In lesions of the superior parietal lobe the stereognostic sense is very often affected. For example, when a coin or a knife is placed in the hand of the affected limb, the patient's eyes being closed, it is not recognized, owing to inappreciation of the form and consistence of the object, and this even though the slightest tactile stimulus applied to the fingers or surface of the hand is felt and may be correctly localized. The sense of touch, pain, and temperature may be lowered, but not markedly unless the superior and inferior parietal lobules are involved in subcortical lesions. Paræsthesias and vaso-motor disturbances are common accompaniments of paralyses of cortical origin.

(*b*) *Irritative lesions* cause localized spasms. The most varied muscle groups corresponding to particular movement forms may be picked out. If the irritation be sudden and severe, typical attacks of Jacksonian epilepsy may occur. These convulsions are often preceded and accompanied by subjective sensory impressions. Tingling or pain, or a sense of motion in the part, is often the *signal symptom* (Seguin), and is of great importance in determining the seat of the lesion.

When lesions are both destructive and irritative, there are combinations of the symptoms produced by each. For instance, certain muscles may be paralyzed, and those represented near them in the cortex may be the seat of localized convulsions, or the paralyzed limb itself may be at times subject to convulsive spasms, or muscles which have been convulsed may become paralyzed. The close observation of the sequence of the symptoms in such cases often makes it possible to trace the progress of a lesion involving the motor cortex. In these cases the most frequent cause is a developing tumor, though sometimes local thickenings of the membranes of the brain, small abscesses, minute hæmorrhages, or fragments of a fractured skull must be held responsible.

Centrum Semiovale.—Lesions may involve either projection fibres (motor or sensory) or association fibres. If the involvement of the motor path causes paralysis, this has the distribution of a cortical palsy when the lesion is near the cortex, and of a paralysis due to a lesion of the internal capsule when it is near that region. Other systems of fibres running in the centrum semiovale may be involved causing sensory disturbances—hemi-anæsthesia and hemianopia—and if the lesion is in the left hemisphere, one of the different forms of aphasia may accompany the paralysis.

Two other features may be associated with a cortical or indeed with any lesion. *Neighborhood symptoms* are produced by pressure. A tumor may cause disturbance of function in adjacent centres, or interrupt motor or sensory paths. A hæmorrhage often causes transient symptoms which clear up after the clot shrinks. Transient disturbances of the speech centres and temporary involvement of the paths in the internal capsule are common effects. *Distal symptoms* are produced in two ways. The pressure of a tumor in the frontal lobe may influence the function of the motor centres or a pituitary growth may affect far distant parts, with localizing symptoms.

Shock symptoms (which have been much studied during the war) arise from functional disturbance of parts distant from the site of the lesion. A blow in the head may abolish the knee-jerks; transient aphasia may be caused by a fall on the right side of the head. The loss of consciousness in apoplexy may be due in part to the shock of the stroke. In the psychic side of war this shock action in causing local or widespread loss of function has played an important rôle. The deleterious effect on neurones or centres far removed from the site of the injury is called *diaschisis* by von Monakow.

Corpus Striatum.—Nothing is known of the functions of the caudate nucleus. The progressive lenticular degeneration (Wilson's disease) is described among the familial nervous affections. The globus pallidus, part of the lenticular nucleus, is involved in paralysis agitans and in Huntington's chorea (Ramsay Hunt).

Corpus Callosum.—It may be absent congenitally. Though often involved in tumors, characteristic symptoms are rare. One of special interest has been noted by Liepmann in connection with Apraxia. The left half of the brain is the dominant partner (as more than 90 per cent. of persons are right-handed) in our manual activities, but through the fibres of the corpus callosum it has guiding influences on the movements controlled by the right hemisphere. Thus a lesion of the left cerebrum above the capsule may cause apraxia of the left arm by cutting the callosal fibres through which influences pass from the left to the right arm centres. The anomalous features of right hemiplegia or monoplegia with apraxia of the non-paralyzed arm are suggestive of a callosal lesion.

The Thalamus.—Much knowledge of its functions has been obtained by a study of local lesions. It is an important sub-station in the sensory path, and, as Nothnagel showed, it is the lower reflex centre for the emotional movements of laughing and crying; and lesions of this part have long been known to be associated with athetoid and choreic movements.

The Thalamic Syndrome, as it is called, consists of: (1) Contra-lateral hemianæsthesia, sometimes with severe pains; (2) irregular movements—ataxic, choreic, or athetoid; and, (3) as the lesion progresses, hemi-paresis, but the plantar reflex may remain flexor. Lesions of the posterior third may involve the optic radiations causing bilateral homonomous hemianopsia. Control of the voluntary movements with loss of the mimic associated movements of the lower half of the face in laughing and crying suggests a thalamic lesion.

Internal Capsule (Fig. 15).—Through this pass within a rather narrow area all, or nearly all, of the projection fibres (both motor and sensory) which are connected with the cerebral cortex. It is divided into an anterior limb, a knee, and a posterior limb, the latter consisting of a thalamo-lenticular portion (its anterior two-thirds) and a retro-lenticular portion (its posterior third). The principal bundle passing through the anterior limb of the capsule is that which connects the frontal gyri and the medial bundle in the base of the peduncle (crus) with the nuclei of the pons. These fibres are centrifugal, and innervate chiefly the lower motor nuclei governing bilaterally innervated muscles, especially those of the eyes, head, neck, and probably those of the mouth, tongue, and larynx. In lower horizontal planes these fibres are situated near the knee of the capsule. It is the region of the knee of the capsule which transmits especially the fibres passing from the cerebral cortex to the nuclei of the facial, hypoglossal, and third nerves. The path which supplies the nuclei governing the muscles used in speech passes through the knee.

The pyramidal tract goes through the thalamo-lenticular portion of the capsule. The motor fibres are arranged according to definite muscle groups, or rather movement forms, those for the movements of the arm being anterior to those for the leg. The number of fibres for a given muscle group corresponds rather to the degree of complexity of the movements than to the size of the muscles concerned. Thus the areas for the fingers and toes are relatively large.

The fibres to the somæsthetic area of the cortex—that is, those from the centro-lateral group of nuclei of the thalamus and the tegmental radiations—carrying impulses concerned in general bodily sensation, pass upward through the posterior part of the thalamo-lenticular portion of the capsule. Some of these fibres pass through the anterior two-thirds of the posterior limb alongside of the fibres of the pyramidal tract.

Through the retro-lenticular portion of the posterior limb, opposite the posterior third of the lateral surface of the thalamus, pass (1) the fibres carrying impulses concerned in the sensations of the opposite visual field (optic radiation from the lateral geniculate body to the visual sense area in the occipital cortex); (2) the fibres carrying impulses concerned in auditory sensations (radiation from the medial geniculate body to the auditory sense area in the cortex of the temporal lobe); (3) the fibres (probably centrifugal) connecting the cortex of the temporal lobe with the nuclei of the pons.

With this preliminary knowledge concerning the internal capsule, it is not difficult to understand the symptoms which result when it is diseased.

Since here all the fibres of the upper motor segment are gathered together in a compact bundle, a lesion in this region is apt to cause complete hemiplegia of the opposite side, followed later by contractures; and if the lesion involves the hinder portion of the posterior limb there is also hemianæsthesia, including even the special senses. As a rule, however, lesions of the internal capsule do not involve the whole structure. The disease usually affects the anterior or posterior portions, and even in instances in which at first the symptoms point to total involvement there is a disappearance often of a large part of the phenomena after a short time. Thus, when the pyramidal tract is destroyed (lesion of the thalamo-lenticular portion of the capsule) the arm may be affected more than the leg, or *vice versa.* The facial paralysis is usually slight, though if the lesion be well forward in the capsule the paralysis of the face and tongue may be marked.

The bilaterally innervated muscles of the upper face, of mastication, of deglutition, phonation, and of the trunk muscles are very slightly involved. The patient can wrinkle the forehead, and close the eye on the affected side, but the muscles may be weak, as shown by lessened respiratory movement on the paralyzed side.

Hemianæsthesia alone without involvement of the motor fibres is rare. There is usually also at least partial paralysis of the leg. When the retro-lenticular portion of the capsule is destroyed the hemianæsthesia is accompanied by hemianopsia, disturbances of hearing, and sometimes of smell and taste. The occurrence of hemianæsthesia with pain, hemichorea, marked tremor, or hemiathetosis—thalamic syndrome—after a capsular hemiplegia points to the involvement of the thalamus or of the hypothalamic region.

Charcot and others have described cases in which as a result of disease of the internal capsule there has been paralysis of the face and leg without involvement of the arm. In such instances the lesion is linear, extending from the posterior part of the anterior limb of the internal capsule backward and lateralward to the leg region in the posterior limb of the capsule, the region for the arm escaping.

Capsular lesions when pure are not usually accompanied by aphasic symptoms, alexia, or agraphia. A "subcortical" motor aphasia may result if the lesion is bilateral, as in pseudo-bulbar paralysis, or if on the left side it is so extensive as to destroy the fibres connecting Broca's convolution with the opposite hemisphere, as well as the pyramidal fibres on the same side.

Crura (Cerebral Peduncles).—From this level through the pons, medulla, and cord the upper and lower motor segments are represented, the first by the fibres of the pyramidal tracts and by the fibres which go from the cortex to the nuclei of the cerebral nerves, the latter by the motor nuclei and the nerve fibres arising from them. Lesions often affect both motor segments, and produce paralyses having the characteristics of each. Thus a single lesion may involve the pyramidal tract and cause a spastic paralysis on the opposite side of the body, and also involve the nucleus or the fibres of one of the cerebral nerves, and so produce a lower segment paralysis on the same side as the lesion—crossed paralysis. In the crus the third and fourth cerebral nerves run near the pyramidal tract, and a lesion of this region is apt to involve them or their nuclei, causing partial paralysis of the muscles of the eye on the same side as the lesions, combined with a hemiplegia of the opposite side (Weber-Gubler syndrome) (Fig. 12, 3).

The optic tract also crosses the crus and may be involved, giving hemianopsia in the opposite halves of the visual fields.

If the tegmentum be the seat of a lesion which does not involve the base of the peduncle (or pes) there may be disturbances of cutaneous and muscular sensibility, ataxia, disturbances of hearing, or oculo-motor paralysis. An oculomotor paralysis of one side, accompanied by a hemi-ataxia of the opposite side, appears to be especially characteristic of a tegmental lesion (Benedikt's syndrome). Or there may be with the crossed paralysis the features of cerebellar ataxia (Nothnagel's syndrome).

Corpora Quadrigemina.—Anatomical studies point to the view that the superior colliculus (anterior quadrigeminal body) represents the most important subcortical central organ for the control of the eye-muscle nuclei. This is supported to a certain extent by clinical evidence, though as yet but few cases have been carefully studied. Sight is only slightly, if at all, disturbed when the superior colliculus is destroyed. The pupil is usually widened, and the pupillary reaction, both to light and on accommodation, interfered with. Apparently actual paralysis of the eye muscles does not occur unless the nucleus of the third nerve ventral to the aqueduct be also injured.

The inferior colliculus (posterior quadrigeminal body) is an important way-station in the auditory conduction-path. A large part of the lateral lemniscus ends in its nucleus, and from it emerge medullated fibres which pass through the brachium quadrigeminum inferius to the medial geniculate body. Thence a large bundle runs through the retro-lenticular portion of the internal capsule to the auditory sense area in the cortex of the temporal lobe.

In 9 of 19 tumors of this region collected by Weinland there were auditory disturbances.

Since the central auditory path of each side receive impulses from both ears, lesion of the colliculus on one side may dull the hearing on both sides, though the opposite ear is usually the more defective. Lesion of the inferior colliculus may be accompanied by disturbance of mastication, owing to paralysis of the descending (mesencephalic) root of the trigeminus. The fourth nerve may also be involved. The ataxia which sometimes accompanies lesions of the corpora quadrigemina is probably to be referred to disturbance in conduction in the medial lemniscus.

Pons and Medulla Oblongata.—Lesions involving the pyramidal tract, together with any one of the motor cerebral nerves of this region, cause crossed paralysis—*hemiplegia alternans*. A lesion in the lower part of the pons causes a lower-segment paralysis of the face on the same side (destruction of the nucleus of the facial nerve or of its root fibres) and a spastic paralysis of the arm and leg on the opposite side (injury to pyramidal tract) (Fig. 12, 4). This is referred to as the alternate hemiplegia or the Millard-Gubler type. The abducens, the motor part of the trigeminus, and the hypoglossus nerves may also be paralyzed in the same manner. When the central fibres to the nucleus of the hypoglossus are involved a peculiar form of anarthria results. If the nucleus itself be diseased, swallowing is interfered with.

When the sensory fibres of the fifth nerve are interrupted, together with the sensory tract (the medial lemniscus or fillet) for the rest of the body, which has already crossed the middle line, there is a crossed sensory paralysis—i. e., disturbed sensation in the distribution of the fifth on the side of the lesion, and of all the rest of the body on the opposite side—*hemianæsthesia cruciata.*

A paralysis of the external rectus muscle of one eye and of the internal rectus of the other eye (conjugate paralysis of the muscles which turn the eyes to one side), in the absence of a "forced position" of the eyeballs, is highly characteristic of certain lesions of the pons. In such cases the internal rectus may still be capable of functioning on convergence, or when the eye to which it belongs is tested independently of that in which the external rectus is paralyzed. This form, known as the Foville type of hemiplegia alternans, is found, as a rule, only when the lesion lies just in front of the abducens or involves the nucleus itself, or includes, besides the root fibres of the abducens, that portion of the formatio reticularis that lies between them and the fasciculus longitudinalis medialis (von Monakow). The facial nerve is often involved in these paralyses.

In lesions of the pons the patient often has a tendency to fall toward the side on which the lesion is, probably on account of implication of the middle peduncle of the cerebellum (brachium pontis). Still more frequent is the simple motor hemi-ataxia consequent upon lesion of the medial lemniscus, and perhaps of longitudinal bundles in the formatio reticularis. This is often accompanied by a dissociated sensory disturbance, pain and temperature being affected, while touch remains normal. The muscular sense may also be involved. Only when the lesion is very extensive are there disturbances of hearing (involvement of the lateral lemniscus or corpus trapezoideum).

So small is the space in which important paths and nuclei are crowded that a lesion of the medulla may involve the motor tract on both sides, causing total bilateral paralysis—tetraplegia, usually due to thrombosis or to a small hæmorrhage. Or the arm on one side and the leg on the other may be involved—hemiplegia cruciata.

Cerebellum.—As "the head ganglion of the proprio-ceptive system" (Sherrington) to this lesser brain converge the impulses of deep sensibility, and from it pass the impulses which control the tone of the muscles and their coördination when in action. The basis of our recent knowledge is in the exhaustive monograph of Luciani, whose conclusions have been confirmed and extended by Horsley and his pupils, Babinski, Thomas, and by the experience of the late war (Gordon Holmes).

In addition to its influence in maintaining equilibrium, the cerebellum has an important rôle in regulating and controlling voluntary movements. This is concerned with the muscular tone, the direction and measurement of movements, the maintenance of attitudes, and the control of coördinated movements. Hence disturbance of coördination, hypotonia, asthenia, ataxia (cerebellar) and volitional tremor result from diseased conditions. The disturbance may affect special functions. Thus Ramsay Hunt has described a condition under the designation *Dyssenergia cerebralis progressiva*, or chronic progressive cerebellar tremor, in which there is a generalized volitional tremor which begins locally and gradually progresses. There is a progressive degeneration of the structures which control and regulate the muscular movements. When at rest and with the muscles relaxed the tremor ceases. Other symptoms of cerebellar disease, such as vertigo, disturbance of equilibrium, nystagmus and seizures are absent.

UNILATERAL LESIONS.—As the functions of each lobe are homolateral, the symptoms are on the same side, and are negative not irritative in character. They may be grouped as follows (Gordon Holmes) :—

1. *Disturbance of Muscle Tone.*—The limbs flop about in an unnatural way, and the muscles are soft and flabby. The hypotonia is so marked that with very little power the thigh can be flexed on the abdomen and the heel placed on the buttock. In walking the arm swings inertly, and if the forearms are held vertically, the wrist on the affected side falls passive in extreme flexion.

2. *Asthenia,* specially dwelt upon by Luciani, was a feature almost constant in the war cases. It is noted when the patient holds the arms outstretched or raises a weight, and is well shown by the dynamometer. The movements are slow, a delay in initiation and in relaxation. The affected limbs tire easily.

3. *Ataxia.*—In direction, force and range the purposive movement errs,

and with the eyes open. With the arm outstretched, asked to touch the nose with the index finger, he will bring it to the chin, and with undue force. Natural movements may be decomposed (Babinski), e. g., when asked to touch the knee with the heel, instead of flexing thigh and leg together, the hip is first flexed and then the knee. This *asynergia* is due to a lack of the proper association of agonists, antagonists and fixating muscles. The movements are ill measured (*dysmetria*), particularly quick movements, in both force and aim, and not along the shortest possible line. Tremor may occur in the moving limb, sometimes "intention" in character, or static, as in slight oscillations of the head when at rest; more characteristic is the tremor occurring in maintaining an attitude and involuntary movement, to which Luciani has given the name *Astasia*.

4. *The Rebound Phenomenon.*—With elbows supported the patient pulls each hand towards his mouth against the resistance of the observer who holds the wrists. If let go suddenly, the hand on the affected side flies to the mouth often with great force, while the other is arrested almost immediately by the antagonists. This is a striking and valuable test.

5. *Adiadochokinesis.*—In executing alternate movements as in rapid pronation and supination of the elbow, the homolateral limb moves more slowly, less regularly, and tires earlier, and there may be adventitious movements of the fingers.

6. *Vertigo,* a common feature, may not be truly cerebellar but labyrinthine. The tendency is to fall towards the affected side, but the sensation of displacement may be of self or of external objects. It seems a more constant symptom in tumor than in injury.

7. *The Pointing Test* (Bárány).—With closed eyes the patient is asked with his extended forefinger to touch the observer's finger held at some distance above the bed, and then as he brings the finger down to the bed and slowly up again the finger deviates outwardly.

8. *Attitude and Gait.*—The head tends to be flexed towards the side of the lesion and rotated to the opposite side; and the body may be concave to the side of the lesion. On standing he is shaky and unsteady, and tends to fall towards the affected side, often with a feeling as if he were pulled over. The attitude may be very striking, the head and trunk inclined to the affected side, the spine concave to it, with the pelvis tilted, the shoulder lifted, the trunk rotated and held stiff. There is no Romberg sign. In walking he mistrusts the affected leg, which is usually rotated outwards, the foot may be dragged or raised unnaturally and brought to the floor with a flop. Stumbling towards the affected side, he makes efforts to control the tendency to fall. When asked to stop, he cannot pull up suddenly. The arm on the affected side hangs inertly, without the normal swing.

9. *Ocular Disturbances.*—In wounds there is early deviation of the eyes to the opposite side—or "skew-deviation," the homolateral eye down and in, the other up and out. Fixation nystagmus is the rule in injury, and the oscillations are slower and larger when the patient looks to the affected side. How far it is due to coexisting labyrinthine lesion is not determined, but Wilson and Pike claim that there are differences, and it is more enduring.

Among minor features to be mentioned are a slow, "sing-song" speech, the words are blurred, and the articulation nasal and the end syllables explosive. The homolateral reflexes may for a time be absent. As a rule the knee jerk is less brisk, and has a pendulum character. The superficial reflexes are not changed. Sensation in any form is unchanged.

Bilateral lesions show disturbances similar to those described above, but speech is more disturbed, the muscles of the trunk and neck are very hypotonic, and naturally when standing the maintenance of equilibrium is much more difficult. The features so characteristic of unilateral lesion are not essentially changed when the *vermis* is involved, unless perhaps the tremor is more marked. The effects of cortical and nuclear lesions do not appear to differ. The war experience does not support the view of special cortical localization, or of the existence of focal centres for movement in different directions (Bárány). The numerous clinical observations confirm Luciani's conclusions that *atonia, asthenia,* and *astasia* form a characteristic cerebellar triad.

II. APHASIA

Under the general term aphasia—with agnosia and apraxia—is included the loss of the memories of the vocal, written, manual and other signs and symbols by which we communicate with our fellows and indicate our knowledge of the nature and use of things.

As in all other voluntary movements speech requires not only a motor but a sensory apparatus, and we have, as composing the speech mechanism, a sensory or receptive part as well as a motor or emissive part. These two parts are associated with the higher centres underlying the intellectual process, and are controlled by them.

The muscles which are used in the production of articulate speech are many and widely distributed; thus, the respiratory muscles, the muscles of the larynx, the pharynx, the tongue, the lips, and those which move the jaws are all brought into play during speech. These muscles are all active in other less complicated movements; for instance, respiration, crying, sucking, etc., and these comparatively simple movements are represented in the gray matter of the lower motor segment in the pons, medulla, and spinal cord. The association of neurones upon which these movements depend is made during fetal life, and is in good working order at the time of birth.

As the child's brain grows and takes control of the spinal centres through the medium of the pyramidal tracts, other more complex movements are developed and special neurones are set apart for this purpose. There is, then, a re-representation (Hughlings Jackson) of the finer movements of these muscles in the upper motor segment. They are localized in the central convolutions about the lower part of the Rolandic fissure.

This group of movements, which are in part congenital and in part acquired during the early months of life, is that from which the delicate movements of articulate speech are developed. The structures upon which these movements depend make the *primary* or *elementary speech mechanism.*

The cortical centres are in the lower third of the central convolution on both sides of the brain. They are bilaterally acting centres, and a lesion limited to either one should not produce marked or permanent defects in speech. This is true for the right side, but on the left Broca's convolution is so closely situated that it or its connecting fibres are usually injured at the same time, and motor aphasia results. The path from the cortical centres is made up of the motor fibres which go to the nuclei of the pons and medulla, and in the internal capsule is situated near the knee. As in the cortex, a unilateral lesion here causes only slight disturbances of speech due to difficult articulation, following weakness of the opposite side of the face and tongue. On the left side, if the lesion is so near the cortex as to involve the fibres which connect Broca's convolution with the primary speech mechanism, *subcortical motor aphasia* is produced. Bilateral lesions (usually in the internal capsule, but at times in the cortex) cause speechlessness, with paralysis of the muscles of articulation—pseudo-bulbar paralysis. To these speech defects Bastian gave the name aphemia and Marie, anarthria.

The lower segment of the primary speech mechanism is made up of the motor nuclei in the medulla, etc., and the peripheral nerves arising from them. Lesions here, if extensive enough—as, for instance, in progressive bulbar paralysis—may cause speechlessness—anarthria (Bastian); but usually they are more limited, giving various disturbances of articulation.

The Auditory Speech Centre.—As the child learns to speak there is developed in the cortex of the brain an association of centres which takes control of the primary speech mechanism. The child is constantly hearing objects called by names, and he learns to associate certain sounds with the look, feel, taste, etc., of certain things. When he hears such a sound he gets a more or less clear mental picture of the object, or, in other words, he has developed certain auditory memories. These memories of the sounds of words are stored in what is called the *auditory speech centre.* This centre, which in the majority of people is the controlling speech centre, is situated on the left side in right-handed people, and on the right side in those who are left-handed. The afferent impressions arising in the ears reach the transverse gyri of the temporal lobes, those from each ear going to both sides of the brain. From each of these primary auditory centres impulses are sent to the auditory speech centre in the temporal lobe of the left hemisphere. The exact location of this so-called centre is not accurately determined, but it is thought to occupy the first and perhaps part of the second temporal convolutions. Marie denies all speech centres, but places the cortical region, which has to do with the intellectual processes underlying language, rather vaguely in the left temporo-parietal lobe. This he designates "Wernicke's zone," a lesion of which alone can produce aphasia. The child endeavors, and by repeated efforts learns, to make the sounds that he hears, and he first becomes able to repeat words, then to speak voluntarily. To do this, he has to learn certain very delicate movements, and so there is developed under the control of the auditory speech centres a special motor centre for speech in which these movements are localized.

The Motor Speech Centre.—This was placed by Broca, and those who immediately followed him, in the posterior part of the left third frontal convolution. It is around this—Broca's centre—that the discussion started by Marie has been most heated. Marie and his followers deny that this portion of the brain has anything to do with speech, and insist that the so-called motor aphasia is merely a "combination of aphasia (of which they admit but one type, that due to lesions of Wernicke's zone) with anarthria." Anarthria they think of as a speech disturbance without any intellectual defect, due to a lesion of their lenticular zone, an ill-defined area in the centre of the brain.

Marie's position has been much discussed, and many excellent observers have come to the rescue of the old view which accepts Broca's convolution as the motor speech centre. The studies of cases of apraxia, which seem to have determined a centre in the left frontal lobe for certain purposive movements, as in the use of objects, gestures, etc., have lent support to the importance of Broca's convolution.

The motor speech centres and the corresponding area in the right brain are connected either directly by special motor fibres with the bulbar nuclei, or, as is more probable, indirectly, through the medium of the cortical centres of the primary speech mechanism in the lower part of the Rolandic region on both sides.

The speech centres are in close connection with the rest of the brain cortex, and in this way they take part in the general mental activities, of which, indeed, the speech processes form a large part. Some authors have assumed that the several sensory elements which go to make a concept are brought together in a special region of the brain, and here, as it were, united by a name. This is called "the centre for concepts," or "naming centre" (Broadbent), but most writers have followed Bastian in considering that the supposition of such a centre is unnecessary.

The mechanism which has been described is that which is developed in uneducated people and in children before they have learned to read and write, and is of primary importance in all speech processes. As the child learns to read he associates certain visual impressions with the speech memories he has acquired, and then adds to his concepts the visual memories of written or printed symbols. These memories are stored in the visual speech centre.

The Visual Speech Centre.—This is placed by nearly all authors in the angular and supramarginal convolutions on the left side, where it is believed visual impressions from both occipital lobes are combined in speech memories. Von Monakow denies such a special centre, but holds that visual speech memories are dependent upon the direct connection of the general visual centres in both occipital lobes with the speech sphere. That speech defects result from injury to the angular and supramarginal convolutions, he admits; but he thinks these are due to an interruption of fibre tracts which lie beneath and not to a destruction of a cortical centre. The distinction is, therefore, of more theoretical than practical importance. Marie includes this region in his Wernicke's zone.

In learning to write, the child develops certain delicate movements of the arm and hand, and thus acquires another method of externalizing his speech activities. Whether or not this requires the development of a separate writing centre, apart from the general Rolandic arm centre, or is brought about by an evolution of the latter through the medium of Broca's convolution, is a vexed question. Gordinier recorded a case of total agraphia, with no sensory or motor speech aphasia, in which a tumor occupying the foot of the second left frontal convolution was found at autopsy. *Agraphia* is a special form of apraxia. The movements of writing are learned under the influence of visual impressions in association with other speech memories, although there is a more direct path, which is used in copying unknown characters. Just as the movements of articulate speech are constantly under the control of auditory memories, so are the movements of writing regulated by visual memories; but in this case the other speech memories are of great importance.

With the development of the associations which underlie reading and writing, the speech mechanism may be said to be complete, although its activities are capable of practically endless extension, as when music or foreign languages are learned.

It will be seen that the cortical speech centres—the speech sphere of the French—occupy the part of the brain near the Sylvian fissure, and that they all receive their blood from the Sylvian artery. Speaking broadly, the posterior part of this region is sensory and the anterior is motor. The sensory areas are near the optic radiation and the motor are near the general motor tracts, and so, with lesions of the posterior part, hemianopia is apt to be associated with the speech disturbance while hemiplegia occurs with disease of the anterior areas. These associations often help to distinguish a sensory from a motor aphasia, but each type has special characteristics.

Auditory Aphasia.—Most people in mentally recalling words do so by means of their auditory speech memories—i. e., they think of the sound of the words, and, in voluntary speech, it is probable that the will acts on the motor centre indirectly through the auditory centre. This centre is also necessary for reading in such persons. There are persons, however, in whom the mental processes are carried on by visual memories, and in these "visuals" the visual speech centres take the predominant place in speech usually occupied by the auditory centres.

Complete abolition of all the auditory speech memories by destruction of the first temporal convolution causes the most extensive disturbances of speech. Such a person is unable to comprehend speech, either spoken or printed. Voluntary speech is much disturbed, and although at first he may talk, his speech is nothing but a jargon of misplaced words, and he soon becomes speechless. Writing is also lost, and he can neither repeat words nor write at dictation. He may be able to copy.

Lesions are often only partial, and the resultant disturbance may be simply a difficulty in speech due to the loss of nouns or to the transposition of words (paraphasia), the writing showing the same defect. The patient usually understands what he hears and reads, and can repeat words and write at dictation. Bastian called this condition "amnesia verbalis." It may be so pronounced that voluntary speech and writing are nearly lost, even when the auditory memories can still be aroused by new afferent impressions and he is able to understand what is said to him and what he reads. He can usually repeat and read aloud.

The afferent paths, which reach the auditory speech centre from the two primary auditory centres, may be destroyed. A lesion to do this must be in the white matter beneath the first temporal convolution on the left side. Such a lesion blocks all auditory impressions coming to the centre, and the patient is not able to understand anything said to him, can not repeat words or write from dictation. As the cortical centres are not disturbed, and the auditory speech memories are still present, there is no disturbance of voluntary speech or writing, and the patient can read perfectly. This is pure word-deafness or subcortical sensory aphasia.

Visual Aphasia.—Destruction of the visual centre in the angular and supramarginal convolutions causes a loss of the visual speech memories, and the patient is unable to read printed or written characters. He is unable to write—agraphia—and he can not copy. His understanding of spoken words is good, and voluntary speech is normal or only slightly paraphasic.

A subcortical lesion involving the afferent fibres going to the visual speech centre causes pure word-blindness (subcortical alexia)—i. e., there is inability to understand written or printed words. Voluntary speech and writing are good. The patient can not read his own writing except by aid of muscle-sense impression, in retracing the letters, either voluntarily or passively. Associated with this is always hemianopia.

Word-deafness and word-blindness are often combined, and at times it is not only the tracts that connect the primary auditory and visual centres with the speech spheres, but also those which associate them with the other sensory centres in the formation of concepts, that are diseased. In this case the patient has lost not only his auditory and visual speech memories, but also all of his memories which have to do with hearing and sight. He has mind-deafness and mind-blindness—i. e., he is unable to recognize objects when he hears or when he sees them. Further, there may be a dissociation of all the sensory centres from each other or from the higher psychical centre, which is practically the same thing, in which case the patient is entirely unable to recognize objects or use them properly—i. e., he has sensory apraxia or agnosia.

Motor Aphasia.—Lesions of the motor speech zone, possibly in rare cases of Broca's convolution alone, more commonly of a wider area, cause loss of the power of speech. The patient may be absolutely dumb, or he may have retained one or two words or phrases, which is believed to be due to the activity of the corresponding region of the right brain. He will make no effort to repeat words. His mind is comparatively clear, and he understands what is said to him, but reads poorly. He has not a clear mental picture of words. This is tested by asking him to squeeze the observer's hand or to make expiratory efforts as many times as there are syllables in a well-known name.

Voluntary writing is usually lost in cortical motor aphasia, and many authors believe that writing movements are controlled from this centre. Others, who believe that there is a special writing centre, contend that a lesion strictly limited to the motor speech centre would not cause agraphia, and cite cases which seem to support their view. If there is much disturbance of internal speech, writing must be impaired.

Subcortical motor aphasia is described as due to the destruction of the fibres which join Broca's convolution to the primary speech mechanism. Lesions which have produced this type of aphasia have been in the white matter of the left hemisphere near Broca's convolution. These would be within Marie's lenticular zone. There is complete loss of the power of speech without any disturbance of internal speech. The patient's mental processes are not disturbed, and he can write perfectly if the hand is not paralyzed.

Cases of aphasia are rarely simple, and it is often impossible to classify them accurately. The problems involved are, in reality, exceedingly complicated, and the student must not for a moment suppose that cases are as straightforward as the various diagrams at first sight would appear to indicate. A majority are very complex, but with patience the diagnosis of the different varieties can often be worked out. The following tests should be applied, after the presence or absence of paralysis has been determined and whether the patient is right- or left-handed: (1) The power of recognizing the nature, uses, and relations of objects—i. e., whether agnosia and apraxia are present or not; (2) the power to recall the name of familiar objects seen, smelled, or tasted, or of a sound when heard, or of an object touched; (3) the power to understand spoken words; (4) the capability of understanding printed or written language; (5) the power of appreciating and understanding music; (6) the power of voluntary speech—in this it is to be noted particularly whether he misplaces words or not; (7) the power of reading aloud and of understanding what he reads; (8) the power to write voluntarily and of reading what he has written; (9) the power to copy; (10) the power to write at dictation; and (11) the power of repeating words.

The *medico-legal aspects* of aphasia are of great importance. No general principle can be laid down, but each case must be considered on its merits. Langdon, in reviewing the whole question, concludes: "Sanity established, any legal document should be recognized when it can be proved that the person making it can understand fully its nature by any receptive channel (viz., hearing, vision, or muscular sense), and can, in addition, express assent or dissent with certainty to proper witnesses, whether this expression be by spoken speech, written speech, or pantomime."

Prognosis.—In young persons the outlook is good, and the power of speech is gradually restored apparently by the development of other portions of the brain. The opposite hemisphere often takes part in this. In adults the condition is less hopeful, particularly in the cases of complete motor aphasia with right hemiplegia. The patient may remain speechless, though capable of understanding everything, and attempts at re-education may be futile. Partial recovery may occur, and the patient may be able to talk, but misplaces words. In sensory aphasia the condition may be only transient, and the different forms rarely persist alone without impairment of the powers of expression.

The *education* of an aphasic person requires the greatest care and patience, particularly if, as so often happens, he is emotional and irritable. It is best to begin by the use of detached letters, and advance, not too rapidly, to words of only one syllable. Children often make rapid progress, but in adults failure is only too frequent, even after the most painstaking efforts. In the cases of right sided hemiplegia with aphasia the patient may be taught to write with the left hand.

III. AFFECTIONS OF THE BLOOD VESSELS

I. ARTERIO-SCLEROSIS—CEREBRAL FEATURES

(1) Transient Paralysis.—With high blood pressure and sclerotic vessels attacks of aphasia, monoplegia and hemiplegia occur, with the following characters:—they are transient, they leave no permanent damage, and they recur. Numbness and tingling may precede the onset. Some of the purest cases of motor aphasia are met with—a twelve to twenty-four hour inability to speak, without any mental disturbance. Monoplegia of the arm alone, or with the face, is more common than hemiplegia. A patient may have scores of attacks over many years. They are often associated with increased blood pressure and headache. Twitching of the angle of the mouth or of the hand may precede an attack. One patient had transient hemianopia. Sudden paraplegia may come on and last part of a day. Coming down the gangway of a steamer, a friend who had had many attacks of monoplegia suddenly lost the power in the legs, and had to be carried. He could walk next day. Another dropped in the street, and when seen twelve hours later, the paralysis was just disappearing and the reflexes obtainable. These are not attacks of intermittent claudication.

(2) **Convulsions**, in association with the above attacks or independently. The attack rarely has the graded features of a true epileptic fit, but there are widespread clonic movements, with unconsciousness lasting from a few minutes to an hour. There may be daily attacks for months and transient paralysis may follow on aphasia. The general condition of the patient may remain good and the mental state undamaged.

(3) **Psychical Changes.**—Following a convulsion, the patient may be dazed and "not himself" for some hours. A remarkable feature in many cases has been the retention of exceptional mental vigor. A transient mental outburst may replace, as it were, the motor attack. One subject of innumerable monoplegias would waken at night, light the candle, stamp about the room, tear up books and papers, all the time talking to himself. He would know nothing about it in the morning. Similar outbursts occurred in the day. Or a transient cloud may pass over the mind before the onset of hemiplegia. Returning from a game of golf, a man did not know his house or recognize his wife and surroundings. After a good night's rest he woke with weakness of the right side and confusion of speech which had gone by the evening.

As the disease progresses, the mental state may fail, but in contradistinction to the presenile and senile types of dementia, many of these patients keep a clear mind to the end, and there are none of the features of Binswanger's *dementia presenilis* or of Alzheimer's disease. An explanation of these attacks is not easy. Their frequency and the rapid restoration of function rule out destructive lesions. Possibly they are due to spasm of the arteries and a temporary ischæmia, a view strongly supported by the occurrence of similar attacks in Raynaud's disease.

Clinically there are three groups of cases:—(1) The arterio-sclerosis of middle-aged men; (2) the senile form; and (3) special presenile forms.

1. Arterio-sclerosis (see p. 837 under diseases of the arteries).

2. Senile Arterio-sclerosis.—Old age is largely a question of the blood vessels, but the wear and tear of life affects different parts in different persons. With the progressive weakening of the mental powers as age advances, widespread changes in the arteries, both basal and cortical, are found. Often it is not a question of the petrol-tank—the blood supply—but the whole machine is worn out. A real mental vigor may exist with advanced arterio-sclerosis. A man of sixty in full practice at the bar died suddenly of angina pectoris. The basal arteries were pipe-stems, and the smaller cortical vessels creaked under the knife!

In a normal old age the convolutions waste, the pigment granules and the lime-salts increase, the meninges become cloudy, the cortical arteries thicken, the glia in the gray matter increases particularly about the smaller vessels, and there are the areas of atrophy, as described by Marie, Peck and others. With these organic changes the mental grip fails, the memory weakens, the emotions are less under control, and year by year in a slow process of devolution the last stage of all is reached, second childhood—babyhood rather—as the man ends as he began, with only a vegetative system.

This happy, normal process with "mild gradations of decay," recognized by all except the senile himself, bears out Plato's dictum that "old age is an easy death." But it may be far otherwise, and "the evening of life may be a stormy and unhappy period." The peculiarities of the individual become more marked and to an unpleasant degree; he may become egotistical, emotional and suspicious, or careless in minor proprieties of life and intensely selfish. The most pathetic of martyrdoms are the miseries endured by children in the unrequited, unappreciated devotion to an irritable, egotistical, self-centred senile parent. But the pity of it is that the worst troubles may not be intensification of any personal peculiarities, but terrible perversions of character of a distressing nature. The man of active useful life may be depressed to distraction by the thoughts of the failure he has been; the godly man is worried over his lost soul; the moral teacher and saintly soul may become a lecher; the loving affectionate husband a brutal tyrant; the millionaire thinks himself a bankrupt.

3. Special Types.—While in normal old age there is nothing local, on the other hand, the senility may be chiefly local and affect the brain at a comparatively early age. The changes are usually those of normal old age, and associated with loss of judgment, emotional perversions, and progressive mental impairment. The cardio-vascular and renal conditions play an important rôle in these cases (Southard). Various forms have been described,—the *presbyophrenia* of Wernicke—characterized by "marked disturbances of the recording faculty, with retention for a long time of orderly thought and judgment . . . and tendency to confabulation" (Barker). Binswanger's *dementia presenilis* begins between the ages of 40 and 50, with loss of memory, apathy, etc., without syphilis or the somatic feature of *general paresis*. *Alzheimer's* disease is a slow dementia with focal symptoms, aphasia and apraxia, and in addition to the regressive changes in the vessels and glia, a peculiar condition of the neuro-fibrils. Southard and Alford called attention to a group of senile dementias (14 of 42 cases specially studied) of obscure etiology, which do not come in these types as the vessels are not sclerotic and the convolutions are not atrophied.

II. HYPERÆMIA AND ANÆMIA

Less and less stress is now laid on these conditions. The symptoms usually referred to active hyperæmia in the infectious diseases, or in association with hypertrophy of the heart accompanying disease of the kidney, are due to the action of toxic agents rather than to changes in the circulation.

Anæmia.—The anatomical condition of the brain is very striking. The membranes are pale, only the large veins are full, the small vessels over the gyri are empty, and an unusual amount of cerebro-spinal fluid is present. On section both the gray and white matter look extremely pale and the cut surface is moist. Very few *puncta vasculosa* are seen.

Symptoms.—The effects of sudden anæmia of the brain are well illustrated by the ordinary fainting fit. When the symptoms are the result of hæmorrhage, there are drowsiness, giddiness, inability to stand; flashes of light, dark spots before the eyes, and noises in the ears; the respiration becomes hurried; the skin is cool and covered with sweat; the pupils are dilated, there may be vomiting, headache, or delirium, and gradually, if the bleeding continues, consciousness is lost and death may occur with convulsions. In the more chronic forms, such as result from impoverishment of the blood, as in protracted illness or starvation, a condition of irritable weakness results. Mental effort is difficult, the slightest irritation is followed by undue excitement, the patient complains of giddiness and noises in the ears, or there may be hallucinations or delirium. These symptoms are met with in an extreme grade as a result of prolonged starvation, and a similar condition is seen in certain cases of arterio-sclerosis when the brain is poorly nourished.

An interesting set of symptoms, to which the term *hydrencephaloid* was applied by Marshall Hall, occurs in the anæmia and debility produced by prolonged diarrhœa in children. The child is in a semi-comatose condition with the eyes open, the pupils contracted, and the fontanelle depressed. In the earlier period there may be convulsions. The coma may gradually deepen, the pupils become dilated, and there may be strabismus and even retraction of the head, symptoms which closely simulate those of basilar meningitis.

III. ŒDEMA OF THE BRAIN

Whether it occurs as a clinical entity is doubtful. The cases reported as such resemble the serous meningitis or anomalous forms of acute polio-myelitis, particularly as skin rashes have been described. As a secondary process it occurs under the following conditions: In general atrophy of the convolutions, in which case the œdema is represented by an increase in the cerebro-spinal fluid and in that of the meshes of the pia. In extreme venous dilatation from obstruction, as in mitral stenosis or in tumors, there may be a condition of congestive œdema, in which, in addition to great filling of the blood vessels, the substance of the brain itself is unusually moist. The most acute œdema is a local process found around tumors and abscesses. The symptoms of compression following concussion or contusion, as shown by Cannon, are frequently attributable to cerebral œdema due to change in osmotic pressure. An intense infiltration, local or general, may occur in nephritis, and to it certain of the uræmic symptoms may be due.

Anatomical Changes.—These are not unlike those of anæmia. When the œdema follows progressive atrophy, the fluid is chiefly within and beneath the membranes. The brain substance is anæmic and moist and has a wet, glistening appearance, which is very characteristic. In some instances the œdema is more intense and local, and the brain substance may look infiltrated with fluid. The amount of fluid in the ventricles is usually increased.

Symptoms.—The symptoms are in great part those of lessened blood flow, and are not well defined. Some of the cerebral features of uræmia may depend upon it. Cases have been reported in which unilateral convulsions or paralysis have occurred in connection with chronic nephritis, and in which the condition appeared to be associated with œdema of the brain. The older writers laid great stress upon an apoplexia serosa, which may really have been a general œdema of the brain. Some of the cases of transient paralysis or aphasia may be caused by œdema.

IV. CEREBRAL HÆMORRHAGE

The bleeding may come from branches of either of the two great groups of cerebral vessels—the *basal,* comprising the circle of Willis and the central arteries passing from it and from the first portion of the cerebral arteries, or the *cortical group,* the anterior, middle, and the posterior cerebral vessels. In a majority of the cases the hæmorrhage is from the central branches, more particularly from those which are given off by the middle cerebral arteries in the anterior perforated spaces, and which supply the corpora striata and internal capsules. One of the largest of these branches which passes to the third division of the lenticular nucleus and to the anterior part of the internal capsule, the lenticulo-striate artery, is so frequently involved in hæmorrhage that it was called by Charcot *the artery of cerebral hæmorrhage.* Hæmorrhages from this and from the lenticulo-thalamic artery include more than 60 per cent. of all cerebral hæmorrhages. The bleeding may be into the substance of the brain, to which alone the term cerebral apoplexy is applied, or into the membranes, in which case it is termed meningeal hæmorrhage; both are usually included under the terms intracranial or cerebral hæmorrhage.

Etiology.—High blood pressure and arterial disease in persons over forty years of age are the main factors.

Age.—After thirty the liability increases with each decade. It may be congenital as in the child of a woman dead of typhoid fever at the Johns Hopkins Hospital. It occasionally occurs in children from rupture of a small aneurism, but before the age of thirty it is very uncommon. In an analysis of the United States Census Report, H. M. Thomas found the increase common in the 7th and 8th decades. Of 154 cases at St. Bartholomew's Hospital traceable to arterial changes there was no case under thirty; the maximum for both sexes was at the fifty-sixth year. After sixty the numbers appear to decline, but if "due correction is made for the age-distribution of a population, the liability of the individual to this form of death increases steadily up to old age" (F. W. Andrewes). Before the fifth decade hæmorrhage is rare; then in the fifth and sixth decades cases progressively increase in number.

Sex.—There is a marked preponderance of males.

Race.—In the United States the death rate from apoplexy in the Report of 1917 was 829 per million population. In England and Wales in 1916 the deaths from apoplexy were 693 per million living. Both apoplexy and paralysis seem to be much more prevalent among the negroes.

Heredity.—Formerly thought to be a very important factor, heredity influences the incidence in rendering members of families in which the blood vessels degenerate early more liable to cerebral hæmorrhage. What was known as the apoplectic habitus, or build, is still spoken of, by which we mean a stout, plethoric person of medium size with a short neck.

Special Factors.—Individuals with progressive renal disease and consecutive arterio-sclerosis and hypertrophy of the heart are particularly liable to cerebral hæmorrhage. Alcohol, immoderate eating, prolonged muscular exertion, syphilis, chronic lead poisoning, and gout are antecedents in many cases. Endocarditis may lead indirectly to apoplexy by causing embolism and aneurism of the vessels of the brain. Cerebral hæmorrhage occurs occasionally in the specific fevers and in such profound alterations of the blood as are met with in leukæmia.

The actual exciting cause is not always evident. The attacks may be sudden without any preliminary symptoms. In other instances straining efforts or overaction of the heart in emotion may cause a rupture. Many cases occur during sleep. Some instances follow slight trauma. The records of University College Hospital analyzed by Ernest Jones indicate that in none of 123 cases did the attack come on through excessive bodily effort.

Morbid Anatomy.—Direct Changes.—The lesions are almost invariably in the cerebral arteries, in which the following changes may lead to it:

(*a*) The production of miliary aneurisms, rupture of which is the most common cause of cerebral hæmorrhage. They occur most frequently on the central arteries, but also on the smaller branches of the cortical vessels. On section of the brain substance they may be seen as localized, small dark bodies, about the size of a pin's head. Sometimes they are seen in numbers upon the arteries when carefully withdrawn from the anterior perforated spaces. In apoplexy after the fortieth year if sought for they are rarely missed.

(*b*) Aneurism of the branches of the circle of Willis. These are by no means uncommon, and will be considered subsequently.

(*c*) Endarteritis and periarteritis in the cerebral vessels most commonly lead to apoplexy by the production of aneurisms, either miliary or coarse. There are instances in which the most careful search fails to reveal anything but diffuse degeneration of the cerebral vessels.

(*d*) Whether hæmorrhage ever occurs by *diapedesis* without actual rupture is doubtful. Possibly it does in purpura.

(*e*) In persons over sixty the hemiplegia may depend upon small areas of softening in the gray matter—the *lacunæ* of Marie—varying in size from a pin's head to a pea or a small bean, grayish red in tint. The lenticular nucleus is particularly apt to be involved. The blood vessels are always diseased.

The hæmorrhage may be meningeal, cerebral, or intraventricular.

Meningeal hæmorrhage may be outside the dura, between dura and arachnoid, or between the arachnoid and the pia mater. The following are the chief causes: Fracture of the skull, in which case the blood usually comes from the lacerated meningeal vessels, sometimes from the torn sinuses. In these cases the blood is usually outside the dura or between it and the arachnoid. The next most frequent cause is rupture of aneurisms on the larger cerebral vessels. The blood is usually subarachnoid. An intracerebral hæmorrhage may burst into the meninges. A special form of meningeal hæmorrhage is found in the new-born, associated with injury during birth. And lastly, meningeal hæmorrhage may occur in the constitutional diseases and fevers. The blood may be in a large quantity at the base; in cases of ruptured aneurism, particularly, it may extend into the cord or upon the cortex. Owing to the greater frequency of the aneurisms in the middle cerebral vessels, the Sylvian fissures are often distended with blood.

Intracerebral hæmorrhage is most frequent in the neighborhood of the corpus striatum, particularly toward the outer section of the lenticular nucleus. The hæmorrhage may be small and limited to the lenticular body, the thalamus, and the internal capsule, or it may extend to the insula. Hæmorrhages confined to the white matter—the centrum semiovale—are rare. Localized bleeding may occur in the crura or in the pons. Hæmorrhage into the cerebellum is not uncommon, and usually comes from the superior cerebellar artery. The extravasation may be limited to the substance or may rupture into the fourth ventricle.

Ventricular Hæmorrhage.—This is rarely primary, coming from the vessels of the plexuses or of the walls. More often it is secondary, following hæmorrhage into the cerebral substance. It is not infrequent in early life and may occur during birth. Of 94 cases collected by Edward Sanders, 7 occurred during the first year, and 14 under the twentieth year. In adults it is almost always caused by rupture of a vessel in the neighborhood of the caudate nucleus. The blood may be found in one ventricle only, but more commonly it is in both lateral ventricles, and may pass into the third ventricle and through the aqueduct of Sylvius into the fourth ventricle, forming a complete mould in blood of the ventricular system. In these cases the clinical picture may be that of *"apoplexie foudroyante."*

Multiple Hæmorrhages.—Of 128 non-traumatic cases at the Cook County Hospital there were 28 with discrete multiple hæmorrhages. The most common form is hæmorrhage into the basal ganglia and into the pons; the next, bilateral basal hæmorrhage. In the brain compression following hæmorrhage, the blood pressure rises; this increased intracranial tension is doubtless the cause of rupture in other vessels weakened by disease. The pontine arteries seem specially susceptible, as the small terminal vessels come off at right angles to a very large trunk (Phyllis Greenacre).

Subsequent Changes.—The blood gradually changes in color, and ultimately the hæmoglobin is converted into hæmatoidin. Inflammation occurs about the apoplectic area, limiting and confining it, and ultimately a definite wall may be produced, inclosing a cyst with fluid contents. In other instances a cyst is not formed, but the connective tissue proliferates and leaves a pigmented scar. In meningeal hæmorrhage the effused blood may be gradually absorbed and leave only a staining of the membranes. In other cases, particularly in infants, when the effusion is cortical and abundant, there may be localized wasting of the convolutions and the production of a cyst in the meninges. Possibly porencephaly may arise in this way. Secondary degeneration follows, varying in character according to the location of the hæmorrhage and the actual damage done by it to nerve cells or their medullated axones. Thus, in persons dying some years after a cerebral apoplexy which has produced hemiplegia (lesion of the motor area in the cortex or of the pyramidal tract leading from it), the degeneration may be traced through the cerebral peduncle, the ventral part of the pons, the pyramids of the medulla, the fibres of the direct pyramidal tract of the cord of the same side, and the fibres of the crossed pyramidal tract on the opposite side. After hæmorrhages in the middle and inferior frontal gyri degeneration of the frontal cerebro-cortico-pontal path follows, going through the anterior limb of the internal capsule and the medial portion of the basis pedunculi to the nuclei pontis; also degeneration of the fibres connecting the nucleus medialis thalami and the anterior part of the nucleus lateralis thalami with the cortex.

When the temporal gyri or their white matter are destroyed by a hæmorrhage the lateral segment of the basis pedunculi degenerates. Cerebellar hæmorrhage, especially if it injure the nucleus dentatus, may lead to degeneration of the brachium conjunctivum.

There may be slow degeneration in the lemniscus medialis, extending as far as the nuclei on the opposite side of the medulla oblongata, after hæmorrhages in the central gyri, hypothalamic region, or dorsal part of the pons. Hæmorrhages destroying the occipital cortex, or subcortical hæmorrhages injuring the optic radiations, occasion slow degeneration (cellulipetal) of the radiations from the lateral geniculate body, and after a time cause marked atrophy or even disappearance of its ganglion cells.

Symptoms.—PRIMARY.—Premonitory indications are rare. As a rule, the patient is seized while in full health or about the performance of some every day action, occasionally an action requiring strain or extra exertion. There may be headache, sensations of numbness or tingling or pains in the limbs, or even choreiform movements in the muscles of the opposite side, the so-called prehemiplegic chorea. In other cases temporary disturbances of vision and of associated movements of the eye-muscles have been noted, but none of the prodromata of apoplexy (the so-called "warnings") are characteristic. Transient aphasia or monoplegia may precede the attack. The onset may be with sudden loss of consciousness and complete relaxation of the extremities. In such instances the name *apoplectic stroke* is particularly appropriate. In other cases it is more gradual and the loss of consciousness may not occur for a few minutes after the patient has fallen, or after the paralysis of the limbs is manifest. In the typical apoplectic attack the condition is as follows: There is deep unconsciousness; the patient can not be roused. The face is injected, sometimes cyanotic, or of an ashen gray hue. The pupils vary; usually they are dilated, sometimes unequal, and always, in deep coma, inactive. If the hæmorrhage be so located that it can irritate the nucleus of the third nerve the pupils are contracted (hæmorrhages into the pons or ventricles). The respirations are slow, noisy, and accompanied with stertor. Sometimes Cheyne-Stokes rhythm may be present. The chest movements on the paralyzed side may be restricted, in rare instances on the opposite side. The cheeks are often blown out during expiration, with spluttering of the lips. The pulse is usually full, slow, and of increased tension. The temperature may be normal, but is often found subnormal, and, as in a case reported by Bastian, may sink below 95°. In cases of basal hæmorrhage the temperature, on the other hand, may be high. The urine and fæces are usually passed involuntarily. Convulsions are not common. It may be difficult to decide whether the condition is apoplexy associated with hemiplegia or sudden coma from other causes. An indication of hemiplegia may be discovered in the difference in the tonus of the muscles on the two sides. If the arm or the leg is lifted, it drops "dead" on the affected side, while on the other it falls more slowly. The lack of muscular tone of the paralyzed limb may be determined by inspection. In this condition the muscle mass of the thigh acts like a semi-fluid sac and takes the shape determined by gravity. In a patient lying or sitting on a firm support, the thigh of the paralyzed limb is broadened or flattened, while that on the normal side has a more rounded contour. Rigidity also may be present. In watching the movements of the facial muscles in the stertorous respiration it will be seen that on the paralyzed side the relaxation permits the cheek to be blown out in a more marked manner. The head and eyes may be turned to one side—conjugate deviation. In such an event the turning is *toward* the side of the hæmorrhage.

In other cases, in which the onset is not so abrupt, the patient may not lose consciousness, but in the course of a few hours there is loss of power, unconsciousness comes on gradually, and deepens into profound coma—ingravescent apoplexy. The attack may occur during sleep. The patient may be found unconscious, or wakes to find that the power is lost on one side. Small hæmorrhages in the territory of the central arteries may cause hemiplegia without loss of consciousness. In old persons the hemiplegia may be slight and follow a transient loss of consciousness, and is usually most marked in the leg. It may be quite slight and difficult to make out. It is associated with other senile changes. This is the form often due to the presence of lacunar softening.

Usually within forty-eight hours after the onset of an attack, sometimes within from two to six hours, there are febrile reaction and more or less constitutional disturbance associated with inflammatory changes about the hæmorrhage and absorption of the blood. The period of inflammatory reaction may continue for from one week to two months. The patient may die in this reaction, or, if consciousness has been regained, there may be delirium or recurrence of the coma. At this period the so-called early rigidity may develop in the paralyzed limbs and trophic changes occur, such as sloughing or the formation of vesicles. The most serious of these is the sloughing eschar of the lower part of the back, or on the paralyzed side, which may appear within forty-eight hours of the onset and is usually of grave significance. The congestion at the bases of the lungs so common in apoplexy is regarded by some as a trophic change.

Conjugate Deviation.—In a right hemiplegia the eyes and head may be turned to the left side; that is to say, the eyes look toward the cerebral lesion. This is almost the rule in hemiplegia. When, however, convulsions or spasm occur or the state of so-called early rigidity, the conjugate deviation of the head and eyes may be in the opposite direction; that is to say, the eyes look away from the lesion and the head is rotated toward the convulsed side. This symptom may be associated with cortical lesions, particularly, according to some authors, when in the neighborhood of the supramarginal and angular gyri. It may also occur in a lesion of the internal capsule or in the pons, but in the latter situation the conjugate deviation is the reverse of that which occurs in other cases, as the patient looks away from the lesion, and in spasm or convulsion looks toward the lesion.

Hemiplegia.—In cases in which consciousness is restored and the patient improves, a unilateral paralysis may persist due to the destruction of the motor area or the pyramidal tract in any part of its course. Hemiplegia is complete when it involves face, arm, and leg, or partial when it involves only one or other of these parts. This may be the result of a lesion (*a*) of the

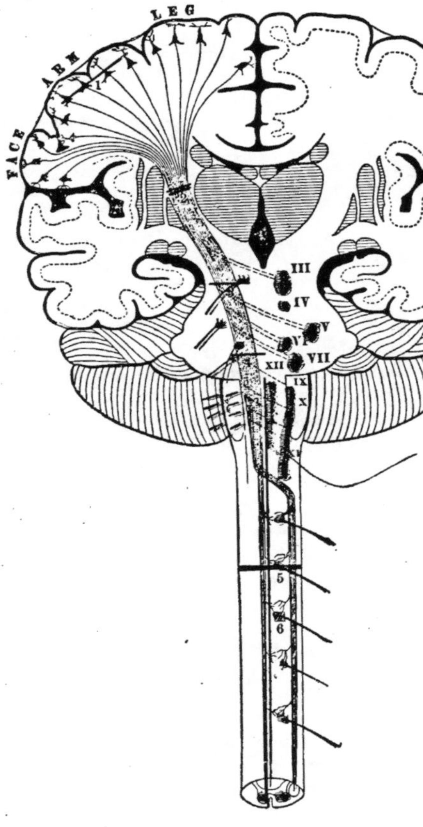

FIG. 20.—DIAGRAM OF MOTOR PATH FROM LEFT BRAIN.

The upper segment is black, the lower red. The nuclei of the motor cerebral nerves are shown on the right side; on the left side the cerebral nerves of that side are indicated. A lesion at 1 would cause upper segment paralysis in the arm of the opposite side—cerebral monoplegia; at 2, upper segment paralysis of the whole opposite side of the body—hemiplegia; at 3 (in the crus), upper segment paralysis of the opposite face, arm, and leg, and lower segment paralysis of the eye-muscles on the same side—crossed paralysis; at 4 (in the lower part of the pons), upper segment paralysis of the opposite arm and leg, and lower segment paralysis of the face and external rectus on the same side—crossed paralysis; at 5, upper segment paralysis of all muscles represented below lesion, and lower segment paralysis of muscles represented at level of lesion—spinal paraplegia; at 6, lower segment paralysis of muscles localized at seat of lesion—anterior poliomyelitis. (Van Gehuchten, modified.)

motor cortex; (*b*) of the pyramidal fibres in the corona radiata and in the internal capsule; (*c*) of a lesion in the cerebral peduncle; or (*d*) in the pons Varolii. The situation of the lesions and their effects are given in Fig. 20. Hæmorrhage is perhaps the most common cause, but tumors and spots of softening may also induce it. The special details of the hemiplegia may here be considered. The face (except in lesions in the lower part of the pons) is involved on the same side as the arm and leg. This results from the fact that the facial muscles stand in precisely the same relation to the cortical centres as those of the arm and leg, the fibres of the upper motor segment of the facial nerve from the cortex decussating just as do those of the nerves of the limbs. The signs of the facial paralysis are usually well marked. There may be a slight difficulty in elevating the eyebrows or in closing the eye on the paralyzed side, or in rare cases, the facial paralysis is complete, but the movements may be present with emotion, as laughing or crying. The facial paralysis is partial, involving only the lower portion of the nerve, so that the orbicularis oculi and the frontalis muscles are much less involved than the lower branch. The hypoglossal nerve also is involved. In consequence, the patient can not put out the tongue straight, but it deviates toward the paralyzed side, inasmuch as the genio-hyo-glossus of the sound side is unopposed. In a few cases the protrusion is toward the side of the lesion, a fact not easily explained. With right hemiplegia there may be aphasia. Even without marked aphasia difficulty in speaking and slowness are common.

The arm is, as a rule, more completely paralyzed than the leg. The loss of power may be absolute or partial. In severe cases it is at first complete. In others, when the paralysis in the face and arm is complete, that of the leg is only partial. The face and arm may alone be paralyzed, while the leg escapes. Less commonly the leg is more affected than the arm, and the face may be only slightly involved.

Certain muscles escape in hemiplegia, particularly those associated in symmetrical movements, as those of the thorax and abdomen, a fact which Broadbent explains by supposing that as the spinal nuclei controlling these movements on both sides constantly act together they may, by means of this intimate connection, be stimulated by impulses coming from only one side of the brain. Hughlings Jackson pointed out that in quiet respiration the muscles on the paralyzed side acted more strongly than the corresponding muscles, but that in forced respiration the reverse condition was true. The degree of permanent paralysis after a hemiplegic attack varies much in different cases. When the restitution is partial, it is always certain groups of muscles which recover rather than others. Thus in the leg the residual paralysis concerns the flexors of the leg and the dorsal flexors of the foot—i. e., the muscles which are active in the second period of walking, shortening the leg, and bringing it forward while it swings. The muscles which lift the body when the foot rests upon the ground, those used in the first period of walking, include the extensors of the leg and the plantar flexors of the foot. These "lengtheners" of the leg often recover almost completely in cases in which the paralysis is due to lesions of the pyramidal tract. In the arms the residual paralysis usually affects the muscle groups which oppose the thumb, those which rotate the arm outward, and the openers of the hand.

As a rule, there is at first no wasting of the paralyzed limbs.

Crossed Hemiplegia.—A paralysis in which there is loss of function in a cerebral nerve on one side with loss of power (or of sensation) on the opposite side of the body is called a crossed or alternate hemiplegia. It is met with in lesions, commonly hemorrhage, in the crus, the pons, and the medulla (Figs. 14, 15 and 20).

(*a*) *Crus.*—The bleeding may extend from vessels supplying the corpus striatum, internal capsule, and optic thalamus, or the hæmorrhage may be primarily in the crus. In the classical case of Weber, on section of the lower part of the left crus, an oblong clot 15 mm. in length lay just below the medial and inferior surface. The characteristic features of a lesion in this locality are paralysis of arm, face, and leg of the opposite side, and oculo-motor paralysis of the same side—the syndrome of Weber or Weber-Gubler. Sensory changes may also be present. Hæmorrhage into the tegmentum is not necessarily associated with hemiplegia, but there may be incomplete paralysis of the oculo-motor nerve, with disturbance of sensation and ataxia on the opposite side. The optic tract or the lateral geniculate body lying on the lateral side of the crus may be compressed, with resulting hemianopia.

(*b*) *Pons and Medulla.*—Lesions may involve the pyramidal tract and one or more of the cerebral nerves. If at the lower aspect of the pons, the facial nerve may be involved, causing paralysis of the face on the same side and hemiplegia on the opposite side. The fifth nerve may be involved, with the fillet (the sensory tract), causing loss of sensation in the area of distribution of the fifth on the same side as the lesion and loss of sensation on the opposite side of the body. The sensory disturbance here is apt to be dissociated, of the syringomyelic type, affecting particularly the sense of pain and temperature.

Sensory Disturbances Resulting from Cerebral Hæmorrhage.—These are variable. Hemianæsthesia may coexist with hemiplegia, but in many instances there is only slight numbing of sensation. When marked, it is usually the result of a lesion in the internal capsule involving the retrolenticular portion of the posterior limb. In a study of sensory localization Dana found that anæsthesia of organic cortical origin was always limited or more pronounced in certain parts, as the face, arm, or leg, and was generally incomplete. Total anæsthesia was either of functional or subcortical origin. Marked anæsthesia was much more common in softening than in hæmorrhage. Complete hemianæsthesia is rare in hæmorrhage. Disturbance of the special senses is not common. Hemianopia may exist on the same side as the paralysis, and there may be diminution in the acuteness of the senses of hearing, taste, and smell. Homonymous hemianopia of the halves of the visual fields opposite to the lesion is very frequent shortly after the onset, though often overlooked (Gowers).

Psychic disturbances, variable in nature and degree, may result from cerebral hæmorrhage.

The Reflexes in Apoplectic Cases.—During the apoplectic coma all the reflexes are abolished, but immediately on recovery of consciousness they return, first on the non-hemiplegic side, later, sometimes only after weeks, on the paralyzed side. As to the time of return, especially of the patellar reflexes, marked differences are observable in individual cases. The deep reflexes later are increased on the paralyzed side, and ankle clonus may be present. Plantar stimulation usually gives an extensor response in the great toe (Babinski's reflex) or dorsal flexion of the foot on irritating the skin over the tibia (Oppenheim's sign). The other superficial reflexes are usually diminished. The sphincters are not affected.

The *course* of the disease depends upon the situation and extent of the lesion. If slight, the hemiplegia may disappear completely within a few days or a few weeks. In severe cases the rule is that the leg gradually recovers before the arm, and the muscles of the shoulder girdle and upper arm before those of the forearm and hand. The face may recover quickly.

Except in the very slight lesions, in which the hemiplegia is transient, changes take place which may be grouped as

SECONDARY SYMPTOMS.—These correspond to the chronic stage. In a case in which little or no improvement takes place within eight or ten weeks it will be found that the paralyzed limbs undergo certain changes. The leg, as a rule, recovers enough power to enable the patient to get about, although the foot is dragged. Occasionally a recurrence of severe symptoms is seen, even without a new hæmorrhage having taken place. In both arm and leg the condition of *secondary contraction* or *late rigidity* comes on and is always most marked in the arm which becomes permanently flexed at the elbow and resists all attempts at extension. The wrist is flexed upon the forearm and the fingers upon the hand. The position of the arm and hand is very characteristic. There is frequently, as the contractures develop, a great deal of pain. In the leg the contracture is rarely so extreme. The loss of power is most marked in the muscles of the foot and, to prevent the toes from dragging, the knee in walking is much flexed, or more commonly the foot is swung round in a half circle.

The reflexes are at this stage greatly increased. These contractures are permanent and incurable, and are associated with a secondary descending sclerosis of the motor path. There are instances, however, in which rigidity and contracture do not occur, but the arm remains flaccid, the leg having regained its power. This *hémiplégie flasque* of Bouchard is found most commonly in children. Among other secondary changes in late hemiplegia may be mentioned the following: Tremor of the affected limbs, post-paralytic chorea, the mobile spasm known as athetosis, arthropathies in the joints of the affected side, and muscular atrophy. The cool surface and thin glossy skin of a hemiplegic limb are familiar to all.

Atrophy of the muscles may occur. It has been thought to be due in some cases to secondary alterations in the gray matter of the ventral horns; but atrophy may follow as a direct result of the cerebral lesion, the ventral horns remaining intact. In Quincke's case atrophy of the arm followed the development of a glioma in the anterior central convolution. The gray matter of the ventral horns was normal. These atrophies are most common in cortical lesions involving the domain of the third main branch of the Sylvian artery, and in central lesions involving the lenticulo-thalamic region. Their explanation is not clear. The wasting of cerebral origin, which occurs most frequently in children, and leads to hemiatrophy of the muscles with stunted growth of the bones and joints, is to be sharply separated from the hemiatrophy of the muscles of the adult following within a relatively short time upon the hemiplegia.

Diagnosis.—There are three groups of cases which offer difficulty.

(1) Cases in which the onset is gradual, a day or two elapsing before the paralysis is fully developed and consciousness completely lost, are readily recognized, though it may be difficult to determine whether the lesion is due to thrombosis or to hæmorrhage.

(2) In the sudden apoplectic stroke in which the patient rapidly loses consciousness the difficulty in diagnosis may be still greater, particularly if the patient is in deep coma when first seen.

The first point to be decided is the existence of hemiplegia. This may be difficult, although, as a rule, even in deep coma the limbs on the paralyzed side are more flaccid and drop instantly when lifted; whereas on the non-paralyzed side the muscles retain some degree of tonus. One cheek may puff or one side of the mouth splutter in expiration. The reflexes may be decreased or lost on the affected side and there may be conjugate deviation of the head and eyes. Rigidity in the limbs on one side is in favor of a hemiplegic lesion. It is practically impossible in a majority of these cases to say whether the lesion is due to hæmorrhage, embolism, or thrombosis.

(3) Large hæmorrhage into the ventricles or into the pons may produce sudden loss of consciousness with complete relaxation, simulating coma from uræmia, diabetes, alcoholism, opium poisoning, or epilepsy.

The previous history and the mode of onset may give valuable information. In *epilepsy* convulsions have preceded the coma; in *alcoholism* there is a history of constant drinking, while in *opium poisoning* the coma develops more gradually; but in many instances the difficulty is practically very great. With *diabetic coma* the breath often smells of acetone. In *ventricular hæmorrhage* the coma is sudden and comes on rapidly. The hemiplegic symptoms may be transient, quickly giving place to complete relaxation. Convulsions occur in many cases, and may be the very symptom to lead astray—as in a case of ventricular hæmorrhage which occurred in a puerperal patient, in whom, naturally enough, the condition was thought to be uræmic. Rigidity is often present. In hæmorrhage into the *pons* convulsions are frequent. The pupils may be strongly contracted, conjugate deviation may occur, and the temperature is apt to rise rapidly. The contraction of the pupils in pontine hæmorrhage naturally suggests opium poisoning. The difference in temperature in the two conditions is a valuable diagnostic point. The apoplectiform seizures of general paresis have usually been preceded by abnormal mental symptoms, and the associated hemiplegia is seldom permanent.

The cerebral attacks in Stokes-Adams disease may resemble apoplexy very closely. One stout patient, the subject of many attacks, had been bled so often that he had a label inside his coat—"Do not bleed me in an attack."

It may be impossible at first to give a definite diagnosis. In admissions to hospitals or in emergency cases the physician should be particularly careful about the following points: The examination of the head for injury or fracture; the urine should be tested for albumin and sugar, and studied microscopically; a careful examination should be made of the limbs with reference to the degree of relaxation or the presence of rigidity, and the condition of the reflexes; the state of the pupils should be noted and the temperature taken. The odor of the breath (alcohol, acetone, chloroform, etc.) should be noted. The most serious mistakes are made in the case of patients who are drunk at the time of the attack, a combination by no means uncommon.

Under these circumstances the case may erroneously be looked upon as one of alcoholic coma. It is best to regard each case as serious and to bear in mind that this is a condition in which, above all others, mistakes are common.

In *meningeal hæmorrhage,* as from ruptured aneurism, the attack is sudden, with pain in the head, rapid loss of consciousness, bilateral flaccidity, or difficulty in determining the existence of hemiplegia, rapid rise in temperature, and the presence of blood under high pressure in the spinal fluid. In one case (death on fourth day) on the second day suggillations and petechiæ complicated the diagnosis.

Prognosis.—From cortical hæmorrhage, unless very extensive, the recovery may be complete without a trace of contracture. This is more common when the hæmorrhage follows injury than when it results from disease of the arteries. Infantile meningeal hæmorrhage, on the other hand, is a condition which may produce idiocy or spastic diplegia.

Large hæmorrhages into the corona radiata, and especially those which rupture into the ventricles, rapidly prove fatal.

The hemiplegia which follows lesions of the internal capsule, the result of rupture of the lenticulo-striate artery, is usually persistent and followed by contracture. When the retro-lenticular fibres of the internal capsule are involved there may be hemianæsthesia, and later, especially if the thalamus be implicated, hemichorea or athetosis. In any case the following symptoms are of grave omen: persistence or deepening of the coma during the second and third day; rapid rise in temperature within the first forty-eight hours after the initial fall. In the reaction which takes place on the second or third day the temperature usually rises, and its gradual fall on the third or fourth day with return of consciousness is a favorable indication. The rapid formation of bed-sores, particularly the malignant decubitus of Charcot, is a fatal indication. The occurrence of albumin and sugar, if abundant, in the urine is an unfavorable symptom.

When consciousness returns and the patient is improving, the question is anxiously asked as to the paralysis. The extent of this can not be determined for some weeks. With slight lesions it may pass off entirely. If persistent at the end of a month some grade of permanent palsy is certain to remain, and gradually the late rigidity supervenes.

V. EMBOLISM AND THROMBOSIS

(*Cerebral Softening*)

Embolism.—The embolus usually enters the carotid, rarely the vertebral artery. In the great majority of cases it comes from the left heart and is either a vegetation of a fresh endocarditis or, more commonly, of a recurring endocarditis, or from the segments involved in an ulcerative process. Less often the embolus is a portion of a clot which has formed in the auricular appendix. Portions of clot from an aneurism, thrombi from atheroma of the aorta, or from the territory of the pulmonary veins, may also cause blocking of the branches of the circle of Willis. In the puerperal condition cerebral embolism is not infrequent. It may occur in women with heart disease, but in other instances the heart is uninvolved, and the condition has been thought to be associated with the development of heart clots, owing to increased coagulability of the blood. A majority of cases of embolism occur in heart disease, 89 per cent. (Saveliew). Cases are rare in the acute endocarditis of rheumatic fever, chorea, and febrile conditions. It is much more common in the secondary recurring endocarditis which attacks old sclerotic valves. The embolus most frequently passes to the left middle cerebral artery and the posterior cerebral and the vertebral are less often affected. A large plug may lodge at the bifurcation of the basilar. Embolism of the cerebellar vessels is rare.

Embolism occurs more frequently in women, owing, no doubt, to the greater frequency of mitral stenosis. Contrary to this general statement, Newton Pitt's statistics of 79 cases at Guy's Hospital indicate, however, that males are more frequently affected; as in this series there were 44 males and 35 females. Saveliew gives 54 per cent. in women.

Thrombosis.—Clotting of blood in the cerebral vessels occurs (1) about an embolus, (2) as the result of a lesion of the arterial wall (either endarteritis with or without atheroma or, particularly, the syphilitic arteritis), (3) in aneurisms, both large and miliary, and (4) as a direct result of abnormal conditions of the blood as in the anæmia of hæmorrhage, chlorosis, septicæmia and the cachexia of cancer. Thrombosis occasionally follows ligation of the carotid artery. The thrombosis is most common in the middle cerebral and in the basilar arteries. It is suggested that softening of limited areas, sufficient to induce hemiplegia, may be caused by sudden collapse of certain cerebral arteries from cardiac weakness.

Anatomical Changes.—Degeneration and softening of the territory supplied by the vessels are the ultimate result in both embolism and thrombosis. Blocking in a terminal artery may be followed by infarction, in which the territory may either be deeply infiltrated with blood (hæmorrhagic infarction) or be simply pale, swollen, and necrotic (anæmic infarction). Gradually the process of *softening* proceeds, the tissue is infiltrated with serum and is moist, the nerve fibres degenerate and become fatty. The neuroglia is swollen and œdematous. The color of the softened area depends upon the amount of blood. The hæmoglobin undergoes gradual transformation, and the early red color may give place to yellow. Formerly much stress was laid upon the difference between *red, yellow,* and *white* softening. The red and yellow are seen chiefly on the cortex. Sometimes the red softening is particularly marked in cases of embolism and in the neighborhood of tumors. The gray matter shows many punctiform hæmorrhages—capillary apoplexy. There is a variety of yellow softening—the *plaques jaunes*—common in elderly persons, occurring in the gray matter, in spots from 1 to 2 cm. in diameter, sometimes angular in shape, the edges cleanly cut, and the softened area represented by a turbid, yellow material or in some instances there is space crossed by fine trabeculæ, in the meshes of which there is fluid. White softening occurs most frequently in the white matter, and is seen best about tumors and abscesses. Inflammatory changes are common in and about the softened areas. When the embolus is derived from an infected focus, as in ulcerative endocarditis, suppuration may follow. The final changes vary very much. The degenerated and dead tissue elements are gradually but slowly removed, and if the region is small may be replaced by a growth of connective tissue and the formation of a scar. If large, the resorption results in the formation of a cyst.

The position and extent of the softening depend upon the obstructed artery. An embolus which blocks the middle cerebral at its origin involves not only the arteries to the anterior perforated space, but also the cortical branches, and in such a case there is softening in the neighborhood of the corpus striatum, as well as in part of the region supplied by the cortical vessels. The freedom of anastomosis between these branches varies. Thus, in embolism of the middle cerebral artery in which the softening has involved only the territory of the central branches, blood may reach the cortex through the anterior and posterior cerebrals. When the middle cerebral is blocked (as is perhaps oftenest the case) beyond the point of origin of the central arteries, one or other of its branches is usually most involved. The embolus may lodge in the vessel passing to the third frontal convolution, or in the artery of the ascending frontal or ascending parietal; or it may lodge in the branch passing to the supramarginal and angular gyri, or enter the lowest branch which is distributed to the upper convolutions of the temporal lobe. These are practically terminal arteries, and instances frequently occur of softening limited to a part, at any rate, of the territory supplied by them. Some of the most accurate focalizing lesions are produced in this way.

There is unquestionably greater freedom of communication in the cortical branches of the different arteries than is usually admitted, although it is not possible, for example, to inject the posterior cerebral through the middle cerebral, or the middle cerebral from the anterior; but the absence of softening in some instances in which smaller branches are blocked shows how complete may be the compensation, probably by way of the capillaries. The dilatation of the collateral branches may take place very rapidly; thus a patient with chronic nephritis died twenty-four hours after the hemiplegic attack. There were recent vegetations on the mitral valve and an embolus in the right middle cerebral artery just beyond the first two branches. The central portion of the hemisphere was swollen and œdematous. The right anterior cerebral was greatly dilated, and its diameter was nearly three times that of the left.

Symptoms.—Extensive thrombotic softening may exist without any symptoms. It is not uncommon in the examination of the bodies of elderly persons to find the *plaques jaunes* scattered over the convolutions. So, too, softening may take place in the "silent" regions, without exciting any symptoms. When the central or cortical branches of the middle cerebral arteries are involved the symptoms are similar to those of hæmorrhage from the same arteries. Permanent or transient hemiplegia results. When the central arteries are involved the softening in the internal capsule is commonly followed by hemiplegia. Certain peculiarities are associated with embolism and with thrombosis respectively.

In *embolism* the patient is usually the subject of heart trouble, or there exist some of the conditions already mentioned. The onset is sudden, without premonitory symptoms but sometimes with intense headache. When the embolus blocks the left middle cerebral artery, the hemiplegia is associated with aphasia. In *thrombosis,* on the other hand, the onset is more gradual; the patient has previously complained of headache, vertigo, tingling in the fingers; the speech may have been embarrassed for some days; the patient has had loss of memory or is incoherent, or paralysis begins at one part, as the hand, and extends slowly, and the hemiplegia may be incomplete or variable. Abrupt loss of consciousness is much less common, and when the lesion is small consciousness is retained. Thus, in thrombosis due to syphilitic disease, the hemiplegia may come on gradually without any disturbance of consciousness.

The hemiplegia following thrombosis or embolism has practically the characteristics, both primary and secondary, described under hæmorrhage.

The following may be the effects of blocking the different vessels: (*a*) *Vertebral.*—The left branch is more frequently plugged. The effects are involvement of the nuclei in the medulla and symptoms of acute bulbar paralysis. It rarely occurs alone; more commonly with

(*b*) Blocking of the *basilar artery.*—When this is entirely occluded, there may be bilateral paralysis from involvement of both motor paths. Bulbar symptoms may be present; rigidity or spasm may occur. The temperature may rise rapidly. The symptoms, in fact, are those of apoplexy of the pons.

(*c*) The *posterior cerebral* supplies the occipital lobe on its medial surface and the greater part of the temporo-sphenoidal lobe. If the main stem be thrombosed there is hemianopia with sensory aphasia. Localized areas of softening may exist without symptoms. Blocking of the main occipital branch (arteria occipitalis of Duret), or of the arteria calcarina, passing to the cuneus may be followed by hemianopia. Hemianæsthesia may result from involvement of the posterior part of the internal capsule. Not infrequently symmetrical thrombosis of the occipital arteries of the two sides occurs, as in Förster's well-known case. Still more frequent is the occurrence of thrombosis of a branch of the posterior cerebral of one hemisphere and a branch of the middle cerebral of the other. It is in such cases that the most pronounced instances of apraxia are met with.

(*d*) *Internal Carotid.*—The symptoms are variable. The vessel is ligated without risk in a majority of cases; in other instances transient hemiplegia follows; in others again the hemiplegia is permanent. These variations depend on the anastomoses in the circle of Willis. If these are large and free, no paralysis follows, but in cases in which the posterior communicating and the anterior communicating vessels are small or absent the paralysis may persist. In No. 7 of the Elwyn series of cases of infantile hemiplegia, the woman, aged twenty-four, when six years old, had the right carotid ligated for abscess following scarlet fever, with the result of permanent hemiplegia. Blocking of the internal carotid within the skull by thrombosis or embolism is followed by hemiplegia, coma, and usually death. The clot is rarely confined to the carotid itself, but spreads into its branches and may involve the ophthalmic artery.

(*e*) *Middle Cerebral.*—This is the vessel most commonly involved, and if plugged before the central arteries are given off, permanent hemiplegia usually follows from softening of the internal capsule. Blocking of the branches beyond this point may be followed by hemiplegia, which is more likely to be transient, involves chiefly the arm and face, and if the lesion be on the left side is associated with aphasia. There may be plugging of the individual branches passing to the inferior frontal (producing motor aphasia if the disease be on the left side), to the anterior and posterior central gyri (usually causing total hemiplegia), to the supramarginal and angular gyri (giving rise, if the thrombosis be on the left side, probably without exception to the so-called visual aphasia (alexia), usually also to right-sided hemianopsia), or to the temporal gyri (in which event with left-sided thrombosis word-deafness results).

(*f*) *Anterior Cerebral.*—No symptoms may follow, and even when the branches which supply the paracentral lobule and the top of the ascending convolutions are plugged the branches from the middle cerebral are usually able to effect a collateral circulation in these parts. Monoplegia of the leg may, however, result. Hebetude and dullness of intellect may occur with obstruction of the vessel.

Treatment of Cerebral Hæmorrhage and of Softening.—The chief difficulty in deciding upon a method of treatment is to determine whether the apoplexy is due to hæmorrhage or to thrombosis or embolism. The patient should be placed in bed, with his head moderately elevated and the neck free. He should be kept absolutely quiet. If there are dyspnœa, stertor, and signs of mechanical obstruction to respiration, he should be turned on his side. This lessens the liability to congestion of the lungs. Venesection seems to be indicated theoretically in cases of hæmorrhage with high pressure, but practically is of little or no value and is not advisable. As Cushing has shown experimentally, a rapid and increasing rise of arterial tension usually indicates an endeavor to counteract an increasing intracranial pressure, in this case due to a continuing hæmorrhage. The indication under these circumstances is the relief of the intracranial pressure by craniotomy and removal of the clot, if this is possible. This is particularly applicable in subdural hæmorrhage. Horsley and Spencer, on experimental grounds, recommended the practice, formerly employed empirically, of compression of the carotid, particularly in the ingravescent form. An ice-bag may be placed on the head and hot bottles to the feet. The bowels should be freely opened, either by calomel or elaterin. Counter-irritation to the neck or to the feet is not necessary. Catheterization of the bladder may be necessary, especially if the patient remains long unconscious.

Special care should be taken to avoid bed-sores; and if bottles are used to the feet, they should not be too hot, since blisters may be readily caused by a much lower temperature than in health. Stimulants are not necessary, unless the pulse becomes feeble and signs of collapse supervene. During recovery the patient should be still kept entirely at rest, even in the mildest attacks remaining in bed for at least fourteen days. The ice-bag should still be kept to the head. The diet should be light. The bowels should be kept freely open. Attention should be paid to the position occupied by the paralyzed limb or limbs, which if swollen may be wrapped in cotton batting or flannel. Small doses of iodide (gr. v, 0.3 gm.) may be given.

The treatment of *softening* from thrombosis or embolism is very unsatisfactory. Venesection is not indicated, as it rather promotes clotting. If, as is often the case, the heart's action is feeble and irregular, small doses of digitalis may be given. The bowels should be kept open, but it is not well to purge actively, as in hæmorrhage.

In the thrombosis which follows syphilitic disease of the arteries, and which is met with most frequently in men between twenty and forty (in whom the hemiplegia often sets in without loss of consciousness), active antisyphilitic treatment is indicated; the iodide should be given in full dosage. Practically these are the only cases of hemiplegia in which we see satisfactory results from treatment.

Very little can be done for the hemiplegia which remains. The damage is too often irreparable and permanent, and it is very improbable that iodide of potassium, or any other remedy, hastens in the slightest degree Nature's dealing with the blood clot.

The paralyzed limbs may be gently rubbed once or twice a day, and this should be systematically carried out, in order to maintain the nutrition of the muscles and to prevent contractures if possible. The massage should not be begun until at least ten days after the attack. The rubbing should be *toward* the body, and should not be continued for more than fifteen minutes at a time. After the lapse of a fortnight, or in severe cases a month, the muscles may be stimulated by the faradic current; faradic stimulation alternating with massage, especially if applied to the antagonists of the muscles which ordinarily undergo contracture, is of service, even when there can be but little hope of any return of voluntary movement. The patient should be encouraged to perform simple movements and exercises himself. When contractures occur, electricity at intervals may be of some benefit along with passive movement and friction, and it has been suggested that tendon transplantation, or indeed cross suture of nerves, may cause some improvement.

In a case of complete hemiplegia the friends should at the outset be frankly told that the chances of full recovery are slight. Power is usually restored in the leg sufficient to enable the patient to get about, but in the majority of instances the finer movements of the hand are permanently lost. The general health should be looked after, the bowels regulated, and the secretions of the skin and kidneys kept active. In permanent hemiplegia in persons above the middle period of life, more or less mental weakness is apt to follow the attack, and the patient may become irritable and emotional.

And, lastly, when hemiplegia has persisted for more than three months and contractures have developed, it is the duty of the physician to explain to the patient, or to his friends, that the condition is past relief, that medicines and electricity will do no good, and that there is no possible hope of cure.

VI. ANEURISM OF THE CEREBRAL ARTERIES

Miliary aneurisms are not included, but reference is made only to aneurism of the larger branches. The condition is not uncommon. There were 12 instances in 800 autopsies in the Montreal General Hospital. This is a considerably larger proportion than in Newton Pitt's collection from Guy's Hospital, 19 times in 9,000 inspections.

Etiology.—Males are more frequently affected than females. Of the 12 cases 7 were males. The disease is most common at the middle period of life. One of the cases was a lad of six. Pitt describes one at the same age. The chief causes are (*a*) endarteritis, either simple or syphilitic, which leads to weakness of the wall and dilatation; and (*b*) embolism. These aneurisms are often found with endocarditis. Pitt, in his study of the subject, concludes that it is exceptional to find cerebral aneurism unassociated with fungating endocarditis. The embolus disappears, and dilatation follows the secondary inflammatory changes in the coats of the vessel.

Morbid Anatomy.—The middle cerebral branches are most frequently involved. In the 12 cases the distribution was as follows: Internal carotid, 1; middle cerebral, 5; basilar, 3; anterior communicating, 3. Except in one case they were saccular and communicated with the lumen of the vessel by an orifice smaller than the circumference of the sac. In 154 cases (statistics of Lebert, Durand, and Bartholow) the middle cerebral was involved in 44, the basilar in 41, internal carotid in 23, anterior cerebral in 14, posterior communicating in 8, anterior communicating in 8, vertebral in 7, posterior cerebral in 6, inferior cerebellar in 3 (Gowers). The size of the aneurism varies from that of a pea to that of a walnut. The hæmorrhage may be entirely meningeal with very slight laceration of the brain substance, but the bleeding may be, as Coats has shown, entirely within the substance.

Symptoms.—The aneurism may attain considerable size and cause no symptoms. In a majority of the cases the first intimation is the rupture and the fatal apoplexy. Distinct symptoms are most frequently caused by aneurism of the internal carotid, which may compress the optic nerve or the commissure, causing neuritis or paralysis of the third nerve. A murmur may be audible. Aneurism in this situation may give rise to irritative and pressure symptoms at the base of the brain or as in the remarkable case reported by Weir Mitchell and Dercum bilateral temporal hemianopia.

Aneurism of the vertebral or of the basilar may involve the nerves from the fifth to the twelfth. A large sac at the termination of the basilar may compress the third nerves or the crura.

The diagnosis is, as a rule, impossible. The larger sacs produce the symptoms of tumor, and their rupture is usually fatal.

VII. THROMBOSIS OF THE CEREBRAL SINUSES AND VEINS

The condition may be primary or secondary. Lebert (1854) and Tonnele were among the first to recognize the condition clinically.

Primary thrombosis of the sinuses and veins is rare. It occurs (*a*) in children, particularly during the first six months of life, usually in connection with diarrhœa. Gowers believed that it is of frequent occurrence, and that thrombosis of the veins is not an uncommon cause of infantile hemiplegia.

(*b*) In connection with chlorosis and anæmia, the so-called *autochthonous sinus-thrombosis*. Of 82 cases of thrombosis in chlorosis, 78 were in the veins and 32 in the cerebral sinuses. The longitudinal sinus is most frequently involved. The thrombosis is usually associated with venous thromboses in other parts of the body, and the patients die, as a rule, in from one to three weeks, but both Bristow and Buzzard, Sen., report recoveries.

(*c*) In the terminal stages of cancer, tuberculosis, and other chronic diseases thrombosis may occur in the sinuses and cortical veins. To the coagulum in these conditions the term marantic thrombus is applied.

Secondary thrombosis is much more frequent and follows extension of inflammation from contiguous parts to the sinus wall. The common causes are disease of the internal ear, fracture, compression of the sinuses by tumor, or suppurative disease outside the skull, particularly erysipelas, carbuncle, and parotitis. In secondary cases the lateral sinus is most frequently involved. Of 57 fatal cases in which ear disease caused death with cerebral lesions, there were 22 in which thrombosis existed in the lateral sinuses (Pitt.). Tuberculous caries of the temporal bone is often directly responsible. The thrombus may be small, or fill the entire sinus and extend into the internal jugular vein. In more than half of these instances the thrombus was suppurating. The disease spreads directly from the necrosis on the posterior wall of the tympanum by way of the petroso-mastoid canal. It is not so common in disease of the mastoid cells.

Symptoms.—*Primary thrombosis* of the longitudinal sinus may occur without exciting symptoms and is found accidentally at the post mortem. There may be mental dullness with headache. Convulsions and vomiting may occur. In other instances there is nothing distinctive. In the chlorosis cases the head symptoms have, as a rule, been marked. Ball's patient was dull and stupid, had vomiting, dilatation of the pupils, and double choked disks. Slight paresis of the left side occurred. An interesting feature in this case was the development of swelling of the left leg. In the cases reported by Andrews, Church, Tuckwell, Isambard Owen, and Wilks the patients had headache, vomiting, and delirium. Paralysis was not present. In Douglas Powell's case, with similar symptoms, there was loss of power on the left side. Bristowe reports a case in an anæmic girl of nineteen, who had convulsions, drowsiness, and vomiting. Tenderness and swelling developed in the position of the right internal jugular vein, and a few days later on the opposite side. The diagnosis was rendered definite by the occurrence of phlebitis in the right leg. The patient recovered.

The onset of such symptoms as have been mentioned in an anæmic or chlorotic girl should lead to the suspicion of cerebral thrombosis. In infants the diagnosis can rarely be made. Involvement of the cavernous sinus may cause œdema about the eyelids or prominence of the eyes.

In the *secondary thrombi* the symptoms are commonly those of septicæmia. For instance, in over 70 per cent. of Pitt's cases the mode of death was by pulmonary pyæmia. This author draws the following important conclusions: (1) The disease spreads oftener from the posterior wall of the middle ear than from the mastoid cells. (2) The otorrhœa is generally of some standing, but not always. (3) The onset is sudden, the chief symptoms being pyrexia, rigors, pains in the occipital region and in the neck, associated with a septicæmic condition. (4) Well-marked optic neuritis may be present. (5) The appearance of acute local pulmonary mischief or of distant suppuration is almost conclusive of thrombosis. (6) The average duration is about three weeks, and death is generally from pulmonary pyæmia. The chief points in the diagnosis may be gathered from these statements.

Associated with thrombosis of the lateral sinus there may be venous stasis and painful œdema behind the ear and in the neck. The external jugular vein on the diseased side may be less distended than on the opposite side, since owing to the thrombus in the lateral sinus the internal jugular vein is less full than on the normal side, and the blood from the external jugular can flow more easily into it.

Treatment.—In marantic individuals stimulants are indicated. The position assumed in bed should favor both the arterial and venous circulation. The clothing should not restrict the neck, and care should be taken to avoid *bending* of the neck. The internal administration of potassium iodide and calomel has been recommended in the autochthonous forms, but no treatment is likely to be of any avail.

The secondary forms, especially those following upon disease of the middle ear, are often amenable to operation, and many lives have been saved by surgical intervention after extensive sinus thrombosis.

VIII. CEREBRAL PALSIES OF CHILDREN

Introduction.—There are three great groups: I. Those due to pre-natal factors, *agenesia cerebri, microcephalus, porencephaly, congenital cysts, etc.* II. *Natal* or *intrapartum* which includes the large group of birth palsies due to meningeal hæmorrhage, etc., and III. The *post-natal* group of which by far the larger proportion is due to acute encephalitis occurring between the second and sixth year, and leading to hemiplegia. In all these cerebral palsies there are three important factors: (1) Disturbance in some degree of the normal mental development, (2) a paralysis disturbing the natural and normal movement of the muscles, and (3) spasticity in greater or less degree.

A number of important conditions may be grouped together for convenience of description—Aplasia cerebri, meningeal hæmorrhage, spastic diplegia, Little's disease, bilateral athetosis, etc.

I. Aplasia (Agenesia) cerebri.—This is due to failure of development of the cerebral cortex due to intra-uterine conditions. Nothing abnormal may be noted at birth, which has not been delayed or assisted by instruments. The head may be small and the sutures may close early. Then it is noticed that the child does not develop normally in the use of the muscles; the movements are irregular but not athetoid. The head wobbles, the child does not sit up, the dentition is delayed, and by the time the second year is reached, the failure of development is evident. The arms and legs may become stiff and the condition of bilateral spastic rigidity supervene. More often the limbs remain relaxed, the child may learn to walk in an awkward way, the full power over the movements is never acquired, and the child settles into a state of idiocy. Anatomically the brain is small, the convolutions ill developed, and there may be areas of lobular sclerosis, sometimes the remarkable tuberose form.

II. Meningeal Hæmorrhage—*with conservative paraplegia spastica cerebralis (Heine); Little's disease; Tetraplegia spastica.*—Heine, one of the founders of modern orthopedics, recognized the cerebral origin of many of the palsies of children; and Little subsequently called attention to the "influence of abnormal parturition, difficult labors, premature birth and asphyxia on the mental and physical condition of the child, especially in relation to deformities." In 1885 Sarah McNutt's careful studies correlated the meningeal hæmorrhage with the subsequent palsies as recognized by Heine and Little.

The causes are: (1) Tearing of the veins due to pressure on the head in a contracted pelvis and in forceps delivery. (2) Asphyxia. The extreme stasis, particularly just after the head is born, causes rupture of the veins at the point of entrance to the longitudinal sinus (Cushing). (3) The hæmorrhage may be in association with the hæmorrhagic condition of the new born.

The hæmorrhage is from the pia, usually over the cortex and widely spread. It may be more on one side than the other, and may extend over the cerebellum. The brain substance may be softened or compressed, and present foci of hæmorrhage. The hæmorrhage may be extradural, and even extend into the spinal cord. First birth, premature birth, foot presentation, but above all, the indiscriminate and careless use of the forceps are the causal factors. There is much wisdom in the dread expressed by Shandy Senior, of the dangers of compression of the delicate and fine web of the brain.

Symptoms. (Early).—The asphyxia may be protracted. Unusual torpor, absence of the natural crying, inability to take the breast, flaccidity of the limbs, sometimes with rigidity on one side or convulsions, unequal and dilated pupils, and slow breathing with signs of atelectasis are the most suggestive features. There may be hæmorrhages elsewhere if the condition is associated with the hæmorrhagic disease of the newborn, as in cases reported by Green and by Margaret Warwick. Lumbar puncture may show blood.

Symptoms (Late).—If the child recovers, nothing may be noticed for a few months. Perhaps there are convulsions. The first thing to attract attention is that when the child should begin to walk the limbs are not used readily, and on examination a stiffness of the legs and arms is found. Even at the age of two the child may not be able to sit up, and often the head is not well supported by the neck muscles. The rigidity, as a rule, is more marked in the legs, and there is an adductor spasm. When supported on the feet, the child either rests on its toes and the inner surface of the feet, with the knees close together, or the legs may be crossed. The stiffness of the upper limbs varies. It may be scarcely noticeable or the rigidity may be as marked as in the legs. When the spastic condition affects the arms as well as the legs, we speak of the condition as diplegia or tetraplegia; when the legs alone are involved, as paraplegia. There seems to be no sufficient reason for considering them separately. The spasticity is probably due to the interruption of the cortico-spinal fibres which exercise an inhibitory influence on the cells of the anterior horns. Constant irregular movements of the arms are not uncommon. The child has great difficulty in grasping an object. The spasm and weakness may be more evident on one side than the other. The mental condition is, as a rule, defective and convulsive seizures are common.

III. Acute Sporadic Encephalitis of Children with Consecutive Hemiplegia.—This is an acute infection characterized by fever, convulsions, coma, and a consecutive hemiplegia. It is possibly the sporadic form of, or related to, epidemic encephalitis or acute polio-myelitis.

History.—Heine first recognized *Hemiplegia spastica cerebralis,* separating it from other forms of infantile paralysis.

Etiology.—Cases of hemiplegia in Children's Homes and Institutions for the Feeble-Minded fall into two groups—(1) a large one, 95 out of 135 in Osler's series, in which the disease began at or shortly after the second year, suddenly, in healthy children; and (2) a small one, with a more advanced age of onset, comprising cases of trauma, heart disease, etc. A certain number in the first group follow the acute infections, 19 of the series. The incidence in relation to acute polio-myelitis is not known. There did not appear to be an increase of cases during the recent outbreaks. Practically nothing is known of the cause. It may be related to polio-myelitis, but it is a much less variable malady.

Pathology.—The motor area of one hemisphere is involved in an acute hæmorrhagic lesion, the convolutions swollen and deeply injected, the veins thrombosed, and on section the substance is moist, deep red, and the limitation of the gray matter ill defined or obliterated. The picture corresponds with Strümpell's encephalitis. No other changes of moment may be present. Years later the cerebral changes depend on the extent of the original lesion—sclerosis with atrophy of the motor area opposite the paralyzed limb is the most common, or there is a sub-meningeal cyst.

Symptoms.—Clinically the disease is very sharply defined. A perfectly healthy child between the second and fifth years has a convulsion, or a series of them, with fever, possibly vomiting, and then becomes comatose. Preliminary indisposition is rare; headache may be complained of, but without warning the fit, as a rule, is the first symptom of the disease. The fever may reach 103°-104°. There may be marked conjugate deviation of the head and eyes: the pupils are usually dilated, and may be unequal. The head may be retracted, and naturally meningitis is suspected. In the deep coma the hemiplegia may be—often is—overlooked, but on careful examination the face is seen to be drawn and the arm and leg of one side limp and paralyzed. One of two things happens—either the coma persists, the convulsions recur, and the child dies from the second to the fifth day, or the fever drops, the coma lessens, and within a couple of days the child seems quite well, but one side is paralyzed.

Complete recovery is rare. The face and arm improve rapidly, the leg lags and drags, as in an ordinary hemiplegia. Speech if disturbed returns. The chief tragedy is a failure to develop mentally, which takes so many of these cases into the Feeble-Minded Homes. The arm of the affected side may not develop but remains shorter and the hand smaller. In other cases recovery is not so complete; both leg and arm are spastic and the latter may present post-hemiplegic movements. Sensation is not disturbed. A very distressing feature is the onset of epilepsy, which may be in the form of pure Jacksonian fits, *petit mal,* or general seizures. Of the 135 cases in the series, 41 had epilepsy.

Post-hemiplegic Movements.—It was in cases of this sort that Weir Mitchell first described the post-hemiplegic movements. They are extremely common, and were present in 34 of the series. There may be either slight tremor in the affected muscles, or incoördinate choreiform movements—the so-called post-hemiplegic chorea—or, lastly,

Athetosis.—This is a remarkable condition in which there is a combination of spasm with the most extraordinary bizarre movements of the muscles. The patient may not be able to walk. The head is turned from side to side; there are continual irregular movements of the face muscles, and the mouth is drawn and greatly distorted. The extremities are more or less rigid, particularly in extension. On the slightest attempt to move, often spontaneously, there are extraordinary movements of the arms and legs. The patients are often unable to help themselves on account of these movements. The reflexes are increased. The mental condition is variable.

Treatment.—Cases with asphyxia and convulsions after difficult labors have been operated upon soon after birth by Cushing and others, and cortical clots have been removed. In some cases there has been a complete restoration to health and the usual spastic sequels have not occurred. As the child grows, conditions have to be met—the mental, requiring the care and training necessary for the grade of feeble-mindedness, and the orthopedic treatment of the spasticity, for which much can be done. The educational care in institutions has shown how much patient training is able to help the development of these defective children. In all these patients the degree of development depends very much upon the thorough, painstaking and systematic training of their minds and muscles.

Surgically much may be done by tenotomy and the use of proper apparatus. For the relief of the spasticity operations on the brain are rarely of any help. Better results have been obtained by injecting drugs into the motor nerves or by their resection, and where there is a high grade of bilateral spasticity, the resection of the posterior nerve roots appears sometimes to have been helpful.

IV. TUMORS, INFECTIONS, GRANULOMATA, AND CYSTS OF THE BRAIN

The following are the most common varieties of new growths within the cranium:

Infectious Granulomata.—(*a*) *Tubercle* may form large or small growths, usually multiple. Tuberculosis of the glands or bones may coexist, but the tuberculous disease of the brain may occur in the absence of other clinically recognizable tuberculous lesions. The disease is most frequent early in life. Three-fourths of the cases occur under twenty, and one-half of the patients are under ten years of age (Gowers). Of 300 cases of tumor in persons under nineteen collected from various sources by Starr, 152 were tubercle. The nodules are most numerous in the cerebellum and about the base.

(*b*) *Syphiloma* is most commonly found on the cortex cerebri or about the pons. The tumors are superficial, attached to the arteries or the meninges, and rarely grow to a large size. They may be multiple. A gummatous meningitis of the base is common and in this process the oculomotor nerves are often affected. The motor nerves of the eye are particularly prone to syphilitic infiltration, and ptosis and squint are common. The pituitary body may be involved with symptoms suggestive of diabetes insipidus.

Tumors.—(*c*) *Glioma and Neuroglioma.*—They may be firm and hard, almost like an area of sclerosis, and not sharply defined or soft and with hæmorrhages. They persist remarkably for many years. Klebs called attention to the occurrence of elements in them not unlike ganglion-cells. Tumors of this character may contain the "Spinnen" or spider cells; enormous spindle-shaped cells with single large nuclei; cells like the ganglion-cells of nerve-centres with nuclei and one or more processes; and translucent, band-like fibres, tapering at each end, which result from a vitreous or hyaline transformation of the large spindle-cells. A separate type is recognizable, in which the cells resemble the ependymal epithelium.

(*d*) *Fibrosarcoma* (endothelioma) occurs most commonly in the membranes covering the hemispheres or brain stem, and for a long time may cause injury by its compression effects alone. Tumors of this kind are particularly common in the cerebello-pontine recess. When sarcoma originates in the brain substance it may become one of the largest and most diffusely infiltrating of intracranial growths. When meningeal in origin, it is the form of tumor most amenable to surgical treatment.

(*e*) *Carcinoma* may be secondary to cancer in other parts. It is seldom primary. Occasionally cancerous tumors have been found in symmetrical parts of the brain.

(*f*) Other varieties are fibroma, usually developing from the membranes; bony tumors, which grow sometimes from the falx, psammoma, cholesteatoma, and angioma. Fatty tumors are occasionally found on the corpus callosum. There is a remarkable condition, originally described by Rokitansky, of brownish-black pigmentation of the brain, partly diffuse, partly focal, associated with pigmented nævi of the skin. The nævi in the brain are in no sense a metastasis from the skin, but are benign tumors arising primarily (MacLachlan).

Cysts.—These occur between the membranes and the brain, as a result of hæmorrhage or of softening. Porencephalus is a sequel of congenital atrophy or of hæmorrhage, or may be due to a developmental defect. Hydatid cysts have been referred to in the section on parasites. An interesting variety of cyst is that which follows severe injury to the skull in early life. Gliomata often undergo cystic degeneration. Dermoid cyst has been described.

Site.—A majority of all tumors occur in the cerebrum and especially in the centrum ovale. The cerebellum, pons, and membranes are next most often involved. Glioma is more common in the hemispheres and grows slowly. It is usually single. Tubercles are usually multiple. Secondary sarcoma and carcinoma are often multiple.

Symptoms.—General.—The following are the most important: *Headache,* either dull, aching, and continuous, or sharp, stabbing, and paroxysmal. It may be diffuse or limited to the back or front. When in the back of the head it may extend down the neck (especially in tumors in the posterior fossa), and when in the front it may be accompanied with neuralgic pains in the face. Occasionally the pain may be very localized and associated with tenderness on pressure.

Choked disk (optic neuritis) should be looked for in every patient presenting cerebral symptoms, for it may be present without impairment of vision. Loss of visual acuity usually indicates that optic atrophy has set in. It is usually double, but occasionally is found in only one eye. Growths may attain considerable size without producing optic neuritis. On the other hand, it may occur with a very small tumor, when this tumor is so situated as to cause internal hydrocephalus. J. A. Martin, from an extensive analysis of the literature with reference to the localizing value, concludes: When there is a difference in the amount of the neuritis in each eye it is more than twice as probable that the tumor is on the side of the most marked neuritis. It is constant in tumors of the corpora quadrigemina, present in 89 per cent. of cerebellar tumors, and absent in nearly two thirds of the cases of tumor of the pons, medulla, and of the corpus collosum. It is least frequent in cases of tuberculous tumor; most common in cases of glioma and cystic tumors.

Paton and Holmes report upon the eyes of 700 cases of cerebral tumor, concluding that the essential feature of the associated optic neuritis is œdema, and in 60 eyes examined histologically the one unfailing change was acute œdema, the origin of which they attribute to the venous engorgement.

Vomiting is a common feature and, with headache and optic neuritis, makes up the characteristic clinical picture of cerebral tumor. An important point is the absence of definite relation to the meals. A chemical examination shows that the vomiting is independent of digestive disturbances. It may be very obstinate, particularly in growths of the cerebellum and the pons.

Giddiness is often an early symptom, on rising suddenly or turning quickly.

Mental Symptoms.—These are usually of progressive mental weakness leading to dementia. Mania, depressive conditions, delusions, hallucinations, confusional states, paranoia, and general paralysis have all been described. The patient may act in an odd, unnatural manner, or there may be stupor and heaviness. The patient may be emotional or silly, or there are symptoms resembling hysteria.

Convulsions, either general and resembling true epilepsy or localized (Jacksonian) in character. Seizures beginning with a gustatory or olfactory aura are common with tumors originating in the infundibular region. There may be *slowing of the pulse,* as in all cases of increased intracranial pressure.

LOCALIZING SYMPTOMS.—The smaller the tumor and the less marked the general symptoms of cerebral compression the more likely is it that any focal symptoms occurring are of *direct* origin. Localizing features are often misleading. A frontal tumor may have cerebellar features due to increased intercranial pressure which has compressed the cerebellum against the base of the skull. The characteristic Bárány cerebellar tests have been present with temporal lobe tumors.

(*a*) *Central Motor Area.*—The symptoms are either irritative or destructive in character. Irritation in the lower third may produce spasm in the muscles of the face, in the angle of the mouth, or in the tongue. The spasm with tingling may be strictly limited to one muscle group before extending to others, and this Seguin terms the *signal symptom.* The middle third of the motor area contains the centres controlling the arm, and here, too, the spasm may begin in the fingers, in the thumb, in the muscles of the wrist, or in the shoulder. In the upper third of the motor areas the irritation may produce spasm beginning in the toes, in the ankles, or in the muscles of the leg. In many instances the patient can determine accurately the point of origin of the spasm, and there are important sensory disturbances, such as numbness and tingling, which may be felt first at the region affected.

In all cases it is important to determine, first, the point of origin, the *signal symptom;* second, the order or march of the spasm; and third, the subsequent condition of the parts first affected, whether it is a state of paresis or anæsthesia.

Destructive lesions in the motor zone cause paralysis, often preceded by local convulsive seizures; there may be a monoplegia, as of the leg, and convulsive seizures in the arm, often due to irritation. Tumors in the neighborhood of the motor area may cause localized spasms and subsequently, as the centres are invaded by the growth, paralysis occurs. With tumors in the left hemisphere the speech mechanism is apt to be involved if the transverse temporal gyrus or the third frontal convolution and their connecting path are implicated.

(*b*) *Prefrontal Region.*—Neither motor nor sensory disturbance may be present. The general symptoms are often well marked. The most striking feature of growths in this region is mental torpor and gradual imbecility. Particularly when the left side is involved mental characteristics may be greatly altered. In its extension downward the tumor may involve on the left side the lower frontal convolution and produce aphasia, or in its progress backward cause irritative or destructive lesions of the motor area. Exophthalmos on the side of the tumor may occur and be helpful in diagnosis.

(*c*) Tumors in the *parieto-occipital lobe,* particularly on the right side, may grow to a large size without causing any symptoms. There may be word-blindness and mind-blindness when the left angular gyrus and its underlying white matter are involved, and paraphasia. Astereognosis may accompany growths in the superior parietal region.

(*d*) Tumors of the *occipital lobe* produce hemianopia, and a bilateral lesion may produce blindness. Tumors in this region on the left hemisphere may be associated with word-blindness and mind-blindness. In all cases of tumor a careful study should be made of the fields of vision. In addition to the lateral hemianopia there may be remarkable visual hallucinations, and in tumors of the left occipital lobe dissociation of the color sense and inability to find the proper colors of various objects presented.

(*e*) Tumors in the *temporal lobe* may attain a large size without producing symptoms. In their growth they involve the lower motor centres. On the left side involvement of the transverse temporal gyri (auditory sense area) may be associated with word-deafness.

(*f*) Tumors growing in the neighborhood of the *basal ganglia* produce hemiplegia from involvement of the internal capsule. Limited growths in either the nucleus caudatus or the nucleus lentiformis of the corpus striatum do not necessarily cause paralysis. Tumors in the thalamus opticus may also, when small, cause no symptoms, but, increasing, they may involve the fibres of the sensory portion of the internal capsule, producing hemianopia and sometimes hemianæsthesia. Growths in this situation are apt to cause early optic neuritis, and, growing into the third ventricle, may cause a distention of the lateral ventricles. What has been termed the thalamic syndrome may be present—hemianæsthesia to pain, touch and temperature, with the loss of deep sensibility. With this there may be a very remarkable type of pain, involving the hand and arm and the foot and leg, on the affected side, a sense of burning discomfort rather than sharp pain. Ataxic features are usually present and astereognosis. Motor hemiplegia may be present, and it is unaccompanied by contractures (Dana).

Growths in the *corpora quadrigemina* are rarely limited, but most commonly involve the crura cerebri as well. Ocular symptoms are marked. The pupil reflex is lost and there is nystagmus. In the gradual growth the third nerve is involved as it passes through the crus, in which case there will be oculo-motor paralysis on one side and hemiplegia on the other, a combination almost characteristic of unilateral disease of the crus.

(*g*) Tumors of the *pons* and *medulla.* The symptoms are chiefly those of pressure upon the nerves emerging in this region. In disease of the pons the nerves may be involved alone or with the pyramidal tract. Of 52 cases analyzed by Mary Putnam Jacobi, in 13 the cerebral nerves were involved alone, in 13 the limbs were affected, and in 26 there were hemiplegia and involvement of the nerves. In 22 of the latter there was alternate paralysis—i. e., involvement of the nerves on one side and of the limbs on the opposite side. In 4 cases there were no motor symptoms. In tuberculosis (or syphilis) a growth at the inferior and inner aspects of the crus may cause paralysis of the third nerve on one side, and of the face, tongue, and limbs on the opposite side (syndrome of Weber). A tumor growing in the lower part of the pons usually involves the sixth nerve, producing internal strabismus, the seventh nerve, producing facial paralysis, and the auditory nerve, causing deafness. Conjugate deviation of the eyes to the side opposite that on which there is facial paralysis also occurs. When the motor cerebral nerves are involved the paralyses are of the peripheral type (lower segment paralyses).

Tumors of the *medulla* may involve the cerebral nerves alone or cause in some instances a combination of hemiplegia with paralysis of the nerves. Paralyses of the nerves are helpful in topical diagnosis, but the fact must not be overlooked that one or more of the cerebral nerves may be paralyzed as a result of a much increased general intracranial pressure. Signs of irritation in the ninth, tenth, and eleventh nerves are usually present, and produce difficulty in swallowing, irregular action of the heart, irregular respiration, vomiting, and sometimes retraction of the head and neck. The hypoglossal nerve is least often affected. The gait may be unsteady or, if there is pressure on the cerebellum, ataxic. Occasionally there are sensory symptoms, numbness and tingling. Toward the end convulsions may occur.

(*h*) Tumors of the *cerebellum* may be latent, but they usually give rise to very characteristic symptoms, headache in the occipital region, giddiness, incoordination, but there is nothing definite in the direction of the swaying, and early optic neuritis. They may be intracerebellar or extracerebellar.

Tumors or enlargements of the *pituitary gland* itself, or growths from a congenital *anlage* in its neighborhood which implicate the pituitary gland secondarily, are very common. The congenital tumors arise presumably from developmental faults, and show either a teratomatous character or are solid or cystic tumors with squamous epithelium, often attaining adamantine characteristics. The most common tumor is a so-called struma (malignant adenoma) of the gland proper. There are characteristic signs of pressure upon the neighborhood structures, bitemporal hemianopia being a frequent though not invariable feature. These lesions may occur in patients who have suffered from acromegaly, or in those who show signs of glandular deficiency or dyspituitarism, and in whom there may or may not be suggestive acromegalic tendencies. The X-rays are most useful in diagnosis.

Diagnosis.—From the general symptoms alone the existence of tumor may be determined, for the combination of headache, optic neuritis, and vomiting is distinctive. As pointed out by R. T. Williamson, progressive hemiplegia, without other symptoms, a paralysis, which gradually becomes more marked day by day and week by week, is almost pathognomonic, even in the absence of optic neuritis, headache, and vomiting. The two exceptions to this rule appear to be in cerebral abscess, and in rare instances a polio-encephalitis. It must not be forgotten that severe headache and neuro-retinitis may be caused by nephritis. The localization must be gathered from the consideration of the symptoms and from the data given in the section on Topical Diagnosis. Mistakes are most likely to occur in connection with uræmia, hysteria, vascular lesions, abscess, serous meningitis, hydrocephalus, and general paresis; but careful consideration of all the circumstances of the case usually enables the practitioner to avoid error. Röntgen ray shadows are noticed with calcification in the tumor or when there is atrophy or thickening of the bones of the skull or the characteristic changes in the sella turcica in pituitary tumors. The pineal gland, which so often shows gritty deposits, may be indicated by a shadow. In about 45 of 100 cases of brain tumor the X-ray picture was of help in the diagnosis (Dandy).

Prognosis.—Syphilitic tumors alone are amenable to medical treatment. Tuberculous growths occasionally cease to grow and become calcified. The gliomata and fibromata, particularly when the latter grow from the membranes, may last for years. The more rapidly growing sarcomata usually prove fatal in from six to eighteen months. Death may be sudden, particularly in growths near the medulla; more commonly it is due to coma in consequence of gradual increase in the intracranial pressure.

Treatment.—(*a*) Medical.—A Wassermann test of the blood and cerebrospinal fluid should always be made before antiluetic measures are instituted. It must not be overlooked that vigorous treatment with potassium iodide often causes a temporary amelioration of pressure symptoms due to a glioma, so that the therapeutic test is not a dependable one. If syphilis is proved the iodide of potassium and mercury should be given. Arsphenamine is sometimes given in repeated small doses. Nowhere do we see more brilliant therapeutical effects than in certain cases of cerebral gummata. The iodide should be given in increasing doses. In tuberculous tumors the outlook is less favorable, though instances of cure are reported, and there is post mortem evidence to show that the solitary tuberculous tumors may undergo changes and become obsolete. A general tonic treatment is indicated in these cases. The headache usually demands prompt treatment. Iodide of potassium in full doses sometimes gives marked relief. An ice-cap for the head or, in the occipital headache, the application of the Paquelin cautery may be tried. The bromides are not of much use in the headache from this cause, and, as the last resort, morphia must be given. For the convulsions bromide of potassium is of little service.

(*b*) Surgical.—Many tumors of the brain have been successfully removed. Though the percentage of cases in which total enucleation is possible is doubtless small, yet in all cases marked amelioration of the pressure symptoms is possible by surgical measures. It is important that they should be instituted early, even in the absence of localizing symptoms, for the sake of preserving vision. The most advantageous cases are the localized fibromata and sarcomata growing from the dura and only compressing the brain substance. There have been numerous successful operations with removal of growths from the cerebellum and cerebello-pontine recess. The safety with which the exploratory operation can be made warrants it in all doubtful cases. For two objects the decompression operation may be performed, to relieve the headache, which it sometimes does promptly and permanently, and to save sight. It is now very generally practised and the reduction of the greatly increased intracranial pressure may cause the choked disk to subside and the risk of subsequent atrophy is much diminished.

V. INFLAMMATION OF THE BRAIN

I. ACUTE ENCEPHALITIS

A focal or diffuse inflammation of the brain substance, usually of the gray matter (polio-encephalitis), is met with (*a*) as a result of trauma; (*b*) in certain intoxications, alcohol, food poisoning, and gas poisoning; (*c*) following the acute infections; and (*d*) as one of the varieties of polio-myelo-encephalitis. The anatomical features are those of an acute hæmorrhagic polio-encephalitis, corresponding in histological details with acute polio-myelitis. Focal forms are seen in ulcerative endocarditis, in which the gray matter may present deep hæmorrhagic areas, firmer than the surrounding tissue. In the fevers there may be more extensive regions, involving two or three convolutions. This acute polio-encephalitis superior was thought by Strümpell to be the essential lesion in infantile hemiplegia. Localizing symptoms are usually present, though they may be obscured in the severity of the general infection. The most typical encephalitis accompanies the meningitis in cerebro-spinal fever.

In acute mania, in delirium tremens, in chorea insaniens, in the maniacal form of exophthalmic goitre, and in the so-called cerebral forms of the malignant fevers the gray cortex is deeply congested, moist, and swollen, and with the finer methods of research will probably show changes which may be classed as encephalitis.

The *symptoms* are not very definite. In severe forms they are those of an acute infection; some cases have been mistaken for typhoid fever. The onset may be abrupt in an individual apparently healthy. Other cases have occurred in the convalescence from the fevers, particularly influenza. One of J. J. Putnam's cases followed mumps. The general symptoms are those which accompany all severe acute affections of the brain—headache, somnolence, coma, delirium, vomiting. etc. The local symptoms are very varied, depending on the extent of the lesions, and may be irritative or paralytic. Usually fatal within a few weeks, cases may drag on for weeks or months and recover, generally with paralysis.

II. ABCESS OF THE BRAIN

Definition.—Purulent encephalitis with abscess formation the result of infection by micro-organisms.

Etiology.—Suppuration of the brain substance is rarely primary, but results, as a rule, from extension of inflammation from neighboring parts or infection from a distance through the blood. The question of idiopathic brain abscess need scarcely be considered, though instances occur in which it is difficult to assign a cause. There are three important etiological factors.

(*a*) *Trauma.* Falls upon the head or blows, with or without abrasion of the skin. More commonly it follows fracture or punctured wounds. In this group meningitis is frequently associated with the abscess. Simple trauma or concussion does not produce abscess but organisms may enter through a laceration of the base opening one of the many sinuses.

(*b*) By far the most important infective foci are those which arise in *direct extension from disease of the middle ear,* of the *mastoid cells,* or of the *accessory nasal sinuses.* From the roof of the mastoid antrum the infection readily passes to the sigmoid sinus and induces an infective thrombosis. In other instances the dura becomes involved, and a subdural abscess is formed, which may readily involve the arachnoid or the pia mater. In another group the inflammation extends along the lymph spaces, or the thrombosed veins, into the substance of the brain and causes suppuration. Macewen thinks that without local areas of meningitis the infective agents may be carried through the lymph and blood channels into the cerebral substance. Infection which extends from the roof of the tympanic cavity is most likely to be followed by abscess in the temporal lobe, while infection extending from the mastoid cells causes most frequently sinus thrombosis and cerebellar abscess.

(*c*) *In septic processes.* Abscess of the brain is not often found in pyæmia. In ulcerative endocarditis multiple foci of suppuration are common. Localized bone disease and suppuration in the liver are occasional causes. Certain inflammations in the lungs, particularly bronchiectasis, may be followed by abscess. It is an occasional complication of empyema. Abscess of the brain may follow the specific fevers. The largest number of cases occur between the twentieth and fortieth years, and the condition is more frequent in men than in women. In children under five years of age, the chief causes are otitis media and trauma.

Morbid Anatomy.—The abscess may be solitary or multiple, diffuse or circumscribed. Practically any one of the different varieties of pyogenic bacteria may be concerned. The bacteriological examination often shows different varieties. Occasionally cultures are sterile. In the acute, rapidly fatal cases following injury the suppuration is not limited; but in long standing cases the abscess is inclosed in a definite capsule, which may have a thickness of from 2 to 5 mm. The pus varies much in appearance, depending upon the age of the abscess. In early cases it may be mixed with reddish *débris* and softened brain matter, but in the solitary encapsulated abscess the pus is distinctive, having a greenish tint, an acid reaction, and a peculiar odor, sometimes like that of sulphuretted hydrogen. The brain substance surrounding the abscess is usually œdematous and infiltrated. The size varies from that of a walnut to that of a large orange. There are cases in which the cavity occupies the greater portion of a hemisphere. Multiple abscesses are usually small. In four-fifths of all cases the abscess is solitary. Suppuration occurs most frequently in the cerebrum, and the temporal lobe is more often involved than other parts, and always on the side of the ear disease. The cerebellum is the next most common seat, particularly in connection with ear disease.

Symptoms.—Following injury or operation the disease may run an *acute* course, with fever, headache, delirium, vomiting, and rigors. The symptoms are those of suppurative meningo-encephalitis, and it may be very difficult to determine, unless there are localizing symptoms, whether there is really suppuration in the brain substance. In the cases following ear disease the symptoms may at first be those of meningeal irritation. There may be irritability, restlessness, severe headache, and aggravated earache. Other striking symptoms, particularly in the more prolonged cases, are drowsiness, slow cerebration, vomiting, and optic neuritis. In the chronic form which may follow injury, otorrhœa, or local lung trouble, there may be a latent period of weeks to several months, or even a year or more. In the "silent" regions, when the abscess becomes encapsulated there may be no symptoms whatever during the latent period. During this time the patient may be under careful observation and no suspicion be aroused of suppuration. Then severe headache, vomiting, and fever set in, perhaps with a chill. So, too, after a blow upon the head or a fracture the symptoms may be transient, and months afterward cerebral symptoms of the most aggravated character may develop.

The localization is often difficult. If situated in or near the motor region there may be convulsions or paralysis, and an abscess in the temporal lobe may compress the lower part of the pre-central convolution and produce paralysis of the arm and face, and on the left side cause aphasia. A large abscess may exist in the frontal lobe without causing paralysis, but in these cases there is almost always some mental dullness. In the temporal lobe, the common seat, there may be no focalizing symptoms. So also in the parieto-occipital region; though early examination may lead to the detection of hemianopia. In abscess of the cerebellum vomiting is common. If the middle lobe is affected there may be staggering—cerebellar incoördination. Localizing symptoms in the pons and other parts are still more uncertain.

Diagnosis.—In the acute cases there is rarely any doubt. A consideration of possible etiological factors is of the highest importance. The history of injury followed by fever, marked cerebral symptoms, the onset of rigors, delirium, and perhaps paralysis, make the diagnosis certain. In chronic ear disease, such cerebral symptoms as drowsiness and torpor, with irregular fever, supervening upon the cessation of a discharge, should excite the suspicion of abscess. Cases in which suppurative processes exist in the orbit, nose, or naso-pharynx, or in which there has been subcutaneous phlegmon of the head or neck, a parotitis, a facial erysipelas, or tuberculous or syphilitic disease of the bones of the skull, should be carefully watched, and immediately investigated should cerebral symptoms appear. It is particularly in the chronic cases that difficulties arise. The symptoms resemble those of tumor of the brain; indeed, they are those of tumor plus fever. Choked disk, however, so commonly associated with tumor, may be absent. In a patient with a history of trauma or with localized lung or pleural trouble, who for weeks or months has had slight headache or dizziness, the onset of a rapid fever, especially if it be intermittent and associated with rigors, intense headache, and vomiting, points strongly to abscess. The pulse rate in cases of cerebral abscess is usually accelerated, but cases are not rare in which it is slowed. Macewen lays stress upon the value of percussion of the skull as an aid in diagnosis. The note, which is uniformly dull, becomes much more resonant when the lateral ventricles are distended in cerebellar abscess and in conditions in which the venæ Galeni are compressed. Tenderness of the skull has been noted over the region of the abscess.

It is not always easy to determine whether the meninges are involved and often in ear disease the condition is a meningo-encephalitis. Sometimes with acute ear disease the symptoms may simulate closely cerebral meningitis or abscess. Indeed, Gowers stated that not only may these general symptoms be produced by ear disease, but even distinct optic neuritis.

Treatment.—In ear disease free discharge of the inflammatory products should be promoted and careful disinfection practised. The treatment of injuries and fractures comes within the scope of the surgeon. The acute symptoms, such as fever, headache, and delirium, must be treated by rest, an ice-cap, and, if necessary, local depletion. In all cases, when a reasonable suspicion exists of the occurrence of abscess, the brain should be explored. The cases following ear disease, in which the suppuration is in the temporal lobe or in the cerebellum, offer the most favorable chances of recovery. The localization can rarely be made accurately in these cases, and the operator must be guided more by general anatomical and pathological knowledge. In cases of injury the exploration should be over the seat of the blow or the fracture. In ear disease the suppuration is most frequent in the temporal lobe or in the cerebellum, and the operation should be performed at the points most accessible to these regions.

VI. HYDROCEPHALUS

Definition.—A condition, congenital or acquired, in which there is a great accumulation of fluid within the ventricles of the brain.

The cases may be divided into three groups—idiopathic internal hydrocephalus (serous meningitis), congenital or infantile, and secondary or acquired.

Serous Meningitis (*Quincke's Disease, Idiopathic Internal Hydrocephalus; Angio-neurotic Hydrocephalus*).—A knowledge of this condition explains many anomalous and puzzling cases. An ependymitis causing a serous effusion into the ventricles, with distention and pressure effects, it may be compared to the serous exudates in the pleura or synovial membranes. It is not certain that the process is inflammatory, and Quincke likens it to the angio-neurotic œdema of the skin. In very acute cases the ependyma may be smooth and natural looking; in more chronic cases thickened and sodden. The exudate does not differ from the normal, and if on lumbar puncture the fluid has a specific gravity above 1.009, with albumin above two tenths per cent., the condition is more likely to be hydrocephalus from stasis, secondary to tumor, etc.

Both children and adults are affected, the latter more frequently. In the acute form the condition is mistaken for tuberculous or purulent meningitis. There are headache, retraction of the neck, and signs of increased intracranial pressure, choked disks, slow pulse, etc. Fever is usually absent, but there are cases with recurring paroxysms of fever. Quincke reported cases of recovery. In the chronic form the symptoms are those of tumor—general, such as headache, slight fever, somnolence, and delirium; and local, as exophthalmos, optic neuritis, spasms, and rigidity of muscles and paralysis of the cerebral nerves. Exacerbations occur, and the symptoms vary in intensity from day to day. Recovery may follow and some of the reported cases of disappearance of all symptoms of brain tumor belong in this category.

A variety of this is the *circumscribed serous meningitis* confined to the cerebello-pontile angle, due to adhesions of the arachnoid to the cerebellum in the region of the flocculus. Fluid accumulates in the cisterna lateralis, which has its own choroid plexus. The increased pressure leads to disturbance in function of the nerves in this region, causing the syndrome described by Bárány—tinnitus with deafness, vertigo, occipital headache, facial paralysis, and the "pointing error." Other lesions of this region, syphilitic meningitis and tumors, may, of course, cause this syndrome.

Congenital Hydrocephalus.—There are two types, one due to obstruction of outflow from the ventricles, the other from decreased absorption from the sub-arachnoid space (Dandy and Blackfan).

The lateral ventricles are enormously distended, but the ependyma is usually clear, sometimes a little thickened and granular, and the veins large. The choroid plexuses are vascular, sometimes sclerotic, but often natural looking. The third ventricle is enlarged, the aqueduct of Sylvius dilated, and the fourth ventricle may be distended. The quantity of fluid may reach several litres. It is limpid and contains a trace of albumin and salts. The changes in consequence of the ventricular distention are remarkable. The cerebral cortex is greatly stretched, and over the middle region the thickness may amount to no more than a few millimetres without a trace of the sulci or convolutions. The basal ganglia are flattened. The skull enlarges, and the circumference of the head of a child of three or four years may reach 25 or even 30 inches. The sutures widen, Wormian bones develop in them, and the bones of the cranium become exceedingly thin. The veins are marked beneath the skin. A fluctuation wave may sometimes be obtained, and Fisher's brain murmur may be heard. The orbital plates of the frontal bone are depressed, causing exophthalmos, so that the eyeballs can not be covered by the eyelids. The small size of the face, widening somewhat above, is striking in comparison with the enormously expanded skull.

The enlarged head may obstruct labor; more frequently the condition is noticed some time after birth. The cause is unknown. It has occurred in several members of the same family. Convulsions may occur. The reflexes are increased, the child learns to walk late, and ultimately in severe cases the legs become feeble and sometimes spastic. Sensation is much less affected than motility. Choked disk is not uncommon. The mental condition is variable; the child may be bright, but, as a rule, there is some grade of imbecility. The congenital cases usually die within the first four or five years. The process may be arrested and the patient may reach adult life. Even when extreme, the mental faculties may be retained, as in Bright's celebrated patient, Cardinal, who lived to the age of twenty-nine, and whose head was translucent when the sun was shining behind him. Care must be taken not to mistake the rachitic head for hydrocephalus. The condition may be associated with other defects, harelip, spina bifida and club-foot.

Dandy has introduced a method of fluoroscopy after the injection of air into the ventricles, the outlines of which are then well seen and the extent but not always the type of hydrocephalus determined.

Acquired Chronic Hydrocephalus.—This is stated to be occasionally primary (idiopathic)—that is to say, it comes on spontaneously in the adult without observable lesion. Dean Swift is said to have died of hydrocephalus, but this seems very unlikely. It is based upon the statement that "he (Mr. Whiteway) opened the skull and found much water in the brain," a condition no doubt of *hydrocephalus ex vacuo,* due to the wasting associated with his prolonged illness and paralysis. In nearly all cases there is either a tumor at the base of the brain or in the third ventricle, which compresses the venæ Galeni. The passage from the third to the fourth ventrical may be closed, either by a tumor or by parasites. More rarely the foramen of Magendie, through which the ventricles communicate with the cerebro-spinal meninges, becomes closed by meningitis. Chronic inflammations of the ependyma may block the foramina of exit of the ventricular fluid. There may be unilateral hydrocephalus from closure of one of the foramina of Monro. In cerebro-spinal fever, particularly in the sporadic form, the foramina of exit of the fluid may be occluded, with great distention of the ventricles. These conditions in adults may produce the most extreme hydrocephalus without any enlargement of the head. Even when the tumor begins early in life there may be no expansion of the skull. In the case of a girl aged sixteen, blind from her third year, the head was not unusually large, the ventricles were enormously distended, and in the Rolandic region the brain substance was only 5 mm. in thickness. A tumor occupied the third ventricle. In other instances the sutures separate and the head gradually enlarges.

The symptoms are curiously variable. In the case mentioned there were headaches and gradual blindness; then a prolonged period in which she was able to attend to her studies. Headaches again supervened, the gait became irregular and somewhat ataxic. Death occurred suddenly. In another case there were prolonged attacks of coma with a slow pulse, and on one occasion the patient remained unconscious for more than three months. Gradually progressing optic neuritis without focalizing symptoms, headache, and attacks of somnolence or coma are suggestive symptoms. These cases of acquired chronic hydrocephalus can not be certainly diagnosed during life, though the condition may be suspected. They simulate tumor very closely.

Treatment.—Medicines are powerless to cause the absorption of the fluid. In the meningitis serosa Quincke advised the use of mercury. Various operations have been devised for conveying the fluid to the subtemporal or subcutaneous regions, and attempts have been made to conduct the fluid to the peritoneum and the pleura, or even connecting the cisterna magna directly with the longtitudinal sinus.

J. DISEASES OF THE PERIPHERAL NERVES

I. NEURITIS

Neuritis may be *localized* in a single nerve, or *general,* involving a large number of nerves—*multiple neuritis* or *polyneuritis.*

Etiology.—*Localized neuritis* arises from (*a*) cold, which is a very frequent cause, as, for example, in the facial nerve. (*b*) Trauma—wounds, blows, direct pressure on the nerves, the tearing and stretching which follow a dislocation or a fracture, and the hypodermic injection of ether. Under this section come the professional palsies, due to pressure in the exercise of certain occupations. (*c*) Extension of inflammation from neighboring parts, as in a neuritis of the facial nerve due to caries in the temporal bone, or in that met with in syphilitic disease of the bones, disease of the joints, and occasionally in tumors.

Multiple neuritis has a very complex etiology, the causes of which may be classified as follows: (*a*) The poisons of infectious diseases, as in leprosy, diphtheria, typhoid fever, small-pox, and occasionally in other forms; (*b*) the organic poisons, comprising the diffusible stimulants, such as alcohol and ether, bisulphide of carbon and naphtha, and metallic bodies, such as lead and arsenic; (*c*) cachectic conditions, such as occur in anæmia, cancer, tuberculosis, or marasmus from any cause; (*d*) the endemic neuritis or beri-beri; and (*e*) lastly, there are cases in which none of these factors prevail, but the disease sets in suddenly after overexertion or exposure to cold.

Morbid Anatomy.—In neuritis due to the extension of inflammation the nerve is usually swollen, infiltrated, and red in color. The inflammation may be chiefly perineural or it may pass into the deeper portion—*interstitial* neuritis—in which form there is an accumulation of lymphoid elements between the nerve bundles. The nerve fibres themselves may not appear involved, but there is an increase in the nuclei of the sheath of Schwann. The myelin is fragmented, the nuclei of the internodal cells are swollen, and the axis-cylinders present varicosities or undergo granular degeneration. Ultimately the nerve fibres may be completely destroyed and replaced by a fibrous connective tissue in which much fat is sometimes deposited—*lipomatous neuritis.*

In other instances the condition is termed *parenchymatous* neuritis, in which the changes are like those met with in the secondary or Wallerian degeneration, which follows when the nerve fibre is cut off from the cell body of the neurone to which it belongs. The medullary substance and the axis-cylinders are chiefly involved, the interstitial tissue being but little altered or only affected secondarily. The muscles connected with the degenerated nerves usually show marked atrophic changes, and in some instances the change in the nerve sheath appears to extend directly to the interstitial tissue of the muscles—the *neuritis fascians* of Eichhorst.

Symptoms.—Localized Neuritis.—As a rule, the constitutional disturbances are slight. The most important symptom is *pain* of a boring or stabbing character, usually felt in the course of the nerve and in the parts to which it is distributed. The nerve itself is sensitive to pressure, probably, as Weir Mitchell suggested, owing to the irritation of its nervi nervorum. The skin may be slightly reddened or even œdematous over the seat of the inflammation. Mitchell described increase in the temperature and sweating in the affected region, and such atrophic disturbances as effusion into the joints and herpes. The function of the muscle to which the nerve fibres are distributed is impaired, motion is painful, and there may be twitchings or contractions. The tactile sensation of the part may be somewhat deadened, even when the pain is greatly increased. In the more chronic cases of local neuritis, such, for instance, as follow the dislocation of the humerus, the localized pain, which at first may be severe, gradually disappears, though some sensitiveness of the brachial plexus may persist for a long time, and the nerve cords may be firm and swollen. The pain is variable—sometimes intense and distressing; at others not causing much inconvenience. Numbness and formication may be present and tactile sensation greatly impaired. The motor disturbances are marked. Ultimately there is extreme atrophy of the muscles. Contractures may occur in the fingers. The skin may be reddened or glossy, the subcutaneous tissue œdematous, and the nutrition of the nails may be defective. In some cases subcutaneous fibroid nodules may develop.

A neuritis limited at first to a peripheral nerve may extend upward—the so-called ascending or migratory neuritis—and involve the larger nerve trunks, or even reach the spinal cord, causing subacute myelitis (Gowers). The condition is rarely seen in the neuritis from cold, or in that which follows fevers; but it occurs most frequently in traumatic neuritis.

J. K. Mitchell, in his monograph on injuries of nerves, concluded that the larger nerve trunks are most susceptible, and that the neuritis may spread either up or down, the former being the most common. The paralysis secondary to visceral disease, as of the bladder, may be due to an ascending neuritis. The inflammation may extend to the nerves of the other side, either through the spinal cord or its membranes, or without any involvement of the nerve-centres, the so-called sympathetic neuritis. The electrical changes in localized neuritis vary a great deal, depending upon the extent to which the nerve is injured. The lesion may be so slight that the nerve and the muscles to which it is distributed may react normally to both currents; or it may be so severe that the typical reaction of degeneration develops within a few days—i. e., the nerve does not respond to stimulation by either current, while the muscle reacts only to the galvanic current and in a peculiar manner. The contraction caused is slow and lazy, instead of sharp and quick as in the normal muscle, and the AC contraction is usually stronger than the KC contraction. Between these extremes there are many grades, and a careful electrical examination is an important aid to diagnosis and prognosis.

The duration varies from a few days to weeks or months. A slight traumatic neuritis may pass off in a day or two, while the severer cases, such as follow unreduced dislocation of the humerus, may persist for months or never be completely relieved.

Multiple Neuritis.—The following are the most important groups:

(*a*) *Acute Febrile Polyneuritis.*—The attack follows exposure to cold or overexertion, or, in some instances, comes on spontaneously. The onset resembles that of an acute infectious disease. There may be a definite chill, pains in the back and limbs or joints, so that the case may be thought to be rheumatic fever. The temperature rises rapidly and may reach 103° or 104° F. There are headache, loss of appetite, and the general symptoms of acute infection. The limbs and back ache. Intense pain in the nerves, however, is by no means constant. Tingling and formication are felt in the fingers and toes, and there is increased sensitiveness of the nerve trunks or of the entire limb. Loss of muscular power, first marked, perhaps, in the legs, gradually comes on and extends with the features of an ascending paralysis. In other cases the paralysis begins in the arms. The extensors of the wrists and the flexors of the ankles are early affected, so that there is foot and wrist drop. In severe cases there is general loss of muscular power, producing a flabby paralysis, which may extend to the muscles of the face and to the intercostals, and respiration may be carried on by the diaphragm alone. The muscles soften and waste rapidly. There may be only hyperæsthesia with soreness and stiffness of the limbs; in some cases, increased sensitiveness with anæsthesia; in other instances the sensory disturbances are slight. The Argyll-Robertson pupil may be present and the pupils may be unequal. Involvement of the cranial nerves is rare, but the oculo-motor, the facial, and the fifth have been involved. The vagus may be attacked and the quickening of the pulse is usually attributed to this cause. Involvement of the bladder and rectum is rare, but it does occur and does not necessarily mean involvement of the cord. The clinical picture is not to be distinguished, in many cases, from Landry's paralysis; in others, from the subacute myelitis of Duchenne.

The course is variable. In the most intense forms the patient may die in a week or ten days, with involvement of the respiratory muscles or from paralysis of the heart. As a rule, in cases of moderate severity, after persisting for five or six weeks, the condition remains stationary and then slow improvement begins. The paralysis in some muscles may persist for many months and contractures may occur from shortening of the muscles, but even when this occurs the outlook is, as a rule, good, although the paralysis may have lasted for a year or more.

(*b*) *Recurring Multiple Neuritis.*—Under the term *polyneuritis recurrens* Mary Sherwood described from Eichhorst's clinic 2 cases in adults—in one case involving the nerves of the right arm, in the other both legs. In one patient there were three attacks, in the other two, the distribution in the various attacks being identical.

(*c*) *Alcoholic Neuritis.*—This, perhaps the most important form of multiple neuritis, was graphically described in 1822 by James Jackson, Sr., of Boston. Wilks recognized it as alcoholic paraplegia, but the starting point of the recent researches dates from the observations of Dumenil, of Rouen. It occurs most frequently in women, particularly in steady, quiet tipplers. Its appearance may be the first revelation of habits of secret drinking. The onset is usually gradual, and may be preceded for weeks or months by neuralgic pains and tingling in the feet and hands. Convulsions are not uncommon. Fever is rare. The paralysis gradually sets in, at first in the feet and legs, and then in the hands and forearms. The extensors are affected more than the flexors, so that there is wrist-drop and foot-drop. The paralysis may be thus limited and not extend higher in the limbs. In other instances there is paraplegia alone, while in some extreme cases all the extremities are involved. In rare instances the facial muscles and the sphincters are also affected. The sensory symptoms are very variable. There are cases in which there are numbness and tingling only, without great pain. In other cases there are severe burning or boring pains, the nerve trunks are sensitive, and the muscles are sore when grasped. The hands and feet are frequently swollen and congested, particularly when held down for a few moments. The cutaneous reflexes, as a rule, are preserved. The deep reflexes are usually lost.

The course of these alcoholic cases is, as a rule, favorable, and after persisting for weeks or months improvement gradually begins, the muscles regain their power, and even in the most desperate cases recovery may follow. The extensors of the feet may remain paralyzed for some time, and give to the patient a distinctive walk, the so-called *steppage* gait, characteristic of peripheral neuritis. It is sometimes known as the pseudo-tabetic gait, although in reality it could not well be mistaken for the gait of ataxia. The foot is thrown forcibly forward, the toe lifted high in the air so as not to trip upon it. The entire foot is slapped upon the ground as a flail. It is an awkward, clumsy gait, and gives the patient the appearance of constantly stepping over obstacles. Among the most striking features are the *mental* symptoms. Delirium is common, and there may be hallucinations with extravagant ideas, resembling somewhat those of general paresis. In some cases the picture is that of delirium tremens, but the most peculiar and almost characteristic mental disorder is that so well described by Wilks, in which the patient loses all appreciation of time and place, and describes with circumstantial details long journeys which, he says, he has recently taken, or tells of persons whom he has just seen. This is the so-called Korsakoff's syndrome.

(*d*) *Multiple Neuritis in the Infectious Diseases.*—This has been already referred to, particularly in diphtheria, in which it is most common. The peripheral nature of the lesion in diphtheria has been shown by post mortem examination. The outlook is usually favorable and, except in diphtheria, fatal cases are uncommon. Multiple neuritis in tuberculosis, diabetes, and syphilis is of the same nature, being probably due to toxic materials absorbed into the blood. It may follow suppuration anywhere, as septic sore throat, and in the recent war multiple neuritis has been seen not infrequently after superficial septic sores.

(*e*) *The Metallic Poisons.*—Neuritis from arsenic may follow: (1) The medicinal use particularly of Fowler's solution. In one case of Hodgkin's disease general neuritis was caused by ℥ j ʒ ij of the solution. In chorea a good many cases have been reported. Changes in the nails are not uncommon, chiefly the transverse ridging. In the case of a young woman who had taken "rough-on-rats," there were remarkable white lines—the leuconychia—running across the nails, without any special ridging. C. J. Aldrich finds that this is not uncommon in chronic arsenical poisoning. (2) The accidental contamination of food or drink. Chrome yellow may be used to color cakes, as in the cases recorded by D. D. Stewart. A remarkable epidemic of neuritis occurred in the Midland Counties of England, which was traced to the use of beer containing small quantities of arsenic, a contamination from the sulphuric acid used in making glucose. Reynolds, who studied these cases, believes that most of the instances of neuritis in drinkers are arsenical, but admits that the slight cases may be due to the alcohol itself. Pigmentation of the skin is an important distinguishing sign. Lead is a much more frequent cause. Neuritis has followed the use of mercurial inunctions. Zinc is a rare cause. In a case seen with Urban Smith neuritis followed the use of two grains of the sulpho-carbolate taken daily for three years. Tea, coffee, and tobacco are mentioned as rare causes.

(*f*) *Endemic neuritis,* beri-beri, is considered elsewhere.

Anæsthesia Paralysis.—Here may most appropriately be considered the forms of paralysis following the use of anæsthetics, or of too long-continued compression during operations. There are two groups of cases:

(*a*) During an operation the nerves may be compressed, either the brachial plexus by the humerus or the musculo-spiral by the table. The pressure most frequently occurs when the arm is elevated alongside the head, as in laparotomy done in the Trendelenburg position, or held out from the body, as in breast amputations. Instances of paralysis of the crural nerves by leg-holders are also reported. The too firm application of a tourniquet may be followed by a severe paralysis.

(*b*) Paralysis from cerebral lesions during etherization. In one of Garrigues' cases paralysis followed the operation, and at the autopsy, seven weeks later, softening of the brain was found. Apoplexy or embolism may occur during anæsthesia. In Montreal a cataract operation was performed on an old man. He did not recover from the anæsthetic and post mortem a cerebral hæmorrhage was found. Epileptic convulsions may occur during anæsthesia, and may even prove fatal. The possibility of paralysis from loss of blood in prolonged operations has to be considered. And, lastly, a paralysis might result from the toxic effects of the ether in a very protracted administration.

Angiopathic Paralysis.—Digital compression, the protracted application of the tourniquet and ligation of the main vessel taught us that normal action of the nerves and muscles of a limb was dependent upon a good blood supply. In sudden blocking of the femoral artery with an embolus, the pain is not simply in the site of the blockage, but is more or less diffuse throughout the limb, which the patient moves very slightly and with the greatest difficulty. In the recent war in the numerous injuries to the arteries, these angiopathic paralyses were not uncommon. In a study of ten cases of severe wounds of the main vessel of a limb Burrows found the chief symptom to be: (*a*) subjective changes, numbness, tingling, etc.; (*b*) anæsthesia, usually of the glove type; (*c*) paralysis, often complete; (*d*) hardness of the muscles, and (*e*) œdema of the limb. With the re-establishment of the collateral circulation these may disappear in a few days.

Diagnosis.—The electrical condition in multiple neuritis is thus described by Allen Starr: "The excitability is very rapidly and markedly changed; but the conditions which have been observed are quite various. Sometimes there is a simple diminution of excitability, and then a very strong faradic or galvanic current is needed to produce contractions. Frequently all faradic excitability is lost and then the muscles contract to a galvanic current only. In this condition it may require a very strong galvanic current to produce contraction, and thus far it is quite pathognomonic of neuritis. In poliomyelitis, where the muscles respond to galvanism only, it does not require a strong current to cause motion until some months after the invasion.

"The action of the different poles is not uniform. In many cases the contraction of the muscle when stimulated with the positive pole is greater than when stimulated with the negative pole, and the contractions may be sluggish. Then the reaction of degeneration is present. But in some cases the normal condition is found and the negative pole produces stronger contractions than the positive pole. A loss of faradic irritability and a marked decrease in the galvanic irritability of the muscle and nerve are therefore important symptoms of multiple neuritis."

There is rarely any difficulty in distinguishing the alcohol cases. The combination of wrist- and foot-drop with congestion of the hands and feet, and the peculiar delirium already referred to, are quite characteristic. The rapidly advancing cases with paralysis of all extremities, often reaching to the face and involving the sphincters, are more commonly regarded as of spinal origin, but the general opinion seems to point strongly to the fact that all such cases are peripheral. The less acute cases, in which the paralysis gradually involves the legs and arms with rapid wasting, simulate closely and are usually confounded with the subacute atrophic spinal paralysis of Duchenne. The diagnosis from tabes is rarely difficult. The *steppage* gait is entirely different. There is rarely positive incoördination. The patient can usually stand well with the eyes closed. Foot-drop is not common in tabes. The lightning pains are absent and there are usually no pupillary symptoms. The etiology is of moment. The patient is recovering from a paralysis which has been more extensive, or from arsenical poisoning, or he has diabetes.

Treatment.—Rest in bed is essential. In the acute cases with fever the salicylates and antipyrin are recommended. To allay the intense pain morphia or the hot applications of lead water and laudanum are often required. Great care must be exercised in treating the alcoholic form, and the physician must not allow himself to be deceived by the statements of the relatives. It is sometimes exceedingly difficult to get a history of drinking. In the alcoholic form it is well to reduce the stimulants gradually. If there is any tendency to bed-sores an air-bed should be used or the patient placed in a continuous bath. Gentle friction of the muscles may be applied from the outset, and in the later stages, when the atrophy is marked and the pains have lessened, massage is probably the most reliable means at our command. Contractures may be gradually overcome by passive movements and extension. Often with the most extreme deformity from contracture, recovery is, in time, still possible. The interrupted current is useful when the acute stage is passed.

Of internal remedies, strychnia is of value and may be given in increasing doses. Arsenic also may be employed, and if there is a history of syphilis the iodide of potassium and mercury should be given.

II. NEUROMATA

Tumors situated on nerve fibres may consist of nerve substance proper, the true neuromata, or of fibrous tissue, the false neuromata. The true neuroma usually contains nerve fibres only, or in rare instances ganglion cells. Cases of ganglionic or medullary neuroma are extremely rare; some of them, as Lancereaux suggests, are undoubtedly instances of malformation of the brain substance. In other instances the tumor is, in all probability, a glioma with cells closely resembling those of the central nervous system. The growths are often intermediate in anatomical structure between the true and the false.

Plexiform Neuroma.—In this remarkable condition the various nerve cords may be occupied by many hundreds of tumors. The cases are often hereditary and usually congenital. The tumors may occur in all the nerves of the body, and, as numbers of them may be made out on palpation, the diagnosis is usually easy. One of the most remarkable cases is that described by Prudden, the specimens of which are in the medical museum of Columbia College, New York. There were over 1,182 distinct tumors distributed on the nerves of the body. These tumors rarely are painful, but may cause symptoms through pressure on neighboring structures.

Generalized Neuro-fibromatosis: von Recklinghausen's Disease: Fibroma Molluscum.—Special attention was directed to this particular form of multiple neuroma by von Recklinghausen in 1882. The disease presents several groups of lesions:

1. Cutaneous.—(*a*) Soft, fibrous nodules, some sessile, others pedunculated, varying in size and greatly in number, are scattered over the skin. They may increase in number as age advances. (*b*) Bluish spots, indicating atrophy of the corium where the fibromata are perforating. (*c*) Pigmentation, in the form of freckles, blotches, or diffuse areas. (*d*) Subcutaneous growths, at times of enormous size, causing the condition known as "elephantiasis neuromatosa." Congenital nævi are frequent.

2. Nervous.—Tumors resembling plexiform neuromata may be present on any of the nerve trunks from the centre to the periphery. The variable situation leads to a variety of sensory or motor phenomena, more especially as they may arise from the nerve roots within the spinal canal or cranium. Cases resembling tabes, syringomyelia and spastic paralysis have been reported. The patients often show mental changes and the speech may be hesitating.

3. Bone Lesions.—Changes similar to those of osteomalacia occur in about 7 per cent. of the cases.

Other features may be mentioned: Three generations have been affected, or two or three members of a family, or a mother and several children. The lesions may develop during pregnancy and disappear after delivery. Brickner, after whom this syndrome has been named, collected 16 cases. The tumors do not always disappear. Adrian reported a case with multiple myomata of the stomach. A sarcomatous change may occur in the central tumors, but not in the optic and olfactory nerves which have not the sheath of Schwann. There may be associated glioma or other brain tumor.

The nature of the disease is unknown. The occurrence of the pigmentation and the osteomalacia suggest an endocrine disturbance; but the familial and hereditary features point rather to an embryonic origin.

The prognosis depends on the possibility of successful removal of such tumors as are causing greatest inconvenience.

"Tubercula Dolorosa."—Multiple neuromata may especially affect the terminal cutaneous branches of the sensory nerves and lead to small subcutaneous painful nodules, often found on the face, breast, or about the joints. They may be associated with tumors of the nerve trunks.

"Amputation Neuromata."—These bulbous swellings may form on the central ends of nerves which have been divided in injuries or operations. They are especially common after amputations. They are due to the tangled coil of axis-cylinder processes growing down from the central stump in an effort to reach their former end structures. They are very painful and usually require surgical removal but may recur.

III. DISEASES OF THE CEREBRAL NERVES

OLFACTORY NERVES AND TRACTS

The functions of the olfactory nerves may be disturbed at their origin, in the nasal mucous membrane, at the bulb, in the course of the tract, or at the centres in the brain. The disturbances may be manifested in subjective sensations of smell, complete loss of the sense, and occasionally in hyperæsthesia.

Subjective Sensations; Parosmia.—Hallucinations of this kind are found in the insane and in epilepsy. The aura may be represented by an unpleasant odor, described as resembling chloride of lime, burning rags, or feathers. In a few cases with these subjective sensations tumors have been found in the hippocampi. In rare instances, after injury of the head, the sense is perverted—odors of the most different character may be alike, or the odor may be changed, as in a patient noted by Morell Mackenzie, who for some time could not touch cooked meat, as it smelt to her exactly like stinking fish.

Increased sensitiveness (hyperosmia) occurs chiefly in nervous, hysterical women, in whom it may sometimes be developed so greatly that, like a dog, they can recognize the difference between individuals by the odor alone.

Anosmia; Loss of the Sense of Smell.—This may be produced by: (*a*) Affections of the origin of the nerves in the mucous membrane, which is perhaps the most frequent cause. It is not uncommon with chronic nasal catarrh and polypi. In paralysis of the fifth nerve, the sense of smell may be lost on the affected side, owing to interference with secretion. It is doubtful whether the cases of loss of smell following the inhalations of foul or strong odors come under this or under the central division.

(*b*) Lesions of the bulbs or of the tracts. In falls or blows, in caries of the bones, and in meningitis or tumor, the bulbs or the olfactory tracts may be involved. After an injury to the head the loss of smell may be the only symptom. Mackenzie noted a case of a surgeon who was thrown from his gig and lighted on his head. The injury was slight, but the anosmia which followed was persistent. In tabes the sense of smell may be lost, possibly owing to atrophy of the nerves.

(*c*) Lesions of the olfactory centres. There are congenital cases in which the structures have not developed. Cases have been reported in which anosmia has been associated with disease in the hemisphere.

To test the sense of smell the pungent bodies, such as ammonia, which act upon the fifth nerve, should not be used, but such substances as cloves, peppermint, and musk. This sense is readily tested as a routine matter in brain cases by having two or three bottles containing the essential oils. In all instances a rhinoscopic examination should be made, as the condition may be due to local, not central causes. The *treatment* is unsatisfactory even in the cases due to local lesions in the nostrils.

OPTIC NERVE AND TRACT

(1) *Lesions of the Retina*

These are of importance to the physician, and information of the greatest value may be obtained by a systematic examination of the eye grounds. Only a brief reference can be made to the more important appearances.

Retinitis.—This occurs in certain general affections, more particularly in nephritis, syphilis, leukæmia, and anæmia. The common feature in all those is the occurrence of hæmorrhage and the development of opacities. There may also be a diffuse cloudiness due to effusion of serum. The hæmorrhages are in the layer of nerve fibres. They vary greatly in size and form, but often follow the course of vessels. When recent the color is bright red, but they gradually change and old hæmorrhages are almost black. The white spots are due either to fibrinous exudate or to fatty degeneration of the retinal elements, and occasionally to accumulation of leucocytes or to a localized sclerosis of the retinal elements. The more important forms of retinitis are:

ALBUMINURIC RETINITIS, which occurs in chronic nephritis, particularly in the interstitial or contracted form. The percentage of cases affected is from 15 to 25. There are instances in which these retinal changes are associated with the granular kidney at a stage when the amount of albumin may be slight or transient; but in all such instances it will be found that there is a marked arterio-sclerosis. Gowers recognized a degenerative form (most common), in which, with the retinal changes, there may be scarcely any alteration in the disk; a hæmorrhagic form, with many hæmorrhages and but slight signs of inflammation; and an inflammatory form, in which there is much swelling of the retina and obscuration of the disk. It is noteworthy that in some instances the inflammation of the optic nerve predominates over the retinal changes, and one may be in doubt for a time whether the condition is associated with renal changes or dependent upon intracranial disease.

SYPHILITIC RETINITIS.—In the acquired form this is less common than choroiditis. In inherited syphilis *retinitis pigmentosa* is sometimes found.

RETINITIS IN ANÆMIA.—A patient may become blind after a large hemorrhage, either suddenly or within two or three days, and in one or both eyes. Occasionally the loss may be permanent and complete. In some of these instances a neuro-retinitis has been found, probably sufficient to account for the symptoms. In the more chronic anæmias, particularly the pernicious form, retinitis is common, as determined first by Quincke.

In MALARIA retinitis or neuro-retinitis may be present, as noted by Stephen Mackenzie. It is seen only in the chronic cases with anæmia, and is not nearly so common proportionately as in pernicious anæmia.

LEUKÆMIC RETINITIS.—In this affection the retinal veins are large and distended; there is also a peculiar retinitis, as described by Liebreich. It is not very common. There are numerous hæmorrhages and white or yellow areas, which may be large and prominent. In one case the retina post mortem was dotted with many small, opaque, white spots, looking like little tumors, the larger of which had a diameter of nearly 2 mm.

Retinitis is also found occasionally in diabetes, in purpura, in chronic lead poisoning, and sometimes as an idiopathic affection.

Functional Disturbances of Vision.—(*a*) TOXIC AMAUROSIS.—This occurs in uræmia and may follow convulsions or come on independently. The condition, as a rule, persists only for a day or two. This form of amaurosis occurs in poisoning by lead, alcohol, and occasionally by quinine. It seems more probable that the poisons act on the centres and not on the retina.

(*b*) TOBACCO AMBLYOPIA.—The loss of sight is usually gradual, equal in both eyes, and affects particularly the centre of the field of vision. The eye-grounds may be normal, but occasionally there is congestion of the disks. On testing the color fields a central scotoma for red and green is found in all cases. Ultimately, if the use of tobacco is continued, organic changes may develop with atrophy of the disk.

(*c*) HYSTERICAL AMAUROSIS.—More frequently this is loss of acuteness vision—amblyopia—but the loss of sight in one or both eyes may apparently be complete. The condition will be mentioned under hysteria.

(*d*) NIGHT-BLINDNESS—NYCTALOPIA—the condition in which objects are clearly seen during the day or by strong artificial light, but become invisible in the shade or in twilight, and *hemeralopia,* in which objects can not be clearly seen without distress in daylight or in a strong artificial light, but are readily seen in a deep shade or in twilight, are rare functional anomalies which may occur in epidemic form.

(*e*) RETINAL HYPERÆSTHESIA is sometimes seen in hysterical women, but is not frequent in actual retinitis. It may occur with albuminuric retinitis, and with aortic insufficiency.

(2) *Lesions of the Optic Nerve*

Optic Neuritis (*Papillitis; Choked Disk*).—In the first stage there is congestion of the disk and the edges are blurred and striated. In the second stage the congestion is more marked; the swelling increases, the striation also is more visible. The physiological cupping disappears and hæmorrhages are not uncommon. The arteries present little change, the veins are dilated, and the disk may swell greatly. In slight grades the swelling gradually subsides and occasionally the nerve recovers completely. In instances in which the swelling and exudate are very great the subsidence is slow, and when it finally disappears there is complete atrophy of the nerve. The retina may participate in the inflammation, which is then a neuro-retinitis.

This condition is of the greatest importance in diagnosis. It may exist in its early stages without any disturbance of vision, and even with extensive papillitis the sight may for a time be good.

Optic neuritis is seen occasionally in anæmia and lead poisoning, more commonly in nephritis as neuro-retinitis. It occurs occasionally as a primary idiopathic affection. The frequent connection with intracranial disease, particularly tumor, makes its presence of great value. The nature of the growth is without influence. In over 90 per cent. of such instances the choked disk is bilateral. It is also found in meningitis, either the tuberculous or the simple form. In meningitis the inflammation may extend down the nerve sheath. In tumor, however, it is probable that mechanical conditions, especially venous stasis, are alone responsible for the œdematous swelling. It often subsides very rapidly after decompression has been performed.

Optic Atrophy.—This may be: (*a*) A primary affection. There is an hereditary form, in which the disease has developed in all the males of a family shortly after puberty. A large number of the cases of primary atrophy are associated with spinal disease, particularly tabes. Other causes which have been assigned for the primary atrophy are cold, sexual excesses, diabetes, the specific fevers, methyl alcohol, and lead.

(*b*) Secondary atrophy results from cerebral diseases, pressure on the chiasma or on the nerves, or, most commonly of all, as a sequence of papillitis.

The ophthalmoscopic appearances are different in the cases of primary and secondary atrophy. In the former the disk has a gray tint, the edges are well defined, and the arteries look almost normal; whereas in the consecutive atrophy the disk has a staring opaque white aspect, with irregular outlines, and the arteries are very small.

The symptom of optic atrophy is loss of sight, proportionate to the damage in the nerve. The change is in three directions: "(1) Diminished acuity of vision; (2) alteration in the field of vision; and (3) altered perception of color" (Gowers). The outlook in primary atrophy is bad.

(3) *Affections of the Chiasma and Tract*

At the chiasma the optic nerves undergo partial decussation. Each optic tract, as it leaves the chiasma, contains nerve fibres which originate in the retinæ of both eyes. Thus, of the fibres of the right tract, part have come through the chiasma without decussating from the temporal half of the right retina, the other and larger portion of the fibres of the tract have decussated in the chiasma, coming as they do from the left optic nerve and the nasal half of the retina on the left side. The fibres which cross are in the middle portion of the chiasma, while the direct fibres are on each side. The following are the most important changes from lesions of the tract and chiasma:

Unilateral Affection of Tract.—If on the right side, this produces loss of function in the temporal half of the retina on the right side, and in the nasal half of the retina on the left side, so that there is only half vision, and the patient is blind to objects on the left side. This is termed homonymous hemianopia or lateral hemianopia. The fibres passing to the right half of each retina being involved, the patient is blind to objects in the left half of each visual field. The hemianopia may be partial and only a portion of the half field may be lost. The unaffected visual fields may have the normal extent, but in some instances there is considerable reduction. When the left half of one field and the right half of the other, or *vice versa,* are blind, the condition is known as heteronymous hemianopia.

Disease of the Chiasma.—(*a*) A lesion involves, as a rule, chiefly the central portion, in which the decussating fibres pass which supply the inner or nasal halves of the retinæ, producing in consequence loss of vision in the outer half of each field, or what is known as temporal hemianopia.

(*b*) If the lesion is more extensive it may involve not only the central portion, but also the direct fibres on one side of the commissure, in which case there is total blindness in one eye and temporal hemianopia in the other.

(*c*) Still more extensive disease is not infrequent from pressure of tumors in this region, the whole chiasma is involved, and total blindness results. The different stages in the process may often be traced in a single case from temporal hemianopia, then complete blindness in one eye with temporal hemianopia in the other, and finally complete blindness.

(*d*) A limited lesion of the outer part of the chiasma involves only the direct fibres passing to the temporal halves of the retinæ and inducing blindness in the nasal field, or, as it is called, nasal hemianopia. This, of course, is extremely rare. Double nasal hemianopia may occur as a manifestation of tabes and in tumors involving the outer fibres of each tract.

(4) *Affections of the Tract and Centres*

The optic tract crosses the crus (cerebral peduncle) to the hinder part of the optic thalamus and divides into two portions, one of which (the lateral root) goes to the pulvinar of the thalamus, the lateral geniculate body, and to the anterior quadrigeminal body (superior colliculus). From these parts, in which the lateral root terminates, fibres pass into the posterior part of the internal capsule and enter the occipital lobe, forming the fibres of the optic radiation, which terminate in and about the cuneus, the region of the visual perceptive centre. The fibres of the medial division of the tract pass to the medial geniculate body and to the posterior quadrigeminal body. The medial root contains the fibres of the commissura inferior of v. Gudden, which are believed to have no connection with the retinæ. It is still held by some physiologists that the cortical visual centre is not confined to the occipital lobe alone, but embraces the occipito-angular region.

A lesion of the fibres of the optic path anywhere between the cortical centre and the chiasma will produce hemianopia. The lesion may be situated: (*a*) In the optic tract itself. (*b*) In the region of the thalamus, lateral geniculate body, and the corpora quadrigemina, into which the larger part of each tract enters. (*c*) A lesion of the fibre passing from the centre just mentioned to the occipital lobe. This may be either in the hinder part of the internal capsule or the white fibres of the optic radiation. (*d*) Lesion of the cuneus. Bilateral disease of the cuneus may result in total blindness. (*e*) There is clinical evidence to show that lesion of the angular gyrus may be associated with visual defect, not so often hemianopia as crossed amblyopia, dimness of vision in the opposite eye, and great contraction in the field of vision. Lesions in this region are associated with mind-blindness, a condition in which there is failure to recognize the nature of objects.

The effect of lesion in the optic nerve in different situations from the retinal expansion to the brain cortex are as follows: (1) Of the optic nerve, total blindness of the corresponding eye; (2) of the optic chiasma, either temporal hemianopia, if the central part alone is involved, or nasal hemianopia, if the lateral region of each chiasma is involved; (3) lesion of the optic tract between the chiasma and the lateral geniculate body produces lateral hemianopia; (4) lesion of the central fibres of the nerve between the geniculate bodies and the cerebral cortex produces lateral hemianopia; (5) lesion of the cuneus causes lateral hemianopia; and (6) lesion of the angular gyrus may be associated with hemianopia, sometimes crossed amblyopia, and the condition known as mind-blindness. (See Fig. 21.)

Diagnosis of Lesions of the Optic Nerve and Tract.—Having determined the presence of hemianopia, the question arises as to the situation of the lesion, whether in the tract between the chiasma and the geniculate bodies or in the central portion of the fibres between these bodies and the visual centres. This can be determined in some cases by the test known as Wernicke's *hemiopic pupillary reaction.* The pupil reflex depends on the integrity of the retina or receiving membrane, on the fibres of the optic nerve and tract which transmit the impulse, and the nerve-centre at the termination of the optic tract which receives the impression and transmits it to the third nerve along which the motor impulses pass to the iris. If a bright light is thrown into the eye and the pupil reacts, the integrity of this reflex arc is demonstrated. It is possible in cases of lateral hemianopia so to throw the light into the eye that it falls upon the blind half of the retina. If when this is done the pupil contracts, the indication is that the reflex arc above referred to is perfect, by which we mean that the optic nerve fibres from the retinal expansion to the centre, the centre itself, and the third nerve are uninvolved. In such a case the conclusion would be justified that the cause of the hemianopia was central; that is, situated beyond the geniculate body, either in the

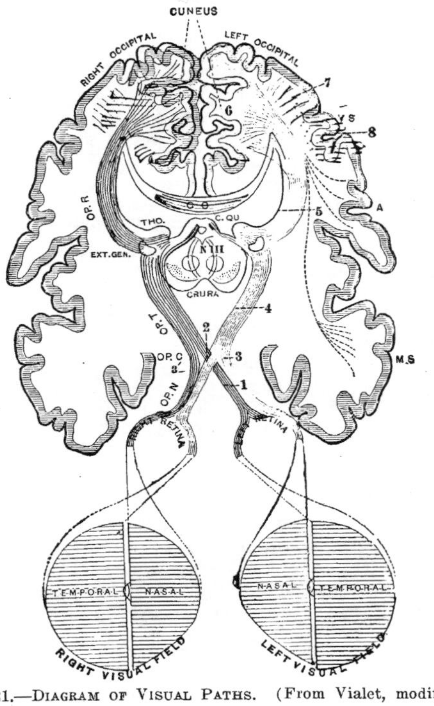

FIG. 21.—DIAGRAM OF VISUAL PATHS. (From Vialet, modified.)

OP. N., Optic nerve. OP. C., Optic chiasm. OP. T., Optic tract. OP. R., Optic radiations. EXT. GEN., External geniculate body. THO., Optic thalamus. C. QU., Corpora quadrigemina. C. C., Corpus callosum. V. S., Visual speech centre. A. S., Auditory speech centre. H. S., Motor speech centre. A lesion at 1 causes blindness of that eye; at 2, bi-temporal hemianopia; at 3, nasal hemianopia. Symmetrical lesions at 3 and 3′ would cause bi-nasal hemianopia; at 4, hemianopia of both eyes, with hemianopic pupillary inaction; at 5 and 6, hemianopia of both eyes, pupillary reflexes normal; at 7, amblyopia, especially of opposite eye; at 8, on left side, word-blindness.

fibres of the optic radiation or in the visual cortical centres. If, on the other hand, when the light is carefully thrown on the hemiopic half of the retina the pupil remains inactive, the conclusion is justifiable that there is interruption in the path between the retina and nucleus of the third nerve, and that the hemianopia is not central, but dependent upon a lesion situated in the optic tract. This test of Wernicke's is sometimes difficult to obtain. It is best performed as follows: "The patient being in a dark or nearly dark room with the lamp or gas-light behind his head in the usual position, I bid him look over to the other side of the room, so as to exclude accommodative iris movements (which are not necessarily associated with the reflex). Then I throw a faint light from a plane mirror or from a large concave mirror, held well out of focus, upon the eye and note the size of the pupil. With my other hand I now throw a beam of light, focussed from the lamp by an ophthalmoscopic mirror, directly into the optical centre of the eye; then laterally in various positions and also from above and below the equator of the eye, noting the reaction at all angles of incidence of the ray of light" (Seguin).

The *significance* of hemianopia varies. There is a functional hemianopia associated with migraine and hysteria. In a considerable proportion of all cases there are signs of organic brain disease. In a certain number of instances of slight lesions of the occipital lobe hemichromatopsia has been observed. The homonymous halves of the retina as far as the fixation point are dulled, or blind for colors. Hemiplegia is common, in which event the loss of power and blindness are on the same side. Thus, a lesion in the left hemisphere involving the motor tract produces right hemiplegia, and when the fibres of the optic radiation are involved in the internal capsule there is also lateral hemianopia, so that objects in the field of vision to the right are not perceived. Hemianæsthesia is not uncommon in such cases, owing to the close association of the sensory and visual tracts at the posterior part of the internal capsule. Certain forms of aphasia also occur in many of the cases.

The *optic aphasia* of Freund may be mentioned here. The patient, after an apoplectic attack, though able to recognize ordinary objects shown to him, is unable to name them correctly. If he be permitted to touch the object he may be able to name it quickly and correctly. Freund's optic aphasia differs from mind-blindness, since in the latter affection the objects seen are not recognized. Optic aphasia, like word-blindness, never occurs alone, but is always associated with hemianopia, or mind-blindness, and often also with word-deafness. In the cases which have thus far come to autopsy there has always been a lesion in the white matter of the occipital lobe on the left side.

MOTOR NERVES OF THE EYEBALL

Third Nerve (*Nervus oculomotorius*).—The nucleus of origin of this nerve is situated in the floor of the aqueduct of Sylvius; the nerve passes through the crus at the side of which it emerges. Passing along the wall of the cavernous sinus, it enters the orbit through the sphenoidal fissure and supplies, by its superior branch, the levator palpebræ superioris and the superior rectus, and by its inferior branch the internal and inferior recti muscles and the inferior oblique. Branches pass to the ciliary muscle and the constrictor of the iris. Lesions may affect the nucleus of the nerve in its course and cause either paralysis or spasm.

Paralysis.—A nuclear lesion is usually associated with disease of the centres for the other eye muscles, producing general ophthalmoplegia. More commonly the nerve itself is involved in its course, either by meningitis, gummata, or aneurism, or is attacked by a neuritis, as in diphtheria. Complete paralysis is accompanied by the following symptoms:

Paralysis of all the muscles, except the superior oblique and external rectus, by which the eye can be moved outward and a little downward and inward. There is divergent strabismus. There is ptosis or drooping of the upper eyelid, owing to paralysis of the levator palpebræ. The pupil is usually dilated. It does not contract to light, and the power of accommodation is lost. The most striking features of this paralysis are the external strabismus, with diplopia or double vision, and the ptosis. In very many cases the affection of the third nerve is partial. Thus the levator palpebræ and the superior rectus may be involved together, or the ciliary muscles and the iris may be affected and the external muscles may escape.

There is a remarkable form of recurring oculo-motor paralysis affecting chiefly women, and involving all the branches of the nerve. In some cases the attacks have come on at intervals of a month; in others a much longer period has elapsed. The attacks may persist throughout life. They are sometimes associated with pain in the head and sometimes with migraine. Mary Sherwood collected 23 cases from the literature.

Ptosis is a common and important sign in nervous affections. We may here briefly refer to the conditions under which it may occur: (*a*) A congenital, incurable form; (*b*) the form associated with definite lesion of the third nerve, either in its course or at its nucleus. This may come on with paralysis of the superior rectus alone or with paralysis of the internal and inferior recti as well. (*c*) There are instances of complete or partial ptosis associated with cerebral lesions without any other branch of the third nerve being paralyzed. The exact position of the cortical centre or centres is as yet unknown. (*d*) Hysterical ptosis, which is double and occurs with other hysterical symptoms. (*e*) Pseudo-ptosis, due to affection of the sympathetic nerve, is associated with symptoms of vaso-motor palsy, such as elevation of the temperature on the affected side with redness and œdema of the skin. Contraction of the pupil exists on the same side and the eyeball appears rather to have shrunk into the orbit. (*f*) In idiopathic muscular atrophy, when the face muscles are involved, there may be marked bilateral ptosis. And, lastly, in weak, delicate women there may be a transient ptosis, particularly in the morning.

Among the most important of the symptoms of the third-nerve paralysis are those which relate to the ciliary muscle and iris.

Cycloplegia, paralysis of the ciliary muscle, causes loss of the power of accommodation. Distant vision is clear, but near objects cannot be properly seen. In consequence the vision is indistinct, but can be restored by the use of convex glasses. This may occur in one or in both eyes; in the latter case it is usually associated with disease in the nuclei. Cycloplegia is an early and frequent sign in diphtheritic paralysis and occurs also in tabes.

Iridoplegia, or paralysis of the iris, occurs in three forms (Gowers):

(*a*) *Accommodation iridoplegia,* in which the pupil does not alter in size during the act of accommodation. To test this the patient should look first at a distant and then at a near object in the same line of vision.

(*b*) *Reflex Iridoplegia.*—The path for the iris reflex is along the optic nerve and tract to its termination, then to the nucleus of the third nerve, and along the trunk of this nerve to the ciliary ganglion, and so through the ciliary nerves to the eyes. Each eye should be tested separately, the other one being covered. The patient should look at a distant object in a dark part of the room; then a light is brought suddenly in front of the eye at a distance of three or four feet, so as to avoid the effect of accommodation. Loss of this iris reflex with retention of the accommodation contraction is known as the Argyll-Robertson pupil.

(*c*) *Loss of the Skin Reflex.*—If the skin of the neck is pinched or pricked the pupil dilates reflexly, the afferent impulses being conveyed along the cervical sympathetic. Erb pointed out that this skin reflex is lost usually in association with the reflex contraction, but the two are not necessarily conjoined. In iridoplegia the pupils are often small, particularly in spinal disease, as in the characteristic small pupils of tabes—spinal myosis. Iridoplegia may coexist with a pupil of medium size.

Inequality of the pupils—anisocoria—is not infrequent in progressive paresis and in tabes. It may also occur in perfectly healthy individuals.

SPASM.—Occasionally in meningitis and in hysteria there is spasm of the muscles supplied by the third nerve, particularly the internal rectus and the levator palpebræ. *Nystagmus* is a rhythmical contraction of the eye muscles met with in many congenital and acquired lesions of the brain, particularly in multiple sclerosis. It may be hereditary and has been traced through four generations in association with head nodding (Yawger). Lid nystagmus may also be present. It is met with in albinos. The nystagmus of miners is apparently due to poor light.

Fourth Nerve (*Nervus trochlearis*).—This supplies the superior oblique muscle. In its course around the outer surface of the crus and in its passage into the orbit it is liable to be compressed by tumors, by aneurism, or in the exudation of basilar meningitis. Its nucleus in the upper part of the fourth ventricle may be involved by tumors or undergo degeneration with the other ocular nuclei. The superior oblique muscle acts in such a way as to direct the eyeball downward and rotate it slightly. The paralysis causes defective downward and inward movement, often too slight to be noticed. The head is inclined somewhat forward and toward the sound side, and there is double vision when the patient looks down.

Sixth Nerve.—Emerging at the junction of the pons and medulla, it passes forward in a long and exposed course to the orbit, and supplies the external rectus muscle. It is often involved in meningeal exudate, compressed by tumors and possibly involved in an independent neuritis. When paralyzed, there is internal squint with diplopia on attempting to look outwards. The true and the false images are parallel, and grow further apart on looking to the paralyzed side. When the nucleus is involved, the internal rectus of the opposite eye may be paralyzed as the nucleus sends fibres up in the pons to that part of the nucleus of the opposite third nerve which supplies the internal rectus. In one symptom-complex there is a combination of otitis media with complete paralysis of the sixth nerve. The inflammation travels to the apex of the petrous bone, then to the sixth nerve. The outlook is usually good.

General Features of Paralysis of the Motor Nerves of the Eye.—Gowers divided them into five groups:

(*a*) *Limitation of Movement.*—Thus, in paralysis of the external rectus, the eyeball can not be moved outward. When the paralysis is incomplete the movement is deficient in proportion to the degree of the palsy.

(*b*) *Strabismus.*—The axes of the eyes do not correspond. Thus, paralysis of the internal rectus causes a divergent squint; of the external rectus, a convergent squint. At first this is evident only when the eyes are moved in the direction of the action of the weak muscle. The deviation of the axis of the affected eye from parallelism with the other is called the primary deviation.

(*c*) *Secondary Deviation.*—If, while the patient is looking at an object, the sound eye is covered, so that he fixes the object looked at with the affected eye only, the sound eye is moved still further in the same direction—e. g., outward, when there is paralysis of the opposite internal rectus. This is known as secondary deviation. It depends upon the fact that, if two muscles are acting together, when one is weak and an effort is made to contract it, the increased effort—innervation—acts powerfully upon the other muscle, causing an increased contraction.

(*d*) *Erroneous Projection.*—"We judge of the relation of external objects to each other by the relation of their images on the retina; but we judge of their relation to our own body by the position of the eyeball as indicated to us by the innervation we give to the ocular muscles" (Gowers). With the eyes at rest in the mid-position, an object at which we are looking is directly opposite our face. Turning the eyes to one side, we recognize that object in the middle of the field or to the side of this former position. We estimate the degree by the amount of movement of the eyes, and when the object moves and we follow it we judge of its position by the amount of movement of the eyeballs. When one ocular muscle is weak the increased innervation gives the impression of a greater movement of the eye than has really taken place. The mind, at the same time, receives the idea that the object is further on one side than it really is, and in an attempt to touch it the finger may go beyond it. As the equilibrium of the body is in a large part maintained by a knowledge of the relation of external objects to it obtained by the action of the eye muscles, this erroneous projection disturbs the harmony of these visual impressions and may lead to giddiness—*ocular vertigo.*

(*e*) *Double Vision.*—This is one of the most disturbing features of paralysis of the eye muscles. The visual axes do not correspond, so that there is a double image—*diplopia.* That seen by the sound eye is termed the true image; that by the paralyzed eye, the false. In simple or homonymous diplopia the false image is "on the same side of the other as the eye by which it is seen." In crossed diplopia it is on the other side. In convergent squint the diplopia is simple; in divergent it is crossed.

Ophthalmoplegia.—Under this term is described a chronic progressive paralysis of the ocular muscles. Two forms are recognized—ophthalmoplegia *externa* and ophthalmoplegia *interna.* The conditions may occur separately or together and are described by Gowers under nuclear ocular palsy.

Ophthalmoplegia externa.—The condition is one of more or less complete palsy of the external muscles of the eyeball, due usually to a slow degeneration in the nuclei of the nerves, but sometimes to pressure of tumors or to basilar meningitis. It is often, but not necessarily, associated with ophthalmoplegia interna. Of 62 cases analyzed by Siemerling in only 11 could syphilis be positively determined. The levator muscles of the eyelids and the superior recti are first involved, and gradually the other muscles, so that the eyeballs are fixed and the eyelids droop. There is sometimes slight protrusion of the eyeballs. The disease is essentially chronic and may last for years. It is found particularly in association with general paresis, tabes, and in progressive muscular atrophy. Mental disorders were present in 11 of the 62 cases. With it may be associated optic atrophy and affections of other cerebral nerves. Occasionally, as noted by Bristowe, it may be functional.

Ophthalmoplegia interna.—Jonathan Hutchinson applied this term to a progressive paralysis of the internal ocular muscles, causing loss of pupillary action and the power of accommodation. When the internal and external muscles are involved the affection is known as total ophthalmoplegia, and in a majority of the cases the two conditions are associated. In some instances the internal form may depend upon disease of the ciliary ganglion.

While, as a rule, ophthalmoplegia is a chronic process, there is an acute form associated with hæmorrhagic softening of the nuclei of the ocular muscles. There is usually marked cerebral disturbance. It was to this form that Wernicke gave the name *poliencephalitis superior*.

Treatment of Ocular Palsies.—It is important to ascertain, if possible, the cause. The forms associated with tabes are obstinate, and resist treatment. Occasionally, however, a palsy, complete or partial, may pass away spontaneously. The cases associated with chronic degenerative changes, as in progressive paresis and bulbar paralysis, are little affected by treatment. On the other hand, in syphilitic cases, specific treatment is often beneficial. Arsenic and strychnia, the latter hypodermically, may be employed. In any case in which the onset is acute with pain, hot fomentations and counter-irritation or leeches applied to the temple give relief. The direct treatment by electricity has been employed, but without any special effect. The diplopia may be relieved by the use of prisms, or it may be necessary to cover the affected eye with an opaque glass.

FIFTH NERVE

(*Nervus trigeminus*)

Etiology.—Paralysis may result from: (*a*) Disease of the pons, particularly hæmorrhage or patches of sclerosis. (*b*) Injury or disease at the base of the brain. Fracture rarely involves the nerve; on the other hand, meningitis, acute or chronic, and caries of the bone are not uncommon causes. (*c*) The branches may be affected as they pass out—the first division by tumors pressing on the cavernous sinus or by aneurism; the second and third divisions by growths which invade the spheno-maxillary fossa. (*d*) Primary neuritis, which is rare.

Symptoms.—(*a*) Sensory Portion.—Disease of the fifth nerve may cause loss of sensation in the parts supplied, including the half of the face, the corresponding side of the head, the conjunctiva, the mucosa of the lips, tongue, hard and soft palate, and of the nose of the same side. The anæsthesia may be preceded by tingling or pain. The muscles of the face are also insensible and the movements may be slower. The sense of smell is interfered with, owing to dryness of the mucous membrane. There may be disturbance of the sense of taste. The salivary, lachrymal, and buccal secretions may be lessened, and the teeth may become loose. Unless properly guarded from injury an ulcerative inflammation of the eye may follow. This was supposed to be due to nutritional changes from paralysis of so-called trophic nerve fibres. This idea has been overthrown by the large number of cases in which the Gasserian ganglion has been removed for obstinate neuralgia without consequent inflammation of the eye. *Herpes* may occur in the region supplied by the nerve, usually the upper branch, and is associated with much pain, which may be persistent, lasting for months or years (Gowers). In herpes zoster with the neuritis there may be slight enlargement of the cervical glands. (See under Neuralgia for Tic Douloureux.)

(*b*) Motor Portion.—The inability to use the muscles of mastication on the affected side is the distinguishing feature of paralysis of this portion of the nerve. It is recognized by placing the finger on the masseter and temporal muscles, and, when the patient closes the jaw, the feebleness of their contraction is noted. If paralyzed, the external pterygoid can not move the jaw toward the unaffected side; and when depressed, the jaw deviates to the paralyzed side. Motor paralysis of the fifth nerve is almost invariably a result of involvement after the nerve has left the nucleus but cases have been associated with cortical lesions. The cortical motor centre for the trigeminus, or for movements effecting closure of the jaw, lies below that for movements of the face at the lower part of the anterior central convolution.

Spasm of the Muscles of Mastication.—Trismus, the masticatory spasm of Romberg, may be tonic or clonic, and is either an association phenomenon in general convulsions or, more rarely, an independent affection. In the tonic form the jaws are kept close together—lock-jaw—or can be separated only for a short space. The muscles of mastication can be seen in contraction and felt to be hard; the spasm is often painful. This tonic contraction is an early symptom in tetanus, and is sometimes seen in tetany. A form of this tonic spasm occurs in hysteria. Occasionally trismus follows exposure to cold, and is said to be due to reflex irritation from the teeth, the mouth, or caries of the jaw. It may also be a symptom of organic disease due to irritation near the motor nucleus of the fifth nerve.

Clonic spasm of the muscles supplied by the fifth occurs in the form of rapidly repeated contractions, as in "chattering teeth." This is rare apart from general conditions, though cases are on record, usually in women late in life, in whom this isolated clonic spasm of the muscles of the jaw has been found. In another form of clonic spasm sometimes seen in chorea there are forcible single contractions. Gowers mentioned an instance of its occurrence as an isolated affection.

(*c*) Gustatory.—There are two views concerning the course of the fibres that carry gustatory impulse from this part of the tongue. According to some they take a devious path, passing with the chorda tympani to the geniculate ganglion, thence by the great superficial petrosal nerve to Meckel's ganglion, and this they leave to reach the maxillary nerve, which they follow through the trigeminal nerve to the brain. A study of clinical cases of disease of the fifth nerve has led to this view. It seems more probable, from the fact that a large number of the trigeminal neurectomies are not followed by loss of taste, that the fibres pass with the facial nerve to the brain directly from the geniculate ganglion by the nervus intermedius of Wrisberg. Possibly there may be more than one course for these fibres.

The *diagnosis* of disease of the trifacial nerve is rarely difficult. It must be remembered that the preliminary pain and hyperæsthesia are sometimes mistaken for ordinary neuralgia. The loss of sensation and the palsy of the muscles of mastication are readily determined.

Treatment.—When the pain is severe morphia may be required and local applications are useful. If there is a suspicion of syphilis, appropriate treatment should be given. Faradization is sometimes beneficial.

FACIAL NERVE

Paralysis (*Bell's Palsy*).—ETIOLOGY.—The facial or seventh may be paralyzed by (*a*) lesions of the cortex—supranuclear palsy; (*b*) lesions of the nucleus itself; or (*c*) involvement of the nerve trunk in its tortuous course within the pons and through the wall of the skull.

(*a*) *Supranuclear paralysis*, due to lesion of the cortex or of the facial fibres in the corona radiata or internal capsule, is, as a rule, associated with hemiplegia. It may be caused by tumors, abscess, chronic inflammation, or softening in the cortex or in the region of the internal capsule. It is distinguished from the peripheral form by the persistence of the normal electrical excitability of both nerves and muscles and the frequent absence of involvement of the upper branches of the nerve, so that the orbicularis palpebrarum, frontalis, and corrugator muscles are spared. In rare instances these muscles are paralyzed. In this form the voluntary movements are more impaired than the emotional. Isolated paralysis—monoplegia facialis—due to involvement of the cortex or of the fibres in their path to the nucleus, is uncommon. In the great majority of cases supranuclear facial paralysis is part of a hemiplegia. Paralysis is on the same side as that of the arm and leg because the facial muscles bear the same relation to the cortex as the spinal muscles. The nuclei of origin on either side of the middle line in the medulla are united by decussating fibres with the cortical centre on the opposite side (see Fig. 20). A few fibres reach the nucleus from the cerebral cortex of the same side, and this uncrossed path may innervate the upper facial muscles.

(*b*) The *nuclear paralysis* caused by lesions of the nerve centres in the medulla is not common alone; but is seen occasionally in tumors, chronic softening, and hæmorrhage. It may be involved in anterior polio-myelitis. In diphtheria this centre may also be attacked. The symptoms are practically similar to those of an affection of the nerve fibre itself—infranuclear paralysis.

(*c*) *Involvement of the Nerve Trunk.*—Paralysis may result from:

(1) Involvement of the nerve as it passes through the pons—that is, between its nucleus in the floor of the fourth ventricle and the point of emergence in the postero-lateral aspect of the pons. The specially interesting feature in connection with involvement of this part is the production of what is called alternating or *crossed paralysis*, the face being involved on the same side as the lesion, and the arm and leg on the opposite side, since the motor path is involved above the point of decussation in the medulla (Fig. 20). This occurs only when the lesion is in the lower section of the pons. A lesion in the upper half of the pons involves the fibres not of the outgoing nerve on the same side, but of the fibres from the hemispheres before they have crossed to the nucleus of the opposite side. In this case there would be paralysis of the face and limbs on the side opposite to the lesion. The palsy would resemble the cerebral form, involving only the lower fibres of the facial nerve.

(2) The nerve may be involved at its point of emergence by tumors, particularly by the cerebello-pontine growths, by gummata, meningitis, or occasionally it may be injured in fracture of the base.

(3) In passing through the Fallopian canal the nerve may be involved in disease of the ear, particularly by caries of the bone in otitis media. This is a common cause.

(4) As the nerve emerges from the styloid foramen it is exposed to injuries and blows which not infrequently cause paralysis. The fibres may be cut in the removal of tumors in this region, or the paralysis may be caused by pressure of the forceps in an instrumental delivery.

(5) Exposure to cold is a common cause, inducing a neuritis of the nerve within the Fallopian canal. Reik believes that in most of these cases there is an acute otitis media from which the nerve is involved.

(6) Syphilis is not an infrequent cause, and the paralysis may appear early with the secondary symptoms.

(7) It may occur in association with herpes.

Facial diplegia is a rare condition occasionally found in affections at the base of the brain, lesions in the pons, simultaneous involvement of the nerves in ear-disease, and in diphtheritic paralysis. Disease of the nuclei or symmetrical involvement of the cortex might also produce it. It may occur as a congenital affection. H. M. Thomas described two cases in one family.

SYMPTOMS.—In the peripheral facial paralysis all the branches of the nerve are involved. The face on the affected side is immobile and can neither be moved at will nor participate in any emotional movements. The skin is smooth and the wrinkles are effaced, a point particularly noticeable on the forehead of elderly persons. The eye can not be closed, the lower lid droops, and the eye waters. On the affected side the angle of the mouth is lowered, and in drinking the lips are not kept in close apposition to the glass, so that the liquid is apt to run out. In smiling or laughing the contrast is most striking, as the affected side does not move, which gives a curious unequal appearance to the two sides of the face. The eye can not be closed nor can the forehead be wrinkled. In long standing cases, when the reaction of degeneration is present, if the patient tries to close the eyes while looking fixedly at an object the lids on the sound side close firmly, but on the paralyzed side there is only a slight inhibitory droop of the upper lid, and the eye is turned upward and outward by the inferior oblique. On asking the patient to show his upper teeth, the angle of the mouth is not raised. In all these movements the face is drawn to the sound side by the action of the muscles. Speaking may be slightly interfered with, owing to the imperfection in the formation of the labial sounds. Whistling can not be performed. In chewing the food, owing to the paralysis of the buccinator, particles collect on the affected side. The paralysis of the nasal muscles is seen on asking the patient to sniff. Owing to the fact that the lips are drawn to the sound side, the tongue, when protruded, looks as if it were pushed to the paralyzed side; but on taking its position from the incisor teeth, it will be found to be in the middle line. The reflex movements are lost in this peripheral form. It is usually stated that the palate is partially paralyzed on the same side and that the uvula deviates. Both Gowers and Hughlings Jackson denied the existence of this involvement in the great majority of cases, and Horsley and Beevor have shown that these parts are innervated by the accessory nerve to the vagus.

The *sensory functions* of the facial nerve, to which much attention has been paid by Cushing, Mills and others, are ministered to by the geniculate ganglion, the intermediary nerve of Wrisberg, and the chorda tympani, which last has chiefly gustatory functions. It seems likely that deep sensibility with sense of pressure, position and passive movement runs in a separate afferent system in the motor nerve of the face. Cutaneous sensibility, both epicritic, by which we localize light touch, and protopathic, by which we recognize degrees of heat and cold, is not ministered to by the facial nerve proper. There are observations that would indicate, however, that the anterior part of the tongue and possibly a little strip of the skin of the auricle have a vestigial supply from this nerve.

When the nerve is involved within the canal between the genu and the origin of the chorda tympani, the sense of taste is lost in the anterior part of the tongue on the affected side. When the nerve is damaged outside the skull the sense of taste is unaffected. Hearing is often impaired in facial paralysis, most commonly by preceding ear disease. The paralysis of the stapedius muscle may lead to increased sensitiveness to musical notes. Herpes is sometimes associated with facial paralysis. Severe *pain* may precede or accompany the paralysis. It is usually in the ear and mastoid region but may radiate to the occipital and trigeminal distribution. The face on the affected side may be swollen.

The *electrical reactions,* which are those of a peripheral palsy, have considerable importance from a prognostic standpoint. Erb's rules are as follows: If there is no change, either faradic or galvanic, the prognosis is good and recovery takes place in from fourteen to twenty days. If the faradic and galvanic excitability of the nerve is only lessened and that of the muscle increased to the galvanic current and the contraction formula altered (the contraction sluggish $AC < KC$), the outlook is relatively good and recovery will probably take place in from four to six weeks; occasionally in from eight to ten. When the reaction of degeneration is present and the mechanical excitability is altered, the prognosis is relatively unfavorable and recovery may not occur for two, six, eight, or even fifteen months.

COURSE.—This is usually favorable. The onset in the form following cold is very rapid, developing perhaps within twenty-four hours, but rarely is the paralysis permanent. Hunt has drawn special attention to *recurrent* facial paralysis which may be on one or alternate sides—"relapsing alternating." In some instances contracture develops as the voluntary power returns, and the natural folds and the wrinkles on the affected side may be deepened, so that on looking at the face one at first may have the impression that the affected side is the sound one. This is corrected at once on asking the patient to smile, when it is seen which side of the face has the more active movement. Aretæus noted the difficulty sometimes experienced in determining which side was affected until the patient spoke or laughed.

PERMANENT FACIAL PARALYSIS.—One of the distressing sequels is permanent loss of power with immobility and the disfigurement resulting from the overaction of the muscles on the sound side. There are three groups of cases: (1) Those due to trauma, especially the birth palsies from injury by forceps. (2) Due to suppurative middle-ear disease, following scarlet fever, diphtheria, or sepsis of any kind, such as puerperal fever. (3) In a few cases following the ordinary Bell's paralysis. Even when paralysis exists from childhood, there may be slight voluntary control, and the muscles may respond to faradic stimulus. The facial nerve in reality may have recovered or regenerated, and the disfigurement and loss of function result from the over-stretching of the degenerated muscles by the action of their opponents on the sound side (Turrell).

DIAGNOSIS.—This is usually easy. The distinction between the peripheral and central form is based on facts already mentioned.

TREATMENT.—In the cases which result from cold and are probably due to neuritis within the bony canal, hot applications should be made; subsequently the thermo-cautery may be used lightly at intervals of a day or two over the mastoid process, or small blisters applied. If the ear is diseased, free discharge should be obtained. The galvanic current may be employed to keep up the nutrition of the muscles. The positive pole should be placed behind the ear, the negative one along the zygomatic and other muscles. The application can be made daily for a quarter of an hour and the patient can make it himself before a looking glass. Massage in the course of the nerve and of the muscles of the face is also useful. A course of iodide of potassium may be given even when there is no indication of syphilis.

In those cases in which the nerve has been destroyed by an injury, during an operation or from disease, and when there has been no evidence of returning function after electric treatment for a few months, a nerve anastomosis should be performed. For this purpose either the spinal accessory or the hypoglossal nerve may be used. Though the normal conditions may never be completely regained after such an operation, the motor power will be largely restored and the deformity lessened. This procedure, based on the results of physiological experimentation, makes one of the most striking of modern operations.

Spasm.—The spasm may be limited to a few or involve all the muscles innervated by the facial nerve, and may be unilateral or bilateral.

It is known also as *mimic spasm* or *convulsive tic.* Several different affections are usually considered under the name of facial or mimic spasm, but we here speak only of the simple spasm of the facial muscles, either primary or following paralysis, and do not include the cases of habit spasm in children, or the *tic convulsif* of the French.

Gowers recognized two classes—one in which there is an organic lesion, and an idiopathic form. It is thought to be due also to reflex causes, such as the irritation from carious teeth or the presence of intestinal worms. The disease usually occurs in adults, whereas the habit spasm and the *tic convulsif* of the French, often confounded with it, are most common in children. True mimic spasm occasionally comes on in childhood and persists. When the result of organic disease, there has usually been a lesion of the centre in the cortex, as in the case reported by Berkley, or pressure on the nerve at the base of the brain by aneurism or tumor.

SYMPTOMS.—The spasm may involve only the muscles around the eye—blepharospasm—in which case there is constant, rapid, quick action of the orbicularis palpebrarum, which, in association with photophobia, may be tonic in character. More commonly the spasm affects the lateral facial muscles with those of the eye, and there is constant twitching of the side of the face with partial closure of the eye. The frontalis is rarely involved. In aggravated cases the depressors of the angle of the mouth, the levator menti, and the platysma myoides are affected. This spasm is confined to one side of the face in a majority of cases, though it may extend and become bilateral. It is increased by emotional causes and by voluntary movements of the face. As a rule, it is painless, but there may be tender points over the course of the fifth nerve, particularly the supraorbital branch. Tonic spasm of the facial muscle may follow paralysis, and is said to result occasionally from cold.

The outlook in facial spasm is always dubious. A majority of the cases persist for years and are incurable.

Treatment.—Sources of irritation should be looked for and removed. When a painful spot is present over the fifth nerve, blistering or the application of the cautery may relieve it. Hypodermic injections of strychnia may be tried, but are of doubtful benefit. Weir Mitchell recommended freezing the cheek for a few minutes daily or every second day with the spray, and this, in some instances, is beneficial. Often the relief is transient and at every clinic patients may be seen who have run the gamut of all measures without material improvement. Severe cases may require surgical interference. The nerve may be divided near the stylomastoid foramen and an anastomosis made between it and the spinal accessory.

AUDITORY NERVE

The eighth, known also as *portio mollis* of the seventh pair, passes from the ear through the internal auditory meatus, and in reality consists of two separate nerves—the cochlear and vestibular roots. These two roots have entirely different functions, and may therefore be best considered separately. The cochlear nerve is the one connected with the organ of Corti, and is concerned in hearing. The vestibular nerve is connected with the vestibule and semicircular canals, and has to do with the maintenance of equilibrium.

The Cochlear Nerve

The cortical centre for hearing is in the temporo-sphenoidal lobe. Primary disease of the auditory nerve in its centre or intracranial course is uncommon. More frequently the terminal branches are affected within the labyrinth.

Affection of the Cortical Centre.—The superior temporal gyrus represents the centre for hearing. In man destruction of this gyrus on the left side results in word-deafness, which may be defined as an inability to understand the meaning of words, though they may still be heard as sounds. The central auditory path extending to the cortical centre from the terminal nuclei of the cochlear nerve may be involved and produce deafness. This may result from involvement of the lateral lemniscus, from the presence of a tumor in the corpora quadrigemina, especially if it involve the posterior quadrigeminal bodies, from a lesion of the internal geniculate body, or it may be associated with a lesion of the internal capsule.

Lesions of the nerve at the base of the brain may result from the pressure of tumors, meningitis (particularly the cerebro-spinal form), hæmorrhage, or traumatism. A primary degeneration of the nerve may occur in tabes. Primary disease of the terminal nuclei of the cochlear nerve (nucleus nervi cochlearis dorsalis and nucleus nervi cochlearis ventralis) is rare. By far the most interesting form results from epidemic cerebro-spinal meningitis, in which the nerve is frequently involved, causing permanent deafness. In young children the condition results in deaf-mutism.

Internal Ear.—In a majority of cases with auditory nerve symptoms the lesion is in the internal ear, either primary or the result of extension of disease of the middle ear. Two groups of symptoms may be produced—hyperæsthesia and irritation, and diminished function or nervous deafness.

(*a*) HYPERÆSTHESIA AND IRRITATION.—This may be due to altered function of the centre as well as of the nerve ending. True hyperæsthesia—hyperacusis—is a condition in which sounds, sometimes even those inaudible to other persons, are heard with great intensity. It occurs in hysteria and occasionally in cerebral disease. In paralysis of the stapedius low notes may be heard with intensity. In dysæsthesia, or dysacusis, ordinary sounds cause an unpleasant sensation, as commonly happens in connection with headache, when ordinary noises are badly borne.

Tinnitus aurium is a term employed to designate certain subjective sensations of ringing, roaring, tickling, and whirring noises in the ear. It is a very common and often a distressing symptom. It is associated with many forms of ear disease and may result from pressure of wax on the drum. It is rare in organic disease of the central connections of the nerve. Sudden intense stimulation of the nerve may cause it. A form not uncommonly met with in medical practice is that in which the patient hears a continual *bruit* in the ear, and the noise has a systolic intensification, usually on one side. It may suggest the presence of an internal aneurism. A systolic murmur may be heard occasionally on auscultation in anæmia and neurasthenia. Subjective noises in the ear may precede an epileptic seizure and are sometimes present in migraine. In whatever form tinnitus exists, though slight and often regarded as trivial, it occasions great annoyance and mental distress, and has even driven patients to suicide.

The *diagnosis* is readily made; but it is often extremely difficult to determine upon what condition the tinnitus depends. The relief of constitutional states, such as anæmia, neurasthenia, or gout, may result in cure. A careful local examination of the ear should always be made. One of the most worrying forms is the constant clicking, sometimes audible many feet away from the patient, and due probably to clonic spasm of the muscles connected with the Eustachian tube or of the levator palati. The condition may persist for years unchanged, and then disappear suddenly. The pulsating forms of tinnitus, in which the sound is like that of a systolic *bruit*, are almost invariably subjective, and it is very rare to hear anything with the stethoscope. It is to be remembered that in children there is a systolic brain murmur, best heard over the ear, and in some instances appreciable in the adult.

(*b*) DIMINISHED FUNCTION OR NERVOUS DEAFNESS.—In testing for nervous deafness, if the tuning fork can not be heard when placed near the meatus, but the vibrations are audible by placing the foot of the tuning fork against the temporal bone, the conclusion may be drawn that the deafness is not due to involvement of the nerve. The vibrations are conveyed through the temporal bone to the cochlea and vestibule. The watch may be used for the same purpose, and if the meatus is closed and the watch is heard better in contact with the mastoid process than when opposite the open meatus, the deafness is probably not nervous. Disturbance of the function of the auditory nerve is not a very frequent symptom in brain disease, but in all cases the function of the nerve should be carefully tested.

The Vestibular Nerve

Our sense of position in space and the control of the balance of the body are functions of the vestibular nerve, and its central associations in the cerebellum and cerebrum. The paths from the labyrinth are not accurately known, beyond the group of Deiters' Nuclei; there is uncertainty, both as to tracts and centres.

Disturbance of the relation of the body to space, or of its balance, produces in consciousness the unpleasant sensation which we call dizziness or vertigo. It results from a discord between the impressions arising in the labyrinth, the cerebellum, the eye muscles and elsewhere, and a failure to coördinate these in the centres (Hughlings Jackson). The controlling factor is the vestibular mechanism. The cochlear nerves are often involved simultaneously, producing tinnitus, and the motor-oculi mechanism, causing nystagmus.

An apprehension, not a true vertigo, is common in looking from a height, and is frequent in neurotic individuals. True dizziness is always accompanied by a sensation of falling or turning, even when the person is in bed, and if standing, there is incoördination of the muscles, with staggering or falling. The patient may feel that he is moving or the objects about him appear to rotate. The direction in which he falls is variable and of special importance. Nystagmus is often associated and the direction and intensity should be studied.

(1) Auditory (Labyrinthine) Vertigo—Méniere's Syndrome.—In 1861 Ménière described an affection characterized by noises in the ear, vertigo (which might be associated with loss of consciousness), vomiting, and, in many cases, progressive loss of hearing. Bárány groups the conditions in which the labyrinth may be affected and vertigo occur under the following heads: (*a*) Acute infectious diseases, influenza, cerebro-spinal meningitis, etc. (*b*) Chronic infectious diseases, syphilis particularly. (*c*) Constitutional conditions and intoxications. Hæmorrhage into the labyrinth (in leukæmia, purpura hæmorrhagica, pernicious anæmia); chlorosis, thyroid intoxications, arterio-sclerosis, etc. (*d*) Tumors and diseases of the central nervous system; tumors of the acoustic nerve, cerebellum, pons, and fourth ventricle, meningitis, cerebellar abscess, multiple sclerosis, tabes, etc. (*e*) Trauma, fracture of the base, etc. (*f*) Hereditary degenerative diseases and malformations of the internal ear. (*g*) Intoxications, alcohol, nicotine, quinine, salicylic acid group, arsenic. To these may be added gas emboli in caisson disease and ordinary emboli.

Symptoms.—The attack usually sets in suddenly with a buzzing noise in the ears and the patient feels as if he was reeling or staggering. He may feel himself to be reeling, or the objects about him may seem to be turning, or the phenomena may be combined. The attack is often so abrupt that the patient falls, though, as a rule, he has time to steady himself by grasping some neighboring object. Consciousness is generally maintained, but may be momentarily lost. Ocular symptoms are usually present. Jerking of the eyeballs, or nystagmus, occurs. The patient becomes pale and nauseated, a clammy sweat breaks out on the face, and vomiting may follow. The duration of the attack varies; it may be very short, but usually the patient has to lie quietly for some time, as any movement of the head brings on another attack. Labyrinthine vertigo is usually paroxysmal, coming on at irregular intervals, sometimes of weeks or months; or several attacks may occur in a day.

Affections of the External and Middle Ears.—Irrigation of the meatus may be followed by giddiness or by a severe Ménière syndrome. *Wax* is one of the commonest causes and the first to be sought for. Removal of a dried fragment pressing against the drum may cure a persistent and distressing vertigo. All forms of *middle ear disease* may cause vertigo, the suppurative as well as the chronic sclerotic. Noises in the ear are usually present as well. The attacks may be of great severity, but apart from gross brain lesions, death is rare. A patient with chronic deafness and tinnitus had severe vertigo in turning in bed on the left side. There was no suggestion of central lesion. Death occurred in one of the attacks.

(2) **Vertigo in Intracranial Tumors.**—The symptom is variable; the largest growths may exist in any region without it—a very small one in a special locality may cause severe attacks. The vestibular fibres may be directly involved in any part of their course or indirectly compressed. Direct involvement is seen in tumors of the cerebello-pontine angle, affecting the eighth and usually the seventh nerves, in tumors of the cerebellum, and in aneurism. Vertigo is rarely a focal symptom as it may follow indirect pressure from tumors of the cerebrum.

(3) **Ocular Vertigo.**—The association of giddiness with ocular defects has long been recognized, and the newly studied ocular reflexes of vestibular nerve origin now play an important rôle in diagnosis. Nystagmus, double vision, and paralysis of accommodation may be ocular associations of vertigo. The central connections of the nuclei of the "space nerve" with those of the ocular muscles is very close. Errors of refraction may cause an irritation and instability of the space nerve centres leading to severe vertigo.

(4) **Cardio-vascular Vertigo.**—Vertigo is a common feature in the group of symptoms known as "soldier's heart." In cardiac insufficiency giddiness is a frequent complaint, particularly with aortic disease. The loss of consciousness in Stokes-Adams' disease may be preceded by distressing symptoms of vertigo. One of the commonest forms is seen in high blood pressure with arterio-sclerosis, very often with tinnitus. It may be slight and noticed only in the morning or on getting up suddenly. In other instances it is one of the most distressing features of progressive sclerosis of the cerebral arteries. Vertigo may precede or accompany the attacks of transient hemi- or monoplegia with asphasia; and with a persistent headache and high blood pressure it may precede an apoplexy. Low blood pressure is also a frequent cause.

(5) **Toxic vertigo** is described as due to alcohol, tobacco and quinine, to the poisons of the specific fevers, and to focal infection. The essential process

is a neuritis of the eighth nerve, or a chronic degenerative change, involving cochlea and labyrinth. A high-pitched tinnitus, with progressive deafness, and transient attacks of vertigo, sometimes of the Ménière type, are the usual symptoms. True toxic neuritis of the vestibular nerve is very rare. Gastric, renal and various types of functional vertigo have diminished progressively in importance since the studies of Bárány.

DIAGNOSIS.—The nervous, anæmic and cardio-vascular groups rarely offer any difficulty but the diagnosis from minor epilepsy is not so easy, particularly in the types without spasm. Tinnitus may be present, but it is rare to have actual loss of consciousness in aural vertigo, in which, also, the actual giddiness is more persistent. The simpler Bárány tests may be applied; the more complicated ones call for the help of the specialist. A full consideration will be found in Barker's "Clinical Diagnosis," vol. iii. The vestibular reflexes are as important in some cases as those of the iris.

PROGNOSIS.—The outlook in Ménière's disease is uncertain. While many cases recover completely, in others deafness results and the attacks recur at shorter intervals. In aggravated cases the patient constantly suffers from vertigo, and may even be confined to his bed.

TREATMENT.—Bromide of potassium, in 20 grain (1.3 gm.) doses three times a day, is sometimes beneficial. If there is a history of syphilis the iodides should be administered. The salicylates are recommended, and Charcot advises quinine to cinchonism. In cases in which there is increase in the arterial tension nitroglycerin may be given, at first in very small doses, but increasing gradually. It is not specially valuable in Ménière's disease, but in the cases of giddiness in middle aged men and women associated with arteriosclerosis it sometimes acts very satisfactorily. Correction of errors of refraction is sometimes followed by prompt relief of the vertigo.

Endemic Paralytic Vertigo.—In parts of Switzerland and France there is a remarkable form of vertigo described by Gerlier, which is characterized by attacks of paretic weakness of the extremities, falling of the eyelids, remarkable depression, but with retention of consciousness. It occurs also in northern Japan, where Miura says it develops paroxysmally among the farm laborers of both sexes and all ages. It is known there as *kubisagari.*

GLOSSO-PHARYNGEAL NERVE

The ninth nerve contains both motor and sensory fibres and is also a nerve of the special sense of taste to the tongue. It supplies, by its motor branches, the stylo-pharyngeus and the middle constrictor of the pharynx. The sensory fibres are distributed to the upper part of the pharynx.

Symptoms.—Of nuclear disturbance we know very little. The pharyngeal symptoms of bulbar paralysis are probably associated with involvement of the nuclei of this nerve. Lesion of the nerve trunk itself is rare, but it may be compressed by tumors or involved in meningitis. Disturbance of the sense of taste may result from loss of function of this nerve, in which case it is chiefly in the posterior part of the tongue and soft palate.

The general disturbances of the sense of taste may be briefly mentioned. Loss of the sense of taste—*ageusia*—may be caused by disturbance of the peripheral end organs, as in affections of the mucosa of the tongue. This is very common in fever or dyspepsia, in which conditions, as the saying is, everything tastes alike. Strong irritants, such as pepper, tobacco, or vinegar, may dull or diminish the sense of taste. Complete loss may be due to involvement of the nerves either in their course or in the centres. Perversion of the sense of taste—*parageusis*—is rarely found, except as an hysterical manifestation and in the insane. Increased sensitiveness is still more rare. There are occasional subjective sensations of taste, occurring as an aura in epilepsy or as part of the hallucinations in the insane.

To test the sense of taste the patient's eyes should be closed and small quantities of various substances applied to the protruded tongue. The sensation should be perceived before the tongue is withdrawn. The following are the most suitable tests: For bitterness, quinine; for sweetness, a strong solution of sugar or saccharin; for acidity, vinegar; and for the saline test, common salt. One of the most important tests is the feeble galvanic current, which gives the well-known metallic taste.

PNEUMOGASTRIC (VAGUS) NERVE

The tenth nerve has an important and extensive distribution, supplying the pharynx, larynx, lungs, heart, œsophagus, and stomach. The nerve may be involved at its nucleus along with the spinal accessory and the hypoglossal, forming what is known as bulbar paralysis. It may be compressed by tumors or aneurism, or in the exudation of meningitis, simple or syphilitic. In its course in the neck the trunk may be involved by tumors or in wounds. It has been tied in ligature of the carotid, and has been cut in the removal of deep-seated tumors. The trunk may be attacked by neuritis.

The affections of the vagus are best considered in connection with the distribution of the separate nerves.

Pharyngeal Branches.—In combination with the glosso-pharyngeal the branches from the vagus form the pharyngeal plexus, from which the muscles and mucosa of the pharynx are supplied. In *paralysis* due to involvement of this either in the nuclei, as in bulbar paralysis, or in the course of the nerve, as in diphtheritic neuritis, there is difficulty in swallowing and the food is not passed on into the œsophagus. If the nerve on one side only is involved the deglutition is not much impaired. In these cases the particles of food frequently pass into the larynx, and, when the soft palate is involved, into the posterior nares.

Spasm of the pharynx is always a functional disorder, usually occurring in hysterical and nervous people. Gowers mentioned a case of a gentleman who could not eat unless alone, on account of the inability to swallow in the presence of others from spasm of the pharynx. This spasm is a well marked feature in hydrophobia, and occurs also in pseudo-hydrophobia.

Laryngeal Branches.—The superior laryngeal nerve supplies the mucous membrane of the larynx above the cords and the crico-thyroid muscle. The inferior or recurrent laryngeal curves around the arch of the aorta on the left side and the subclavian artery on the right passes along the trachea and supplies the mucosa below the cords and all the muscles of the larynx except the crico-thyroid and the epiglottidean. Experiments have shown that these motor nerves of the pneumogastic are all derived from the spinal accessory. The remarkable course of the recurrent laryngeal nerves renders them liable to pressure by tumors within the thorax, particularly by aneurism. The following are the most important forms of paralysis:

(*a*) Bilateral Paralysis of the Abductors.—In this condition the posterior crico-arytenoids are involved and the glottis is not opened during inspiration. The cords may be close together in the position of phonation, and during inspiration may be brought even nearer together by the pressure of air, so that there is only a narrow chink through which the air whistles with a noisy stridor. This dangerous form of laryngeal paralysis occurs occasionally as a result of cold, or may follow a laryngeal catarrh. The posterior muscles have been found degenerated when the others were healthy. The condition may be produced by pressure upon both vagi, or upon both recurrent nerves. As a central affection it occurs in tabes and bulbar paralysis, but may be seen also in hysteria. The characteristic symptoms are inspiratory stridor with unimpaired phonation. Possibly, as Gowers suggested, many cases of so-called hysterical spasm of the glottis are in reality abductor paralysis.

(*b*) Unilateral Abductor Paralysis.—This frequently results from the pressure of tumors or involvement of one recurrent nerve. Aneurism is the most common cause, though on the right side the nerve may be involved in thickening of the pleura. The symptoms are hoarseness or roughness of the voice, as is so common in aneurism. Dyspnœa is not often present. The cord on the affected side does not move in inspiration. Subsequently the adductors may become involved, in which case phonation is still more impaired.

(*c*) Adductor Paralysis.—This results from involvement of the lateral crico-arytenoid and the arytenoid muscle itself. It is common in hysteria, particularly of women, and causes the hysterical aphonia, which may come on suddenly. It may result from catarrh of the larynx or from overuse of the voice. In laryngoscopic examination it is seen, on attempting phonation, that there is no power to bring the cords together.

(*d*) Spasm of the Muscles of the Larynx.—In this the adductor muscles are involved. It is not uncommon in children, and has been referred to as laryngismus stridulus. Paroxysmal attacks of laryngeal spasm are rare in the adult, but cases are described in which the patient, usually a young girl, wakes at night in an attack of intense dyspnœa, which may persist long enough to produce cyanosis. Liveing states that they may replace attacks of migraine. They occur in a characteristic form in tabes, the so-called laryngeal crises. There is a spastic aphonia, in which, when the patient attempts to speak, phonation is completely prevented by a spasm.

Disturbance of the sensory nerves of the larynx is rare.

(*e*) Anæsthesia may occur in bulbar paralysis and in diphtheritic neuritis—a serious condition, as portions of food may enter the windpipe. It is usually associated with dysphagia and is sometimes present in hysteria. Hyperæsthesia of the larynx is rare.

Cardiac Branches.—The cardiac plexus is formed by the union of branches of the vagi and of the sympathetic nerves. The vagus fibres subserve motor, sensory and probably trophic functions.

Motor.—The fibres which inhibit, control, and regulate the cardiac action pass in the vagi. Irritation may produce slowing of the action. Czermak could slow or even arrest the heart's action for a few beats by pressing a small tumor in his neck against one pneumogastric nerve, and it is said that the same can be produced by forcible bilateral pressure on the carotid canal. There are instances in which persons appear to have had voluntary control over the action of the heart. Cheyne mentions the case of Colonel Townshend, "who could die or expire when he pleased, and yet by an effort or somehow come to life again, which it seems he had sometimes tried before he had sent for us." Retardation of the heart's action has also followed accidental ligature of one vagus. Irritation of the nuclei may also be accompanied with a neurosis of this nerve. On the other hand, when there is complete paralysis of the vagi, the inhibitory action may be abolished and the acceleratory influences have full sway. The heart's action is then greatly increased. This is seen in some instances of diphtheritic neuritis and in involvement of the nerve by tumors, or its accidental removal or ligature. Complete loss of function of one vagus, however, may not be followed by any symptoms.

Sensory symptoms on the part of the cardiac branches are very varied. Normally, the heart's action proceeds regularly without the participation of consciousness, but the unpleasant feelings and sensations of palpitation and pain are conveyed to the brain through this nerve. How far the fibres of the pneumogastric are involved in angina it is impossible to say.

Pulmonary Branches.—We know very little of the pulmonary branches of the vagi. The motor fibres are stated to control the action of the bronchial muscles. The various alterations in the respiratory rhythm are probably due more to changes in the centre than in the nerves themselves.

Gastric and Œsophageal Branches.—The muscular movements of these parts are presided over by the vagi and vomiting is induced through them, usually reflexly, but also by direct irritation, as in meningitis. Spasm of the œsophagus generally occurs with other nervous phenomena. Gastralgia may be due to cramp of the stomach or to sensory disturbance of this nerve, due to irritation of the peripheral ends, or a neuralgia of the terminal fibres. Some forms of nervous dyspepsia probably depend upon disturbed function of this nerve. The severe gastric crises which occur in tabes are due to central irritation of the nuclei. Vagotonia is an important element in many disorders of the digestive tract.

SPINAL ACCESSORY NERVE

Paralysis.—The smaller or internal part of this nerve joins the vagus and is distributed through it to the laryngeal muscles. The larger external part is distributed to the sterno-mastoid and trapezius muscles.

The nuclei of the nerve, particularly of the accessory part, may be involved in bulbar paralysis. The nuclei of the external portion, situated as they are in the cervical cord, may be attacked in progressive degeneration of the motor nuclei of the cord. The nerve may be involved in the exudation of meningitis, or be compressed by tumors, or in caries. The *symptoms* of paralysis of the accessory portion which joins the vagus have already been given in the account of the palsy of the laryngeal branches of the pneumogastric. Disease or compression of the external portion is followed by paralysis of the sterno-mastoid and of the trapezius on the same side. In paralysis of one sterno-mastoid the patient rotates the head with difficulty to the opposite side, but there is no torticollis, though in some cases the head is held obliquely.

As the trapezius is supplied in part from the cervical nerves, it is not completely paralyzed, but the portion which passes from the occipital bone to the acromion is functionless. The paralysis of the muscle is well seen when the patient draws a deep breath or shrugs the shoulders. The middle portion of the trapezius is also weakened, the shoulder droops a little, and the angle of the scapula is rotated inward by the action of the rhomboids and the levator anguli scapulæ. Elevation of the arm is impaired, for the trapezius does not fix the scapula as a point from which the deltoid can work.

In progressive muscular atrophy we sometimes see bilateral paralysis of these muscles. Thus, if the sterno-mastoids are affected, the head tends to fall back; when the trapezii are involved, it falls forward, a characteristic attitude of the head in many cases of progressive muscular atrophy. Gowers suggested that lesions of the accessory in difficult labor may account for those cases in which during the first year of life the child has great difficulty in holding up the head. In children this drooping of the head is an important symptom in cervical meningitis, the result of caries.

The TREATMENT of the condition depends much upon the cause. In the central nuclear atrophy but little can be done. In paralysis from pressure the symptoms may gradually be relieved. The paralyzed muscles should be stimulated by electricity and massage.

Accessory Spasm (*Torticollis; Wryneck*).—The forms of spasm affecting the cervical muscles are best considered here, as the muscles supplied by the accessory are chiefly, though not solely, responsible for the condition. The following forms may be described in this section:

(*a*) CONGENITAL TORTICOLLIS.—This condition, also known as fixed torticollis, depends upon the shortening and atrophy of the sterno-mastoid on one side. It occurs in children and may not be noticed for several years on account of the shortness of the neck, the parents often alleging that it has only recently come on. It affects the right side almost exclusively. A remarkable circumstance in connection with it is the existence of facial asymmetry noted by Wilks, which appears to be an essential part of this congenital form. In congenital wryneck the sterno-mastoid is shortened, hard and firm, and in a condition of more or less advanced atrophy. This must be distinguished from the local thickening in the sterno-mastoid due to rupture, which may occur at the time of birth and produce an induration or muscle callus. Although the sterno-mastoid is almost always affected, there are rare cases in which the fibrous atrophy affects the trapezius. This form of wryneck in itself is unimportant, since it is readily relieved by tenotomy, but Golding-Bird states that the facial asymmetry persists, or may become more evident. With reference to the pathology of the affection, Golding-Bird concludes that the facial asymmetry and the torticollis are integral parts of one affection which has a central origin, and is the counterpart in the head and neck of infantile paralysis with talipes in the foot.

(*b*) SPASMODIC WRYNECK.—Two varieties of this spasm occur, the tonic and the clonic, which may alternate in the same case; or, as is most common, they are separate and remain so from the outset. The disease is most frequent in adults and, according to Gowers, more common in females. In America it is certainly more frequent in males. In females it may be an hysterical manifestation. There may be a marked neurotic family history, but it is usually impossible to fix upon any definite etiological factor. Some cases have followed cold; others a blow. Brissaud described what he calls mental torticollis. It is usually met with in neurasthenic patients and in elderly persons, and consists of a clonic spasm of the rotators of the head.

The *symptoms* are well defined. In the tonic form the contracted sterno-mastoid draws the occiput toward the shoulder of the affected side; the chin is raised, and the face rotated to the other shoulder. The sterno-mastoid may be affected alone or in association with the trapezius. When the latter is implicated the head is depressed still more toward the same side. In long-standing cases these muscles are prominent and very rigid. There may be some curvature of the spine, the convexity of which is toward the sound side. The cases in which the spasm is clonic are much more distressing and serious. The spasm is rarely limited to a single muscle. The sterno-mastoid is almost always involved and rotates the head so as to approximate the mastoid process to the inner end of the clavicle, turning the face to the opposite side and raising the chin. When with this the trapezius is affected, the depression of the head toward the same side is more marked. The head is drawn somewhat backward; the shoulder, too, is raised by its action. According to Gowers, the splenius is associated with the sterno-mastoid about half as frequently as the trapezius. Its action is to incline the head and rotate it slightly toward the same side. Other muscles may be involved, such as the scalenus and platysma myoides; and in rare cases the head may be rotated by the deep cervical muscles, the rectus and obliquus. There are cases in which the spasm is bilateral, causing a backward movement—retro-colic spasm. This may be tonic or clonic; in extreme cases the face is horizontal and looks upward.

These clonic contractions may come on without warning, or be preceded by irregular pains or stiffness of the neck. The jerking movements recur every few moments, and it is impossible to keep the head still for more than a minute or two. In time the muscles undergo hypertrophy and may be distinctly larger on one side than the other. In some cases the pain is considerable; in others there is simply a feeling of fatigue. The spasms cease during sleep. Emotion, excitement, and fatigue increase them. The spasm may extend from the neck muscles and involve those of the face or arms.

The disease varies much; cases occasionally get well, but the majority persist, and, even if temporarily relieved, the disease frequently recurs. The affection is usually regarded as a functional neurosis, but it is possibly due to disturbance of the cortical centres presiding over the muscles.

Treatment.—Temporary relief is sometimes obtained; a permanent cure is exceptional. Various drugs have been used, but rarely with benefit. Occasionally, large doses of bromide lessen the intensity of the spasms. Morphia, subcutaneously, has been successful in some cases, but there is great danger of establishing the habit. Galvanism may be tried. Counter-irritation is probably useless. Fixation of the head mechanically can rarely be borne by the patient. These obstinate cases come ultimately to the surgeon, and the operations of stretching, division, and excision of the accessory nerve and division of the muscles have been tried. Temporary relief may follow, but, as a rule, the condition returns. Risien Russell thinks that resection of the posterior branches of the upper cervical nerves is most likely to give relief.

(*c*) The NODDING SPASM of children may here be mentioned as involving chiefly the muscles innervated by the accessory nerve. It may be a simple trick, a form of habit spasm, or a phenomenon of epilepsy (*E. nutans*), in which case it is associated with transient loss of consciousness. A similar nodding spasm may occur in older children. In women it sometimes occurs as an hysterical manifestation, commonly as part of the so-called salaam convulsion.

HYPOGLOSSAL NERVE

This is the motor nerve of the tongue and for most of the muscles attached to the hyoid bone. Its cortical centre is probably the lower part of the anterior central gyrus.

Paralysis.—(*a*) CORTICAL LESION.—The tongue is often involved in hemiplegia, and the paralysis may result from a lesion of the cortex itself, or of the fibres as they pass to the medulla. It does not occur alone and is considered with hemiplegia. There is this difference, however, between the cortical and other forms, that the muscles on both sides of the tongue may be more or less affected but do not waste, nor are their electrical reactions disturbed.

(*b*) NUCLEAR and INFRA-NUCLEAR lesions result from slow progressive degeneration, as in bulbar paralysis or tabes; occasionally there is acute softening from obstruction of the vessels. The nuclei of both nerves are usually affected together, but may be attacked separately. Trauma and lead poisoning have also been assigned as causes. The fibres may be damaged by a tumor, and at the base by meningitis; or the nerve is sometimes involved in the condylar foramen by disease of the skull. It may be involved in its course in a scar, as in Birkett's case, or compressed by a tumor in the parotid region. As a result, there is loss of function in the nerve fibres and the tongue undergoes atrophy on the affected side. It is protruded toward the paralyzed side and may show fibrillary twitching.

The *symptoms* of involvement of one hypoglossal, either at its centre or in its course, are those of unilateral paralysis and atrophy of the tongue. When protruded, it is pushed toward the affected side, and there are fibrillary twitchings. The atrophy is usually marked and the mucous membrane on the affected side is thrown into folds. Articulation is not much impaired in the unilateral affection. When the disease is bilateral, the tongue lies almost motionless in the floor of the mouth; it is atrophied, and can not be protruded. Speech and mastication are extremely difficult and deglutition may be impaired. If the seat of the disease is above the nuclei, there may be little or no wasting. The condition is seen in progressive bulbar paralysis and occasionally in progressive muscular atrophy.

The *diagnosis* is readily made and the situation of the lesion can usually be determined, since when supra-nuclear there is associated hemiplegia and no wasting of the muscles of the tongue. Nuclear disease is only occasionally unilateral; most commonly bilateral and part of a bulbar paralysis. It should be borne in mind that the fibres of the hypoglossal may be involved within the medulla after leaving their nuclei. In such a case there may be paralysis of the tongue on one side and paralysis of the limbs on the opposite side, and the tongue, when protruded, is pushed toward the sound side.

Spasm.—This rare affection may be unilateral or bilateral. It is most frequently a part of some other convulsive disorder, such as epilepsy, chorea, or spasm of the facial muscles. In some cases of stuttering, spasm of the tongue precedes the explosive utterance of the words. It may occur in hysteria, and is said to follow reflex irritation in the fifth nerve. The most remarkable cases are those of paroxysmal clonic spasm, in which the tongue is rapidly thrust in and out, as many as forty or fifty times a minute. The prognosis is usually good.

COMBINED PARALYSIS OF THE LAST THREE AND FOUR CRANIAL NERVES

The war experience has widened our knowledge of these cases. There may be: (*a*) *Avelli's syndrome,* palato-laryngeal paralysis from involvement of the ninth and eleventh. With this there may be involvement of the tenth with paralysis of the superior constrictor of the pharynx. When the outer fibres of the spinal accessory are involved, the sterno-cleido-mastoid may be paralyzed on the same side (*Schmidt syndrome*). (*b*) *Hughlings-Jackson syndrome.* Involvement of the ix, x, xi, and xii—disturbance of taste and paralysis of the superior constrictor of the pharynx (ix and x); hemi-anæsthesia of the palate and pharynx, sometimes with cough and dyspnœa and salivation which may be profuse (x and xi); hemi-paralysis of the larynx (xi) with hemi-paralysis of the tongue (xii). In wounds of the retro-parotidean space or after a parotid bubo, in addition to the hypoglossal, the sympathetic nerves with fibres of the ix, x, and xi may be involved, causing exophthalmos, myosis, and sweating, with the combined paralyses known as Villaret's syndrome. These combined paralyses may be nuclear, caused by gummatous or tuberculous meningitis, by tumor or by injury. In the war cases the lesions have often been more extensive, and symptoms of involvement of the vagus have been more common than in the ordinary instances from tumor or meningitis.

IV. DISEASES OF THE SPINAL NERVES

CERVICAL PLEXUS

Occipito-cervical Neuralgia.—This involves the nerve territory supplied by the occipitalis major and minor, and the auricularis magnus nerves. The pains are chiefly in the back of the head and neck and in the ear. The condition may follow cold and is sometimes associated with stiffness of the neck or torticollis. Unless disease of the bones exists with it or it is due to pressure of tumors, the outlook is usually good. There are tender points midway between the mastoid process and the spine and just above the parietal eminence, and between the sterno-mastoid and the trapezius. The affection may be due to direct pressure in carrying heavy weights.

Affections of the Phrenic Nerve.—Paralysis may follow a lesion in the anterior horns at the level of the third and fourth cervical nerves, or may be due to compression of the nerve by tumors or aneurism. More rarely paralysis results from neuritis, diphtheritic or saturnine.

When the *diaphragm* is paralyzed respiration is carried on by the intercostal and accessory muscles. When the patient is quiet and at rest little may be noticed, but the abdomen retracts in inspiration and is forced out in expiration. On exertion or even on attempting to move there may be dyspnœa. If the paralysis sets in suddenly there may be dyspnœa and lividity, which is usually temporary (W. Pasteur). Intercurrent attacks of bronchitis seriously aggravate the condition. Difficulty in coughing, owing to the impossibility of drawing a full breath, adds greatly to the danger of this complication.

When the phrenic nerve is paralyzed on one side the paralysis may be scarcely noticeable, but careful inspection shows that the descent of the diaphragm is much less on the affected side.

The *diagnosis* of paralysis is not always easy, particularly in women, who habitually use this muscle less than men, and in whom the diaphragmatic breathing is less conspicuous. Immobility of the diaphragm is not uncommon, particularly in diaphragmatic pleurisy, in large effusions, and in extensive emphysema. The muscle itself may be degenerated.

Owing to the lessened action of the diaphragm, there is a tendency to stasis at the bases of the lungs, and there may be impaired resonance and signs of œdema. As a rule, however, the paralysis is not confined to this muscle, but is part of a general neuritis or an anterior polio-myelitis, and there are other symptoms of value in determining its presence. The outlook is usually serious. Pasteur states that of 15 cases following diphtheria only 8 recovered. The treatment is that of the neuritis or polio-myelitis.

Hiccough.—Here may be considered this remarkable symptom, caused by intermittent, sudden contraction of the diaphragm. The mechanism, however, is complex, and while the afferent impressions to the respiratory centre may be peripheral or central the efferent are distributed through the phrenic nerve to the diaphragm, causing the intermittent spasm, and through the laryngeal branches of the vagus to the glottis, causing sudden closure as the air is rapidly inspired. There are various groups:

(*a*) INFLAMMATORY, seen particularly in affections of the abdominal viscera, gastritis, peritonitis, hernia, internal strangulation, appendicitis, suppurative pancreatitis, and in the severe forms of typhoid fever.

(*b*) IRRITATIVE, as in the direct stimulation of the diaphragm when very hot substances are swallowed, in disease of the œsophagus near the diaphragm, and in many conditions of gastric and intestinal disorder, more particularly those associated with flatus.

(*c*) TOXIC.—In these cases there is usually some general disease, as gout, diabetes, or chronic nephritis. Hiccough may be very obstinate in the later stages of chronic nephritis.

(*d*) NEUROTIC, cases in which the primary cause is in the nervous system; hysteria, epilepsy, shock, or cerebral tumors. Of these cases the hysterical are, perhaps, the most obstinate.

The TREATMENT is often very unsatisfactory. Sometimes in the milder forms a sudden reflex irritation will check it at once. A pinch of snuff may be effective. Readers of Plato's Symposium will remember that the physician Eryximachus recommended to Aristophanes, who had hiccough from eating too much, either to hold his breath (which for trivial forms of hiccough is very satisfactory) or to gargle with a little water; but if it still continued, "tickle your nose with something and sneeze; and if you sneeze once or twice even the most violent hiccough is sure to go." The attack must have been of some severity, as it is stated subsequently that the hiccough did not disappear until Aristophanes had resorted to the sneezing.

Ice, a teaspoonful of salt and lemon juice, or salt and vinegar, or a teaspoonful of raw spirits may be tried. When the hiccough is due to gastric irritation, lavage is sometimes promptly curative. Alkali should be given freely. A hypodermic injection of gr. 1/8 (0.008 gm.) of apomorphia may give prompt relief. In obstinate cases the various antispasmodics have been used in succession. Pilocarpine has been recommended. The ether spray on the epigastrium may be promptly curative. Hypodermics of morphia, inhalations of chloroform, the use of nitrite of amyl and of nitroglycerin have been beneficial in some cases. Galvanism over the phrenic nerve, or pressure on the nerves, applied between the heads of the sterno-cleido-mastoid muscles may be used. Strong traction upon the tongue may give immediate relief. Of all measures morphia used freely is the best.

BRACHIAL PLEXUS

Cervical Rib.—FREQUENCY.—The anomaly is much more common than indicated in the literature. Sometimes bilateral, it may be complete with bony attachment to the second rib; incomplete, forming a short stump of variable length, or—and this is important—there may be a fibrous band-like attachment from a short rib to the first. It is more common on the left side. Symptoms usually appear between the fifteenth and thirtieth years.

The ribs may be visible, one more plainly than the other, and the subclavian artery, lifted up, may pulsate high in the supraclavicular fossa. This abnormal pulsation and the fullness in the fossa may suggest the presence of the extra rib. The throbbing may be marked enough to suggest aneurism. The rib may be felt, often more marked on one side; even the bifid extremity may be palpable, and the artery felt above the rib sometimes appears longer and larger than normal.

SYMPTOMS.—In a large proportion the patients are unaware of the anomaly; the symptoms, which may come on suddenly, may be grouped as follows:

1. *Local.* (*a*) Supraclavicular swelling. (*b*) Pulsation. (*c*) Palpable tumor and aneurism.

2. *Neuritic.* (*a*) Neuralgic pains (supraclavicular, cervical, brachial). (*b*) Paræsthesia. (*c*) Local anæsthesia. (*d*) Sympathetic nerve features.

3. *Muscular.* (*a*) Atrophy, in ulnar distribution. (*b*) Spasm. (*c*) Intermittent claudication.

4. *Vascular.* (*a*) Vaso-motor changes (ischæmia, hyperæmia, swelling). (*b*) Local gangrene. (*c*) Aneurism, (i) spurious, (ii) true. (*d*) Thrombosis.

Neuralgic pains occur in the cervical region, sometimes passing up the back of the head; more commonly the pain is in the distribution of the eighth cervical and first dorsal nerve, sometimes only a dull pain and aching with numbness and tingling or even anæsthesia. Dissociation of cutaneous sensation, loss of tactile and thermic with retention of pain sense, may be present. The cervical sympathetic may be involved with the usual features. *Muscular atrophy* is usually in the region of distribution of the ulnar nerve. The difference between the two arms may be marked and the interossei wasted, as in progressive muscular atrophy, for which, when bilateral, cases may be mistaken. With pressure on and narrowing of the subclavian, intermittent claudication is present, characterised by numbness, tingling and swelling, sometimes by redness of the arm and muscular disability on exertion. At rest the arm is normal and comfortable, but on exertion these features occur: spasm, tonic or clonic, in the muscles of the hand is occasionally seen.

Vaso-motor Changes.—Redness with swelling, sometimes cyanosis and mottling, may be present, with changes resembling Raynaud's disease; in a few cases gangrene of the finger tips has followed.

Aneurism.—The subclavian artery may be tilted by the ribs and give a wide area of supraclavicular pulsation. There may be: (1) slight narrowing from pressure, with feeble pulse on the affected side; (2) manifest enlargement of the vessel, fusiform or uniform; or (3) a definite cylindrical aneurism. In 27 of 525 clinical cases collected by Halsted these local changes were present. The dilatation is distal to the point of constriction made by the rib and the scalenus anticus, which Halsted explains by the abnormal play of the blood in the relatively dead pocket beyond the constriction, and the absence of the normal pulse pressure necessary to maintain the integrity of the arterial wall. The nervi arteriorum may be involved.

Thrombosis.—This may occur in the vessels beyond the point of constriction, in one case involving suddenly the brachial and gradually extending to the axillary and subclavian, with the gradual development of an effective collateral circulation.

The relative distribution of the symptoms as given by Halsted from an exhaustive review of the literature was in 63.3 per cent. nerve symptoms alone, in 29.4 per cent. nervous and vascular symptoms, while 5.3 per cent. have only vascular symptoms.

Diagnosis.—This is easy as a rule even without the X-rays. A serious difficulty arises when disease of the cord occurs in the subjects of cervical rib, e. g., syringomyelia and progressive muscular atrophy. In cases of prolonged discomfort or pain with vascular or trophic disturbance in the arm, cervical rib should be considered.

Treatment.—When accidentally discovered, it is best not to tell the patient. Elevation of the shoulders may give relief. Massage, electricity and other forms of local treatment may be tried. The rib may be removed, but only as a last resort, as the results are not always satisfactory.

Combined Paralysis.—The plexus may be involved in the supraclavicular region by compression of the nerve trunks as they leave the spine, or by tumors and other morbid processes in the neck. Below the clavicle lesions are more common and result from injuries following dislocation or fracture, sometimes from neuritis. A cervical rib may lead to a pressure paralysis of the lower cord of the plexus. A not infrequent form of injury in this region follows falls or blows on the neck, which by lateral flexion of the head and depression of the shoulder seriously stretch the plexus. The entire plexus may be ruptured and the arm be totally paralyzed. The rupture may occur anywhere between the vertebræ and the clavicle, and involve all the cords of the plexus, or only the upper ones. The so-called "obstetrical palsy" usually results from the forcible separation of the head and neck from the shoulder during delivery, with the result of tearing the deep cervical fascia and the nerves, involving the roots from above and downwards, so that the injury may vary from a slight lesion of the upper root to complete rupture of the plexus or the tearing of the roots from the cord itself. In the complete lesion the arm is flaccid and immobile, does not grow, and there is displacement of the head of the humerus; sensory disturbances are rare. The prognosis is bad; only mild cases recover completely. Suturing the broken cords and planting them in the neighboring roots have been followed by good results, but complete recovery rarely if ever follows. Another common cause of lesion of the brachial plexus is luxation of the head of the humerus, particularly the subcoracoid form.

A primary neuritis of the brachial plexus is rare. More commonly the process is an ascending neuritis from a lesion of a peripheral branch, involving first the radial or ulnar nerves, and spreading upward to the plexus, producing gradually complete loss of power in the arm.

Lesions of Individual Nerves of the Plexus.—(*a*) LONG THORACIC NERVE. —*Serratus paralysis* follows injury to this nerve in the neck, usually by direct pressure in carrying loads, and is very common in soldiers. It may be due to a neuritis following an acute infection or exposure. Isolated serratus paralysis is rare. It usually occurs in connection with paralysis of other muscles of the shoulder girdle, as in the myopathies and in progressive muscular atrophy. Concomitant trapezius paralysis is the most frequent. In the isolated paralysis there is little or no deformity with the hands hanging by the sides. There are slight abnormal obliquity of the posterior border of the scapula and prominence of the inferior angle, but when, as so commonly happens, the middle part of the trapezius is also paralyzed the deformity is marked. The shoulder is at a lower level, the inferior angle of the scapula is displaced inward and upward, and the superior angle projects upward. When the arms are held out in front at right angles to the body the scapula becomes winged and stands out prominently. The arm can not, as a rule, be raised above the horizontal. The outlook of the cases due to injury or to neuritis is good.

(*b*) CIRCUMFLEX NERVE.—This supplies the deltoid and teres minor and may be involved in injuries, in dislocations, bruising by a crutch, or sometimes by extension of inflammation from the joint. Occasionally the paralysis arises from a pressure neuritis during an illness. As a consequence of loss of power in the deltoid, the arm can not be raised. The wasting is usually marked and changes the shape of the shoulder. Sensation may be impaired in the skin over the muscle. The joint may be relaxed and there may be a distinct space between the head of the humerus and the acromion.

(*c*) MUSCULO-SPIRAL PARALYSIS; RADIAL PARALYSIS.—This is one of the most common of peripheral palsies, and results from the exposed position of the musculo-spiral nerve. It is often bruised in the use of the crutch, by injuries of the arm, blows, or fractures. It is frequently injured when a person falls asleep with the arm over the back of a chair, or by pressure of the body upon the arm when a person is sleeping on a bench or on the ground. It may be paralyzed by sudden violent contraction of the triceps. It is sometimes involved in a neuritis from cold, but this is uncommon in comparison with other causes. The paralysis of lead poisoning is the result of involvement of certain branches of this nerve.

A lesion when high up involves the triceps, the brachialis anticus, and the supinator longus, as well as the extensors of the wrist and fingers. In lesions just above the elbow the arm muscles and the supinator longus are spared. The most characteristic feature is the wrist-drop and the inability to extend the first phalanges of the fingers and thumb. In the pressure palsies the supinators are usually involved and the movements of supination can not be accomplished. The sensations may be impaired, or there may be marked tingling, but the loss of sensation is rarely so pronounced as that of motion.

The affection is readily recognized, but it is sometimes difficult to say upon what it depends. The sleep and pressure palsies are, as a rule, unilateral and involve the supinator longus. The paralysis from lead is bilateral and the supinators are unaffected. Bilateral wrist-drop is a very common symptom in many forms of multiple neuritis, particularly the alcoholic; but the mode of onset and the involvement of the legs and arms make the diagnosis easy. The duration and course of the musculo-spiral paralyses are very variable. The pressure palsies may disappear in a few days. Recovery is the rule, even when the affection lasts for many weeks. The electrical examination is of importance in prognosis, and the rules laid down under paralysis of the facial nerve hold good here. The *treatment* is that of neuritis.

(*d*) Ulnar Nerve.—The motor branches supply the ulnar half of the deep flexor of the fingers, the muscles of the little finger, the interossei, the adductor and the inner head of the short flexor of the thumb, and the ulnar flexor of the wrist. The sensory branches supply the ulnar side of the hand—two and a half fingers on the back, and one and a half fingers on the front. Paralysis may result from pressure, usually at the elbow joint, although the nerve is here protected. Possibly the neuritis in the ulnar nerve in some cases of acute illness may be due to this cause. Owing to paralysis of the ulnar flexor of the wrist, the hand moves toward the radial side; adduction of the thumb is impossible; the first phalanges can not be flexed, and the others can not be extended. In long standing cases the first phalanges are over-extended and the others strongly flexed, producing the claw-hand; but this is not so marked as in the progressive muscular atrophy. The loss of sensation corresponds to the sensory distribution just mentioned.

(*e*) Median Nerve.—This supplies the flexors of the fingers except the ulnar half of the deep flexors, the abductor and the flexors of the thumb, the two radial lumbricales, the pronators, and the radial flexor of the wrist. The sensory fibres supply the radial side of the palm and the front of the thumb, the first two fingers and half the third finger, and the dorsal surfaces of the same three fingers.

This nerve is seldom involved alone. Paralysis results from injury and occasionally from neuritis. The signs are inability to pronate the forearm beyond the mid-position. The wrist can be flexed only toward the ulnar side; the thumb can not be opposed to the tips of fingers. The second phalanges can not be flexed on the first; the distal phalanges of the first and second fingers can not be flexed; but in the third and fourth fingers this action can be performed by the ulnar half of the flexor profundus. The loss of sensation is in the region corresponding to the sensory distribution already mentioned.

The wasting of the thumb muscles, which is usually marked in this paralysis, gives to it a characteristic appearance.

Volkmann's Paralysis.—Ischæmic paralysis, as it is called, usually follows the pressure of splints and bandages in children with fracture in the region of the elbow-joint. The changes are thought to be due to arrest of the circulation in the muscles, which are hardened and stiff and the flexors of the forearm are contracted. The hand is claw-like with the metacarpo-phalangeal joints strongly extended and the middle and terminal phalanges strongly flexed. The condition may come on with great rapidity and appears to be a muscular lesion though it is not always possible to exclude pressure on the nerves. The prognosis is good with judicious treatment.

LUMBAR AND SACRAL PLEXUSES

Lumbar Plexus.—The lumbar plexus is sometimes involved in growths of the lymph glands, in psoas abscess, and in disease of the bones of the vertebræ. The *obturator nerve* is occasionally injured during parturition. When paralyzed the power is lost over the adductors of the thigh and one leg can not be crossed over the other. Outward rotation is also disturbed. The *anterior crural nerve* is sometimes involved in wounds or in dislocation of the hip-joint, less commonly during parturition, and sometimes by disease of the bones and in psoas abscess. The special symptoms of affection of this nerve are paralysis of the extensors of the knee with wasting of the muscles, anæsthesia of the antero-lateral parts of the thigh and of the inner side of the leg to the big toe. This nerve is sometimes involved early in growths about the spine, and there may be pain in its area of distribution. Loss of the power of abducting the thigh results from paralysis of the *gluteal nerve,* which is distributed to the gluteus medius and minimus muscles.

External Cutaneous Nerve.—A peculiar form of sensory disturbance, confined to the territory of this nerve, was first described by Bernhardt in 1895, and a few months later by Roth, who gave it the name of *meralgia parœsthetica.* The disease is probably due to a neuritis which seems to originate in that part of the nerve where it passes under Poupart's ligament, just internal to the anterior superior iliac spine. The nerve is usually tender on pressure at this point. The disease is more common in men. Musser and Sailer in 1900 collected 99 cases, of which 75 were in men. A large number of the cases are attributable to direct traumatism or to simple pressure on the nerve by the aponeurotic canal through which it passes. Pregnancy is among the more common causes in women. The sensory disturbances consist of various forms of paræsthesia located over the outer side of the thigh, oftentimes with some actual diminution in the acuity of sense perception. The symptoms may persist for years, and the discomfort in some cases be so great, and so exaggerated by the mere touch of the clothing, that patients may be greatly incapacitated. Excision of the nerve as it passes under Poupart's ligament has given good results.

Sacral Plexus.—The sacral plexus is frequently involved in tumors and inflammations within the pelvis and may be injured during parturition. Neuritis is common, usually an extension from the sciatic nerve.

Goldthwaite calls attention to the fact that the lumbo-sacral articulation varies very greatly in its stability, and actual displacement of the bones may result with separation of the posterior portion of the intervertebral disc. The cauda equina, or the nerve roots, may be compressed. With displacement on one side the spine is rotated and the articular process of the fifth is drawn into the spinal canal, with such narrowing that paraplegia may result, and he reports a remarkable case in which the paralysis came on during the application of a plaster jacket. Weakness of the joints or displacements may cause irritation of the nerves inside and outside the canal with resulting sciatica.

Of the branches, the *sciatic nerve,* when injured at or near the notch, causes paralysis of the flexors of the legs and the muscles below the knee, but injury below the middle of the thigh involves only the latter muscles. There is also anæsthesia of the outer half of the leg, the sole, and the greater portion of the dorsum of the foot. Wasting of the muscles and trophic disturbances may follow. In paralysis of one sciatic the leg is fixed at the knee by the action of the quadriceps extensor and the patient is able to walk.

Paralysis of the *small sciatic nerve* is rarely seen. The gluteus maximus is involved and there may be difficulty in rising from a seat. There is a strip of anæsthesia along the back of the middle third of the thigh.

External Popliteal Nerve.—Paralysis involves the peronæi, the long extensor of the toes, tibialis anticus, and the extensor brevis digitorum. The ankle can not be flexed, resulting in a condition known as foot-drop, and as the toes can not be raised the whole leg must be lifted, producing the characteristic *steppage* gait seen in so many forms of peripheral neuritis. In long-standing cases the foot is permanently extended and there is wasting of the anterior tibial and peroneal muscles. The loss of sensation is in the outer half of the front of the leg and on the dorsum of the foot.

Internal Popliteal Nerve.—When paralyzed, plantar flexion of the foot and flexion of the toes are impossible. The foot can not be adducted, nor can the patient rise on tiptoe. In long standing cases talipes calcaneus follows and the toes assume a claw-like position from secondary contracture, due to over-extension of the proximal and flexion of the second and third phalanges.

SCIATICA

Definition.—The term sciatica is applied to any painful condition referred to the sciatic nerve. It may be defined as an interstitial inflammation of the sciatic nerve, causing severe pain in the branches of distribution and, if long continued, atrophy of the muscles.

Etiology.—Primary neuritis of this nerve is very rare and is seen chiefly in men who have diabetes and gout. In the vast majority the condition is *secondary* to a process elsewhere which affects the component cords or the trunk itself. Among the causal factors are: (1) arthritis which may be of the lower spine, lumbo-sacral, sacro-iliac or hip joints. In this case the arthritic lesion is often due to a focus of infection. (2) Anatomical anomalies, as an unusually long transverse process of the fifth lumbar vertebra. (3) Disease of the bones of the lower spine or pelvis, e. g., tuberculosis. (4) Strain, which may be acute or chronic, especially of the sacro-iliac joint. Exposure to cold after heavy muscular exertion is said to be a cause. In trench warfare the men were not as subject to sciatica as the officers. (5) Pelvic conditions, such as a solid ovarian or fibroid tumor in women and prostatic disease in men. Constipation is said to be a cause and the pressure of the fetal head in labor. (6) Syphilis is responsible in a few cases. (7) It may be due to a focus of infection. Sciatica occurs most often in adult males, just as do spondylitis and sacro-iliac joint disease to which it is most often secondary.

Symptoms.—Pain is the most constant and troublesome symptom. The onset may be severe, with slight pyrexia, but, as a rule, it is gradual, and for a time there is only slight pain in the back of the thigh, particularly in certain positions or after exertion. Soon the pain becomes more intense and, instead of being limited to the upper portion of the nerve, extends down the thigh, reaching the foot and radiating over the entire distribution of the nerve. The patient can often point out the most sensitive spots, usually at the notch or in the middle of the thigh; and on pressure these are exquisitely painful. The pain is described as gnawing or burning, and is usually constant, but in some instances is paroxysmal, and often worse at night. On walking it may be very great; the knee is bent and the patient treads on the toes, so as to relieve the tension on the nerve. In protracted cases there may be much wasting of the muscles, but the reaction of degeneration can seldom be obtained. In these chronic cases cramp may occur and fibrillary contractions. Herpes may develop but this is unusual. In rare instances the neuritis ascends and involves the spinal cord.

Duration and Course.—The duration and course are extremely variable. As a rule, it is an obstinate affection, lasting for months, or even, with slight remissions, for years. Relapses are not uncommon, and the disease may be relieved in one nerve only to appear in the other. In the severer forms the patient is bedridden, and such cases prove among the most distressing and trying which the physician is called upon to treat.

Diagnosis.—In the diagnosis it is important, in the first place, to determine whether the disease is primary, or secondary to some affection elsewhere. The diagnosis should determine the cause; lesions of the lower spine and sacro-iliac joints should be searched for especially. A careful rectal examination should be made, and, in women, pelvic tumor should be excluded. "Lumbago" may be confounded with it. Affections of the hip-joint are easily distinguished by the absence of tenderness in the course of the nerve and the sense of pain on movement of the hip-joint or on pressure in the region of the trochanter. Pressure on the nerve trunks of the cauda equina, as a rule, causes bilateral pain and disturbances of sensation, and, as double sciatica is rare, these always suggest lesion of the nerve roots. Between the severe lightning pains of tabes and sciatica the differences are usually well defined. It is not to be forgotten that in a certain number of cases the condition is a fibrositis. There is no tenderness along the course of the sciatic nerve, but there is pain in the gluteal region, with disability and Lasègue's sign, i. e., inability to extend the leg completely when the thigh is flexed on the abdomen.

Treatment.—If the cause can be determined, treatment should be directed to correcting this as soon as possible. So many are due to bone conditions which themselves are secondary to disease elsewhere (such as foci of infection) that a very complete study is necessary. The removal of an infected tooth may cause a rapid improvement. In cases associated with diabetes or gout the usual treatment for these should be carried out. In all cases certain palliative measures are indicated and may be the only ones available in some cases. The most important is *rest* which should be absolute and in the position which gives the most relief. Fixation of the leg by a splint may be of aid. The patient should not be allowed up for any purpose. The application of heat in some form is helpful. An electric pad, the hot water bag or the cautery may be used. Hot bottles are sometimes of value. Counter-irritation, especially by blisters, sometimes gives relief. Acupuncture is worth a trial in obstinate cases. Injections into the nerve have been frequently used and various solutions have been employed, e. g., sterile water or novocaine. Stretching of the nerve has gone out of fashion. Electricity may give temporary relief but is often disappointing. In some cases time, usually months, seems necessary.

As to drugs, sedatives are usually necessary, the simple ones being preferred, and morphia avoided if possible. The coal-tar products and salicylates in full doses are worth a trial and often give relief when combined with codeine. The use of suppositories is often especially helpful. If there is any suspicion of syphilis, active treatment should be given.

V. HERPES ZOSTER

(*Acute Posterior Ganglionitis*)

Definition.—An acute disease with localization in the cerebral ganglia and in the ganglia of the posterior nerve roots, associated with a vesicular inflammation of the skin of the corresponding cutaneous areas.

Distribution.—Herpes most frequently occurs in the region of the dorsal roots and extends in the form of a half girdle, on which account the names "zona" and "zoster" have been given. The trigeminal region is very often involved, particularly the first branch. Common forms also are the herpes sterno-nuchalis, cervico-subclavicularis and dorso-ulnaris.

Etiology.—A curious association of occurrence with chicken-pox has been noted. It occurs with the acute infections, particularly pneumonia, malaria and cerebro-spinal fever. Epidemics have been described. In some cases, especially those in the lower part of the body, syphilis co-exists. Even in non-syphilitic cases the spinal fluid may show increase in the cells. The globulin is rarely much increased. Herpes zoster may occur with traumatic paraplegia or injury to the ganglia (fracture) or tumors may be responsible.

Pathology.—Bärensprung first showed that there was involvement of the spinal ganglia. The disease is an acute hæmorrhagic inflammation of the ganglia of the posterior nerve roots and of the homologous cranial ganglia (Head and Campbell). It is analogous to acute anterior poliomyelitis. There are inflammatory foci, hæmorrhage in and destruction of certain of the ganglion cells leading to degeneration of the axis-cylinders. In herpes facialis accompanying pneumonia W. T. Howard has shown that similar lesions are demonstrable in the Gasserian ganglion, and Hunt found the same changes in the otic ganglion in herpes auricularis.

Symptoms.—In ordinary zona there is often a slight prodromal period in which the patient feels ill, has moderate fever, and pain in the side, sometimes of such severity as to suggest pleurisy. On the third or fourth day the rash appears. The characteristic group of vesicles has a segmental distribution limited to one side of the body. One or more of the adjoining skin fields is usually affected. With involvement of the cervical, lumbar, or sacral ganglion the zonal or girdle form of the vesicular crop is naturally lost owing to the distortion of the skin fields from the growth of the limbs. The typical zonal form is only seen in involvement of the thoracic ganglia. Groups of vesicles are regularly arranged on the hyperæmic skin, at first filled with a clear or sometimes bloody serum, which later becomes purulent. The crop varies greatly, and the individual vesicles may be superficial, in which case they leave no scar, or they may be deep and in healing leave superficial scars. By far the most serious form is that seen in the upper division of the fifth. The fever may be high and the eruption very profuse with great swelling and much pain. Permanent disfigurement may follow the scarring.

It seems not improbable, as Chauffard suggests, that there may be extension of the disease from the posterior ganglia to the neighboring meninges as there may be pains down the spine, the girdle sensation, exaggerated knee-jerks, the Kernig sign, and lymphocytosis in the cerebro-spinal fluid.

Complications.—Perhaps the most serious of these is that occasionally seen in ophthalmic zoster, when there is intense inflammation of the conjunctiva and cornea with consecutive panophthalmitis and destruction of the eye.

In a few cases the eruption becomes gangrenous. Swelling of the lymph glands has been noted. A bilateral distribution has occurred. A generalized herpes zoster is occasionally seen with a widespread vesicular rash on the face, neck, trunk, and thighs. A facial paralysis may develop during or after ophthalmic or cervical herpes. Swelling of the parotid gland on the same side may occur. In rare cases paralysis of the extremities has occurred. By far the most distressing complication is *post-zonal neuralgia*. After recovery from the herpes, hot burning sensations are not uncommon in the cutaneous distribution. In other instances, particularly in old people, the pain persists and for years may be a terrible affliction resisting all treatment. The victim may commit suicide.

Treatment.—Care should be taken to protect the vesicles; a one per cent. cocaine ointment with lanolin carefully applied on lint gives relief to the pain. In very severe involvement of the ophthalmic division of the fifth nerve the greatest care should be taken to keep the conjunctiva clean. For the severe post-zonal neuralgia, injections into the spinal cord have been tried, and in cases of great severity the posterior nerve roots may be cut.

K. GENERAL AND FUNCTIONAL DISEASES.

I. PARALYSIS AGITANS

(*Parkinson's Disease; Shaking Palsy*)

Definition.—A chronic affection of the nervous system, characterized by disturbance of certain automatic and associated movements, tremors, and rigidity. The globus pallidus mechanism is affected.

Etiology.—By no means uncommon, the disease affects men more than women. It rarely occurs under forty, but instances have been reported in which the disease began about the twentieth year. Direct heredity is rare, but the patients often belong to families in which there are other nervous affections. In some cases it may be caused by senile degeneration and arterio-sclerotic changes. Among exciting causes may be mentioned business worries and anxieties; in some instances the disease has followed directly upon severe mental shock or trauma. Cases have been described after the specific fevers.

Morbid Anatomy.—There are changes in the efferent motor system of the globus pallidus mechanism. In the juvenile type there are atrophy and decrease in number of the large motor cells of the globus pallidus system. These are regarded as a primary atrophy (abiatrophy). In the globus pallidus system the large cells are motor and the small ganglia cells are inhibitory and co-ordinating. If this destructive lesion involves both types of cells in the caudate nucleus and putamen, the Vogt syndrome results, that is double athetosis with spastic contractures and pseudo-bulbar palsy. If the caudate nucleus and lenticular nucleus are the seat of this destructive lesion there results progressive lenticular degeneration—Wilson's disease—that is the paralysis agitans syndrome with rigidity, tremor, clonic and tonic spasms and perhaps choreic and athetoid movements (Gowers' tetanoid chorea).

Symptoms.—The disease begins gradually, usually in one or other hand, and the tremor may be either constant or intermittent. With this may be associated weakness or stiffness. At first these symptoms may be present only after exertion. Although the onset is slow and gradual in nearly all cases, there are instances in which it sets in abruptly after fright or trauma. When well established the disease is very characteristic. The following are the prominent features.

The face—Parkinson's mask.—Even before the tremor begins the expressionless face, slow movement of the lips, the elevated eyebrows, and general facial immobility suggest the disease. When well developed it is the most characteristic—and pathetic—feature.

Tremor.—This may be in the four extremities or confined to hands or feet; the head is not so commonly affected. The tremor is usually marked in the hands, and the thumb and forefinger display the motion made in the act of rolling a pill. At the wrist there are movements of pronation and supination, and, though less marked, of flexion and extension. The upper-arm muscles are rarely involved. In the legs the movement is most evident at the ankle-joint, and less in the toes than in the fingers. Shaking of the head is less frequent, but does occur, and is usually vertical, not rotatory. The rate of oscillation is about five per second. Any emotion exaggerates the movement. The attempt at a voluntary movement may check the tremor (the patient may be able to thread a needle), but it returns with increased intensity. The tremors cease, as a rule, during sleep, but persist when the muscles are not in use. The writing of the patient is tremulous and zigzag. For months or years the chief tremor may be in one arm or one leg.

Weakness.—Loss of power is present in all cases, and may occur before the tremor, but is not very striking, as tested by the dynamometer, until the late stages. The weakness is greatest where the tremor is most developed. The movements are remarkably slow. There is rarely complete loss of power.

Rigidity may early be expressed in a slowness and stiffness in the voluntary movements, which are performed with some effort and difficulty, and all the actions of the patient are deliberate. This rigidity is in all the muscles, and leads ultimately to the characteristic attitude.

Attitude and Gait.—The head is bent forward, the back bowed, and the arms held away from the body, somewhat flexed at the elbow-joints. The fingers are flexed and in the position assumed when the hand is at rest; in the late stages they can not be extended. Occasionally there is overextension of the terminal phalanges. The hand is usually turned toward the ulnar side and the attitude somewhat resembles that of advanced cases of arthritis deformans. In the late stages there are contractures at the elbows, knees, and ankles. The movements of the patient are characterized by great deliberation. He rises from the chair slowly in the stooping attitude, with the head projecting forward. In attempting to walk the steps are short and hurried, and, as Trousseau remarks, he appears to be running after his centre of gravity. This is termed festination or propulsion, in contradistinction to a peculiar gait observed when the patient is pulled backward, when he makes a number of steps and would fall over if not prevented—retropulsion.

The *voice,* as pointed out by Buzzard, is at first shrill and piping, and there is often a hesitancy in beginning a sentence; then the words are uttered with rapidity, as if the patient was in a hurry.

The reflexes are normal in most cases, but in a few they are exaggerated.

Of sensory disturbances Charcot noted alterations in the temperature sense. The patient may complain of subjective sensations of heat, either general or local—which may be present on one side only and associated with an actual increase of the surface temperature. In other instances, patients complain of cold. Localized sweating may be present. The skin, especially of the forehead, may be thickened. The mental condition rarely shows any change.

Variations in the Symptoms.—The tremor may be absent, but the rigidity, weakness, and attitude are sufficient to make the diagnosis. The disease may be hemiplegic in character, involving only one side or even one limb. Usually these are but stages of the disease.

Diagnosis.—In well developed cases the disease is recognized at a glance. The attitude, gait, stiffness, and mask-like expression are points of as much importance as the oscillations, and usually serve to separate the cases from senile and other forms of tremor. Disseminated sclerosis develops earlier, and is characterized by the nystagmus and the scanning speech, and does not present the *attitude* so constant in paralysis agitans. Yet Schultze and Sachs have reported cases in which the signs of multiple sclerosis have been associated with those of paralysis. The hemiplegic form might be confounded with post-hemiplegic tremor, but the history, the mode of onset, and the greatly increased reflexes distinguish the two. The Parkinsonian face is of great importance in the diagnosis of the obscure and anomalous forms.

The disease is incurable. Periods of improvement may occur, but the tendency is for the affection to proceed progressively downward. It is a slow, degenerative process and the cases last for years.

Treatment.—There is no method which can be recommended as satisfactory in any respect. Slowly performed muscular movements, with strong mental concentration, are sometimes useful in controlling the tremor. Arsenic, opium and the extract of the parathyroid gland may be tried and sometimes give relief, but are not curative. Hyoscine seems helpful in some cases. The friends should be told frankly that the disease is incurable, and that nothing can be done except to attend to the physical comforts of the patient.

OTHER FORMS OF TREMOR

Simple Tremor.—This is occasionally found in persons in whom it is impossible to assign any cause. It may be transient or persist for an indefinite time. It is often extremely slight, and is aggravated by all causes which lower the vitality.

Hereditary Tremor.—C. L. Dana has reported remarkable cases of hereditary tremor. It occurred in all the members of one family, and beginning in infancy continued without producing any serious changes.

Senile Tremor.—With advancing age tremulousness during muscular movements is extremely common, but is rarely seen under seventy. It is always a fine tremor, which begins in the hands and often extends to the muscles of the neck, causing slight movement of the head.

Toxic tremor is seen chiefly as an effect of tobacco, alcohol, lead, or mercury; more rarely in arsenical or opium poisoning. In elderly men who smoke much it may be entirely due to tobacco. One of the commonest forms is the alcoholic tremor, which occurs only on movement and has considerable range. Lead tremor is considered under lead poisoning, of which it constitutes a very important symptom.

Hysterical tremor, which usually occurs under circumstances which make the diagnosis easy, will be considered in the section on hysteria.

II. ACUTE CHOREA

(*Sydenham's Chorea; St. Vitus's Dance*)

Definition.—A disease, probably an acute infection, chiefly affecting children, characterized by irregular, involuntary contraction of the muscles, a variable amount of psychical disturbance, and a remarkable liability to acute endocarditis.

Etiology.—Sex.—Of 554 cases analyzed at the Philadelphia Infirmary for Nervous Diseases, 71 per cent. were in females and 29 per cent. in males (Osler). Of 808 Johns Hopkins Hospital cases, 71.2 per cent. were females (Thayer and Thomas).

Age.—The disease is most common between the ages of five and fifteen. Of 522 cases, 380 occurred in this period; 84.5 per cent. in Thayer and Thomas' series. It is rare among the negroes and native races of America. Only 25 of the Johns Hopkins Hospital cases were in negroes.

Rheumatic Fever.—Of the 554 cases, in 15.5 per cent. there was a history of rheumatism in the family. In 88 cases, 15.8 per cent., there was a history of articular swelling, acute or subacute. In 33 cases there were pains, sometimes described as "rheumatic," in various parts, but not associated with joint trouble. Adding these to those with manifest articular trouble, the percentage is raised to nearly 21. It is rather remarkable that in the Baltimore series the percentage with a history of rheumatism was the same—21.6.

In one group of cases the arthritis antedates by some months or years the onset of the chorea, and does not recur before or during the attack. In the other the chorea sets in with or follows immediately upon the acute arthritis. It is difficult to differentiate the cases of irregular pains without definite joint affection. It is probable that many of them are rheumatic, but it is a mistake to regard as such all cases in children in which there are complaints of vague pains in the bones or muscles—so-called growing pains. It should never be forgotten, however, that there may be no acute arthritis with rheumatic fever in a child.

Heart-disease.—Endocarditis is believed by some writers to be the cause of the disease. On this view chorea is the result of an embolic process occurring in the course of a rheumatic endocarditis.

Infectious Diseases.—Scarlet fever with arthritic manifestations may be a direct antecedent. With the exception of rheumatic fever, there is no intimate relationship between chorea and the acute diseases incident to childhood. It may be noted in contrast to this that the so-called canine chorea is a common sequel of distemper. Chorea may follow gonorrhœa, puerperal fever, and other forms of sepsis. The tonsils are frequently diseased.

Syphilis.—There is a small group, with features much like those of chorea, in which congenital syphilis is apparently the cause. The clinical features of chorea may be typical and specific treatment result in rapid improvement.

Anæmia is less often an antecedent than a sequence, and though cases occur in children who are anæmic and in poor health, this is by no means the rule. Chorea may come on during chlorosis.

Pregnancy.—A choreic patient may become pregnant; more frequently the disease occurs during pregnancy; sometimes after delivery. Buist, of Dundee, has tabulated 226 cases: in 6 the chorea preceded and in 105 it occurred during the pregnancy; in 31 in recurrent pregnancies; 45 cases terminated fatally, and in 16 cases the attack developed post partum. The alleged frequency in illegitimate primiparæ is not borne out by his figures. Beginning in the first three months were 108 cases, in the second three months 70 cases, in the last three months 25 cases. The disease is often severe, and maniacal symptoms may occur.

A tendency to the disease is found in certain families. In 80 cases there was a history of attacks of chorea in other members. In one instance both mother and grandmother had been affected. High-strung, excitable, nervous children are especially liable. *Fright* is considered a frequent cause, but in a large majority of the cases no close connection exists between the fright and the onset of the disease. Occasionally the attack sets in at once. Mental worry, trouble, a sudden grief, or a scolding may apparently be the exciting cause. The strain of *education,* particularly in girls during the third hemidecade, appears to be an important factor. Bright, intelligent, active minded girls from ten to fourteen, ambitious to do well at school, often stimulated in their efforts by teachers and parents, form a large contingent of the cases—the so-called *school-made* chorea. *Imitation,* which is mentioned as an exciting cause, is extremely rare, and did not appear to have influenced the onset in a single case in the Infirmary records.

The disease may rapidly follow an injury or a slight surgical operation. Reflex irritation was believed to play an important rôle, particularly the presence of worms or genital irritation, but this is very doubtful. Ocular defects do not occur in greater proportion in choreic than in other children, and a majority of the cases in which operation has been followed by relief have been instances of *tic,* local or general.

Pathology.—Two anatomical changes are found: (1) *Endocarditis,* usually simple (and of the mitral valve), which was present in 62 of 73 fatal cases recorded.* In a few instances the lesion was ulcerative. (2) Foci of softening in the basal ganglia, regarded as embolic by Kirkes, but in the situation and with the appearance of an acute encephalitis. Minute hæmorrhages have been found elsewhere in the brain. Connected with the endocarditis there are on record seven cases of embolism of the central artery of the retina (H. M. Thomas) and cerebral embolism has been found.

The *pathology* is still obscure. That it is an acute infection is suggested by (1) the frequent association with rheumatic fever; (2) the character of the acute febrile cases; (3) the frequency of involvement of the tonsils; (4) the seasonal relations; (5) the presence of endocarditis; (5) the finding of micro-organisms—though the diplococcus of Poynton is not generally accepted as the cause; and (7) the occurrence of a chorea type in the epidemic encephalitis in which the lesions are very similar to and in the same situation, basal ganglia, as in simple chorea. It seems not improbable that it is a form of infective encephalitis with a special localization.

Symptoms.—Three groups of cases may be recognized—the mild, severe, and maniacal chorea.

Mild Chorea.—In this the affection of the muscles is slight, the speech is not seriously disturbed, and the general health not impaired. Premonitory symptoms are shown in restlessness and inability to sit still, a condition well characterized by the term "fidgets." There are emotional disturbances, such as crying spells, or sometimes night terrors. There may be pains in the limbs and headache. Digestive disturbances and anæmia may be present. A change in the temperament is frequently noticed, and a docile, quiet child may become cross and irritable. After these symptoms have persisted for a week or more the characteristic involuntary movements begin, and are often first noticed at the table, when the child spills a tumbler of water or upsets a plate. There may be only awkwardness or slight incoördination of voluntary movements, or constant irregular clonic spasms. The jerky, irregular character of the movements differentiates them from almost every other disorder of motion. In the mild cases only one hand, or the hand and face, are affected, and it may not spread to the other side.

In the second grade, the *severe form,* the movements become general and the patient may be unable to get about or to feed or undress herself, owing to the constant, irregular, clonic contractions of the various muscle groups. The speech is also affected, and for days the child may not be able to talk. Often with the onset of the severer symptoms there is loss of power on one side or in the limb most affected.

* Osler, "Chorea and Choreiform Affections," Philadelphia, 1894.

The third and most extreme form, the so-called maniacal chorea, or *chorea insaniens,* is truly a terrible disease, and may arise out of the ordinary form. These cases are more common in adult women and may develop during pregnancy.

Chorea begins, as a rule, in the hands and arms, then involves the face, and subsequently the legs. The movements may be confined to one side—hemichorea. The attack begins oftenest on the right side, though occasionally it is general from the outset. One arm and the opposite leg may be involved. In nearly one-fourth of the cases speech is affected; this may amount only to an embarrassment or hesitancy, but in other instances it becomes an incoherent jumble. In very severe cases the child will make no attempt to speak. The inability is in articulation rather than in phonation. Paroxysms of panting and of hard expiration may occur, or odd sounds may be produced. As a rule the movements cease during sleep.

Weakness.—A prominent symptom is muscular weakness, usually no more than a condition of paresis. The loss of power is slight, but the weakness may be shown by an enfeebled grip or by a dragging of the leg or limping. In his original account Sydenham refers to the "unsteady movements of one of the legs, which the patient drags." There may be extreme paresis with but few movements—the paralytic chorea of Todd. Occasionally a local paralysis or weakness remains after the attack.

Mutism is an interesting feature; for weeks the child may not speak. It is more common in severe cases, but is not marked by special choreic unrest of the muscles of speech; it is probably a motor weakness. Complete recovery follows.

HEART SYMPTOMS.—*Neurotic.*—As so many of the subjects of chorea are nervous girls, it is not surprising that a common symptom is a rapidly acting heart. Irregularity is not so special a feature in chorea as rapidity. The patients seldom complain of pain about the heart.

Hæmic Murmurs.—With anæmia and debility, not uncommon associates of chorea in the third or fourth week, we find a corresponding cardiac condition. The impulse is diffuse, perhaps wavy in thin children. The carotids throb visibly, and in the recumbent posture there may be pulsation in the cervical veins. On auscultation a systolic murmur is heard at the base, perhaps, too, at the apex, soft and blowing in quality.

Endocarditis.—Acute valvulitis rarely gives evidence of its presence by symptoms. It must be sought, and it is usually associated with murmurs at one or other of the cardiac orifices.

For the guidance of the practitioner these statements may be made:

(*a*) In thin, nervous children a systolic murmur of soft quality is extremely common at the base, with accentuation of the second sound, particularly at the second left costal cartilage, and is probably of no moment.

(*b*) A systolic murmur of maximum intensity at the apex, and heard also along the left sternal margin, is not uncommon in anæmic, enfeebled states, and does not necessarily indicate either endocarditis or insufficiency.

(*c*) A murmur of maximum intensity at the apex, with rough quality, and transmitted to the axilla or angle of the scapula, indicates an organic lesion of the mitral valve, and is usually associated with enlargement of the heart.

(*d*) When in doubt it is much safer to trust to the evidence of eye and hand than to that of the ear. If the apex beat is in the normal position, and the area of dulness not increased vertically or to the right of the sternum, there is probably no serious valvular disease.

The *endocarditis* of chorea is almost invariably of the simple or warty form, and in itself not dangerous; but it leads to those sclerotic changes in the valve which produce incompetency. Of 140 patients examined more than two years after the attack, the heart was normal in only 51; in 17 there was functional disturbance, and 72 presented signs of organic heart-disease. In an analysis of the cases at the Johns Hopkins Hospital, Thayer found evidence of involvement of the heart in 25 per cent. of the out-patients and in more than 50 per cent. of the cases in the wards. Cardiac involvement was more common in the cases with a history of rheumatism, and was much more frequent in the relapses. Pericarditis is an occasional complication.

Sensory Disturbances.—Pain in the affected limbs is not common. Occasionally there is soreness on pressure. There are cases, usually of hemichorea, in which pain in the limbs is a marked symptom. Weir Mitchell has spoken of these as *painful choreas*. Tender points along the lines of emergence of the spinal nerves or along the course of the nerves of the limbs are rare.

Psychical disturbances are common. Irritability of temper, marked wilfulness, and emotional outbreaks may indicate a complete change in the character. There is deficiency in the powers of concentration, the memory is enfeebled, and the aptitude for study is lost. Rarely there is progressive impairment of the intellect with termination in actual dementia. Acute melancholia has been described. Hallucinations of sight and hearing may occur. Patients may behave in an odd and strange manner and do all sorts of meaningless acts. By far the most serious manifestation of this character is the maniacal delirium, occasionally associated with the very severe cases—*chorea insaniens*. Usually the motor disturbance in these cases is aggravated, but it has been overlooked and patients have been sent to an asylum.

The psychical element is apt to be neglected and it is always a good plan to tell the parents that it is not the muscles alone which are affected, but that the general irritability and change of disposition really form part of the disease.

The condition of the reflexes is usually normal, but they may show much variation. Trophic lesions rarely occur unless, as some writers have done, the joint troubles are regarded as arthropathies occurring in the course of a cerebrospinal disease.

Fever, usually slight, was present in all but one of 110 cases (Thayer). Endocarditis may occur with little if any rise in temperature; but, on the other hand, with an acute arthritis, severe endocarditis or pericarditis, and in the maniacal cases the fever may range from 102° to 104°.

Cutaneous Affections.—The pigmentation, which is not uncommon, is due to the arsenic. Herpes zoster occasionally occurs. Erythema nodosum and a purpuric urticaria have been described. There may, indeed, be the more aggravated condition of rheumatic purpura, known as Schönlein's *peliosis rheumatica*. Subcutaneous fibrous nodules may be present.

Duration and Termination.—From eight to ten weeks is the average duration of an attack of moderate severity. Cases described as chronic chorea following an acute attack are usually instances of cerebral sclerosis or Friedreich's ataxia; but occasionally an attack which has come on in the ordinary way persists for months or years, and recovery ultimately takes place. A slight grade, particularly noticeable under excitement, may persist for months in nervous children.

The tendency to recur has been noticed by all writers since Sydenham first made the observation. Of 410 cases analyzed for this purpose, 240 had one attack, 110 had two attacks, 35 three attacks, 10 four attacks, 12 five attacks, and 3 six attacks. The recurrence is apt to be vernal.

Recovery is the rule. The statistics of out-patient departments are not favorable for determining the mortality. A reliable estimate is that of the Collective Investigation Committee of the British Medical Association, in which 9 deaths were reported among 439 cases, about 2 per cent. There were 102 deaths in the U. S. registration area in 1917.

The paralysis rarely persists. Mental dulness may be present for a time, but usually passes away; permanent impairment of the mind is exceptional.

Diagnosis.—In a majority of instances the nature of the trouble is recognized at a glance; but there are several affections which may simulate and be mistaken for it.

(*a*) *Multiple and diffuse cerebral sclerosis.* The cases are often mistaken for ordinary chorea, and have been described as *chorea spastica.* As a rule, the movements are readily distinguishable from those of true chorea, but the simulation is sometimes very close; the onset in infancy, the impaired intelligence, increased reflexes and in some instances rigidity with the chronic course separate them sharply from true chorea.

(*b*) *Friedreich's ataxia.* Cases of this well-characterized disease were formerly classed as chorea. The slow, irregular, incoördinate movements, the scoliosis, the scanning speech, the early talipes, the nystagmus, and the family character of the disease are points which render the diagnosis easy.

(*c*) In rare cases the paralytic form of chorea may be mistaken for *poliomyelitis* or, when both legs are affected, for paraplegia of spinal origin; but this can be the case only when the choreic movements are very slight.

(*d*) *Hysteria* may simulate chorea minor most closely, and unless there are other manifestations it may be impossible to make a diagnosis. Most commonly, however, the movements in the so-called hysterical chorea are rhythmic and differ entirely from those of ordinary chorea.

(*e*) The *mental symptoms* in maniacal chorea may mask the true nature of the disease and patients have been sent to an asylum.

Treatment.—Abnormally bright, active minded children belonging to families with pronounced neurotic taint should be carefully watched from the ages of eight to fifteen and not allowed to overtax their mental powers. So frequently in children of this class does the attack of chorea date from the worry and stress incident to school examinations that the competition for prizes or places should be emphatically forbidden.

The treatment of the attack consists largely in attention to hygienic measures, with which alone, in time, a majority of the cases recover. Parents should be told to scan gently the faults and waywardness of choreic children. The psychical element, strongly developed in so many cases, is best treated by quiet and seclusion. The child should be confined to bed in the recumbent posture, and mental as well as bodily quiet enjoined. In private practice this is often impossible, but with well-to-do patients the disease is always serious enough to demand the assistance of a skilled nurse. Toys and dolls should not be allowed at first, for the child should be kept amused without excitement. The rest allays the hyper-excitability and reduces to a minimum the possibility of damage to the valve segments should endocarditis exist.

The child should be kept apart from other children and, if possible, from other members of the family, and should see only those persons directly concerned with the nursing of the case. In the latter period of the disease daily rubbings may be resorted to with great benefit.

The medical treatment is unsatisfactory; with the exception of arsenic, no remedy seems to have any influence in controlling the progress of the affection. Without any specific action, it certainly does good in many cases, probably by improving the general nutrition. It is conveniently given in the form of Fowler's solution, and the good effects are rarely seen until maximum doses are taken. It may be given as Martin originally advised (1813); he began "with five drops and increased one drop every day, until it might begin to disagree with the stomach or bowels." When the dose of 15 minims is reached, it may be continued for a week, and then again increased, if necessary, every day or two, until physiological effects are manifest. On the occurrence of these the drug should be stopped for three or four days. The practice of resuming the administration with smaller doses is rarely necessary, as tolerance is usually established and we can begin with the dose which the child was taking when the symptoms of saturation occurred. Usually the signs of saturation are trivial but plain, but in very rare instances more serious symptoms develop. A fatal arsenical neuritis followed in the case of a child, aged eight, who took seven drops of Fowler's solution three times a day for ten days, then stopped for a week, and then took seven drops three times a day for fourteen days (Cary Gamble).

Sedatives are useful in the severe attacks. Chloral is the most useful and may be begun in doses of five grains (0.3 gm.), gradually increased if necessary. Sodium bromide in the same dosage may be added. Belladonna has been found useful in some cases. Syphilis, if present, should be actively treated.

Electricity is of doubtful value. The question of gymnastics is an important one. Early in the disease, when the movements are active, they are not advisable; but during convalescence carefully graduated exercises are undoubtedly beneficial. It is not well, however, to send a choreic child to a school gymnasium, as the stimulus of other children and the excitement of the violent play are very prejudicial.

Other points may be mentioned. Food should be simple and some children do best on a milk diet, the amount being rapidly increased. It is important to regulate the bowels and to attend carefully to the digestive functions. For the anæmia so often present preparations of iron are indicated.

In the severe cases with incessant movements, sleeplessness, dry tongue, and delirium, the important indication is to procure rest, for which purpose chloral may be freely given, and, if necessary, morphia. Chloroform inhalations may be necessary to control the intensity of the paroxysms, but the high rate of mortality in this class of cases illustrates how often our best endeavors are fruitless. The wet pack is sometimes very soothing and should be tried.

As these patients are apt to sink rapidly into a low typhoid state with heart weakness, a supporting treatment is required from the outset.

There are cases which drag on from month to month without getting better or worse and resist all modes of treatment. In such cases a combination of suggestion and passive movements, followed by voluntary movements under control, and later simple exercises, may be useful. Change of air and scene is sometimes followed by rapid improvement, and in these cases the treatment by rest and seclusion should always be given a full trial.

Diseased tonsils should be removed and nasal trouble corrected. Glaring ocular defects should be properly corrected by glasses or, if necessary, by operation.

After the child has recovered, the parents should be warned that return is by no means infrequent, and is particularly liable to follow overwork at school or debilitating influences. These relapses are apt to occur in the spring. Sydenham advised purging in order to prevent the recurrence.

III. HABIT SPASMS AND TICS

Habit Spasm (*Habit Chorea*) ; **Convulsive Tic.**—Two groups of cases may be recognized under the designation of habit spasm—one in which there are simply localized spasmodic movements, and the other in which, in addition to this, there are explosive utterances and psychical symptoms, a condition to which French writers have given the name *tic convulsif*.

(*a*) Habit Spasm.—This is found chiefly in childhood, most frequently in girls from seven to fourteen years of age (Mitchell). In its simplest form there is a sudden, quick contraction of certain of the facial muscles, such as rapid winking or drawing of the mouth to one side, or the neck muscles are involved and there are unilateral movements of the head. The head is given a sudden, quick shake, and at the same time the eyes wink. A not infrequent form is the shrugging of one shoulder. The grimace or movement is repeated at irregular intervals, and is much aggravated by emotion. A short inspiratory sniff is not an uncommon symptom. The cases are found most frequently in children who are "out of sorts," or who have been growing rapidly, or who have inherited a tendency to neurotic disorders. Allied to or associated with this are some of the curious tricks of children. A boy was in the habit every few moments of putting the middle finger into the mouth, biting it, and at the same time pressing his nose with the forefinger. Hartley Coleridge is said to have had a somewhat similar trick, only he bit his arm. In all these cases the habits of the child should be examined carefully, the nose and vault of the pharynx thoroughly inspected, and the eyes accurately tested. As a rule the condition is transient, and after persisting for a few months or longer gradually disappears. Occasionally a local spasm persists—twitching of the eyelids, or the facial grimace.

Spasmus nutans, head nodding, is a coördinated tic in young infants usually of a harmless nature; it may be associated with nystagmus.

(*b*) Impulsive Tic (Gilles de la Tourette's Disease.)—This remarkable affection, often mistaken for chorea, more frequently for habit spasm, is really a psychosis allied to hysteria, though in certain of its aspects it has the features of monomania. The disease begins, as a rule, in young children, occurring as early as the sixth year, though it may occur after puberty. There is usually a neurotic family history. The special features are:

(1) Involuntary muscular movements, usually affecting the facial or brachial muscles, but in aggravated cases all the muscles of the body may be involved and the movements may be extremely irregular and violent.

(2) Explosive utterances, which may resemble a bark or an inarticulate cry. A word heard may be mimicked at once and repeated over and over again, usually with the involuntary movements. To this the term *echolalia* has been applied. A much more distressing disturbance in these cases is *coprolalia,* or the use of bad language. A child of eight or ten may shock its mother and friends by constantly using the word *damn* when making the involuntary movements, or by uttering all sorts of obscene words. Occasionally actions are mimicked—*echokinesis.*

(3) Associated with some of these cases are curious mental disturbances; the patient becomes the subject of a form of obsession or a fixed idea. In other cases the fixed idea takes the form of the impulse to touch objects, or it is a fixed idea about words—onomatomania—or the patient may feel compelled to count a number of times before doing certain actions—arithmomania. The disease is readily distinguished from ordinary chorea. The movements have a larger range and are explosive in character. Tourette regards the coprolalia as the most distinctive feature. The prognosis is doubtful, but recovery may follow.

Saltatory Spasm (*Latah; Myriachit; Jumpers*).—Bamberger has described a disease in which when the patient attempted to stand there were strong contractions in the leg muscles, which caused a jumping or springing motion. This occurs only when the patient attempts to stand. The affection has occurred in both men and women, more frequently in the former, and the subjects have usually shown marked neurotic tendencies. In many cases the condition has been transitory; in others it has persisted for years. Remarkable affections similar to this in certain points occur as a sort of epidemic neurosis. One of the most striking of these occurs among the "jumping Frenchmen" of Maine and Canada. As described by Beard and Thornton, the subjects are liable on any sudden emotion to jump violently and utter a loud cry or sound, and will obey any command or imitate any action without regard to its nature. The condition of echolalia is present in a marked degree. The "jumping" prevails in certain families.

A very similar disease prevails in parts of Russia and in Java and Borneo, where it is known by the names of myriachit and latah, the chief feature of which is mimicry by the patient of everything he sees or hears.

Rhythmic Chorea.—This is readily recognized by the rhythmical character of the movements. It may affect the muscles of the abdomen, producing the salaam convulsion, or involve the sterno-mastoid, producing a rhythmical movement of the head, or the psoas, or any group of muscles. In its orderly rhythm it resembles the canine chorea.

IV. INFANTILE CONVULSIONS

Convulsive seizures similar to those of epilepsy are not infrequent in children. The fit may be identical with epilepsy, from which the condition differs in that when the cause is removed there is no tendency for the fits to recur. Occasionally, however, the convulsions continue and pass into true epilepsy.

Etiology.—A convulsion may be due to many causes, all of which lead to an unstable condition of the nerve centres, permitting sudden, excessive, and temporary nervous discharges. The following are the most important:

(1) *Debility*, resulting usually from gastro-intestinal disturbance. Convulsions frequently supervene toward the close of an attack of entero-colitis and recur, sometimes proving fatal. The death-rate in children from eclampsia rises steadily with that of gastro-intestinal disorders (M. J. Lewis).

(2) *Peripheral Irritation.*—Dentition alone is rarely a cause, but is often one of several factors in a feeble, unhealthy infant. The greatest mortality from convulsions is during the first six months, before the teeth have really cut through the gums. Other irritative causes are the overloading of the stomach with indigestible food. It has been suggested that some of these cases are toxic. Worms, to which convulsions are so frequently attributed, probably have little influence. Among other sources possible are phimosis and otitis.

(3) *Rickets.*—Rickets and convulsions are often associated (Jenner). The spasms may be laryngeal, the so-called child-crowing, which, though convulsive in nature, can scarcely be reckoned under eclampsia. The influence of this condition is more apparent in Europe than in the United States, although rickets is a common disease, particularly among the colored people. Spasms, local or general, in rickets are probably associated with the condition of debility and malnutrition and with craniotabes.

(4) *Fever.*—In young children the onset of the infectious diseases is frequently with convulsions, which may take the place of a chill in the adult. It is not known upon what they depend. Scarlet fever, measles, and pneumonia are most often preceded by convulsions.

(5) *Congestion of the Brain.*—That extreme engorgement of the blood-vessels may produce convulsions is shown by their occasional occurrence in severe whooping-cough, but their rarity in this disease really indicates how small a part mechanical congestion plays in the production of fits.

(6) *Severe convulsions* usher in or accompany many of the serious diseases of the nervous system in children. The acute encephalitis of children, which is followed by hemiplegia, usually has severe convulsions at the onset. They less frequently precede a spinal paralysis. They occur with meningitis, tuberculous or simple, and with tumors and other lesions of the brain.

And, lastly, convulsions may occur immediately after birth and persist for weeks or months. In such instances there has probably been meningeal hæmorrhage or serious injury to the cortex.

The relation of convulsions in children to true epilepsy is important. In Gowers' figures of 1,450 cases of epilepsy, the attacks began in 180 during the first three years of life. Of 460 cases of epilepsy in children, in 187 the fits began within the first three years and the greatest number, 74, was in the first year (Osler). In nearly all these instances there was no interruption in the convulsions. J. L. Morse regards as the dangerous forms those in which the convulsions occur over a considerable period or in which there are repeated attacks suggesting *petit mal.*

Symptoms.—The attack may come on suddenly without any warning; more commonly it is preceded by restlessness, twitchings and perhaps grinding of the teeth. The convulsion is rarely so complete in its stages as true epilepsy. The spasm begins usually in the hands, most commonly in the right hand. The eyes are fixed and staring or are rolled up. The body becomes stiff and breathing is suspended for a moment or two by tonic spasm of the respiratory muscles, in consequence of which the face becomes congested. Clonic convulsions follow, the eyes are rolled about, the hands and arms twitch, or are fixed and extended in rhythmical movements, the face is contorted, and the head is retracted. The attack gradually subsides and the child sleeps or passes into a state of stupor. Following indigestion the attack may be single, but in rickets and intestinal disorders it is apt to be repeated. Sometimes the attacks follow each other with great rapidity, so that the child never rouses but dies in a deep coma. If the convulsion has been limited chiefly to one side there may be slight paresis after recovery, or if the convulsions usher in infantile hemiplegia, when the child arouses, one side is completely paralyzed. During the fit the temperature is often raised. Death rarely occurs from the convulsion itself, except in debilitated children or when the attacks recur with great frequency. In the so-called hydrocephaloid state in connection with protracted diarrhœa convulsions may close the scene.

Diagnosis.—Coming on when the subject is in full health, the attack is probably due either to an overloaded stomach, to some peripheral irritation, or occasionally to trauma. Setting in with high fever and vomiting, it may indicate the onset of an exanthem, or occasionally be the primary symptom of encephalitis, or whatever the condition is which causes infantile hemiplegia. When the attack is associated with debility and with rickets the diagnosis is easily made. The carpopedal spasms and pseudo-paralytic rigidity which are often associated with rickets, laryngismus stridulus, and the hydrocephaloid state are usually confined to the hands and arms and are intermittent and usually tonic. The convulsions associated with tumor or those which follow infantile hemiplegia are usually at first Jacksonian in character. After the second year convulsive seizures which come on irregularly without apparent cause and recur while the child is apparently in good health, are likely to prove true epilepsy.

Prognosis.—Convulsions play an important part in infantile mortality. In chronic diarrhœa convulsions are usually of ill omen. Those ushering in fevers are rarely serious, and the same may be said of the fits associated with indigestion and peripheral irritation.

Treatment.—Every source of irritation should be removed. If associated with indigestible food, a prompt emetic should be given, followed by an enema. The teeth should be examined, and if the gum is swollen, hot, and tense, it may be lanced; but never if it looks normal. When seen at first, if the paroxysm is severe, no time should be lost by giving a hot bath, but chloroform should be given at once, and repeated if necessary. A child is so readily put under chloroform and with such a small quantity that this procedure is quite harmless and saves much valuable time. The practice is almost universal of putting the child into a warm bath, and if there is a fever the head may be douched with cold water. The temperature of the bath should not be above 95° or 96°. The very hot bath is not suitable, particularly if the fits are due to indigestion. After the attack an ice-cap may be placed upon the head. If there is much irritability, particularly in rickets and in severe diarrhœa, small doses of opium will be found efficacious. When the convulsions recur after the child comes from under the influence of chloroform it is best to place it rapidly under the influence of opium, which may be given as morphia hypodermically, in doses of gr. 1/25 to 1/30 (0.0026 to 0.0022 gm.) for a child of one year. Other remedies recommended are chloral by enema, in 5 grain (0.3 gm.) doses, and nitrite of amyl. After the attack has passed the bromides are useful, of which 5 to 8 grains (0.3 to 0.5 gm.) may be given in a day to a child a year old. Recurring convulsions, particularly if they come on without special cause, should receive careful treatment with bromides. When associated with rickets the treatment should be directed to improving the general condition.

V. EPILEPSY

Definition.—An affection of the nervous system characterized by attacks of unconsciousness, with or without convulsions. The transient loss of consciousness without convulsive seizures is known as *petit mal;* the loss of consciousness with general convulsive seizures is known as *grand mal.* Localized convulsions, occurring usually without loss of consciousness, are known as epileptiform, or more frequently as Jacksonian or cortical epilepsy.

Etiology.—Idiopathic or essential epilepsy, the form with an unknown or indefinite etiology, appears to depend upon a congenital tendency in the individual. Coarse anatomical changes in the brain are not present, but with the development of technique alterations have been determined in an increasing proportion of cases, particularly a gliosis of the superficial layers of the cortex described by Alzheimer. Apart from this, the common variety, is the large group of *symptomatic* epilepsies due to toxæmias, trauma, growths, chronic infections and arterio-sclerosis.

Age.—In a large proportion of cases the disease begins before puberty. Of 1,450 cases observed by Gowers, in 422 the disease began before the tenth year, and three-fourths of the cases began before the twentieth year. Of 427 cases of epilepsy in children, the age of onset was as follows: First year, 74; second year, 62; third year, 51; fourth year, 24; fifth year, 17; sixth year, 18; seventh year, 19; eighth year, 23; ninth year, 17; tenth year, 27; eleventh year, 17; twelfth year, 18; thirteenth year, 15; fourteenth year, 21; fifteenth year, 34. Arranged in hemidecades the figures are as follows: From the first to the fifth year, 229; from the fifth to the tenth year, 104; from the tenth to the fifteenth year, 95 (Osler). These figures illustrate in a striking manner the early onset in a large proportion of cases. It is well always to be suspicious of "epilepsy" beginning in adult life, for in a majority of such cases the convulsions are due to a local lesion.

Sex.—No special influence appears to be discoverable, certainly not in children. Of 435 cases, 232 were males and 203 were females, showing a slight predominance of the male sex. After puberty unquestionably, if a large number of cases are taken, the males are in excess.

HEREDITY.—Gowers remarks "there are few diseases in the production of which inheritance has a more marked influence." Of 2,523 epileptics, 16 per cent. were due to heredity (Spratling). The study of the American Eugenics Bureau (Bulletin No. IV), analyzing the data of 206 epileptics, shows how potent are inherited factors. Pierce Clark considers that there are more or less definite essential defects in epileptics which account in part for the predisposition. These are "egocentricity, supersensitiveness, an emotional poverty and an inherent lack of adaptability to normal social life." Stress and annoyance, and an intensive regression to day-dreaming, lethargy and somnolence are precipitating factors. "The attack occurs at the final break of a too severe tension."

Chronic alcoholism in the parents is regarded by many as a potent predisposing factor. Echeverria analyzed 572 cases bearing upon this point and divided them into three classes, of which 257 cases could be traced directly to alcohol as a cause; 126 cases in which there were associated conditions, such as syphilis and traumatism; 189 cases in which the alcoholism was probably the result of the epilepsy. Figures equally strong are given by Martin, who in 150 insane epileptics found 83 with a marked history of parental intemperance. Spratling found 15 per cent. with marked alcoholic history in the parents.

Syphilis.—This in the parents is probably less a predisposing than an actual cause of epilepsy, which is the direct outcome of local cerebral manifestations. There is no reason for recognizing a special form of syphilitic epilepsy. On the other hand, convulsive seizures due to acquired syphilitic disease of the brain are very common.

Alcohol.—Severe epileptic convulsions may occur in steady drinkers.

Of exciting causes fright is believed to be important, but probably less so than is usually stated. Trauma is present in a certain number of instances. An important group depends upon a local disease of the brain existing from childhood, as seen in the post-hemiplegic epilepsy. Occasionally cases follow the infectious fevers. Masturbation is stated to be a cause but its influence is probably overrated. A large group of convulsive seizures allied to epilepsy are due to some toxic agent, as in lead poisoning and uræmia.

REFLEX CAUSES.—Eye strain, dentition, and worms, the irritation of a cicatrix, some local affection, such as adherent prepuce, or a foreign body in the ear or the nose, are given as causes. In some of these cases the fits cease after the removal of the cause, so that there can be no question of the association. In others the attacks persist. Genuine cases of reflex epilepsy are rare. A remarkable instance occurred at the Philadelphia Infirmary for Nervous Diseases, in a man with a testis in the inguinal canal, pressure upon which would cause a typical fit. Removal of the organ was followed by cure.

Cardio-vascular "epilepsy" is usually a manifestation of advanced arteriosclerosis, and is associated with slow pulse (see Stokes-Adams Disease). There may be palpitation and uneasy sensations about the heart prior to the attack. The passage of a gall-stone or the removal of pleuritic fluid may induce a fit. Gastric troubles are extremely common in epilepsy, and the eating of indigestible articles seems often to precipitate an attack. And lastly, epileptic seizures may occur in old people without obvious cause.

Symptoms.—(*a*) Grand Mal.—Preceding the fits there is usually a localized sensation, known as an *aura,* in some part of the body. This may be somatic, in which the feeling comes from some particular region in the periphery, as from the finger or hand, or is a sensation felt in the stomach or about the heart. The peripheral sensations preceding the fit are of great value, particularly those in which the aura always occurs in a definite region, as in one finger or toe. It is the equivalent of the signal symptom in a fit from a brain tumor. The varieties of these sensations are numerous. The epigastric sensations are most common. In these the patient complains of an uneasy sensation in the epigastrium or distress in the intestines, or the sensation may not be unlike that of heartburn and may be associated with palpitation. These groups are sometimes known as pneumogastric auræ or warnings.

Of *psychical* auræ one of the most common, as described by Hughlings Jackson, is the vague, dreamy state, a sensation of strangeness or sometimes of terror. The auræ may be associated with special senses; of these the most common are the visual, consisting of flashes of light or sensations of color; less commonly, distinct objects are seen. The auditory auræ consist of noises in the ear, odd sounds, musical tones, or occasionally voices. Olfactory and gustatory auræ, unpleasant tastes and odors, are rare.

Occasionally the fit may be preceded not by an aura, but by certain movements; the patient may turn round rapidly or run with great speed for a few minutes, the so-called epilepsia procursiva. In an Elwyn case the lad stood on his toes and twirled with extraordinary rapidity, so that his features were scarcely recognizable. It is stated that the pulse sometimes stops just before the fit. The studies of Gibson and Good show that no alteration in the pulse occurred up to the point of clonic convulsions, and there was no lowering of the blood pressure suggesting anæmia of the brain. At the onset of the attack the patient may give a loud scream or yell, the so-called epileptic cry. The patient drops as if shot, making no effort to guard the fall. In consequence, epileptics frequently injure themselves, cutting the face or head or burning themselves. In the attack, as described by Hippocrates, "the patient loses his speech and chokes, and foam issues from the mouth, the teeth are fixed, the hands are contracted, the eyes distorted, he becomes insensible, and in some cases the bowels are affected. And these symptoms occur sometimes on the left side, sometimes on the right, and sometimes on both." The fit may be described in three stages:

(1) *Tonic Spasm.*—The head is drawn back or to the right, and the jaws are fixed. The hands are clinched and the legs extended. This tonic contraction affects the muscles of the chest, so that respiration is impeded and the initial pallor of the face changes to a dusky or livid hue. The muscles of the two sides are unequally affected, so that the head and neck are rotated or the spine is twisted. The arms are usually flexed at the elbows, the hand at the wrist, and the fingers are tightly clinched in the palm. This stage lasts only a few seconds, and then the clonic stage begins.

(2) *Clonic Stage.*—The muscular contractions become intermittent; at first tremulous or vibratory, they gradually become more rapid and the limbs are jerked and tossed about violently. The muscles of the face are in constant

clonic spasm, the eyes roll, the eyelids are opened and closed convulsively. The movements of the muscles of the jaw are very forcible and strong, and at this time the tongue is apt to be caught between the teeth and lacerated. The cyanosis, marked at the end of the tonic stage, gradually lessens. A frothy saliva, which may be blood stained, escapes from the mouth. The fæces and urine may be discharged involuntarily. The duration of this stage is variable. It rarely lasts more than one or two minutes. The contractions become less violent and the patient passes into the condition of coma.

(3) *Coma.*—The breathing is noisy or even stertorous, the face congested, but no longer intensely cyanotic. The limbs are relaxed and the unconsciousness is profound. After a variable time the patient can be aroused, but if left alone he sleeps for some hours and then awakes, complaining only of slight headache or mental confusion. If the attack has been severe, petechial hæmorrhages may be scattered over the neck and chest. In the case of a young man in good health in a severe convulsion both subconjunctival spaces were entirely filled with blood, and free blood oozed from them (Walter James). Hæmoptysis is a rare sequel.

(4) *Status Epilepticus.*—This is the climax of the disease, in which attacks occur in rapid succession, and the patient does not recover consciousness. The pulse, respiration, and temperature rise in the attack. It is a serious condition, and often proves fatal.

After the attack the reflexes are sometimes absent; more frequently they are increased and the ankle clonus can usually be obtained. The state of the urine is variable, particularly as regards the solids. The quantity is usually increased after the attack, and albumin is not infrequently present.

(5) *Post-epileptic symptoms* are of great importance. The patient may be in a trance-like condition, in which he performs actions of which subsequently he has no recollection. More serious are the attacks of mania, in which the patient is often dangerous and sometimes homicidal. It is held by some that an outbreak of mania may be substituted for the fit. And, lastly, the mental condition of an epileptic patient is often seriously impaired.

(6) *Paralysis,* which rarely follows the epileptic fit, is usually hemiplegic and transient. Slight disturbances of speech may occur; in some instances, forms of sensory aphasia. Scripture draws attention to an inflexibility of speech of the epileptic which sounds "expressionless or wooden" and can be recognized by a trained ear. The absence of flexibility can be demonstrated by graphic records.

The attacks may occur at night, and a person may be epileptic for years without knowing it. As Trousseau truly remarks, when a person tells us that in the night he has incontinence of urine and awakes in the morning with headache and mental confusion, and complains of difficulty in speech owing to the fact that he has bitten his tongue, if also there are purpuric spots on the skin of the face and neck, the probability is very strong indeed that he is subject to nocturnal epilepsy.

(b) Petit Mal.—Epilepsy without the convulsions consists of transient unconsciousness, which may come on at any time, with or without a feeling of faintness and vertigo. Suddenly, for example, at the dinner table, the subject stops talking and eating, the eyes become fixed, and the face slightly pale. Anything which may have been in the hand is usually dropped. In a moment or two consciousness is regained and the patient resumes conversation as if nothing had happened. In other instances there is slight incoherency or the patient performs some almost automatic action. He may begin to undress himself and on returning to consciousness find that he has partially disrobed. He may rub his beard or face, or may spit about in a careless way. In other attacks the patient may fall without convulsive seizures. A definite aura is rare. Though transient, unconsciousness and giddiness are the most constant manifestations of *petit mal;* there are many other equivalent manifestations, such as sudden jerkings in the limbs, sudden tremor, or a sudden visual sensation. Gowers gave no less than seventeen different manifestations of *petit mal.* Occasionally there are cases in which the patient has a sensation of losing his breath and may even get red in the face.

After the attack the patient may be dazed for a few seconds and perform certain automatic actions, which may seem to be volitional. As mentioned, undressing is a common action, but all sorts of odd actions may be performed, some of which are awkward or even serious. One patient after an attack was in the habit of tearing anything he could lay hands on, particularly books. Violent actions have been committed and assaults made, frequently giving rise to questions which come before the courts. This condition has been termed masked epilepsy, or *epilepsia larvata.* In a majority of the cases of *petit mal* convulsions finally occur, at first slight, but ultimately the *grand mal* becomes well developed, and the attacks may then alternate.

(*c*) Jacksonian Epilepsy.—This is also known as cortical, symptomatic, or partial epilepsy. It is distinguished from the ordinary epilepsy by the important fact that consciousness is retained or is lost late. The attacks are usually the result of irritative lesions in the motor zone, though there are probably also sensory equivalents of this motor form. In a typical attack the spasm begins in a limited muscle group of the face, arm, or leg. The zygomatic muscles, for instance, or the thumb may twitch, or the toes may first be moved. Prior to the twitching the patient may feel a sensation of numbness or tingling in the part affected. The spasm extends and may involve the muscles of one limb only or of the face. The patient is conscious throughout and watches, often with interest, the march of the spasm.

The onset may be slow, and there may be time for the patient to place a pillow on the floor, so as to be as comfortable as possible during the attack. The spasms may be localized for years, but there is a great risk that the partial epilepsy may become general. The condition is due, as a rule, to an irritative lesion in the motor zone. Thus of 107 cases analyzed by Roland, there were 48 of tumor, 21 instances of inflammatory softening, 14 instances of acute and chronic meningitis, and 8 cases of trauma. The remaining instances were due to hæmorrhage or abscess, or were associated with sclerosis cerebri. Two other conditions may cause typical Jacksonian epilepsy—uræmia and general paresis. A considerable number of the cases of Jacksonian epilepsy are found in children following hemiplegia, the so-called post-hemiplegic epilepsy. The convulsions usually begin on the affected side, either in the arm or leg, and the fit may be unilateral and without loss of consciousness. Ultimately they become more severe and general.

Diagnosis.—In *major epilepsy* the suddenness of the attack, the abrupt loss of consciousness, the order of the tonic and clonic spasm, and the relaxation of the sphincters at the height of the attack are distinctive features. The convulsive seizures due to uræmia are epileptic in character and usually readily recognized by the existence of greatly increased tension and the condition of the urine. Practically in young adults hysteria causes the greatest difficulty, and may closely simulate true epilepsy. A careful study and observation of an attack usually make the diagnosis clear.

Recurring epileptic seizures in a person over thirty who has not had previous attacks is always suggestive of organic disease, usually syphilis.

Petit mal must be distinguished from attacks of syncope, and the vertigo of Ménière's disease, of a cardiac lesion, and of indigestion. In these cases there is no actual loss of consciousness, which forms a characteristic though not an invariable feature of *petit mal.*

Jacksonian epilepsy has features so distinctive and peculiar that it is at once recognized. It is, however, by no means easy always to determine upon what the spasm depends. Irritation in the motor centres may be due to a great variety of causes, among which tumors and localized meningo-encephalitis are the most frequent; but in uræmia localized epilepsy may occur. The most typical Jacksonian spasms are not infrequent in general paresis.

Prognosis.—This may be given to-day in the words of Hippocrates: "The prognosis in epilepsy is unfavorable when the disease is congenital, and when it endures to manhood, and when it occurs in a grown person without any previous cause. . . . The cure may be attempted in young persons, but not in old." Of cases beginning under ten years few are arrested, whereas of those beginning at puberty the opposite is true (W. A. Turner).

Death during the fit rarely occurs, but it may happen if the patient falls into water or if the fit comes on while he is eating. Occasionally the fits stop spontaneously. This is particularly the case in the epilepsy in children which has followed the convulsions of teething or of the fevers. Frequency of the attacks and marked mental disturbance are unfavorable indications. Hereditary predisposition is apparently of no moment in the prognosis. The outlook is better in males than in females. The post-hemiplegic epilepsy is rarely arrested. Of the cases coming on in adults, those due to syphilis and to local affections of the brain allow a more favorable prognosis.

Treatment.—General.—In the case of children the parents should be made to understand from the outset that epilepsy in the great majority of cases is an incurable affection, so that the disease may interfere as little as possible with the education of the child. The subjects need firm but kind treatment. Indulgence and yielding to caprices and whims are followed by weakening of the moral control, which is so necessary in these cases. The disease does not incapacitate a person for all occupation. It is much better for epileptics to have some definite pursuit. The individual should take up an out-of-door occupation, or have manual training suited to his condition. This is best done in an institution where he is carefully watched and studied. Psychoanalysis, with re-education, over a prolonged period is of value in some patients. There are many instances in which they have been persons of extraordinary mental and bodily vigor, as, for example, Julius Cæsar and Napoleon. One of the most distressing features is the mental impairment which follows in a certain number of cases. If such patients become extremely irritable or show signs of violence they should be placed under supervision in an institution. Marriage should be forbidden to epileptics. During the attack a cork or bit of rubber should be placed between the teeth and the clothes should be loosened. The patient should be in the recumbent posture. As the attack usually passes off with rapidity, no special treatment is necessary, but in cases in which the convulsion is prolonged a few whiffs of chloroform or nitrite of amyl or a hypodermic of a quarter of a grain of morphia may be given.

DIETETIC.—The old authors laid great stress upon regimen in epilepsy. The important point is to give the patient a light diet at fixed hours, and on no account to permit overloading of the stomach. Meat should not be given more than once a day. There are cases in which animal food seems injurious. A strict vegetable diet is sometimes useful. The patient should not go to sleep until the completion of gastric digestion. The bowels should be kept freely open and colon irrigations are useful.

MEDICINAL.—The bromides have been extensively used. They act as a motor depressant and therefore should be used only after a careful study of each patient. Sodium bromide is probably less irritating than the potassium salt and is better borne for a long period. It may be given in milk, in which it is scarcely tasted. In all instances the dilution should be considerable. The dose for an adult should be from half a dram to a dram and a half (2 to 6 gm.) daily. The diet should be salt-free. It is often best to give but a single dose daily, about four to six hours before the attacks are most likely to occur. For instance, in the case of nocturnal epilepsy a dram should be given an hour or two after the evening meal. If the attack occurs early in the morning, the patient should take a full dose when he awakes. When given three times a day it is less disturbing after meals. Each case should be carefully studied to determine how much bromide should be used. The individual susceptibility varies and some patients require more than others. Fortunately, children take the drug well and stand proportionately larger doses than adults. Saturation is indicated by certain unpleasant effects, particularly drowsiness, mental torpor, and gastric and cardiac distress. Loss of palate reflex is one of the earliest indications. A very unpleasant feature is the development of acne, which, however, is no indication of bromism. The tendency to this is much diminished by giving the drug largely diluted in alkaline waters and administering arsenic from time to time. Written directions should be given to the mother or to the friends of the patient, and he should not be held responsible for the administration of the medicine. The addition of belladonna to the bromide is warmly recommended by Black, of Glasgow. Luminal has proved useful in some cases, beginning with doses of gr. i (0.065 gm.) and gradually increased. In very obstinate cases Flechsig uses opium, 5 or 6 grains (0.35 gm.), in three doses daily; then at the end of six weeks opium is stopped and the bromides in large amounts, 75 to 100 grains (4 to 6 gm.) daily, are used for two months.

Among other remedies recommended are chloral, cannabis indica, and nitroglycerin. Nitroglycerin is sometimes advantageous in *petit mal,* but is not of much service in the major form. To be beneficial it must be given in full doses, from 2 to 5 drops of the 1 per cent. solution, and increased until the physiological effects are produced. Calcium lactate in 20 grain (1.3 gm.) doses daily has been recommended. Counter-irritation is rarely advisable. When the aura is very definite and constant in its onset, as from the hand or from the toe, a blister about the part or a ligature tightly applied may stop the oncoming fit. In children, care should be taken that there is no source of peripheral irritation. In boys, an adherent prepuce may occasionally be the cause.

The subjects of a chronic and, in most cases, a hopelessly incurable disease, epileptic patients form no small portion of the unfortunate victims of charlatans and quacks, who prescribe to-day, as in the time of the father of medicine, "purifications and spells and other illiberal practices of like kind."

Surgical.—In Jacksonian epilepsy the propriety of surgical interference is universally granted. It is questionable, however, whether in the epilepsy following hemiplegia, considering the anatomical condition, it is likely to be of any benefit. In idiopathic epilepsy, when the fit starts in a certain region —the thumb, for instance—and the signal symptom is invariable, the centre controlling this part may be removed. Operation in the traumatic epilepsy, in which the fit follows fracture, is much more hopeful.

The operation, *per se,* appears in some cases to have a curative effect. The operations have not been always on the skull, and White collected an interesting series in which various surgical procedures have been resorted to, often with curative effect, such as ligation of the carotid artery, castration, excision of the superior cervical ganglia, incision of the scalp, circumcision, etc.

VI. MIGRAINE

(*Hemicrania; Sick Headache*)

Definition.—A paroxysmal affection characterized by severe headache, usually unilateral, and often associated with disorders of vision.

Etiology.—Heredity plays an important rôle in 90 per cent. of cases according to Möbius. Women and members of neurotic families are most frequently attacked. Many distinguished men have been its victims, and the astronomer Airy gave a classical account of his case. The nature of the disease is unknown, and many views have been entertained:

(*a*) That it is a toxæmia from disorder of the intestinal digestion or from some self-manufactured poison.

(*b*) That it is a vasomotor affection with spasm of the arteries, in favor of which are the facts that in the attack the temporal arteries on the affected side may be felt to be small, the retinal arteries may sometimes be seen in spasm, and sclerosis of the arteries on the same side is found in a certain number of cases of hemicrania. A still more striking confirmation is the temporary paralysis which may be associated with an attack of monoplegic or hemiplegic character. Mitchell Clarke has reported a history of recurring motor paralysis in eleven members in three generations of the same family. The characteristic visual phenomena preceded the unilateral headache, especially the hemiopia. In most of the attacks the hemiplegia was on the right side. It lasted from a few hours to a day and disappeared completely, leaving no damage. It is difficult to explain such cases except on the view of a transient spasm of the arteries.

(*c*) Others regard the affection as of reflex origin arising from a refractiv error in the eyes, or from troubles in the nose or sexual organs.

(*d*) The disease has been attributed to transient plugging of the foramen of Monro with increased pressure in the ventricles (Spitzner).

The majority of cases begin in young adults, but Sinclair refers to a case in a child of two years. Many circumstances bring on the attack: a powerful emotion of any sort, mental or bodily fatigue, digestive disturbances, or the eating of some particular article of food. The paroxysmal character is one of the most striking features of the attacks which may occur on the same day every week, every fortnight, or every month. Headaches of the migraine type may occur for years in connection with chronic nephritis, and it is well to remember that attacks may occur in connection with tumors and other lesions of the base of the brain.

Symptoms.—Premonitory signs are present in many cases, and the patient can tell when an attack is coming on. Remarkable prodromata have been described, particularly in connection with vision. Apparitions may appear—visions of animals, such as mice, dogs, etc. Transient hemianopia or scotoma may be present. In other instances there is spasmodic action of the pupil on the affected side, which dilates and contracts alternately, the condition known as *hippus*. Frequently the disturbance of vision is only a blurring, or there are balls of light, or zigzag lines, or the so-called fortification spectra (teichopsia), which may be illuminated with gorgeous colors. Disturbances of the other senses are rare. Numbness of the tongue and face and occasionally of the hand may occur with tingling. More rarely there are cramps or spasms in the muscles of the affected side. Transient aphasia may occur and be intermittent. The *paralysis* may be (1) of cerebral origin—hemiplegia or aphasia, or (2) due to lesions of cranial nerves—optic nerve and ophthalmoplegias; the oculomotor most often, abducens rarely, trochlearis very rarely. The supposed involvement of the facial is relapsing facial palsy in migraine (Ramsay Hunt). Some patients show marked psychical disturbance, either excitement or, more commonly, mental confusion or great depression. Dizziness occurs in some cases. The headache follows a short time after the prodromal symptoms have appeared. It is cumulative and expansile in character, beginning as a localized small spot, which is generally constant either on the temple or forehead or in the eyeball. It is usually described as of a penetrating, sharp, boring character. The pain gradually spreads and involves the entire side of the head, sometimes the neck, and may pass into the arm. In some cases both sides are affected. Nausea and vomiting are common and if the attack comes on when the stomach is full vomiting usually gives relief. Vasomotor symptoms may be present. The face may be pale, and there may be a marked difference between the two sides. Subsequently the face and ear on the affected side may become a burning red from the vasodilator influences. The pulse may be slow. The temporal artery on the affected side may be firm and hard, and in a condition of arterio-sclerosis—a fact confirmed anatomically by Thoma. Few affections are more prostrating and during the paroxysm the patient may scarcely be able to raise the head from the pillow. The slightest noise or light aggravates the condition.

The duration of the attack is variable. The severer forms usually incapacitate the patient for at least three days. In other instances the entire ttack is over in a day. The disease recurs for years, and in cases with a marked hereditary tendency may persist throughout life. In women the attacks often cease after the climacteric, and in men after the age of fifty.

Treatment.—The patient is usually aware of the causes which precipitate an attack. Avoidance of excitement, regularity in the meals, and moderation in diet are important rules. Some patients are benefited by a strict vegetable diet. The treatment should be directed toward the removal of the conditions upon which the attacks depend. In children much may be done by watchfulness and care on the part of the mother in regulating the bowels and watching the diet. Errors of refraction should be adjusted. On no account should such children be allowed to compete in school for prizes. A prolonged course of bromides sometimes proves successful. If anæmia is present, iron and arsenic should be given. When the arterial tension is increased a course of nitroglycerin may be tried. Not too much, however, should be expected from preventive treatment as in a large proportion of cases the headaches recur in spite of all we (including the refractionists) can do. Lavage of the stomach with water at 105°, a brisk saline cathartic and irrigation of the colon with hot saline solution are sometimes of value at the onset. Alkaline water should be taken freely by mouth. During the paroxysm the patient should be kept in bed and absolutely quiet. If the patient feels faint and nauseated a small cup of strong coffee may give relief. A prolonged course of cannabis indica may be tried. Antipyrin, antifebrin, and phenacetin have been much used. When given early, at the very outset of the paroxysm, they are sometimes effective. Small, repeated doses are more satisfactory. Of other remedies, caffein, in 5-grain doses of the citrate, nux vomica, and ergot have been recommended. Electricity does not appear to be of much service.

Ophthalmoplegic Migraine.—This term was applied by Charcot to a special form in which there is weakenss or paralysis of one or more eye muscles, with or after a migraine attack. The oculo-motor nerve is usually involved. Ptosis, loss of certain movements, and double vision are the common features, which may persist for some days. Local causes, especially syphilis, should be excluded before the diagnosis is established. The treatment is the same as for migraine.

VII. NEURALGIA

Definition.—A painful affection of the nerves, due to functional disturbance of their central or peripheral extremities or to neuritis in their course.

Etiology.—Members of neuropathic families are most subject to the disease. It affects women more than men. Children are rarely attacked. Of all causes debility is the most frequent. It is often the first indication of an enfeebled nervous system. The various forms of anæmia are frequently associated with neuralgia. It may be a prominent feature at the onset of certain acute diseases, particularly typhoid fever. It has not been shown that neuralgia is more frequent in malarial districts, but it occasionally occurs in malarial cachexia. Exposure to cold is a cause in very susceptible persons. Reflex irritation, particularly from carious teeth, and disease of the antrum and frontal sinuses are common causes of neuralgia of the fifth nerve. The disease occurs sometimes in gout, lead poisoning, and diabetes. Persistent neuralgia may be a feature of latent nephritis.

Symptoms.—Before the onset of the pain there may be uneasy sensations, sometimes tingling in the part which will be affected. The pain is localized to a certain group or division of nerves, usually affecting one side. The pain is not constant, but paroxysmal, and is described as stabbing, burning, or darting in character. The skin may be exquisitely tender in the affected region, particularly over certain points along the course of the nerve, the so-called tender points. Movements, as a rule, are painful. Trophic and vaso-motor changes may accompany the paroxysm; the skin may be cool, and subsequently hot and burning; occasionally local œdema or erythema occurs. More remarkable still are the changes in the hair, which may become blanched (canities), or even fall out. Fortunately, such alterations are rare. Twitchings of the muscles, or even spasms, may be present during the paroxysm. After lasting a variable time—from a few minutes to many hours—the attack subsides. Recurrence may be at definite intervals—every day at the same hour, or at intervals of two, three, or even seven days. Occasionally the paroxysms develop only at the catamenia. This periodicity is quite as marked in non-malarial as in malarial regions.

CLINICAL VARIETIES, DEPENDING ON THE NERVE ROOTS AFFECTED

Trigeminal Neuralgia; Tic Douloureux.—A distinction must be drawn between the minor and major neuralgias of the fifth cranial nerve. The former may merely be symptomatic of the involvement of one or another of its peripheral branches in some disease process—the pressure of a tumor, carious teeth, or a neuritis due to the proximity of suppurative processes in the bony sinuses, etc. There may be referred neuralgic pains in this area from morbid processes within the cranium, or from visceral disease elsewhere. A painful neuralgia may follow an attack of zoster in any division of the fifth nerve.

The *major* trigeminal neuralgia is a primary affection of the Gasserian ganglion. The designation *tic* is not descriptive; there is usually immobility. The sex incidence is about equal; the majority of cases begin between the ages of forty and sixty. No definite etiological factor is evident. The right side is involved in about two-thirds of the cases. Patrick's figures show that the second and the third branches are involved more often than the first. It begins most often in the second branch and later two or all three branches may be involved. The *pain* is of sudden onset, usually excruciating and in paroxysms, which may recur, usually not lasting longer than two minutes. The attacks are excited by any external irritation which may be very slight, such as a draught of air, touching the skin, and the movements in speaking, eating or swallowing. The areas over which irritation excites the pain are termed doloro-genetic or "trigger" zones. These do not always correspond to the pain zone. The pain may radiate into the cervical nerves or down the arms. The attacks tend to be of increasing severity and in advanced cases the paroxysms may recur at short intervals in steady succession.

The *diagnosis* is rarely in doubt but minor forms should not be mistaken for the major. The pain is paroxysmal, so that a steady pain about the face is probably not trifacial neuralgia. If the area has been rubbed or massaged, or the patient touches it to show where the pain is, the disease is probably not the major form. The disease may be remittent but tends to progress and increase in severity so that the patient's life is almost insufferable.

Cervico-occipital neuralgia involves the posterior branches of the first four cervical nerves, particularly the inferior occipital, at the emergence of which there is a painful point about half-way between the mastoid process and the first cervical vertebra. It may be caused by cold, or be due to cervical caries. Surgical measures may be required if the pain is severe.

Cervico-brachial neuralgia involves the sensory nerves of the brachial plexus, particularly in the cubital division. When the circumflex nerve is involved the pain is in the deltoid. The pain is most commonly about the shoulder and down the course of the ulnar nerve. There is usually a marked tender point upon this nerve at the elbow. This form rarely follows cold, but more frequently results from arthritis and trauma.

Neuralgia of the phrenic nerve is rare. It is sometimes found in pleurisy and in pericarditis. The pain is chiefly at the lower part of the thorax on a line with the insertion of the diaphragm, and here may be painful points on deep pressure. Full inspiration is painful, and there is great sensitiveness on coughing or any movement by which the diaphragm is suddenly depressed.

Intercostal Neuralgia.—This is most frequent in women and common in hysteria. Post-zoster neuralgias are common in this situation. The possibility of spinal disease, of tumor, spondylitis, caries, or aneurism must be borne in mind.

Lumbar Neuralgia.—The posterior fibres of the lumbar plexus, particularly the ilio-scrotal branch, are affected. The pain is in the region of the iliac crest, along the inguinal canal, in the spermatic cord, and in the scrotum or labium majus. The affection known as irritable testis, probably a neuralgia of this nerve, may be severe and accompanied by syncopal sensations.

Coccydynia.—This is regarded as a neuralgia of the coccygeal plexus. It is most common in women, and is aggravated by the sitting posture. It is very intractable, and may necessitate the removal of the coccyx, an operation, however, which is not always successful.

Neuralgias of the Nerves of the Feet.—Many of these cases accompany varying degrees of flat-foot. The condition is brought about by weakness or fatigue of the muscles supporting the arches of the foot, which consequently settle until the strain of the superimposed body-weight falls upon the ligamentous and aponeurotic attachments between the metatarsal and tarsal bones. Rest, massage, exercises, and orthopædic measures are indicated.

PAINFUL HEEL.—Both in women and men there may be about the heel severe pains which interfere seriously with walking—the pododynia of S. D. Gross. There may be little or no swelling, no discoloration, and no arthritis. Some cases follow a gonococcus infection and are due to a bony spur.

PLANTAR NEURALGIA.—This is often associated with a definite neuritis, such as follows typhoid fever, and has been seen in an aggravated form in caisson disease (Hughes). The pain may be limited to the tips of the toes or to the ball of the great toe. Numbness, tingling, and hyperæsthesia or sweating may occur with it. In typhoid fever it is not uncommon for patients to complain of great sensitiveness in the toes.

METATARSALGIA.—Thomas G. Morton's "painful affection of the fourth metatarso-phalangeal articulation" is a peculiar and very trying disorder, seen most frequently in women, and usually in one foot. Morton regards it as due to a pinching of the metatarsal nerve. The condition usually requires operation. The red, painful neuralgia—erythromelalgia—is described under the vaso-motor and trophic disturbances.

Causalgia (*Thermalgia*).—A form of neuralgia following gunshot wounds, most frequently of the median and of the sciatic branches, characterized by burning pains of the greatest intensity, glossy skin, vaso-motor disturbances, and at last a condition of general hyperæsthesia and nervousness that makes life unbearable. Nothing has been added to Weir Mitchell's classical description (1864), and later he gave the above name from the Greek words for burning and pain. Many cases have been seen in the late war, and Stopford has suggested the name thermalgia. An explanation of causalgia is difficult. The median and post-tibial nerves have a large number of vaso-motor fibres, interference with which may cause the peculiar character of the pain; indeed, it has been suggested that the pain is caused by irritation of the peri-arterial sympathetic fibres and not by the wound of the nerve itself. Anatomically partial division and intra-neural fibrosis are present, but these are found in scores of cases in which causalgia is not present.

Visceral Neuralgias.—The more important of these have been noted in connection with the cardiac and the gastric neuroses. They are most frequent in women, often with neurasthenia and hysteria. The pains are common in the pelvic region, particularly about the ovaries. Nephralgia is of great interest, as the symptoms may closely simulate those of stone.

TREATMENT OF NEURALGIA

Causes of reflex irritation should be carefully removed. The neuralgia, as a rule, recurs unless the general health improves; so that tonic and hygienic measures of all sorts should be employed. Often a change of air or surroundings will relieve a severe neuralgia. Obstinate cases may be cured by a prolonged residence in the mountains, with an out-of-door life and plenty of exercise. A strict vegetable diet will sometimes relieve the neuralgia or headache of a gouty person. Of general remedies, iron is often a specific in the cases associated with chlorosis and anæmia. Arsenic, too, is very beneficial in these forms, and should be given in ascending doses. The value of quinine has been much overrated. It probably has no more influence than any other bitter tonic, except in the rare instances in which the neuralgia is definitely associated with malaria. Strychnine, cod-liver oil, and phosphorus are advantageous. Of remedies for the pain, antipyrin, antifebrin, phenacetin and acetyl-salicylic acid should first be tried, for they are sometimes of service. Morphia should be given with great caution, and only after other remedies have been tried in vain. On no consideration should the patient be allowed to use the hypodermic syringe. Gelsemium is highly recommended. Of nerve stimulants, valerian and ether, which often act well together, may be given. In the minor form of trigeminal neuralgia nitroglycerin in large doses may be tried. Dana has seen good results follow rest with large doses of strychnia given hypodermically. Aconitin in doses of one two-hundredth of a grain (0.00032 gm.) may be tried. Diathermy may be useful.

Of local applications, the thermo-cautery is invaluable, particularly in zona and the more chronic forms of neuralgia. Acupuncture may be used. Chloroform liniment, camphor and chloral, menthol, the oleates of morphia, atropia, and belladonna used with lanolin may be tried. Freezing over the tender point with ether spray is sometimes successful. The continuous current may be used. The sponges should be warm, and the positive pole should be placed near the seat of the pain. The strength of the current should be such as to cause a slight tingling or burning, but not pain.

For trigeminal neuralgia there are two successful measures, (1) injection of alcohol into the branch, the trunk or the ganglion itself, often satisfactory in skilled hands; and (2) removal of the ganglion. Cushing's results show the remarkable benefit which may result.

VIII. PROFESSIONAL SPASMS; OCCUPATION NEUROSES

The continuous and excessive use of the muscles in performing a certain movement may be followed by an irregular, involuntary spasm or cramp, which may completely check the performance of the action. The condition is found most frequently in writers, hence the term writer's cramp or scrivener's palsy; but it is also common in piano and violin players and in telegraph operators. The spasms occur in many other persons, such as milkmaids, weavers, and cigarette-rollers.

The most common form is *writer's cramp,* which is much more frequent in men than in women. Of 75 cases of impaired writing power reported by Poore, all of the instances of undoubted writer's cramp were in men. An investigation by Thompson and Sinclair into telegraphist cramp in England shows that the disease is rare, only 13 cases among between 7,000 and 8,000 employees. Persons of a nervous temperament are more liable to the disease. Occasionally it follows slight injury. In a majority of the cases a faulty method of writing has been employed, using either the little finger or the wrist as the fixed point. Persons who write with the middle of the forearm or the elbow as the fixed point are rarely affected.

No anatomical changes have been found. The most reasonable explanation of the disease is that it results from a deranged action of the nerve centres presiding over the muscular movements involved in the act of writing, a condition which has been termed irritable weakness.

Symptoms.—These may be described under five heads (Lewis).

(*a*) Cramp or Spasm.—This is often an early symptom and most commonly affects the forefinger and thumb; or there may be a combined movement of flexion and adduction of the thumb, so that the pen may be twisted from the grasp and thrown to some distance. Weir Mitchell described a lock-spasm, in which the fingers become so firmly contracted upon the pen that it can not be removed.

(*b*) Paresis and Paralysis.—This may occur with the spasm or alone. The patient feels a sense of weakness and debility in the muscles of the hand and arm and holds the pen feebly. Yet the grasp of the hand may be strong and there may be no paralysis for ordinary acts.

(*c*) Tremor.—This is most commonly seen in the forefinger and may be a premonitory symptom of atrophy. It is not an important symptom, and is rarely sufficient to produce disability.

(*d*) Pain.—Abnormal sensations, particularly a tired feeling in the muscles, are very constantly present. Actual pain is rare, but there may be irregular shooting pains in the arm. Numbness or soreness may exist. If, as sometimes happens, a subacute neuritis develops, there may be pain over the nerves and numbness or tingling in the fingers.

(*e*) Vaso-motor Disturbances.—These may occur in severe cases. There may be hyperæsthesia. Occasionally the skin becomes glossy, or there is a condition of local asphyxia resembling chilblains. In attempting to write, the hand and arm may become flushed and the veins increased in size. Early the electrical reactions are normal, but in advanced cases there may be diminution of faradic and sometimes increase in the galvanic irritability.

Diagnosis.—A well marked case of writer's cramp or palsy could scarcely be mistaken for any other affection. Care must be taken to exclude the existence of any cerebro-spinal disease, such as progressive muscular atrophy or hemiplegia, or local affection, such as cervical rib. The physician is sometimes consulted by nervous persons who fancy they are becoming subject to the disease and complain of stiffness or weakness without displaying any characteristic features.

Prognosis.—The course of the disease is usually chronic. If taken in time and if the hand is allowed perfect rest, the condition may improve rapidly, but too often there is a strong tendency to recurrence. The patient may learn to write with the left hand, but this also may after a time be attacked.

Treatment.—Various prophylactic measures have been advised. It is important that a proper method of writing be adopted. Gowers suggested that if all persons wrote from the shoulder writer's cramp would practically not occur. Various devices have been invented for relieving the fatigue, but none of them are very satisfactory. The use of the type-writer has diminished the frequency of scrivener's palsy. Rest is essential and no measures are of value without it. Massage and manipulation, when combined with systematic gymnastics, give the best results. The patient should systematically practise the opposite movements to those concerned in the cramp. This muscle training often gives good results. Poore recommends the galvanic current applied to the muscles, which are at the same time rhythmically exercised. In very obstinate cases the condition remains incurable.

IX. HYSTERIA

Definition.—A disorder of personality manifested by a heightened and perverted suggestibility, a change in character, together with certain mental and bodily states induced by suggestion—auto or hetero—and cured by persuasion.

Etiology.—Persons with mobile emotional dispositions, especially women, are the chief subjects. In periods of great stress, as in the recent war, it becomes a widespread and serious disorder. A community disease, often spreading widely in institutions, such as schools and convents, it may behave like an epidemic, as in the dancing mania. The essential element under the above definition is the first—*heightened suggestibility.*—(*a*) With the chameleon we take the color of our surroundings. The company, physical conditions, the weather, etc., send our spirits up and down like the mercury in a barometer. Suggestion, deliberate by speech, unconscious through imitation, is the most important part of education, and to free the mind as far as possible from the mastery of these external influences has been the goal from the days of the Greeks. Love, hate and fear, the three powerful emotions, control us individually or sway us in herds as the cattle on the plains. The dominant influence of suggestion is everywhere in the story of human progress; just as it is in the black chapters of superstition, folly, and crime. Unconscious imitation, or an imitation against which the individual is powerless to fight, has been the important factor in outbreaks of hysteria as the dancing mania, the epidemic chorea, and such tragedies as led to the persecutions for witchcraft.

(*b*) Right judgments are indispensable conditions to right action in mind or muscle and it is in this Stoic doctrine of the control of the will—the will to do and the will to avoid—that we find the key to many of the problems of hysteria. It may be a knee "locked" for months. An injury or pain induces the fixed belief that the joint can not be moved, loss of muscle judgment—there have been scores of such war cases—but ten minutes at Seale-Hayne or a trip to Lourdes and the joint is flexible. After the shock of an explosion a man is blind (without a lesion), the condition persists—the visual judgment has been lost—to be restored months afterwards at a temple of Æsculapius or by some modern Galen. An emotional girl takes an aversion to her mistress. The moral judgment is lost and she begins to play pranks, sometimes harmless, but often serious as entailing great inconvenience and loss, as in the recent Norfolk case in which the walls of a house were so covered with paraffin, sandal oil and water that it had to abandoned. Or craving sympathy, she will inflict all sorts of injuries, even wound herself to such an extent as to necessitate amputation of a limb. Loss of right judgment then in muscle action, sense action, and conduct are essential factors. As the impulse—suggestion—is spontaneous we speak of it as auto-suggestion—and in direct proportion to the feebleness of control by the will is the readiness with which muscles, sense and mind yield to impulses not prompted by right judgment.

Charcot and his followers regarded hysteria as a psychosis, in which morbid states are induced by ideas. The capability of responding to suggestion is the test of its existence. It is a disturbance in the sphere of personality, in which the emotions have an exaggerated influence on the sensory, motor and secretory functions. Babinski holds that hysteria is a mental condition with certain primary phenomena and certain secondary accidental symptoms. The essence of the primary features is that they may be produced by suggestion, and may be made to disappear by persuasion (pithiatism). The primary symptoms include hemi-anæsthesia, paralysis, contractures, etc.; secondary features, as muscular atrophy, are directly dependent upon the primary and cannot themselves be induced by suggestion.

In the Breuer-Freud theory we return to the days of Aretæus, who originated (?) the views of sexual hysteria and believed the womb, "like an animal within an animal" and altogether erratic, caused all sorts of trouble in its wanderings. Freud's view is thus analyzed by Jelliffe in his article in our "System of Medicine" (2nd Ed., Vol. V.). "There develop usually on a constitutional basis, in the period before puberty, definite sexual activities which are mostly of a perverse nature. These activities do not, as a rule, lead to a definite neurosis up to the time of puberty, which in the psychic sphere appears much earlier than in the body, but sexual phantasy maintains a perverse constellated direction by reason of the infantile sexual activities. On constitutional (affect) grounds the increased fantasy of the hysteric leads to the formation of complexes which are not taken up by the personality and by reason of shame or disgust remain buried. There, therefore, results a conflict between the characteristic normal libido and the sexual repressions of these buried infantile perversions. These conflicts give rise to the hysterical symptoms. It is in his contributions to the sexual theory that Freud develops his later thoughts of the sexual origin of the hysterical reaction. By sexual it is important to remember that Freud is not speaking of sensual.

"The significance of Freud's theory is the tracing of every case to sexual traumata during early childhood. Sexual experiences differ, however, from ordinary experiences—the latter have a tendency to fade out, while the idea of the former grows with increasing sexual maturity. There results a disproportionate capacity for increased reaction which takes place in the subconscious. This is the cause of the mischief.

"There must be, however, a connecting link between the infantile sexual traumata and the later manifestations. This connection Freud finds in the so-called 'hysterical fancies.' These are the day-dreams of erotic coloring, wish-gratifications, originating in privation and longing. These fancies hark back to the original traumatic moment, and, either originating in the subconscious or shortly becoming conscious, are transformed into hysterical symptoms. They constitute a defence of the ego against the revival, as reminiscences, of the repressed traumatic experiences of childhood" (White).

The affection is most common in women, and usually appears first about the time of puberty, but the manifestations may continue until the menopause, or even until old age. Men are by no means exempt, and hysteria in the male is not rare. It occurs in all races, but is much more prevalent, particularly in its severer forms, in members of the Latin race. In England and the United States the milder grades are common, but the graver forms are rare in comparison with the frequency with which they are seen in France.

Children under twelve years of age are not very often affected, but the disease may be well marked as early as the fifth or sixth year. One of the saddest chapters in the history of human deception, that of the Salem witches, might be headed *hysteria in children,* since the tragedy resulted directly from the hysterical pranks of girls under twelve years of age.

Of predisposing causes, two are important—*heredity* and *education.* The former acts by endowing the child with a mobile, abnormally sensitive nervous organization. We see cases most frequently in families with marked neuropathic tendencies, the members of which have suffered from neuroses of various sorts. Education at home too often fails to inculcate habits of self-control. A child grows to girlhood with an entirely erroneous idea of her relations to others, and accustomed to have every whim gratified and abundant sympathy lavished on every woe, however trifling; she reaches womanhood with a moral organization unfitted to withstand the cares and worries of every-day life. At school, between the ages of twelve and fifteen, when the vital energies are absorbed in the rapid development of the body, she is often cooped in close school rooms for six or eight hours daily. The result too frequently is an active, bright mind in an enfeebled body, ill adapted to subserve the functions for which it was framed, easily disordered, and prone to react abnormally to the ordinary stimuli of life. Among the more direct influences are emotions of various kinds, fright occasionally, more frequently love affairs, grief, and domestic worries. Physical causes less often bring on hysterical outbreaks, but they may follow an injury or develop during the convalescence from an acute illness or be associated with disease of the generative organs.

"Chorea Major": "Pandemic Chorea."—The common name, St. Vitus's dance, applied to chorea has come to us from the middle ages, when under the influence of religious fervor there were epidemics characterized by great excitement, gesticulations, and dancing. For the relief of these symptoms, when excessive, pilgrimages were made, and, in the Rhenish provinces, particularly to the Chapel of St. Vitus in Zebern. Epidemics of this sort occurred also during the nineteenth century, and descriptions of them among the early settlers in Kentucky have been given by Robertson and Yandell. It was unfortunate that Sydenham applied the term chorea to an affection in children totally distinct from this chorea major, which is in reality an hysterical manifestation under the influence of religious excitement.

Symptoms.—A useful division is into the convulsive and non-convulsive varieties.

CONVULSIVE HYSTERIA.—(*a*) *Minor Forms.*—The attack, commonly following emotional disturbance, sets in suddenly or may be preceded by symptoms, called by the laity "hysterical," such as laughing and crying alternately, or a sensation of constriction in the neck, or of a ball rising in the throat—the *globus hystericus*. Sometimes, preceding the convulsive movements, there may be painful sensations arising from the pelvic, abdominal, or thoracic regions. From the description these sensations resemble auræ. They become more intense with the rising sensation of choking in the neck and difficulty in getting breath, and the patient falls into a more or less violent convulsion. The fall is not sudden, as in epilepsy, but the subject goes down, as a rule, easily, often picking a soft spot, like a sofa or an easy-chair, and in the movements apparently exercises care to do herself no injury. Yet at the same time she appears to be unconscious. The movements are clonic and disorderly, with the head and arms thrown about in an irregular manner. The paroxysm after a few minutes slowly subsides, then the patient becomes emotional, and gradually regains consciousness. When questioned the patient may confess to having some knowledge of the events which have taken place, but, as a rule, has no accurate recollection. During the attack the abdomen may be much distended with flatus, and subsequently a large amount of clear urine may be passed. These attacks vary greatly; there may be scarcely any movements of the limbs, but after a nerve storm the patient sinks into a torpid, semi-unconscious condition, from which she is roused with difficulty. In some cases the patient passes from this state into a condition of catalepsy.

(*b*) *Major Forms; Hystero-epilepsy.*—Typical instances are very rare in the United States and in England. The attack is initiated by certain prodromata, chiefly minor hysterical manifestations, either foolish or unseemly behavior, excitement, sometimes dyspeptic symptoms with tympanites, or frequent micturition. Areas of hyperæsthesia may be marked, the so-called hysterogenic spots so elaborately described by Richet. These are usually symmetrical and situated over the upper dorsal vertebra, and in front in a series of symmetrically placed areas on the chest and abdomen, the most marked being over the ovaries. Painful sensations or a feeling of oppression and a *globus* rising in the throat may be complained of prior to the onset of the convulsion, which, according to French writers, has four distinct stages: (1) Epileptoid condition, which closely simulates a true epileptic attack with tonic spasm (often leading to opisthotonos), grinding of the teeth, congestion of the face, followed by clonic convulsions, gradual relaxation, and coma. (2) Succeeding this is the period which Charcot has termed *clownism,* in which there is an emotional display and a remarkable series of contortions or of cataleptic poses. (3) Then in typical cases there is a stage in which the patient assumes certain attitudes expressive of the various passions—ecstasy, fear, beatitude, or erotism. (4) Finally consciousness returns and the patient enters upon a stage in which she may display very varied symptoms, chiefly manifestations of a delirium with extraordinary hallucinations. Visions are seen, voices heard, and conversations held with imaginary persons. In this stage patients will relate with the utmost solemnity imaginary events, and make extraordinary and serious charges against individuals. This sometimes gives a grave aspect to these seizures, for not only does the patient make and believe the statements, but when recovery is complete the hallucination sometimes persists. After an attack a patient may remain for days in a state of lethargy or trance.

Non-convulsive Forms.—So complex and varied is the picture that the manifestations are best considered according to the systems involved.

(*a*) *Disorders of Motion.*—(1) *Paralysis.*—These may be hemiplegic, paraplegic, or monoplegic. Hysterical diplegia is extremely rare. The paralysis either sets in abruptly or gradually, and may take weeks to attain its full development. *There is no type or form of organic paralysis which may not be simulated in hysteria.* Sensation is either lessened or lost on the affected side. The hysterical paraplegia is more common than hemiplegia. The loss of power is not absolute; the legs can usually be moved, but do not support the patient. The reflexes may be increased, though the knee-jerk is often normal. A spurious ankle clonus may sometimes be present. The feet are usually extended and turned inward in the equino-varus position. The muscles do not waste and the electrical reactions are normal. Other manifestations, such as paralysis of the bladder or aphonia, are usually associated. Hysterical monoplegias may be facial, crural, or brachial. A condition of ataxia sometimes occurs with paresis. Incoördination may be a marked feature, and there are usually sensory manifestations.

The following points are important in deciding between functional and organic hemiplegia. The absence of epigastric and cremasteric reflexes with Babinski's sign suggests organic disease. If the patient folds the arms and attempts to rise from the recumbent to the sitting posture the thigh on the affected side flexes at the hip and the whole extremity will be raised, to fall back later. This does not occur in the functional cases. Another test is made with the patient lying on the back. When asked to raise the unaffected leg, the opposite leg, paralyzed for voluntary effort, is strongly pressed down (Hoover).

(2) *Contractures and Spasms.*—The hysterical contractures may attack almost any group of voluntary muscles and be of the hemiplegic, paraplegic, or monoplegic type. They may come on suddenly or slowly, persist for months or years, and disappear rapidly. The contracture is most commonly seen in the arm, which is flexed at the elbow and wrist, while the fingers tightly grasp the thumb in the palm of the hand; more rarely the terminal phalanges are hyperextended. It may occur in one or in both legs, more commonly in one. The ankle clonus is present; the foot is inverted and the toes are strongly flexed. These cases may be mistaken for lateral sclerosis and the difficulty in diagnosis may really be very great. The spastic gait is typical, and with the exaggerated knee-jerk and ankle clonus the picture may be characteristic. Other forms of contracture may be in the muscles of the hip, shoulder, or neck; more rarely in those of the jaws—hysterical trismus—or in the tongue. Remarkable indeed are the local contractures in the diaphragm and abdominal muscles, producing a phantom tumor, in which just below and in the neighborhood of the umbilicus is a firm, apparently solid growth. According to Gowers, this is produced by relaxation of the recti and a spasmodic contraction of the diaphragm, together with inflation of the intestines with gas and an arching forward of the vertebral column. They are apt to occur in middle-aged women about the menopause, and are frequently associated with symptoms of spurious pregnancy—*pseudo-cyesis.* The resemblance to a tumor may be striking. The only safeguard is to be found in complete anæsthesia, when the tumor entirely disappears. Mitchell reported an instance of a phantom tumor in the left pectoral region just above the breast, which was tender, hard, and dense.

Rhythmic Hysterical Spasm.—The movements may be of the arm, either flexion and extension, or, more rarely, pronation and supination. Clonic contractions of the sterno-cleido-mastoid or of the muscles of the jaws or of the rotatory muscles of the head may produce rhythmic movements of these parts. The spasm may be in one or both psoas muscles, lifting the leg in a rhythmic manner eight or ten times in a minute. In other instances the muscles of the trunk are affected, and every few moments there is a bowing movement—salaam convulsions—or the muscles of the back may contract, causing strong arching of the vertebral column and retraction of the head.

Tremor may be a purely hysterical manifestation, occurring either alone or with paralysis and contracture. It most commonly involves the hands and arms; more rarely the head and legs. The movements are small and quick. In the type described by Rendu the tremor may or may not persist during repose, but it is increased or provoked by volitional movements. Volitional or intention tremor may exist, simulating closely that of insular sclerosis. Many instances of this disease are mistaken for hysteria.

(*b*) *Disorders of Sensation.*—*Anæsthesia* is most common, and usually confined to one half of the body. It may not be noticed by the patient. Usually it is accurately limited by the middle line and involves the mucous surfaces and deeper parts. The conjunctiva, however, is often spared. There may be hemianopsia. This symptom may come on slowly or follow a convulsive attack.

Sometimes the various sensations are dissociated and the anæsthesia may be only to pain and to touch. The skin of the affected side is usually pale and cool, and a pin-prick may not be followed by blood. With the loss of feeling there may be loss of muscular power. Curious trophic changes may be present, such as unilateral swelling of the hemiplegic side.

By metallotherapy, the application of certain metals, the anæsthesia or analgesia can be transferred to the other side of the body. This phenomenon may be caused by the electro-magnet and by wood and various other agents, and is an effect of suggestion.

Hyperæsthesia.—Increased sensitiveness and pains occur in various parts of the body. One of the most frequent complaints is of pain in the head, usually over the sagittal suture, less frequently in the occiput. This is described as agonizing, and is compared to the driving of a nail into the part; hence the name *clavus hystericus.* Neuralgias are common. Hyperæsthetic areas, the hysterogenic points, exist on the skin of the thorax and abdomen, pressure upon which may cause minor manifestations or even a convulsive attack. Increased sensitiveness in the ovarian region is not peculiar to hysteria. Pain in the back is an almost constant complaint. The sensitiveness may be limited to certain spinous processes, or may be diffuse. In hysterical women the pains in the abdomen may simulate those of gastric ulcer, or the condition may be almost identical with that of peritonitis; more rarely the abdominal pains closely resemble those of appendix disease.

Special Senses.—Disturbances of taste and smell are not uncommon and may cause much distress. Of ocular symptoms, retinal hyperæsthesia is common, and the patients prefer to be in a darkened room. Retraction of the field of vision is common and usually follows a convulsive seizure. It may persist for years. The color perception may be normal even with complete anæsthesia. Hysterical deafness may be complete and alternate or come on with hysterical blindness. Hysterical amaurosis may occur in children. One must distinguish between functional loss of power and simulation.

(*c*) *Visceral Manifestations.*—*Respiratory Apparatus.*—Of disturbances in the respiratory rhythm, the most frequent, perhaps, is an exaggeration of the deeper breath, which is taken normally every fifth or sixth inspiration, or there may be a "catching" breathing, such as is seen when cold water is poured over a person. In hysterical *dyspnœa* there is no special distress and the pulse is normal. In what is known as the syndrome of Briquet there are shortness of breath, suppression of the voice, and paralysis of the diaphragm. The anhelation is extreme. In rare instances there is bradypnœa. Among laryngeal manifestations *aphonia* is frequent and may persist for months or even years without other special symptoms. Spasm of the muscles may occur with violent inspiratory efforts and great distress, and even lead to cyanosis. Hiccough, or sounds resembling it, may be present for weeks or months at a time. Among the most remarkable of the respiratory manifestations are the hysterical cries. These may mimic the sounds produced by animals, such as barking, mewing, or grunting, and in France epidemics of them have been observed. Attacks of gaping, yawning, and sneezing may also occur.

The hysterical *cough* is a frequent symptom, particularly in young girls. It may occur in paroxysms, but is often a dry, persistent, croaking cough, extremely monotonous and unpleasant to hear. Sir Andrew Clark has called attention to a loud, barking cough (*cynobex hebetica*) occurring about the time of puberty, chiefly in boys belonging to neurotic families. The attacks, which last about a minute, recur frequently. A form of hysterical *hæmoptysis* may be deceptive and lead to a diagnosis of pulmonary disorder. The sputum is a pale-red fluid, not so bright in color as in ordinary hæmoptysis, and contains particles of food, pavement epithelium, red corpuscles, and micrococci, but no cylindical or ciliated epithelium. It probably comes from the mouth or pharynx.

Digestive System.—Disturbed or depraved appetite, dyspepsia, and gastric pains are common. The patient may have difficulty in swallowing, apparently from spasm of the gullet. There are instances in which the food seems to be expelled before it reaches the stomach. In other cases there is incessant gagging. In the hysterical vomiting the food is regurgitated without much effort and without nausea. This feature may persist for years without great disturbance of nutrition. The most striking and remarkable digestive disturbance in hysteria is the *anorexia nervosa* described by Sir William Gull. "To call it loss of appetite—anorexia—but feebly characterizes the symptom. It is rather an annihilation of appetite, so complete that it seems in some cases impossible ever to eat again. Out of it grows an antagonism to food which results at last and in its worst forms in spasm on the approach of food, and this in turn gives rise to some of those remarkable cases of survival for long periods without food" (Mitchell). There are three special features in anorexia nervosa: *First,* and most important, a psychical state, usually depressant, occasionally excited and restless. It is not always hysterical. *Secondly,* stomach symptoms, loss of appetite, regurgitation, vomiting, and the whole series of phenomena associated with nervous dyspepsia. *Thirdly,* emaciation, which reaches a grade seen only in cancer and dysentery. The patient finally takes to bed, and in extreme cases lies upon one side with the thighs and legs flexed, and contractures may occur. Food is either not taken at all or only upon urgent compulsion. The skin becomes wasted, dry, and covered with bran-like scales. No food may be taken for several weeks at a time, and attempts to feed may be followed by severe spasms. Although the condition looks so alarming, these patients, when removed from their home surroundings and treated by isolation, sometimes recover in a remarkable way. It may take many months before any improvement is noted. Death, however, may follow with extreme emaciation. In one fatal case the girl weighed only 49 pounds. No lesions were found post mortem.

Hysterical *tympanites* is common, caused usually by tonic contraction of the diaphragm and retraction of the abdominal muscles. It may be associated with peristaltic unrest. Frequent discharges of fæces may be due to disturbance in the small or large bowel. An obstinate form of diarrhœa is found in some hysterical patients, which proves very intractable and is associated especially with the taking of food. It seems an aggravated form of the looseness of bowels to which many nervous people are subject on emotion or of the tendency which some have to diarrhœa immediately after eating. An entirely different form is that produced by what Mitchell calls the irritable rectum, in which scybala are passed frequently, sometimes with great violence. Constipation is more frequent and may be due to lack of attention to the need for defecation or to spasm (Vagotonia). In extreme cases the bowels may not be moved for two or three weeks. Other disturbances are ano-spasm or intense pain in the rectum apart from any fissure. Hysterical ileus and fæcal vomiting are among the most remarkable of hysterical phenomena. Following a shock there are constipation, tympanites, vomiting, sometimes hæmatemesis. The constipation grows worse, everything taken by the mouth is rejected, the vomitus becomes fæcal in character, even scybala are brought up, and suppositories and enemata are vomited. The symptoms may continue for weeks and then gradually subside. Laparotomy—even thrice in one patient—has shown a perfectly normal-looking condition of the bowels (Parkes Weber).

Cardio-vascular.—Rapid action of the heart on slight emotion, with or without the subjective sensation of palpitation, is often a source of great distress. A slow pulse is less frequent. Pains about the heart may simulate angina. Flushes in various parts are common. Sweating may occur, or the *seborrhœa nigricans,* causing a darkening of the skin of the eyelids.

Among the more remarkable vaso-motor phenomena are the so-called stigmata or hæmorrhages in the skin, such as were present in the celebrated case of Louise Lateau. In many cases these are undoubtedly fraudulent, but if, as appears credible, such bleeding may occur in the hypnotic trance, there seems no reason to doubt its possibility in the trance of religious ecstasy.

(*d*) *Joint Affections.*—To Sir Benjamin Brodie and Sir James Paget we owe the recognition of these extraordinary manifestations. Perhaps no single affection has brought more discredit upon the profession, for the cases are very refractory, and often fall into the hands of a charlatan or faith-healer, under whose touch the disease may disappear at once. Usually it affects the knee or the hip, and may follow a trifling injury. The joint is usually fixed, sensitive, and swollen. The surface may be cool, but sometimes the local temperature is increased. To the touch it is very sensitive and movement causes great pain. In protracted cases the muscles are somewhat wasted, and in consequence the joint looks larger. The pains are often nocturnal, at which time the local temperature may be increased. While, as a rule, neuromimetic joints yield to proper management, there are instances in the literature in which organic change has succeeded the functional disturbance. Intermittent hydrarthrosis may be a manifestation of hysteria, sometimes with transient paresis.

(*e*) *Mental Symptoms.*—Mental perversions of all kinds are common in hysterical patients and not much dependence can be placed on statements either about themselves or about others. A morbid craving for sympathy may lead to the commission of all sorts of bizarre and foolish acts.

Hallucinations and delirium may alternate with emotional outbursts of an aggravated character. There is a condition which may be spoken of as the *status hystericus.* For weeks or months they may be confined to bed, entirely oblivious to their surroundings, with a delirium which may simulate that of delirium tremens, particularly in being associated with loathsome and unpleasant animals. The nutrition may be maintained, but there is a heavy, foul breath. With seclusion and care recovery usually takes place within three or four months. At the onset of these attacks and during convalescence the patients must be incessantly watched, as a suicidal tendency is not uncommon.

Of hysterical manifestations in the higher centres that of *trance* is the most remarkable. This may develop spontaneously without any convulsive seizure, but more frequently it follows hysteroid attacks. Catalepsy may be present, a condition in which the limbs are plastic and remain in any position in which they are placed.

(*f*) *Manifestations.*—(1) Œdema. Puffiness of the face, even unilateral, and swelling of the hands are not uncommon and the features of Raynaud's disease may be met with. A white and a blue type of œdema is recognized, and either may be associated with paralyses, motor and sensory. (2) *Stigmata.*—Local bleedings have been described, sometimes, as in the so-called marks of the cross, on forehead, hands, feet and side, as in the famous case of Louise Lateau. Organic lesions of the skin (blisters) are claimed to have been produced by hypnotic suggestion (Hadfield) and the stigmata are probably produced by auto-suggestion in the trance state. (3) *Pathomimia,* the self-inflicted injuries, usually of the skin, by caustics, etc. In a case seen at the Hôtel Dieu with Dieulafoy, the patient, supposed to be the subject of severe trophic disorder, submitted to amputation of the arm before a confession was obtained that the lesions were self-inflicted.

(*g*) *Hysterical Fever.*—In hysteria the temperature, as a rule, is normal. The cases with fever may be grouped as follows: (1) Instances in which the fever is the sole manifestation. These are rare, but there are cases in which the chronic course, the retention of nutrition, and the entirely negative condition of the organs leaves no other diagnosis possible. In one case the patient had for four or five years an afternoon rise of temperature, usually to 102° or 103°. She was well nourished and had no pronounced hysterical symptoms, beyond the interrupted sighing respiration so often seen.

(2) Cases of hysterical fever with spurious local manifestations. These are very troublesome and deceptive cases. The patient may be suddenly taken ill with pain in various regions and elevation of temperature. The case may simulate meningitis. There may be pain in the head, vomiting, contracted pupils, and retraction of the neck—symptoms which may persist for weeks—and some anomalous manifestation during convalescence may alone indicate to the physician that he has had to deal with hysteria, and has not, as he perhaps flattered himself, cured a case of meningitis. Mary Putnam Jacobi, in an article on hysterical fever, mentions a case in the service of Cornil which was admitted with dyspnœa, slight cyanosis, and a temperature of 39° C. The condition proved to be hysterical. There is also an hysterical pseudo-phthisis with pain in the chest, slight fever, and the expectoration of a blood-stained mucus. The cases of hysterical peritonitis may also show fever.

(3) *Hyperpyrexia.*—It is a suggestive fact that the cases of paradoxical temperatures in which the thermometer has registered 112° to 120° have been in women. Fraud has been practised in nearly all these cases.

Astasia; Abasia.—These terms, indicating respectively inability to stand and inability to walk, have been applied by Charcot and Blocq to conditions characterized by loss of the power of standing or of walking, with retention of muscular power, coördination, and sensation. Blocq's definition is as follows: "A morbid state in which the impossibility of standing erect and walking normally is in contrast with the integrity of sensation, of muscular strength, and of the coördination of the other movements of the lower extremities." The condition forms a symptom group, not a morbid entity, and is a functional neurosis. Knapp analyzed 50 cases, of which half were in women. In 21 cases hysteria was present; in 3, chorea; in 2, epilepsy; and in 4, intention psychoses. As a rule, the patients, though able to move the feet and legs perfectly when in bed, are either unable to walk properly or can not stand at all. The disturbances have been very varied, and different forms have been recognized. The commonest, according to Knapp's analysis of the recorded cases, is the paralytic, in which the legs give out as the patient attempts to walk and "bend under him as if made of cotton." "There is no rigidity, no spasm, no incoördination. In bed, sitting, or even while suspended, the muscular strength is found to be good." Other cases are associated with spasm or ataxia; thus there may be movements which stiffen the legs and give to the gait a somewhat spastic character. In other instances there are sudden flexions of the legs, or even of the arms, or a saltatory, spring-like spasm. The condition is a manifestation of hysteria.

Diagnosis.—Inquiry into the occurrence of previous manifestations and the mental conditions may give important information. These questions, as a rule, should not be asked the mother, who of all others is least likely to give satisfactory information. The occurrence of the globus hystericus, of emotional attacks, of weeping and crying is always suggestive. The points of difference between the convulsive attacks and true epilepsy may give difficulty at first. The hysterical paralyses are very variable and apt to be associated with anæsthesia. The contractures may be deceptive, but the occurrence of areas of anæsthesia, of retraction of the visual field, and the development of minor hysterical manifestations give valuable indications. The contractures disappear under full anæsthesia. Special care must be taken not to confound the spastic paraplegia of hysteria with lateral sclerosis.

The visceral manifestations are usually recognized without much difficulty.

The practitioner has constantly to bear in mind the strong tendency in hysterical patients to practise deception.

Treatment.—The prophylaxis may be gathered from the remarks on the relation of education to the disease. The successful treatment of hysteria demands qualities possessed by few physicians. The first element is a due appreciation of the nature of the disease on the part of the physician and friends. It is pitiable to think of the misery which has been inflicted on these unhappy victims by the harsh and unjust treatment which has resulted from false views of the nature of the trouble; on the other hand, worry and ill health, often the wrecking of mind, body, and estate, are entailed upon the near relatives in the nursing of a protracted case. The minor manifestations, attacks of the vapors, the crying and weeping spells, are not of much moment and rarely require treatment. The physical condition should be carefully looked into and the mode of life regulated so as to insure system and order in everything. A congenial occupation offers the best remedy for many of the manifestations. Any functional disturbance should be attended to and tonics prescribed. Special attention should be paid to the action of the bowels.

PSYCHOTHERAPY, in which the important features are hypnosis, suggestion, and reëducation.

Hypnosis.—The majority of hysterical patients can be hypnotized, but the general opinion of those who know most on the subject is that by hypnosis alone hysteria is rarely cured. Sometimes a brilliant miracle is wrought in the case of hysterical paraplegia or hemiplegia, but as a routine treatment it has fallen into disfavor even in France.

Suggestion.—Babinski defines suggestion as "the action by which one endeavors to make another accept or realize an idea which is manifestly unreasonable." On the other hand, persuasion is applied when the ideas are reasonable, or at least are not in opposition to good sense. Most writers, however, use the word "suggestion" as meaning the introduction of mental associations and modifications of the patient's mental state leading to betterment. In proper hands it is a most powerful instrument, particularly when the patient has faith in the person who makes it. After a careful and sympathetic examination and testing the electrical reactions of the muscles of a paralyzed limb the suggestion to the hysteric, "Now you will be able to move it" may be all-sufficient. A strong, imperative command may have the same effect.

Reëducation.—In both hysteria and neurasthenia this should be the aim of all reasonable practice, but it is not always feasible: some of our patients would have to be rebuilt from the blastoderm. With patience and method much may be done, and the special merit of Weir Mitchell's work and of his system (which is not simply a rest cure, as many suppose) is that it is an elaborate plan of reëducation. The essentials are that the patient should be isolated from his friends and under the charge of an intelligent nurse. The physical condition is carefully studied and a rigid daily régime carried out: A milk diet of three to four quarts daily, rising to five or six, varying the food as the patient improves, and as the weight increases. This may be followed by a rapid gain in weight and the disappearance of the unpleasant abdominal symptoms. Massage, hydrotherapy, and electricity are adjuncts, but very much depends upon the tact, patience, and, above all, the personality of the physician; the man counts more than the method. The mental condition has to be carefully studied and the patient's attitude toward life influenced by specially selected literature, careful conversation, and suggestion.

THE ANALYTICAL METHOD.—Introduced by Breuer and extended by Freud, it is partly the method of the confessional, in which the sinner poured out his soul in the sympathetic ear of the priest, but it also enables the patient to bring out into the open what he may not consciously know. It is a difficult procedure, not for all to attempt, exhausting alike to patient and doctor, and, when thoroughly carried out, time consuming. In the hands of those who have practised it, very good results have been obtained, particularly in young and carefully selected cases. This statement of the method is taken from Jelliffe ("System of Medicine," 2nd Ed., vol. v.):

"His (Freud's) general procedure is to place the patient in a recumbent position, the physician sitting behind the patient's head at the end of the lounge. The physician thus remains practically out of sight of the patient, who is then asked to give a detailed account of his troubles, and to say everything that comes to the mind irrespective of its seeming logic or sense, and apart from disturbing, mortifying, or unnice suggestions. In all such histories gaps are inevitable. These the patient is urged to fill in by thinking closely of the attendant circumstances, speaking aloud all of the flitting thoughts that pass during this search ('free association'). All the thoughts are requested to be uttered, notwithstanding their disagreeable nature. The patient must exercise no critique and remain passive. It will be found that the disagreeable thoughts are pushed back with the greatest resistance. This is made all the more striking since the hysterical reaction, i. e., the symptom, is the symbolic expression of the realization of a repressed wish and gives the patient some gratification. A great effort is made to retain the symptom, especially as its origin is not really perceived, and since it represents, in symbol, the individual's former conscious strivings. In psycho-analysis one attempts to overcome all of these resistances, and by a series of judicious and tactful probings reconduct into the patient's consciousness the hidden thoughts which underlie these symptoms. Every symptom has some meaning; behind it there lies some associated mechanism, the origin of which the patient unconsciously or partly consciously represses. In the psycho-neurotic symbol may be read the cryptic expression of the original thought driven back and hidden.

"To slowly analyze and pick apart the mechanism is the object of the analytical method. One needs not only special tact for such excursions into the subtleties of the mental life of some individuals, but also a developed method of interpretation. Every act, every symbolic expression or action, lapse in speech, mannerism, needs to be carefully noted and its bearing coördinated. Freud lays particular emphasis on the analysis of dreams, since he believes that in the dream the subconscious, or the 'repressed conscious' is more apt to reveal itself. Hence a careful reading of Freud's 'Significance of Dreams' is of the greatest value in this study, also his 'Psychopathology of Every-day Life.' In his work on dreams he has developed to the full the chief directions along which his mind has traveled in the psychoanalytical method.

"It is of the utmost importance to trace back into the earliest years the striking emotional influences that have come into experience, as, for Freud, the hysterical reaction consists in a perverted type of reaction to these experiences. As is known, the blurring, or loss of an emotional influence—an affect, in short—is due to a number of factors. In normal life forgetting is the commonest type of a corrective adaptation, and forgetting is carried out with special ease if the emotional stress has not been excessive. Forgetting, however, is only a secondary phenomenon, and usually is more successful if the immediate reaction has been an adequate one. Such immediate reactions express themselves as tears, as anger, as impulsive acts, etc., and in such reactions the effect is discharged. In every-day life one calls it giving vent to one's feelings. If, however, the reaction is suppressed, the effect becomes united to the memory of the experience, and an emotional complex, or, to use a rather broad simile, a psychic boil, results, which must heal by absorption, by discharge, or by other means. Freud uses the term ab-react (abreagieren) to signify the adequate reaction, or discharge of such effects or their resulting complexes. Talking the whole thing over, giving vent to one's secrets and confessions are well-known abreactions.

"In hysteria certain of these complexes remain prominent; they are neither reacted too promptly, nor is their unpleasant feeling tone diminished by the blurring process of forgetting, although it is characteristic of the Freud point of view that the actual experience which gives rise to them becomes forgotten and the cause of the affect disturbance which becomes later converted, it may be into physical signs, remains apparently unknown to the patient. It must be dug out by psycho-analysis, and when once discovered catharsis takes place and the patient becomes cured."

HYDROTHERAPY is of great value, especially wet packs, salt baths, and various douches. General tonics, such as arsenic and iron, may be helpful, especially if the patients are nervous and anæmic. Sedatives are rarely indicated. Occasionally bromides may be necessary, but for the relief of sleeplessness all possible measures should be resorted to before the employment of drugs. The wet pack given hot or cold at night will usually suffice.

X. NEURASTHENIA

(*Psychasthenia*)

Definition.—A condition of weakness or exhaustion of the nervous system, giving rise to various forms of mental and bodily inefficiency.

The term, an old one, but first popularized by Beard, covers an ill-defined, motley group of symptoms, which may be either general and the expression of derangement of the entire system, or local, limited to certain organs; hence, the terms cerebral, spinal, cardiac, and gastric neurasthenia.

Etiology.—The causes may be grouped as hereditary and acquired.

(*a*) HEREDITARY.—We do not all start in life with the same amount of nerve capital. Parents who have led irrational lives, indulging in excesses of various kinds, or who have been the subjects of nervous complaints or of mental trouble, may transmit to their children an organization which is defective in what, for want of a better term, we must call "nerve force." Such individuals start handicapped with a neuropathic predisposition, and furnish a considerable proportion of our neurasthenic patients. As van Gieson sonorously puts it, "the potential energies of the higher constellations of their association centres have been squandered by their ancestors." So long as these individuals are content to transact a moderate business with their life capital, all may go well, but there is no reserve, and in the exigencies of modern life these small capitalists go under and come to us as bankrupts.

(*b*) ACQUIRED.—The functions, though perverted most readily in persons who have inherited a feeble organization, may also be damaged in persons with no neuropathic predisposition by exercise which is excessive in proportion to the strength—i. e., by strain. The cares and anxieties attendant upon the gaining of a livelihood may be borne without distress, but in many persons the strain becomes excessive and is first manifested as *worry*. The individual loses the distinction between essentials and non-essentials, trifles cause annoyance, and the entire organism reacts with unnecessary readiness to slight stimuli, and is in a state which the older writers called "irritable weakness." If such a condition be taken early and the patient given rest, the balance is quickly restored. In this group may be placed a large proportion of the neurasthenia which we see among business men, teachers, and journalists. Neurasthenia may follow the infectious diseases, particularly influenza, typhoid fever, and syphilis. The abuse of certain drugs, alcohol, tobacco, morphine may lead to neurasthenia, though the drug habit is more often a result than a cause.

(*c*) SEXUAL CAUSES.—Undoubtedly the part played in the production of hysteria and allied neurosis by sexual factors is of the first importance. As already stated, Freud regards sexual trauma as the basis of hysteria, and he also regards neurasthenia as largely a product of disturbance in the sexual sphere. For him and his school the sexual impulses furnish the basis of the psychoneuroses. Repressed as they have to be in so many in our modern civilization, without normal outlet, the thought formations, retained in the unconscious state, express themselves by means of somatic phenomena—the objective features of hysteria and neurasthenia. *Cherchez la femme* is a safe rule in investigating a neurotic case. Freud may have ridden his hobby too hard, particularly in the insistence upon the importance of infantile sexuality, but in recognizing the rôle of the younger Aphrodite in the lives of men and women he has but followed the great master, Plato, who saw, while he deplored, the havoc wrought by her universal dominance.

The traumatic forms will be considered separately.

Symptoms.—These are extremely varied, and may be general or localized; more often a combination of both. The appearance of the patient is suggestive, sometimes characteristic, but difficult to describe. Important information can be gained by the physician if he observes the patient closely as he enters the room—the way he is clothed, the manner in which he holds his body, his facial expression, and the humor which he is in. Loss of weight and slight anæmia may be present. The physical debility may reach a high grade and the patient may be confined to bed. Mentally the patients are usually low-spirited and despondent; women are frequently emotional.

The *local* symptoms may dominate the situation, and there have accordingly been described a whole series of types of the disease—cerebral, spinal, cardio-vascular, gastric, and sexual. In all forms there is a striking lack of accordance between the symptoms of which the patient complains and the objective changes discoverable by the physician. In nearly every clinical type of the disease the predominant symptoms are referable to pathological sensations and the psychic effects of these. Imperfect sleep is complained of by a majority of patients, or, if not complained of, is found to exist on inquiry.

In the *cerebral* or psychic form the symptoms are chiefly connected with an inability to perform the ordinary mental work. Thus, a row of figures can not be correctly added, the dictation or the writing of a few letters is a source of the greatest worry, the transaction of petty details in business is a painful effort, and there is loss of power of fixed attention. With this condition there may be no headache, the appetite may be good, and the patient may sleep well. As a rule, however, there are sensations of fulness and weight or flushes, if not actual headache. Sleeplessness is frequent in this form, and may be the first manifestation. Some patients are good-tempered and cheerful but a majority are moody, irritable, and depressed.

Hyperæsthesia, especially to sensations of pain, is one of the main characteristics of almost all neurasthenic individuals. The sensations are nearly always referred to some special region—the skin, eye muscles, the joints, the blood-vessels, or the viscera. It is frequently possible to localize a number of points painful to pressure (Valleix's points). In some patients there is marked vertigo, occasionally resembling that of Ménière's disease.

If such pathological sensations continue for a long time the mood and character of the patient gradually alter. The so-called "irritable humor" develops. Many obnoxiously egoistic individuals met with in daily life are in reality examples of psychic neurasthenia. Everything is complained of. The patient demands the greatest consideration for his condition; he feels that he has been deeply insulted if his desires are not always immediately granted. He may at the same time have but little consideration for others. Indeed, in the severer forms he may show a malicious pleasure in attempting to make people who seem happier than himself uncomfortable. Such patients complain frequently that they are "misunderstood" by their fellows.

In many cases the so-called "anxiety conditions" gradually come on; one scarcely ever sees a case of advanced neurasthenia without the existence of some form of "anxiety." In the simpler forms of anxiety (nosophobic) there may be only a fear of impending insanity or of approaching death or of apoplexy. More frequently the anxious feeling is localized somewhere in the body—in the præcordial region, in the head, in the abdomen, in the thorax, or more rarely in the extremities.

In some cases the anxiety becomes intense and the patients are restless, and declare that they do not know what to do with themselves. They may throw themselves upon a bed, crying and complaining, and making convulsive movements with the hands and feet. Suicidal tendencies are not uncommon in such cases, and the patients may in desperation actually take their own lives.

Involuntary mental activity may be very troublesome; the patient complains that when he is overtired thoughts which he cannot stop or control run through his head with lightning-like rapidity. In other cases there is marked absence of ideas, the individual's mind being so filled up owing to the overexcitability of latent memory pictures that he is unable to form the proper associations for ideas called up by external stimuli. Sometimes a patient complains that a definite word, a name, a number, a melody, or a song keeps running in his head in spite of all he can do to abolish it.

In the severer cases the so-called *"phobias"* are common. A frequent form is *agoraphobia,* in which patients when they come into an open space are oppressed by a feeling of anxiety. They seem "frightened to death," and commence to tremble; they complain of compression of the thorax and palpitation of the heart. They may break into profuse perspiration and assert that they feel as though chained to the ground or that they can not move a step. It is remarkable that in some such cases the open space can be crossed if the individual be accompanied by some one, even by a child, or if he carry a stick or an umbrella! Other people are afraid to be left alone (monophobia), especially in a closed compartment (claustrophobia).

The fear of people and of society is known as anthropophobia. A whole series of other phobias has been described—batophobia, or the fear that high things will fall; pathophobia, or fear of disease; siderodromophobia, or fear of a railway journey; siderophobia or astrophobia, fear of thunder and lightning. Occasionally we meet with individuals who are afraid of everything and every one—victims of the so-called pantophobia. By psycho-analysis it is possible to explain the mechanism of these fears.

The *special senses* may be disturbed, particularly vision. An aching or weariness of the eyeballs after reading a few minutes or flashes of light are common symptoms. The "irritable eye," the so-called nervous or neurasthenic asthenopia, is familiar to every physician. There may be acoustic disturbances —hyperalgesia and even true hyperacusia.

One of the most common symptoms is *pressure in the head.* This symptom, variously described, may be diffuse, but is more frequently referred to some one region—frontal, temporal, parietal, or occipital.

When the *spinal symptoms* predominate—spinal irritation or spinal neurasthenia—in addition to many of the features just mentioned, the patients complain of weariness on the least exertion, of weakness, pain in the back, intercostal neuralgiform pains, and of aching pains in the legs. There may be spots of local tenderness on the spine. The rachialgia may be spontaneous, or may be noticed only on pressure or movement. Occasionally there may be disturbances of sensation, particularly numbness and tingling, and the reflexes may be increased. Visceral neuralgias, especially in connection with the genital organs, are frequent. The aching pain in the back or in the back of the neck is the most constant complaint. In women it is often impossible to say whether the condition is neurasthenia or hysteria. It is in these cases that the disturbances of muscular activity are most pronounced, and in the French writings *amyosthenia* plays an important rôle. The symptoms may be irritative or paretic, or a combination of both. Disturbances of coördination are not uncommon in the severer forms. These are particularly prone to involve the associated movements of the eye muscles, leading to asthenopic lack of accommodation. Drooping of one eyelid is common, probably owing to insufficient innervation on the part of the sympathetic rather than to paresis of the oculomotor nerve. Occasionally Romberg's symptom is present, and the patient, or his physician, may fear a beginning tabes. More rarely there is disturbance of such coördinated acts as writing and articulation, not unlike those seen at the onset of general paresis. Such symptoms are always alarming, and the greatest care must be taken in establishing a diagnosis. That they may be the symptoms of pure neurasthenia can not be doubted.

The *reflexes* are usually increased, the deep reflexes especially never being absent. The condition of the superficial reflexes is less constant, though these, too, are usually increased. The pupils are often dilated, and the reflexes are usually normal. There may be inequality of the pupils. Errors in refraction are common, the correction of which may give great relief.

In another type the muscular weakness is extreme, and may go on to complete motor helplessness. Very thorough examination is necessary before deciding as to the nature of the affection, since in some instances serious mistakes have been made. Here belong the *atremia* of Neftel, the *akinesia algera* of Möbius, and the neurasthenic form of *astasia abasia* described by Binswanger.

In other cases the *cardio-vascular* symptoms are the most distressing, and may occur with only slight disturbance of the cerebro-spinal functions, though the conditions are nearly always combined. Palpitation of the heart, irregular and very rapid action (neurasthenic tachycardia), and pains and oppressive feelings in the cardiac region are the most common symptoms. Some of these are due to the "dropped" heart which may be dilated. The slightest excitement may be followed by increased action of the heart, sometimes associated with sensations of dizziness and anxiety, and the patients frequently have the idea that they suffer from serious disease of this organ. Attacks of "pseudo-angina" may occur.

Vaso-motor disturbances constitute a special feature of many cases. Flushes of heat, especially in the head, and transient hyperæmia of the skin may be very distressing symptoms. Profuse sweating may occur, either local or general, and sometimes nocturnal. The pulse may show interesting features, owing to the extreme relaxation of the peripheral arterioles. The arterial throbbing may be everywhere visible, almost as much as in aortic insufficiency. The pulse, too, may have a somewhat collapsing quality and the capillary pulse may be seen. A characteristic symptom in some cases is the *throbbing aorta.* This "preternatural pulsation in the epigastrium," as Allan Burns calls it, may be extremely forcible and suggest abdominal aneurism. The subjective sensations associated with it may be very unpleasant, particularly when the stomach is empty.

In women especially, and sometimes in men, the peripheral blood-vessels are contracted, the extremities are cold, the nose is red or blue, and the face has a pinched expression. These patients feel much more comfortable when the cutaneous vessels are distended, and resort to various means to favor this (wearing of heavy clothing, use of diffusible stimulants).

The general features of *gastro-intestinal neurasthenia* have been dealt with under the section on nervous dyspepsia. The connection with dilatation of the stomach, floating kidney, and *enteroptosis* has been mentioned.

In *sexual neurasthenia* there is an irritable weakness of the sexual organs manifested by nocturnal emissions, unusual depression after intercourse, and often by a dread of impotence. The mental condition of these patients is most pitiable, and they fall an easy prey to quacks and charlatans. In males these symptoms are frequently due to diseased conditions in the deep urethra, especially of the verumontanum, and prostate. Spermatorrhœa is the bugbear of the majority. They complain of continued losses especially with defecation or micturition. Microscopic examination sometimes reveals the presence of spermatozoa. Actual nervous impotence is not uncommon. The "painful testicle" is a well-known neurasthenic phenomenon. In the severer cases, especially those bearing the stigmata of degeneration, there may be sexual perversion. In females it is common to find a tender ovary, and painful or irregular menstruation. There may be disturbances in the sexual sphere.

Diagnosis.—*Psychasthenia.*—Under this term Janet would separate from neurasthenia the cases characterized by mental, emotional, and psychical disturbances, imperative ideas, phobias of all sorts, doubts, enfeebled will, uncontrollable movements, and many of the borderland features of the insanity of young persons. It is really an inherited psychoneurosis, while neurasthenia is usually acquired. Obsessions of all sorts characterize the condition and there may be a feeling of unreality and even of loss of personality. How complicated the condition may be is shown from the following varieties distinguished by Janet: (1) The *doubter,* in whom obsessive ideas are not very precise, more of the nature of a general indication rather than a specific idea, such as a craze for research, for explanation, for computing. (2) The *scrupulous,* whose obsessions are of a moral nature. Their manias are of literalness of statement, of exact truth, of conjuration, of reparation, of symbols, etc. (3) The *criminal,* whose obsessive ideas are of homicide, theft, and other overt acts. The impulsive idea is stronger in this than in the other varieties. (4) The *inebriates,* morphinomaniac, etc., in whom the impulse seems to be least resistible. (5) The *genesically perverted.* (6) *Delirious psychasthenia,* in which a delirious state of mind occurs, connected with the obsession.

Neurasthenia is a disease above all others which has to be diagnosed from the subjective statements of the patient, and from an observation of his general behavior rather than from the physical examination. The physical examination is of the highest importance in excluding other diseases likely to be confounded with it. That somatic changes occur and that physical signs are often to be made out is very true, but there is nothing typical or pathognomonic in these objective changes.

The *hypochondriac* differs from the neurasthenic in the excessive psychic distortion of the pathological sensations to which he is subject. He is the victim of actual delusions regarding his condition.

The confusion of neurasthenia with *hysteria* is still more frequent; in women especially a diagnosis of hysteria is often made when in reality the condition is one of neurasthenia. In the absence of hysterical paroxysms, of crises, and of those marked emotional and intellectual characteristics of the hysterical individual the diagnosis of hysteria should not be made. If hysterical stigmata (paralyses, convulsions, contractures, anæsthesias, alterations in the visual field, etc.) are present, the diagnosis is not difficult.

Epilepsy is not likely to be confounded with neurasthenia if there be definite epileptic attacks, but the cases of *petit mal* may be puzzling.

The onset of *exophthalmic goitre* may be mistaken for neurasthenia, especially if there be no exophthalmos at the beginning. The emotional disturbances and the irritability of the heart may mislead the physician. Tuberculosis should always be excluded and careful search made for signs of any internal secretion disturbance. In pronounced cases of nervous prostration the differential diagnosis from the various psychoses may be extremely difficult.

The two forms of *organic disease* of the nervous system with which neurasthenia is most likely to be confounded are tabes and general paresis. The symptoms of the spinal form of neurasthenia may resemble those of the former disease, while the symptoms of the psychic or cerebral form of neurasthenia may be very similar to those of general paresis. The diagnosis, as a rule, presents no difficulty if the physician makes a thorough routine examination. It is only the superficial study of a case that is likely to lead one astray. In tabes a consideration of the sensory disturbances, of the deep reflexes, and of the pupillary findings will establish the presence or absence of the disease. In general paresis there is sometimes more difficulty. The onset is often characterized by symptoms quite like those of ordinary neurasthenia, and the physician may overlook the grave nature of the malady. The mistake in the other direction is, however, perhaps just as common. A physician who has seen a case of general paresis arise out of what appeared to be one of pronounced neurasthenia is too prone afterward to suspect every neurasthenic to be developing the malign affection. The most marked symptoms of psychic exhaustion do not justify a diagnosis of general paresis even when the history is suspicious, unless along with it there is a definite paresis of the pupils, of the facial muscles, or of the muscles of articulation. The physician should be sharply on the lookout for intellectual defects, paraphasia, facial paresis, and sluggishness of the pupils. The examination of the spinal fluid will remove any doubt.

Treatment.—Prophylaxis.—Many patients come under our care a generation too late for satisfactory treatment, and it may be impossible to restore the exhausted capital. The greatest care should be taken in the rearing of children of neuropathic predisposition. From a very early age they should be submitted to a process of "psychic hardening," every effort being made to strengthen the bodily and mental condition. Even in infancy the child should not be pampered. Later on the greatest care should be exercised with regard to food, sleep, and school work. Complaints of children should not be too seriously considered. Much depends upon the example set by the parents. An emotional, constantly complaining mother will rack the nervous system of a delicate child. In some instances, for the welfare of a developing boy or girl, the physician may find it necessary to advise removal from home.

Neurotic children are especially liable during development to fits of temper and of emotional disturbance. These should not be too lightly considered. Above all, violent chastisement in such cases is to be avoided, and loss of temper on the part of the parent or teacher is particularly pernicious for the nervous system of the child. Where possible, in such instances, the best treatment is to put the obstreperous child immediately to bed, and if the excitement and temper continue a warm bath followed by a cool douche may be effective. If he be put to bed after the bath sleep soon follows.

Special attention is necessary at puberty in both boys and girls. If there be at this period any marked tendency to emotional disturbance or to intellectual weakness the child should be removed from school and every care taken to avoid unfavorable influences.

Personal Hygiene.—Throughout life individuals of neuropathic predisposition should obey scrupulously certain hygienic and prophylactic rules. Intellectual work especially should be judiciously limited and alternate frequently with periods of repose. Excitement of all kinds should be avoided, and such individuals will do well to be abstemious in the use of tobacco, tea, coffee, and alcohol, if, indeed, they be permitted to use them at all. The habit of taking at least once a year a prolonged holiday in the woods, in the mountains, or at the seashore, should be urgently enjoined upon every neuropathic individual. In many instances it is found to be the greatest relief and rest if the patient can take his holiday away from his relatives.

During ordinary life nervous people should, during some portion of each day, pay rational attention to the body. Cold baths, swimming, exercises in the gymnasium, gardening, golf, lawn tennis, cricket, hunting, shooting, rowing, sailing, and bicycling are of value in maintaining the general nutrition. Such exercises are to be recommended only to individuals physically equal to them. If neurasthenia be once well established the greatest care must be observed in the ordering of exercise. Many nervous girls have been completely broken down by following injudicious advice with regard to long walks.

Treatment.—The treatment of neurasthenia when once established presents a varied problem to the thoughtful physician. Every case must be handled upon its own merits, no two, as a rule, requiring exactly the same methods. In general it will be the aim to remove the patient as far as possible from the influences which have led to his downfall, and to restore to normal the nervous mechanisms which have been weakened by injurious influences. The general character of the individual, his physical and social status, must be considered and the therapeutic measures carefully adjusted to these.

The diagnosis having been settled, the physician may assure the patient that with prolonged treatment, during which his coöperation is absolutely essential, he may expect to get well. He must be told that much depends upon himself and that he must make a vigorous effort to overcome certain of his tendencies, and that all his strength of will will be needed to further the progress of the cure. In business or professional men, in whom the condition develops as a result of overwork or overstudy, it may be sufficient to enjoin absolute rest with change of scene and diet. A trip abroad or, if there are symptoms of nervous dyspepsia, a residence at one of the Spas will usually prove sufficient. The excitement of large cities should be avoided. The longer the disease has lasted and the more intense the symptoms have been, the longer the time necessary for the restoration of health. In cases of any severity the patient must be told that at least six months' complete absence from business, under strict medical guidance, will be necessary. Shorter periods may be of benefit, which, however, as a rule, will be only temporary.

It will often be found advisable to make out a daily programme, which shall occupy almost the whole time of the patient. At first he need know nothing about this, the case being given over entirely to the nurse. As improvement advances, moderate physical and intellectual exercises, alternating frequently with rest and the administration of food, may be undertaken. Some one hour of the day may be left free for reading, correspondence, conversation, and games. In some instances the writing of letters is particularly harmful and must be prohibited or limited. Cultured individuals may find benefit from attention to drawing, painting, modelling, translating from a foreign language, the making of abstracts, etc., for short periods in the day.

In some cases, including a large proportion of neurasthenic women, a systematic rest treatment rigidly carried out should be tried. The patient must be isolated from her friends, and any regulations undertaken must be strictly adhered to, the consent of the patient and the family having first been gained. The treatment of the gastric and intestinal symptoms has been considered. For the irregular pains, particularly in the back and neck, the cautery is invaluable.

Hydrotherapy is indicated in nearly every case if it can be properly applied. Much can be done at home or in an ordinary hospital, but for systematic hydrotherapeutic treatment residence in a suitable sanitarium is necessary. The wet pack is of especial value and, particularly at night, in cases of sleeplessness, is perhaps the best remedy against insomnia we have. Salt baths are more helpful to some patients. The various forms of douches, partial packs, etc., may be valuable in individual cases. Electrotherapy is of some value, though only in combination with psychic treatment and hydrotherapy.

Special care should be given to the recognition of local disease and proper measures instituted. Attention to the eyes is important. Infection of the naso-pharynx, teeth or tonsils, sinus disease, visceroptosis, or anæmia should be corrected. In women the pelvic organs and in men the deep urethra and prostate may require treatment.

Treatment by drugs should be avoided as much as possible. They are of benefit chiefly in the combating of single symptoms. Alcohol, morphia, chloral, or cocaine should never be given. General tonics may be helpful, especially if the individual be anæmic, when arsenic and iron are indicated. For the severer pains and nervous attacks some sedative may be necessary, especially at the beginning of the treatment. The bromides may be given with advantage. An occasional dose of phenacetin or acetyl salicylic acid may be required, but the less of these substances we can get along with the better. For the relief of sleeplessness all possible measures should be resorted to before the employment of drugs. The wet pack will usually suffice. If absolutely necessary to give a drug, sulphonal, trional, or barbital may be employed.

In cases in which the anxiety conditions are disturbing the cautious use of opium in pill form may be necessary, since, as in the psychoses, opium here will sometimes yield permanent relief. A prolonged treatment with opium is, however, never necessary in neurasthenia.

PSYCHOTHERAPY.—Hypnotism is rarely indicated. Carefully practised suggestion is most helpful and psycho-analysis is of value.

The use of religious ideas and practices may be most helpful, and this has come into vogue in various forms, as Christian Science, Mental Healing, etc. It is an old story. In all ages, and in all lands, the prayer of faith, to use the words of St. James, has healed the sick; and we must remember that amid the Æsculapian cult, the most elaborate and beautiful system of faith healing the world has seen, scientific medicine took its rise. As a profession, consciously or unconsciously, more often the latter, *faith* has been one of our most valuable assets, and Galen expressed a great truth when he said, "He cures most successfully in whom the people have the greatest confidence." It is in these cases of neurasthenia and psychasthenia, the weak brothers and the weak sisters, that the personal character of the physician comes into play, and once let him gain the confidence of the patient, he can work just the same sort of miracles as Our Lady of Lourdes or Ste. Anne de Beaupré. Three elements are necessary: first, a strong personality in whom the individual has faith—Christ, Buddha, Æsculapius (in the days of Greece), one of the saints, or, what has served the turn of common humanity very well, a physician. Secondly, certain accessories—a shrine, a sanctuary, the services of a temple, or for us a hospital or its equivalent, with a skillful nurse. Thirdly, suggestion, either of the "only believe," "feel it," "will it" attitude of mind, which is the essence of every cult and creed, or of the active belief in the assurance of the physician that the precious boon of health is within reach.

XI. THE TRAUMATIC NEUROSES

(*Railway Brain and Railway Spine; Traumatic Hysteria*)

Definition.—A morbid condition following shock which presents the symptoms of neurasthenia or hysteria or of both.

Erichsen regarded the condition as the result of inflammation of the meninges and cord, and gave it the name "railway spine." Walton and J. J. Putnam, of Boston, were the first to recognize the hysterical nature of many of the cases, and to Westphal's pupils we owe the name traumatic neurosis.

Etiology.—The condition follows an accident, often in a railway train, in which injury has been sustained, or succeeds a shock or concussion, from which the patient may apparently not have suffered in his body. A man may appear perfectly well for several days, or even a week or more, and then develop the symptoms of the neurosis. Bodily shock or concussion is not necessary. The affection may follow a profound mental impression; thus, an engine-driver ran over a child, and received thereby a very severe shock, subsequent to which the most pronounced symptoms of neurasthenia developed. Severe mental strain combined with bodily exposure may cause it, as in a case of a naval officer who was wrecked in a violent storm and exposed for more than a day in the rigging before he was rescued. A slight blow, a fall from a carriage or on the stairs may suffice. The possibility of actual injury of the spine should always be considered.

Symptoms.—The cases may be divided into three groups: simple neurasthenia, cases with marked hysterical manifestations, and cases with severe symptoms indicating or simulating organic disease.

(1) Simple Traumatic Neurasthenia.—The first symptoms usually develop a few weeks after the accident, which may or may not have been associated with an actual trauma. The patient complains of headache and tired feelings. He is sleepless and finds himself unable to concentrate his attention properly upon his work. A condition of nervous irritability develops, which may have a host of trivial manifestations, and the entire mental attitude of the person may for a time be changed. He dwells constantly upon his condition, gets very despondent and low-spirited, and in extreme cases melancholia may develop. He may complain of numbness and tingling in the extremities, and in some cases of much pain in the back. The bodily functions may be well performed, though such patients usually have, for a time at least, disturbed digestion and loss in weight. The physical examination may be entirely negative. The reflexes are slightly increased, as in ordinary neurasthenia. The pupils may be unequal; cardio-vascular changes may be present in a marked degree.

(2) Cases with Marked Hysterical Features.—Following an injury of any sort, neurasthenic symptoms, like those described above, may develop, and in addition symptoms regarded as characteristic of hysteria. The emotional element is prominent, and there is but slight control over the feelings. The patients have headache, backache, and vertigo. A violent tremor may be present, and constitute the most striking feature. In an engineer who developed subsequent to an accident a series of nervous phenomena the most marked feature was an excessive tremor of the entire body, which was specially manifest during emotional excitement. The most pronounced hysterical symptoms are the sensory disturbances. As first noted by Putnam and Walton, hemianæsthesia may occur as a consequence of trauma. This is a common symptom in France, but rare in England and the United States. Achromatopsia may exist on the anæsthetic side. A second, more common, manifestation is limitation of the field of vision, similar to that in hysteria.

(3) Cases in which the Symptoms Suggest Organic Disease of the Brain and Cord.—As a result of spinal concussion, without fracture or external injury, there may subsequently develop symptoms suggestive of organic disease, which may come on rapidly or at a late date. In a case reported by Leyden the symptoms following the concussion were at first slight and the

patient was regarded as a simulator, but finally the condition became aggravated and death resulted. The post mortem showed a chronic pachymeningitis, which had doubtless resulted from the accident. The cases in this group about which there is so much discussion are those which display marked sensory and motor changes. Following an accident in which the patient has not received external injury a condition of excitement may develop within a week or ten days; he complains of headache and backache, and on examination sensory disturbances are found, either hemianæsthesia or areas in which the sensation is much benumbed; or painful and tactile impressions may be distinctly felt in certain regions, and the temperature sense is absent. The distribution may be bilateral and symmetrical in limited regions or hemiplegic in type. Limitation of the field of vision is usually marked, and there may be disturbance of the senses of taste and smell. The superficial reflexes may be diminished; usually the deep reflexes are exaggerated. The pupils may be unequal; the motor disturbances are variable. The French writers describe cases of monoplegia with or without contracture, symptoms upon which Charcot laid great stress as a manifestation of profound hysteria. The combination of sensory disturbances—anæsthesia or hyperæsthesia—with paralysis, particularly if monoplegic, and the occurrence of contractures without atrophy and with normal electrical reactions, may be regarded as distinctive of hysteria.

In rare cases following trauma and succeeding to symptoms which may have been regarded as neurasthenic or hysterical there are organic changes which may prove fatal. That this occurs is demonstrated clearly by post mortem examinations. The features upon which the greatest reliance can be placed as indicating organic change are optic atrophy, bladder symptoms, particularly in combination with tremor, paresis, and exaggerated reflexes.

The anatomical changes in this condition have not been very definite. When death follows spinal concussion within a few days there may be no apparent lesion, but in some instances the brain or cord has shown punctiform hæmorrhages. Edes reported 4 cases in which a gradual degeneration in the pyramidal tracts followed concussion or injury of the spine; but in all these cases there was marked tremor and the spinal symptoms developed early, or followed immediately upon the accident.

Diagnosis.—A condition of fright and excitement following an accident may persist for days or even weeks, and then gradually pass away. The symptoms of neurasthenia or of hysteria which subsequently develop present nothing peculiar and are identical with those which occur under other circumstances. Care must be taken to recognize simulation, and, as in these cases the condition is largely subjective, this is sometimes extremely difficult. In a careful examination a simulator will often reveal himself by exaggeration of certain symptoms, particularly sensitiveness of the spine, and by increasing voluntarily the reflexes. Maunkopff suggests as a good test to take the pulse rate before, during, and after pressure upon an area said to be painful. If the rate is quickened, it is held to be proof that the pain is real. This is not, however, always the case. It may require careful study to determine whether the individual is honestly suffering from the symptoms of which he complains. A still more important question is, Has the patient organic disease? The symptoms given under the first two groups of cases may exist in a marked degree and may persist for several years without the slightest evidence of organic change.

Hemianæsthesia, limitation of the field of vision, monoplegia with contracture, may all be present as hysterical manifestations, from which recovery may be complete. The diagnosis of an organic lesion should be limited to those cases in which optic atrophy, bladder troubles, and signs of sclerosis of the cord are well marked—indications either of degeneration of the lateral columns or of multiple sclerosis. Examination by the X-rays is an important aid and has showed in some cases definite injury to the spine.

Prognosis.—A majority of patients with traumatic hysteria recover. In railway cases, so long as litigation is pending and the patient is in the hands of lawyers, the symptoms usually persist. Settlement is often the starting-point of a speedy and perfect recovery. On the other hand, there are a few cases in which the symptoms persist even after the litigation has been closed; the patient goes from bad to worse and psychoses develop, such as melancholia, dementia, or occasionally progressive paresis. And, lastly, in extremely rare cases organic lesions may result as a sequence.

The function of the physician acting as medical expert in these cases consists in determining (*a*) the existence of actual disease, and (*b*) its character, whether simple neurasthenia, severe hysteria, or an organic lesion. The outlook for ultimate recovery is good except in cases which present the more serious symptoms above mentioned. Nevertheless it must be borne in mind that traumatic hysteria is one of the most intractable affections which we are called upon to treat. In the treatment of the traumatic neuroses the practitioner may be guided by the principles laid down for the treatment of hysteria and neurasthenia.

L. VASO-MOTOR AND TROPHIC DISEASES

I. RAYNAUD'S DISEASE

Definition.—A vascular change, without organic disease of the vessels, chiefly seen in the extremities, but occurring also in the internal parts, in which a persistent ischæmia or a passive hyperæmia leads to disturbance of function or to loss of vitality with necrosis.

Etiology.—It is a comparatively rare disease. There were only 19 cases in about 20,000 medical patients admitted to the Johns Hopkins Hospital. Women are more frequently attacked than men—62.5 to 37.5 per cent. in Monro's series. Sixty per cent. of the cases occurred in the second and third decades, but no age is exempt. A case has been reported in a six-months-old child and in a woman of 77 years.

Several members of a family may be affected. Neurotic and hysterical patients are more prone to the disease. Damp and cold weather, as in Great Britain, appears to favor its occurrence. Severe chilblain leading to superficial necrosis represents a type of the malady. In the infectious diseases areas of multiple necrosis occur, but, as a rule, the distribution is very different, and such cases should not be included under Raynaud's disease, nor should the local gangrene associated with arteritis.

Pathology.—According to the definition, cases are excluded in which organic disease of the vessels is present. In advanced cases sclerosis of the blood-vessels has been found; and neuritis has been described, but neither is an essential factor. Changes in the spinal cord have been reported, but in a majority of all cases the examination has been negative. The local syncope is an expression of a widespread constrictor influence causing spasm of the arteries and arterioles, so that not a drop of blood enters a part. This may be followed in an hour or two, or less, by active hyperæmia; the arteries and arterioles dilate widely and the dead-white finger becomes a bright pink. While hyperæmia may follow the ischæmia directly, more commonly there is an intervening period of asphyxia in which the finger becomes blue. In frost-bite, active hyperæmia, cyanosis, and local syncope is the order. In Raynaud's disease the order is usually syncope, asphyxia, and hyperæmia. In frost-bite it seems clear that the asphyxia is due to a backward flow from the veins, to which the local syncope yields as the part thaws, before the arteries passing to the part can be felt to pulsate. The asphyxia of Raynaud's disease may be due to the same cause; contraction of the veins has been seen by Barlow and by Weiss, but that was when the asphyxia already existed. The first thing must be the relaxation of the spasm of the venules and veins to permit of the blood entering the empty capillaries. In moderate grades of asphyxia some little blood trickles through the sluice gates, but in the deep purple skin of a typical example of Raynaud's disease the circulation has ceased and death of the part is imminent. The necrosis is a simple matter, as simple as if a string is tied tightly about the finger-tip.

The disease is the result of some as yet unknown instability of the vaso-motor system.

Symptoms.—There are various grades of the disease, of which mild, moderate, and severe types may be recognized. In the mild forms the disease never gets beyond the stage of such vascular disturbance as is frequently seen in chilblains. The hands alone may be affected. In the winter, on the slightest exposure, there is acro-cyanosis, which gives place in the warmth to active hyperæmia, sometimes with swelling, throbbing, and aching. The so-called "beefsteak" hand is often a great annoyance to women. It is a vaso-motor disturbance representing a potential case of Raynaud's disease. In these mild attacks one finger may be white and the adjacent ones red and blue.

The condition may persist for years and never pass on to necrosis. In a case of moderate severity a woman, aged say twenty or twenty-five, after a period of worry or ill health, has pains in the fingers, or a numbness or tingling; then she notices that they are white and cold, and in an hour or so they become red and hot. Within a day or two a change occurs; they remain permanently blue perhaps as far as the second joint or to the knuckles. There is pain, sometimes severe enough to require morphia. The cyanosis persists and the tip of one finger or the terminal joint of another gets darker and a few blebs form. The other fingers show signs of restored circulation, but necrosis has occurred in the pad of one finger and perhaps the terminal inch of another. The necrotic parts gradually separate, and the patient may never have another attack, or in a year or two there is a recurrence.

The severer form is a terrible malady, and may affect fingers and toes at once and with them sometimes the tip of the nose and the ears. The pain is of great severity. Both feet may be swollen to the ankle with the toes black. It may look as if both feet would become gangrenous, but as a rule the process subsides, and in a case even of great severity only the tips of the toes are lost. A severe attack of this sort may last three or four months, when the patient recovers with the loss of two or three fingers or toes, a snip off the edge of both ears and a scar on the tip of the nose. Attacks of this severity may occur year by year, and there are terrible instances in which the patients have lost both hands and feet.

Of the parts affected Monro states that in 43 per cent. of the cases one or both of the upper extremities is involved. Parts other than the extremities may be attacked, as the chin, lips, nates, and eyelids.

Complications.—Temporary amblyopia due to spasm of the retinal vessels, transient aphasia, and transient hemiplegia have been met with. In one case there were three attacks of aphasia with hemiplegia from which complete recovery took place. Associated with these were the features of Raynaud's disease. The patient died in a severe attack with pain in the right hand, gangrene to the elbow, and coma. Epilepsy has been reported in a great number of cases, and in one case, reported by Thomas, the attacks only occurred in the winter when he had Raynaud's disease.

Albuminuria may occur during the attacks. Hæmoglobinuria has been present in a number of cases, and was well studied by the well-known surgeon, Druitt, in his own case. It is of the same nature as the paroxysmal hæmoglobinuria already described.

Scleroderma of the fingers may follow recurring attacks. Occasionally true generalized scleroderma begins with the features of Raynaud's disease. Arthritis has been present in certain cases.

Diagnosis.—There is rarely any difficulty in the diagnosis. One condition closely simulates it, namely, local gangrene of the toes associated with obliterative arteritis; but this occurs most frequently in older persons, in diabetic subjects, or in connection with well marked arterio-sclerosis. As a rule, the pulse in such cases is not to be felt in the dorsal artery. Allied to this form is an affection described by Buerger, thrombo-angeitis obliterans. In the early stages the resemblance to Raynaud's disease is very close.

In the acute infections, particularly typhus fever, occasionally in epidemics of typhoid fever, and in malaria, areas of multiple gangrene occur. The distribution is usually different, and there is rarely any difficulty in distinguishing this form from Raynaud's disease.

Lastly, there are cases of multiple neurotic skin gangrene met with in hysterical and nervous patients, in the majority of which the lesions are self-inflicted. In military recruits local gangrene of the big toe has been caused by carbolic acid, and it seems probable that all of those so-called trophic and hysterical lesions are simulated.

Treatment.—In many cases the attacks recur for years uninfluenced by treatment. Mild attacks require no treatment. In the severer forms of local asphyxia, if in the feet, the patient should be kept in bed with the legs elevated. The toes should be wrapped in cotton wool. The pain is often very intense and may require morphia. Carefully applied, systematic massage of the extremities is sometimes of benefit. Galvanism may be tried. Nitroglycerin has been warmly recommended. Calcium lactate in 15 grain (1 gm.) doses, three or four times a day, is sometimes very effectual. It often relieves chilblains. Small doses of thyroid extract sometimes are useful. Cushing introduced a plan of treatment with the tourniquet which has proved very successful in several cases. The elastic bandage, or, better, a pneumatic tourniquet, is applied to an extremity tight enough to shut off the arterial circulation and left for some minutes. On releasing the constriction the member flushes brightly, owing to the vaso-motor relaxation. The application in cases of severe spasm may have to be repeated at frequent intervals before the vascular constriction in the affected parts will be overcome, and the normal temperature and color return in them.

II. ERYTHROMELALGIA

(Red Neuralgia)

Definition.—"A chronic disease in which a pai or parts—usually one or more extremities—suffer with pain, flushing, and local fever, made far worse if the parts hang down" (Weir Mitchell). The name signifies a painful, red extremity.

Symptoms.—In 1872 (Phila. Med. Times, November 23d), in a lecture on certain painful affections of the feet, Weir Mitchell described the case of a sailor, aged forty, who after an African fever began to have "dull, heavy pains, at first in the left and soon after in the right foot. There was no swelling at first. When at rest he was comfortable and the feet were not painful. After walking the feet were swollen. They scarcely pitted on pressure, but were purple with congestion; the veins were everywhere singularly enlarged, and the arteries were throbbing visibly. The whole foot was said to be aching and burning, but above the ankle there was neither swelling, pain, nor flushing." As the weather grew cool he got relief. Nothing seemed to benefit him. This brief summary of Mitchell's first case gives an accurate clinical picture of the disease. His second communication, On a Rare Vaso-Motor Neurosis of the Extremities, appeared in the Am. Jour. of the Medical Sciences for July, 1878, while in his Clinical Lessons on Nervous Diseases, 1897, will be found additional observations.

The disease is rare. The feet are much more often affected than the hands. The pain may be of the most atrocious character. It is usually, but not always, relieved by cool weather; in one case the winter aggravated the trouble.

Mitchell speaks of it as a "painful nerve-end neuritis." Dehio suggests that there may be irritation in the cells of the ventral horns of the cord at certain levels. Excision of the nerves passing to the parts has been followed by relief. In one of Mitchell's cases gangrene of the foot followed excision of four inches of the musculo-cutaneous nerve and stretching of the posterior tibial. Sclerosis of the arteries was found. Of 9 cases in which the local conditions were studied anatomically, the only constant change was a chronic endarteritis (Batty Shaw).

III. ANGIO-NEUROTIC ŒDEMA

(*Quincke's Disease*)

Definition.—An affection characterized by the occurrence of local œdematous swellings, more or less limited in extent, and of transient duration. Severe colic is sometimes associated with the outbreak. There is a marked hereditary disposition in the disease. Some cases appear to be due to hypersusceptibility to certain food.

Symptoms.—The œdema appears suddenly and is usually circumscribed. It may appear in the face; the eyelid is a common situation; or it may involve the lips or cheek. The backs of the hands, the legs, or the throat may be attacked. Usually the condition is transient, associated perhaps with slight gastro-intestinal distress, and the affection is of little moment. There may be a remarkable periodicity in the outbreak of the œdema. In Matas' case this periodicity was very striking; the attack came on every day at eleven or twelve o'clock. The disease may be hereditary through many generations In one family five generations had been affected, including twenty-two members (Osler). The swellings appear in various parts; only rarely are they constant in one locality. The hands, face, and genitalia are the parts most frequently affected. Itching, heat, redness, or in some instances urticaria, may precede the outbreak. Sudden œdema of the larynx may prove fatal. Two members of the family just referred to died of this complication. In one member of this family the swellings came on in different parts; for example, the under lip would be swollen to such a degree that the mouth could not be opened. The hands enlarge suddenly, so that the fingers can not be bent. The attacks recur every three or four weeks. Accompanying them are usually gastro-intestinal attacks, severe colic, pain, nausea, and sometimes vomiting. It is quite possible that some of the cases of Leyden's intermittent vomiting may belong to this group. The colic is of great intensity and usually requires morphia. Arthritis apparently does not occur. Periodic attacks of cardialgia have also been met with during the outbreak of the œdema. Hæmoglobinuria has occurred in several cases. There is a hysterical variety in which the œdema affects geometrical areas, has abrupt edges and may be accompanied by sensory disturbances but not by gastro-intestinal attacks.

The disease has affinities with urticaria, the giant form of which is probably the same disease, and with Henoch's purpura. Quincke regards the condition as a vaso-motor neurosis, under the influence of which the permeability of the vessels is suddenly increased.

The **treatment** is unsatisfactory. In the cases associated with anæmia and general nervousness, tonics, particularly large doses of strychnia, do good. Improvement may follow the prolonged use of nitroglycerin; and calcium lactate may be tried, in doses of 15 grains (1 gm.) thrice daily. Epinephrine (♏ vii, 0.5 c. c.) given hypodermically and repeated in fifteen minutes has been helpful. In cases proved to be due to food susceptibility, a small dose of the causal material may be given an hour before the usual feeding is taken. In one case in which there was susceptibility to any albumin, the administration of peptone was successful.

IV. PERSISTENT HEREDITARY ŒDEMA OF THE LEGS

(*Milroy's Disease*)

This remarkable condition, first described by Milroy of Omaha, is characterized by persistent œdema of the legs, without any traceable cause or any constitutional features. It is a fairly common complaint, affecting males and females equally. As many as 22 persons in Milroy's series were affected among 97 in six generations; in Hope and French's series 13 of 42 persons in five generations. The œdema is strictly limited to the lower limbs and varies very slightly. In some instances there are remarkable acute attacks, with chill, fever, and increase of swelling. Except mechanically the condition does not seriously interfere with health.

Here may be mentioned a remarkable familial affection described by Edgeworth of Bristol (*Lancet,* July 22, 1911), of a general subcutaneous œdema. Of six infants born of healthy parents, all but one died within the first few months, with general œdema, following upon diarrhœa. The cases differ essentially from those of œdema neonatorum.

V. FACIAL HEMIATROPHY

A rare affection characterized by progressive wasting of the bones and soft tissues of one side of the face. The atrophy starts in childhood, but in a few cases has not come on until adult life. Perhaps after a trifling injury or disease the process begins, either diffusely or more commonly at one spot on the skin. It gradually spreads, involving the fat, then the bones, more particularly the upper jaw, and last and least the muscles. The wasting is sharply limited at the middle line, and the appearance of the patient is very remarkable, the face looking as if made up of two halves from different persons. There is usually change in the color of the skin and the hair falls. Owing to the wasting of the alveolar processes the teeth become loose and ultimately drop out. The eye on the affected side is sunken, owing to loss of orbital fat. There is usually hemiatrophy of the tongue on the same side. Disturbance of sensation and muscle twitching may precede or accompany the atrophy. In a majority of the cases the atrophy has been confined to one side of the face, but there are instances on record in which the disease was bilateral, and a few cases in which there were areas of atrophy on the back and on the arm of the same side.

In Mendel's case there was found the terminal stage of an interstitial neuritis in all the branches of the trigeminus, from its orgin to the periphery, most marked in the superior maxillary branch.

The disease is recognized at a glance. The facial asymmetry associated with congenital wryneck must not be confounded with progressive facial hemiatrophy. Other conditions to be distinguished are: Facial atrophy in anterior polio-myelitis, and in the hemiplegia of infants and adults; the atrophy following nuclear lesions and sympathetic nerve paralysis; acquired facial hemihypertrophy, which may by contrast give to the other side an atrophic appearance; and scleroderma (a closely related affection), if confined to one side of the face. The precise nature of the disease is doubtful, but it is a suggestive fact that in many cases the atrophy followed the acute infections. It is incurable.

VI. SCLERODERMA

Definition.—A condition of localized or diffuse induration of the skin.

Varieties.—Two forms are recognized: the circumscribed, which corresponds to the keloid of Addison, and to morphœa; and the diffuse, in which large areas are involved.

The disease affects females more frequently than males. The cases occur most commonly at the middle period of life. The *sclerema neonatorum* is a different affection. The disease is more common in the United States than statistics indicate. The senior author saw 20 cases in sixteen years.

In the *circumscribed form* there are patches, ranging from a few centimetres in diameter to the size of the hand or larger, in which the skin has a waxy or dead-white appearance, and to the touch is brawny, hard, and inelastic. Sometimes there is a preliminary hyperæmia of the skin, and subsequently there are changes in color, either areas of pigmentation or of complete atrophy of the pigment—leucoderma. The sensory changes are rarely marked. The secretion of sweat is diminished or entirely abolished. The disease is more common in women than in men, and is situated most frequently about the breasts and neck, sometimes in the course of the nerves. The patches may develop with great rapidity, and may persist for months or years; sometimes they disappear in a few weeks.

The *diffuse form,* though less common, is more serious. It begins in the extremities or in the face, and the patient notices that the skin is unusually hard and firm, or that there is a sense of stiffness or tension in making accustomed movements. Gradually the skin becomes firm and hard, and so united to the subcutaneous tissues that it cannot be picked up or pinched. It may look natural, but more commonly is glossy, drier than normal, and unusually smooth. With reference to the localization, in Lewin and Heller's statistics in 66 observations the disease was universal; in 203, regions of the trunk were affected; in 193, parts of the head or face; in 287, portions of one or other of the upper extremities; and in 122, portions of the lower extremities. In 80 cases there were disturbances of sensation. The disease may gradually extend and involve the skin of an entire limb. When universal, the face is expressionless, the lips can not be moved, mastication is hindered, and it may become extremely difficult to feed the patient. The hands become fixed and the fingers immobile, on account of the extreme induration of the skin over the joints. Remarkable vaso-motor disturbances are common, as extreme cyanosis of the hands and legs. Tachycardia may be present. The disease is chronic, lasting for months or years. There are instances on record of its persistence for more than twenty years. Recovery may occur, or the disease may be arrested. One patient, with extensive involvement of the face, ears, and hands, improved very much. The patients are apt to succumb to pulmonary complaints or to nephritis. Arthritic troubles have been noticed in some instances; in others, endocarditis. Raynaud's disease may be associated with it. The pigmentation of the skin may be as deep as in Addison's disease, for which cases have been mistaken; scleroderma may occur as a complication of exophthalmic goitre.

The remarkable dystrophy known as *sclerodactylie* belongs to this disorder. There are symmetrical involvements of the fingers, which become deformed, shortened, and atrophied; the skin becomes thickened, of a waxy color, and is sometimes pigmented. Multiple calcareous nodules, not unlike tophi, but not uratic, occur about the fingers. Bullæ and ulcerations have been met with in some instances, and a great deformity of the nails. The disease has usually followed exposure, and the patients are much worse during the winter, and are curiously sensitive to cold. There may be changes in the skin of the feet, but the deformity similar to that which occurs in the hand has not been noted. Some of the cases present in addition diffuse sclerodermatous changes of the skin of other parts. In Lewin and Heller's monograph there are 35 cases of isolated sclerodactylism, and 106 cases in which it was combined with scleroderma.

The **pathology** is unknown. It is usually regarded as a tropho-neurosis, probably dependent upon changes in the arteries of the skin leading to connective tissue overgrowth. The thyroid has been found atrophied.

Treatment.—The patients require to be warmly clad and to be guarded against exposure, as they are particularly sensitive to changes in the weather. Warm baths followed by frictions with oil should be systematically used. Thyroid feeding should be tried thoroughly in the diffuse form. In one case the disease appeared to be arrested; the patient took the extract for seven years. In a second case, after a year the face became softer, and there was permanent improvement. In a case of quite extensive localized scleroderma the patches became softer and the pigmentation much less intense. Salol in 15 grain (1 gm.) doses three times a day is stated to have been helpful.

VII. AINHUM

This is a disease of the fifth, rarely of the fourth and other toes in which a groove forms at the digito-plantar fold and deepens until the toe drops off. Described first by Da Silva Lima in 1852, it has since been met with in many tropical regions, in the southern states of America, and very rarely in temperate regions, as Canada and Italy. Nothing has been determined as to the *etiology*. It may occur in families, and is more common in males. There is endarteritis, with proliferation of the epidermis. Parasites have not been found. It is a local disease without symptoms and in the affected toe there is no disability and rarely any pain, except when the skin of the groove ulcerates. The toe drops off in about two years. In about 10 per cent. of cases the fourth toe is affected. It is said that the affection may occur in the fingers. A longitudinal section across the groove will sometimes stop the progress.

VIII. LIPODYSTROPHIA PROGRESSIVA

A rare affection, possibly confined to females, in which the subcutaneous fat gradually disappears from the face, arms, and trunk. The cause of the condition is unknown. Beginning usually about the tenth to thirteenth year, the wasting is progressive, but limited to the parts mentioned. The buttocks and legs remain normal and look by contrast abnormally plump. The breasts are spared. In the early stages it resembles the "bilateral atrophy of the face."

SECTION XIII

DISEASES OF THE LOCOMOTOR SYSTEM

A. DISEASES OF THE MUSCLES

I. MYOSITIS

Definition.—Inflammation of the voluntary muscles.

A primary myositis occurs as an acute, subacute, or chronic affection. It is seen in two chief forms—the suppurative and non-suppurative.

I. Suppurative myositis (infectious myositis) is especially frequent in Japan, where, according to Miyake, some 250 cases have been reported; but he claims that some of these belong to other affections. Miyake personally saw 33 cases in Japan in twenty-one months, and took cultures from all but one of them. In 2 cases the results were negative, but in 27 a pure culture of the staphylococcus pyogenes aureus was obtained, while in another the streptococcus and in 2 more the albus with the aureus was grown. The malady may involve one or many muscles, and is usually sudden in its onset with high fever and marked prostration. Subsequently abscesses occur in the indurated muscles, and pyæmia may ensue if the implicated areas are not thoroughly evacuated.

II. Dermato-myositis.—An acute or subacute inflammation of the muscles of unknown origin associated with œdema and dermatitis. Steiner collected 28 cases from the literature and reported two cases from the Hopkins clinic. The muscle inflammation is multiple, and associated with œdema and a dermatitis. The case of E. Wagner may be taken as a typical example. A tuberculous but well-built woman entered the hospital, complaining of stiffness in the shoulders and a slight œdema of the back of the hands and forearms. There was paræsthesia, the arms became swollen, the skin tense, and the muscles felt doughy. Gradually the thighs became affected. The disease lasted about three months. The post mortem showed slight pulmonary tuberculosis; all the muscles except the glutei, the calf, and abdominal muscles were stiff and firm, but fragile, and there were serous infiltration, great proliferation of the interstitial tissue, and fatty degeneration. The duration is usually from one to three months, though there are instances in which it has been longer. The swelling and tenderness of the muscles, the œdema, and the pain naturally suggest trichinosis, and Hepp speaks of it as a pseudo-trichinosis. The nature of the disease is unknown. Of the 28 cases collected by Steiner 17 died. The anatomical changes are those mentioned as found in Wagner's cases. One of Senator's cases presented marked disorders of sensation and has been named neuro-myositis. Wagner suggests that some of these cases were examples of acute progressive muscular atrophy. The differentiation from trichinosis is possible only by removing a portion of the muscle. It has not been determined whether eosinophilia is peculiar to the trichinosis myositis.

III. Polymyositis Hæmorrhagica.—This form resembles the dermatomyositis in general features, but differs in the presence of hæmorrhages into and between the muscles. Of the ten cases analyzed by Thayer four recovered. Purpura and hæmorrhages from the mucous membranes may occur.

II. MYOSITIS OSSIFICANS PROGRESSIVA

This is a progressive inflammatory affection of the locomotor system of unknown origin, characterized by the gradual formation of bony masses in the fasciæ, muscles, aponeuroses, tendons, ligaments, and bones, with resulting ankylosis of most of the articulations (Steiner). About 100 cases have been reported. The process begins in the neck or back, usually with swelling of the affected muscles, redness of the skin, and slight fever, or with small nodules in the muscles which appear and disappear. After subsiding an induration remains, which becomes progressively harder as the transformation into bone takes place. The disease may ultimately involve a majority of the skeletal muscles. Nothing is known of the etiology. Malformation, microdactylism of the thumbs and big toes, is present in 75 per cent. of the cases.

III. FIBROSITIS

(Myalgia, Myositis)

Definition.—A painful affection of the voluntary muscles and of the fasciæ and periosteum to which they are attached. It is probable that the fibrous tissue is especially affected—a fibrositis. It is by no means certain that the muscular tissues are involved. Many writers claim that in some cases it is a neuralgia of the sensory nerves of the muscles.

Etiology.—The attacks follow cold and exposure, and trauma is often a factor. It is most commonly met with in men, particularly those exposed to cold and whose occupations are laborious. It is apt to follow exposure to a draft of air, as from an open window in a railway carriage. A sudden chilling after heavy exertion may bring on an attack of lumbago. Persons of a gouty habit are more prone to this affection, and one attack renders an individual more liable to another. It is usually acute, but may become subacute or even chronic, the last being more common in later life. In many cases the condition is secondary to an area of focal infection.

Pathology.—The changes are usually in the white fibrous tissue and are of an inflammatory nature. In acute cases there is a serous exudation in the affected parts and following this there may be proliferation of the fibrous tissue. This may extend between the muscle fibres and cause stiffness and pain. Disability with muscular atrophy may result from this. Nodules sometimes form which may be painful.

Symptoms.—In the acute forms the affection is entirely local. The constitutional disturbance is slight, and, even in severe cases, there may be no fever. *Pain* is a prominent feature and may be constant or occur only when the muscles are in certain positions. It may be a dull ache, like the pain of a bruise, or sharp, severe, and cramp-like. It is often sufficiently intense to cause the patient to cry out. Pressure on the affected part usually gives relief. As a rule, pain is transient, lasting from a few hours to a few days, although occasionally it is prolonged for weeks. It is very apt to recur.

Much attention has been given to a form occurring chiefly in the muscles of the head and neck, causing at first swelling and puffiness, later indurations. They are found particularly in the muscles at the back of the neck, but they are occasionally present in the muscles of the abdomen and limbs. The affection of the muscles of the head and neck may be associated with headache, the so-called indurative headache. Some are very similar to migraine. In the abdominal muscles these limited swellings may cause pain and suggest appendicitis.

The following are the principal varieties:

(1) *"Lumbago,"* a term which means nothing more than pain in the lower back, is due to many causes. (*a*) *Fibrositis* is a common cause and may recur at short intervals. It comes on suddenly and may incapacitate the patient, any movement, particularly stooping or turning, causing severe pain. (*b*) *Ischæmic lumbago,* described as a type of intermittent claudication, may be bilateral or unilateral and is excited by movement. The pain is between the twelfth rib and the crest of the ilium and may radiate forward. The area is not tender and the pain is dependent on muscular exertion. (*c*) *Static* conditions, due to faulty posture, which may be lateral (one leg shorter) or antero-posterior, flat feet, stooping, occupation, etc. (*d*) *Anatomical variations* of the transverse processes of the fifth lumbar vertebra. (*e*) *Arthritis* of the spine. (*f*) *Sacro-iliac* joint strain or relaxation. (*g*) *Neuritis* of the posterior nerve roots. (*h*) Pain due to *pelvic disease* in males (prostate, etc.) or females. (*i*) *Trauma,* especially with lifting in a stooped position. The diagnosis of "backache" as being due to fibrositis should only be made after other possibilities are excluded. In every case the effort should be made to arrive at an etiological diagnosis as only then is proper treatment possible. For the cases due to strain some form of fixation is useful; faulty posture should be corrected and flat feet receive attention.

(2) Stiff neck or *torticollis* affects the muscles of the antero-lateral or back region of the neck. It is very common, often unilateral, and occurs most frequently in the young. The patient holds the head in a peculiar manner turned to one side, and rotates the whole body in attempting to turn it.

(3) *Pleurodynia* involves the intercostal muscles on one side, and in some instances the pectorals and serratus magnus. This is, perhaps, the most painful form of the disease, as the chest can not be at rest. It is more common on the left than on the right side. A deep breath, or coughing, causes a very intense pain on pressure, sometimes over a very limited area. It may be difficult to distinguish from intercostal neuralgia, in which, however, the pain is usually more circumscribed and paroxysmal, and there are tender points along the course of the nerves. It is sometimes mistaken for pleurisy, but careful examination readily distinguishes between the two affections.

(4) Among other forms are cephalodynia, affecting the muscles of the

head; scapulodynia, omodynia, and dorsodynia, affecting the muscles about the shoulder and upper part of the back. Fibrositis may also occur in the abdominal muscles and in the muscles of the extremities. In the legs it causes tenderness and pain, increased by use. Areas of infiltration may be palpated. Nodules are sometimes felt in the sole of the foot. The chronic forms are distinguished by soreness or pain associated with varying degrees of disability. There may be marked stiffness of the muscles, which are sometimes painful on pressure and may show definite tender areas of induration.

Treatment.—Rest of the affected muscles is of the first importance, and it is well to protect them from cold by a covering of flannel. Strapping of the side will sometimes completely relieve pleurodynia. No belief is more widespread among the public than in the efficacy of porous plasters for muscular pains of all sorts. If the pain is severe and agonizing, a hypodermic of morphia gives immediate relief. For lumbago acupuncture is, in acute cases, an efficient treatment. Needles of from three to four inches in length (ordinary bonnet-needles, sterilized, will do) are thrust into the lumbar muscles at the seat of pain, and withdrawn after five or ten minutes. The constant current is sometimes beneficial. In many forms of myalgia the thermocautery gives great relief and in obstinate cases blisters may be tried. Heat or counter-irritation in any form is useful and at the outset a Turkish bath may cut short the attack. The bowels should be freely opened and large amounts of water taken. The salicylates are usually effectual; sodium salicylate (gr. x to xv, 0.6 to 1 gm.), acetyl-salicylic acid (gr. x, 0.6 gm.), or salol (gr. v, 0.3 gm.) may be given. Some patients respond well to colchicum (♏ xv, 1 c. c. of the wine). In chronic cases potassium iodide may be used. Persons subject to this affection should be warmly clothed, and avoid, if possible, exposure to cold and damp. Massage sometimes gives relief; it should be given gently at first and more vigorously later. For the lumbar form, fixation is most useful by strapping, or some form of support.

IV. MYOTONIA

(*Thomsen's Disease*)

Definition.—An affection characterized by tonic cramp of the muscles on attempting voluntary movements. The disease received its name from the physician who first described it, in whose family it existed for five generations.

While the disease is in a majority of cases hereditary, hence the name myotonia congenita, there are other forms of spasm very similar which may be acquired, and others still which are quite transitory.

Etiology.—All the typical cases have occurred in family groups; a few isolated instances have been described in which similar symptoms have been present. Males are much more frequently affected than females. In 102 recorded cases, 91 were males and only 11 females (Hans Koch). The disease is rare in America and in England; it seems more common in Germany and in Scandinavia.

Symptoms.—The disease comes on in childhood. It is noticed that on account of the stiffness the children are not able to take part in ordinary games. The peculiarity is noticed only during voluntary movements. The contraction which the patient wills is slowly accomplished; the relaxation which the patient wills is also slow. The contraction often persists for a little time after he has dropped an object which he has picked up. In walking, the start is difficult; one leg is put forward slowly, it halts from stiffness for a second or two, and then after a few steps the legs become limber and he walks without any difficulty. The muscles of the arms and legs are those usually implicated; rarely the facial, ocular, or laryngeal muscles. Emotion and cold aggravate the condition. In some instances there is mental weakness. The sensation and reflexes are normal. G. M. Hammond reported three remarkable cases in one family, in which the disease began at the eighth year and was confined entirely to the arms. It was accompanied with some slight mental feebleness. The condition of the muscles is interesting. The patients appear and are muscular, and there is sometimes definite muscular hypertrophy. The force is scarcely proportionate to the size. Erb described a characteristic reaction of the nerve and muscle to the electrical currents—the so-called myotonic reaction, the chief feature of which is that normally the contractions caused by either current attain their maximum slowly and relax slowly, and vermicular, wave-like contractions pass from the cathode to the anode.

The disease is incurable, but may be arrested temporarily. The nature of the affection is unknown. Dejerine and Sottas found hypertrophy of the primitive fibres with multiplication of the nuclei of all the muscles, including the diaphragm, but not the heart. The spinal cord and the nerves were intact. From Jacoby's studies it is doubtful whether these changes in the muscles are in any way characteristic or peculiar to the disease. J. Koch found, in addition to the muscle hypertrophy, degenerative and regenerative changes, which he considers sufficient to account for the myotonic disorder. Karpinsky and von Bechterew regard the affection as due to an auto-intoxication of the muscle tissue, caused by some faulty metabolism. No treatment is known.

V. PARAMYOCLONUS MULTIPLEX

(*Essential Myoclonia*)

Definition.—An affection described by Friedreich, characterized by irregular clonic contractions, chiefly of the muscles of the extremities, occurring either constantly or in paroxysms.

Etiology.—The subjects are usually degenerate young males. Hysteria, emotion, fright, trauma, sexual excesses and parathyroid disease have been suggested as possible causes. The disease may occur in several generations.

Pathology.—The nature of the disease is unknown. Pierce Clark suggests that it is an abiotrophy of the *corpus striatum*—the region of control of the automatic and associated movements.

Symptoms.—The characteristic features are the short, sudden and lightning-like contractions, not rhythmic and of equal intensity, and without the synergic quality of a purposive movement. The two sides may be unequally involved, and single muscles may be affected. The face and fingers are not often affected. Sensation is not involved; the reflexes are increased. The movements are usually absent during sleep.

Diagnosis.—The disease may be confounded with the various symptomatic myoclonias seen in the tics, chronic chorea, and the rhythmic movements associated with mid-brain lesions. The myoclonia with epilepsy (Unverricht) is described elsewhere.

Treatment.—Various forms of suggestion may be tried, but the disease may prove very resistant. The movements may cease spontaneously.

VI. MYASTHENIA GRAVIS

(*Asthenic Bulbar Paralysis; Erb-Goldflam's Symptom-Complex*)

Definition.—A disease with fatigue symptoms referable to the muscular system, due to failure of innervation without definite changes in muscles or nerves.

Of 180 cases collected by McCarthy, 83 were males and 96 females. In women the disease usually occurs before the age of twenty-five, in males in middle life. Of 56 autopsies since 1901, in 17 there was hyperplasia or persistence of the thymus and in 10 a thymic tumor, only one of which was malignant. Examination of the nervous system has revealed no abnormality. Hun, Bloomer, and Streeter described an infiltration of the muscles and of the thymus gland with lymphoid cells and a proliferation of the glandular elements of the thymus.

The muscles innervated by the bulb are first affected—those of the eyes, the face, of mastication, and of the neck. After effort the muscles show fatigue, and if persisted in they fail to act and a condition of paresis or complete paralysis follows. All the voluntary muscles may become involved. After rest the power is recovered. In severe cases paralysis may persist. The *myasthenic reaction* of Jolly is the rapid exhaustion of the muscles, by faradism, not by galvanism. There are marked remissions and fluctuations in the severity of the symptoms.

The *diagnosis* is easy—from the ptosis, the facial expression, the nasal speech, the rapid fatigue of the muscles, the myasthenic reaction, the absence of atrophy, tremors, etc., and the remarkable variations in the intensity of the symptoms. Of 180 collected cases 72 proved fatal; sudden death may occur. The patient may live many years; recovery may take place. Rest, strychnia in full doses, massage, and alternate courses of iodide of potassium and mercury may be tried.

VII. AMYOTONIA CONGENITA

(*Oppenheim's Disease*)

A congenital affection characterized by general or local hypotonus of the voluntary muscles. Oppenheim called the disease *myatonia*, but this is phonetically so similar to *myotonia* (Thomsen's disease) that the name amyotonia of English writers is preferable. Collier and Wilson give the following definition: "A condition of extreme flaccidity of the muscles, associated with an entire loss of the deep reflexes, most marked at the time of birth and always showing a tendency to slow and progressive amelioration. There is great weakness, but no absolute paralysis of any of the muscles. The limbs are most affected; the face is almost always exempt. The muscles are small and soft, but there is no local wasting. Contractures are prone to occur in the course of time. The faradic excitability in the muscles is lowered and strong faradic stimuli are borne without complaint. No other symptoms indicative of lesions of the nervous system occur."

Faber has collected 115 cases (1917). Recovery has not been reported, but improvement was noted in 41 cases. The post-mortem changes are variable —increase in the muscle nuclei, and in the fat and connective tissue; defective myelinization of the peripheral nerves; absence of the nerve endings in the muscle fibres, without changes in the central nervous system. The disease seems to come in the group of Gowers' abiotrophies—a failure in the proper development of the lower motor neurone.

B. DISEASES OF THE JOINTS

I. ARTHRITIS DEFORMANS

Definition.—A disease of the joints, the result of infection, characterized by changes in the synovial membranes, cartilage, and peri-articular structures, and in some cases by atrophic and hypertrophic changes in the bones. A tendency to a chronic course is the rule.

Long believed to be intimately associated with gout and rheumatism (whence the names rheumatic gout and rheumatoid arthritis), this relationship seems disproved. There is a difference of opinion as to whether there are two distinct diseases or varying forms of the same disease included under this heading. Those who hold the former view consider that in one disease the synovial membranes and the peri-articular tissues are particularly affected (rheumatoid arthritis) and in the other disease the cartilage and bone (osteo-arthritis). The disease occurs frequently and to it belong many of the cases termed "chronic rheumatism."

Etiology.—Age.—A majority of the cases are between the ages of twenty and fifty. In A. E. Garrod's analysis of 500 cases there were only 25 under twenty years of age. In 40 per cent. of our series of 500 cases, the onset was before the age of thirty years. In the group with peri-articular changes predominating the age of onset is usually lower than in the group with special cartilaginous and bony changes.

Sex.—Among Garrod's cases there were 411 in women. Practically half of our series were males. The incidence as to sex is influenced by the inclusion of the cases of spondylitis, of which a large majority is in males. In women a close association with the menopause has been noted.

Predisposition.—Two or three children in a family may be affected. In America the incidence in the negro is relatively much less than in the white.

Occupation and the station in life do not seem to have any special influence.

Exposure to cold, wet and damp, errors in diet, worry and care, and local injuries are spoken of as possible exciting causes, but probably play but a small part.

Arthritis Deformans as a Chronic Infection.—This view is steadily gaining ground and the evidence suggests certain varieties of streptococci as the causal organism. This seems more probable than that the disease is due to a specific organism. The work of Hastings suggests *Streptococcus viridans* as the organism in many cases. The arthritis is secondary to a focus of infection somewhere. The possible sources are many but infection of the mouth and throat probably takes first place. Abscesses about the teeth should always be searched for (X-ray study) and the tonsils carefully examined. Other sources are: infection of the nose or sinuses, pyorrhœa alveolaris, otitis media, chronic bronchitis, infection of the biliary or urinary tract, pelvic disease in women, and infection of the prostate and seminal vesicles in men. The possibility of chronic infection from the intestinal tract must be considered although this is difficult to prove.

The acute onset, with fever in many cases, the polyarthritis, the presence of enlarged glands, the frequent enlargement of the spleen, the occurrence of pleurisy, endocarditis, and pericarditis in some cases are all suggestive of an infection. The likeness of the lesions to those due to arthritis from a specific cause, such as the gonococcus, is suggestive, and also the association of the arthritis with definite foci of infection in many cases.

Metabolic.—While the nutrition suffers in many cases there does not seem any evidence to support the view that the disease is primarily due to disturbance of metabolism. Metabolic changes are probably secondary just as are the trophic changes.

Morbid Anatomy.—The usual descriptions are of the late stages when extensive damage has occurred, for there have been few opportunities to study the early changes, although more frequent operations have extended our knowledge of them and radiographs have aided much. There are three main forms of change: (1) Lesions principally in the synovial membranes and peri-articular tissues (the so-called rheumatoid arthritis), (2) with atrophic changes in the cartilage and bones predominating, and (3) with hypertrophy and overgrowth of bone (so-called osteo-arthritis). The first and second are seen most frequently in the joints of the extremities, the third in the spine. In many cases all forms of change are found, which speaks against the view that there are two distinct diseases. The changes in general are: (1) Effusion, which is not constant and shows no special features. (2) Changes in the synovial membrane. These are inflammatory and often hæmorrhagic at the onset. There may be marked thickening and proliferation of the synovial fringes with the formation of villi—*villous arthritis.* (3) The capsule and surrounding tissues may be infiltrated and much swollen. The peri-articular tissues show infiltration and swelling, and the enlargement of the joint is more often due to swelling about it than to bony changes. (4) *Cartilage.* This may show erosion, ulceration, atrophy, or proliferation. The cartilage may disappear entirely, but the changes are often very irregular and uneven and the cartilage may be replaced by fibrous tissue or by bone, the latter being most common at the edge of the cartilage. The cartilages may be soft and gradually absorbed or thinned (this often begins opposite the point of greatest involvement of the synovial membrane). (5) *Bone*. This may show atrophy of varying grade. If the cartilage is completely absorbed the surface of the bone often becomes hard and eburnated. In the form spoken of as *hypertrophic* there is new bone formation which is most common at the edge of the articular surfaces. In the hip joint this may form an irregular ring of bone about the joint cavity. The commonest example of overgrowth of bone is seen in the so-called "Heberden's nodes," which are bony outgrowths at the terminal interphalangeal joints. There may be deposit of new bone in the ligaments, particularly in the spine. Proliferation of bone usually occurs at the margins of the joints in the form of irregular nodules—the osteophytes. The formation of bone may also occur in ligaments, especially of the spine, which may be converted into a rigid bony column. Bony ankylosis rarely occurs in the peripheral joints, but is common in the spine.

There may be extensive *secondary* changes. Muscular atrophy is common and may appear with great rapidity. Subluxation may occur, especially in the knee and finger joints. The hands often show great deformity, particularly ulnar deflection. Contractures may follow and the joints become fixed in a flexed position. Neuritis and trophic disturbances may be associated; the neuritis is sometimes due to direct extension of the inflammatory process. Subcutaneous nodules occasionally occur.

The radiographs show the changes very well. Erosion of the cartilage is easily seen. In the type with predominant peri-articular changes the cartilage and bone often show little alteration. The occurrence of various changes in different joints or even in the same joint is common and bony change may occur with marked involvement of the peri-articular tissues.

Symptoms.—The onset may be acute or gradual. In the acute form a number of joints may be involved, there may be high fever and the whole condition be suggestive of rheumatic fever. In other cases the onset is acute in one joint and others are involved a few days later. With the gradual onset one joint is attacked and others follow. Some cases are between and may be termed subacute. In cases with an acute onset the attack may not persist very long; with the chronic onset the duration is usually prolonged. The acute onset occurs more frequently in the form in which changes in the soft parts predominate.

Arthritis.—In the acute form the joints are swollen, tender, and hot to the touch, but do not often show marked redness. There may be effusion in the larger joints. Pain is a marked feature and is increased by movement, the patient usually taking the position in which he has the greatest ease. When a joint is once attacked, the process does not subside quickly, and when the arthritis lessens some change remains in the joint which, however, may be very slight. The joints of the spine, especially in the cervical region, are often involved in the more acute forms, and in these there is rarely any permanent change. The temporo-maxillary joint is often involved, and arthritis here is always suggestive of this disease. The hands, when involved, show very characteristic changes. The knuckle joints are red, swollen, tender, and show limitation of motion. The fingers are often involved; swelling of the interphalangeal joints is common with a resulting thickening which gives a fusiform appearance to the finger. Partial dislocation, particularly at the terminal joint, is common. The knee-joints are often affected, with pain, effusion, limitation of motion, and later villous arthritis or subluxation. Thickening of the capsule usually occurs early.

In the hypertrophic (osteo-arthritis form) the process is rarely as acute as when the peri-articular parts are particularly involved (rheumatoid arthritis), but is usually polyarticular. The terminal finger joints, the hip joint, and the spine are especially affected. Pain is usually severe and the local features are not so marked. This form is more likely to be chronic.

HEBERDEN'S NODES.—These are small bony outgrowths ("little hard knobs"—Heberden) at the terminal phalangeal joints, which develop gradually at the sides of the distal phalanges. They are much more common in women than in men. Heberden says "they have no connection with gout, being found in persons who have never had it," yet they are often regarded as indicating gout. In the early stage the joints may be swollen, tender, and slightly red, particularly when injured. The attacks of pain and swelling may come on at long intervals or follow injury. Sometimes they are the first manifestation of a general arthritis. Their distribution is not always regular and they are often largest on the fingers most used. They may be found in patients in whose other joints the arthritis is of the other form. The condition is not curable; but there is this hopeful feature—the subjects whose arthritis begins in this way rarely have severe involvement of the larger joints.

The MON-ARTICULAR FORM affects chiefly old persons, and is seen particularly in the hip and shoulder. It is identical with the general disease in its anatomical features. The muscles show wasting early and in the hip the condition ultimately becomes that described as *morbus coxæ senilis*. These cases seem not infrequently to follow an injury. They differ from the polyarticular form in occurring chiefly in men and at a later period of life.

THE VERTEBRAL FORM (*Spondylitis*).—This may occur alone or with involvement of the peripheral joints. With the acute polyarthritis of the peripheral joints the spine may be involved, but there is usually no permanent change. With the hypertrophic form there is often bony proliferation and some spinal rigidity results which may involve the whole spine or only a part; in the latter case the lower dorsal and lumbar regions suffer most frequently. The condition may not involve more than a few vertebræ. The features are as variable as in the peripheral joints and there may be repeated acute attacks or a steady progressive process. In the general spine involvement the ribs may be fixed, the thorax immobile, and the breathing abdominal. There are two varieties of the general involvement which are sometimes regarded as special diseases. In one (von Bechterew) the spine alone is involved, and there are pronounced nerve-root symptoms—pain, anæsthesia, atrophy of the muscles, and ascending degeneration of the cord. Von Bechterew thinks it begins as a meningitis, leads to compression of the nerve roots, loss of function of the spinal muscles, atrophy of the intervertebral disks, and gradually ankylosis of the spine. In the other—Strümpell-Marie type—the hip and shoulder joints may be involved (spondylose rhizomélique), and the nervous symptoms are less prominent. Both appear to be forms of arthritis deformans, and should neither be regarded nor described as separate diseases. Spondylitis deformans is more frequent in males, and trauma probably plays an important part in its etiology.

Local involvement is particularly common in the lumbar region and may cause sciatica and a great variety of referred pains. Pressure on the nerve-roots causes pain, paræsthesia, and atrophy of the muscles. Movement of the spine is usually restricted.

Arthritis Deformans in Children.—Some cases resemble closely the disease in adults, in others there are very striking differences. A variety has been differentiated by Still, in which the general enlargement of the joints is associated with swelling of the lymph glands and the spleen. The onset is almost always before the second dentition, and girls are more frequently affected than boys. At first there is usually slight stiffness in one or two joints; gradually others become involved. The onset may be acute with fever or even with chills. The enlargement of the joints is due rather to a general thickening of the soft tissues than to bony enlargement. The limitation of movement may be extreme, and there may be much muscular wasting. The enlargement of the lymph glands is striking, increases with fever, and may be general; even the epitrochlear glands may be as large as hazel nuts. The spleen can usually be felt below the costal margin. Sweating is often profuse and there may be anæmia, but heart complications are rare. The children look puny and generally show arrest of development.

General Features.—*Temperature.*—In the acute attacks this may rise to 102° or 103° F., but is frequently lower and often persists for weeks with a maximum about 100° F. The *pulse* is rapid in proportion to the fever, the most frequent range being from 90 to 110. Cardiac changes are found in a small proportion of cases. *Glandular enlargement* is common and may be general or especially marked in the glands related to the affected joints. The *spleen* is enlarged in some cases, the frequency being greater in the younger patients. *Subcutaneous nodules* occur in a few cases and are sometimes tender. The *blood* often shows a slight anæmia, which is not as marked as might be expected from the appearance of the patients. There is rarely much increase in the leucocytes and the differential count shows no peculiarity. The *urine* does not show any change of moment. The *skin* sometimes shows irregular areas of yellow pigmentation, especially on the face and arms. It may have a glossy appearance over the affected joints. Profuse sweating of the hands and feet is common. The *reflexes* are usually increased in acute cases and a return to normal is of good significance. They are sometimes absent. Muscular *atrophy* is common and sometimes advances very rapidly. It is most marked in the hands. Twitching of the muscles is not uncommon.

In some patients the bony atrophy is very marked. This is most common in females. In these disorganization of the joints occurs and the cartilage rapidly disappears. These cases usually progress rapidly downward. This atrophy is to be distinguished from that due to disuse.

Course.—*General Progressive Form.*—This occurs in two varieties, acute and chronic. The *acute* form may resemble, at its outset, rheumatic fever. There is involvement of many joints; swelling, particularly of the synovial sheaths and bursæ, but not often redness; there is moderate fever which is often persistent and may be from 99° to 100° F. for weeks. The pulse rate is usually high in proportion to the fever. In this form there may be repeated acute attacks, perhaps at intervals of years, or there may be repeated attacks in various joints. These usually leave definite changes, which may be slight at first, but tend to increase with subsequent attacks. Acute cases may occur at the menopause. Some cases progress very rapidly; they lose weight and strength; atrophy and arthritic deformity are marked; and they suggest a progressive septic process without suppuration.

The *chronic* form is the most common, although most of these have had at some time an acute attack, especially at the onset. The first symptoms are pain on movement and slight swelling, which may be in the joint itself or in the peri-articular sheaths. In some cases the effusion is marked, in others slight. The local conditions vary greatly, and periods of improvement alternate with attacks of swelling, redness, and pain. At first only one or two joints are affected; gradually others are involved, and in extreme cases every joint in the body is affected. Pain is a variable symptom. Some cases proceed to the most extreme deformity without severe pain; in others the suffering is very great, particularly at night and during exacerbations of the disease. There are cases in which pain of an agonizing character is almost constant, quite apart from the occurrence of acute disturbances. Pain has an important influence in the production of deformity, as it hinders movement and the joints are kept in the position of greatest ease.

Gradually the shape of the joints is greatly altered, partly by the thickening of the capsule and surrounding tissues, perhaps by osteophytes, and often by muscular contraction. Crepitus may be felt in the affected joint. Ultimately the joints may be completely immobile, not by a true bony ankylosis, although it may be by the osteophytes which form around the articular surfaces, but more often from adhesions and peri-articular thickening. There is often an acute atrophy of the muscles and atrophy from disuse supervenes, so that contractures tend to flex the thigh upon the abdomen and the leg upon the thigh. Numbness, tingling, pigmentation or glossiness of the skin, and onychia may be present. In extreme cases the patient is completely helpless, and lies with the legs drawn up and the arms fixed. Fortunately, it often happens in these severe general cases that the joints of the hand are not so much affected, and the patient may be able to knit or write, though unable to walk or use the arms. In many cases, after involving two or three joints, the disease becomes arrested. A majority of the patients finally reach a quiescent stage, in which they are free from pain and enjoy fair health, suffering only from the inconvenience and crippling associated with the disease. Coincident affections are not uncommon. A small percentage show cardiac lesions, and the pulse rate is usually higher than normal.

Diagnosis.—The cases with an acute onset may be difficult to distinguish from *rheumatic fever*. The affected joints are rarely as tender as in rheumatic fever, and the smaller joints are more often involved. The presence of thickening in a joint, rapid muscular atrophy, a relatively high pulse rate in relation to the fever (in the absence of endocarditis), and the absence of marked response to salicylate medication speak against rheumatic fever. The diagnosis from *gonorrhœal arthritis* may be difficult, but in this the small joints are usually not attacked so often, and after an onset with polyarthritis the majority of the affected joints usually clear, leaving one joint particularly involved. This rarely occurs in arthritis deformans. A careful search for gonococci is a great aid in diagnosis. In the chronic stage there may be considerable difficulty in distinguishing this disease from *gout*. This is particularly marked in either disease without marked joint changes. The study of the radiographs is particularly helpful and marked peri-articular changes speak for arthritis deformans. The finding of tophi or the estimation of the uric acid content of the blood may give the diagnosis of gout. It is important to distinguish *sub-deltoid bursitis* from the mon-articular form in the shoulder; the radiographs are a great aid. They are also important in the recognition of disease of the *sacro-iliac* joint and *tuberculosis* of the *hip-joint*. Special importance attaches to the diagnosis of the spinal forms. There is no difficulty in the case of general involvement, but with local changes in the lower spine it is not so easy. Pain on and restriction of movement are important; the patient is careful to limit any motion of the spine. Tuberculosis of the spine rarely offers any difficulty, especially with skiagrams.

Prognosis.—The age, general circumstances, character of the patient, the extent of arthritis, and the variety are all important. The outlook is not as dark as is usually described. If the source of infection can be found early and properly treated the prognosis is encouraging. In many patients the disease runs a certain course, and, if they can be brought through it with a minimum of damage, the ultimate outlook is good. In the form with peri-articular changes predominating, early diagnosis, treatment of the point of infection, the preservation of good nutrition, and a patient who is willing to fight are all encouraging factors. The outlook in the cases with the acute attacks is usually better than in those with a more chronic progressive course. Rapid muscular atrophy is of grave import. Cases in women beginning about the menopause should always have a grave prognosis. Rapid advancement in the joint changes is serious. In the form in children the outlook is not good, but some recover entirely. The group with marked hypertrophic changes (osteo-arthritis) usually do well. Heberden's nodes are permanent, but in the larger joints it is rare for the condition to advance to absolute crippling, although there may be considerable interference with function. Spondylitis rarely advances to complete immobility of the whole spine. The outlook is good in the local cases, but depends somewhat on the occupation and possibility of trauma. The general condition is of importance in estimating the outlook. In those with marked nervous features the prognosis is not good.

Treatment.—Much depends on proper management and the pessimistic attitude is not justified. Certain things are important: early diagnosis so that treatment can be begun early, the avoidance of harmful measures, careful attention to the general condition, and every effort to limit the damage in the joints. Too much stress can not be placed on the need of early diagnosis; the disease is often regarded as "rheumatic" and the treatment directed to this (especially restriction of diet and the giving of salicylates for long periods) is usually harmful.

Source of Infection.—Every effort should be made to find any such and prompt treatment carried out. Infection of the teeth and tonsils has always to be excluded. The possibility of infection of the bile passages should be considered. Whenever possible an autogenous vaccine should be prepared and used if the removal of the focus is not enough. Serums have not been of benefit in our experience.

General Measures.—The patient should be kept out of doors as much as possible and every effort made to improve the general health. The *diet* should be the most nourishing possible. The mistake of cutting down the proteins is often made. Regard must be had to the digestion, and it is more often the carbohydrates which should be reduced. Water should be freely given, as elimination is important. The bowels should be kept open, and for this the salines are useful. It is important to see that the patients are warmly clad in cold weather and guarded against chilling. *Hydrotherapy* is useful locally in the form of compresses, but the hot bath treatment, so often given, more frequently does harm than good, particularly in acute cases. Baths, when taken, should be of very short duration. In more chronic cases bathing is sometimes of value. *Massage* is especially useful in the cases with synovial and peri-articular changes, and in them passive motion should be used early. *Climate* is of value in so far as patient is able to be out of doors and is saved from rapid changes of temperature.

MEDICINAL.—There is no drug which essentially influences the disease. The salicylates may aid in relieving pain, but should not be given for long periods. Iron, arsenic, and iodine are often useful. Iodine may be given as the tincture in doses of five to ten drops. Potassium iodide is sometimes of value when given for a long period. Thyroid and thymus gland extracts given persistently are sometimes beneficial. For the *pain* it is necessary to give drugs, although local measures should be used as much as possible. There are many which are available. Acetyl-salicylic acid (gr. x, 0.6 gm.), guaiacol carbonate (gr. v, 0.3 gm.), antipyrin (gr. iii, 0.2 gm.), and sometimes codein (gr. ½, 0.03 gm.), are useful. Morphia should not be given on account of the danger of a habit.

LOCAL.—(*a*) Use of the joints must be governed by the condition. When the cartilage and bones are not involved, passive motion and massage are useful, followed later by active motion. The patient should be taught simple exercises. When the cartilages and bones are involved, *rest* is usually advisable for a time. Every effort should be made to avoid contracture and displacement, and in this the use of splints during the night is often valuable. Caution should be exercised in advising complete fixation. This is sometimes useful for short periods in the osteo-arthritic form, but may result in fixation in the other form and is usually not advisable for it. (*b*) *Counter-irritation.* This is usually an aid, and the Paquelin cautery, blisters, mustard, and iodine may be used. It is usually better to use light counter-irritation frequently than severe at longer intervals. (*c*) *Hyperæmia.* This may be active, and baking is a favorite method, but it should not be given for more than thirty minutes at a time. The temperature should be as high as the patient can stand. Passive hyperæmia may be used for a short period at first, and later for many hours at a time. (*d*) *Hydrotherapy.* The persistent use of compresses is often of value. They may be put on in the evening and left on all night.

SURGICAL MEASURES.—These are useful for the correction of deformities. In the case of villous arthritis operation is usually indicated. In the group with marked hypertrophy of bone removal of the outgrowths may be helpful.

SPECIAL FORMS.—(*a*) *Heberden's nodes.* Avoidance of irritation and injury is important, and in the case of pain the use of compresses is helpful. (*b*) *Spondylitis.* During the acute stages rest is essential and should be secured by a plaster jacket or simple apparatus. In the milder forms firm strapping may give relief. Trauma should be especially avoided. (*c*) *Knee joint.* In many cases a simple elastic support is useful and may save the joint from injury.

Foreign Protein.—This has proved useful in some cases, given intravenously in the form of proteose (1-2 c.c. of a 4 per cent. solution) or as typhoid vaccine (75-150 millions). A sharp reaction is necessary if any benefit is to result.

Arthritis Secondary to Acute Infection.—While the majority of cases of arthritis are secondary to some form of infection, it is important to recognize various forms. (1) Those with a definite bacterial cause, such as gonorrhœal or tuberculous arthritis. These usually have fairly well defined features. (2) Those secondary to infections of doubtful etiology, such as scarlet fever or measles. In some of these the arthritis is due to a secondary infection, but in others it appears to be due to the specific cause of the disease. (3) Arthritis secondary to definite infections in which there is no evidence of any organism in the joint. These are comparatively common and are difficult to designate. For example, arthritis, which may not be severe and subsides rapidly, occurs with an attack of tonsillitis. It has been suggested that these might be termed "toxic" or "toxæmic" arthritis. The term "infectious" arthritis, sometimes applied, is not a satisfactory one. The cases in this group usually clear without leaving permanent damage, but if long continued they may result in the changes included under the heading of arthritis deformans.

"Chronic Rheumatism."—This term deserves mention because it is so commonly used, but it is a question whether its retention is justified. There is no uniformity in its usage and it is applied without discrimination to all kinds of arthritis and frequently to conditions which have nothing to do with the joints. Painful conditions of the joints, muscles, fasciæ, bones, and nerves are all termed "rheumatism." There is no disease entity to which the term can be applied, and it would be an advantage to give it up entirely.

II. INTERMITTENT HYDRARTHROSIS

The condition was described by Perrin in 1845. The affection is characterized by a remarkable periodic swelling of one or several of the joints without fever. The swelling may take place with great rapidity, and there may even be a sensation of water rushing into the joint. There are usually pain and stiffness. The periods may be from ten to twelve days, or a month or even three months. Many of the cases have been in women and sometimes with marked hysterical symptoms. While some of the cases are secondary and only represent a phase in the evolution of various articular lesions, there appears to be a primary form characterized by a periodic swelling and nothing else. It is sometimes the joint equivalent to Quincke's œdema and may be associated with erythema, with angio-neurotic œdema, and in one of Garrod's patients there was at the same time circumscribed œdema of the lips and eyelids. Some cases are due to anaphylaxis. A mother and daughter have been affected. The prognosis is not good; the attacks are apt to recur in spite of all forms of treatment.

C. DISEASES OF THE BONES

I. HYPERTROPHIC PULMONARY ARTHROPATHY

Definition.—A symmetrical enlargement of the bones of the hands and feet, and of the distal ends of the long bones, occurring in association with certain chronic diseases, particularly affections of the lungs.

Bamberger in 1889 reported a condition of abnormal thickening of the long bones in bronchiectasis, and the next year Marie described other cases and named the condition.

Etiology.—*Clubbing* of the fingers, or the Hippocratic fingers, represent a minor manifestation of this condition. Many varieties occur; indeed, there is a monograph with sketches of some thirty or forty forms. It is met with perhaps most constantly in congenital disease of the heart, in tuberculosis and in other affections of the lungs, particularly bronchiectasis, in congenital syphilis, in chronic jaundice, and in other chronic affections. In thoracic aneurism it may involve only the fingers of one hand. It usually comes on very slowly, but cases have been described of an acute appearance within a week or a fortnight. It may disappear. There is no bony alteration, but there is a fibrous thickening of the connective tissues with turgescence of the vessels. The condition is by no means easy to explain. The mechanical effect of congestion, the usual feature, explains the heart and lung cases, but not those of congenital syphilis and diseases of the liver, in which this is not present. Others have attributed it to a toxin.

Marie's syndrome is met with: (1) In diseases of the lungs and pleura. This was the case in 43 out of 55 cases collected by Thayer, and in 68 of Wynn's 100 cases. Bronchiectasis is the most common, then pulmonary tuberculosis and empyema. (2) Other affections, such as chronic diarrhœa, chronic jaundice, nephritis, and congenital syphilis.

Marie regards the process as resulting from the absorption of toxins causing a periostitis; others have regarded it as a low form of tuberculous infection. The bones most frequently involved are the lower ends of the radius and ulna and the metacarpals, more rarely the lower end of the humerus, and the lower ends of the tibia and fibula.

Symptoms.—The affection comes on gradually, unnoticed by the patient. In other cases there is great sensitiveness of the ends of the long bones and of the fingers and toes. In one of our cases this was present in an extreme degree. The fully developed condition is easily recognized. The hands are large, the terminal phalanges swollen, the nails large and much curved. Similar changes occur in the toes, and the feet look large, especially the toes and the malleoli. The bones of the fore-arms are diffusely thickened, particularly near the wrist, and the tibiæ and fibulæ are greatly enlarged. Sometimes in advanced cases both ankles and knee-joints stand out prominently. The hypertrophy rarely affects the other long bones, though occasionally the extremities of the humerus and femur may be involved. The bones of the head are not attacked. Kyphosis may occur.

Diagnosis.—There is rarely any difficulty, as the picture presented by the hands and feet differs from that in acromegaly, and in practically all cases it is a secondary condition.

II. OSTEITIS DEFORMANS

(*Paget's Disease*)

Definition.—A chronic affection of the bones characterized by enlargement of the head, dorso-cervical kyphosis, enlargement of the clavicles, spreading of the base of the thorax and an outward and forward bowing of the legs.

The affection was described first by Sir James Paget, in 1877.

Etiology.—In the generalized form it is a rare disease, only two cases occurring among about 20,000 medical cases at the Johns Hopkins Hospital. The etiology is unknown. Mother and daughter have been affected. Some have regarded it as luetic, others as due to the arterio-sclerosis, which is a constant lesion. It may possibly be due to perversion of some internal secretion.

Pathology.—The skull, spine, and long bones are chiefly affected; those of the face, hands and feet are less involved. The skull may be as much as three quarters of an inch in thickness, and its circumference is increased. In one of Paget's cases it measured 71 cm. The shafts of the long bones are greatly thickened and they may weigh twice as much as a healthy bone of the same length. The femur is bent, the convexity forward; the tibiæ may be huge and very much bowed anteriorly. The bones of the upper extremities are less often involved, the spine shows a marked kyphosis, sometimes partial ankylosis; the pelvis is broadened.

The process is a rarefying osteitis which gradually involves the centre of the bones with the formation of Howship's lacunæ, Haversian spaces, and perforating canals. There is also new bone formation, both subperiosteal and myelogenous; the latter process gradually gains, and so the bones thicken.

Symptoms.—The disease begins, as a rule, in the sixth decade, sometimes with indefinite pains, but more frequently the patient notices first that the head begins to enlarge, so that he has to buy a larger hat. Then his friends notice that he is growing shorter, and that the legs are getting more and more bowed. There is a painful variety with great soreness of the arms and legs, which may be much worse at night. Headache, bronchitis, pigmentation of the skin, have been noted. The reduction in stature is very remarkable; one patient lost 13 inches in height.

Diagnosis.—The disease is readily recognized. The face differs from acromegaly, in which it is ovoid or egg-shaped with the large end down, while in Paget's disease the face is triangular with the base upward. In a few cases the disease may be limited to a few bones. There is a variety involving the tibiæ and fibulæ alone, and in some the femurs to a slight extent. These bones gradually enlarge, are bowed anteriorly and laterally, so that the only obvious features are a reduction in height with bowing of the legs. There is also a variety, sometimes known as tumor-forming osteitis deformans, in which the bones are much deformed with multiple hyperostosis and new growths. The relation of this to Paget's disease is doubtful.

III. LEONTIASIS OSSEA

In a remarkable condition known as *leontiasis ossea* there is hyperostosis of the bones of the cranium, and sometimes those of the face. The description is largely based upon the skulls in museums, but Allen Starr reported an instance in a woman, who presented a slowly progressing increase in the size of the head, face, and neck, the hard and soft tissues both being affected. He applied the term *megalo-cephaly* to the condition. Putnam states that the disease begins in early life, often as a result of injury. There may be osteophytic growths from the outer or inner tables, which in the latter situation may give the symptoms of tumor.

IV. OSTEOGENESIS IMPERFECTA

(*Fragilitas Ossium, Osteopsathyrosis, Lobstein's Disease*)

Definition.—A prenatal and postnatal defective activity of the osteoblasts, rendering the bones abnormally brittle. The condition is often hereditary and is sometimes associated with a peculiar shape of the head and blue sclerotics.

History.—Lobstein described the disease as osteopsathyrosis in 1833, while Vrolik in 1849 described the prenatal idiopathic type as *osteogenesis imperfecta*. Recklinghausen and others have thought the conditions were not identical, but the general opinion now seems to be that they are the same, and that *idiopathic fragilitas ossium,* whether prenatal or postnatal, is due to a deficient activity of the osteoblasts, whether in sub-periosteal or chondral ossification (Bronson). The terms *osteogenesis imperfecta congenita* and *tarda* best describe the two conditions.

Etiology.—Nothing is known except the single factor of heredity which occurs in a variable number of cases. Davenport and Conrad state that the heredity is typically direct and that the factor determining the irregular bone formation is a dominant one. The younger half of the family of an osteopsathyrotic parent will be affected, "but if neither parent, though of affected stock, has shown the tendency, then the expectation is that none of the children will have brittle bones." Biotypes occur, in some families the femur only, in some the humerus only is affected, and in some any pressure causes a break, while others show a much greater resistance.

Symptoms.—In the prenatal cases the child is often premature and stillborn, the extremities short and thick with many fractures in all stages of healing. The head may feel like a crepitant bag of bones. The characteristic bitemporal enlargement has been described by Cameron. In the postnatal cases the onset is usually after infancy. While the liability to fracture, as a rule, decreases with years, it may persist until the age of fifty. Slight blows may cause a fracture, of which a child may have a score or more before puberty. As a rule, they are painless and heal readily.

Blue Sclerotics.—Eddowes first described this remarkable condition which is more common in the inherited form. It may occur in individuals of the family who have never had fractures. It is not due to any color in the sclera itself but to increased transparency, possibly depending upon the absence of lime salts in the connective tissue.

V. OSTEOMALACIA

(*Mollities Ossium*)

This disease is characterized by pain, muscular weakness, and softness of the bones, due to decalcification, resulting in fractures and deformity. The great majority of the cases are in women; repeated pregnancies may play a part. A relationship to rickets is doubtful. Disturbance of internal secretions may be responsible. The onset is usually between the ages of twenty and thirty. The bones are soft and show both decalcification and new formation. The earliest *symptom* is pain, especially in the back and sacral regions, increased by movement. Weakness is marked and there may be stiffness with contractures. The gait may be uncertain, sometimes spastic. The bony deformity is usually first in the spine or pelvis. Later there is marked deformity with fractures, callus formation and muscular wasting. The course is usually over some years and death may result from exhaustion or a terminal infection. The early *diagnosis* is difficult and may only be made when deformities appear. The X-rays are of value. In *treatment,* phosphorus in oil should be given (gr. 1/20-1/12, 0.003-0.005 gm.). The removal of the ovaries has been useful in some cases. Proper treatment for the symptoms should be given.

VI. ACHONDROPLASIA

(*Chondrodystrophia Fetalis*)

Definition.—A dystrophy of the epiphyseal cartilages due to connective tissue invasion from the periosteum, in consequence of which the epiphyses and diaphyses are prematurely united and there is failure of the normal growth of the long bones. In consequence the subjects become dwarfs with normal heads and trunks, but short, stumpy extremities.

Description.—Achondroplasic dwarfs are easily recognized. They are well nourished and strong, and of average intelligence. Their height varies from 3 to 4 feet; the head and trunk are of about normal size, but the extremities are very short, the fingers, when the arms are at the sides, reaching little below the crest of the ilium. The important point is that in the shortness of the limbs it is the proximal segments which are specially involved, the humerus and femur being even shorter than the ulna and tibia (rhizomelia). The limbs are considerably bent, but this is more an exaggeration of normal curves and abnormalities in the joints than pathological curves. The features of rickets are absent. The hand is short, and has a trident shape, since the fingers, which are of almost equal length, often diverge somewhat. The root of the nose is depressed, the back flat, and the lumbar lordosis abnormally deep, owing to a tilting forward of the sacrum. The scapulæ are short, the fibulæ longer than the tibiæ, and the pelvis is contracted; hence, the number of these cases reported by obstetricians. Heredity plays little part.

Pathology.—Anatomically it is a dystrophy of the epiphyseal cartilages. the cells of which are irregularly scattered, and the ground substances invaded by connective tissues from the periosteum, which sends in bands of tissues across the end of the diaphysis. The development of the bones with a membranous matrix seems normal.

Virchow described the disease as fetal cretinism, others as fetal rickets. Of late naturally its origin has been associated with disturbance of the pituitary function, or of its hormonic relations. On the other hand, Jansen of Leyden, in a monograph (1912), brings forward evidence to show that it results from a disturbance of the direct and indirect amniotic pressure, and brings it into relationship with a number of other fetal malformations. He states that the anatomical evidence is against changes in the sella turcica. But it is an argument in favor of some associated disturbance of the pituitary gland that achondroplasics often show precocious sexual development.

VII. HEREDITARY DEFORMING CHONDRODYSPLASIA

(*Multiple Cartilaginous Exostoses*)

The disease is characterized by the occurrence of multiple, usually symmetrical, cartilaginous or osteo-cartilaginous growths, generally benign, which result from proliferation and ossification of bone-forming cartilage, and cause bony deformities. The disease is hereditary in many instances; in one family there were 26 cases in four generations. The American cases have been collected by Ehrenfried, who found that males were more often affected (3 to 1). The changes begin in infancy or early childhood, increase with skeletal growth and cease about the age of 22 years. The height is often less than normal. There are "irregular juxta-epiphyseal hyperostoses" most marked at the hips, knees, ankles, shoulders and wrists. There is often knock-knee and pes valgus, and the ulna may be relatively shortened. There may be symptoms due to pressure of the exostoses on nerves or vessels. Removal of the exostoses is indicated if they cause troublesome symptoms.

VIII. OXYCEPHALY

Definition.—A cranial deformity associated with exophthalmos and impairment of vision.

Description.—The condition, known as *tower* or *steeplehead,* is characterized by great height of the forehead, sloping to a pointed vertex, with feebly marked supra-orbital ridges, and the hairy scalp may be raised above the normal level, looking as if perched on the top of a comb. The intelligence is unimpaired. The condition is usually present at birth, though in some instances it develops from the second to the sixth year. As this curious growth of the head proceeds, headache may be present, exophthalmos develops, and the vision becomes impaired, due to progressive optic atrophy. Smell is often completely lost. The deformity appears to be due to premature synostosis of certain sutures, notably the sagittal and coronal. As a result of the premature union of these two sutures the growth of the vault of the skull is restricted in both its antero-posterior and transverse diameters, and to accommodate the increasing bulk of the brain a compensatory increase in height takes place. Eventually the anterior fontanelle closes, but there is reason to think that this occurs at a later date than the normal, and its former site is marked by a slight protuberance with thinning of the bone. (Morley Fletcher, *Quarterly Jour. Med.*, IV, 1911.)

The optic neuritis and atrophy are the result of pressure exerted by the growing brain and may be compared to that of cerebral tumor. As yet we do not know the cause of this premature synostosis. The condition is one for which a decompression operation with ventricular puncture is indicated.

INDEX

B

D

E

F

H

I

J

K

L

M

P

Q

R

T

U

V